W9-AGZ-781

OBSTETRIC NURSING

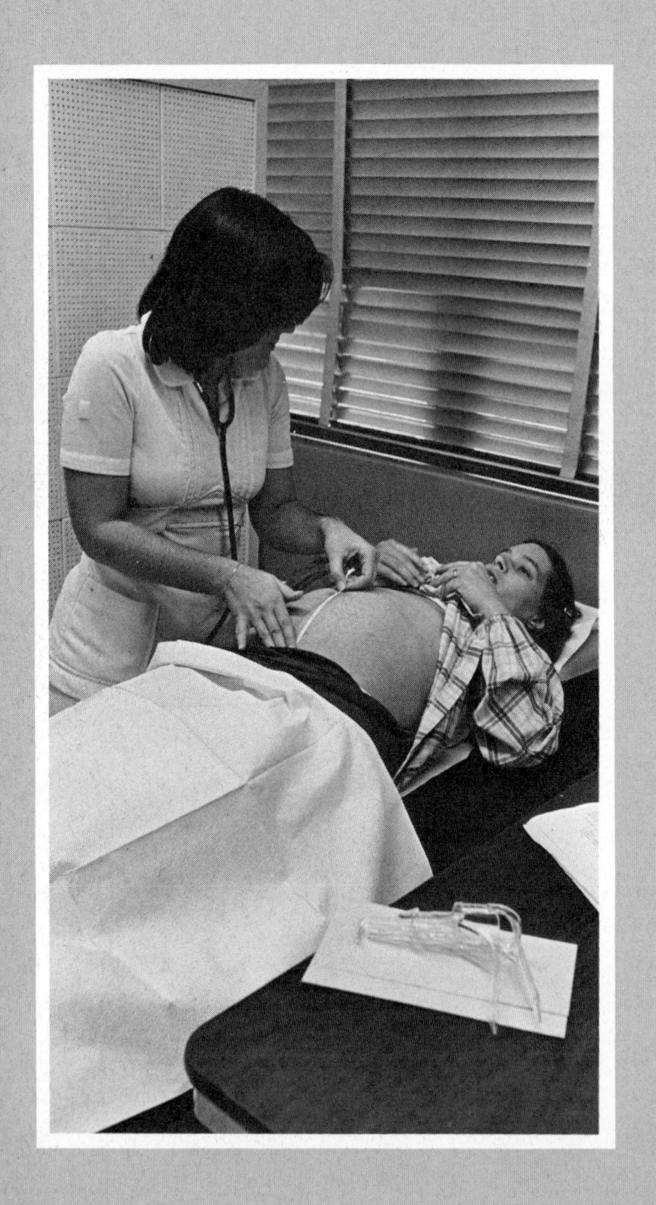

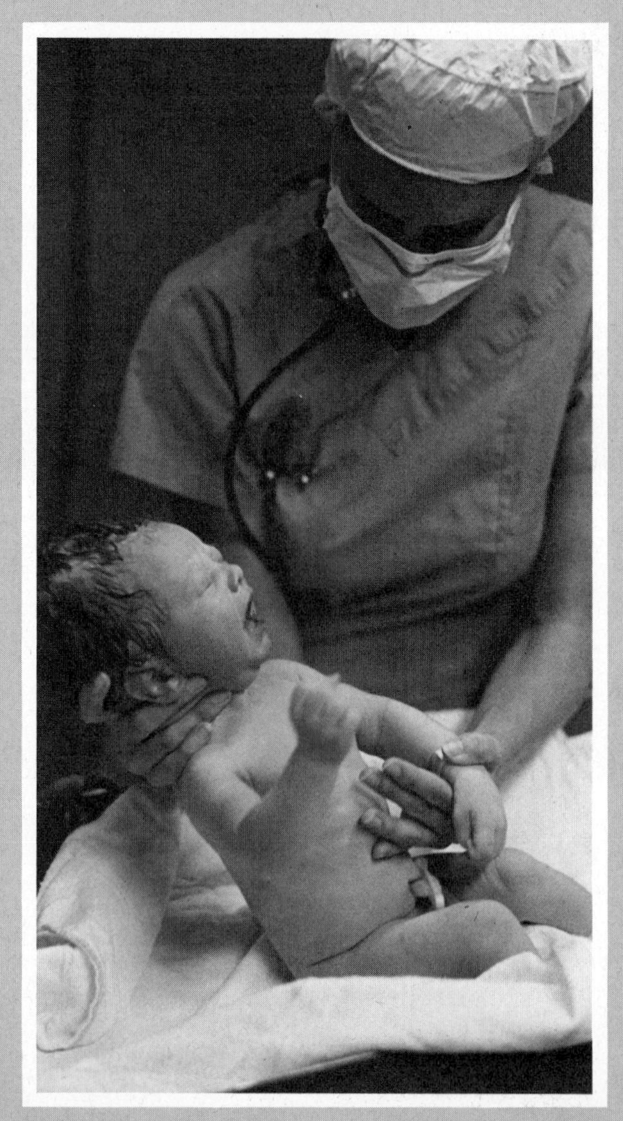

OBSTETRIC NURSING

Sally B. Olds, R.N., B.S.N., M.S.

Marcia L. London, R.N., B.S.N., M.S.N.

Patricia A. Ladewig, R.N., B.S., M.S.N.

Sharon V. Davidson, R.N., B.S.N., M.Ed.

Addison-Wesley Publishing Company
Medical/Nursing Division, Menlo Park, California
Reading, Massachusetts • London • Amsterdam • Don Mills, Ontario • Sydney

Sponsoring Editor: James Keating
Developmental Editor and Production Coordinator: Deborah Gale
Production Editor: Nancy Sjoberg
Copyeditors: Jackie Estrada, Rebecca Smith
Cover Design: Michael A. Rogondino
Book Design: Linda S. Stinchfield
Artists: Jack Tandy, Mike Ivester
Photographer: George B. Fry III

Library of Congress Cataloging in Publication Data

Main entry under title
Obstetric nursing.

Bibliography: p.
Includes index.
1. Obstetrical nursing. I. Olds, Sally B., 1940–
RSG951.026 610.73'678 79-25158
ISBN 0-201-02718-6

ABCDEFGHIJ-MU-83210

The authors and publishers have exerted every effort to ensure that drug selection and dosage set forth in this text are in accord with current recommendations and practice at the time of publication. However, in view of ongoing research, changes in government regulations and the constant flow of information relating to drug therapy and drug reactions, the reader is urged to check the package insert for each drug for any change in indications of dosage and for added warnings and precautions. This is particularly important where the recommended agent is a new and/or infrequently employed drug.

Addison-Wesley Publishing Company
Medical/Nursing Division
2725 Sand Hill Road
Menlo Park, California 94025

To our families, who were patient, supportive, and always there.
Joe, Scott, and Allison Olds
David and Craig London
Tim, Ryan, and the littlest Ladewig who is due in 1980

To the memory of my godfather, James H. Grandy, for his inspiration *(S.V.D.)*

PREFACE

Today's maternity nurse must have in-depth knowledge about the physical and psychologic aspects of childbearing, many technical and clinical skills, and the ability to assess and satisfy the needs of the childbearing patient and her family. It is not enough to merely "do for" people; nurses must work with them to provide truly effective health care.

We believe that the nursing care that a family receives during childbearing can influence its attitudes about future health care. With this in mind, it is essential that maternity nurses consider all aspects about the childbearing family. Additionally, we feel that other maternity nursing textbooks have not fully explored the influence (potential or realized) that the nursing profession has on the well-being of the childbearing family.

Obstetric Nursing was written with these beliefs in mind. Our purpose is to present the vast amount of information available about maternal-child care in a cogent, applicable manner.

Organization

Unit I provides an introduction to the historical highlights of maternity nursing and current trends in the field. An introduction to family dynamics provides the basis for the family-centered approach utilized throughout the text.

Unit II focuses on the reproductive process, including spermatogenesis, oogenesis, nidation, and fetal development. The problem of infertility and available treatment measures is explored, and methods of family planning are presented. Genetics and the role of the nurse in genetic counseling are also thoroughly examined.

Unit III considers the prenatal family both physiologically and psychologically. Signs and symptoms of pregnancy, maternal changes during each trimester, and prenatal nutrition are explored in depth. An entire chapter is devoted to nursing assessment during the prenatal period. The concept of parenting is explored in depth and the nursing care needs of the childbearing family are detailed. Common prenatal complications, the maternal-fetal-neonatal implications, and therapeutic interventions are also included, as are cross-cultural aspects of prenatal maternity care.

Unit IV utilizes a similar approach to consider the intrapartal needs of the childbearing family during normal labor and delivery and in the event of complications. The chapter on alternative birth methods is both fascinating and enlightening in its consideration of birth options available today.

In Unit V the focus shifts to the newborn. The nursing assessment of the neonate is followed by a consideration of the needs and care of both the normal and the high-risk newborn. We also explore the psychologic responses of parents to the birth of a newborn with complications.

Unit VI considers the family during the postpartal period. Assessment, normal nursing care, and care of the postpartal patient with complications are examined. In addition, an in-depth discussion of the process of attachment and its ramifications for parenthood is presented. The final chapter deals with families in crisis and the role of the nurse.

Integration of the Nursing Process

The theory of the nursing process provides the framework for this text. Each of the components of the nursing process is applied. Chapters dealing with nursing assessment skills have been developed for the prenatal, intrapartal, postpartal, and neonatal periods. The information has been consolidated into tabular physical and psychologic assessment guides. The application of the assessment function is illustrated in the nursing care plans that are provided for the major nursing situations in maternal-newborn care.

The nursing care plans further serve as models for the other components of the nursing process: planning, implementation, and evaluation. Intelligent planned care begins with a data base, including the patient's history, laboratory data, and physical examination findings. This permits the establishment of nursing priorities and the formulation of a plan to achieve these objectives. The nursing care plans are based on a problem-solving approach; after a problem has been identified, the appropriate nursing actions are delineated, and the rationale for these actions is explained. The final step of the nursing process, evaluation, is demonstrated in the evaluation criteria given at the end of each nursing care plan.

Family-Centered Nursing

We have emphasized a family approach to maternity nursing in this textbook. The family is presented using a developmental approach, after an in-depth examination of family dynamics. Our study of the family follows the family along a continuum, from its beginning structure and role through its changes during pregnancy, childbirth, and childrearing. The physiologic and psychologic aspects of parenthood are considered, as are parenting techniques, care of the newborn, and family adjustments to its altered state. Throughout the text, we highlight the various ways that nurses can impact on the family's well-being.

An integrated approach to the family is offered with appropriate considerations of cultural aspects, nutrition, and socioeconomic factors affecting nursing care. In addition, we examine those family situations that may be critical, such as adolescent pregnancy and single parenthood.

Pedogogical Aids

Learning objectives have been developed for each chapter to guide the efforts of the nursing student. Suggested activities at the end of each chapter offer an opportunity for related clinical application and experiences. In addition, the correct method of performing common obstetric procedures as well as the rationale for the actions have been incorporated throughout the text. The glossary and appendices at the end of the book are in essence a reference bank. Numerous illustrations and original photographs have been developed to enhance the text and assist the student in visualizing various aspects of nursing care.

To aid the nursing educator in making full use of the text, an *Instructor's Manual* is also available. This manual, keyed to the chapters, can function as a detailed syllabus or can supplement the instructor's planned approach.

Applications

Its logical organization and clear presentation of nursing skills make *Obstetric Nursing* suitable for all types of nursing programs. In addition, this text is eminently valuable to practicing nurses. A description of common obstetric procedures provides quick reference for the practitioner, and the assessment chapters will be invaluable to nurses seeking to upgrade their assessment skills. The material on families, parenting, attachment, and crisis intervention will broaden the psychosocial base of knowledge of both students and nurses, and the material on genetics and prenatal diagnostic testing will provide state of the art information in those areas.

Clarification of Terms

Although many men are now functioning as registered nurses, women still comprise the majority of nurses in maternity care, and consequently the feminine pronoun has primarily been used when referring to the nurse in this text. Although a variety of life-styles exist and unmarried individuals often choose to become parents, for the sake of simplicity, throughout this book the male partner in a relationship is usually referred to as "the husband" or "the father," and the female partner is usually referred to as "the wife" or "the mother."

Acknowledgments

We wish to thank the nursing educators and numerous clinical practitioners from all areas of the country who have contributed to this text or provided assistance in reviewing material. Their contributions have enabled us to produce a comprehensive text, one that avoids regionalization in focus or approach.

Our appreciation goes to Dr. Eva Sandusky, who reviewed the chapter on genetics. A special thanks goes to Deborah Gale for her unfailing support, encouragement, and developmental editing skills. We also want to express our appreciation to the individuals, families, nurses, and other health care personnel who allowed us to photograph them.

We are especially grateful for the support, encouragement, and assistance of our families during the long hours spent in preparing the manuscript. Without them, we might not have persevered.

Sally B. Olds
Marcia L. London
Patricia A. Ladewig
Sharon V. Davidson

EDITORS

Sally B. Olds, R.N., B.S.N., M.S.
Instructor, Maternal-Child Nursing, Beth-El School of Nursing, Memorial Hospital, Colorado Springs, Colorado.

Marcia L. London, R.N., B.S.N., M.S.N.
Pediatric Clinical Specialist, Coordinator of Maternal-Child Nursing, Beth-El School of Nursing, Colorado Springs, Colorado.

Patricia A. Ladewig, R.N., B.S., M.S.N.
Instructor, Associate Degree Nursing Program, Pikes Peak Community College, Colorado Springs, Colorado.

Sharon V. Davidson, R.N., B.S.N., M.Ed.
President, C.P.E., Inc. Colorado Springs, Colorado.

Martha Cox Bailey, R.N.
Vice Chairman, District VIII, NAACOG; Head Nurse, Labor and Delivery, Swedish Medical Center, Englewood, Colorado. Contributed to Chapter 20.

Elizabeth M. Bear, C.N.M., M.S.
Associate Professor and Coordinator of Nurse-Midwifery, Graduate Program, College of Nursing, University of Kentucky, Lexington, Kentucky. Contributed to Chapter 1.

Irene Bobak, R.N., M.N., M.S.N., C.N.P.
Associate Professor, San Francisco State University, San Francisco, California. Contributed to Chapters 12 and 26.

Sallye P. Brown, M.N.
Associate Professor and Level II Coordinator, Florida State University School of Nursing, Tallahassee, Florida. Contributed to Chapter 27.

Penelope Childress, R.N.
Head Nurse, Newborn Nursery, Swedish Medical Center, Englewood, Colorado. Contributed to Chapter 23.

Pamela Crispin, R.N.
Formerly Assistant Director of Nursing, Colorado Springs Community Hospital, Colorado Springs, Colorado. Contributed to Chapter 23.

CONTRIBUTORS

Marilynn Doenges, R.N., M.A.
Private Consultant, Parenting and Sexuality, Colorado Springs, Colorado. Contributed to Chapter 12.

Nancy Donaldson, R.N., B.S.N., M.S.N.
Parent-Child Clinical Nurse Specialist, Childrens Hospital of Orange County, Orange, California; National Continuing Education Faculty, NAACOG. Contributed to Chapter 27.

Mildred R. (Holly) Emrick, R.N., B.S., M.S.N.
Pediatric Nurse Consultant, Handicapped Children's Program, Colorado Department of Health, Denver, Colorado. Contributed to Chapter 25.

Jack Ford, M.D., F.A.C.O.G.
Obstetrician-Gynecologist, Colorado Springs, Colorado; Volunteer Instructor, University of Colorado, Denver, Colorado. Contributed to Chapter 9.

Laurel Freed, R.N., M.N., P.N.P.
Chairperson and Associate Professor, Department of Nursing, Sonoma State University, Rohnert Park, California. Contributed to the development of the Assessment Guide format.

Sandra L. Gardner, R.N., M.S., P.N.P.
Perinatal/Neonatal/Pediatric Consultant, Professional Outreach Consultation, Denver, Colorado. Contributed to Chapter 24.

Pauline Goolkasian, R.N., M.S.N.
Formerly Assistant Professor, University of Maryland, School of Nursing; Parent Education Specialist, Greater Baltimore Medical Center, Baltimore, Maryland. Contributed to Chapters 13 and 23.

Ann Kelley Havenhill, R.N., B.S.N., M.N.
Assistant Professor, Graceland College, Division of Nursing, Lamoni, Iowa. Contributed to Chapter 16.

Loretta C. Cermely Ivory, C.N.M., M.S.
Director, Midwifery Services, Denver Birth Center, Denver, Colorado; Clinical Faculty, University of Utah, Salt Lake City, Utah; Clinical Faculty, Yale University, Nurse-Midwife Program, New Haven, Connecticut. Contributed to Chapters 27 and 29.

L. Jean Johns, R.N., B.S., M.S.
Director of Nursing Education, Beth-El School of Nursing, Memorial Hospital, Colorado Springs, Colorado. Contributed to Chapter 12.

E. JoAnne Jones, R.N., A.B., M.Ed., M.S.N.
Doctoral Candidate, College of William and Mary, Williamsburg, Virginia. Contributed to Chapter 18.

Emma K. Kamm, R.N.
Assistant Head Nurse, Newborn Nursery, Swedish Medical Center, Englewood, Colorado. Contributed to Chapter 23.

Janet Kennedy, B.S., M.S., D.N.Sc.
Formerly Assistant Professor, Boston University School of Nursing, Maternal-Child Health Graduate Program, Boston, Massachusetts. Contributed to Chapter 28.

Jean Theirl King, R.D., B.S.
Clinical Dietitian, Memorial Hospital; Nutrition Instructor, Beth-El School of Nursing, Memorial Hospital, Colorado Springs, Colorado. Contributed to Chapter 11.

Virginia Gramzow Kinnick, B.S.N., M.S.N., C.N.M.
Assistant Professor, University of Northern Colorado School of Nursing, Greeley, Colorado. Contributed to Chapters 11 and 12.

Eleanor Latterell, R.D., B.S., M.S.
Dietetic Consultant, Nutrition Clinic and Consultant Service, Eugene, Oregon. Contributed to Chapter 11.

Eileen Leaphart, R.N.C., B.S.N., M.N.
Ob-Gyn Clinical Nurse Specialist, Presbyterian Hospital, Charlotte, North Carolina; formerly Assistant Professor and Maternity Coordinator, Baccalaureate Program, School of Nursing, University of North Carolina at Greensboro, Greensboro, North Carolina; Vice-President and National Continuing Education Faculty, NAACOG. Contributed to Chapter 15.

Anne Lamphier Matthews, R.N., M.S.
Assistant Professor and Nurse Geneticist, School of Nursing, University of Colorado Health Services Center, Denver, Colorado. Contributed to Chapter 8.

Mary Ann McClees, B.Sc., M.S.
Assistant Professor, University of Calgary, Alberta, Canada. Contributed to Chapter 28.

Nancy McCluggage, R.N., B.S.N., C.N.M.
Formerly Perinatal Nurse Clinician, Kansas Regional Perinatal Program, University of Kansas Medical Center; Clinical Services Director of Maternal and Child Health, Bethany Medical Center, Kansas City, Kansas. Contributed to Chapter 14.

Caryl E. Mobley, B.S.N., M.S.N.
Formerly Assistant Professor, College of Nursing, University of North Carolina, Charlotte, North Carolina. Contributed to Chapter 3.

Irene L. Nielsen, R.N., B.S., M.S., C.N.M.
Director, Birth Center-Lucinia, Cottage Grove, Oregon; Director, Birth Center-Meleah, Harrisburg, Oregon. Contributed to Chapter 15.

Lovena L. Porter, R.N.C., B.A., M.S.N.
Clinical Nurse Specialist, Colorado Springs Medical Center, Colorado Springs, Colorado. Contributed to Chapter 9.

Carol Freeman Rosenkranz, R.N., B.S.N., M.N.
Associate Professor, University of Mississippi School of Nursing, Jackson, Mississippi. Contributed to Chapters 15, 17, and 19.

Joanne F. Ruth, R.N., M.S.
Instructor, Maternal-Child Nursing, Beth-El School of Nursing, Memorial Hospital, Colorado Springs, Colorado. Contributed to Chapter 11.

Paula Shearer, R.N., B.S.N., M.S.N.
Associate Professor, Graceland College, Lamoni, Iowa. Contributed to Chapter 30.

Mari Lou Fifield Steffen, R.N., M.S.
Maternal-Child Health Nurse Consultant, Division of Family Health Services, Utah State Department of Health, Salt Lake City, Utah. Contributed to Chapters 6 and 26.

Marie Swigert, R.N., M.S.N.
Maternal Health Nursing Consultant and Acting Nursing Director, Colorado Department of Health, Denver, Colorado. Contributed to Chapter 2.

Teresa Van Sell, R.N., B.S.N.
Labor and Delivery Nurse, Dale General Hospital, Bedford, Indiana

Marcia Vavich, R.N., B.S., M.A.
Formerly Assistant Professor, Maternal-Child Nursing, College of Nursing, University of Arizona, Tucson, Arizona. Contributed to Chapter 30.

Janet Veatch, R.N., B.S.N., M.N.
Assistant Clinical Professor, University of California at San Francisco School of Nursing, San Francisco, California. Contributed to procedures for newborn.

Bette Blome Winyall, R.N., B.A., B.S.N., M.S.N.
Assistant Professor, University of Maryland School of Nursing, Baltimore, Maryland. Contributed to Chapters 4 and 5.

CONTENTS IN BRIEF

UNIT I INTRODUCTION TO FAMILY-CENTERED OBSTETRIC NURSING 1

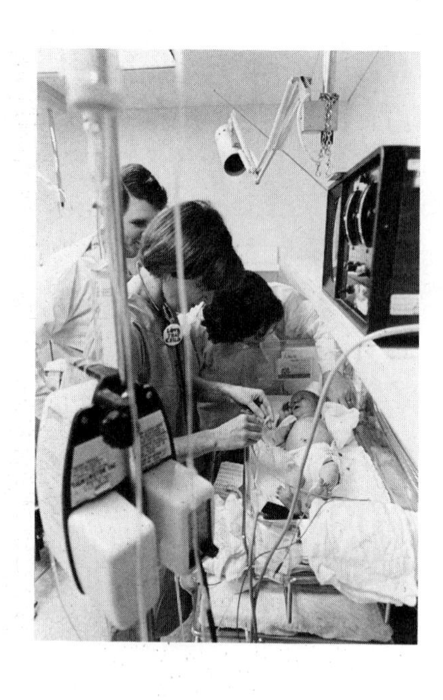

CONTENTS IN DETAIL

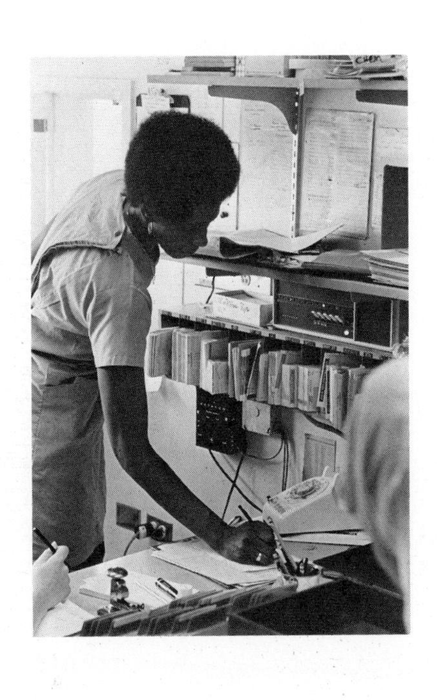

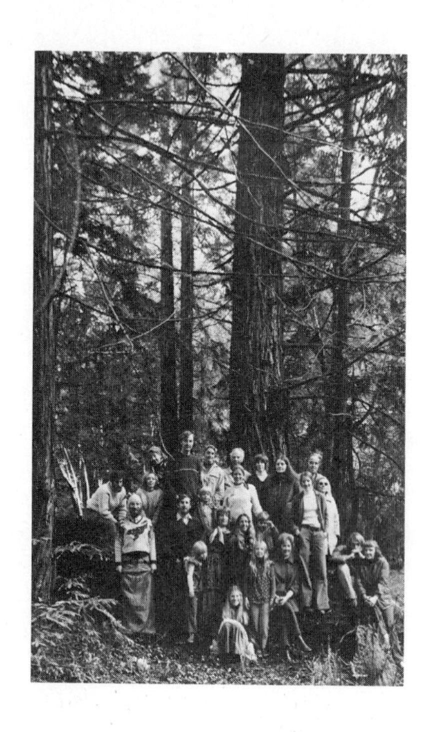

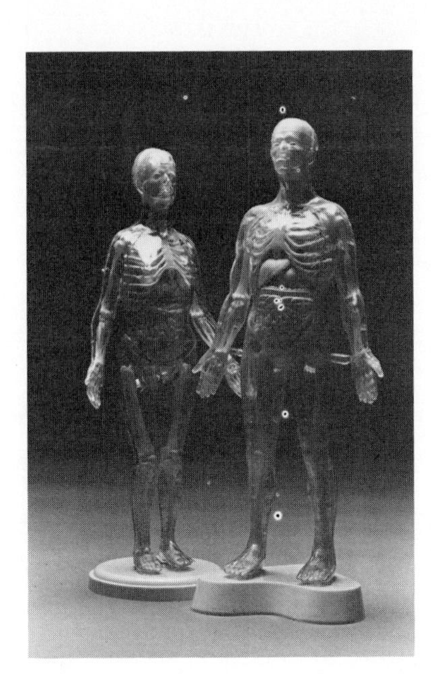

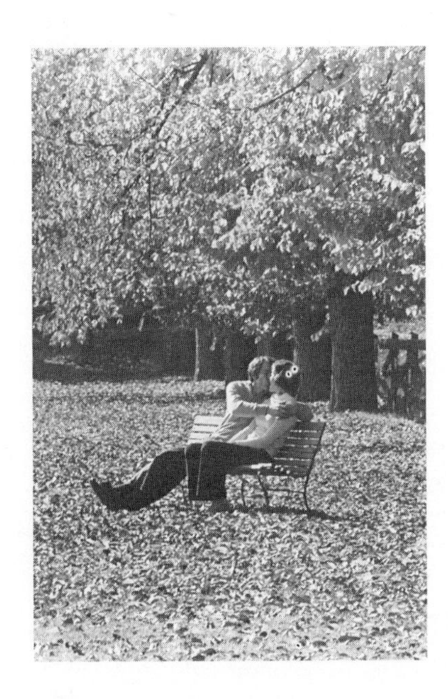

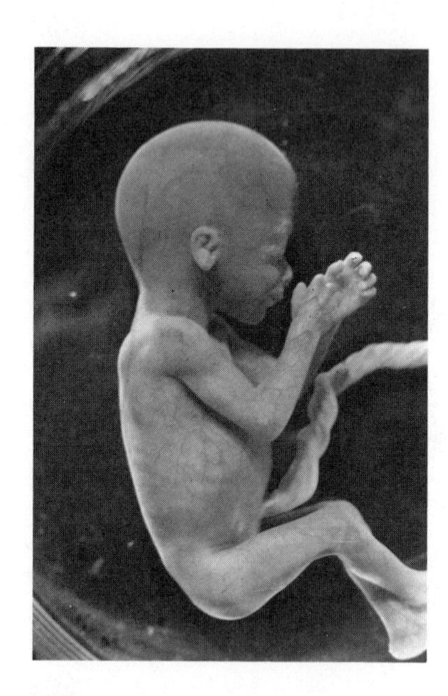

UNIT III PREGNANCY 211

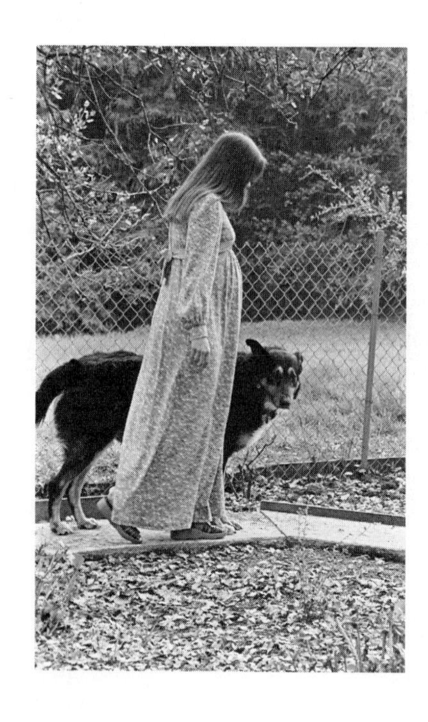

Chapter 9 PHYSICAL AND PSYCHOLOGIC CHANGES OF PREGNANCY 213

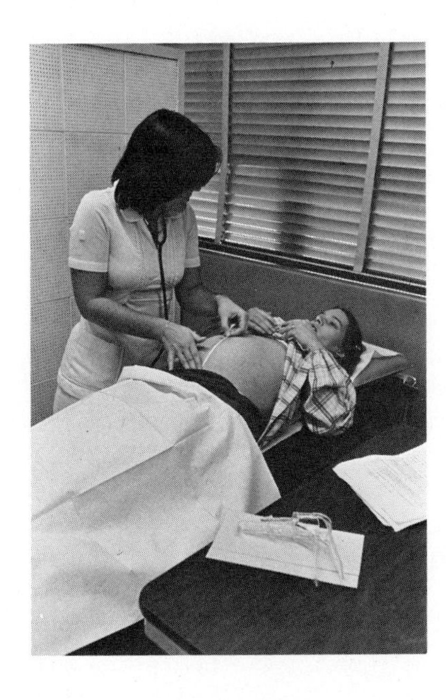

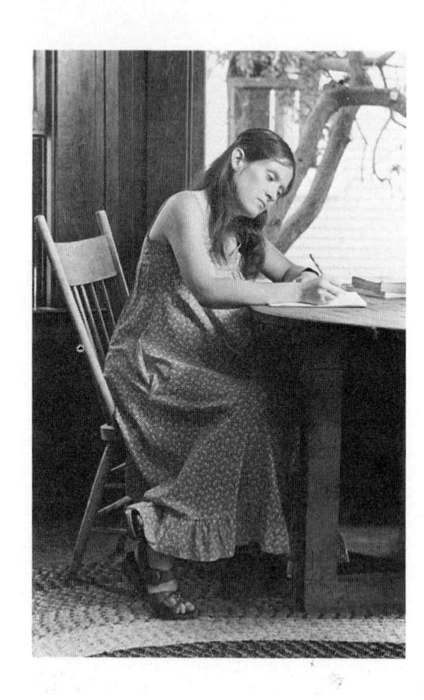

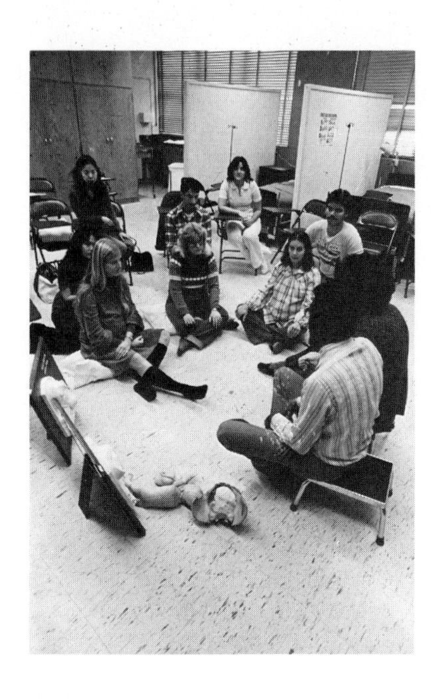

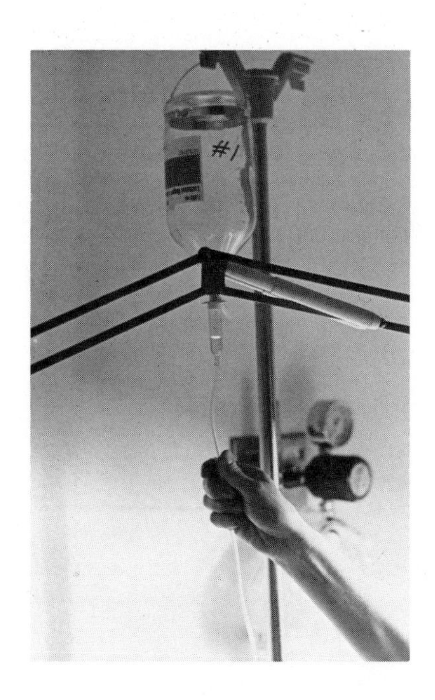

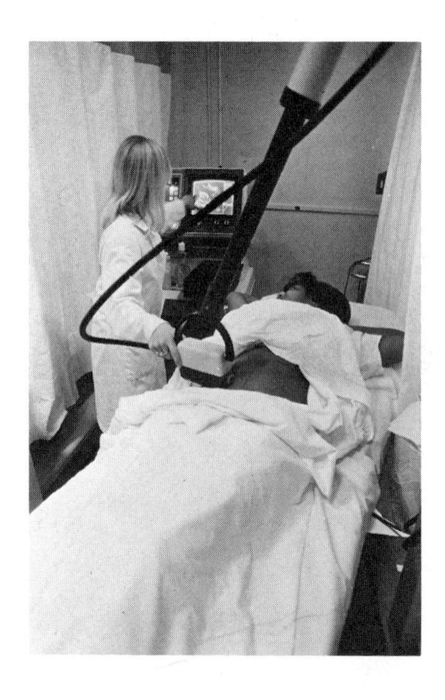

UNIT IV LABOR AND DELIVERY 409

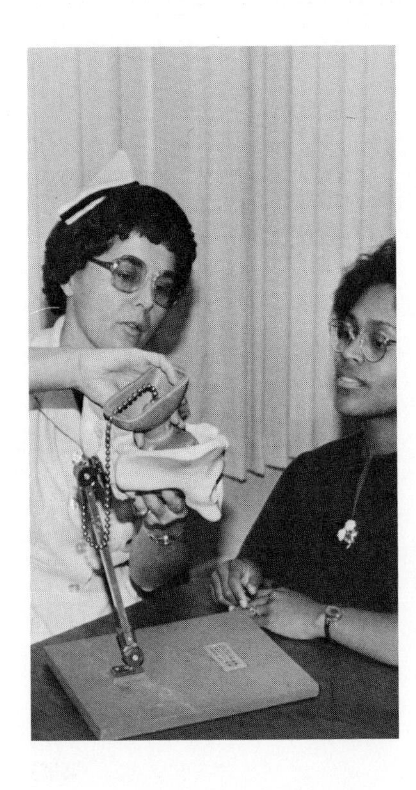

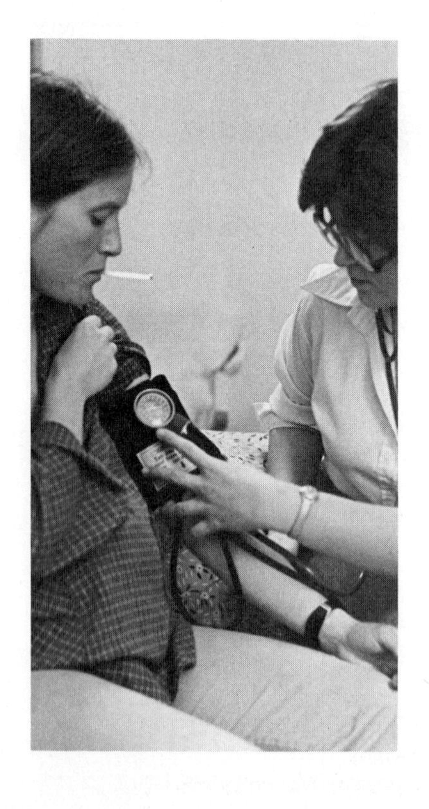

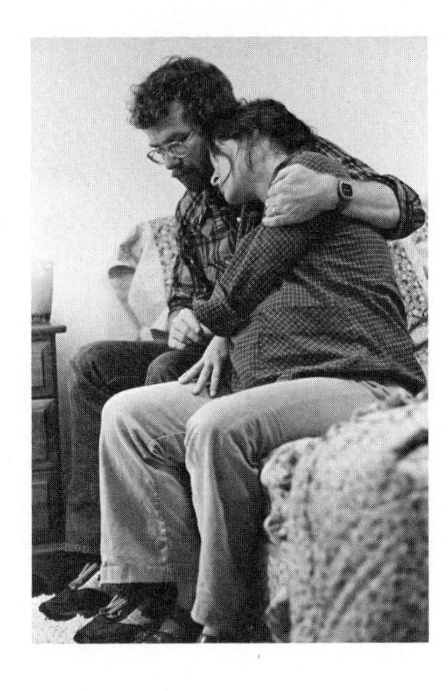

Chapter 17 THE PARENTS IN CHILDBIRTH: NEEDS AND CARE 479

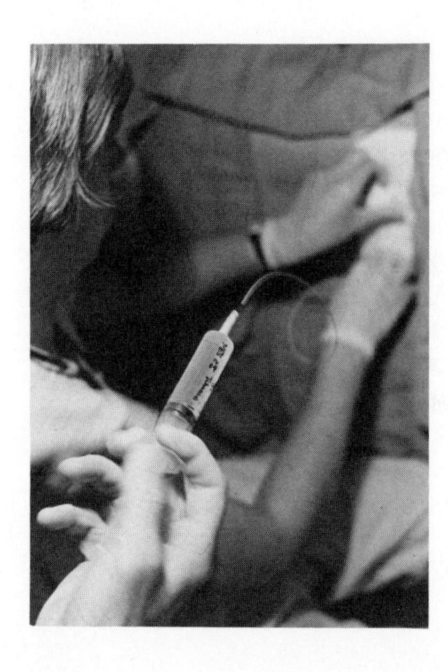

Chapter 18 PAIN RELIEF AND OBSTETRIC ANESTHESIA 515

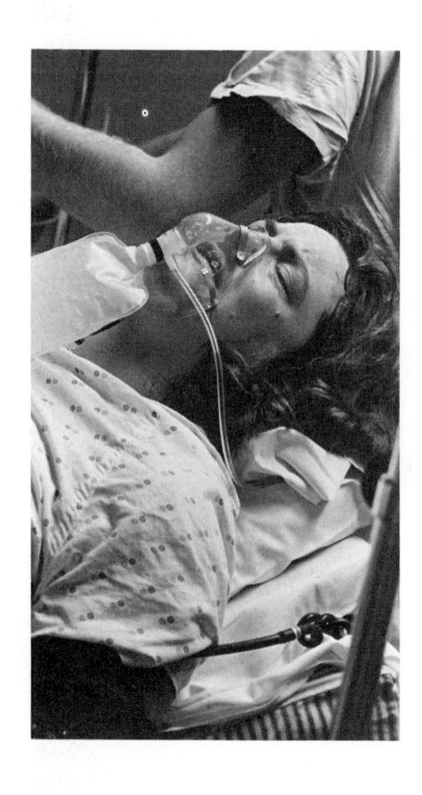

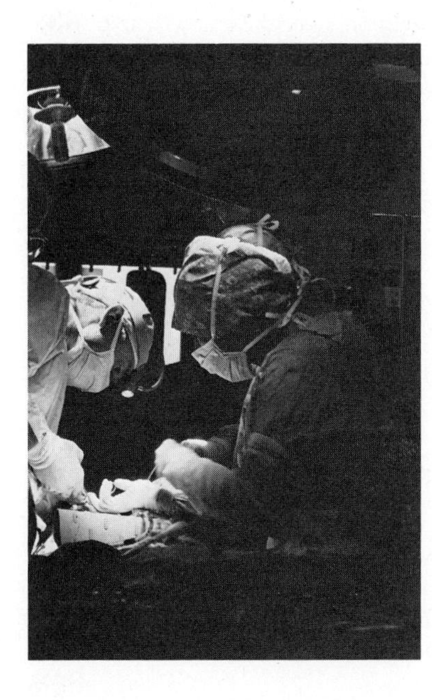

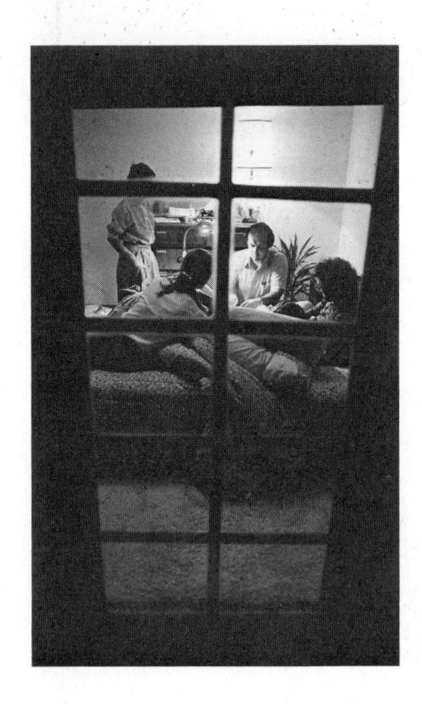

Chapter 21 BIRTH ALTERNATIVES AND EMERGENCY DELIVERIES 629

UNIT V THE NEONATE 649

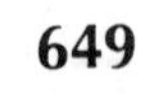

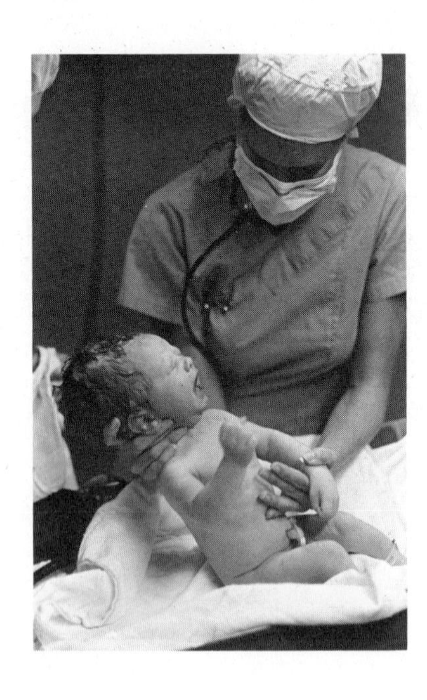

Chapter 22 NURSING ASSESSMENT OF THE NEWBORN 651

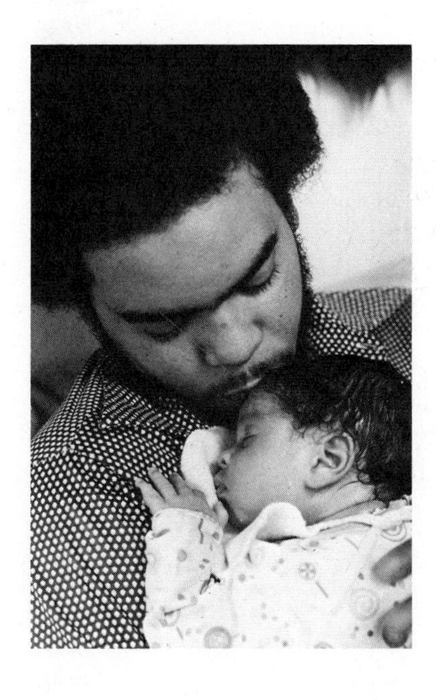

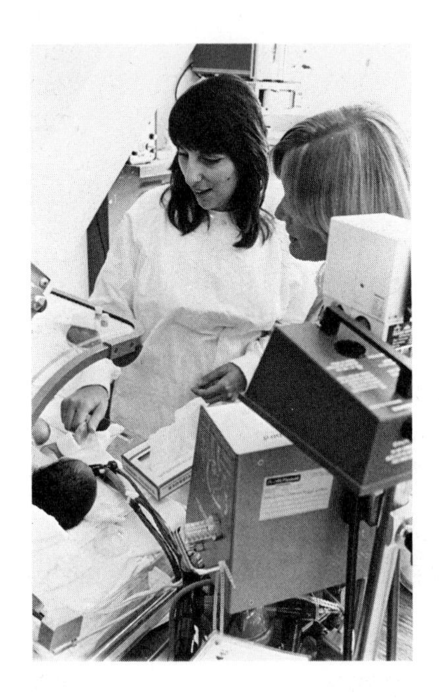

Chapter 24 THE HIGH-RISK NEWBORN: NEEDS AND CARE 729

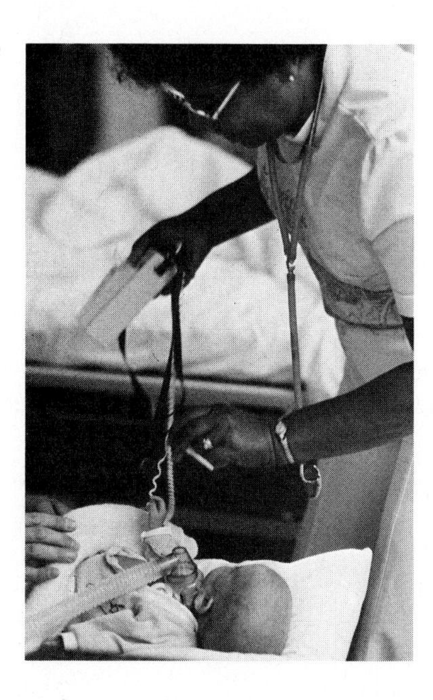

Chapter 25 COMPLICATIONS OF THE NEONATE 779

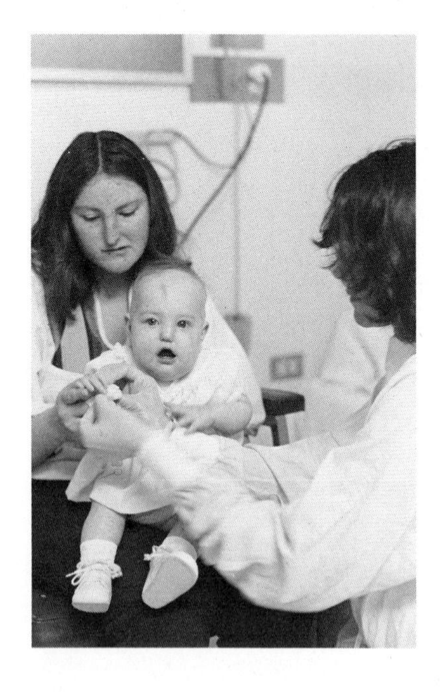

UNIT VI THE PUERPERIUM 899

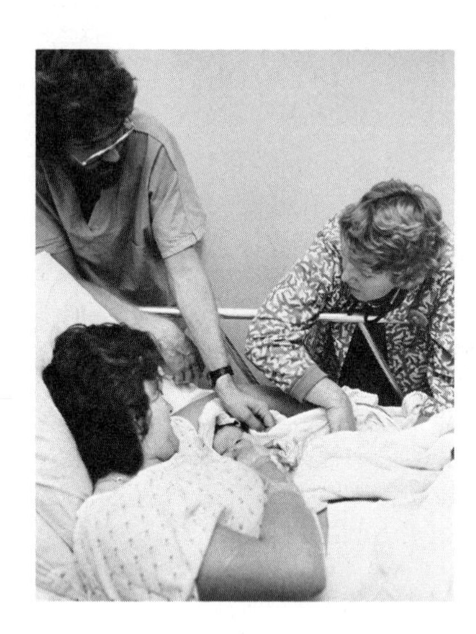

Chapter 27 THE POSTPARTAL FAMILY: ASSESSMENT, NEEDS, AND CARE 901

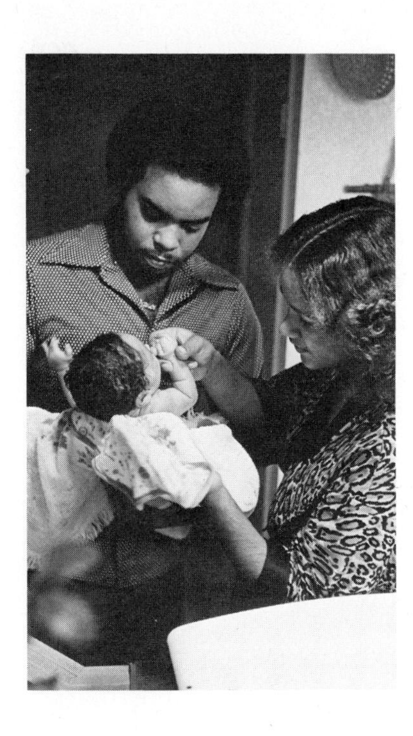

Chapter 28 ATTACHMENT 941

Chapter 29 COMPLICATIONS OF THE PUERPERIUM 963

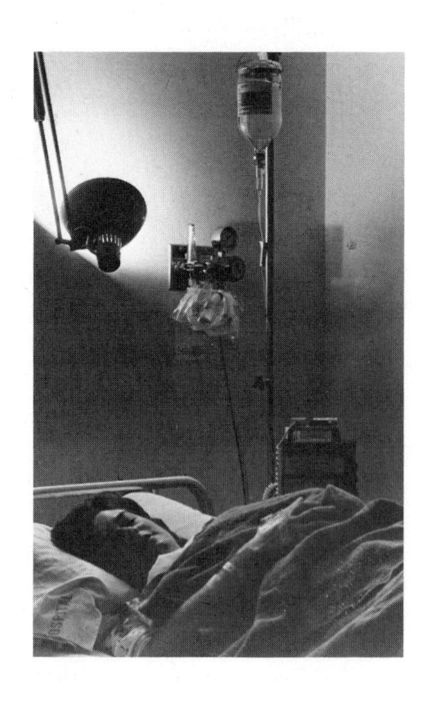

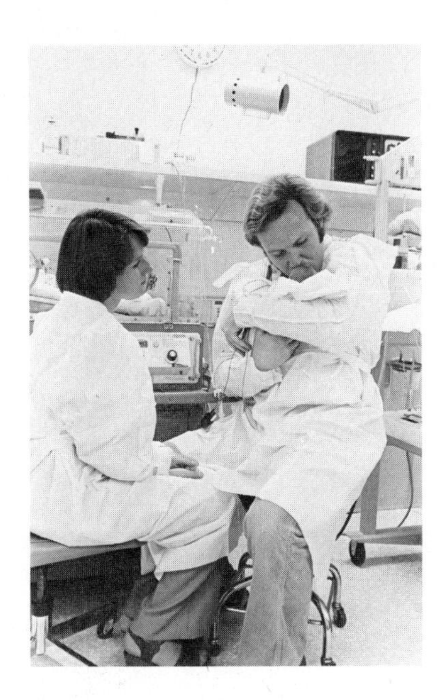

Obstetric Nursing is a comprehensive textbook that delineates the nursing knowledge and skills necessary to care for the childbearing family. Thus, current nursing practice is the primary focus of this textbook. It is imperative, however, that nursing students be aware of the professional issues and trends that ultimately will determine the future of nursing. The purpose of this introduction, therefore, is to explore these issues and trends.

The controversies and questions affecting the direction of nursing are well represented by those arising in obstetric practice. Here we take three of these issues and their effects on obstetric nursing into consideration. The first issue we consider is the increasing use of technology in obstetrics, the controversies that surround its use, and its effect on nursing practice. The second issue is consumerism in obstetrics and its implications for the professional nurse. Finally, we examine the expanded role of the obstetric nurse and consider the responses of physicians and patients to this trend. Although these issues are discussed as separate entities, they are in fact interrelated. The implications for nurses in one area certainly influence the outcomes in the other areas.

OBSTETRIC TECHNOLOGY

Scientific Advances or Medical Excesses?

In the past few years, tremendous technologic strides have been made in obstetrics and neonatalogy. The medical and nursing knowledge base is increasing, and as a result more services are available to health care consumers. For example, amniotic fluid analysis provides information concerning the fetus during the critical intrapartal period, and intensive care units are equipped with sophisticated machinery that can maintain the physiologic functions of critically ill infants when they are unable to do so independently.

The "good" that these technologic advances have done is undeniable. More lives, maternal and neonatal, are being saved daily; more families are being helped to live qualitative lives. Yet there is a growing concern that the reliance on technology in obstetrics is excessive and that in some cases the risks of certain procedures outweigh the advantages of their use. For example, amniocentesis is fatal to fetuses in 1.5% of cases (*Science News,* 1979a). Elective induction of labor may lead to maternal and fetal morbidity. Other medical procedures are also being scrutinized for their potential negative effects.

The controversy about electronic fetal monitoring is representative of the larger issue of excessive technological involvement in obstetrics. In the United States, nearly 65% of all labors are monitored by electronic equipment (*Science News,* 1979b). Some health care professionals advocate monitoring all labors (Butler and Parer, 1976). In this way, cases can be identified that were prenatally categorized as low risk but that are adversely affected by labor.

Yet there are situations in which external or internal electronic monitoring physically adversely affects the laboring woman or her fetus. Although data about maternal and fetal complications due to invasive fetal monitoring are conflicting, there have been reports of maternal infection, uterine perforation, and other soft tissue trauma. The newborn may suffer scalp abscesses from clipping of the electrode on soft tissue (Gee and Ledger, 1976).

And what of the effects of electronic monitoring on the psyches of the expectant couple whose delivery is considered low risk? Fetal monitoring equipment may interfere with the childbirth experience. The couple who have prepared for the childbirth may find the equipment and the staff's concern with the technical aspects of labor and delivery limiting and a symbol of their lack of control in this matter. In addition, the couple may suffer from unwarranted anxiety about the well-being of the fetus because of the complexity and noise of the machinery.

The increasing incidence of cesarean births has been attributed to the routine use of fetal monitoring. When fetal distress is indicated by abnormal fetal heart rate patterns, the infant is delivered immediately by cesarean section. However, the National Institutes of Health warns that "abnormal fetal heart rate patterns do not always mean that a fetus is in distress" (*Science News*, 1979b). Thus, the decision to perform a cesarean section may in fact be based on misleading data from the electronic monitoring equipment. The woman is then subjected to a surgical procedure that is not really needed, and the couple are deprived of the emotional satisfaction of a shared, natural delivery.

Do intrapartal fetal monitoring or similar procedures in cases of low-risk labor and delivery constitute excessive medical practice? There are those who argue that every pregnancy and delivery carries with it potential medical problems, and therefore maternity patients must be managed intensively to prevent complications and to ensure the well-being of both mother and child. To that end, the use of any tool in the medical repetoire is justified. Others support the notion that pregnancy and childbirth are natural, normal processes and should not be managed in the same rigorous way as pathophysiologic abnormalities. Medical intervention is perceived as an unnecessary and costly interference in low-risk cases.

Opinion is growing that there should be more stringent screening of patients receiving certain services. Because of the high cost of certain procedures, insurance companies are becoming involved in this issue, as are consumers who are questioning the necessity and compulsory nature of particular medical procedures. Many expectant couples are responding to the increase in technologic interventions by seeking alternatives to the health care system's traditional management of childbirth (see Chapters 12 and 21).

Implications for Nursing

Consumers and health care professionals are increasingly supportive of the idea that medical and nursing actions should be dependent on the maternity patient's level of risk. Nursing has recognized the need for rigorous evaluation of all patients, and all nurses are being encouraged to develop their assessment skills. In this textbook, entire chapters are devoted to assessment during the maternity cycle, and in-depth physical and psychologic assessment guides and high-risk screening tools are provided.

The increasing technology of the health care system has had an additional effect on the educational and occupational aspects and opportunities available to nurses. Many nurses are participating in medical research; others are administering highly specialized services that require stringent training. This trend will probably continue, since the need for highly skilled staff is growing.

Those nurses who choose to provide general health maintenance services to maternity patients must be aware of the current "state of the art" if they are to provide optimum care to these women and their families. To that end, information about obstetric technology and related nursing actions is provided in this textbook.

The increasing sophistication of high-risk obstetric technology raises several questions regarding the direction of nursing, however, and today's student—tomorrow's nurse—may be called upon to answer these questions. For example, will this trend toward specialization result in further fragmentation of patient care? If the nurse becomes a technician, who will provide continuity of care to the maternity patient and her family? Does the concept of specialization run counter to the nursing philosophy of caring for the whole patient? Indeed, these are difficult questions, but they should be kept in mind by nursing educators as they further refine the theories and philosophy of the profession.

CONSUMERISM IN OBSTETRICS

In the past 20 years, attitudes of those utilizing health care services have changed radically. No longer do patients and their families believe that "the doctor always knows best." People are asking for complete information about medical practices—what, why, and how much. Entrants into the health care system are looking at traditional medical methodology and philosophy with new eyes. They are finding that the costly services offered by the system are not always meeting their needs.

Obstetrics may be one of the most highly criticized specialties because of the traditional methods of management of pregnancy and labor and delivery. In the past, labor and delivery was treated as a medical problem. The conduct of labor and delivery was controlled by the obstetrician and the hospital staff. Many types of analgesic agents were given during labor, and general anesthesia was administered for delivery. During labor and delivery, the father sat in the waiting room. After the delivery the father saw his child through the window of the nursery. Frequently, the mother was separated from her infant for hours after the delivery, and maternal-infant contact was dependent on hospital routine and schedule. Postpartal stays for mother and child were usually about ten days, and infant care classes were unknown.

Research of health care professionals has shown that traditional labor and delivery practices do not necessarily provide the optimum childbirth experience for the family. Nor are these practices the most healthful for every woman. For example, there is substantial evidence that certain analgesic and anesthetic agents may be harmful to the fetus. In addition, a rigid hospital routine that requires separation of family members is detrimental to the family bonding process (see Chapter 1).

More and more it is being recognized that obstetric patients do not fit the medical model. Typically, the maternity patient enters the health care system not because of ill health but because she and the expectant father want to optimize their chances of having a healthy child. Many couples are seeking assistance from physicians and nurses—not control. Fathers often desire to be participants, not passive by-standers. Each couple wants their childbearing experience to be special and meaningful.

The outcry from obstetric consumers and health care professionals regarding the management of pregnancy and childbirth has resulted in the "Pregnant Patient's Bill of Rights," a document delineating the rights of every pregnant woman who is able to participate in decisions involving herself and her unborn child. This document appears on p. xlvi.

Obstetricians, nurses, and hospital administrators are gradually responding to consumers' demands and complaints about traditional maternity care. Certain policies and practices are being modified, and facilities are being constructed in an attempt to satisfy the request for family-centered maternity care. The consumers' demand for complete information is being met by an increase in prenatal and postpartal educational opportunities.

Birth Alternatives

Alternatives to conventional institutional childbirth are being offered to low-risk patients by some hospitals. Labor and delivery rooms are being remodeled to convey a homelike atmosphere. Some hospitals are establishing outpatient birth centers.

The goal of birth rooms within hospitals is to promote a meaningful experience for the family. The father and persons important to the mother are permitted to participate in the birth. Medical intervention is minimal. In a few in-hospital birth rooms, siblings are permitted to be present during the labor and delivery.

Those birth facilities that are being established outside the hospital are usually associated with a nearby hospital and are often managed jointly by physicians and nurse-midwives (Lubec and Ernst, 1978; Norwood, 1978). Occasionally the birth center is established and managed by nurse-midwives solely, and support services include physician consultation. Nurse-midwives are the staff in attendance during labor and delivery. If a complication arises during labor or delivery, patients are transferred quickly to a health care facility that is equipped to handle the situation. These birth centers attempt to offer high-quality care to low-risk patients at low cost. Medical interventions such as episiotomies and anesthetics are not standard procedures. Fathers are permitted to assist during the delivery. The family and health care staff work together.

Despite the changes in maternity services, some expectant families feel that the health care system has not responded suitably or quickly enough to their demands. They object to the increase in technologic interventions and regard certain conventional medical practices more a matter of physician convenience than patient safety. These families may choose to deliver their children at home and may engage a midwife or nurse-midwife to attend the birth. It is infrequent that a physician will perform an elected home delivery, since many regard home birth as a potentially dangerous practice.

The data concerning the safety of home births are conflicting. One study has found that the risk of fetal mortality is two to five times greater for babies born out of the hospital than those born in a hospital (*J. Obstet. Gynecol. Neonatal Nurs.*, 1978). Other evidence suggests that home birth is a safe alternative for medically screened healthy women (Mehl et al., 1977).

A primary focus of this textbook is nursing care during in-hospital births, simply because the majority of births occur in hospitals. However, we do consider the alternative modes of childbirth in Chapter 21.

Implications for Nurses

Traditionally, the phrase "patient-physician relationship" has implied a specific pattern of interaction. The patient placed faith and trust in the professional's expertise, and the professional assumed the role of primary decision-maker for the patient in matters of health and sickness (Reeder, 1978).

The phrase "consumer–health care provider" denotes a different perspective. A consumer purchases services or goods from the providers of these services or goods and expects quantity and quality for his or her money. Faith and trust are not the bases of the relationship between consumer and the providers of health care. Satisfaction with services rendered determines the continuation of this relationship. The formerly unquestioned expertise of the professional is no longer sufficient justification for certain actions. Patients are demanding explanations about medical actions.

Thus, the relationship between patient and nurse has also been altered. *Nurses are as accountable for their actions as physicians are* and must accept the legal consequences of malpractice as a physician must.

In obstetrics the nurse is ultimately accountable to two patients—the mother and child. It is therefore extremely important that the nurse explain her actions to the expectant parents and clearly delineate all the options available to the maternity patient, as well as any risks. Ideally, the nurse counsels the obstetric patient and provides appropriate referrals depending on patient decisions. The nurse is thereby meeting two consumer needs by acting as patient educator and advocate.

The nursing profession is meeting consumer demands in obstetrics in other important ways. Nurses are usually the instructors of prenatal and postpartal education classes. Many nurse practitioners and nurse-midwives are providing the kind of alternatives to conventional institutional obstetric management that many families are seeking. Nurses are frequently the primary caregivers in clinics and birth centers that emphasize family-centered health. Maternity patients and their families are finding that nursing's orientation toward education, self-care, and health maintenance meshes with their desire for participation in and decision-making about the childbirth experience.

The expanded role of nurses in obstetrics is discussed further in the next section, but it is important to note that the obstetric consumer's demand for alternatives has aided the nursing profession in its striving for autonomy and recognition for its unique role in the health care system. The demand for choices by patients and their families has provided nurses with choices of specialization, work setting, and degree of involvement in patient care.

In *Obstetric Nursing* we emphasize the nurse's role as educator of the maternity patient and her partner. The nurse must prepare the expectant couple for the physical and psychologic rigors of pregnancy and childbirth, and this text offers complete information about these subjects. In addition, we provide an in-depth discussion about communication skills (Chapter 12), which can be taught to expectant parents to enhance their parenting abilities and their relationship as a couple. Nurses will also find these skills useful when dealing with patients and their families.

THE PREGNANT PATIENT'S BILL OF RIGHTS*

The Pregnant Patient has the right to participate in decisions involving her well-being and that of her unborn child, unless there is a clearcut medical emergency that prevents her participation. In addition to the rights set forth in the American Hospital Association's "Patient's Bill of Rights," the Pregnant Patient, because she represents TWO patients rather than one, should be recognized as having the additional rights listed below.

1. *The Pregnant Patient has the right,* prior to the administration of any drug or procedure, to be informed by the health professional caring for her of any potential direct or indirect effects, risks or hazards to herself or her unborn or newborn infant which may result from the use of a drug or procedure prescribed for or administered to her during pregnancy, labor, birth or lactation.

2. *The Pregnant Patient has the right,* prior to the proposed therapy, to be informed, not only of the benefits, risks and hazards of the proposed therapy but also of known alternative therapy, such as available childbirth education classes which could help to prepare the Pregnant Patient physically and mentally to cope with the discomfort or stress of pregnancy and the experience of childbirth, thereby reducing or eliminating her need for drugs and obstetric intervention. She should be offered such information early in her pregnancy in order that she may make a reasoned decision.

3. *The Pregnant Patient has the right,* prior to the administration of any drug, to be informed by the health professional who is prescribing or administering the drug to her that any drug which she receives during pregnancy, labor and birth, no matter how or when the drug is taken or administered, may adversely affect her unborn baby, directly or indirectly, and that there is no drug or chemical which has been proven safe for the unborn child.

4. *The Pregnant Patient has the right* if cesarean birth is anticipated, to be informed prior to the

*Prepared by Doris Haire, Chair, Committee on Health Law and Regulation, International Childbirth Education Association, Inc., Rochester, N.Y.

administration of any drug, and preferably prior to her hospitalization, that minimizing her and, in turn, her baby's intake of nonessential pre-operative medicine will benefit her baby.

5. *The Pregnant Patient has the right,* prior to the administration of a drug or procedure, to be informed of the areas of uncertainty if there is NO properly controlled follow-up research which has established the safety of the drug or procedure with regard to its direct and/or indirect effects on the physiological, mental and neurological development of the child exposed, via the mother, to the drug or procedure during pregnancy, labor, birth or lactation—(this would apply to virtually all drugs and the vast majority of obstetric procedures).

6. *The Pregnant Patient has the right,* prior to the administration of any drug, to be informed of the brand name and generic name of the drug in order that she may advise the health professional of any past adverse reaction to the drug.

7. *The Pregnant Patient has the right* to determine for herself, without pressure from her attendant, whether she will accept the risks inherent in the proposed therapy or refuse a drug or procedure.

8. *The Pregnant Patient has the right* to know the name and qualifications of the individual administering a medication or procedure to her during labor or birth.

9. *The Pregnant Patient has the right* to be informed, prior to the administration of any procedure, whether that procedure is being administered to her for her or her baby's benefit (medically indicated) or as an elective procedure (for convenience, teaching purposes or research).

10. *The Pregnant Patient has the right* to be accompanied during the stress of labor and birth by someone she cares for, and to whom she looks for emotional comfort and encouragement.

11. *The Pregnant Patient has the right* after appropriate medical consultation to choose a position for labor and for birth which is least stressful to her baby and to herself.

12. *The Obstetric Patient has the right* to have her baby cared for at her bedside if her baby is normal, and to feed her baby according to her baby's needs rather than according to the hospital regimen.

13. *The Obstetric Patient has the right* to be informed in writing of the name of the person who actually delivered her baby and the professional qualifications of that person. This information should also be on the birth certificate.

14. *The Obstetric Patient has the right* to be informed if there is any known or indicated aspect of her or her baby's care or condition which may cause her or her baby later difficulty or problems.

15. *The Obstetric Patient has the right* to have her and her baby's hospital medical records complete, accurate and legible and to have their records, including Nurses' Notes, retained by the hospital until the child reaches at least the age of majority, or to have the records offered to her before they are destroyed.

16. *The Obstetric Patient,* both during and after her hospital stay, has the right to have access to her complete hospital medical records, including Nurses' Notes, and to receive a copy upon payment of a reasonable fee and without incurring the expense of retaining an attorney.

It is the obstetric patient and her baby, not the health professional, who must sustain any trauma or injury resulting from the use of a drug or obstetric procedure. The observation of the rights listed above will not only permit the obstetric patient to participate in the decisions involving her and her baby's health care, but will help to protect the health professional and the hospital against litigation arising from resentment or misunderstanding on the part of the mother.

THE EXPANDING ROLE OF NURSES IN OBSTETRICS

Professional options are growing for nurses. In Chapter 1 the various roles and settings for nurses in obstetrics are discused in depth. Here we would like to explore some of the issues that have developed from the expansion of nursing practice.

Nurses and Physicians

The nurse-midwife and nurse practitioner are becoming major providers of health services during the prenatal, intrapartal, and postpartal periods. Family planning and general health clinics are being established and run by nurse practitioners. These nurses are assuming the responsibilities of genetic counseling, family planning guidance, and health maintenace. Patients are referred to physicians as necessary.

Nurse-midwives are often the primary caregivers in birth centers. Frequently, the facility is run independently of physician control, although physicians are consulted when necessary. The nurse-midwives provide education to clients and serve as the delivery attendants. In addition, nurse-midwives are called upon to attend the family during home births.

Many physicians are supporting the increasing autonomy of nursing professionals. Joint practices in which physicians and nurse practitioners or nurse-midwives are equal partners have been established. Physicians serve as consultants and provide support services to clinics and birth centers. These physicians are showing their endorsement of the expanded role of nurses by their participation in and encouragement of this development.

Other physicians support the theory behind expansion of nursing roles but find the practice less palatable. In theory, the physician will have more time to care for seriously ill patients if other health care professionals assume the responsibility of caring for individuals who are not seriously ill or who are essentially healthy and want to maintain that state (Tomich, 1978). The low-risk maternity patient fits this last category, and nurse practitioners and nurse-midwives are adequately trained to care for this person.

The reaction of many physicians to actual independent nursing practice is less than supportive. Physician organizations have blocked clinics run by nurse practitioners (Beason, 1978; *RN*, 1979). Birth centers have also been under attack. Physicians in New York petitioned the state government unsuccessfully to deny a license to a birth center in Manhattan (Norwood, 1978). Regulations have been proposed in New Jersey that would hamper home birth by nurse-midwives and that would make physician presence necessary during certain procedures performed by nurse-midwives in birth centers (*New York Times*, April 1978).

The reason usually cited for the negative reaction of many physicians is the threat that these alternatives pose to patient safety. Certainly this is a legitimate concern, and quality control is a necessity in all health care facilities. However, other reasons for this negative response by physicians have been proposed. As Tomich (1978) points out, "The emergence of new roles in nursing may be considered as a set of challenges to the primacy of the physician." Consumers are also challenging the status of the medical profession and are making choices between conventional physician management and nursing services. Some physicians may feel threatened economically, which may provide further motivation for their nonsupportive attitude.

It is only natural that those desiring change will be opposed by those fearful of it. In obstetrics, the role of nurses is expanding and some physicians are opposing this change. Even so, physicians and nurses are becoming colleagues in the health care system, and nurses are continuing their development as autonomous professionals.

Legal Implications for Nurses

Nurses are legally bound to perform their duties according to specified standards of care and their recognized level of skill and training. Standards of care and the scope of nursing functions are determined by each employing institution and by each state's licensure laws.

As the role of nurses expands, so do their legal accountabilities. Nurses who are careless, who perform their professional duties below the acceptable standards of care, or who behave unprofessionally place their patients at risk. If a patient suffers loss or damage because of faulty nursing action, the nurse and employing institution may be held liable in a civil suit action.

Nursing responsibilities include assuring the accurate functioning of equipment (such as drainage tubes and oxygen and infusion equipment), assuring that the patient receives prescribed treatment, and observing and reporting changes in a patient's condition. The nurse is responsible for observing and reporting an incorrectly prescribed or performed medical intervention (for example, an incorrect drug or incorrect dosage of the right drug). Failure to carry out these responsibilities and other duties that conform to an established standard of care and that are within the scope of nursing practice may result in a charge of negligence or malpractice.

The importance of clear, concise, and complete nursing records cannot be overemphasized. These records are evidence that a nurse performed prescribed treatments, reported important patient observations to the appropriate staff, and adhered to acceptable standards of care.

The obstetric nurse must be able to perform certain professional duties depending on the employing institution's standards of care and on the nurse's recognized level of skill and training. The in-hospital labor and delivery nurse's accountabilities may be somewhat different from the nurse-midwife's or the nurse practitioner's. The labor and delivery nurse is not expected to have the same knowledge or specialized skills as the nurse practitioner or the nurse-midwife. This is not to say that the labor and delivery nurse is not subject to legal scrutiny, however. The hospital staff nurse must be able to perform certain actions depending on hospital requirements; he or she must be aware of the risks of these and physician-performed interventions; and the nurse must be observant of the patient's response to these actions and report and record all pertinent information. If the maternity patient or fetus suffers damage because of alleged faulty medical practice, these individuals or any other person who suffers loss from the incident can sue the physicians and nurses in attendance, as well as the institution.

Nurse practitioners and nurse-midwives are also at risk for civil action in the event of injury or loss to patients. The definitions of negligence and malpractice for these nurses depend on each state's determination of scope of practice. These nurses are specialists performing duties similar to those of physicians in some cases. It is interesting to speculate what standard of care these nurses will be measured against in a court of law. Will they be evaluated according to the standards of care established for physicians or to those established for nurses?

In summary, the nurse's role in the health care system is growing. Underlying the concept of professional autonomy is the concept of responsible, thoughtful action. Clearly, nurses must render care of the highest quality to every patient. However, they must do so with their legal limitations in mind.

SUMMARY

Increasing medical technology, consumerism, and the expanding role of the nurse are issues with interrelated ramifications throughout the health care system. The future of nursing in general and obstetric nursing in particular will be determined by the resolution of the controversies discussed here. Certainly nursing educators will affect the outcomes of these issues as they continue to delineate the direction of professional nursing.

Clearly, the nursing student is faced with many professional challenges and choices. The ultimate challenge, however, is to learn how to provide quality care to those seeking their services. This textbook offers to the nursing student the comprehensive knowledge and skills necessary to promote the health of maternity patients and their families.

REFERENCES

Beason, C. Oct. 1978. Nurse practitioners: the flak from doctors is getting heavier. *RN.* 41:27.

Butler, J. M., and Parer, J. T. Sept.–Oct. 1976. Is intensive intrapartum monitoring necessary? *J. Obstet. Gynecol. Neonatal Nurs.* 5(supp.):45.

Gee, C. L., and Ledger, W. J. Sept.–Oct. 1976. Maternal and fetal morbidity associated with intrapartum monitoring. *J. Obstet. Gynecol. Neonatal Nurs.* 5(supp.):65.

J. Obstet. Gynecol. Neonatal Nurs. May–June 1978. Editorial. 7:5.

Lubec, R. W., and Ernst, E. K. N. 1978. The childbearing center: an alternative to conventional care. *Nurs. Outlook.* 26:754.

Mehl, L. E., et al. 1977. Outcome of elective home births: a series of 1,146 cases. *J. Reproduc. Med.* 19:281.

Norwood, C. May 1978. Birth centers: a humanizing way to have a baby. *Ms.* p. 89.

New York Times. April 6, 1978 (II:24); April 20, 1978 (XI:6).

Reeder, S. J. 1978. The social context of nursing. In *The nursing profession: views through the mist,* ed. N. L. Chaska. New York: McGraw-Hill Book Co.

RN. Feb. 1979. Nursing news. 42:14.

Science News. 1979a. A safer alternative to amniocentesis. 115:230.

Science News. 1979b. NIH on electronic fetal monitoring. 115:183.

Tomich, J. H. 1978. The expanded role of the nurse: current status and future prospects. In *The nursing profession: views through the mist,* ed. N. L. Chaska. New York: McGraw-Hill Book Co.

UNIT I

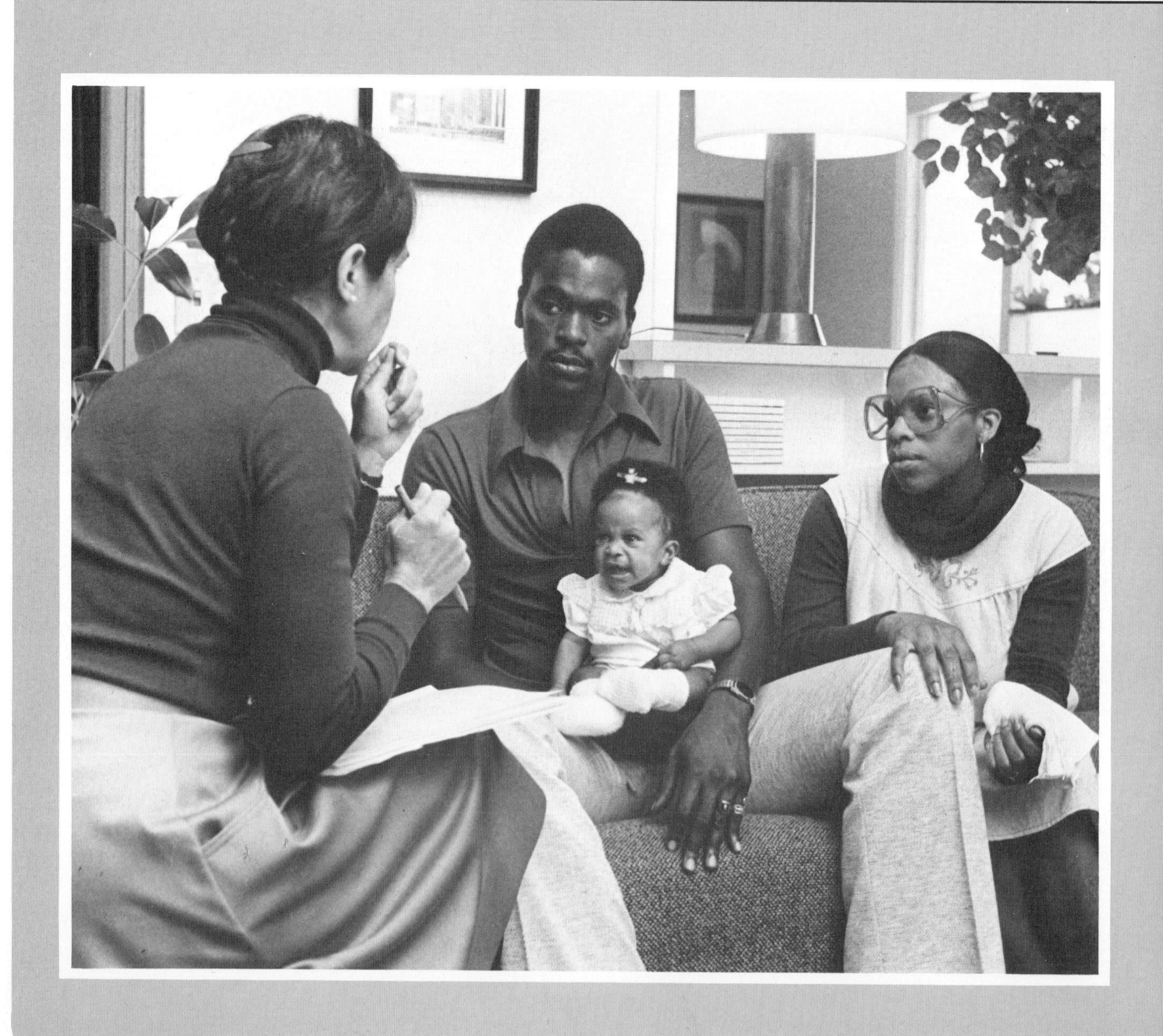

INTRODUCTION TO FAMILY-CENTERED OBSTETRIC NURSING

CHAPTER 1

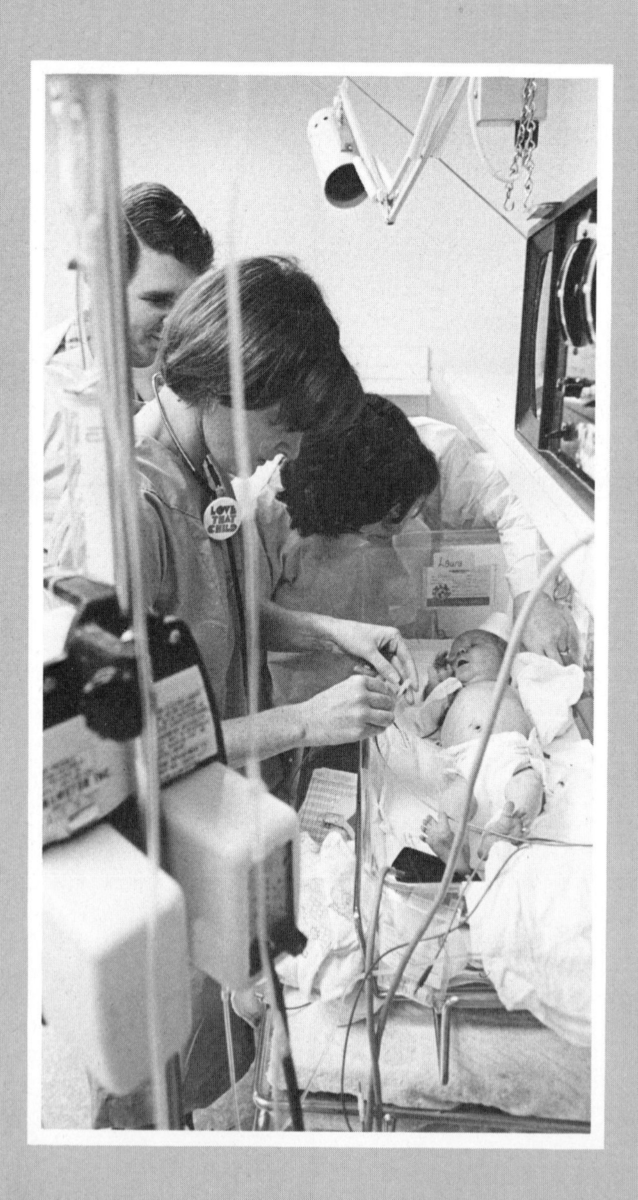

NURSING THE CHILDBEARING FAMILY: HISTORICAL AND CURRENT PERSPECTIVES

DEVELOPMENT OF FAMILY-CENTERED CARE

NURSING AND THE CHILDBEARING FAMILY

- **Roles and Settings for Nurses**
- **Application of the Nursing Process**

OBJECTIVES

- Identify pertinent historical developments in obstetrics.
- Describe the role of the midwife in providing obstetric care.
- Identify present obstetric nursing roles.
- Discuss the components of the nursing process and its application to maternity nursing.

At the moment a child is born, the quality of his or her future depends on many factors, not the least of which are the physical and psychologic health of the parents. The maternity nurse contributes to the optimum quality of the child's life by providing expert care to both parents and child throughout the entire time that the family is expanding.

The quality of care provided to the childbearing family is a product of the professional's skill and knowledge. The empirical knowledge of primitive ages provided the basis for discovery of the facts, theories, and concepts used today in the scientific approach to the nursing process. Knowing the significant events in childbearing and childrearing customs throughout history provides the practicing nurse of the present with increased awareness of and sensitivity to the consumer's need for care that both maintains the integrity of the family and preserves the uniqueness of the individual.

The beginnings of today's family-centered approach to nursing care can be traced back to prehistoric times, when groups of families struggled to survive and to maintain the most basic of human needs. Childbirth was regarded as a natural part of life, requiring no special care or assistance. Women usually delivered alone, without difficulty or interference. Anthropologic studies indicate that primitive women were of physical statures that allowed for easy delivery; only abnormal presentations proved fatal to mother and infant. Sepsis was virtually unknown because a clean environment, good nutrition, abundant exercise, and lack of fear in bearing young predominated.

As primitive tribes grew and clustered together, other members of the community began to assist in birth. Mutual support came from experienced and wise women who had already borne their children. Their loving and nurturing care welcomed the new mother and infant into a close symbiotic relationship. This was the beginning of midwifery and obstetric nursing in its simplest form.

HISTORICAL OVERVIEW OF OBSTETRICS AND MATERNITY CARE

Early Developments

The earliest known medical records are the Egyptian papyruses. Papyrus scrolls written about 2200 BC give guidelines on treatments to relieve pain in labor, a method for determining the sex of the unborn child, and ways to diagnose pregnancy. The Ebers papyrus (circa 1550 BC), a more comprehensive papyrus scroll dealing primarily with obstetrics and gynecology, documents practices relating to abortion, augmentation of labor, menstruation, diseases peculiar to women, and methods of treatment.

Egyptian religious beliefs prohibited the practice of dissecting the dead body; knowledge of anatomy was therefore scant. Despite this limitation, the Egyptians developed an embalming skill that has yet to be duplicated. Their ability to see causal relationships is illustrated by their tests to determine pregnancy and fetal sex. The woman's urine was used to water wheat and barleycorns. If the plants grew rapidly, pregnancy was confirmed; if the barley grew faster than the wheat, the unborn child was a female. Modern-day replication of this practice, based on knowledge of pituitary and ovarian hormonal influences on growth and germination, has produced results with an 85% accuracy.

The medical history of ancient India comes from the Sacred Books of Brahma and from the Veda, which were the bases for Hindu medicine from 1400 BC to AD 1000. Charaka and Susruta were the most widely recognized of the Indian physician-priests, and their classifications of diseases, theories on body humors, and therapeutic regimens were followed for centuries.

Operative obstetrics had its beginnings in these ancient times. Like those of the Egyptians, Hindu religious edicts forbade the mutilation of a dead body. However, it was thought that an unborn child possessed no spirit until some time after birth, so the baby could be extracted by crude forceps or by severing various limbs until the entire infant was removed. Although women from royal families or with malpresentations were attended by a physician, most deliveries were handled by midwives, and birth stools were common (Figure 1–1).

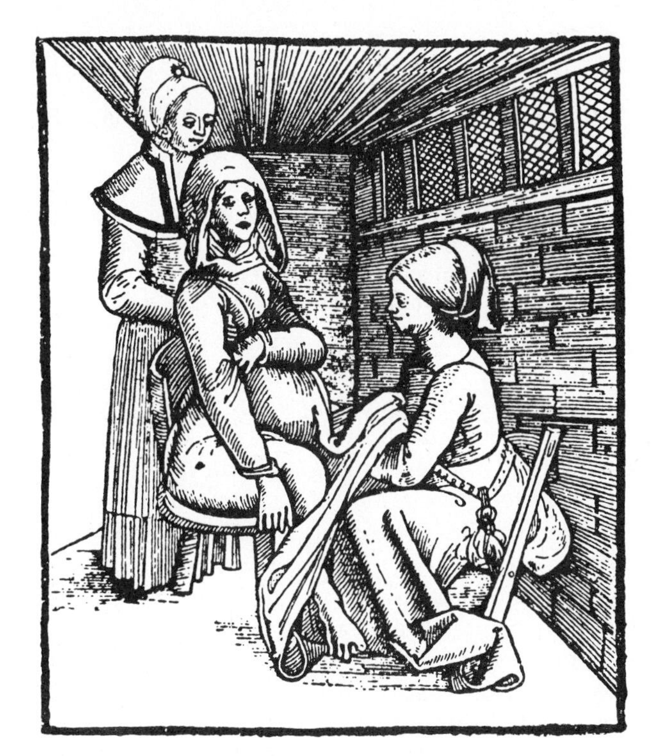

Figure 1–1. Reproduction of a sixteenth-century woodcut illustrating a birth chair (stool) in use. (From Culver Pictures, Inc. New York, N.Y.)

The scientific approach to medicine came from ancient Greece. Hippocrates, the father of medicine, was born on the Greek island of Cos around 460 BC. Born in an era of great men of ethics, philosophy, and creativity, Hippocrates laid the foundation of the medical model: objectivity, cleanliness, respect, judgment, and dignity. He believed that there was an art to the practice of medicine and that it was essential to consider the whole patient, the patient's way of life, and the natural processes of life. Only essential surgical interventions and a few medications were used in this era. Diet and exercise were paramount; observation and prognosis were the premises upon which care and cure could be effected.

Little is written about obstetrics in Greek history. Athenian law required pregnant women to be attended by midwives—Greek women who had borne children and were past the childbearing age. Midwives and physicians performed abdominal palpations and vaginal examinations, noted cervical changes during pregnancy, and used vaginal speculums, irrigations, and dilators. Pessaries were commonly used for uterine support and other gynecologic problems but could not be used to induce an abortion, which was absolutely forbidden under the Hippocratic oath.

As in our day, the issue of abortion went unresolved. Plato and Aristotle believed abortion should be used to limit the population, Lysias said the question was one of when the fetus reaches viability, and Hippocrates felt it had no place in healing.

The belief that a woman is "unclean" after childbirth is ancient. There are numerous Biblical references to this effect, but Chapter 12 of Leviticus clearly states the law concerning postpartal treatment of women and specifically implies that the female is inferior and less desirable than the male:

> The Lord said to Moses: Tell the Israelites: When a woman has conceived and has given birth to a boy, she shall be unclean seven days, unclean as at the time of her menstruation. On the eighth day the flesh of his foreskin shall be circumcised. She shall then continue for 33 days in the blood of purification. She shall contact nothing holy and shall not attend the sanctuary till the days of her purification are completed. If she gives birth to a girl, then she shall be unclean for two weeks as in her monthly separation and for yet 66 days, while bleeding, she shall stay at home, during the purification period. (Lev. 12:2–5)

It is still common practice to advise couples to abstain from intercourse for six weeks (42 days) after childbirth, even though research by Masters and Johnson (1966) has proved that there is no physiologic reason for this limitation of sexual activity.

We next come to ancient Rome, where a Greek physician named Soranus specialized in gynecology and obstetrics. His writings on the subject were extensive, and he became known as the father of obstetrics. He is best known for the use of podalic version.

With the decline of Rome, interest in the medical sciences also waned. Smallpox invaded the land, and fear of demons and evil spirits pervaded the populace. Christian priests and monks assumed the care of the sick, and superstition and punishment for sin were declared the cause of most ills. During the ensuing Dark Ages, all aspects of progress were paralyzed until the fifteenth century, when the transition from the medieval to the modern world began in Europe.

European Developments

The invention of movable type by Gutenberg in 1450 heralded the end of the oral tradition, which had limited knowledge as well as misinterpreted it. Renaissance art became the forerunner of the new scientific age. Artists such as Leonardo da Vinci (1452–1519) and Michelangelo Buonarroti (1475–1564) did human dissections and accurately illustrated every aspect of the human body.

The anatomic studies of Andreas Vesalius (1514–1564) radically changed medical science. He discovered that early anatomists used only animals for evaluation. His subsequent studies of the human body influenced the development of obstetrics. As a result of his continued research, Vesalius produced a seven-volume work on anatomy and established Padua as the medical center of Europe.

Ambroise Paré (1517–1590), a French physician profoundly influenced by Vesalius, wrote two books on obstetrics and in one described the technique of podalic version, which had been lost from the time of Soranus. It replaced the crude and usually fatal practice of cesarean section (Figure 1–2). Paré used cervical dilatation to induce labor in women who were bleeding, described fetal movement on abdominal palpation, and proposed the use of a nipple shield. His contribution to the science of obstetrics was perhaps the turning point that shifted the responsibility of the management of pregnancy and birth from untrained midwives to physicians.

The sixteenth and seventeenth centuries produced several men whose influence on obstetrics is still felt. Peter Chamberlen (1560–1631) is credited with the invention of the obstetric forceps, but he kept it a family secret for a generation. Not until the eighteenth century did the secret become known when Leuret and Smellie modified the Chamberlen model for practical use.

William Harvey (1578–1657), the discoverer of the circulatory system, studied the blood and its function in the body, leading him to develop the scientific field of embryology. Furthermore, Harvey set the pattern for the evolution of the midwifery schools in England; he is thus often referred to as the father of British midwifery.

Francois Mauriceau (1637–1709) of Paris was the first to observe that puerperal fever was epidemic. He described a mechanism for breech extraction, refuted the idea that the pubic bones separated during labor, advocated suturing tears of the perineum, instituted the routine use of a bed for delivery rather than a birth stool, and tried to dispel the ancient idea that a fetus had some control over birth. It was believed that the fetus would attempt to be born at seven months' gestation; if unsuccessful, it would attempt again at eight months' gestation but would be weakened by the first efforts. The general belief was that a fetus born at seven months was stronger and would be healthier than a fetus delivered at eight months. Some lay people still believe this myth.

It was the studies of Hendrik van Deventer (1651–1724), a Dutch physician specializing in or-

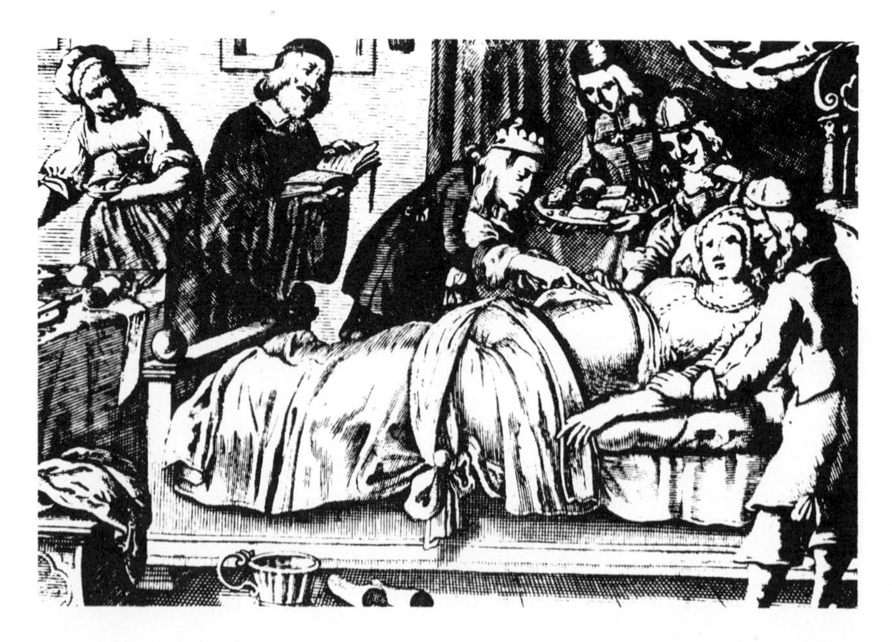

Figure 1–2. Cesarean operation. The surgeon is surrounded by his helpers and is preparing the woman for the operation. (After Scultetus.) (From Bettmann Archives, Inc., New York, N.Y.)

thopedics and obstetrics, that resulted in the first accurate description of the pelvis. He identified several different types of pelves and the axis of the birth canal and noted deformities that could delay or impede delivery of the infant. His writings on midwifery were widely accepted, and he is known as the father of modern midwifery.

During the 1700s, two British physicians, William Smellie (1697–1763) and William Hunter (1718–1783), had significant influence on obstetric practice. Smellie's many contributions included observation and recording of the mechanisms of labor, the use of manikins for teaching, measurement of the diagonal conjugate, the invention of curved and locked forceps, and the advocacy of a conservative third stage of labor. Hunter, a pupil of Smellie, discovered the separate nature of maternal and fetal circulations and established the first lying-in ward in London.

Sir Fielding Ould introduced the episiotomy in the middle of the eighteenth century, despite the lack of anesthetics. It was used sparingly and only when indicated.

During the nineteenth century European advances in medical practice were significant (Figure 1–3). Hospitals were built and enlarged, the germ theory was established, vaccination was introduced, and records of vital statistics were being compiled. And, of major importance to obstetrics, anesthesia was discovered.

In 1847, shortly after William Morton reported the use of ether in the United States, James Simpson administered chloroform, first to a woman in labor, then to a child needing surgery. The use of anesthesia was extremely controversial. Scientists viewed it as an end to pain; moralists declared it the work of the devil and a violation of scripture. The arguments continued for several years and finally ceased when Queen Victoria delivered Prince Leopold after receiving chloroform from Dr. John Snow. Simpson was subsequently knighted and internationally acclaimed for his contribution to mankind.

Many techniques, procedures, and clinical findings used in modern practice bear the names of Europeans who devoted their practice to obstetrics and gynecology: John Braxton Hicks (Braxton Hicks sign, p. 215), Friedrich Wilhelm Scanzoni (Scanzoni's maneuver or operation, p. 570), Alfred Hegar (Hegar's sign, p. 215), Franz Nägele (Nägele's rule, p. 263), and Karl Credé (Credé's method).

Credé and his contemporary, Ignaz Philipp Semmelweis (1818–1865), used their clinical observations, the newly established germ theory, and independent research to produce two simple techniques with overwhelming significance: eye prophylaxis and hand-washing.

A paper published by Credé in 1884, called "The Prophylactic Treatment of Ophthalmia Neonatorum," described in detail the administration of a 2% silver nitrate solution to a newborn infant's eyes. Only the advent of antibiotic ointments and the use of 1% silver nitrate solution have altered the basic procedure, which has prevented blindness due to gonorrhea in countless numbers of newborns.

The story of Semmelweis is legend. During the 1840s, while serving as a physician at Vienna General Hospital, he noted the low mortality rate in the ward run by midwives and the high number of deaths in the ward managed by obstetricians. Then a colleague died of septicemia after receiving a cut from an infected scalpel used to examine a woman who had died from puerperal fever. This incident confirmed for Semmelweis his belief that puerperal sepsis was passed from one woman to another by the contaminated hands of physicians and medical students coming from the cadaver laboratory. Semmelweis immediately instituted a policy of hand scrubbing in a chloride of lime solution before examining any patient in labor or performing a delivery or postpartum examination. The results were conclusive: the incidence of sepsis dropped from almost 12% to 3.8% in a year and to 1.2% the following year. Later, in a controlled study at another hospital, Semmelweis further reduced deaths to 0.39% (Graham, 1951).

Semmelweis continued to replicate his studies, moving from one institution to another, trying to gain acceptance for his discovery. Despite his dramatic findings, Semmelweis could not convince his colleagues to wash their hands. He continued to be ridiculed and ignored by the majority of physicians throughout Europe.

United States Developments

During the early colonization period, maternity care was based on the different traditions and practices of the European settlers. Midwives or neighbors helped with deliveries, breast-feeding was assumed, and home care was the only option.

There are conflicting opinions as to when the first hospitals were established in this country;

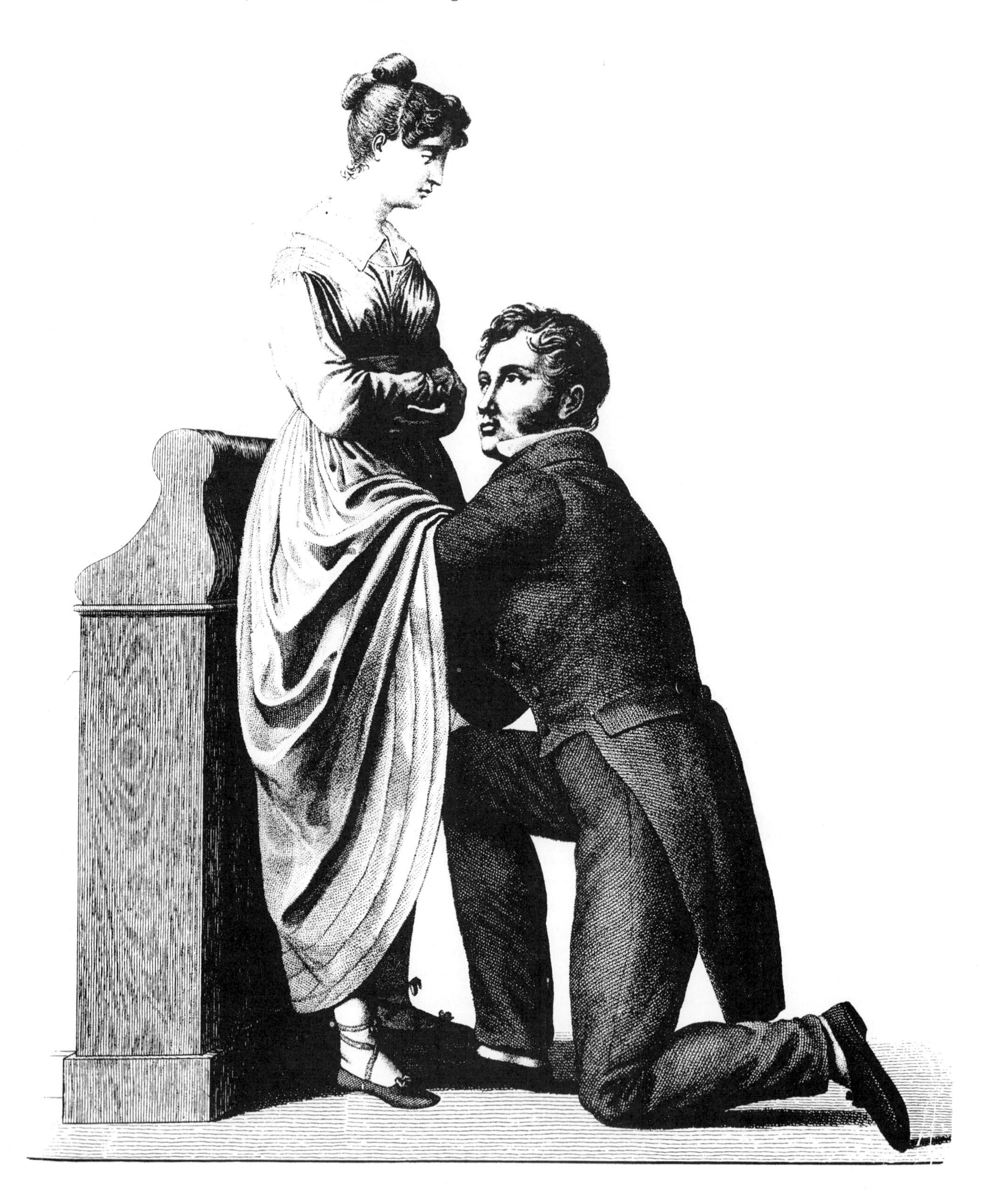

Figure 1–3. Physician examining a woman during pregnancy. (Lithograph, 1822.) (From Bettmann Archives, Inc., New York, N.Y.)

the dates range from 1658 to 1736, when Charity Hospital in New Orleans was built. Most of the early hospitals were associated with poorhouses, wards for the insane, and the homeless. As in Europe, the "sick houses" were poorly run, dirty, and managed by inept personnel. Efforts were begun in the mid-1700s to improve the status of these institutions so that physicians and nurses could receive adequate training.

William Shippen, a pupil of Smellie and Hunter, established a school for midwifery in Philadelphia in 1762, designed to be attended by both men and women. However, few, if any, women entered the school, and "man-midwifery" had its start in the United States. Shippen's school eventually became part of the University of Pennsylvania, and the curriculum became known as "obstetrics" rather than midwifery.

Samuel Bard, educated abroad and trained in midwifery, was a respected American medical educator who helped establish King's Medical College (known today as Columbia University) and who wrote the first American obstetrics textbook. Valentine Seaman established the first school of nursing in New York in 1798 to train women in midwifery and the care of children. A Philadelphia physician, Joseph Warrington, also began a school of midwifery but soon extended it to all kinds of care of patients with medical and surgical conditions.

During the nineteenth century, obstetrics and midwifery were greatly influenced by William Dewees. He brought into practice the lithotomy position for delivery, insisted on relieving pain during labor, and advocated judicious use of forceps. Many consider him the person who made obstetrics a science in the United States and refer to him as the father of American obstetrics.

The American Medical Association, founded in 1847, established a section on obstetrics, women's diseases, and children in 1873.

As in Europe, the need for hand-washing prior to obstetric procedures was viewed with skepticism and doubt by physicians in the United States. A paper written in 1843 by a young Harvard physician, Oliver Wendell Holmes, titled "On the Contagiousness of Puerperal Fever," was not well received by the medical world. However, eventually the importance of asepsis was recognized, and hand-washing and other aseptic measures became standard procedures.

By the end of its first hundred years, the United States was well on the way to having an organized system of medical and nursing care that would leave the European tradition and become institutionally oriented.

The concept of health maintenance was in its embryonic stage, as was the idea of prevention as a primary force in creating a state of continual well-being.

Prior to 1900 few babies were delivered in hospitals. Only the very poor or unwed mothers went to a hospital for confinement. After a hospital delivery, newborn babies remained with their mothers; hammocklike cribs were placed at the foot of the bed where, with some help from a nurse, the mother could tend her infant. However, wards became noisy and crowded, and many women were too ill to care for their babies. To remedy this situation, the Boston Lying-in Hospital established a night nursery in 1898 to prevent infants from disturbing the patients and personnel on the ward. This proved satisfactory. Indeed, many of the physicians and nurses were of the opinion that babies should remain in a nursery at all times to maintain the quiet and tidiness of the ward.

Early in the twentieth century, a real need for newborn nurseries appeared. Outbreaks of diarrhea, scarlet fever, diphtheria, and other communicable diseases caused a large number of infant and maternal deaths. Physicians stressed the need for separate care as a control method for preventing the spread of infection, and nurseries became essential.

By mid-century, hospital deliveries had steadily increased, with a concomitant decrease in mortality rates. The newborn nursery—and thus the separation of mother and child—became a firmly entrenched practice, heralding an era of rigid schedules, formula feedings, and strict asepsis. Minimal thought was given to the psychologic effects of this practice on the childbearing family.

About 50 years ago, the federal government became involved in improving the quality of maternity care. The Sheppard-Towner Act of 1921 was the first federal legislation to provide funds for state programs in maternal and child health; this act was in force until 1929. In 1935 came the Social Security Act, which provides federal grants for health and welfare programs, with extensive services in the maternal-child health area.

In 1964, as a result of an amendment to Title V of the Social Security Act, the Maternity and

Infant (M&I) Care Projects were begun by the Public Health Service of the Department of Health, Education, and Welfare in 56 areas where maternal and infant mortality rates were significantly higher than the national average. The states recently assumed management of these projects, although they are still federally funded.

The purpose of these projects is to provide good maternity care to high-risk mothers, thereby reducing mortality rates and preventing or decreasing prematurity, birth traumas, and mental retardation. Services include medical care, dental care, social services, infant care, nutrition services, patient education, family planning services, nursing care, and special services to adolescent mothers. The efficacy of the program has been demonstrated by reduced rates of prematurity and maternal and infant mortality (Wallace, 1975). The most significant contributions of the M&I Care Projects for the professional have been the emphasis on early prenatal care, a humanizing approach to public clinics, and utilization of the health team as a functional unit.

NURSE-MIDWIFERY

Throughout history, most societies have used some form of birth attendant or midwife. Midwifery is an honored profession, evolving distinct characteristics as it has developed throughout the ages. Even today, 80% of the world's population is attended in childbirth by a midwife.

Midwifery and nursing are distinct disciplines; in fact, the training, regulation, and practice of the professional midwife were instituted before organized professional nursing came into existence in 1871. However, they are complementary disciplines, and this has led to the development of another health professional—the nurse-midwife.

The history of the establishment of nurse-midwifery as an accepted and respected profession is briefly reviewed here. It is interesting to note how the professional development of midwifery and nurse-midwifery have differed in Europe and the United States.

European Milestones

The Scandinavian countries led Europe in providing a sound basis for the development of the professional midwife. In 1673 a well-known anatomist, Thomas Bartholin, gave the first examination to Danish midwives to determine their competency. In 1774 the King of Denmark declared that all midwives should be examined prior to starting practice and established the Midwives Examination Board, which still exists. In 1752 Finland initiated a plan of maternity care that used the first trained Finnish midwife. The Swedish Midwifery Organization had its beginning in 1886.

By the early 1800s schools of nursing were being established throughout Europe. In 1860 Florence Nightingale founded St. Thomas School of Nursing in London. She advocated the training of a "better class" of women as nurses and midwives to provide services to women, and she even wrote a book on the subject, *Introductory Notes on Lying-in Institutions Together with a Proposal for Organizing an Institution for Training Midwives and Midwifery Nurses.* She probably influenced the founding of the Ladies' Obstetrical College (1864), which was attended by women who were daughters of professional men and who wished to become midwives.

Nightingale attempted to establish a school of nurse-midwifery in 1867, but an unfortunate epidemic of puerperal sepsis forced the closing of the program. Her emphasis on training had its effect, however, and in 1872 the Obstetrical Society of London began issuing certificates to qualified midwives. In 1881, Miss Rosalind Paget, one of "Miss Nightingale's Young Ladies," founded the Midwives Institute (now the Royal College of Midwives) to register midwives and promoted a bill to ensure proper education and control. In 1902 the English Midwives Act was passed, and state registration became mandatory. The act also brought into existence the Central Midwives Board, a statutory body controlling the training and practice of midwives in England. The original act of 1902 has been revised several times, most recently in 1951. It requires the training period for midwives to be one year for trained nurses and two years for those untrained. The act clearly states that it gives "statutory recognition to the position of the midwife as a professional practitioner in her own right" (Central Midwives Board, 1962).

Throughout the Continent, the option still exists to become either a midwife or nurse-midwife; each is considered a professional. The settings for practice vary extensively from nation to nation, with births being conducted in family dwellings, maternity homes, and hospitals.

At the end of the nineteenth century, midwives in Europe began to propose the establishment of an organization that would strive to improve maternity care. In 1922 representatives from eight European countries met to discuss common aims. The International Midwives Union was established in 1928, later changing its name to the International Confederation of Midwives in 1954, during its first International Congress. At the most recent triennial Congress, held in 1975, 48 member countries were present, and more than 100 countries were represented in the Confederation. The goals of the organization are to work toward greater international cooperation in the professional practice of midwifery and to assist other organizations in improving standards of maternal and infant care, including family planning.

Development of Nurse-Midwifery in the United States

Historical Status of Midwifery

Early records indicate that the midwife was an important person in settlements and towns throughout the colonies. However, in strongly Puritan communities she was frequently suspected of witchcraft. The most infamous midwife of the time was Anne Hutchinson. She came to Boston from England in 1634 and soon established her skill as a midwife, but she was suspect because of her so-called heretical religious views. When she delivered an anencephalic child, the community had its confirmation that she was a witch. Hutchinson was banished from Massachusetts by the General Court and was excommunicated as well.

Midwifery was unattractive in America as a result of economic problems related to educating midwives and of strong religious pressures affecting the practice of midwifery. There were no effective licensing regulations or training programs (recall that Shippen established a school for midwifery in 1762 that attracted only men). The different ethnic groups had their own traditions and myths about childbirth. It also became the fashion for middle-class women to seek the care of a physician or male attendant. All these factors made midwifery a less than highly esteemed profession in the United States.

Although great numbers of midwives were practicing in the United States, no professional advances occurred in over 200 years. In 1905 there were over 3000 midwives delivering approximately 40% of all the babies born in New York City. Only a small percentage of these midwives had any formal training, and even fewer had medical support. This prompted an investigation of midwifery in New York City in 1906 by the Public Health Commission of the Association of Neighborhood Workers in conjunction with the New York City Health Department. The report described midwives as ignorant, untrained, incompetent, and dirty women. The published results were devastating to midwifery throughout the United States. States passed laws prohibiting or restricting the practice of midwifery and placed the control of midwives under physicians within state health departments.

By state law (1907) the New York City Board of Health became responsible for the regulation and practice of midwifery, and in 1911 a school for midwives was opened at Bellevue Hospital. The city's Sanitary Code of 1914 required that all midwives applying for a permit to practice must graduate from a school approved by the Board of Health. Thus in New York City the number of practicing midwives decreased from 3000 in 1905 to approximately 850 licensed midwives in 1932. The Bellevue School was forced to close in 1936, and three decades later no more licensed midwives were practicing in New York City.

Growth of Nurse-Midwifery

Despite the prevailing attitudes toward midwifery, women in public health and obstetric nursing recognized their responsibility to provide services and care to pregnant women, newly delivered mothers, and their infants. One such nurse was Mary Breckinridge, who had graduated from St. Luke's School of Nursing in 1910. The deaths of a premature daughter and 4-year-old son gave impetus to her plan of preparing herself to work in remote, rural areas and to provide a sound basis of child care beginning before birth and continuing through school age. She did public health and visiting nursing in Boston and, after World War I, went to Europe with the American Committee for Devastated France. There she was introduced to French midwives and saw how effectively they provided care in villages, small farm communities, and areas destroyed by the war. She found that although competent midwives in France were not nurses and competent nurses in the United States were not midwives, the English had combined the two successfully. Breckinridge realized that nurse-midwifery was the answer in the rural areas of the United States.

She received training as a nurse-midwife in 1923 in England and returned to the United States to practice in rural Kentucky. In 1925 she established the first nurse-midwifery program in this country, the Kentucky Committee for Mothers and Babies. The name was changed to the Frontier Nursing Service in 1928, and a 28-bed hospital was constructed in Hyden, Kentucky, that year.

The excellent work and accomplishments of the nurse-midwives of the Frontier Nursing Service were soon recognized. Infant and maternal mortality dropped significantly, and the families received quality health care.

The Frontier Graduate School of Midwifery was founded in 1939. In 1970 a certificate program to prepare family nurses was developed in coordination with the nurse-midwifery curriculum to produce a broadly prepared primary care nurse for rural areas. The school changed its name to the Frontier School of Midwifery and Family Nursing. Since its inception the school has trained approximately 500 nurse-midwives. In 1975 the new 40-bed Mary Breckinridge Hospital and Health Center was dedicated and opened.

While Breckinridge was proving the value of nurse-midwives in a rural setting, women's groups, nurses, and physicians joined forces in New York City in an attempt to reduce the high number of maternal and infant deaths. In 1918 the Maternity Center Association was founded. The goal of this organization was and still is to work "to assure that every baby born will be wanted and welcomed, and will have the high quality of care needed before, during and after birth" (Maternity Center Association, 1975). Dr. Ralph W. Lobenstein was the first chairman of the Medical Advisory Board for the Maternity Center Association, and it was his name that was given to a midwifery clinic and to the first nurse-midwifery school established in the United States. The Lobenstein School began in 1931 under the auspices of the Association for the Promotion and Standardization of Midwifery and merged (along with the clinic) with the Maternity Center Association in 1934. The intent of this educational program was "to teach midwifery to qualified public health nurses so they might supervise the untrained midwives now practicing throughout the country and, also, under the direction of obstetricians, bring skilled care to the mothers in isolated rural areas" (Maternity Center Association, 1975). In the early years, the Maternity Center Association program graduated approximately a dozen nurse-midwives a year. The Maternity Center Association became allied with the State University of New York at Downstate Medical Center about 20 years ago.

The third educational program in nurse-midwifery to open was the Tuskegee School in Alabama, a short-lived venture lasting from 1941 to 1945. Apparently, the community and the professionals of that area were not ready for nurse-midwives.

In 1943 Catholic Maternity Institute in Santa Fe, New Mexico, was established under the auspices of the Medical Mission Sisters at the request of the New Mexico State Health Department and the United States Children's Bureau. In 1945 New Mexico became the first state to license nurse-midwives, and in 1948 Catholic Maternity Institute became affiliated with Catholic University and became the first degree-granting nurse-midwifery program within a university.

The impact of this program on maternal and infant death rates was most significant. In 1939 maternal mortality in the United States was 48 per 10,000 live births, but in New Mexico the rate was a staggering 109.1 per 10,000 live births; Santa Fe County had a rate of 87.6. By 1967 the figures had dropped to 24.8 statewide, 15.1 in Santa Fe County, and 22.1 nationally. Despite its remarkable success, the program eventually closed after almost 30 years of family-centered care in the Southwest.

In the late 1950s and early 1960s additional nurse-midwifery schools opened. Currently there are 24 nurse-midwifery programs in the United States approved by the American College of Nurse-Midwives (see accompanying list). Some are certificate programs, which provide additional training for RNs; the others are master's degree programs. Approximately 150 nurse-midwives graduate each year from these schools, bringing the number of nurse-midwives in the United States to about 2000.

NURSE-MIDWIFERY PROGRAMS IN THE UNITED STATES

Booth Maternity Center, Philadelphia, Pa.
College of Medicine and Dentistry of New Jersey, Newark, N.J.
Columbia University, New York, N.Y.
Cuyahoga County Hospital, Cleveland, Ohio
Emory University, Atlanta, Ga.
Frontier School of Midwifery and Family Nursing, Hyden, Ky.
Georgetown University, Washington, D.C.
Johns Hopkins University, Baltimore, Md.
Medical University of South Carolina, Charleston, S.C.
Meharry Medical College, Nashville, Tenn.
University of Southern California, Los Angeles, Calif.
St. Louis University, St. Louis, Mo.
State University of New York, Brooklyn, N.Y.
United States Air Force, Andrews Air Force Base, Md.
University of Arizona, Tucson, Ariz.
University of California at San Diego, San Diego, Calif.
University of California at San Francisco, San Francisco, Calif.
University of Florida, Miami, Fla.
University of Illinois Medical Center, Chicago, Ill.
University of Kentucky, Lexington, Ky.
University of Minnesota, Minneapolis, Minn.
University of Mississippi, Jackson, Miss.
University of Utah, Salt Lake City, Utah
Yale University School of Nursing, New Haven, Conn.

Certificate programs are usually 8 to 12 months and the master's programs, 12 to 24 months. As of 1977 the American College of Nurse-Midwives determined that all educational programs preparing a nurse-midwife must be within or affiliated with an institution of higher learning. This reinforces the nurse-midwife's need for increased knowledge for a practice base.

Current Status of Nurse-Midwives

A certified nurse-midwife (CNM) is an individual educated in the two disciplines of nursing and midwifery and who possesses evidence of certification according to the requirements of the American College of Nurse-Midwives. Nurse-midwifery practice is the independent management of care of essentially normal newborns and women, antepartally, intrapartally, postpartally, and/or gynecologically, occurring within a health care system that provides for medical consultation, collaborative management, or referral and is in accord with the *Functions, Standards, Qualifications* for nurse-midwifery practice as defined by the American College of Nurse-Midwives (1979).

The nurse-midwife practices within the framework of a medically directed health service. She functions as a member of the obstetric team in medical centers, institutions, universities, and community health projects with active programs of nurse-midwifery. The nurse-midwife is prepared to provide prenatal, intrapartal, and postpartal care geared to the individual needs of each mother and family. She cares for the mother during pregnancy and stays with her during labor, providing continuous physical and emotional support. The nurse-midwife evaluates the progress of and manages labor and delivery, watchful for signs requiring medical attention, and provides immediate care for the newborn. She then helps the mother to care for herself and the infant, to adjust the home situation to the new child, and to lay a healthful foundation for future pregnancies by providing such care as family planning, yearly breast and cervical examinations, and treatment for minor gynecologic problems.

The nurse-midwife is prepared to teach, interpret, and provide support to families as an integral part of her service. Furthermore the nurse-midwife prepared in a graduate program leading to a master's degree is equipped to teach, to do beginning research, and to work in an administrative position as well as to give expert care. The person trained in a program leading to a certificate generally functions primarily as a staff nurse-midwife in a clinical service.

The official professional organization is the American College of Nurse-Midwives. It evolved from the desire of nurse-midwives for an organization that would meet the needs of the practitioner, that would assure quality of care, and that would maintain standards for safe, effective care that meet the individual needs of childbearing families.

In 1928 the Kentucky State Association of Midwives became the first nurse-midwifery organization in the United States. The name was changed in 1941 to the American Association of Nurse-Midwives. At this time there were only two schools open and very few nurse-midwives in the country. The National Organization for Public Health Nursing, established in 1912 by Lillian Wald, eventually created a section for nurse-midwives in 1944 with three specific objectives: (a) to study and set standards of practice for nurse-midwives, (b) to study and promote new opportunities in the field of nurse-midwifery, and (c) to study and evaluate standards of schools of nurse-midwifery.

However, The National Organization for Public Health Nursing was absorbed by the National League for Nursing when it was founded in 1952. After this merger there was no designated place for nurse-midwifery. As a result, the American College of Nurse-Midwifery was established in New Mexico in 1955. In 1969 the American Association of Nurse-Midwives joined with the American College of Nurse-Midwifery, becoming the American College of Nurse-Midwives.

Not only does this professional body determine the functions, standards, and qualifications for the practice of nurse-midwifery, but it also is the official agency for approving educational programs and certifying graduates of these programs. The National Certification Examination, first administered in 1971, assures that an individual is capable of safe, effective practice as a nurse-midwife. The initials CNM indicate that one is a certified nurse-midwife.

The basic beliefs and commitments of nurse-midwives are well reflected in the philosophy of the American College of Nurse-Midwives:

> Every childbearing family has a right to a safe, satisfying experience with respect for human dignity and worth; for variety in cultural forms; and for the parents' right to self-determination.
>
> Comprehensive maternity care, including educational and emotional support as well as management of physical care throughout the childbearing years, is a major means for intercession into, and improvement and maintenance of, the health of the nation's families. Comprehensive maternity care is most effectively and efficiently delivered by interdependent health disciplines.
>
> Nurse-midwifery is an interdependent health discipline focusing on the family and exhibiting responsibility for insuring that its practitioners are provided with excellence in preparation and that those practitioners demonstrate professional behavior in keeping with these stated beliefs.*

DEVELOPMENT OF FAMILY-CENTERED CARE

As medical skill and technology developed in North America, home deliveries, especially in urban areas, decreased. Hospitalization for labor and delivery became a common practice.

Childbirth was no longer an experience shared by the parents. Hospital rules insisted on the isolation of maternity patients to prevent and control infections. Thus parents were separated during labor and delivery, and mothers and infants were separated at birth. Infants were placed in newborn nurseries where routine care was provided primarily by nurses. The pattern of infant care established in the nurseries was characterized by strict aseptic procedures, rigid feeding schedules, and formula feedings.

In the early 1940s, parents began to question the necessity of the rigid rules and routines of the hospital. Social scientists and health care professionals began analyzing the effects of these practices on family relationships and on individual members. Studies revealed that the quality of the early mother-child relationship was a critical factor in child development. Psychologists and psychiatrists stated that it was important to a new mother's emotional security that she handle her infant and meet his physical and psychologic needs. Breast-feeding, which was thought to provide psychologic satisfaction for both mother and infant, had decreased with the separation of mother and infant in the hospital, and it was believed that the rigid feeding schedules in newborn nurseries contributed to many of the feeding problems that later developed.

Increasingly, psychologic and social problems were being attributed to the rigid practices advocated by hospitals. It became evident to some

*Philosophy of the American College of Nurse-Midwives. 1972. Washington, D.C.: American College of Nurse-Midwives.

individuals that more personalized and family-oriented maternity care was essential, and they began advocating changes in the kind of care given during the childbearing experience.

The concept of *natural childbirth* was introduced to this country by Grantly Dick-Read around 1944. He published his classic book, *Childbirth Without Fear,* in 1944. Educational classes were devised to give expectant parents an understanding of the normal birth process and to provide them with some emotional support. This method of childbirth preparation is still used (Chapter 12). Expectant parents are taught what to anticipate before, during, and after delivery. Under the natural childbirth regimen, the husband stays with his wife during labor, giving her needed support and assurance; he assumes the role of participant in and contributor to the birth of their child.

Rooming-in was advocated by Arnold Gesell and others as a way of achieving satisfactory postpartal adjustment of the mother to her child. The concept of rooming-in was not totally new or revolutionary. As discussed on page 9, this practice was common prior to 1900, although for different reasons than those discussed here.

Rooming-in means that newborn infants remain with their mothers during the hospital stay instead of being removed to nurseries. It focuses attention on the family unit, and both mother and father are permitted to care for the baby in the hospital. Parents learn how to properly hold, feed, and care for their infants, and the hospital staff provides emotional support and guidance, a prime factor in satisfactory postpartal care.

From 1941 to 1946, experimental rooming-in units were developed. The most widely known of these were the Detroit, Yale, Jefferson, and Duke programs. The first two programs were on an elective basis, but the others were mandatory for nonprivate patients for the purpose of preventing infection during a shortage of nursing staff. Since 1946, rooming-in units have been established in hospitals throughout the country. Modifications to the original programs have been made to meet the needs of the individual hospital and families.

One of the early advocates of change was John Bowlby, a psychiatrist who described the tragic effects of maternal deprivation on children, their parents, and the mental health of both (Bowlby, 1953). This study had great impact on motivating health care professions to implement change. Since this early work, the results of other studies in child development have also emphasized the importance of establishing sound early mother-child relationships. Focus on the family was now viewed as essential; the orientation of hospital care needed to be redirected to become patient-centered rather than hospital-centered.

The movement toward family-centered care during the childbearing experience was furthered in the late 1950s by the Family-Centered Maternity Care Program established at St. Mary's Hospital in Evansville, Indiana. This program was based on the notion that a hospital could provide professional services to mothers, fathers, and infants in a homelike environment that would enhance the integrity of the family unit. Seven basic principles underlay the project (Wooden, 1961):

1. Precautionary measures would be taken to safeguard the physical safety of the mother and infant.
2. Family members would not be separated during the mother's stay.
3. Human differences would be recognized from both physical and psychocultural standpoints.
4. The infant's growth dynamics would be recognized.
5. The parents' needs for information would be met.
6. Parental involvement would be encouraged.
7. Emotional preparation would be provided to personnel and staff, and their personal growth would be supported.

The success of St. Mary's Hospital's maternity program has been followed by a movement in other hospitals to extend the family-oriented approach to other areas besides the maternity unit. For example, many hospitals allow and even encourage parents or other family members to participate in the care of sick children in pediatric units.

Nurses and other health professionals are well aware that a patient's needs generally go beyond the purely physical and that these other needs must be met for the patient to achieve optimum health. Others who are affected by that individual's life, such as family members, also have needs that must be satisfied. Because the physical and emotional status of a patient is strongly influenced by that of his family, and because improving the health of its consumers is a goal of the health care system, family-centered care would seem to be an effective method of achieving this goal. During periods of change in a family, the nurse provides direct service to individuals, families, and the community, combining technical skills with professional competencies for a family-centered approach to maternity nursing.

NURSING AND THE CHILDBEARING FAMILY

Expectant parents must cope both as individuals and as a couple with first the crisis of childbearing and then the task of childrearing. Nurses can provide effective care to all members of the childbearing family by using their unique skills and implementing the principles of the nursing process.

Roles and Settings for Nurses

Many different titles have evolved to describe the professional requirements of the nurse in various maternity care roles. The most widely accepted definitions were developed by the Nurses Association of the American College of Obstetrics and Gynecology (NAACOG) Committee on Practice, approved by the NAACOG Executive Board, and recently published in the *Journal of Obstetric, Gynecologic, and Neonatal Nursing*. The definitions of nursing titles are as follows:

Professional Nurses

Qualifications. Graduates of an accredited basic nursing program and licensed to practice nursing.

Role/Function. Professional nurses provide direct care to patients, utilizing the nursing process in arriving at decisions. They work in a collegial and collaborative relationship with other health professionals to determine health care needs and assume responsibility for nursing care. In the course of their practice, they identify and carry out systematic investigations of clinical problems, assess the effectiveness of actions taken, and engage in periodic review of their contribution to health care and those of their professional peers.

On entry into the profession of nursing, it is recognized that the new graduate needs an extensive orientation period or internship to provide an opportunity for assimilation of knowledge and application of clinical skills.

Nurse Clinicians

Qualifications. Professional nurses who demonstrate expertise in nursing practice and insure ongoing development of expertise through clinical experience and continuing education. At the present time, this attainment is by means of certification for excellence.

Role/Function. Nurse clinicians have well-developed competencies in utilizing the nursing process for both direct and indirect nursing care. Knowledge and clinical expertise are utilized to provide care aimed at returning the patient to the highest level of health in the shortest period of time. Nurse clinicians coordinate actions of other health team members to provide continuous physical care and emotional support for the patient.

Nurse Practitioners

Qualifications. Professional nurses prepared in a specialized education program with emphasis on the expanded nursing role. This preparation shall be either in the context of a formal continuing education program or an advanced degree nursing program.

Role/Function. Nurse practitioners provide nursing care as primary health care providers; nurse practitioners assess the physical and psychological status of patients by means of interview, health history, physical examination, and diagnostic test. The nurse practitioners interpret data, develop and implement therapeutic plans, and follow through on the continuum of care of the patient. The practitioners implement these plans through independent action, appropriate referrals, health counseling, and collaboration with other members of the health care team.

Clinical Nurse Specialists

Qualifications. Professional nurses with advanced knowledge, skill, and competence in a specialized area of nursing. Clinical nurse specialists are prepared at the Master's level with emphasis in specific areas of clinical nursing.

Role/Function. The role of clinical nurse specialists is defined by the needs of a select patient population, the expectations of a larger society, and the clinical expertise of the nurse. By exercising judgments and demonstrating leadership ability, clinical nurse specialists function within a field of practice that focuses on the needs of the patient and system and encompasses interaction with others in the nursing and health care system serving the patient.

Clinical nurse specialists effect change by direct nursing care or indirectly by planning and guiding care with other health team members. Their roles include participating in activities designed to continue self-development, advance the goals of the nursing profession, and promote effective collaborative relationships with members of the other health care disciplines.*

An additional nursing role requiring definition is the *certified nurse-midwife* (CNM). Qualifications for a CNM include successful completion of an approved midwifery program at an institution of higher learning that awards a certificate or master's degree. This added knowledge and skill has extended the CNM practice into the management of care for mothers and infants throughout the normal maternity cycle. The nurse-midwife practices within the framework of a medically directed health service as a member of the obstetric team. The CNM provides antepartal, intrapartal, and postpartal care geared to the needs of each mother and family (refer to p. 13 for more information about the nurse-midwife).

Nursing is unique in its adaptability and flexibility in providing maternity care in various settings. Maternity nurses are found in the obstetric department of acute care facilities, in physicians' offices, in public health department clinics, in college health services, in family planning clinics, in school nursing programs dealing with sex education or adolescent pregnancies, in volunteer community health services, in abortion clinics, and in any other setting where a patient has a need for maternity care. The depth of nursing involvement in various settings is determined by the qualifications and role/function of the nurse employed. For example, the nurse practitioner may provide primary health care, identifying problems and recommending treatment, whereas the professional nurse provides direct nursing care, carrying out the treatment directives for the maternity patient.

*From NAACOG Committee on Practice. Jan.-Feb. 1978. Definitions of nursing titles. *J. Obstet. Gynecol. Neonatal Nurs.* 7:45.

Application of the Nursing Process

Nursing care is more than merely following medical orders and as such requires thoughtful assessment of nursing problems, identification of solutions for the problems, actions to correct problems, and evaluation of the services rendered. A logical, organized, systematic method incorporating a problem-solving approach has evolved to assist the professional nurse in providing nursing care. It is referred to as the *nursing process.*

The nursing process has four components: assessment, planning, implementation, and evaluation. The various tasks of each component are as follows:

Assessment

Establish patient data base by completing nursing history and assessment.
Review medical information.
Analyze patient information.
Identify patient problems.

Planning

Recognize possible solutions to problems.
Establish objectives for dealing with problems.
Identify nursing intervention (or nursing actions) for each problem.
Determine priorities for problems and interventions.
Establish goals and time parameters.
Communicate the plan of care to other members of the health team.
Complete a written nursing care plan.

Implementation

Provide nursing actions according to the written nursing care plan.
Record results of care in a medical record.
Direct other members of the health team.
Teach the patient and family.

Evaluation

Evaluate the effectiveness of nursing care and resolution of problems.
Review and update the nursing care plan.

Since the nursing process has clinical application and is evident in every hospital, the student is encouraged to develop the skills necessary for the utilization of this approach. Its application ensures that a high quality of care will be rendered to assigned patients.

This textbook offers several tools, based on the components of the nursing process, that will assist the maternity nurse in providing care. Assessment guides demonstrate an effective means of determining patient problems; they are provided for the antepartal, intrapartal, postpartal, and neonatal periods. Nursing care plans are provided for major obstetric and newborn conditions; they serve as models for the planning and implementation components of the nursing process. Evaluation of nursing care can be accomplished by using the outcome criteria provided at the conclusion of each nursing care plan. These tools will assist the student in developing a familiarity with the application of the nursing process.

SUMMARY

Integration of historical data about obstetrics and maternity care allows the professional nurse to understand the evolution of modern-day nursing care. The foundation for modern family-centered maternity care was laid in ancient times, and the difficulties experienced by midwives through the ages have influenced the current practice of midwifery and obstetric nursing. As the nursing role has expanded, the qualifications, practice, and settings for providing maternity care have been modified. Only through careful evaluation can the continued effects of past, present, and future approaches to maternity nursing be monitored and used for the improvement of nursing care.

SUGGESTED ACTIVITIES

1. As an independent study project, trace the historical developments that have affected obstetrics from ancient times.
2. In small group discussion, compare the role of the ancient midwife with the role of the present-day certified nurse-midwife.
3. During a postclinical conference, discuss the various responsibilities of the nurse practitioner and the nurse clinician.

REFERENCES

American College of Nurse-Midwives. 1972. *Statement of philosophy.* Washington, D.C.: The College.

Bowlby, J. 1953. *Child care and the growth of love.* Baltimore: Penguin Books.

Central Midwives Board. 1962. *Midwives Act, 1951: handbook.* London: Wm. Clowes & Sons, Ltd.

Dick-Read, G. 1953. *Childbirth without fear.* Rev. New York: Harper & Row Publishers, Inc.

Graham, H. 1951. *Eternal Eve.* New York: Doubleday and Co., Inc.

Masters, W., and Johnson, V. 1966. *Human sexual response.* Boston: Little, Brown & Co.

Maternity Center Association. 1975. *Log 1915–1975.* New York: The Association.

NAACOG Committee on Practice. Jan.–Feb. 1978. Definitions of nursing titles. *J. Obstet. Gynecol. Neonatal Nurs.* 7:45.

Wallace, H., ed. 1975. *Health care of mothers and children in national health services.* Philadelphia: Ballinger Publishing Co.

Wooden, H. 1961. *Hospital maternity care: family centered.* U.S. Public Health Service Research Project. Washington, D.C.: U.S. Government Printing Office.

ADDITIONAL READINGS

American College of Nurse-Midwives. 1979. *What is a nurse-midwife?* Washington, D.C.: The College.

American Nurses' Association. 1973. *Standards of maternal and child health nursing practice.* Kansas City: The Association.

Bear, E. 1957. *A study of the development of rooming-in in the United States of America and implications for nursing care.* Unpublished master's thesis. Detroit: Wayne State University.

Bettmann, O. L. 1956. *A pictorial history of medicine.* Springfield, Ill.: Charles C Thomas, Publisher.

Breckinridge, M. 1951. *Wide neighborhoods.* New York: Harper & Row Publishers, Inc.

Cutter, I. S., and Viets, H. R. 1964. *A short history of midwifery.* Philadelphia: W. B. Saunders Co.

Dietz, L., and Lehozky, A. 1967. *History of modern nursing.* 2nd ed. Philadelphia: F. A. Davis Co.

Fair, H. D. 1925. An epitome of the history of obstetrics. *Am. J. Obstet. Gynecol.* 10:747.

Ford, L., and Silver, H. 1967. The expanded role of the nurse in child care. *Nurs. Outlook.* 15:43.

Forman, A., ed. 1973. *New horizons in midwifery.* London: The International Confederation of Midwives.

Fox, C. Aug. 1969. Toward a sound historical basis for nurse-midwifery. *Bull. Am. Coll. Nurse-Midwifery.* 14:76.

Frontier Nursing Service, Inc. 1976. *A demonstration in family centered primary health care.* Wendover, Ky.: The Service.

Haggard, H. W. 1929. *Devils, drugs and doctors.* New York: Harper & Row Publishers, Inc.

Harris, D. Feb. 1969. The development of nurse-midwifery in New York City. *Bull. Am. Coll. Nurse-Midwifery.* 14:4.

Leff, S., and Leff, V. 1957. *From witchcraft to world health.* New York: The Macmillan Co.

Lieberman, J. May–June 1976. Childbirth practices: from darkness into light. *J. Obstet. Gynecol. Neonatal Nurs.* 5:41.

McCleary, E. 1974. *New miracles of childbirth.* New York: David McKay Co., Inc.

The midwife in the United States. 1968. New York: Josiah Macy, Jr, Foundation.

Myles, M. 1974. *Textbook for midwives.* 8th ed. London: E & S Livingstone, Ltd.

Parker, E. 1960. *The seven ages of woman.* Baltimore: Johns Hopkins University Press.

Prevention of fragmentation of patient care: the coordinative role of the registered professional nurse. May–June 1978. *J. Obstet. Gynecol. Neonatal Nurs.* 7:51.

Roberts, J. E. May–June 1976. Priorities in prenatal education. *J. Obstet. Gynecol. Neonatal Nurs.* 5:17.

Smith, C. March–April 1977. The maternity clinical specialist: an academic viewpoint. *J. Obstet. Gynecol. Neonatal Nurs.* 6:57.

Thomas, M. 1965. *The practice of nurse midwifery in the U.S.* Children's Bureau Publication No. 436. Washington, D.C.: U.S. Department of Health, Education, and Welfare.

Venzmer, G. 1972. *Five thousand years of medicine.* London: Macdonald & Co.

Wallace, H. 1962. *Health services for mothers and children.* Philadelphia: W. B. Saunders Co.

Wooden, H. Spring 1962. The family centered approach to maternity care. *Nurs. Forum.* 1:61.

CHAPTER 2

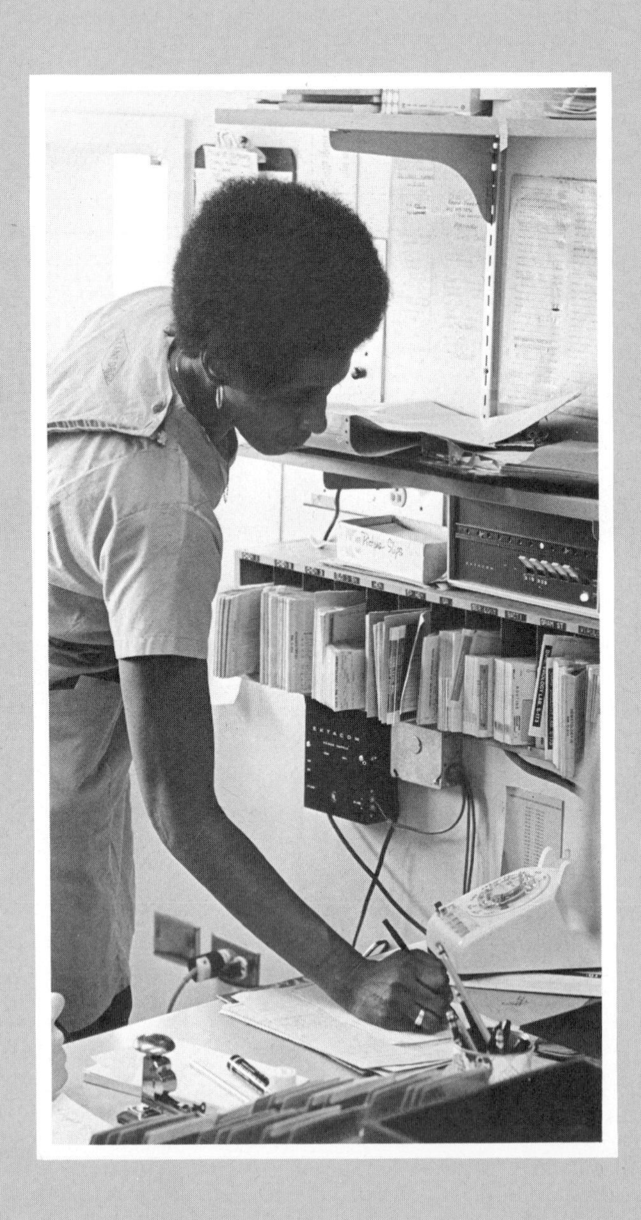

BIRTH RATES

MORTALITY (DEATH RATES)

Infant Mortality

Maternal Mortality

MATERNAL-INFANT STATISTICS

SOCIOECONOMIC STATISTICS

Educational Level

Income Level

Age

STATISTICS AND MATERNITY NURSING

OBJECTIVES

- Identify methods by which the nurse may use statistical data in planning patient care.
- Define selected statistical terms used in maternal-child health.
- Utilizing statistical data provided, list the principal causes of infant mortality in the United States.
- Utilizing statistical data provided, discuss the influence of age on childbearing.

Evaluation of the health care system relies on *statistics,* the collection and analysis of pertinent numerical data. Health-related statistics provide an objective basis for projecting patient needs, planning for utilization of resources, and analyzing data for evaluation of effectiveness.

The successful implementation of the nursing process depends on the appropriate application of statistics. Nurses can make use of statistics in a number of ways:

- To determine populations at risk.
- To determine the relationship between specific factors.
- To help establish a data base for different patient populations.
- To determine the levels of care needed by particular patient populations.
- To evaluate the success of specific nursing interventions.
- To determine priorities in case loads.
- To estimate staffing and equipment needs of hospital units and clinics.

Statistical data directly related to maternity nursing include birth rates, maternal and infant mortality and morbidity, and the relationship of these rates to such socioeconomic factors as race, age, and economic status. This chapter briefly examines current data in each of these areas.

BIRTH RATES

Birth rate refers to the number of live births per 1000 population. A related statistic, the *fertility rate,* is the number of births per 1000 women age 15 to 44 in a given population.

Figure 2-1 graphs live births and fertility rates in the United States from 1910 to 1976. The birth rate remained constant in 1975 and 1976—14.8 live births per 1000 population. This is the lowest recorded birth rate in the history of the United States. Fertility rates have also been decreasing, and in 1976, for the fifth consecutive year, a record low was reached—65.8 live births per 1000 women age 15 to 44. In 1975 the rate was 66.7, a significant drop since 1957, during the post-Korean War baby boom, when the rate was 122.7 (U.S. Department of Health, Education, and Welfare, March 29, 1978).

Provisional data from 1977 suggest a slight change in these trends, however. As Table 2-1 shows, births in the United States numbered approximately 3,313,000 in 1977, about a 5% increase over the final figures for 1976. The 1977 provisional birth rate was 15.3 and the fertility rate was 67.4, representing the first increase in the fertility rate since 1970. Research suggests that these increases may be attributed to both an increase in the number of women of childbearing age (15–44) and an increase in the rate of previously postponed births. These trends are demonstrated by an increase in first births to women age 25 to 29 and by an increase in first- through third-order births for women in the age ranges of 30–34 and 35–39 (U.S. Department of Health, Education, and Welfare, Dec. 7, 1978).

Table 2-2 compares live births, birth rates, and fertility rates by race for 1970–1976. The fertility rate was 87.2 for black women and 62.2 for white women in 1976. Although the fertility rate is significantly higher for black women, the differential between white and black birth rates is decreasing, chiefly because of the greater decline in the birth rate for black women.

Table 2–1. Live Births, Birth Rates, and Fertility Rates: United States, 1976 and 1977*

Year	Number	Birth rate†	Fertility rate†
1976	3,167,788	14.8	65.8
1977	3,313,000	15.3	67.4

*Modified from U.S. Department of Health, Education, and Welfare. Dec. 7, 1978. Provisional statistics annual summary for the United States, 1977. *Monthly Vital Statistics Report,* Publication No. (PHS) 79-1120, Vol. 26, No. 13.

†Rates on an annual basis. Birth rates per 1000 population and fertility rates per 1000 women age 15–44 years.

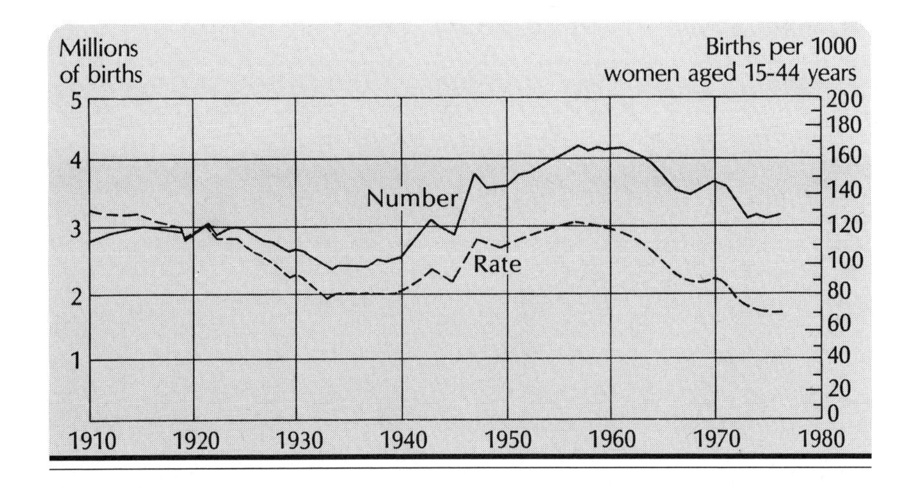

Figure 2-1. Live births and fertility rates, United States, 1910-1976.

MORTALITY (DEATH RATES)

Mortality is the ratio of the number of deaths in a specified area to the population. Mortality statistics of particular significance to maternity nursing include infant mortality data and maternal mortality data.

Infant Mortality

The *infant death rate* is the number of deaths of infants under 1 year of age per 1000 live births in a given population. *Neonatal mortality* is the number of deaths of infants less than 28 days of age per 1000 live births. *Perinatal mortality* encompasses both neonatal deaths and fetal deaths per 1000 live births. (Fetal death is death in utero at 20 weeks' or more gestation.) For statistical purposes the period from 28 days to 11 months of age is designated the *postneonatal period.* Table 2-3 delineates infant mortality by age and race. Although the United States ranked fifteenth among nations in infant deaths in 1970, with few exceptions there has been a steady decline in neonatal and postneonatal deaths within the United States since 1940.

Table 2-2. Live Births, Birth Rates, and Fertility Rates by Race: United States, 1970-1976*

	Number				Birth rate[†]				Fertility rate[†]			
			All other				All other				All other	
Year	Total	White	Total	Black	Total	White	Total	Black	Total	White	Total	Black
1976[‡]	3,167,788	2,567,614	600,174	514,479	14.8	13.8	21.1	20.8	65.8	62.2	87.6	87.2
1975[‡]	3,144,198	2,551,996	592,202	511,581	14.8	13.8	21.2	20.9	66.7	63.0	89.3	89.2
1974[‡]	3,159,958	2,575,792	584,166	507,162	14.9	14.0	21.4	21.0	68.4	64.7	91.0	90.8
1973[‡]	3,136,965	2,551,030	585,935	512,597	14.9	13.9	21.9	21.5	69.2	65.3	94.3	94.3
1972[‡]	3,258,411	2,655,558	602,853	531,329	15.6	14.6	22.9	22.6	73.4	69.2	100.3	100.5
1971[††]	3,555,970	2,919,746	636,224	564,960	17.2	16.2	24.7	24.5	81.8	77.5	109.5	110.1
1970[††]	3,731,386	3,091,264	640,122	572,362	18.4	17.4	25.1	25.3	87.9	84.1	113.0	115.4

*From U.S. Department of Health, Education, and Welfare. March 29, 1978. Advance report: final natality statistics, 1976. *Monthly Vital Statistics Report,* Publication No. (PHS) 78-1120, Vol. 26, No. 12 (supplement).

[†]Birth rates per 1000 population in specified group. Fertility rates per 1000 women aged 15-44 years in specified group. Excludes births to nonresidents of the United States.

[‡]Based on 100% of births in selected states and on a 50% sample of births in all other states.

[††]Based on a 50% sample of births.

Table 2–3. Infant Mortality by Age and Race: United States 1950 and 1960–1977*

Year†	Total			White			All other		
	Under 1 year	Under 28 days	28 days to 11 months	Under 1 year	Under 28 days	28 days to 11 months	Under 1 year	Under 28 days	28 days to 11 months
1977 (est.)	14.0	9.8	4.2	12.4	8.7	3.7	21.0	14.5	6.5
1970	20.0	15.1	4.9	17.8	13.8	4.0	30.9	21.4	9.5
1965	24.7	17.7	7.0	21.5	16.1	5.4	40.3	25.4	14.9
1960	26.0	18.7	7.3	22.9	17.2	5.7	43.2	26.9	16.4
1950	29.2	20.5	8.7	26.8	19.4	7.4	44.5	27.5	16.9
1940	47.0	28.8	18.2	-	-	-	-	-	-

*Modified from U.S. Department of Health, Education, and Welfare. Dec. 7, 1978. Provisional statistics: annual summary for the United States, 1977. *Monthly Vital Statistics Report,* Publication No. (PHS) 79-1120, Vol. 26, No. 13, and *Colorado Vital Statistics 1977.* Colorado Department of Health, Health Statistics, and Vital Records Division, Public Health Statistics Section, Denver, Colorado.

†For 1977, based on a 10% sample of deaths; for all other years, based on final data. Rates per 1000 live births.

Among the principal causes of infant death are congenital anomalies, immaturity, asphyxia, influenza and pneumonia, birth injury, and gastrointestinal diseases (Table 2-4). With the advent of neonatal intensive care nurseries and perinatal care centers, many of the problems of prematurity have been ameliorated. In addition, access to early and ongoing prenatal care appears to reduce the rate of prematurity and its inherent complications.

Maternal Mortality

Maternal mortality is the number of deaths from any cause during the pregnancy cycle (including the 42-day postpartal period) per 100,000 live births. Obstetric death, a term less frequently used, identifies deaths directly related to pregnancy and its complications. For example, obstetric death may be caused by amniotic fluid embolism, hemorrhage, or preeclampsia-eclampsia,

Table 2–4. Infant Mortality by Age and Selected Causes: United States, 1973–1977*

Age and cause of death†	1977 (est.)	1976	1975	1974	1973
Total, under 1 year	14.0	15.2	16.1	16.7	17.7
Under 28 days	9.8	10.9	11.6	12.3	13.0
28 days to 11 months	4.2	4.3	4.5	4.4	4.8
Certain gastrointestinal diseases	0.2	0.2	0.3	0.2	0.2
Influenza and pneumonia	0.5	0.6	0.7	0.8	1.1
Congenital anomalies	2.4	2.6	2.7	2.7	2.9
Birth injuries	0.4	0.6	0.6	0.6	0.6
Asphyxia of newborn, unspecified	0.9	1.1	1.3	1.5	1.7
Immaturity, unqualified	1.2	1.3	1.4	1.5	1.7
Other diseases of early infancy	4.5	4.9	5.2	5.5	5.6
All other causes	3.9	3.9	3.9	3.8	3.8

*U.S. Department of Health, Education, and Welfare. Dec. 7, 1978. Provisional statistics: annual summary for the United States, 1977. *Monthly Vital Statistics Report,* Publication No. (PHS) 79-1120, Vol. 26, No. 13.

†For 1977, based on a 10% sample of deaths; for all other years, based on final data. Rates per 1000 live births.

while maternal death includes other causes as well, such as deaths from accidents or from peritonitis following a ruptured appendix.

The maternal death rate in the United States has decreased steadily in the last 25 years (Table 2-5). The 1977 estimated maternal mortality of 9.4 is almost two-thirds less than the 1967 rate of 28.0. In 1977, 310 women died of causes listed as complications of pregnancy, childbirth, and puerperium (U.S. Department of Health, Education, and Welfare, Dec. 7, 1978). Factors influencing the decrease in maternal mortality include development of obstetrics and gynecology as a recognized medical specialty; the increased use of hospitals and specialized health care personnel for antepartum, intrapartum, and postpartum care of the maternity patient; the establishment of high-risk centers for mother and infant care; the prevention and control of infection with antibiotics and improved techniques; the availability of blood and blood products for transfusions; decreased anesthesia-related deaths; and the application of research for the prevention of maternal deaths (Danforth, 1977).

SOCIOECONOMIC STATISTICS

Maternal and child health statistics can be delineated in relation to the educational level, income level, and age of the parents.

Educational Level

In 1976, reporting of the educational attainment of parents of newborns was required by 44 states and the District of Columbia (Table 2-6). Since these data first became available in 1969, there has been a decrease in the proportion of births to individuals with eight years or less of schooling and an increase in the proportion of births to persons with twelve or more years. In 1976, 5.4% of all births were to mothers in the less-educated category, and fathers in this category accounted for 5.6% of births. During the same year, 72.6% of births were to mothers who had completed twelve or more years of formal education and 79.4% were to fathers in this category.

Table 2-6 also shows that disparity exists in educational attainment by race, although the degree of difference is diminishing and has been since 1969. In 1976 white mothers with twelve years or more schooling gave birth to 76.1% of the white infants born, but black mothers in the same category gave birth to only 56.7% of black infants born that year. The difference for fathers based on education and race was somewhat smaller. Fathers with at least twelve years of formal education accounted for 80.7% of white births, whereas 69.7% of the black births were to fathers at this educational level.

Statistical data also revealed that as the median number of years of formal education decreased, the number of children (or birth order) of the mother increased. For instance, the average educational level was 12.5 years for first births and 12.6 years for second births. However, from that point it decreased to a median of 10.8 years schooling for women having eight or more births (U.S. Department of Health, Education, and Welfare, March 29, 1978).

Table 2-5. Maternal Mortality Rate per 100,000 Live Births*

Year	Rate	Year	Rate
1977 (est.)	9.4	1967	28.0
1976	12.3	1966	29.1
1975	12.8	1965	31.6
1974	14.6	1964	33.3
1973	15.2	1963	35.8
1972	18.8	1962	35.2
1971	18.8	1961	36.9
1970	21.5	1960	37.1
1969	22.2	1950	83.3
1968	24.5		

*From U.S. Department of Health, Education, and Welfare. Dec. 7, 1978. Provisional statistics: annual summary for the United States, 1977. *Monthly Vital Statistics Report,* Publication No. (PHS) 79-1120, Vol. 26, No. 13.

Income Level

Poverty income ranges used by vital statistics agencies in the United States are based on such factors as family size, sex of family head, number of children under 18 years of age, farm or nonfarm residence, and use of a nutritionally adequate food plan as designated by the Department of Agriculture. Income ranges are utilized in research related to maternal trends, care-seeking trends, nutrition, and health practices (Colorado Vital Statistics, 1975).

Age

Two high-risk maternity populations are age related: adolescents (14 to 19 years old) and middle-aged childbearing women (35 years or older). Table 2-7 gives birth rates by age of mother, live-birth order, and race in the United States for 1976. Teenagers in the 15-19 age group had a total birth rate for first births of 53.5. White girls age 15 to 17 had a birth rate of 26.7, whereas the total birth rate for all other races was 77.1. Interestingly, the birth rate for all other races was higher for 15- to 17-year-olds than for 30- to 34-year-olds. Although the incidence of births to mothers age 10-14 is low, its existence is of concern to health care providers and educators.

During this same year the illegitimacy rate decreased slightly from 24.8 to 24.7. This rate has been declining yearly since 1970, except during 1975. The illegitimacy rate for adolescents age 15-19 decreased in 1976. This was the first decrease for this adolescent age group since 1962. Table 2-8 provides illegitimacy figures for 1976. In 1976 the rate for white teenagers increased 2% and the rate for black teenagers decreased 4%, accounting for the overall decline. However, there was an increase of nearly 4% in the total illegitimacy rate for other races. It will be interesting to evaluate statistical data for the last years of the

Table 2-6. Live Births by Educational Attainment of Mother and Father and by Race: 44 Reporting States and District of Columbia, 1976*

Years of school completed	Mother			Father		
	Total	White	Black	Total	White	Black
Total[†]	2,485,820	1,991,875	436,631	2,485,820	1,991,875	436,631
0-5 years	17,414	13,391	2,552	19,317	15,336	3,054
6 years	13,891	10,151	2,681	14,624	11,832	2,282
7 years	19,731	13,474	5,691	15,517	12,388	2,766
8 years	79,169	59,348	17,302	70,001	60,329	8,148
9 years	124,448	88,915	32,559	70,242	58,657	10,216
10 years	197,083	139,492	53,341	116,706	94,829	19,691
11 years	211,284	138,621	67,966	129,956	98,140	29,154
12 years	1,084,688	894,422	170,835	873,106	738,725	116,481
13 years	165,636	140,962	21,473	126,766	111,084	12,851
14 years	148,598	125,855	19,132	177,549	156,374	16,965
15 years	64,365	55,611	7,013	66,718	58,312	6,741
16 years	208,867	188,300	14,428	242,673	224,442	12,527
17 years or more	83,858	73,954	5,888	192,986	177,987	7,746
Not stated	66,788	49,379	15,770	369,659	173,440	188,009

*From U.S. Department of Health, Education, and Welfare. March 29, 1978. Advance report: final natality statistics, 1976. *Monthly Vital Statistics Report,* Publication No. (PHS) 78-1120, Vol. 26, No. 12 (supplement).

[†]Based on 100% of births in selected states and on a 50% sample of births in all other states. Excludes data for Arkansas, California, Idaho, New Mexico, Texas, and Washington, which did not require reporting of educational attainment of mother and father. Refers only to births occurring within the areas reporting educational attainment to residents of these areas.

1970s to determine whether the 1976 decline in illegitimacy rates continues.

Since the 1960s teenage girls have become more active sexually, resulting in increased numbers of pregnancies and births. The incidence of prematurity, low-birth-weight infants, pre-eclampsia-eclampsia, and maternal morbidity and mortality in this group is high (Moore, 1978).

Women age 35 years and older also represent a high-risk population for complications during pregnancy. As Table 2-9 shows, the greatest incidence of low-birth-weight infants occurs in this age group and in adolescents under age 19.

As a woman becomes older, changes occur in her hormonal regulation that decrease her body's ability to provide an optimal internal environ-

Table 2-7. Birth Rates by Age of Mother, Live-Birth Order, and Race: United States, 1976*

Children by birth order and race†	15–44 years‡	Age of mother in years									
		10–14	15–19 Total	15–19: 15–17	15–19: 18–19	20–24	25–29	30–34	35–39	40–44	45–49
Total	65.8	1.2	53.5	34.6	81.3	112.1	108.8	54.5	19.0	4.3	0.2
First	27.9	1.2	42.0	30.6	58.8	53.8	32.5	8.9	1.9	0.3	0.0
Second	21.1	0.0	9.9	3.7	18.9	41.1	41.8	16.1	3.2	0.4	0.0
Third	9.6	0.0	1.4	0.3	3.1	12.9	21.8	13.8	3.7	0.5	0.0
Fourth	3.8	0.0	0.2	0.0	0.4	3.3	8.0	7.7	3.2	0.6	0.0
Fifth	1.7	-	0.0	0.0	0.1	0.8	2.9	3.9	2.4	0.6	0.0
Sixth and seventh	1.2	-	0.0	0.0	0.0	0.2	1.5	3.0	2.7	0.8	0.0
Eighth and over	0.6	-	0.0	-	0.0	0.0	0.2	1.1	1.9	1.1	0.1
White	62.2	0.6	44.6	26.7	70.7	107.0	108.4	53.5	17.7	3.8	0.2
First	26.5	0.6	36.1	24.2	53.5	53.9	33.5	8.9	1.9	0.3	0.0
Second	20.4	0.0	7.5	2.3	15.1	39.4	42.8	16.2	3.1	0.4	0.0
Third	9.0	0.0	0.9	0.1	1.9	10.9	21.4	14.0	3.6	0.5	0.0
Fourth	3.4	0.0	0.1	0.0	0.2	2.3	7.2	7.5	3.1	0.5	0.0
Fifth	1.4	-	0.0	0.0	0.0	0.5	2.3	3.6	2.3	0.5	0.0
Sixth and seventh	1.0	-	0.0	-	0.0	0.1	1.0	2.6	2.4	0.8	0.0
Eighth and over	0.4	-	0.0	-	0.0	0.0	0.1	0.7	1.4	0.8	0.1
All other	87.6	4.3	102.4	77.1	141.5	141.7	111.6	60.7	27.0	7.0	0.5
First	35.9	4.2	74.1	64.4	89.2	53.3	26.7	8.6	2.4	0.4	0.0
Second	25.3	0.1	22.8	11.3	40.5	51.0	35.7	15.5	4.2	0.6	0.1
Third	13.1	0.0	4.7	1.3	9.9	24.7	24.5	12.7	4.3	0.7	0.0
Fourth	6.2	0.0	0.7	0.1	1.7	9.0	13.2	8.7	3.7	0.6	0.0
Fifth	3.0	-	0.1	0.0	0.2	2.7	6.5	5.8	3.0	0.7	0.0
Sixth and seventh	2.5	-	0.0	0.0	0.0	0.9	4.2	6.1	4.6	1.4	0.1
Eighth and over	1.5	-	0.0	-	0.0	0.1	0.8	3.1	4.8	2.7	0.2
Black	87.2	4.7	107.0	81.5	146.8	143.4	105.5	54.7	24.6	6.8	0.5
First	35.8	4.5	77.0	67.9	91.3	52.0	21.7	6.4	1.8	0.3	0.0
Second	24.8	0.1	24.1	12.2	42.7	51.9	33.1	12.3	3.2	0.5	0.0
Third	13.1	0.0	5.0	1.4	10.7	25.9	24.6	11.5	3.7	0.6	0.0
Fourth	6.3	0.0	0.8	0.1	1.8	9.6	13.7	8.7	3.4	0.6	0.0
Fifth	3.1	-	0.1	0.0	0.2	2.9	6.9	6.0	3.0	0.7	0.0
Sixth and seventh	2.6	-	0.0	0.0	0.0	1.0	4.6	6.5	4.6	1.4	0.1
Eighth and over	1.6	-	0.0	-	0.0	0.1	0.9	3.4	4.9	2.6	0.2

*From U.S. Department of Health, Education, and Welfare. March 29, 1978. Advance report: final natality statistics, 1976. *Monthly Vital Statistics Report*, Publication No. (PHS) 78-1120, Vol. 26, No. 13 (supplement).

†Based on 100% of births in selected states and on a 50% sample of births in all other states. Rates are live births per 1000 women in specified age and racial groups. Live-birth order refers to number of children born alive to mother. Figures for age of mother and live-birth order not stated are distributed.

‡Rates computed by relating total births, regardless of age of mother, to women age 15-44.

Table 2–8. Estimated Number of Illegitimate Live Births, Illegitimacy Rates, and Illegitimacy Ratios by Age of Mother and by Race: United States, 1976*

Age of mother in years	Number (in thousands)[†]				Rates per 1000 unmarried[‡] women in specified group				Ratio per 1000 live births			
			All other				All other				All other	
	Total	White	Total	Black	Total	White	Total	Black	Total	White	Total	Black
All ages	468.1	197.1	271.0	258.8	24.7[‖]	12.7[‖]	78.1[‖]	83.2[‖]	147.8	76.8	451.5	503.0
Under 15	10.3	3.5	6.8	6.6	-	-	-	-	863.5	692.5	989.2	990.8
15–19	225.0	97.6	127.4	122.7	24.0	12.4	84.6	91.6	402.7	248.2	769.9	797.1
15	22.9	9.2	13.7	13.2	19.3 (ages 15–17)	9.9 (ages 15–17)	69.0 (ages 15–17)	74.6 (ages 15–17)	719.0	528.1	949.3	956.0
16	41.7	17.9	23.8	22.9					585.6	399.2	902.8	917.0
17	51.9	22.9	29.0	28.0					461.6	295.0	833.4	857.6
18	55.9	24.6	31.3	30.2	32.5 (ages 18–19)	17.0 (ages 18–19)	112.4 (ages 18–19)	121.6 (ages 18–19)	363.5	221.9	728.8	761.1
19	52.6	23.0	29.6	28.4					277.6	161.4	630.7	663.1
20–24	145.4	58.9	86.5	82.4	32.2	16.0	103.1	109.3	133.2	66.3	425.3	460.6
25–29	55.4	22.8	32.7	30.8	27.5	14.4	76.8	81.1	57.0	27.3	239.2	284.9
30–34	21.0	9.4	11.6	10.7	17.8	10.2	44.3	45.9	53.6	28.3	194.8	239.9
35–39	8.6	3.9	4.7	4.4	8.9	5.5	18.8	19.0	74.4	41.8	209.5	251.2
40 and over	2.3	1.0	1.3	1.2	2.5[‡‡]	1.4[‡‡]	6.9[‡‡]	7.0[‡‡]	89.1	49.8	226.2	252.8

*Modified from U.S. Department of Health, Education, and Welfare. March 29, 1978. Advance report: final natality statistics, 1976. *Monthly Vital Statistics Report*, Publication No. (PHS) 78–1120, Vol. 26, No. 12 (supplement).

[†]Due to rounding estimates to the nearest hundred, figures by race may not add to totals.

[‡]National estimates based on births occurring in the 38 states and District of Columbia that require reporting of legitimacy status. Based on 100% of births in selected reporting states and on a 50% sample of births in all other reporting states. Figures for age of mother not stated are distributed.

[‖]Rates computed by relating total illegitimate births, regardless of age of mother, to unmarried women 15–44 years.

[‡‡]Rates computed by relating illegitimate births to mothers aged 40 years and over to unmarried women aged 40–44 years.

ment for the development of the ovum. Incidence of multiple pregnancy also increases with age, as does risk of certain chromosomal anomalies, most notably Down's syndrome. After age 35, the risk of Down's syndrome increases dramatically (Table 2–10). It is therefore considered appropriate to use amniocentesis to screen for Down's syndrome in women over 35 (Moore, 1978).

STATISTICS AND MATERNITY NURSING

Statistical information is available through many sources, including professional literature; state and city health departments; vital statistics sections of private, county, state, and federal agencies; special programs or agencies (family planning agencies); demographic profiles of specific geographic areas. The nurse who makes use of this information will find herself well prepared to project the health care needs of maternity patients and their families. The community health nurse can evaluate the adequacy of maternal health services and resources in her area by statistical analysis. Hospital staffs can use statistics to plan for high-risk maternal labor and delivery units, intensive care nurseries, postpartal beds, staffing, and use of health resources. The maternity nurse can use these data as a basis for determining health priorities and for planning patient care activities.

Table 2-9. Percent Low Birth Weight and Live Births by Birth Weight, by Age and Race of Mother: United States, 1976*

Age of mother and race	Percent low birth weight	Total[1]	Birth weight (in grams) 500 or less	501–1000	1001–1500	1501–2000	2001–2500	2501–3000	3001–3500	3501–4000	4001 or more
Total	7.3	3,167,788	3,301	13,602	19,546	44,691	148,235	543,549	1,185,890	886,433	313,295
Under 15 years	14.8	11,928	36	171	212	337	996	3,021	4,586	2,110	406
15–19 years	9.9	558,744	702	3,537	5,209	11,331	34,414	118,666	219,138	130,544	33,572
20–24 years	7.1	1,091,602	1,094	4,499	6,544	14,710	50,772	192,131	417,903	302,249	98,629
25–29 years	6.0	972,130	938	3,259	4,637	10,863	38,263	149,253	359,423	292,731	109,965
30–34 years	6.5	391,896	371	1,513	2,020	5,041	16,385	58,664	137,891	118,052	50,758
35–39 years	7.9	115,662	141	483	741	1,910	5,871	17,752	38,788	33,475	16,118
40–44 years	9.2	24,383	19	130	170	455	1,451	3,832	7,691	6,883	3,653
45–49 years	10.5	1,443	–	10	13	44	83	230	470	389	194
White	6.1	2,567,614	2,032	8,461	12,836	30,424	103,224	397,951	954,073	768,354	282,832
Under 15 years	11.8	5,054	11	49	81	142	308	1,029	2,022	1,135	252
15–19 years	8.1	393,275	370	1,894	2,878	6,590	19,909	72,196	154,527	104,704	29,017
20–24 years	6.0	888,219	679	2,835	4,387	9,971	35,514	141,997	338,168	262,632	89,570
25–29 years	5.3	835,398	624	2,264	3,395	8,222	29,507	119,652	306,250	262,060	101,032
30–34 years	5.8	332,359	236	1,019	1,471	3,841	12,620	46,751	115,930	103,804	45,710
35–39 years	7.0	93,229	100	309	495	1,311	4,266	13,374	30,938	28,133	13,992
40–44 years	8.3	19,014	12	83	118	319	1,047	2,774	5,911	5,587	3,094
45–49 years	9.4	1,066	–	8	11	28	53	168	327	299	165
Black	13.0	514,479	1,209	4,850	6,276	13,207	40,964	128,323	197,202	96,767	24,153
Under 15 years	17.1	6,661	25	121	129	189	668	1,967	2,482	915	140
15–19 years	14.7	153,936	322	1,593	2,248	4,571	13,879	44,118	59,968	22,988	3,845
20–24 years	12.6	178,902	399	1,578	2,055	4,423	14,068	45,205	69,831	33,526	7,294
25–29 years	11.3	108,124	289	913	1,116	2,356	7,525	23,689	41,497	23,588	6,820
30–34 years	11.6	44,596	127	438	468	1,021	3,083	9,012	15,910	10,514	3,860
35–39 years	13.1	17,514	40	158	216	521	1,350	3,410	5,955	4,104	1,703
40–44 years	12.8	4,436	7	47	42	110	361	870	1,455	1,057	465
45–49 years	16.3	310	–	2	2	16	30	52	104	75	26

*Modified from U.S. Department of Health, Education, and Welfare. March 29, 1978. Advance report: final natality statistics, 1976. *Monthly Vital Statistics Report.* Publication No. (PHS) 78-1120, Vol. 26, No. 12 (supplement).

[1]Based on 100% of births in selected states and on a 50% sample of births in all other states.

Table 2-10. Risk of Down's Syndrome*

Age of mother	Risk in any pregnancy	Risk after birth of baby with Down's syndrome
29 and under	1 in 3000	1 in 1000
30-34	1 in 600	1 in 200
35-39	1 in 280	1 in 100
40-44	1 in 70	1 in 25
45-49	1 in 40	1 in 15
All mothers	1 in 665	1 in 200

*From Moore, M. L. 1978. *Realities in childbearing.* Philadelphia: W. B. Saunders Co., p. 295.

SUMMARY

Statistical information is an important resource from which the professional nurse derives knowledge necessary for successful implementation of the nursing process. The use of information such as the identification of adolescents as at risk for pregnancy, the increase in educational level of parents as being related to number of births, and the relation of race to fertility illustrates the application of statistics for the nursing process.

SUGGESTED ACTIVITIES

1. Through small group discussion identify

ways in which maternity nurses may use statistical data in planning nursing care.

2. Establish a small maternity population using classmates and friends and formulate statistical tables and graphs based on selected aspects of their childbearing experiences.

REFERENCES

Colorado Vital Statistics, 1975. Colorado Department of Health, Health Statistics, and Vital Records Division, Public Health Statistics Section, Denver, Colorado.

Colorado Vital Statistics, 1977. Colorado Department of Health, Health Statistics, and Vital Records Division, Public Health Statistics Section, Denver, Colorado.

Danforth, D. N., ed. 1977. *Obstetrics and gynecology.* 3rd ed. New York: Harper & Row Publishers, Inc.

Moore, M. L. 1978. *Realities in childbearing.* Philadelphia: W. B. Saunders Co.

U.S. Department of Health, Education, and Welfare. March 29, 1978. Advance report: final natality statistics, 1976. *Monthly Vital Statistics Report,* Publication No. (PHS) 78-1120, Vol. 26, No. 12 (supplement).

U.S. Department of Health, Education, and Welfare. Dec. 7, 1978. Provisional statistics: annual summary for the United States, 1977. *Monthly Vital Statistics Report,* Publication No. (PHS) 79-1120, Vol. 26, No. 13.

CHAPTER 3

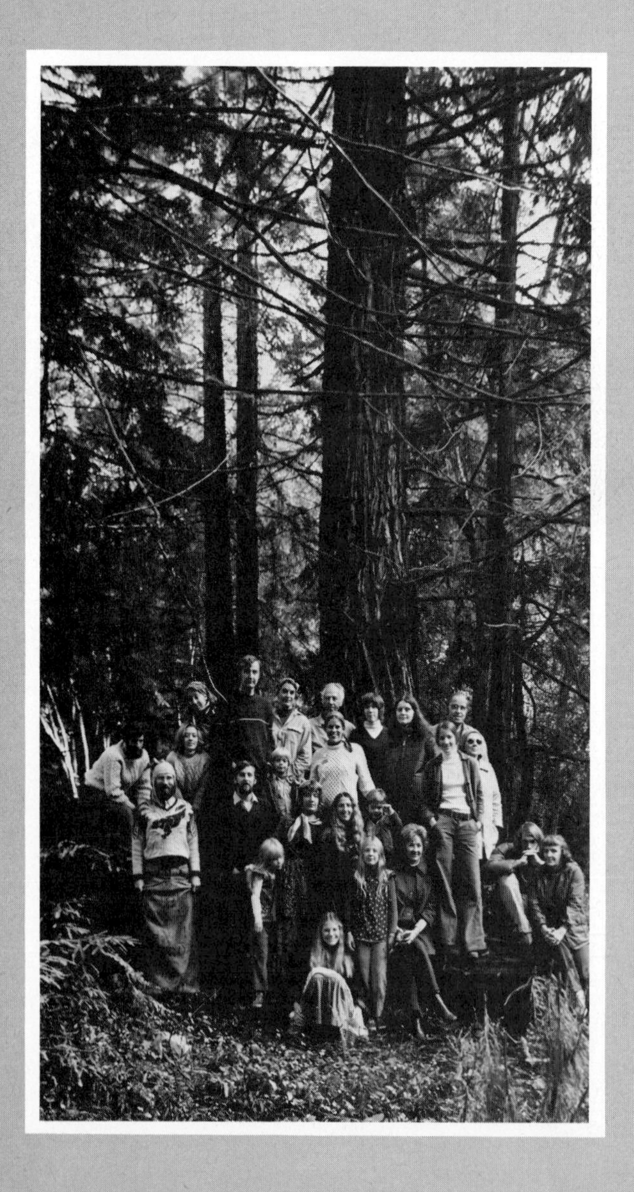

THE FAMILY

TYPES OF FAMILIES

- Traditional versus Democratic Families
- Structural Configurations

FEATURES OF THE FAMILY

- Characteristics
- Functions
- Roles

SOCIOCULTURAL AND SOCIOECONOMIC INFLUENCES ON THE FAMILY

- Life-style and Socioeconomic Levels
- Changing Status of Women
- Value of Children

DYNAMICS OF FAMILY LIFE

OBJECTIVES

- Discuss the application of family theory as it relates to the interaction and communication between the nurse and various family members.
- Explain the best measures that a nurse can use in determining the degree of family wellness.
- Identify the main features of a family.
- Compare various family interactions.
- Contrast the family's developmental stages with the psychosocial stages of family members.

The family-centered concept of health care has been widely endorsed by educators and health practitioners. Professionals recognize that the family is the primary influence on a child's development. Because the individual develops as an independent and intradependent component of the family unit, the health care professional must acquire a comprehensive understanding of the family as a prerequisite to understanding the individual.

Family nursing, long the bastion of the public health nurse, is now evolving as an essential part of the total health care delivery system. Until recently, the family was excluded from the acute phase of hospitalization, even in cases of young children, by restrictive visiting hours, lack of privacy and accommodations for families, and covert or overt discouragement of family visiting by health team members. With the recent awareness of the family as a potential resource of physical and emotional support to a patient, the role of the nurse has expanded to encompass functions that maintain health through family involvement.

Interaction with the family and with each family member provides the nurse with clues about the factors that contribute to or detract from health maintenance and restoration and helps the nurse assess problems associated with illness prevention. Information about the family's culture and community and about the availability of facilities within the community aids the nurse in determining the family's potential for acquiring and using health care services within the environment.

The development of family nursing is a result of our changing society. As people have become better educated, their desire for knowledge about themselves and how they function has expanded. Changing value systems and the high cost of health care have generated an increase in home care for the sick and elderly. Philosophies of humanitarianism and equality have led health workers to make care available to all people, regardless of values, race, or ability to pay. Concerns for population control and the environment have made working with the entire family a necessity. With increased medical knowledge, acute illness and infections have become less of a problem for the population in general. However, increased longevity has led to an increase in chronic illness and to the necessity for greater emphasis on health teaching, on clarification of medical and surgical regimen, and on coordination of health care activities. These changes in societal attitudes have had a strong impact on the belief in the right of the individual and the family to concerned, comprehensive, conscientious delivery of health care by nurses.

According to Dunn (1961), a high level of wellness within the family means a high degree of well-being in family members and in social groups composed of such families. The best measures of family wellness are a positive direction of family movement, the availability of opportunities for the family to reach its highest potential, and the operation of the family as an integrated whole. A high level of wellness within the family can be achieved if the family works toward protection and security for its members and helps them grow in their confidence in the esteem and worth of themselves and others (Dunn, 1961). The family is important because generally it is that group in which a person is given love, trust, and response consistently so that he or she may mature into an individual who is able to give these qualities to others.

THE FAMILY

Traditionally, *family* is defined as a group of people united by marriage, blood, or adoption, residing in the same household, maintaining a common culture, and interacting with one another depending on their roles within the group. The middle-class family in our culture is commonly depicted as comprising husband, wife, and one to four children.

However, the concept of family is changing. Many conceptual and structural differences can be found among groups calling themselves families. As a result, a broader definition of family has emerged: The family is a constantly changing natural organization that consists of one or more people who live in close proximity.* The interre-

*One person can live as a separate unit and fulfill the roles and functions of a family that are pertinent to his needs.

lationships among family members are determined by culture and by the individuals. Each member has roles and functions defined by the individual and the group. The goal of the family is for each member to develop independently and yet to retain characteristics that identify him or her as part of the culture and the family group.

A family is a small group with a discernible structure that has many facets. Figure 3–1 is a conceptual diagram of a family and its field of influence. The center, or nucleus, is the small group that makes up the *nuclear family*, with one or more adults and possibly one or more children. The arrows between family members denote interaction—emotional and intellectual communication. This interaction is necessary for the maintenance of the family unit.

On the outside of the wheel are the concrete and abstract forces that exert power and influence over the family. Culture has the greatest impact, as it prescribes expected behaviors, including family traditions, childrearing practices, and methods of handling illness. Social changes that bring about changes within the family include moving to a new home, assuming a new social status, birth, death, and marriage. Interaction with the environment takes place as people change their surroundings to meet their needs. Friends and relatives outside the nuclear family also have direct and indirect influences on it. In many cases they are the ones who impart cultural and social standards to the family. And if certain members of the family are not present, some of their roles may be assumed by friends or relatives. The indirect influence of such individuals is exemplified by the relative who gives a family member a gift that broadens his or her interests and motivation.

Between the nucleus and the outside of the wheel are spokes representing facets of the family that are influenced by culture, social change, environmental interaction, and friends and relatives. Roles, status, and behavior are specific to each family member, and a member's change in any one area can effect a like change in another member. Routines and rituals, interactional patterns, childrearing patterns, and adaptation to health and illness are behaviors used by an individual or by the entire family. Although the responsibility for leadership and authority usually

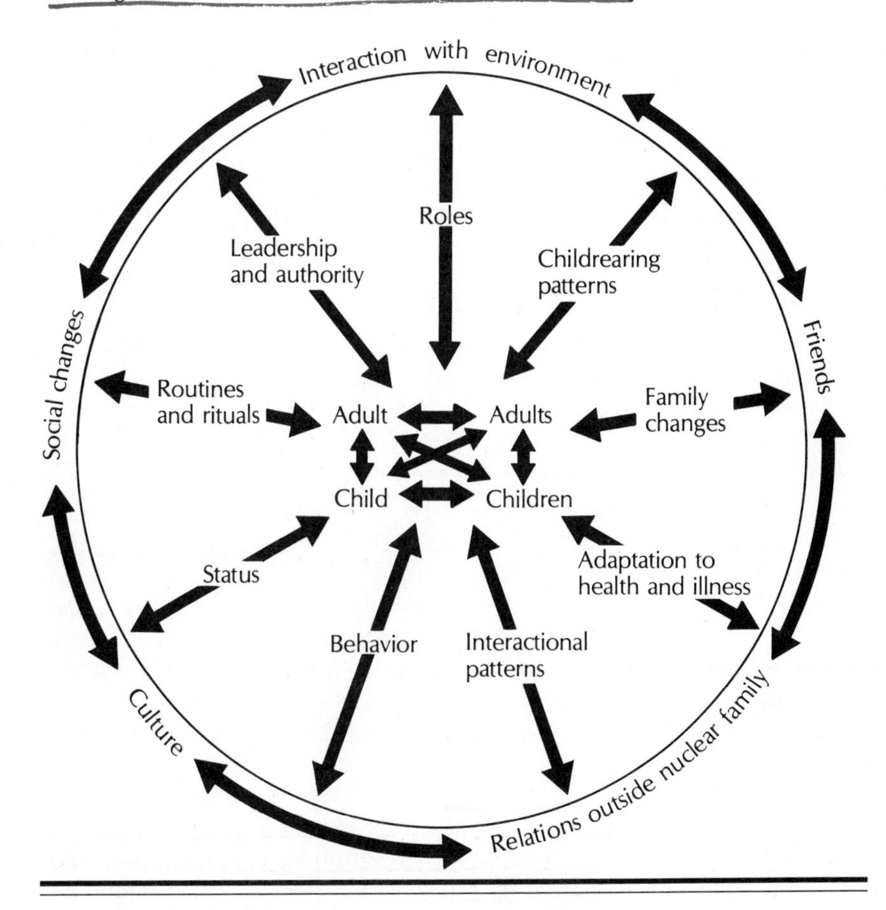

Figure 3–1. Conceptual framework of a family unit. Arrows indicate interactional patterns and the influence of the family on its environment and the influences of the environment on the family.

rests on one or two family members, other individuals within the family may occasionally take on this role. Family change can cause like changes in the roles and status of family members; some roles that were dominant in one person may become recessive as they become dominant in another family member. One principle to remember is that the larger the family, the greater the possibilities for change and the more interpersonal relationships to help or hinder the family structure.

TYPES OF FAMILIES

Traditional versus Democratic Families

Families are often categorized on the basis of two types: the *traditional* and the *democratic*. These two types represent opposite ends of a continuum that is based on certain philosophical and political characteristics of the family.

The traditional family prevails in many countries. This family type draws its strength from the *autocratic* and *authoritarian* patriarchal line, with power ensconced in the eldest male, and women and children subordinate to him. Marriages are frequently arranged by the parents, who base their selection on the economic and social status of the prospective mate. Among the major expectations within the family are compliance with duty and following tradition. The interrelationships of family members tend to be dictated by custom, tradition, and law. The family's culture and social status depend on highly stylized economic, educational, recreational, health, protective, and religious roles and traditions.

The democratic type of family is marked by a high degree of equality and mutuality between husband and wife as they work out an acceptable division of labor. Decisions are reached by consensus rather than dictum. As children get older, they become less subordinate and increasingly participating members of the family. Selection of marriage partners is made by the children, with affection and personality compatibility being the major factors influencing their decision. Achievement of happiness, personal growth, and economic security are the major expectations. Family functions are highly influenced by individual needs and wishes.

The democratic family is bound together by a desire to remain together and by affection. Ideally, each family member is accepted as an individual with unique talents, strengths, weaknesses, and desires; family members work together for the good of all, recognizing the differences among individuals and according each one personal security. Family members also help each other with unique personal, mental, and emotional needs, and they achieve satisfaction and a sense of purpose through the family unit.

The transition from the traditional family to the democratic family in the twentieth century has resulted in changes in attitudes and has brought about many new trends (Kantor and Lehr, 1975). The average age of individuals marrying has increased, with most marriages occurring between persons in their early twenties. Fewer children are resulting from the marriages, particularly in middle- and upper-class families. Concerns about population control and the economic costs of providing children with educational and social opportunities have made large families unfeasible. In addition, many women are extending their interests and energies to situations outside the home and thus are less tied to the traditional mother role. Another major change that has occurred with the transition from traditional to democratic families has been a decrease in the control that the kinship group and the community have over the family.

Structural Configurations

Most people belong to one of the following six types of family configurations (Hymovich and Barnard, 1973):

1. *Single adult living alone*. This type of living arrangement is often not considered a family configuration, because the interaction and support that are considered part of family life are not present. However, the single person living alone must perform functions typically ascribed to the family, such as finding suitable housing and income and organizing relationships with his or her extended family and community.

2. *Nuclear dyad*. Frequently referred to as the *beginning family*, this structure consists of a husband and wife living in a single family residence (Figure 3-2). One or both partners have a career, and

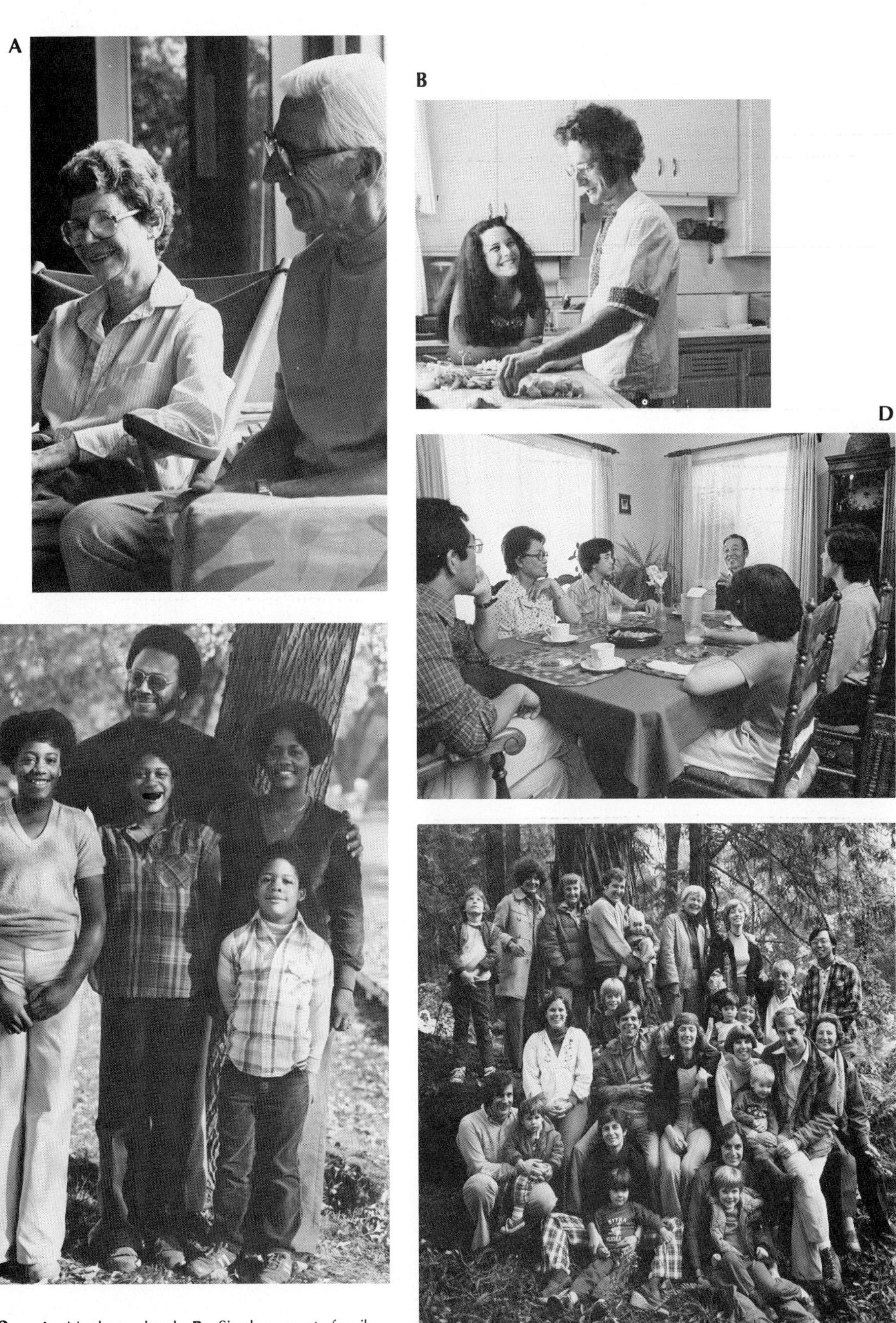

Figure 3–2. **A,** Nuclear dyad. **B,** Single-parent family. **C,** Nuclear family. **D,** Three-generation family. **E,** Kin network.

either there are no children or, in the case of an older couple, there are no children at home.

3. *Single-parent families.* This family type is becoming far more prevalent as the rate of divorces and separations continues to rise. One adult is left alone (by separation, divorce, or death) to raise minor children in a separate household from other adults. If no other source of family income exists or if the adult prefers, he or she may seek a career, adding additional responsibilities to family life.

4. *Nuclear family.* This is the most common family configuration in our society. It includes husband, wife, and all minor children living together in a single household. In this chapter the nuclear family is generally the unit referred to, although many of the concepts discussed can be applied to other family types.

5. *Three-generation family.* In this structure, one or more dependent grandparents live in a single household with either a single-parent family or a nuclear family. The parents have authority over the household and care for the grandparents.

6. *Kin network (or extended family).* This family type includes two or more nuclear households of any of the previously described configurations living in close proximity, exchanging goods, and looking to each other for interaction and support. Although the adults have authority within their single household, the elder adults are looked to for advice, support, and authority in intrafamily affairs.

People by choice or by circumstance move from one family configuration to another. The nuclear dyad becomes a nuclear family when the first child is born and returns to the nuclear dyad as the last child leaves the household. Each family has its own role systems, socialization patterns, interaction patterns, and relationship style with other relatives and with the environment. These will be discussed in greater depth later in this chapter.

In North America great value is placed on the husband-wife-minor children configuration. Adult children are expected to leave the family center and form families of their own. Much of our society continues to hold this idea as being the most viable form of the family. But family structures that break from the more traditional ones have emerged in recent years. Some authorities theorize that they are the outgrowth of disorganization within the traditional family units. The causes of this disorganization seem to be increased mobility, movement to cities, increased economic independence of women, and decreased control of the kin network and the traditional family style (Mowrer, 1927). The resulting emerging family structures include the communal family, the unmarried single-parent family, the common-law family, and the homosexual family (Hymovich and Barnard, 1973):

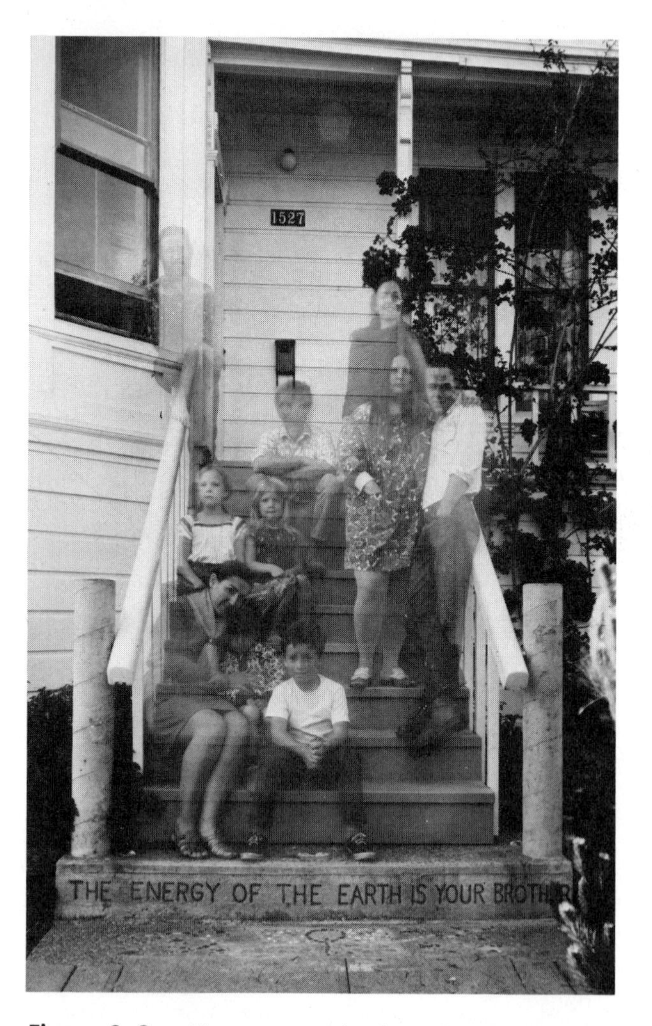

Figure 3–3. The commune family is often thought of as a transient entity, and the communes of the later 1960s were stereotyped as casual, sexually liberal, and politically radical. However, many commune organizations are well-established, long-lived structures, and their membership is governed by the same principles governing most families.

1. *The communal family.* This type of family can vary in its organization and philosophy. One type of communal family is made up of more than one married couple, with or without children, sharing a common household with its facilities and resources and participating in common experiences and childrearing responsibilities. Each family retains its legal identity within the larger community. This style is best typified by the kibbutzim in Israel. In another type, adults and their offspring, living in a common household, merge in a type of "group marriage" arrangement (Figure 3–3). All adults are considered parents to all children and share childrearing responsibilities.

2. *Unmarried parent family.* One family structure that has become more prevalent in recent years is the unmarried parent with one or more children. The adult is usually a woman who either does not choose to marry or for some reason cannot marry the father of her child. As attitudes toward sexuality have become more liberal, the option of keeping a child rather than giving it up for adoption is being chosen by a greater number of young women. In addition, an increasing number of single adults are adopting children.

3. *Common-law family.* The common-law marriage, in which a man and woman live together sharing companionship and responsibilities without the legal commitment of marriage, is not a recent form of family structure. However, the number of couples choosing this arrangement is increasing. Children can be conceived by the couple or can be informally adopted.

4. *Homosexual family.* This type of family, in which two adults of the same sex choose to live together in a sexual relationship and share responsibilities, has received a great deal of publicity within recent years. Children from a previous marriage may live with the couple, or children may not be present.

No matter what type of structure a family has, its primary objective generally is to support the emotional and physical health of its members through stability, comfort, reassurance, encouragement, and empathy and to provide warm and intimate relationships.

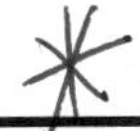

FEATURES OF THE FAMILY

Characteristics

The following characteristics are typically attributed to the family:

1. The relationships among the members are loving and affectionate.

2. The family provides a long-term environment for the sharing of ideas, experiences, and companionship.

3. The family is usually organized to provide interaction between members of at least two generations, allowing for the transmission of cultural traits and values from one generation to the next.

4. In the family group, each member is a unique individual, separate from stereotypes imposed by people outside the family. Achievements and other individual characteristics are observed and accepted as part of the member's personal role within the family.

Functions

The primary functions of the family include:

1. *Care and rearing of children.* This function has become less important in some families as a result of population control and individual desires not to have children. Nevertheless, many young couples continue to bear children and to rear them in the traditions and values of their parent cultures.

2. *Transmission of cultural values and/or rituals from one generation to the next.* Traditions are passed from generation to generation as children are told about and participate in cultural activities. Children learn to accept the values of their parents as they are taught to distinguish right from wrong. In addition, children learn much of their behavior by imitating their parents or other persons they respect and admire.

3. *Socialization and provision for physiologic needs.* The family provides food, shelter, clothing, and

comfort and promotes the safety of its members. In addition, the family prepares its children to take their place in society by *socialization,* the formal or informal teaching of physical, intellectual, and social skills. This process includes the learning of social group mores, traditions, and standards, and conforming to them (Kenkel, 1966).

Socialization begins in infancy and continues throughout childhood and adolescence. The infant learns through others' responses to his or her needs and demands, and the child learns through a system of rewards and punishments and by imitation of those around him or her. Schools and other social institutions also participate in the socialization of the individual. Even as a person marries and begins his own family, the process of socialization continues as his background is meshed with that of his spouse to derive the patterns and values they will teach their own children.

The desired outcome of socialization is "an adult whose personality characteristics are compatible with the demands and expectations of the society of which he is a member" (Kenkel, 1966).

Roles

A *role* is a cluster of interpersonal behaviors, attitudes, and activities that are associated with an individual in a certain situation or position. The behaviors tend to be learned through interactions with parents and with siblings. *Attitudes* are expectations of the society in which the child is raised; they affect and can be modified by the individual's behaviors. Role activities are governed by expectations and behavior patterns of friends, relatives, and others outside the individual (Burgess, 1971). Role behaviors, attitudes, and activities are learned to a large extent through the process of socialization.

Each family must define its role in the community and the roles of its individual members within the family unit. These roles are learned through interaction and imitation.

Each member has a number of positions: the woman may be wife, mother, teacher, nurse, housekeeper, and cook, with additional positions in the community; the man's roles may include husband, father, wage earner, gardener, and mechanic; each offspring is a child and perhaps a sister or brother, with responsibilities for some household or family tasks. These roles, determined partially by culture and partially by the family and the individual, prescribe what persons do, to whom they are obligated, and upon whom they have a rightful claim (Robischon and Scott, 1969). For each role in the family there is a complementary role: husband-wife, parent-child, sister-brother. Each individual must learn about the role of his or her complement to understand and perform his or her own role properly. Children learn the roles of their parents while learning their own roles and thus form concepts about parental authority. Children form their self-concepts on the basis of how well they execute their roles.

Roles are not static; they change from time to time as circumstances and events precipitate a change. Within the family a person may change roles many times; a woman becomes a wife with marriage and adds the role of mother when she has her first child.

Once the roles of family members are developed, family processes usually continue in a predictable pattern. If there are interruptions in the expected personal roles, family processes will also be interrupted. In most cases, one person will assume the other's role. For example, when the wage earner is disabled for a period, the spouse may need to find a job to replace the lost income and the children may have to add more household duties and responsibilities to their roles.

Specific roles within the family warrant further discussion. First, the adult relationship, on which the success of the nuclear family is based, is determined by the roles the partners assume. In our discussion, for the sake of simplicity, we will assume that the couple is married. Second, the roles that the children assume affect their psychosocial development to adulthood.

Adult Roles

People have expectations of their marriage partners before and during marriage. These expectations are developed from observation of parents and others in the husband and wife roles. Each person sees others interact in ways he or she considers beneficial to a marriage relationship and strives to imitate these behaviors. Because the background of each marriage partner is different, the expectations of each will differ. Adjustment to these varying expectations begins during the courtship period. As soon as a couple meets, differentiation of behaviors and allocation of role sets begins. Each person reinforces those behaviors that meet his or her criteria for a mate and reacts negatively to those that do not. The behaviors that are reinforced become a permanent part of each person's actions when he or she is with the other.

If the role expectations of each person are too divergent, the couple may choose to terminate their relationship. People tend to select mates who are physically, mentally, emotionally, socially, and culturally like themselves. The adage that opposites attract usually does not apply to successful marriages unless the roles of the individuals are complementary and the partners are flexible, allowing variety in the roles assumed.

Burgess (1971) places marital role relationships on a continuum. At one end of this continuum are segregated conjugal relationships, and at the other end are joint conjugal relationships. In the *segregated conjugal relationship,* the roles of the husband and wife are distinct, are usually sexually delineated, and are highly defined by culture; the male and female partners do not assume each other's functions for fear of disdain of peers and friends. The wife usually fulfills traditional roles in the home, there is little cooperation in accomplishing household tasks, and the husband retains strong authority over the family. Husband and wife have separate interests, frequently with separate groups of friends. Segregated conjugal role relationships frequently occur when ties with family or friendship groups are close. The expectations of family and friends for the individual may be different from those of the partner, leading to elements of discord within the marriage, thereby perpetuating the separateness of the couple. This type of relationship is seen most often in lower-income families.

In the *joint conjugal relationship,* roles are not as strictly delineated. The partners share interests and activities. The division of labor to meet occupational and domestic responsibilities is established through mutual satisfaction of both parties, and joint involvement in most activities sets the theme. There is usually less contact with relatives outside the nuclear family than in the segregated conjugal relationship. This type of couple is seen most often in the upper middle class, where affluence and mobility cause the family to draw close as a unit, because the opportunity to lay down many roots is lacking.

The relationships of most couples lie somewhere between these two extremes. Marital partners share many activities but also retain their individual interests. Division of labor in the home, a reflection of the roles assumed by the couple, is usually agreed on by both partners and is largely executed according to physical strength. Although the family is involved with and visits relatives outside the household, the partners recognize that their primary allegiance is to each other and make joint decisions accordingly.

Children's Roles

The economic role that children perform in largely agrarian societies is extremely important. However, in our society children are usually not needed as laborers.

Murphree (1975) has identified three roles of children in families of the postindustrialized United States: (a) to act as messenger, (b) to serve as an ego extension of parents, and (c) to participate in social rituals. The messenger role is exemplified by the common occurrence of a child being sent to borrow a needed object from a neighbor. When children are thought to reflect the characteristics and training of their parents, they are seen as ego extensions of their parents. This particular role carries with it the danger of overidentifying with another person, resulting in a lack of development of one's "selfness." Children also participate in social or cultural rituals, which in turn reinforce certain values and provide status. Baptisms or christenings, confirmations, bar mitzvahs, and weddings are all cultural rituals that recognize the changing developmental status of the child and his or her parents.

The role of a child as a sibling is an important one in the family. For example, older siblings serve important functions in the sex-role development of younger children and assist in the discrimination of what is appropriate at various ages (Burgess, 1968). However, each child has to work out his or her own identity within the network of family relationships.

Earlier research on birth order tended to focus on the characteristics of children in different positions in the family, but it does not appear that any position is especially preferable. The primary value of examining the influence of birth order and the roles of children in the family is to enhance one's sensitivity to the subtle patterning of relationships within the family.

SOCIOCULTURAL AND SOCIOECONOMIC INFLUENCES ON THE FAMILY

The family does not function in isolation. The well-being of a family can be promoted or hindered by the policies or acts of other persons or institutions. For example, inherent characteristics such as race may have implications for the family in terms of social status, income level, and so on. Some of the factors affecting the family include:

1. *Local, state, and federal governments.* Laws are enacted to protect the rights of parents and children. Frequently, the government also assumes functions usually ascribed to families, such as providing food, shelter, or income to those with insufficient resources. The government promotes the health of families by establishing standards for health care, by investigating and regulating the use of substances such as drugs and food additives, and by protecting family members from other dysfunctional members (for example, by removing battered or neglected children from the custody of their parents).

2. *Schools.* As mentioned earlier, the socialization of children that begins in the family is assumed to a large degree by the schools.

3. *Religion.* The church has a strong influence on the values, beliefs, and moral concepts of the family. Many religions also dictate behavioral codes, rituals, and traditions of family life.

4. *Culture.* Different cultures prescribe different patterns of behavior, modes of eating and dressing, language, religion, response to authority, values, and attitudes. For example, the Mexican-American culture is characterized by a strong emphasis on family life, by the use of the Spanish language, by respect for authority, by pride in one's heritage, and by specific attitudes and beliefs regarding health and health care (Hymovich and Barnard, 1973). A central focus of Mexican-American culture is social identification, with emphasis on the family as a whole rather than on the individual member. The extended family is the prevalent configuration, with the father or eldest son having the authority.

5. *Race.* Prevailing societal attitudes about certain races of people are often reflected in economic terms. Thus, in the United States, opportunities and resources have generally not been as available to black families as to white families.

The implications of these and other factors differ for each family. In addition, members within each family can be affected to varying degrees by these factors.

Life-style and Socioeconomic Levels

Although the class system among whites and blacks is similar, there are some basic differences in orientations, values, and beliefs. In general, values in the middle class focus on self-direction, whereas those in the working class emphasize conformity.

The following description of the class system, based on Schultz (1972), uses life-style as a basis rather than income. This analysis focuses on general characteristics; note that within these broad categories there are many persons whose life-styles or beliefs do not necessarily correspond to those typically ascribed to their socioeconomic level.

In the white upper class, family groupings are usually made up of extended patriarchal families. Men carry high prestige, and sons are highly desired to carry on the family name. Women have lower prestige and usually no career, but they are highly refined and maintain an influential style of life through household management and entertaining.

The white upper middle class is populated with professionals who are achievement- and college-oriented. Families think in terms of long-term goals. Because of the high degree of mobility in this group, the nuclear family predominates. However, there is strong extended family support despite the distance separating the nuclear family from the family of origin. The wife may work, but the husband is still considered head of the household. Children are raised to value self-discipline, to take responsibility, and to show initiative; aggression is permitted only as needed for self-defense.

White-collar, skilled, and semiskilled workers comprise the white middle class. Most middle-class adults achieve a high school education but desire more for their children. They live in nuclear families, but mobility is less than in the upper middle class, and close relatives frequently live in the same community. Women often work to supplement their husband's income, but few have actual careers. The husband continues to be the head of the household, but the wife keeps the budget and maintains finances.

The white lower class is also divided into two segments. The upper lower class comprises semiskilled and skilled laborers, many of whom are foreign born and some of whom have high school educations. This group is characterized by nuclear families with strong kinship ties, and women fulfill the traditional tasks of homemaking and child care. Success for the upper lower class is thought of in terms of material goods and possessions; job security is of greater priority than upward mobility—an attitude that leads to job stagnation and dissatisfaction. Children are expected to work and supplement the family income after high school; a college education is considered of little value.

Impoverishment, poor housing with inadequate health and safety facilities, poor education, and unskilled, sometimes seasonal, jobs mark the lives of the poverty-level white family. Life takes on an aura of hopelessness and despair, leading to distrust of the social system. Families are larger, with more children being born out of wedlock than in the other classes. There is no motivation to marry, and fatherless children are readily accepted into the mother's family. Although the number of one-parent families in this class is large, a high proportion of two-parent families is still prevalent. Extended families supply emotional support but are unable to give economic aid.

Among black people, the upper class consists of professionals, many of whom become wealthy with the help of the wife's income. Many blacks enter this class from the middle and lower classes through fame in athletics, entertainment, or other highly paid endeavors. Black upper-class families live in nuclear households and have close relations with their extended families, but these relationships are not as close as in the white upper class.

The black middle class is patriarchal or egalitarian, with both partners working in many cases. They occupy the same types of occupations as the white middle class and are widely involved in community affairs. The black lower class is very similar to the white lower class but is highly matriarchal.

Changing Status of Women

The traditional role for a woman in our society gave her dominance in the home, especially in the kitchen. This role had value for the family but did not have prestige. The lack of prestige made it a safe role for women, one in which their husbands would not intervene. Thus the home became the stronghold for women. However, division of labor within the home changed greatly as women found that they were able to fulfill other roles without being subjected to culturally defined boundaries.

Similarly, the husband has traditionally been considered the head of the household, and the status and life-style of those within the home have depended to a large extent on him. But now more women are becoming part of the work force to supplement family income in the lower and middle classes, to satisfy chosen career goals in the upper middle class, or to work voluntarily in charitable organizations in the upper class. As women move out into the working world and find fulfillment, they are gaining more status for themselves within their family and the community, in addition to supplementing the income so that their family can enjoy a higher standard of living. Their increase in status has confirmed the importance of women in the household and is increasing their privileges and responsibilities, especially for women in the middle and upper classes.

Value of Children

The value of children varies greatly, depending on the meaning each society attaches to children. In addition, the reaction of individual family members to a child is personalized and subjective. Historically, the motivations for having children have been religious, political, and cultural. Some individuals want children for their own gratification—to have someone to guide and control, to reap economic gains, to improve one's status, to ensure one is cared for in old age, to satisfy cultural requirements, or to provide a means of personal immortality (Berelson, 1976).

In industrial societies the degree to which children are wanted seems to depend somewhat on the state of the economy. For example, during the economic recession of the 1970s, the birth rate in the United States dropped and continued to decline until zero population growth was reached in 1976. This trend can be contrasted to the post-World War II "baby boom," which occurred in a thriving economy.

Many historical changes have influenced the importance of children in society. In agrarian societies, children are valued for the economic gain they bring to their family and society. Industrialization and urbanization in North America have reduced the economic necessity of having children. As a result, children have become less "valuable" and more valued.

Among the events that have stimulated many persons to reevaluate their childbearing function are (a) lower death rates, which threaten to drastically accelerate population growth; (b) the "sexual revolution," which has resulted in the separation of sexuality from reproduction and has liberalized sex roles; and (c) the women's liberation movement, which promoted the realization that childbearing and childrearing are not necessarily the only roles for women.

The decision for many couples today is not *when* to have a child but *whether* to have a child. They are thoughtful about the consequences of childbearing—the effects that the presence of children will have on their relationship or career goals and the cost of children in terms of money and time—and about their ability to raise a well-adjusted, well-provided-for child.

INTERACTION WITHIN FAMILIES

Burgess (1971) theorizes that the family is viable as long as there is interaction among members; the family ceases to be a united group when interaction ceases. Rodgers (1973) views the study of interactions within the family as an aid to understanding its internal functioning. Such studies allow for analysis of members' behavior on both an individual and a one-to-one basis. Interactional patterns in the family can also be used to examine the family in relationship to other organizations in society.

Interactions have two major ingredients: content and process. *Content* is related to the tasks the group is working on or the subject matter the group is dealing with. *Process* is concerned with the inner workings and interrelationships among group members. In most daily interactions, people focus on content—what is being said and what the reply will be—rather than on process. Within the family, process can be dealt with in greater depth because the relationships are long term and family members are deeply involved in the activities of others within the group. Close attention to the family process can help members assess and deal with problems as they arise rather than allow them to fester until they have grown out of proportion.

Family process has nine basic components: verbal participation, social influence, decision-making, task functions, maintenance functions, group atmosphere, group membership, individual feelings, and norms. Observations in all these areas must focus on nonverbal as well as verbal behavior, as the strength of the message is frequently contained in the nonverbal communication.

Verbal participation in the family is one indication of the involvement of a member in the family group. Some individuals are verbal about their feelings, whereas others need to be encouraged to participate. A shift in participation may occur as the topic of conversation increases or decreases in interest. The manner in which low participators are treated may affect their participation in the future; a quiet person who is encouraged to express his or her viewpoint and who receives positive feedback for doing so is more likely to increase his or her participation in future family interactions than the person who does not receive positive feedback for interacting.

Culture and society have set up the patterns of *influence* within the traditional family to a large degree. Although the mother has a strong influence over the children, the father's authority over the entire family is recognized. In the democratic family, in which husband and wife share decision-making responsibilities, they also share influence. Within the family group, members may become rivals, struggling to exert the greatest influence. This struggle is frequently apparent between children vying for their parents' love and affection.

It should be noted that the amount of influence one has within the family does not necessarily correspond to one's participation level. A low participator may have more influence than one who is outspoken.

Decision-making procedures are the key to the success of family interaction. In some families, members may make decisions and carry them out without regard to their effects on the rest of the group. Or the family group may move from one circumstance to the next without making any decisions. Within the democratic family, decision-making may rest on the entire family, particularly if the children are old enough for such responsibility. There may be a specific mechanism for resolving problems, such as a family council, or the process may be informal, such as an impromptu discussion during mealtime. The more the decision-making responsibility is shared by all family members, the more likely it is that the decision will be accepted by everyone.

Behaviors that occur for the purpose of working through certain content are termed *task functions.* They may be initiated by anyone within the family and they require the work of one or more members of the family. Task functions include cleaning the house, mowing the lawn, running errands, and providing income.

The purpose of *maintenance functions* is to preserve the morale of the family unit. Harmonious working relationships among all members are paramount to proper functioning of the group. Maintenance functions include helping all members to participate in the family and meeting their needs. Some family members can impede the group functioning by not listening or by being preoccupied with themselves or with events outside the group. The effectiveness of the functioning of the family is determined by the actions of its members to maintain the internal unity of the group.

The *atmosphere* of the family group can differ from family to family. General impressions of the group usually reveal much about its atmosphere. The family can take on an atmosphere of work or play, satisfaction or dissatisfaction, vivaciousness or sluggishness, contentment or discontent. Some families provide a friendly, congenial atmosphere in which conflict and unpleasant feelings can be expressed calmly. But the atmosphere may also be one of tension and unrest, in which members avoid or are in conflict with one another. The kinds of interactions encouraged by the atmosphere can aid in maintaining close friendly relationships among family members or can alienate them from one another.

Membership within the family group is determined by birth and roles. However, certain persons may not feel accepted by other members of the family. There may be a subgrouping of two or more people who always support each other. Parents may create in their children feelings that they have no influence in the group. Family members need a sense of inclusion in their family unit; this acceptance is important to their feelings of self-esteem.

Interactions among family members frequently generate *feelings* that may be seldom discussed but that set the mood for group and person-to-person interactions. Feelings can be easily observed in a person's facial expression, body movements, tone of voice, and other nonverbal behaviors. Feelings expressed in the family group can vary from anger, irritation, frustration, boredom, defensiveness, and competitiveness to excitement, warmth, and affection. Certain family members may attempt to block the expression of feelings, particularly negative ones, by changing the subject, by negatively reacting to the person expressing the feelings, or by other suppressive methods.

Family groups establish *norms,* which are ground rules or standards that all members are expected to follow. The views of the majority are expressed in the norms, although some group members may not be aware of all the group norms. Some norms, such as use of the democratic method for decision-making, help the family process, whereas others, such as the suppression of negative feelings, tend to hinder the family process.

Investigations have demonstrated that interactions between parents and children have a significant effect on the psychologic well-being of children (Burgess, 1971). Interactions in the homes of emotionally disturbed children are characterized by more tension and less warmth, affection, and mutuality than those in homes where the children grow up emotionally healthy. Fewer problems are found in children of warm mothers than in those of less affectionate mothers; coolness of mothers toward their children is associated with feeding and toilet-training problems, aggressive behavior, and slower development of conscience in the child. Mothers who have a permissive view toward aggression have more aggressive children, but mothers who allow their children to demonstrate dependency behaviors do not produce any effect on the amount of dependency behavior manifested by their children.

DEVELOPMENTAL APPROACH TO THE FAMILY

The study of family development involves tracing the family from its inception with the newly married couple, through its developmental stages, to the family's termination by the death of one or both spouses or by divorce if no children are involved. The developmental pattern is not rigid. For example, some families may decide not to have children, thus skipping those stages that deal with childbearing and childrearing; in other families, adoption of older children may result in omission of particular steps in the developmental process.

The following principles govern family development, according to Duvall (1971):

1. Development tends to be orderly, regular, and predictable. Life in the traditional family follows a regular pattern in most cases, from marriage, to bearing children, to raising children, to having them establish homes of their own, to eventual death. This pattern is alterable by family crisis, although most crises are weathered and family development continues.

2. Developmental rates vary within certain stages according to the individual family's needs. The duration of many of Duvall's developmental stages (for example, the length of time between marriage and the birth of the first child) can vary depending on the desire of the couple or on acts of nature.

3. The family sets the pace that is appropriate for itself at its particular stage of development in its environment. Family members can determine to a large extent the speed at which they will complete the tasks of a specific stage.

4. Development is sequential, with each stage based on the accomplishments of earlier stages. Just as a child learns to sit, crawl, and stand before he walks, a family establishes relationships, bears children, and raises them prior to launching them into families of their own.

5. Development occurs most rapidly in the early stages. A family generally moves through the early stages in a few years, with each successive stage becoming longer.

6. Socially prescribed expectations order the major events of development. Although marriage is certainly not a biologic prerequisite for bearing and rearing children, it is expected in society that a couple will have a courtship period followed by a period of adjustment to marriage prior to bringing children into the world.

7. Family development proceeds in a specific direction from a known beginning to an expected end. Development of the traditional family begins with marriage, and the expected end is death of one or both spouses, although divorce may occur and extinguish a family without children. However, when children are involved, one of the parents usually retains custody, and the family continues as a single-parent family.

8. Anticipated endpoints of the developmental stages serve as family goals. Many goals are set along the way and may be achieved within a relatively short period. However, such anticipated endpoints as the successful launching of children into independence or the establishment of economic security for the parents in their old age become long-term goals toward which the family works.

9. Attainment of family goals brings a sense of fulfillment and success, as when the children become well-established members of society and the parents face retirement with a sense of ego integrity.

10. When certain developmental tasks are successfully accomplished, further tasks evolve. For example, after the birth of a child, the couple must prepare for the task of rearing that child.

11. Only the family can complete the developmental tasks it faces. An outsider cannot set the goals or direct the movement toward these goals for the family. Within the family are the resources and knowledge necessary to deal with the tasks it faces.

12. Most family developmental tasks require social interaction. Tasks for the family are not determined and accomplished in isolation. The society imposes its expectations and delineates acceptable modes of behavior. Families act and direct the actions of their children within this framework.

Developmental Stages and Tasks

According to Duvall (1971), eight family tasks are essential for the survival of the family unit, for continuity of family development, and for growth of the individual and his family. The specific manner in which the following goals are met is determined by each family in reference to the developmental stage in which it finds itself:

1. *Physical maintenance.* Providing shelter, food, clothing, and health care and meeting other fundamental physiologic needs of the family.
2. *Allocation of resources.* Ascertaining which family needs will be met and how they will be cared for financially, and distributing material goods, space, authority, and affection.
3. *Division of labor.* Determining who will procure needed income, manage the household, and care for the children.
4. *Socialization of family members.* Guiding the internalization of acceptable patterns of behavior and physical functioning.
5. *Reproduction, recruitment, and release of family members.* Bearing of children, adoption of children, adding new members by marriage, and establishing policies for the inclusion of other family members or friends into the family circle.
6. *Maintenance of order.* Devising and using effective means of communication and patterns of interaction and affection, determining and clearly defining right and wrong, and attaining a certain degree of conformity within the group.
7. *Placement of members into the larger society.* Determining which social institutions family members wish to participate in (church, school activities, political and social groups) and protecting the family from undesirable outside influences.
8. *Maintenance of motivation and morale.* Satisfying needs of family members, providing rewards as positive feedback, giving encouragement when needed, dealing with crises, and inculcating a sense of family loyalty.

Duvall (1971) has also identified stages in the family life cycle in which these eight tasks are accomplished by a variety of methods. The two major phases in the family life cycle are the *expanding family,* from the beginning of the marriage until the children leave home, and the *contracting family,* from the launching of children to the death of one or both spouses. These two major stages are further divided into the following eight stages, which are based on the age group of the eldest child:

1. Establishment phase
   a. Settling-in period
   b. Expectant family period
2. Childbearing families
3. Families with preschool children
4. Families with schoolchildren
5. Families with teenagers
6. Families launching young adults
7. Middle-aged parent families
8. Aging families

Table 3-1 summarizes Duvall's stages of the family with the tasks of each. The first two stages, establishment and childbearing, will be discussed in detail to give maternity nurses a more complete picture of the new family.

Establishment Phase

The first stage of Duvall's developmental family life cycle is the establishment phase, which begins when the couple enters marriage and ends with the birth or adoption of the first child. Prior to marriage each couple has started to work on the tasks involved in the first stage; however, the intimate relationship of marriage accentuates the importance of these tasks and their evolution. A great deal is involved in this transition from single to married life—new roles to learn, new situations to deal with, and new relationships with people. Success in this period depends on completion of developmental tasks as a single person and in large measure on past family experience.

Settling-in Period

The first task of the young couple is to establish a first home. They sometimes find it necessary to have a room in one of their parents' homes. The more affluent find a house that they furnish themselves. Living with relatives may be particularly difficult, because couples in this situation must establish relationships with other people as well as with each other. However, having their own home may present financial problems.

Table 3–1. Duvall's Family Life Cycle and Developmental Tasks*

Overall family tasks	Establishment phase Settling-in period	Expectant family period	Childbearing families	Families with preschool children
Physical maintenance	Establishing home base to call their own	Arranging for physical care of baby	Adapting housing arrangements for life with baby	Supplying adequate space, facilities, and equipment for expanding family
Allocation of resources	Establishing mutually satisfactory system of getting and spending money	Developing earning and spending patterns to meet costs of having baby	Meeting costs of family living	Meeting predictable and unexpected costs of family life with small children
Division of labor	Establishing mutually acceptable system of work loads and accountability	Determining work loads for expectant wife and husband	Reworking patterns of mutual responsibility and accountability for care of child	Sharing responsibilities within expanding family
Socialization of family members	Establishing systems of emotional and intellectual communication	Expanding communication as expectant parents	Refining communication for childbearing and rearing	Creating and maintaining effective communications within family
Reproduction, recruitment, and release of family members	Establishing continuity of mutually satisfying sexual relationship	Adapting patterns of sexual relationships to pregnancy	Reestablishing mutually satisfying sexual relationships	Maintaining mutually satisfying sexual relationship and planning for future children
	Facing possibility of children and planning for their coming	Acquiring knowledge about pregnancy, childbirth, and parenthood	Planning for further children	
Maintenance of order	Establishing workable relationships with relatives	Reorienting relationships with relatives to birth of baby	Reestablishing working relationships with relatives	Cultivating relationships within extended family
Placement of members in larger society	Establishing ways of interacting with friends, associates, and community organizations	Adapting relationships with friends and community to realities of pregnancy	Fitting into community life as young family	Tapping resources and serving needs outside family
Maintenance of motivation and morale	Establishing workable philosophy of life as couple	Maintaining morale and workable philosophy of life during pregnancy	Reworking suitable philosophy of life as family	Facing dilemmas and reworking philosophy of life

*Modified from Duvall, E. 1971. *Family development.* Philadelphia: J. B. Lippincott Co.

Families with schoolchildren	Families with teenagers	Families launching young adults	Middle-aged parent families	Aging families
Providing for children's activities and parents' privacy	Providing facilities for widely different needs	Rearranging physical resources and facilities as family contracts	Maintaining pleasant and comfortable home	Finding satisfying home for later years
Remaining financially solvent	Working out money matters with teenagers	Meeting expenses of launching children	Assuring security for later years	Adjusting to retirement income
Cooperating to get things done	Sharing responsibilities for family living	Reallocating responsibilities among grown and growing children	Carrying out household responsibilities	Establishing comfortable household routines
Utilizing family communication systems effectively	Bridging communication gap	Maintaining open systems of communication within family	Maintaining contact with grown children's families	Maintaining contact with children and grandchildren
			Keeping in touch with siblings' families and aging parents	Caring for elderly relatives
Continuing to satisfy each other as married partners	Putting marriage relationship in focus	Coming to terms with each other as husband and wife	Drawing closer together as couple	Nurturing each other as husband and wife
		Widening the family circle through release of young adult children and recruitment of new members by marriage		
Feeling close to relatives in larger family system	Keeping in touch with relatives			Facing bereavement and death of spouse
Tying in with life outside family	Widening horizons of teenagers and their families		Participating in community life	Keeping an interest in people outside the family
Testing and retesting family philosophy of life	Reworking and maintaining philosophy of life	Reconciling conflicting loyalties and philosophies of life	Reaffirming meaningful values in life	Finding meanings in life

Another task faced by young couples after marriage is setting up a system of obtaining and spending money. If one or both spouses are in school, they may have to take on part-time work or one may have to drop out of school to secure employment. In recent years it has become increasingly necessary for wives to work to earn the family income. When both partners are working to the extent that they have little time together to adjust to their new relationship, stress may develop. However, these stressful circumstances can work to the advantage of the young couple if they make mutually agreeable decisions about the responsibilities they will accept in their home life, in social activities, and in budgeting and financial planning.

Along with finding appropriate resources and budgeting, couples must make decisions about who will handle household and other tasks and about their accountability to each other. Tradition and societal values generally give direction to these decisions. However, with more women entering the working world and more men participating in household chores, the young couple has a greater number of options open to them. Conflicts may arise in the performance of this developmental task. The husband may be caught between the traditional role of being head of the household and his desire to include his wife in the decision-making process. The wife may have similar conflicts about home planning and execution of responsibilities.

Communication on both the emotional and intellectual levels must also be worked out to the satisfaction of the couple. Marriage is an intimate relationship charged with intense emotions. Feelings that may be suppressed when dealing with others outside the family may be directed at the marriage partner. Frustrations at work or in the day-to-day routines of managing the household may build up and not be apparent until a minor crisis provokes them. Appropriate methods for dealing with these feelings must be found, or they can divert the marriage relationship. Many couples find that nonverbal gestures can reveal thoughts and feelings, although the skill to interpret them frequently takes months and even years to develop. Couples who have differences in their reactions to certain situations can mesh their behaviors so that they complement rather than detract from each other.

Another significant task is the establishment of a mutually satisfying sexual relationship. The degree of sexual experience and knowledge one brings to marriage affects one's adjustment to the relationship. There is evidence that prior experience does not necessarily facilitate sexual adjustment, but factual knowledge can increase the couple's understanding of sexual functioning. The marriage partners may have varying levels of needs and expectations, conscious and unconscious, and they must work together to achieve a relationship that is fulfilling to both.

The couple's families of origin continue to be important, but relationships with them change. No longer is each partner a member of one family; each now has relationships with three families—the family of origin of each partner and the couple's own developing family. The accountability that they once had to their parents now has turned to each other. The young couple may maintain close ties with their original families, may choose to keep distant from their families for fear of interference, or may choose a satisfying degree of involvement with both families.

The couple must also establish patterns of interaction with friends and others in their community. Young married people may find that they have less in common with single friends and may seek out groups or other couples for companionship. Demands from the work group of the husband or wife may put pressure on the couple. Religious affiliation may be a major concern of the couple. If both partners are of the same religion and participate similarly, there will be little problem; but if different religions are involved, agreement must be reached about continuing affiliations.

Married couples face the decision about bearing children. Family planning and the use of contraceptives have received widespread acceptance in our society. Many couples are choosing not to have children; many more are limiting the size of their families because of economic concerns or the desires of the woman to pursue a career or other interests. A small proportion of couples are unable to conceive a child despite their desire to have one and may seek medical help for a solution to their reproduction problem.

The final task of the establishment phase is to work out a philosophy of life as a couple. Optimally, each individual enters marriage with a philosophy of life, which must be correlated with that of the partner. The young couple is faced with decisions about religion, political affiliations, social groups, and recreational activities.

They may disagree on particular issues, but they may be able to live with these differences with little concern. The philosophy they develop will identify them and reflect their attitudes and priorities. In addition, it will provide a framework for later decision-making.

The settling-in stage is a precarious period when the marriage is vulnerable to many stresses that could potentially destroy it. The tasks just described may not be completed within the first few years of marriage or indeed may never be completed. However, the greater the accomplishment in meeting the demands of these tasks, the more likely the marriage is to be mutually satisfying to both partners.

Expectant Family Period

In the latter part of the first stage in the family life cycle, the family's expectations of having their own child may be fulfilled. Although the expectant phase may cover the shortest time span in the cycle, this period is filled with many intense and diverse feelings. When the couple is told that conception has occurred, they may either accept or reject the pregnancy. Some pregnancies are unplanned, although the woman may subconsciously desire to become pregnant. Others are planned and may even have been of concern for months or years before conception actually takes place.

After their initial reactions to the fact that the wife is pregnant, the couple must accomplish certain tasks that are an offshoot of those from the earlier part of the establishment phase. For example, arrangements must be made for the physical care of the baby. These arrangements may mean drastic changes for the family if they have to move into larger quarters or to a place where children are accepted. Within their living space they must set aside a special area for the baby, whether it is a corner of a room or a separate nursery. Sleeping accommodations for the infant and parents, as well as arrangements for feeding, bathing, and playing, must be given consideration.

In the expectant family period, the couple must make adjustments in patterns of earning and spending. Generally, the man is in the early phase of his career, when his salary may be low. His wife's salary, which may be a necessary part of the family income, may come to an end during the pregnancy. Many women who have worked during the early part of their marriage stop work during pregnancy or when the baby is born—a time when there is greater monetary outlay for shelter, food, clothing, and other supplies for the baby. Even if the mother chooses to return to work after the baby is born, child care is a costly item in the budget. Health care during the pregnancy and birth also requires large amounts of money, especially with rising medical costs.

Work loads and designation of authority also change out of necessity during pregnancy. The husband may assume more of the heavy household chores, as it is difficult for his pregnant wife to bend and move about. At the same time, pregnant women do not find that their physical state prohibits them from pursuing many of the activities they enjoy, such as working, entertaining, or even participating in sports. The physician and nurse take on more authority as the couple seeks their advice at this time, anticipating the birth of a healthy baby.

Sexual activities are another aspect of marital interaction that must be altered to accommodate both physical and emotional changes of pregnancy. The pregnancy may have positive, negative, or no effects on the couple's sexual relationship. Husbands are as likely to feel changes in their sexual responses as their wives are. Because of changes in breast and abdominal size, the couple will need to reorient their normal sexual activities.

As soon as the couple knows they are expecting a child, a new focus of interaction becomes evident, enlarging their need for and use of communication. The couple is about to enter Erikson's developmental stage of generativity versus stagnation (p. 54), and with this stage come the motivations that will help them work together to prepare for their child. Most couples feel a sense of fulfillment as they feel pride in their ability to conceive a child, as the wife starts to show signs of pregnancy, and as they make plans for the child's arrival. Husband and wife undergo changes in self-concepts in terms of masculinity, femininity, and parenthood. All of these tasks are accomplished with greater ease if the husband and wife develop communication patterns that help them cope with new responsibilities.

Communication with relatives also takes on a new perspective. Close relatives can take a prominent role in helping the young couple with their baby after birth; they can give physical and emotional support to the wife as she undertakes the new tasks of child care. On the other hand, family members can interfere with the couple's adjustment to pregnancy and childbirth with the telling of "old wives' tales" and possibly frightening myths. Reorienting relatives to the kind of relationship that is most desirable for new parents and their child is a major task of the expectant family.

Reorientation must also occur in relationships to friends and in community activities. Recreational and social activities can continue to be a major part of the couple's life and may be curtailed only to the extent that the pregnancy decreases the woman's ability to participate. The mother-to-be may be more sensitive to her husband's activities because his mobility is not affected. She may believe that he is seeking outside interests as she becomes more introspective about the birth of the child. The man may feel left out of many activities of his wife as she has frequent visits to the physician and attends groups that discuss the care and rearing of children. If they plan joint activities that help them remain with each other while continuing to respect each other's needs for autonomy, the couple can make a comfortable transition to the complementary relationship that will be needed in future years.

The expectant parents need to acquire a great deal of knowledge about pregnancy, labor and delivery, and child care. Their background knowledge may be based more on hearsay than on fact. They may have had little or no experience with infants and small children. Pregnancy is a period when expectant parents are open to and anxious for knowledge. The more highly educated the couple, the more likely that they desire in-depth knowledge about this event. Classes for expectant parents are offered by hospitals, physicians, and community organizations such as the Red Cross to prepare couples for childbirth and parenthood.

The final task of the expectant couple—maintenance of morale and a workable philosophy—can be accomplished if each partner meets the other's needs for acceptance, support, and affection. They must deal with questions of whether they are prepared to bring a child into their lives, of how the baby will fit into their pattern of living, and of how they will alter their life-style for their child. As mentioned earlier, both partners feel emotions that are new to them and seek understanding from their partners. The more one partner is able to meet the other's emotional needs, the more love each will be able to give to their child.

These tasks of the expectant family parallel those of the newly married couple, although the intensity and sense of urgency is heightened as the expectant couple prepare for the impending birth. If the parents-to-be have successfully completed the tasks in the settling-in period, they are ready to build on them and enlarge their horizons as their family expands. They may face difficulties along the way, such as finding suitable housing within their income, adjusting to emotional changes in each other, or not receiving needed support from within and outside their families. However, as young families find themselves on their own, coping with new experiences away from their families of origin, they begin to look to available community resources to provide support.

Childbearing Family Stage

The arrival of the first child marks a time of both great joy and crisis for the young family. Again, the family faces a period of reorganization. During the childbearing family stage (from the birth of the first child until that child is 30 months old), the baby and family become stabilized in their schedules and relationships to each other. The parents have great joy about the birth of their first child and share their joy with their family and friends; the new mother feels a sense of accomplishment and is ready to relax and let others care for her and her baby for a few days. At the same time, the young family has a feeling of great responsibility for their child's growth and development.

The first task of the childbearing family is to arrange the home to meet the needs of the infant. The reality of the baby in the home setting necessitates tailoring the already-prepared accommodations to most easily meet the needs of the infant and parents. The primary responsibility of the parents is to provide a safe, comfortable environment for the child. A primary need of the newborn infant is a quiet, clean place to sleep. As the child grows and becomes more mobile, his immediate environment enlarges, even though he is still unable to protect himself from many of its dangers. Eventually his curiosity leads him to explore, and his parents have to "childproof" the home, setting limits within which the child can function safely.

Costs of raising a child are drastically increasing, creating additional problems for a couple who are already dealing with the increased costs of daily living. Even in the United States, where prosperity is relatively common, many families are below poverty level and children are raised with a minimum of economic expenditure.

The husband in the childbearing family probably still has low earning power and may have to take on an additional part-time job to make ends meet; this takes away from the time he can spend supplementing the mother's care in meeting the child's needs. Some young families choose to live with a minimum of income, hoping their purchasing power will increase in the near future; other couples borrow money to obtain what they want and hope that eventual salary increases will make payment of bills easier.

The crisis of the first child's birth requires a reworking of responsibility and accountability patterns. A baby requires round-the-clock care, some of which is assumed by the mother, particularly if she is breast-feeding the child. The husband must assume more of the household tasks, such as shopping and running errands outside the home, during the mother's confinement with child care. Both partners share in seeking solutions to problems arising during the day. The child also has accountability to parents as he grows older. The approval or disapproval of his parents teaches him what his parents consider good and bad, and he recognizes good acts as pleasing ones. While the young child is in Erikson's stage of autonomy versus shame and doubt (see p. 54), he develops a sense of accountability to himself as he learns to control his bodily functions.

Reestablishing a satisfying sexual relationship with one's partner is another task of the childbearing family stage. Sex life usually decreases or ceases during the postnatal period. The new mother becomes absorbed in her child, and her close physical relationship with the baby may decrease her sexual needs. Her husband may feel rejected as the new mother focuses on the baby's needs and frequently misses those of her husband. A great deal of mutual patience and understanding is necessary as the couple strives to reunite to meet each other's needs.

Two stresses occur in the childbearing family period that can hinder or further the development of effective communication. The first stress comes from the type of communication that a newborn brings into the world to express his needs—crying. Until the new parents can interpret what the various types of cries mean and until they learn to anticipate their infant's needs, the crying can be extremely disconcerting. When the parents believe they have met the needs of their child and the crying continues for no apparent reason, their frustration increases. However, as the parents attempt to meet the baby's needs lovingly, his trust in them increases, and other methods of communication emerge, such as smiling, cooing, and eventually talking. The other stress to effective communication is decreased sharing between the parents. Their tasks may be more separately defined as the husband works outside the home while his wife remains busy caring for their new baby and the house. They participate in different activities and have less time to be alone together. Instead of the one relationship of husband-wife, three relationships have developed to include the infant in the family circle. However, even though the parents may have distinct tasks, they can share more as they watch their baby grow.

Dealing with relationships with relatives is also a facet of the development of the family with a very young child. The coming of the first child may be a major signal that a new, separate family has indeed emerged. The new parents will receive a great deal of advice on how to care for the child. If they are mature and have successfully completed their previous developmental tasks, they are able to sift through this information and use what is most meaningful to them. The greater the difference between the two parental families, the greater the likelihood of conflicting advice, because each set of grandparents will want the child to be raised according to the traditions of their family. And, of course, the parental families can also supply a great deal of support and comfort to the new parents who are endeavoring to establish their own traditions.

The young family must participate in community activities to establish relationships outside the home. They are more involved in their home life than they were prior to their baby's birth and must find suitable babysitting arrangements if they desire to go out together. Their interests may change as they seek out congenial couples with young children who can share similar experiences.

A further task of the childbearing family is to decide whether or when to have more children and to take appropriate measures. Having children too close may prove to be a tremendous strain for both parents, or parents may choose to have their children close together to allow the mother to resume her career as soon as possible. If the first child is defective or dies shortly after birth, the decision about whether or when to have another child becomes paramount.

Maintenance of morale and the philosophy of life of the childbearing family may become difficult. The repetitious tasks of everyday child care may overshadow the basic satisfactions of parenthood. Values placed on material objects may need to be changed, becoming dependent on what is good for the young child. The parents need to continue their independence as a couple while recognizing the child's dependence on them. The developmental needs of the child and those of the parents may be in conflict, so priorities must be set. The young family may need to accept assistance from relatives and friends at a time when they are still striving to be a separate unit.

The early childbearing and childrearing years have a significant influence on the ultimate strength of the family unit. Many crises occur that can either divide or unite the family. A division or conflict may not be evident while the children are still dependent but may manifest itself when the children have left home and there is little else to hold the parents together. Yet these same stresses can unite the family more solidly if they are faced as mutual problems and if individual needs and priorities are taken into account in family interrelationships.

Psychosocial Development of Family Members

Erikson (1963) has described the psychosocial development of an individual as occurring in eight stages. Successful resolution of each of these stages results in the emergence of a predominant positive quality, whereas unsuccessful handling of each stage produces negative qualities. These stages are as follows:

1. *Basic trust versus basic mistrust (early infancy: birth to 1 year).* If the infant's needs are met consistently and if there is constancy in his surroundings and of his caretakers, he will develop a sense of certainty and predictability about his external and internal environment.

2. *Autonomy versus shame and doubt (late infancy: 1–3 years).* As a result of muscular maturation, the child develops a sense of control over his bodily functions and environment. The child begins to realize that he is a person apart from the parents. Overcontrol by others can result in a loss of self-esteem.

3. *Initiative versus guilt (early childhood: 4–5 years).* During this stage, the quality of purpose emerges. The child undertakes or plans to achieve activities that seem desirable. Depending on external influences or parental sanctions, the child may feel guilt about the goals or acts he contemplates.

4. *Industry versus inferiority (middle childhood: 6–11 years).* The child develops skills and learns to use tools to a productive end. Feelings of inadequacy may arise about his abilities or about what he produces.

5. *Identity versus role confusion (puberty and adolescence: 12–20 years).* The major developmental task at this stage is to integrate how one sees oneself with how one is perceived by others. The adolescent's attempt to determine his place in the world may lead to overidentification with groups, ideologies, or individuals.

6. *Intimacy versus isolation (early adulthood: 20–40 years).* The young adult manifests a readiness to commit himself to others and to situations. The individual who is afraid of ego loss avoids such experiences, leading to separation and isolation.

7. *Generativity versus stagnation (early and middle adulthood: 40 to 64 years).* Primary motivations during this period of life are productivity and creativity. For many persons, this involves reproduction and readying the next generation for its life.

8. *Ego integrity versus despair (late adulthood: 65 years and older).* The person accepts how he has lived his life, how he will continue to live it, and the fact that it will end.

In Table 3–2 the stages of the family life cycle are listed with the probable corresponding developmental stages of the individual members. It is clear that development of the individual and of the family are interdependent phenomena and that one influences the well-being of the other.

Just as Erikson's stages serve as guidelines for

Table 3–2. Stages of Individual and Family Development

Erik Erikson's stages	Evelyn Duvall's stages
1. Adult: intimacy vs. isolation	Establishment phase
2. Adult: generativity vs. stagnation Child: trust vs. mistrust autonomy vs. shame and doubt	Childbearing family phase
3. Adult: generativity vs. stagnation Child: initiative vs. guilt	Families with preschool children stage
4. Adult: generativity vs. stagnation Child: industry vs. inferiority	Families with schoolchildren stage
5. Adult: generativity vs. stagnation Child: identity vs. role confusion	Families with teenagers stage
6. Adult: generativity vs. stagnation Child: intimacy vs. isolation	Families launching young adults stage
7. Adult: generativity vs. stagnation Child: generativity vs. stagnation	Middle-aged parent families stage
8. Adult: integrity vs. despair Child: generativity vs. stagnation	Aging families stage

evaluating the development of the individual, those for the family serve as guidelines for analyzing the nuclear family. During each stage, certain key needs of the family must be met. The differences among these needs are a result of the varying developmental stages of the individuals within the family. As Duvall (1971) points out, the success of the family and the developmental stages of the individuals within it depends on close, nurturing interrelationships among all members of the family.

The developmental approach is useful to nurses dealing with expectant and childbearing families. Nurses can better identify the goals of the maternity patient and her family, anticipate family crises, and meet patient and family needs after determining the developmental stage of the family and its members.

NURSING IMPLICATIONS FOR FAMILY CARE

A major goal of nursing is to help families and individuals within them achieve optimal health by preventive, maintenance, and restorative measures. In addition, nurses have a role in helping families to accomplish the appropriate developmental tasks at each family stage. The success of the family depends on the achievement of these tasks. At times the family may find that success comes easily; at other times, they must overcome failure. Since failure tends to follow failure as success follows success, the nurse may need to intervene to break a family's cycle of failures in performing tasks and to guide them toward success.

When an individual within the family becomes ill, he becomes dependent on others, thereby increasing stress and perhaps temporarily or permanently impeding the ability of the family to perform its tasks, depending on the severity and length of the illness. The nurse can help the other family members devise methods of taking on added responsibilities and of finding outside resources to support family functioning; by doing so the nurse may prevent further complications for the sick individual or his family.

When giving care to a patient, the nurse should keep in mind the long-term, intimate relationships among family members. That person has performed a unique role within the family group that must be accounted for if the family is to function optimally. Thus, families have the right to examine the kind of care and service a family member is receiving, to complain when the service is unsatisfactory, and to seek other sources of services when they are dissatisfied.

When working with families, a nurse performs many roles, including teacher, counselor, coordinator, and advocate. These roles fulfill many of the needs of expanding and contracting families.

The nurse acts primarily as a teacher, counselor, and advocate in helping a couple determine their family-planning needs. The nurse offers information in a manner that the family can understand and use, demonstrating understanding and respect for needs. The family may be hesitant to use family planning because of fears of, dislike for, or misconceptions about contraception; because of worries that they cannot afford family planning; or because of beliefs that others are trying to limit the size of their social group.

The nurse's responsibilities to the expectant family include assessing the mother's physical and emotional status and needs and the father's desires for involvement, teaching parents about pregnancy and labor and delivery, and counseling them about child care and the parental role.

After the child is born, a primary concern of the nurse is to make sure that the family can meet the needs of the newborn infant. The nurse assumes the roles of teacher and counselor when she discusses the needs of the infant and demonstrates infant care to the parents. In addition, the nurse acts as the family advocate by giving emotional support to new parents and by providing guidance on effective use of health care professionals.

The nurse can serve as a resource person to parents with children of various ages who need guidance and who desire knowledge about their children's developmental tasks, appropriate toys for each age group, safety in the household, health care needs, adjustment to school or the mother's return to work, and the child's gradual separation from the family.

Families with an elderly member may require counseling on his or her physical and emotional needs and their responsibilities to meet these needs. The nurse can help coordinate health care for the older family member and can teach the family how to meet his or her health care needs.

Application of the Nursing Process

Adhering to the concepts of the nursing process is important in caring for the family. Assessment of the family's health status is the first step toward optimal family functioning. The assessment data can be gathered in any setting, including home visits.

The initiation of a good relationship with the family is necessary to the collection of pertinent data and to the validation of data gathered. The nurse must use all her interpersonal and intellectual skills when collecting data.

Basic information that should be obtained include the names, ages, relationships, and sex of all family members. Data about members of the extended family who are closest to the nuclear family should be included—names, ages, sex, where they live, and what kind of relationship they have with the family.

A health history of the entire family should be taken. The nurse should gather information about both the extended and nuclear family regarding past acute and chronic illness, mental health, and such alterations in health status as obesity or occurrence of accidents. Past experiences of family members with health care delivery or hospitalization are important in ascertaining the approach to the family that will be most helpful.

Data about the current health status of each family member must be obtained. Important information includes data on each member's allergies, present illnesses, and defects; the family's knowledge about these disorders; and treatments and recommendations that have been made and carried through. Assessing the competency of family members to care for ill members and to carry out instructions is vital in determining the nurse's role with the family. Many families use preventive health measures such as routine medical, dental, and ophthalmic examinations; receive immunizations; and participate in other screening programs. If the family does not use such measures, the question arises as to their availability or the family's attitudes about them. It may be necessary to discover what health care facilities are available to the family and how they are utilized.

A complete assessment of the family requires a visit to the home. Families may feel that a home visit by a health team member is an invasion of privacy but may become more amenable as rapport is established. The nurse should observe living conditions objectively; she should not allow personal standards and values to block true assessment. Living space providing all family members private, comfortable sleeping arrangements and permitting each person to pursue interests and needs is important. Facilities for ill and convalescent family members should also be evaluated. Adequate heat, light, cooking facilities, water, storage facilities, and hygienic equipment are necessary for maintaining the well-being of all family members. Toys, books, and other recreational and educational equipment should be available for the children. Play areas should be away from safety hazards and should be adequately supervised. Safety hazards such as peeling paint, exposed electrical wiring, rugs that are not held in place, and exposed heating equipment can be of great danger, particularly to small children and the elderly. The distance of the home from health care facilities and the availability of transportion to them should also be investigated.

Appraisal of the home environment will give only some indication of the economic status of the family. Knowledge about the sources and amounts of family income and about the work skills of individual members will aid in the appraisal of health behavior and needs. Information about the allocation of income to shelter, clothing, food, savings, insurance, education, recreation, and health care reveals the family's economic priorities and their ability to meet the needs of all family members.

As discussed earlier in this chapter, interaction among members is vital to the maintenance of a healthy, well-adjusted family. Observing the roles that various members have in the family, the flexibility of these roles, and the sources of authority and influence within the family reveals the underlying relationships among its members. Other important aspects of family interaction include the parents' childrearing practices, rationales for using particular procedures, attitudes toward health and the health care delivery system, intellectual interests, religious practices and beliefs, and sociocultural reference groups. Interactions with members of the extended family and the types and amount of support they give each other should be explored.

The assessment must also include observations of the population characteristics and resources of the community in which the family lives and of the family's involvement in community activities. Certain health problems can affect many within a community; for example, diseases can be transmitted by children to other children in schools and from them to the rest of the family. After identifying such situations, nurses can make recommendations that will help families to reduce or eliminate such problems.

After the nurse has made her observations, has assessed the family, and has determined behavior patterns and patterns of interaction, she is prepared to select and order the data that are most pertinent. She must then formulate a nursing diagnosis to set goals for the family. These should be divided into short- and long-range goals and should be a joint enterprise between the family and the nurse. Without this cooperative interaction, the goals may not meet those needs that the family believes are important, may not be realistic for the family, or may not be accepted by the family as their responsibility.

The priority of these goals must then be determined. This is a highly individualized process in which input from the family continues to have great importance. A severe illness, a safety hazard in the home, and lack of funds for a needed purchase can all be important matters. However, the family may consider obtaining funds to be the most important goal, the nurse may believe that correction of the safety hazard should receive immediate attention, and the physician may think that the treatment of the illness should be given top priority. Factors that affect the setting of priorities include the family's perceptions of their needs, the number of problems that require attention, the feasibility of goals set, the readiness of the family to meet the goals, and the amount of preparation or education necessary before the goals can be met (Sobol and Robischon, 1970). With the family the nurse must validate the goals and their importance to gain the family's support in working toward them.

Planning interventions is the next step in the nursing process. The nursing care plan must be based on the goals set in consultation with the family. There are generally a variety of approaches to every problem, and the nurse must identify the one that seems most likely to work in the family's particular framework of attitudes, beliefs, and values. Family participation in the decision about the approach can be valuable, because the family is aware of its ability to deal with the situation. In any event, the nursing plan must be accepted by the family prior to putting it into action.

During the planning stage, decisions must be made about those health care workers, other professionals, and community agencies that will be of greatest value to the family. The services available from these agencies must be explained to the family. The family's needs may be best satisfied through the participation of several agencies, which requires interagency cooperation and coordination of efforts. The nurse may serve as the coordinator of these activities, assuring continuity of services to the family. One long-term goal for the family should be to strengthen its knowledge of community resources to meet its own health needs.

In implementing a plan of care, the nurse must constantly be aware of the short- and long-term goals that have been set for the family. Therapeutic interaction continues to be of primary importance. Needs of the family often produce stress on some or all members. The recommendations and teaching of the nurse or other professionals may cause more stress, as any change will always cause some tension and anxiety. Family members may feel guilty about having certain needs and may be concerned about how these needs will be accepted by others. Any serious problems have probably already disrupted the family, and its members may have had to take on roles and responsibilities with which they are unfamiliar; this can change the life-style of the family. The family nurse must be aware of any situations that arise as the nursing plan is implemented. Further resources may need to be consulted to help in dealing with any problems.

In working with the family, the nurse should strive to present material in a manner that is understandable. Knowledge of the family's cultural background helps in determining the most effective manner to be used.

To interpret the success or failure of the nursing care plan, the nurse must evaluate her effectiveness. The evaluation should be in terms of the goals set for the family and the effects produced. Again, the family should play an important part in this evaluation, as it has in other steps of the nursing process. Members must be encouraged to respond freely and openly. If a goal has been fully achieved, the nursing interventions have been successful. If a goal has not been attained, the nurse should explore the reasons for the failure and devise a new plan that might meet with greater success. If a goal has been partially achieved, the nurse and family must ascertain whether the plan is realistic and simply needs more time or whether modifications are necessary. The nurse may find that changes in the family necessitate adjustments and adaptations in the nursing care plan at any point during its implementation. Even when all goals appear to have been attained, periodic reevaluation and encouragement are necessary for the family to continue to function maximally (Figure 3-4).

Let us look at the example of the Johnston family to demonstrate the effective use of the nursing process with a family. Mr. Johnston is 30 years old and his wife is 27. They have two children, Jeffrey, 3 years old, and Jennifer, 7 months. Mrs. Johnston and Jennifer were attending a well-baby examination when Mrs. Johnston mentioned that she was concerned that Jennifer was not yet sitting by herself. She noted that Jeffrey was sitting by 6½ months of age and that several neighbors had been surprised at Jennifer's inability to sit alone. Through further exploration the nurse learned that Mrs. Johnston was concerned that Jeffrey had been caught several times treating Jennifer roughly and had tried to pick her up by her legs several times. The nurse's plan was to allow Mrs. Johnston to express her anxieties freely and to ask pertinent questions about Jeffrey's behavior and other family members' reaction to it. The nurse discovered that this behavior began shortly after Jennifer was born. At first Jeffrey ignored his new baby sister, but he began to pat her after about a week. His parents accompanied his touching her with remarks that he should pat her gently because she was only a baby and could be easily harmed. Jeffrey was usually kept away from Jennifer, but several times he got into her room and was caught hitting her. When his parents found him holding her up by the legs, they were afraid that her spine had been injured; this fear seemed validated by Jennifer's slow motor development. Punishing Jeffrey did not seem to alleviate his problem but rather accentuated it.

The nurse explained to Mrs. Johnston that all babies develop at their own rate, even within the same family. A Denver Developmental Screening Test showed that Jennifer was functioning within the normal limits for her age. These results were explained to Mrs. Johnston, and several books on child development were suggested to her. Mrs. Johnston was advised that although Jennifer's motor development was fine and the physician had determined that there were no residual effects from Jeffrey's rough treatment, they both might enjoy infant physical stimulation classes that were offered through a local agency.

Mrs. Johnston was still concerned about Jeffrey's possible future physical harm to Jenni-

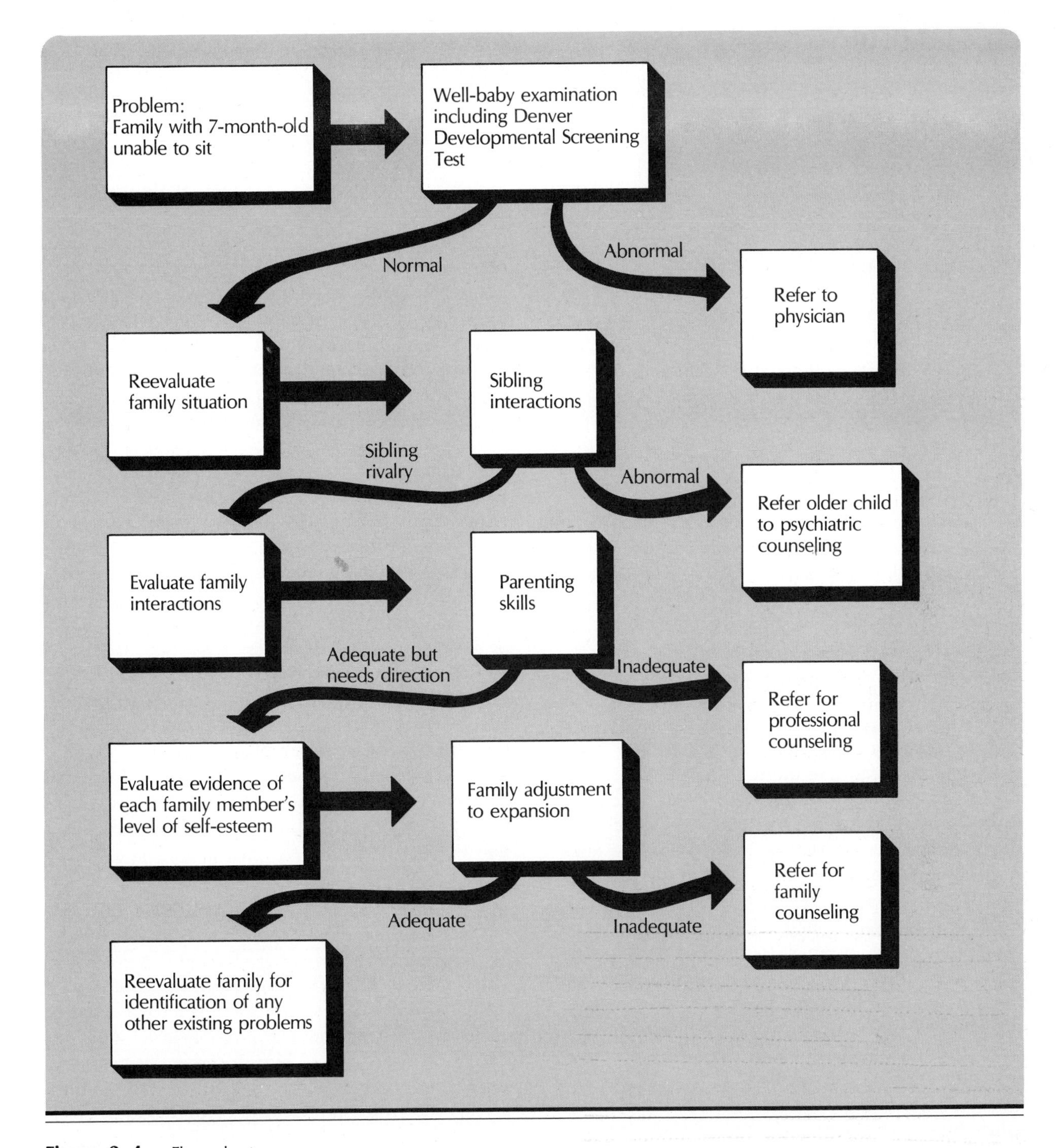

Figure 3–4. Flow chart.

fer. The nurse explained that behavior like Jeffrey's is a frequent reaction of an older sibling to the birth of a baby and that he probably felt that Jennifer had usurped his place of importance within the family. Mrs. Johnston was asked to bring Jeffrey in, as it was time for his routine examination. His developmental abilities were assessed, along with his sleep and activity patterns, eating, elimination, communication, temperament, and dependence-independence patterns. He was found to have occasional temper tantrums when he was tired and to wet his bed at night. Otherwise, he demonstrated no difficulties in adapting to his surroundings. The nurse suggested that Jeffrey be included in the care of Jennifer when possible and that the parents set aside a special time period each night, possibly after Jennifer was in bed, to devote entirely to Jeffrey's needs and desires. Mrs. Johnston was advised to set up an area in Jeffrey's room with a hammering board and tools where he could retreat to take out his frustrations in a more acceptable manner.

Several weeks later, during Jennifer's next routine examination, the nurse evaluated the effectiveness of her suggestions. Mrs. Johnston reported that Jeffrey continued to have angry outbursts but that he was sent to his room, where he had learned to work out his feelings. He seemed to enjoy playing with Jennifer now that she was able to appreciate his antics; he had not been caught being overly rough with her in the previous month, although he liked to jostle her while she laughed back at him. Jennifer had shown progress in sitting and remained sitting for indefinite periods and had also started crawling. The nurse's role of support, encouragement, and reassurance had worked well through planned, thoughtful intervention.

Legal Considerations

In dealing with families, the nurse must be aware of legal and governmental regulations and practices that affect families and children and must be ready to support those that will be beneficial to them. Among the legal aspects with which the nurse may have to deal at some point are marriage, divorce, adoption, child abuse, and juvenile court (Hymovich and Barnard, 1973). The legal aspects of marriage stipulate that spouses have the right to support, company, affection, and service from each other and the responsibility to fulfill these needs for the other partner. If one partner does not fufill his or her part of the marriage contract, the marriage can be terminated by annulment or divorce.

An annulment of the marriage is granted when one of the partners has been under the influence of drugs or alcohol at the time of the marriage and has not voluntarily cohabited with his or her partner, when either partner is impotent, when the marriage took place by force, or when one partner is mentally incompetent.

Legal grounds for divorce include cruelty, adultery, conviction of a felony, and abandonment. In some states, one party must be blamed for the failure of the marriage. Many states are now taking a more humanistic view of divorce, recognizing that incompatibility can be caused by both partners, and they are allowing a divorce decree to be granted after a certain period of separation. When children are involved in a divorce action, the case is more complicated; in finding a suitable home for the children, their welfare is placed above that of either parent.

Adoption is a legal process for bringing children into the family. Each state has its own laws about the rights of adoptive parents, natural parents, and adopted children that specify the degree to which an adopted child is considered the same as a natural-born child. In most states the adopted child is granted full rights and privileges.

All states have laws that require the reporting of suspected cases of child abuse. Actual conviction of an adult for battering a child is difficult; parents are expected to discipline their children, and there is a fine line between what is considered reasonable and unreasonable punishment.

Juvenile courts handle cases that would normally be considered criminal if the perpetrator were an adult. The child (anyone under 18 years of age) is not treated as a criminal but rather as a person needing education and protection. To this end, his or her name and crime are not published. Juvenile courts also handle neglected or abandoned children, who are placed in custodial institutions or foster homes until the parents have demonstrated their ability and willingness to care for them or until they have been adopted by other families.

SUMMARY

The family is a unit of simple origin but complex makeup. Many of the family's needs for assistance in accomplishing developmental tasks and for health care can be met by the nurse. By means of supportive intervention, the nurse can assume therapeutic roles that maintain or restore health as well as prevent illness within families.

SUGGESTED ACTIVITIES

1. Observe three families and identify which developmental phase is currently in progress.
2. Describe the behaviors that might be exhib-

ited by children of different cultures while learning the traditions of their family.

3. For single-person families, how would the nurse identify completion of family roles?
4. Develop a questionnaire that could be used to obtain a meaningful family history as it relates to maternity nursing care. Assess three families and explain the usefulness of the family history tool.
5. Interact with three families and identify the type of family structure exhibited.
6. List the variations in family roles that the nurse might expect to find in a black family, a hispanic family, a single-parent family, a white family, a Japanese-American family, a Vietnamese refugee family, and a Native American (Indian) family.

REFERENCES

Berelson, B. 1976. The value of children: a taxonomical essay. In *Raising children in modern America: problems and prospective solutions,* ed. N. B. Talbot. Boston: Little, Brown & Co.

Burgess, E. 1968. The family as a unit of interacting personalities. In *Family roles and interactions: an anthology,* ed. J. Heiss. Chicago: Rand McNally & Company.

Burgess, E. 1971. *The family: from traditional to companionship.* New York: Van Nostrand Reinhold Company.

Dunn, H. L. 1961. *High level wellness.* Arlington, Va.: R. W. Beatty, Ltd.

Duvall, E. 1971. *Family development.* Philadelphia: J. B. Lippincott Co.

Erikson, E. H. 1963. *Childhood and society.* 2nd ed. New York: W. W. Norton & Co., Inc.

Hymovich, D. P., and Barnard, M. U. 1973. *Family health care.* New York: McGraw-Hill Book Co.

Kantor, D., and Lehr, W. 1975. *Inside the family.* San Francisco: Jossey-Bass, Inc., Publishers.

Kenkel, W. 1966. *The family in perspective.* New York: Appleton-Century-Crofts.

Mowrer, E. R. 1927. *Family disorganization: an introduction to a sociological analysis.* Chicago: The University of Chicago Press.

Murphree, A. M. 1975. Cultural influences on development. In *Comprehensive pediatric nursing,* ed. G. M. Scipien et al. New York: McGraw-Hill Book Co.

Robischon, P., and Scott, D. 1969. Role theory and its application in family nursing. *Nurs. Outlook.* 17:52.

Rodgers, R. H. 1973. *Family interaction and transaction: the developmental approach.* Englewood Cliffs, N.J.: Prentice-Hall, Inc.

Schultz, D. A. 1972. *The changing family: its function and future.* Englewood Cliffs, N.J.: Prentice-Hall, Inc.

Sobol, E. G., and Robischon, P. 1970. *Family nursing: a study guide.* St. Louis: The C. V. Mosby Co.

ADDITIONAL READINGS

Brandes, N. S. 1972. Family togetherness and other fairy tales. *Clin. Pediatr.* 115:516.

Burton, G. 1975. Families in crisis: knowing when and how to help. *Nursing 75.* 5:36.

Clark, A. L. 1966. The beginning family. *Am. J. Nurs.* 66:802.

Eiduson, B. T., et al. Oct. 1973. Alternatives in childrearing in the 1970s. *Am. J. Orthopsychiatry.* 43:720.

Folta, J., and Deck, E., eds. 1966. *A sociological framework for patient care.* New York: John Wiley & Sons, Inc.

Heiss, J., ed. 1968. *Family roles and interactions: an anthology.* Chicago: Rand McNally & Company.

Klein, C. 1972. *The single parent experience.* New York: Walker & Company.

Rising problems of "single parents." July 16, 1973. *U.S. News and World Report,* pp. 32–35.

Storlie, F. 1976. The family: thirteen years of observation. *Super. Nurse.* 7:10.

Thamm, R. 1975. *Beyond marriage and the nuclear family.* San Francisco: Canfield Press.

Turner, R. H. 1970. *Family interaction.* New York: John Wiley & Sons, Inc.

UNIT II

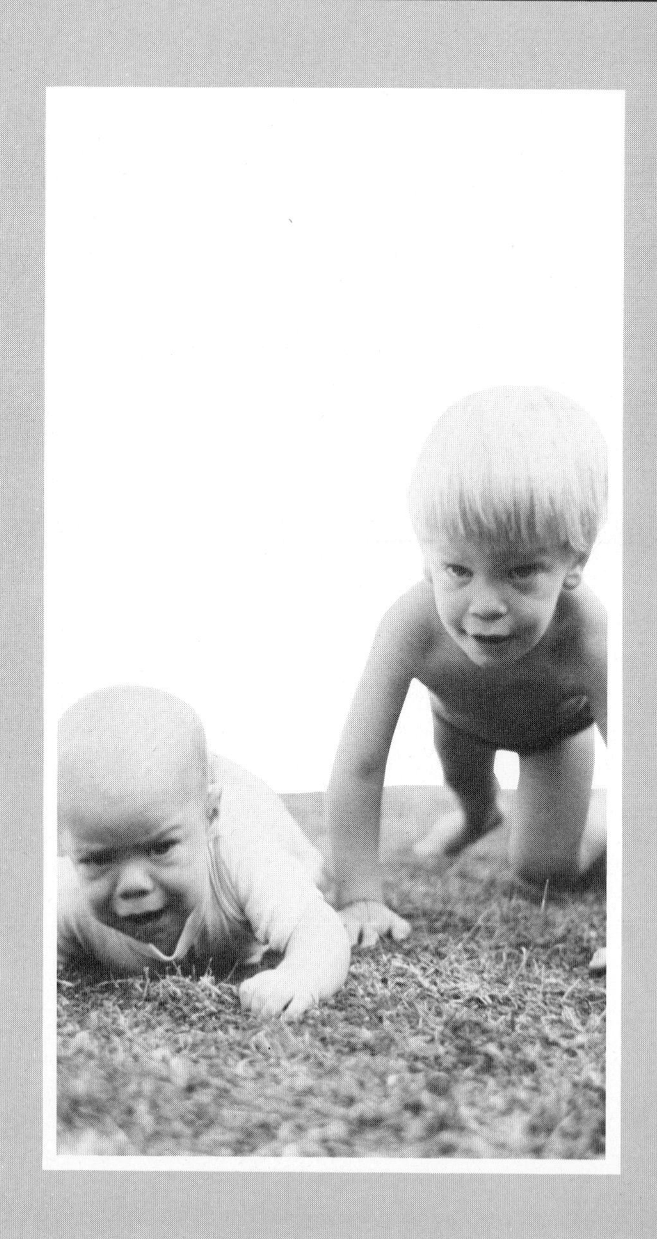

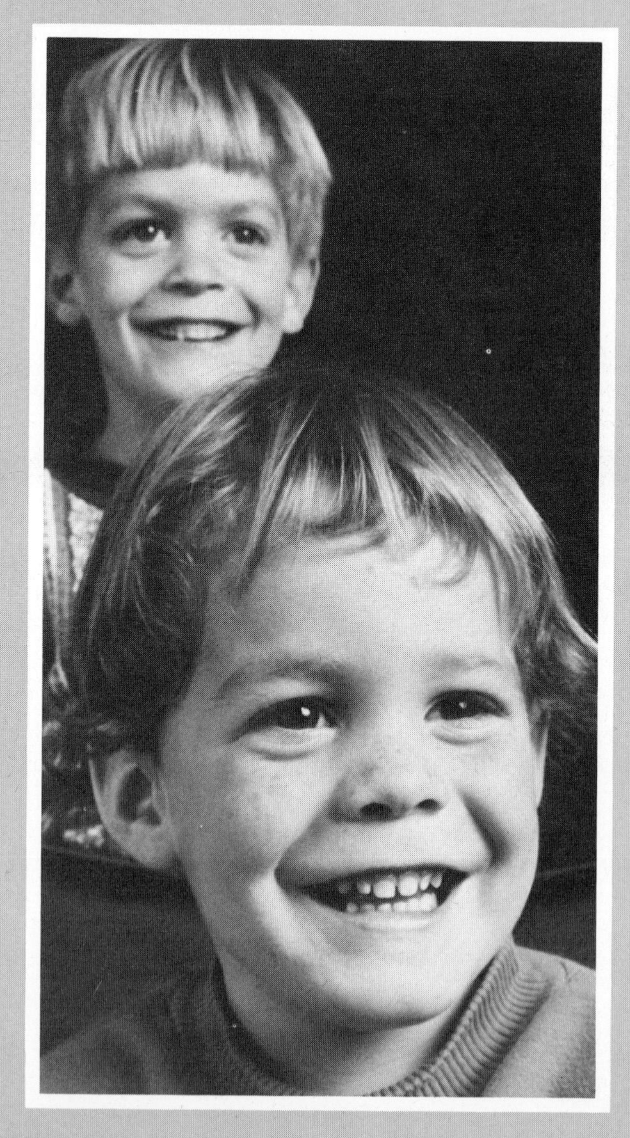

HUMAN REPRODUCTION AND DEVELOPMENT

CHAPTER 4

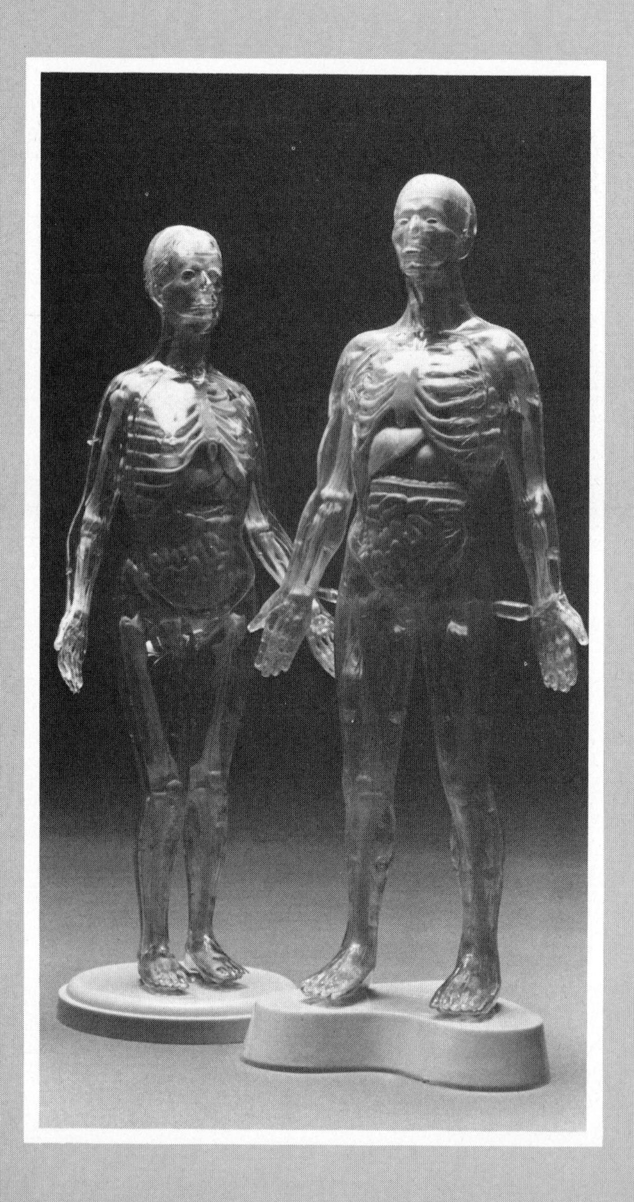

HUMAN REPRODUCTIVE SYSTEM

FEMALE REPRODUCTIVE SYSTEM

- **Bony Pelvis**
- **External Genitals**
- **Internal Genitals**
- **Breasts**

OBJECTIVES

- Relate information about the embryologic development of the human reproductive system to reproductive functions.
- Review the anatomy and physiology of the male and female reproductive systems.
- Correlate anatomic and physiologic information with pathology and obstetric nursing care.

Any logical account of prenatal development must start with a consideration of the phenomena that initiate it. Understanding life before birth requires more than knowledge of the structure of the conjugating sex cells. One needs information about germ cell production and the extraordinary provisions that ensure the union of egg and sperm in a given place and at such a time that each is capable of discharging its function. One also needs an understanding of the changes in the mother's body that provide for the embryo's nutrition during its intrauterine existence and for breast-feeding after birth. But before proceeding to these matters, it is necessary for one to become familiar with the embryologic development and main structural features of the male and female reproductive organs.

EMBRYOLOGIC DEVELOPMENT OF THE REPRODUCTIVE SYSTEM

Knowledge of the embryologic development of the human reproduction system greatly facilitates understanding of the correlations among anatomy, physiology, and function. This section provides a brief overview of the development of the internal and external genitals. Chapter 6 contains a more complete discussion of fetal development.

The male and female reproductive organs are homologous; that is, they are fundamentally similar in structure and function. The genetic sex of the embryo is determined at fertilization (Chapter 6). However, the developing fetus exhibits no sexual differentiation until the eighth week. This early period is known as the *indifferent stage*.

Ovaries and Testes

A *gonad* is an organ that produces sex cells. The female gonad is the ovary, which produces ova; the male counterpart is the testis, which produces sperm. During the fifth week of gestation, a primitive gonad arises from the medial aspect of the urogenital ridge. The gonads develop a medulla and cortex as primary sex cords appear in the underlying mesenchyme. In genetic males, during the seventh and eighth week the medulla develops into a testis, and the cortex regresses. In genetic females, the cortex develops into an ovary, recognizable about the tenth week, and the medulla regresses. All primordial follicles, which contain the primitive ovarian eggs (oogonia), are formed during prenatal life.

Figure 4–1 illustrates the embryologic development of the gonads and other internal reproductive organs.

Other Internal Genitals

During the indifferent period, two pairs of genital ducts develop: the *mesonephric* and *paramesonephric* ducts. These ducts are complete at the seventh week. The paramesonephric ducts meet in midline to form the Y-shaped uterovaginal primordium. At its dorsal end is the urogenital tubercle or sinus. In genetic males, the fetal testes secrete two hormones: testosterone stimulates the mesonephric ducts to develop into the male genital tract, and the other hormone (müllerian regression factor) suppresses development of the paramesonephric ducts, which would otherwise develop into the female genital tract.

With further differentiation of the mesonephric ducts comes development of the efferent ductules, ductus deferens, epididymides, seminal vesicles, and ejaculatory ducts. Both the prostate and the bulbourethral glands develop from endodermal outgrowths of the urethra (see Figure 4–1).

In genetic females, the paramesonephric ducts develop and the mesonephric ducts regress. The uterine tubes are formed from the unfused portions of the ducts, and the fused portions give rise to the epithelium and uterine glands. The endometrial stroma and the myometrium develop from the adjacent mesenchyme.

The vagina is derived from more than one embryologic structure. The vaginal epithelium develops from the endoderm of the urogenital sinus, and the musculature, from the uterovaginal primordium.

The urethral and paraurethral glands develop from outgrowths of the urethra into the surrounding mesenchyme. Bartholin's glands arise from similar structures.

External Genitals

In the fourth week a genital tubercle develops ventrally to the cloacal membrane. On each side of the cloacal membrane, labioscrotal swellings

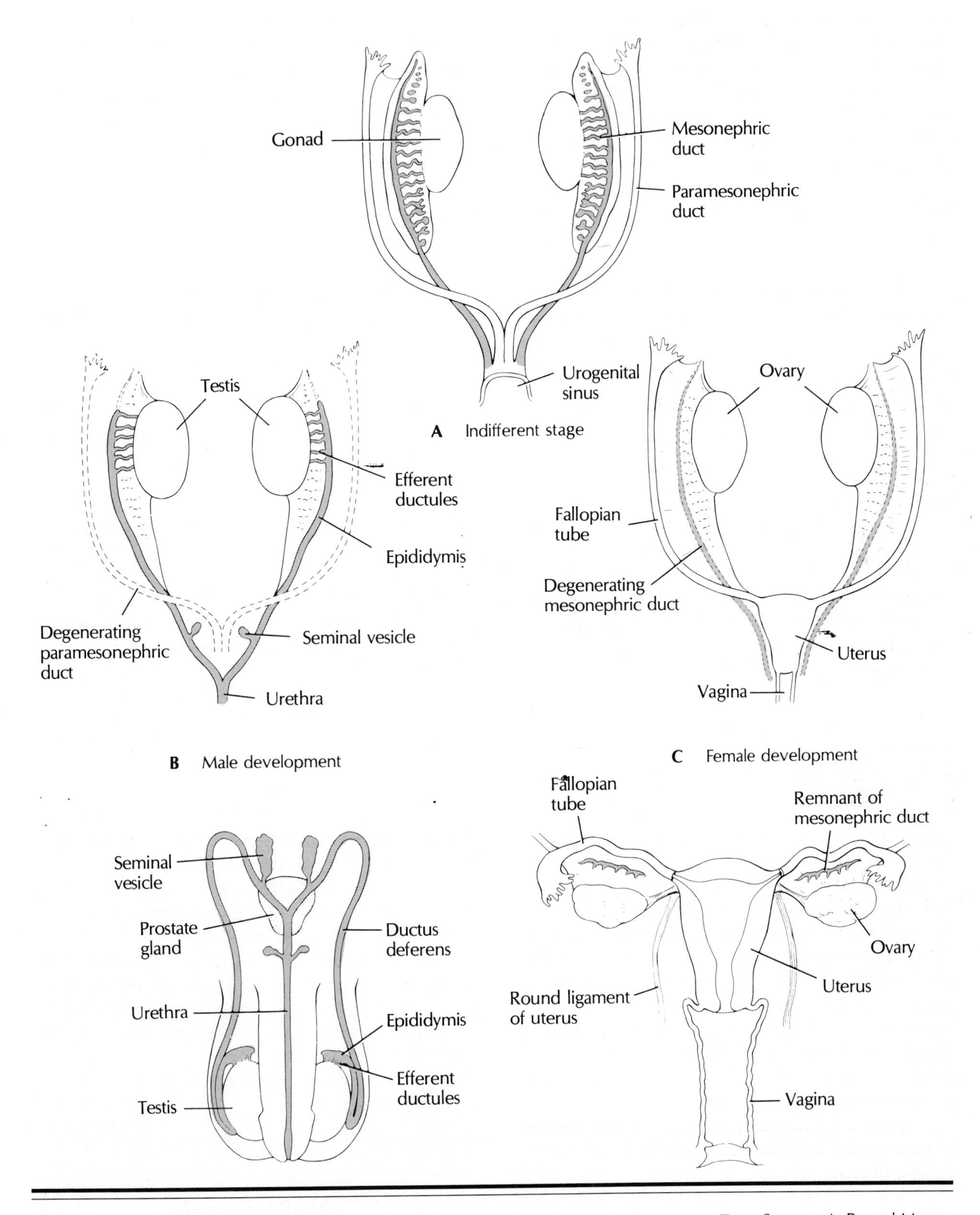

Figure 4–1. Embryologic differentiation of male and female internal reproductive organs. (From Spence, A. P., and Mason, E. B. 1979. *Human anatomy and physiology.* Menlo Park, Calif.: Benjamin/Cummings Publishing Co., p. 756.)

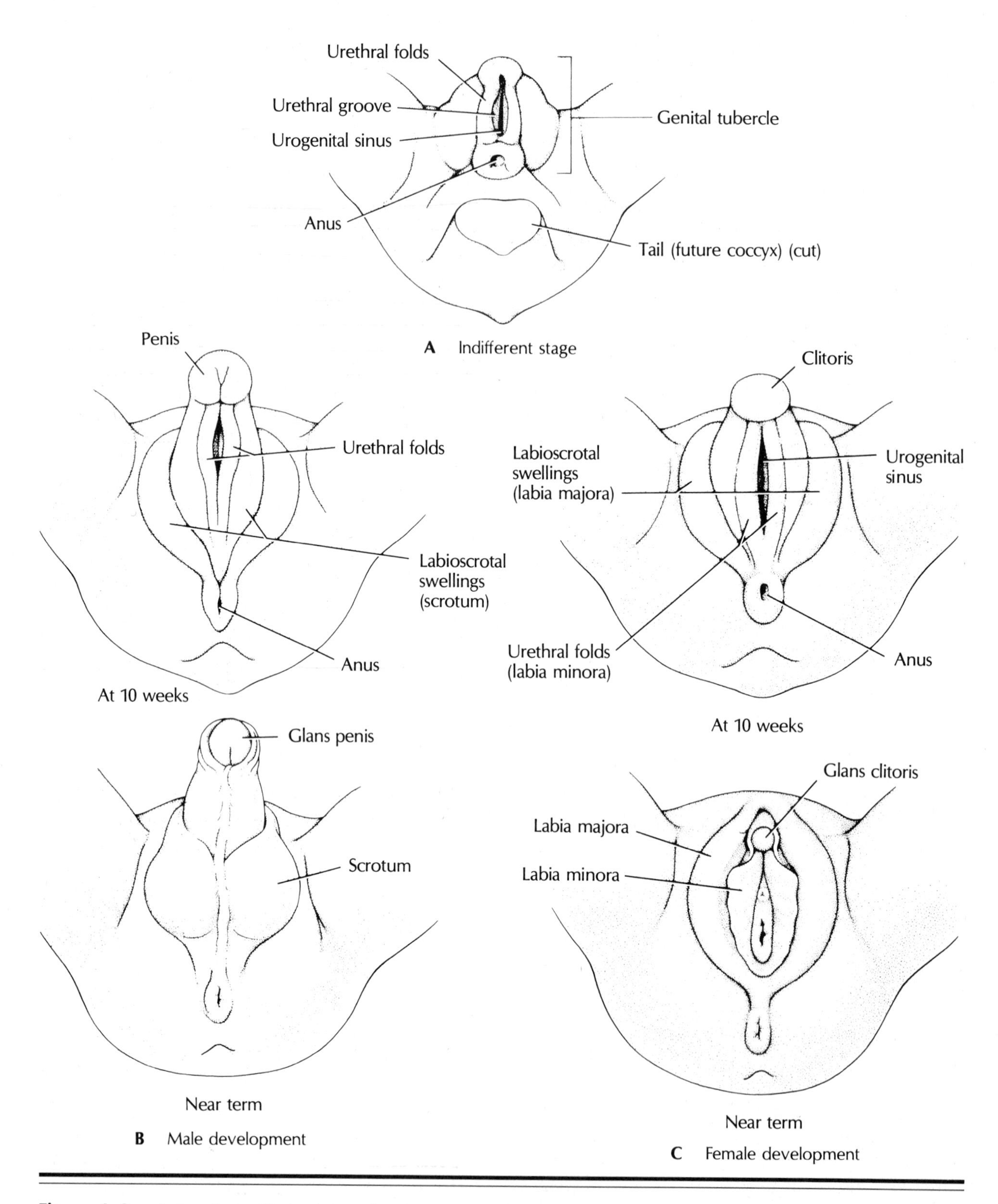

Figure 4–2. Embryologic differentiation of male and female external genitals. (From Spence, A. P., and Mason, E. B. 1979. *Human anatomy and physiology.* Menlo Park, Calif.: Benjamin/Cummings Publishing Co., p. 758.)

and urogenital folds develop. The genital tubercle lengthens and is called a *phallus* in both males and females. On the ventral side of the phallus, a urethral groove develops. Genetic males and fe-

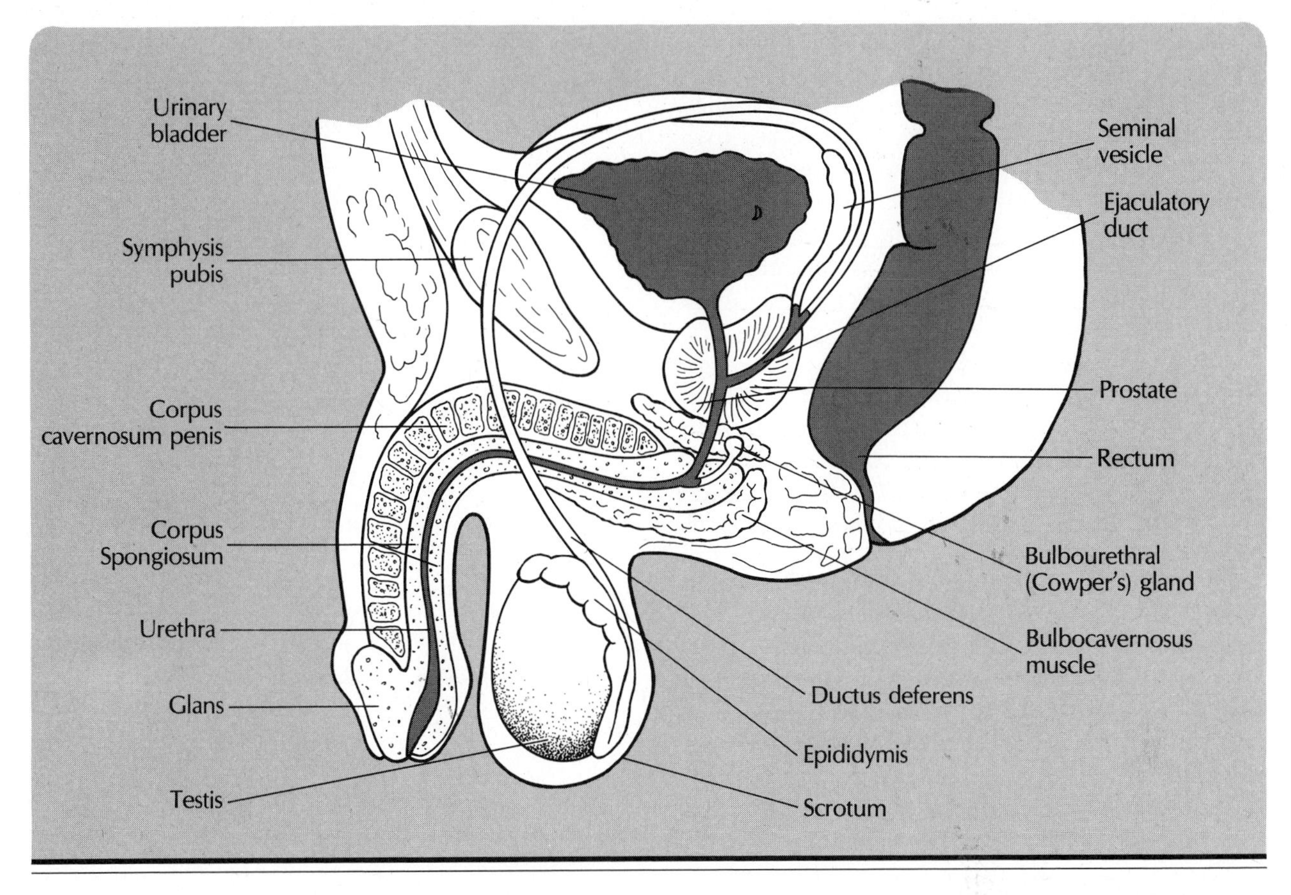

Figure 4–3. Male reproductive system.

males possess the same external genitals until the end of the ninth week. By the twelfth week, differentiation of the external genitals is complete (Figure 4–2).

Under the influence of the fetal testes' production of testosterone, the indifferent external genitals become masculine. The phallus elongates, forming the penis. The fusion of the urogenital folds on the ventral surface of the penis forms the penile urethra, with the urethral meatus moving forward toward the glans penis.

In the absence of fetal testosterone, feminization of the indifferent external genitals occurs. The phallus becomes the clitoris, and the urogenital folds remain open, forming the labia minora. The labioscrotal folds form the labia majora (Figure 4–2).

MALE REPRODUCTIVE SYSTEM

Andrology is the study of the male reproductive organs. To date, the male organs have not been studied to the same depth as their female counterparts. As appropriate techniques become available for clinical study and research, the role of males in such areas as infertility, contraception, congenital anomalies, and reproduction in general will be made more clear (Hafez, 1976).

The male reproductive system consists of the external and internal genitals (Figure 4–3). Because the breasts seem related to the purely sexual aspects of the reproductive system, they will be considered as accessory organs.

External Genitals

The two external reproductive organs are the penis and the scrotum.

Penis

The *penis,* or copulatory organ, is an elongated, pendant structure consisting of a body, termed the *shaft*, and the *glans* (Figure 4-4). It is attached to the front and sides of the pubic arch and lies anterior to the scrotum.

The shaft of the penis is made up of three longitudinal columns of erectile tissue: the paired *corpora cavernosa penis* and a third, the *corpus spongiosum penis*. These columns are covered by a dense fibrous connective tissue called the *tunica albuginea* and then enclosed by an elastic areolar tissue, the *fascia penis*. The penis is covered by an outer layer of skin with a very thin epithelium continuous with that covering the pubic region anteriorly, the perineum laterally, and the scrotum posteriorly.

The paired corpora cavernosa penis are side by side on the dorsal surface of the organ. The third column, the corpus spongiosum penis (also known as the corpus cavernosum urethra), lies ventral to the others, contains the urethra, and extends beyond the corpora cavernosa to become the glans at the distal end of the penis. The urethra widens within the glans to form the *fossa navicularis* and terminates in a slitlike orifice, located in the tip of the glans, called the *urethral meatus*. A circular fold of skin arises just behind the glans and covers it. Known as the *prepuce*, or foreskin, it is frequently removed by the surgical procedure of circumcision (Chapter 23). If the corpus spongiosum does not surround the urethra completely, the urethral meatus may occur on the ventral aspect of the penile shaft (hypospadias) or on the dorsal aspect (epispadias).

At the proximal end of the penis, the paired corpora cavernosa penis diverge into two tapering processes known as the *crura*, which are attached to the rami of the ischium and pubic bones by the ischiocavernous muscle. The corpus spongiosum penis is fixed to the inferior urogenital diaphragm. At its point of attachment it expands into a circular structure, the *bulb*, which surrounds the initial portion of the penile urethra. In turn, the bulb is surrounded by the bulbocavernous muscle.

The suspensory ligament is the main attachment and support for the penis. It extends from the symphysis pubis and merges with the deep fascia of the penis. Additional support is given by the urethra, the muscles around the crura, and the bulb.

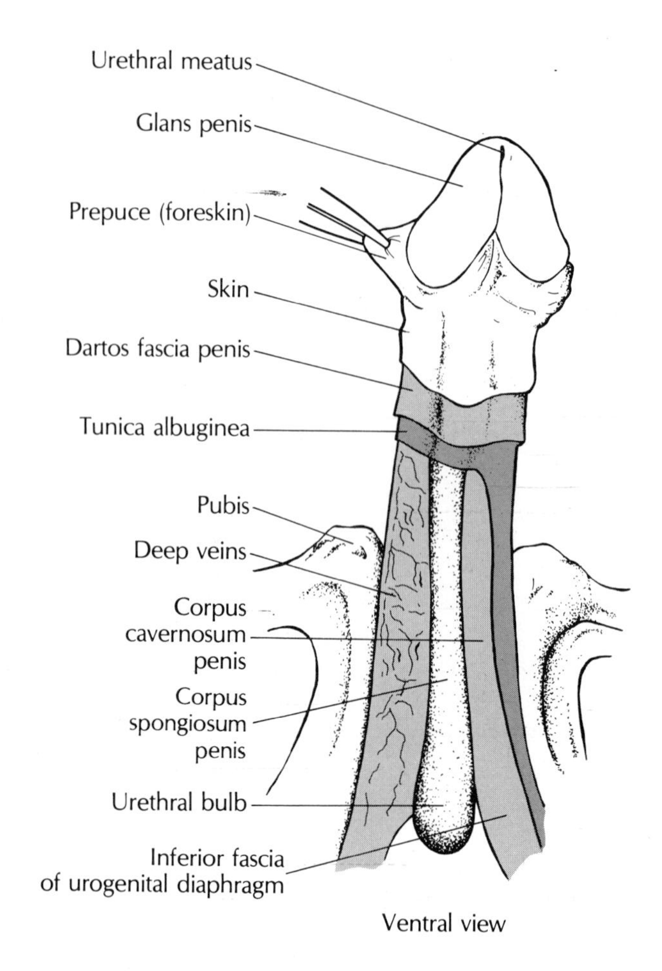

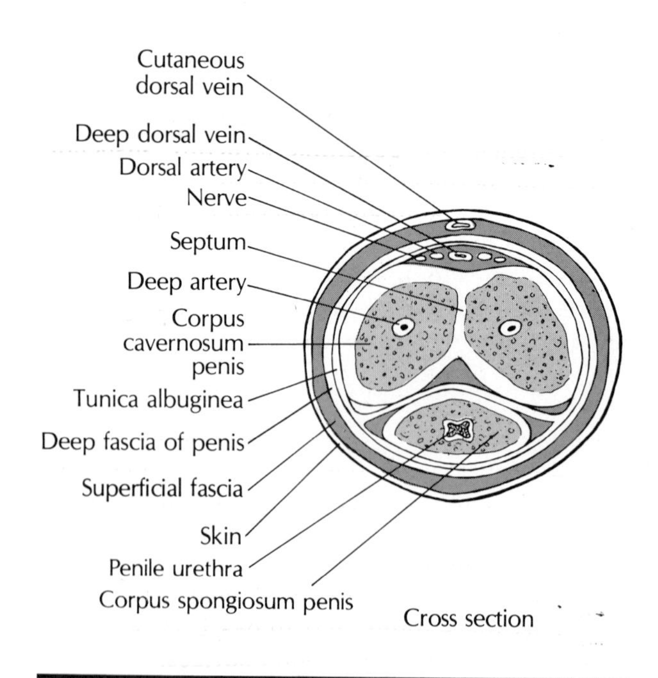

Figure 4-4. Anatomy of the penis.

The blood supply to the penis is a parallel system of internal and external pudendal arteries and veins. Blood to the cavernous sinuses is provided by two branches of the penile artery.

The penile substance is supplied by the dorsal nerve of the penis from the pudendal nerve. Sympathetic fibers come from the hypogastric and pelvic plexuses, while parasympathetic fibers from the third and fourth sacral nerves form the splanchnic nerves. When the parasympathetic fibers are stimulated, the penis becomes erect because the contraction of the ischiocavernous muscle prevents the return of venous blood from the cavernous sinuses, resulting in engorgement of the blood vessels.

The penis serves both the urinary and reproductive systems. Urine is expelled through the urethral meatus. However, the primary function of the penis is the depositing of sperm in the female vagina during sexual intercourse to provide for fertilization of the ovum.

As the procreative functions of men and women have become minimized, the penis has assumed increasing importance as provider of sexual pleasure. To many men, the penis is a symbol of virility and masculinity, and its loss or altered function results in a lessening of their self-esteem.

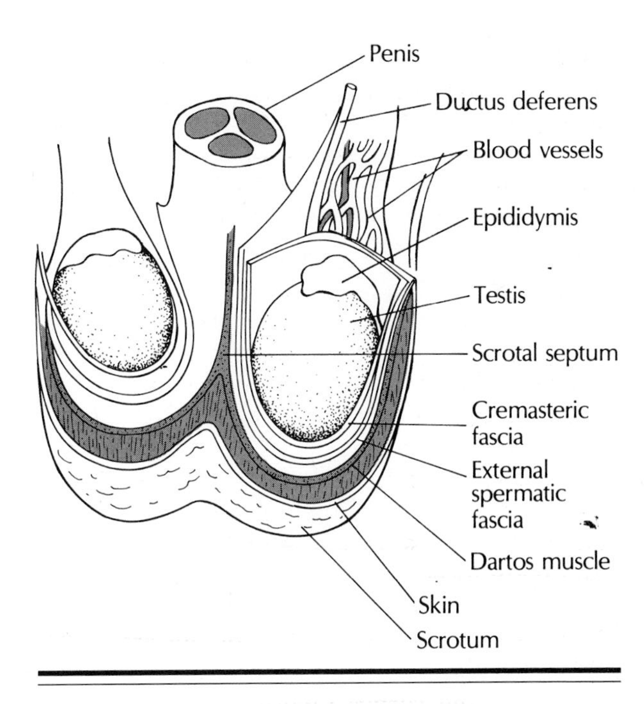

Figure 4–5. Anatomy of the scrotum.

Scrotum

The *scrotum* is a pouchlike structure suspended from the perineal region (Figure 4–5). It hangs anterior to the anus and posterior to the penis and may extend below it. Composed of skin and the *dartos*, which contains fascial connective tissue with smooth muscle fibers, the scrotum shows increased pigmentation and scattered hairs. The sebaceous glands open directly onto the scrotal surface; their secretion has a distinctive odor. Because of the rugae caused by the dartos and the cremasteric muscle, the scrotum appears rough and wrinkled. The degree of wrinkling is greatest in young men and at cold temperatures and is least in older men and at warm temperatures. Contraction of the dartos and cremasteric muscles shortens the scrotum and draws it closer to the body, thus wrinkling its outer surface.

Inside the scrotum are two lateral compartments separated by a medial septum derived from the dartos muscle. In each compartment is a testis with its related structures. Because the left spermatic cord grows longer during embryologic development, the left testis and its scrotal sac hang lower than the right. A ridge (raphe) on the external scrotal surface marks the position of the medial septum. This raphe continues anteriorly on the urethral surface of the penis but disappears in the perineal area.

Scrotal innervation is concentrated and is derived from the genitofemoral, pudendal, posterior femoral cutaneous, and ilioinguinal nerves and the hypogastric plexus.

The function of the scrotum is to protect the testes and the sperm by maintaining a temperature lower than that of the body. Spermatogenesis will not occur if the testes fail to descend, thus remaining at body temperature. By being sensitive to touch, pressure, temperature, and pain, the scrotum serves as a defense against potential harm to the testes. Innervation of the anterior third of the scrotum is supplied mainly from the first lumbar segment of the spinal cord, whereas the posterior two-thirds are supplied mainly from the third sacral segment. Thus spinal anesthetic agents must be injected much higher up to anesthetize the anterior rather than the posterior portion of the scrotum.

Internal Genitals

The male internal reproductive organs include the gonads (testes or testicles), a system of ducts (epididymis, ductus deferens, ejaculatory duct, and urethra), and accessory glands (seminal vesicles, prostate gland, bulbourethral glands, and urethral glands).

Testes

The *testes* are a pair of bilateral, oval, compound glandular organs contained in the scrotum (Figure 4-6). The testes are abdominal organs, whereas the penis is a pelvic organ. Each testis is 4–6 cm long, 2–3 cm wide, and 3–4 cm deep and weighs about 10–15 gm. It is covered by a serous membrane known as the *tunica vaginalis.* Under this membrane is the *tunica albuginea,* which is a tough, white, fibrous capsule covering each testis. The tunica albuginea sends projections inward to form septa, thereby dividing the testis into 250 to 400 lobules. Each lobule contains one to three tightly packed, convoluted seminiferous tubules containing sperm cells in all stages of development, arranged in layers. The seminiferous tubules are surrounded by loose connective tissue, which houses abundant blood and lymph vessels and the Leydig's (interstitial) cells, producers of testosterone.

The connective tissue septa extend from the tunica albuginea to the posteriorly positioned mediastinum. In this area a system of collecting ducts begins, with smaller ducts forming larger ducts, which in turn form even larger ducts. The multitudinous seminiferous tubules come together to form the 20 or 30 straight tubules, or tubuli recti, which in turn form an anastomosing network of thin-walled spaces, the *rete testis.* At the upper border of the mediastinum, the rete testis forms 10 to 15 efferent ducts that perforate the tunica albuginea and empty into the duct of the epididymis. Prior to this, the efferent ducts enlarge and become convoluted.

Most of the cells lining the seminiferous tubules undergo a process of maturation called *spermatogenesis.* The successive stages of differentiation of these cells are: spermatogonia, primary spermatocytes, secondary spermatocytes, spermatids, and spermatozoa. (See Chapter 6 for further discussion of spermatogenesis.) These cells are located between the basement membrane and the lumen of the tubule, with the most immature cells on the basal membrane. Sperm production varies among and within the tubules, with cells in different areas of the same tubule undergoing different stages of spermatogenesis.

After the onset of puberty, spermatogenesis occurs continually to provide the large numbers of sperm necessary for unlimited ejaculations over the mature life span. Estimates of the time required for the complete process range from two to ten weeks. Spermatogenesis is primarily under the control of the central nervous system. The process is complex. Briefly, afferent impulses are integrated in the hypothalamus, which in turn secretes releasing factors. These stimulate the anterior pituitary to release the gonadotropins, hormonal substances that stimulate the activity of the gonads (see Chapter 5 for further discussion of hormonal activity and the reproductive system). These hormones in turn cause the testes to produce testosterone, which maintains spermatogenesis, increases sperm production by the tubules, and stimulates production of seminal plasma. The mature sperm is discussed on p. 135.

The seminiferous tubules also contain Sertoli's cells, which provide nutrients and protection for the germ cells. Sertoli's cells undergo specific cyclic changes with each generation of spermatozoa, beginning with the spermatogonia and ending as the mature sperm are released into the lumen.

The blood supply of the testes originates at the kidney level. Each testis is supplied by the internal spermatic artery, which branches from the dorsal aorta near the kidney. The spermatic veins lead from the testes, the right entering the vena cava, the left entering the left renal view. Both artery and vein pass through the inguinal canal and reach the testis by way of the spermatic cord.

Lymphatic vessels are prolific in the interstitial tissue and drain with those of the epididymis into those in the spermatic cord. They eventually empty into the lumbar nodes near the kidney or into those surrounding the aorta.

The testes are supplied with parasympathetic fibers from the vagus nerve and with sympathetic fibers from the tenth thoracic spinal cord segment via the testicular plexus. Visceral afferent fibers transmit impulses to the central nervous system.

In summary, the testes are the site of spermatogenesis and the production of testosterone. The

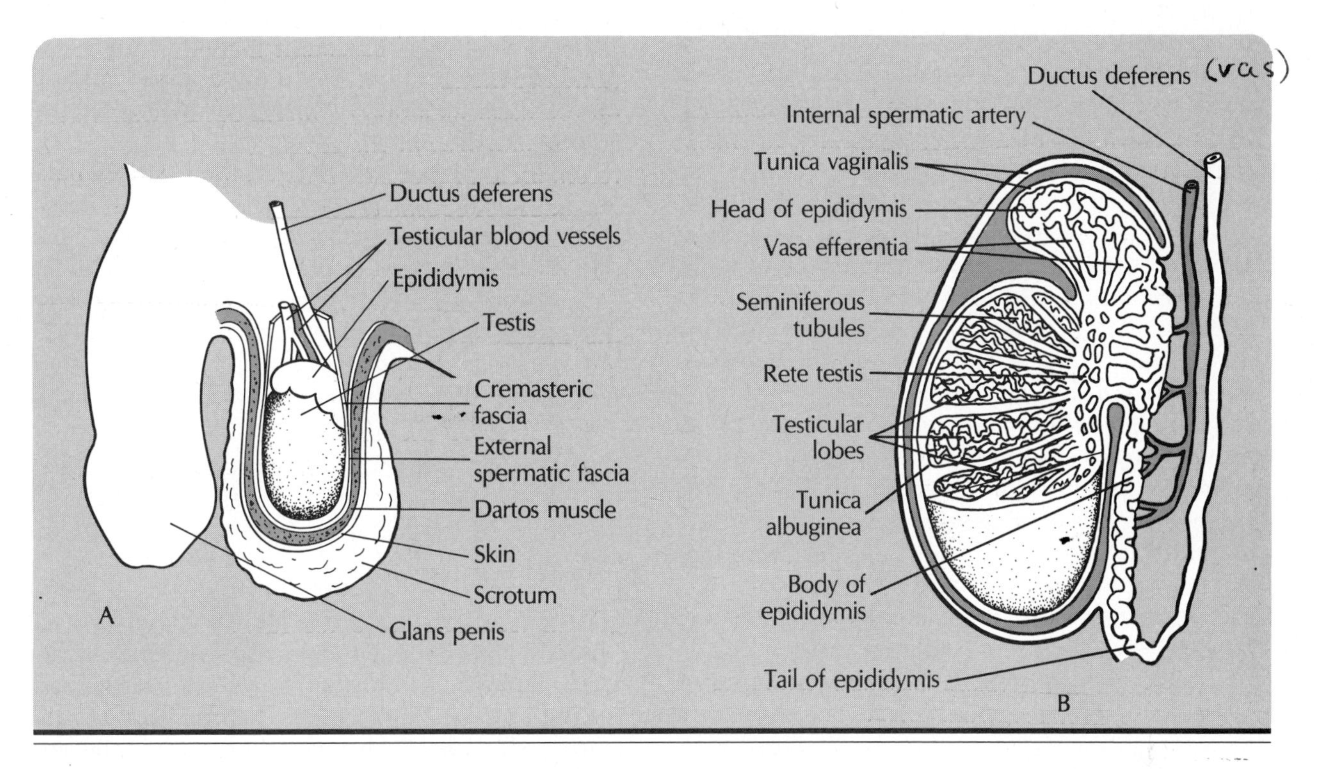

Figure 4–6. The testes. **A,** External view. **B,** Sagittal section showing internal anatomy.

spermatozoa that are released from the testes must undergo a process of maturation in the duct system before ejaculation.

Epididymides

As the initial part of the excretory duct system of the testis, an *epididymis* lies posterior to each testis (Figure 4–6). Consisting of a head, body, and tail, the epididymis is about 5.6 meters long, although it is convoluted into a compact structure about 3.75 cm long. The head sits on top of the superior aspect of the testis, firmly attached to it by the efferent ductules. The body, made up of the tightly coiled portion, descends posteriorly along the testis. The tail narrows slightly, becomes less convoluted with a wider lumen, and turns back on itself to become the ductus deferens (discussed in the next section).

The tail of the epididymis provides a reservoir where spermatozoa can survive for a long period of time. The secretory epithelium of the epididymis provides a nutritional fluid for the maturing sperm. When discharged from the seminiferous tubules into the epididymis, the sperm are immotile and incapable of fertilizing an ovum. The spermatozoa remain in the epididymis for two to ten days, until the process of maturation is complete.

Ductus Deferens (vas deferens)

The *ductus deferens,* also known as the *vas deferens,* is about 40 cm long and connects the epididymal lumen with the prostatic urethra. There is one ductus deferens ascending the posterior border of each testis (Figure 4–6). It joins the spermatic cord, passing through the inguinal canal and entering the abdominal cavity. The ductus deferens passes over the bladder, and between the ureter and the posterior surface of the bladder, then bends medially along the seminal vesicle until it meets the ductus deferens from the opposite side. Turning downward to the base of the prostate gland, it forms the ejaculatory duct as it joins the duct from the seminal vesicle. Prior to its entrance into the prostate, the ductus deferens becomes enlarged and tortuous. This enlargement is called the *terminal ampulla* and serves as the primary storehouse for spermatozoa and tubule secretions.

The ductus deferens can be divided into five portions: the sheathless epididymal portion within the tunica vaginalis; the scrotal portion; the inguinal portion; the retroperitoneal or pelvic portion; and the ampulla. The scrotal portion is usually the surgical site of a vasectomy, the male sterilization procedure.

The three layers of smooth muscle that make up the ductus deferens are the middle circular and the outer and inner longitudinal layers. The duct is capable of vigorous peristaltic motion. The ductal lumen is lined with epithelium lying on a basement membrane. Thick connective tissue surrounds the muscle layers.

Stored sperm remain relatively immotile, although mature. No doubt this is because of the metabolic production of carbon dioxide by the sperm, creating an acidic environment that inhibits motility. Also, the ductus deferens secretions do not provide high-energy nutrients (which can be metabolized into lactic acid) (Odell and Moyer, 1971).

Innervation is through the hypogastric plexus of the autonomic nervous system. There are pain receptors in the sheath of the vas deferens in the scrotal portion.

The spermatic cord is made up of the ductus deferens and the pampiniform plexus of veins, arteries, lymphatic vessels, and nerves. Held together by connective tissue, this cord extends from the tail of the epididymis to the abdominal inguinal ring and is enclosed by the cremaster muscle and layers of fascia issuing from the abdominal wall.

Ejaculatory Ducts

The ductus deferens and a seminal vesicle duct unite to form the *ejaculatory duct*. Each of the two ejaculatory ducts enters the posterior surface of the prostate gland. After a distance of about 2.5 cm, they terminate in the prostatic urethra. These ducts serve as passageways for semen and for fluid secreted by the seminal vesicles.

Urethra

The male urethra is a common passageway for urine and semen. The epithelium tissue throughout the urethra is specific to the urethral section.

The urethra begins a little posterior to the midpoint of the inferior aspect of the bladder and courses through the prostate gland, where it is called the *prostatic urethra*. The surrounding connective tissue is highly vascular and contains glands, elastic fibers, and smooth muscles arranged in an inner longitudinal layer and an outer circular layer. These circular fibers form the internal urethral sphincter.

The urethra emerges from the prostate gland to become the *membranous urethra*. As it passes through the urogenital diaphragm, skeletal muscle fibers form the external urethral sphincter.

The *spongy urethra* is contained in the corpus spongiosum penis. In the penile urethra, discussed on p. 71, goblet secretory cells are present, and smooth muscle is replaced by erectile tissue.

Accessory Glands

Seminal Vesicles

The *seminal vesicles* are two lobulated glands, each about 7.5 cm long, situated between the bladder and rectum and immediately superior to the base of the prostate. A fold of peritoneum forming the rectovesical pouch separates them from the rectum, and nerves are supplied from the hypogastric plexus. Secretory columnar epithelium lines the diverticula of the seminal vesicles and secretes an alkaline, viscid, clear fluid rich in high-energy fructose and proteins that becomes mixed with the sperm during ejaculation. This fluid assists in providing an environment favorable to optimal sperm motility and metabolism.

Prostate Gland

The *prostate gland* surrounds the upper part of the urethra and lies inferior to the neck of the urinary bladder and superior to the fascia of the urogenital diaphragm. Made up of several lobes, it measures about 4 cm in diameter and weighs 20–30 gm. A dense capsule of muscle fibers encloses this gland, which is made up of both glandular and muscular tissue.

The two ejaculatory ducts are located between the middle and lateral lobes of the prostate gland and join the prostatic urethra.

Prostatic glandular tissue consists of 30 to 50 branched tubular glands with ducts opening into the prostatic urethra. There are mucosal, submucosal, and external (main) glands. The mucosal glands are the smallest and frequently hypertrophy in older men, causing urinary distress because of pressure on the prostatic urethra. The submucosal glands circle the mucosal glands, and the external glands form the major portion of the prostate.

The prostate secretes a thin, milky, slightly acidic fluid (pH 6.5) containing high levels of zinc, calcium, citric acid, and acid phosphatase. The daily secretion averages 4-6 ml. This fluid protects the sperm from the acidic environment of the female vagina and male urethra (Polakoski et al., 1976). The enzyme fibrinolysin, capable of dissolving fibrin, is also present. Unlike the seminal vesicle ejaculate, the prostate fluid does not contain fructose (Eliasson and Lindholmer, 1976).

Bulbourethral and Urethral Glands

The *bulbourethral* or *Cowper's glands* are a pair of small round lobulated structures within the urogenital diaphragm on either side of the membranous urethra. Each gland, about 1 cm in diameter, has a terminal excretory duct, about 2.5 cm long, opening into the base of the corpus spongiosum penis. These glands secrete a clear, viscous, alkaline fluid rich in mucoproteins that becomes part of the seminal plasma. It is thought that this secretion also lubricates the penile urethra during sexual excitement as well as neutralizing the acid in the male urethra and the female vagina, thereby enhancing sperm motility.

The *urethral* or *Littre's glands* are tiny mucus-secreting glands found throughout the membranous lining of the penile urethra. Their secretions add to those of the bulbourethral glands.

In summary, the male accessory glands are specialized structures under endocrine and neural control. Each secretes a unique and essential component of the total seminal plasma in an ordered sequence. The continuing study of the physiology of these ejaculates will lead to an increased understanding of male fertility and infertility and to potential methods of modifying both.

Semen

The male ejaculate *semen* is made up of spermatozoa and seminal plasma, which is composed of the secretions of the accessory sex glands in a specific pattern. The bulbourethral and urethral glands, prostate, epididymides, and seminal vesicles contribute components to the seminal plasma, which serves to transport viable and motile sperm to the female reproductive tract. Effective transportation of sperm requires adequate nutrients, a pH of 7.4, a specific concentration of sperm to fluid, and an optimal osmolarity (Polakoski et al., 1976).

Sperm may be stored in the male genital system for a period of several hours to 42 days, depending primarily on the frequency of ejaculations. Table 4-1 lists the physiologic parameters of the migration and survival of human sperm.

The average volume of ejaculate following continence for several days is 2.5-4 ml but may vary from 1-10 ml. Repeated ejaculation results in decreased volume. Sterility always results when sperm counts are less than 20 million/ml, and about half the men with sperm counts of between 20 and 40 million/ml are sterile.

Table 4-1. Physiologic Parameters of Migration and Survival of Human Spermatozoa*

Physiologic parameters	Values
Spermatozoan transport time, measured from their release by Sertoli's cells to appearance in ejaculate	
^{3}H-thymidine following irradiation	12 days
Recovery after illness	19-23 days
After castration	19-23 days
Ductular depletion after high temperature	35 days
Propagation of mucus secretion from cells by ciliary action	1-7 mm/min
Wave frequency of sperm flagellum at 32C	14-16 beats/sec
Number of spermatozoa per ejaculate	200-400 million
Period from ejaculation to semen coagulation	< 1 min
Period required for complete or partial liquefaction of coagulum	5-15 min
Velocity of sperm progression in cervical mucus during preovulatory stage	0.2-3.1 mm/min
Duration of sperm motility	
Motile sperm in vagina	0.5 day
Motile sperm in cervical mucus	2-8 days
Motile sperm in cervical mucus following artificial insemination	7 days
Motile sperm in uterus and oviduct	2-2.5 days

*Hafez, E. S. E., ed. 1976. *Human secretion and fertility regulation in men.* St. Louis: The C. V. Mosby Co., p. 114.

The chemical composition of semen is complex and still under investigation. Over 60 components have been identified. Semen tends to clot and then liquefies in about 15 minutes. This liquefaction is thought to be due to the presence of fibrinolysin.

Once deposited in the female vagina, sperm travel at about 3 mm/min through the female genital tract. Sperm transport is complex, and Table 4–2 summarizes the major physiologic phenomena associated with sperm transport in both the male and female reproductive tracts.

A spermatozoon is made up of a head and a tail that is divided into the middle piece, principal piece, and endpiece (Figure 4–7). The head's main components are the acrosome, nucleus, and nuclear vacuoles. The head carries the haploid number of chromosomes (23), and it is the part that enters the egg at fertilization (Chapter 6). The tail, or flagellum, is uniquely specialized for opti-

Table 4–2. Summary of Sequence of Events of Major Physiologic Phenomena Associated with Sperm Transport in Male and Female Reproductive Tracts*

Site	Physiologic phenomena	Mechanisms involved
Male reproductive tract	1. Sperm undergo maturation in epididymides	Neuromuscular
	2. At ejaculation, sperm released from epididymis are mixed with male accessory secretions	Metabolic
	3. Semen deposited in several ejaculatory pulsations	
Vagina	4. Semen mixed with vaginal and cervical secretions	Copulatory motor activities
Cervix	5. Sperm migrate through micelles of cervical mucus	Biophysical
	6. Abnormal sperm filtered (gross selection of sperm) through cervical canal	Biochemical
	7. Cervical crypts establish "sperm reservoir" or reject excessive sperm, causing massive reduction in sperm number	Mechanical (kinocilia of epithelium)
Uterus	8. Sperm separated from seminal plasma and transported to oviduct	Myometrial contraction
	9. Surface plasma of sperm removed	Agglutination of sperm
	10. Metabolic changes and capacitation of sperm	Leukocytes; enzymatic
	11. Acrosomal proteinase (trypsinlike enzyme) inactivated by trypsin inhibitors from seminal plasma	
Uterotubal junction	12. Quantitative selection of sperm	Mechanical
Isthmus	13. Sperm numbers reduced	
	14. Control of egg transport in oviduct	Neural
	15. Sperm plasma membrane changes (acrosome reaction); sperm capacitation	Biochemical
Ampulla	16. Sperm motility increases in oviductal fluid to permit penetration of corona radiata and zona pellucida	Mechanical; metabolic
	17. Reduction division of gametes completed	Enzymatic
	18. Acrosomal proteinase released	Biophysical
	19. Selection at egg surface (receptors?) by sperm	
Fimbriae	20. Excessive sperm lost into peritoneal cavity	Sperm motility

*From Hafez, E. S. E., ed. 1976. *Human secretion and fertility regulation in men.* St. Louis: The C. V. Mosby Co., p. 114.

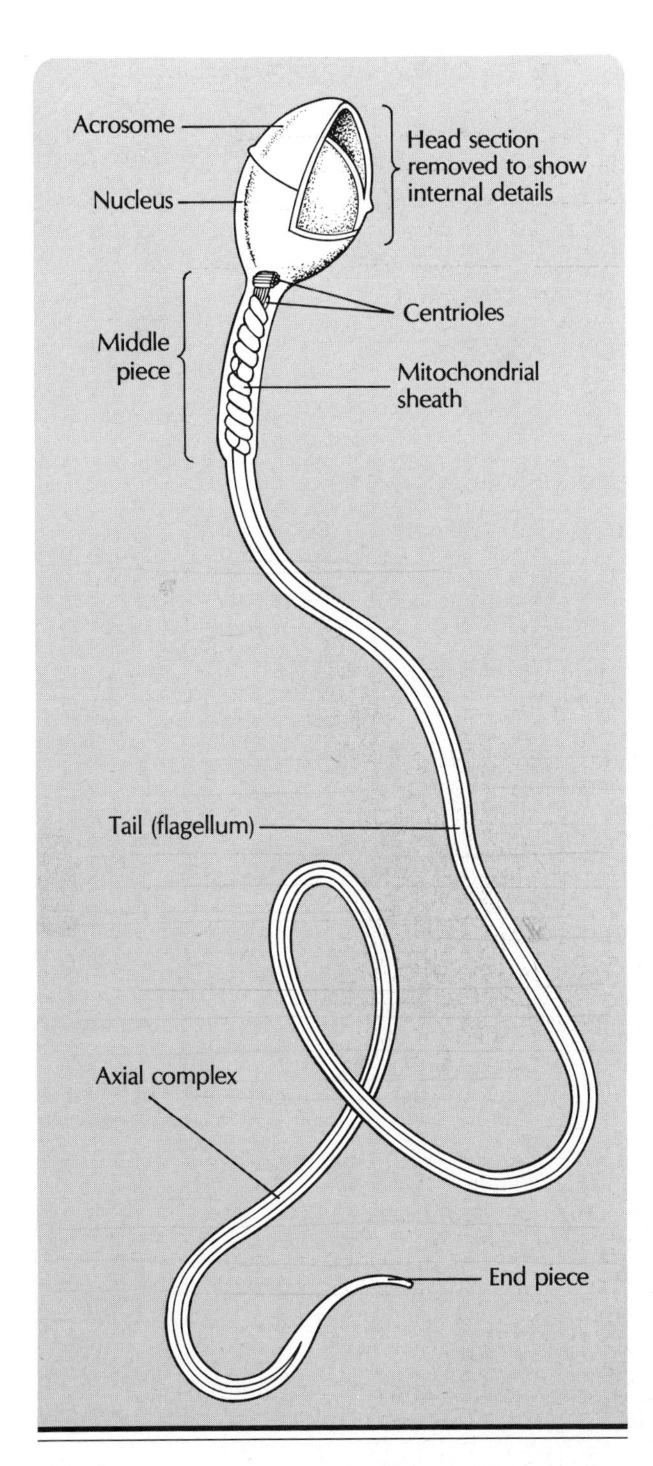

Figure 4–7. Schematic representation of mature spermatozoon.

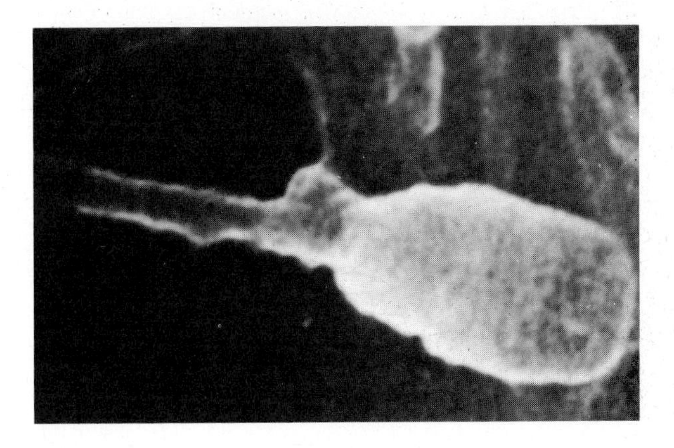

Figure 4–8. Scanning electron micrograph of human spermatozoa. (Courtesy Landrum B. Shettles.)

mal motility in each of its parts. Figure 4–8 shows a scanning electron micrograph of human spermatozoa.

Breasts

Although the male breast remains dormant throughout the life span (Donovan, 1977), it is a site of sexual arousal and pleasure for the male. Given no particular sexual connotation in American society, male breasts are bared without notice. They can provide exquisite sensation if stimulated during sexual activity. Such stimulation is frequently accompanied by spontaneous erection of the penis.

Occasionally, bilateral or unilateral gynecomastia will occur during adolescence. This hypertrophy of rudimentary mammary tissue occurs in response to increased hormonal levels and may cause embarrassment. If spontaneous remission does not occur, reduction surgery usually achieves excellent cosmetic and psychologic results (Donovan, 1977).

Less than 1% of all breast cancer in the United States occurs in men (Urban, 1977). Inspection of the breasts for dimpling, discharge, inverted nipples, or other unusual changes should be routine, and abnormalities should be investigated immediately.

FEMALE REPRODUCTIVE SYSTEM

The female reproductive system consists of the external and internal genitals and the accessory organs of the breasts, or mammary glands. Also important to the female system is the bony pelvis and its structures, which have important obstetric implications.

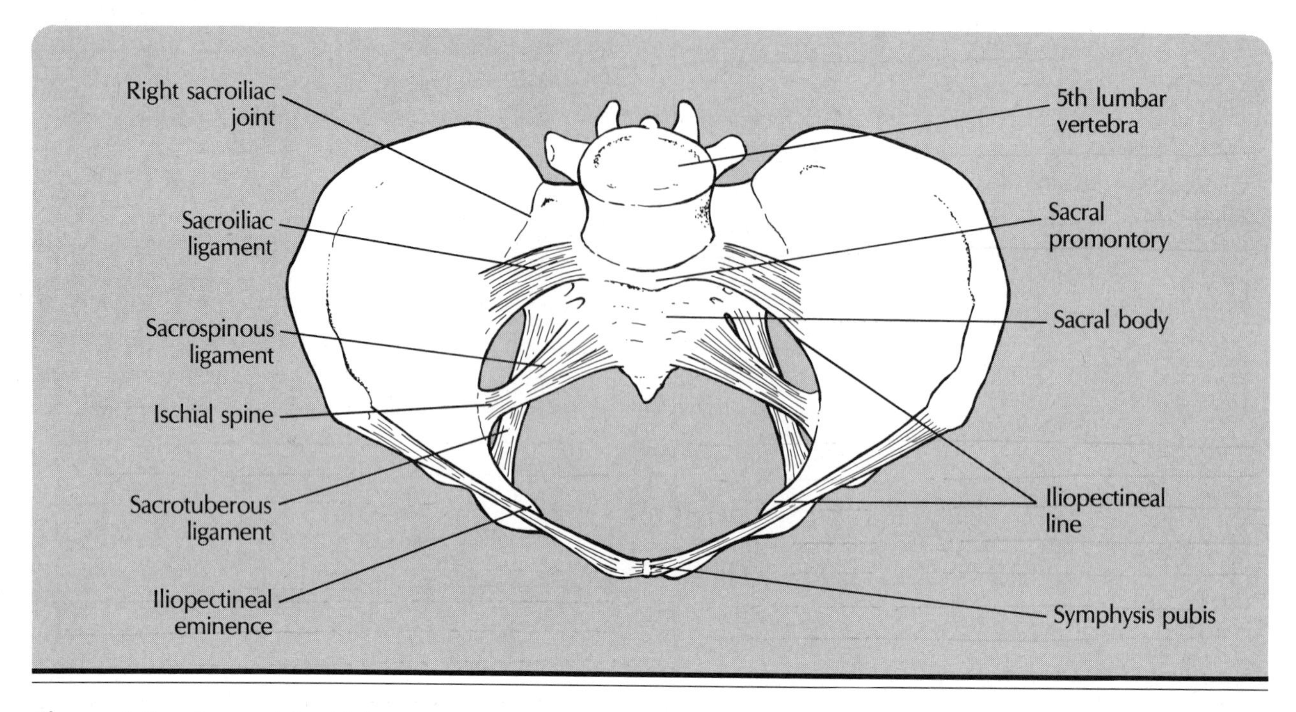

Figure 4–9. Bony pelvis with ligaments.

Bony Pelvis

In addition to supporting the weight of the upper torso and distributing it to the lower body, the female *bony pelvis* has the unique functions of supporting and protecting the pelvic contents as well as forming the relatively fixed axis of the birth passage. For these reasons, structural aspects of the pelvis important to childbearing must be understood clearly.

Bony Stucture

The pelvis, which resembles a bowl or basin, is made up of four bones: two innominate bones (os coxae), the sacrum, and the coccyx. The innominate or hip bones comprise the anterior and lateral framework, and the sacrum and coccyx provide the posterior section. Lined with fibrocartilage and held tightly together by ligaments, the four bones articulate at the symphysis pubis, the two sacroiliac joints, and the sacrococcygeal joints (Figure 4–9).

The *innominate bones* are made up of three separate bones whose junctions are calcified at puberty: the ilium, the ischium, and the pubis. The fusion of these bones forms an articular circular cavity, the *acetabulum*, which articulates with the head of the femur.

The *ilium*, which makes up a large portion of the acetabulum, is the broad upper part of the innominate bone. Its anterior prominence, palpated as the foremost angle of the innominate bone, is the anterior iliac spine. The iliac crest extends backward and is convex, thickened, and rough.

The *ischium* is the strongest bone and is inferior to the ilium and below the acetabulum. It consists of a body and a ramus. The ramus joins the inferior ramus of the pubis. At its posterior point the ischium terminates in a marked protuberance, the ischial tuberosity, upon which the weight of the body rests when in a seated position. The ischial spines arise from the posterior border of the ischium and jut into the pelvic cavity. Between the ischial spines is the shortest diameter of the pelvic cavity. The ischial spines can be palpated during rectal or vaginal examination, and they can serve as a guide during labor to evaluate the descent of the fetal head into the birth canal.

The *pubis* consists of a superior ramus, body, and inferior ramus and forms the slightly bowed anterior portion of the innominate bone. It contributes to the anteromedial one-fifth of the acetabulum. The ischial and pubic inferior rami form a large triangular aperture, the *obturator foramen*,

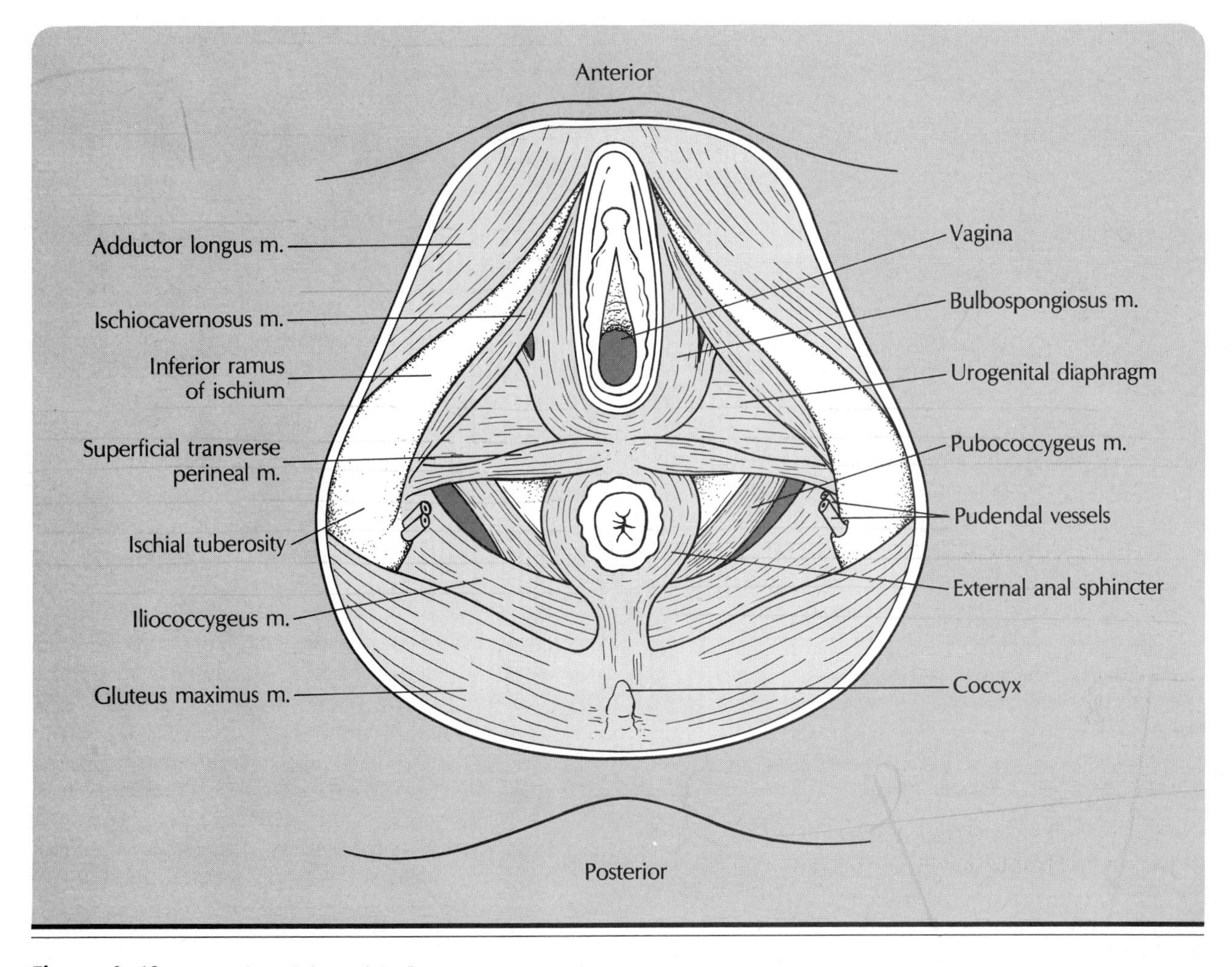

Figure 4–10. Muscles of the pelvic floor.

in the lower half of the hip bone. A strong membrane of thin fibrous tissue is attached to its boundary. The pubis extends medially from the acetabulum to the midpoint of the bony pelvis, where it forms the symphysis pubis at its junction with the other pubis. The triangular space below this junction is known as the pubic arch. The baby's head passes under this arch during birth. The symphysis pubis is formed by heavy fibrocartilage and the superior and inferior pubic ligaments, with the latter designated as the *arcuate pubic ligament*. The mobility of the arcuate pubic ligament increases during pregnancy and to a greater extent in multiparas than in primigravidas.

The sacroiliac joints also have a degree of mobility that increases at term as the result of an upward gliding movement. The pelvic outlet may be increased by 1.5–2 cm in the dorsal lithotomy position. These relaxations of the joints are induced by the hormones of pregnancy.

The *sacrum*, a wedge-shaped bone formed by the fusion of five vertebras, becomes smaller toward the inferior portion. On the anterior upper portion of the body of the first sacral vertebra is a marked projection into the pelvic cavity, known as the *sacral promontory*, that can be palpated vaginally and is another obstetric guide in determining pelvic measurements. The inner surface of the sacrum is concave in both the lateral and vertical aspects.

The *coccyx*, a small triangular bone that is the last on the vertebral column, is formed by the union of four rudimentary vertebras. Its course is downward and slightly forward from the lower sacral border, and it articulates with the sacrum at the sacrococcygeal joint. Generally, there is an intervertebral disk between the sacrum and the coccyx. In its absence, there is partial or complete fusion between the two bones, making them immovable. The coccyx usually moves backward during labor to provide the fetus with more room.

Pelvic Floor

A complementary structure of the bony pelvis is its muscular *pelvic floor,* which is designed to overcome the force of gravity exerted on the pelvic viscera and, to a lesser extent, on the abdominal viscera. It acts as a buttress to the outlet of the pelvis, thereby providing stability and support to surrounding structures and organs. Three groups of musculature and fascia make up the pelvic floor (Figure 4–10): the levator ani and coccygeal muscles, which form the pelvic diaphragm; the deep transverse perineal muscle, which forms the urogenital triangle; and the muscles of the external genitals and anus. Together they form the *perineum* (Table 4–3).

The sheetlike *levator ani muscle* makes up the major portion of the pelvic diaphragm and is comprised of three parts: the iliococcygeal, pubococcygeal, and puborectal muscles. Forming a sling for the pelvic structures, the levator ani is interrupted by the urethra, vagina, and rectum. The coccygeal muscle also contributes to the pelvic floor; it is a thin muscular sheet overlying the sacrospinous ligament and assists the levator ani in giving support to the abdominal and pelvic viscera.

The *urogenital triangle* (diaphragm) is found in the hollow of the pubic arch and is made up of superficial and deep perineal membranes extending from the rami of the ischial and pubic bones. Most important in this region are the deep transverse perineal muscles, which are flat bands of muscle arising from the ischiopubic rami and intertwining in the midline to form a seam, or raphe. These muscles are modified to encircle both the urinary meatus and the vaginal orifice, forming the urethral and vaginal sphincters.

The ischiocavernosus and bulbocavernosus are the muscles of the external genitals and form external coverings for the vestibular bulbs and crus of the clitoris. The fibers of the bulbocavernous muscle do not articulate with each other on either side of the vagina; they are separate.

Table 4–3. Muscles of the Perineum*

Muscle/Nerve†	Origin	Insertion	Action
Bulbocavernosus	Male, median raphe over bulb of penis, central tendon of perineum; female, central tendon of perineum	Male, corpus cavernosus, root of penis; female, dorsum of clitoris, urogenital diaphragm	Male, compresses bulb; female, compresses vaginal orifice
Deep transverse perineus‡	Inferior ramus of ischium	Central tendon, external anal sphincter	Fixes central tendon
External anal sphincter	Skin and fascia of anus, tip of coccyx	Central tendon of perineum	Closes anus
External urethral sphincter	Inferior ramus of ischium	Fibers interdigitate around urethra	Closes urethra
Ischiocavernosus	Ischium adjacent to crus of penis or clitoris	Crus near pubic symphysis	Maintains turgescence of penis or clitoris
Superficial transverse perineus	Ramus of ischium near tuberosity	Central tendon of perineum	Supports central tendon

*From Langley, L. L., et al. 1974. *Dynamic anatomy and physiology.* New York: McGraw-Hill Book Co.

†All are supplied by pudendal nerve, except that external anal sphincter is supplied by inferior rectal nerve.

‡In females a portion of deep transverse perineal muscle is specialized to form constrictor vaginae, which acts to compress vaginal orifice and greater vestibular glands.

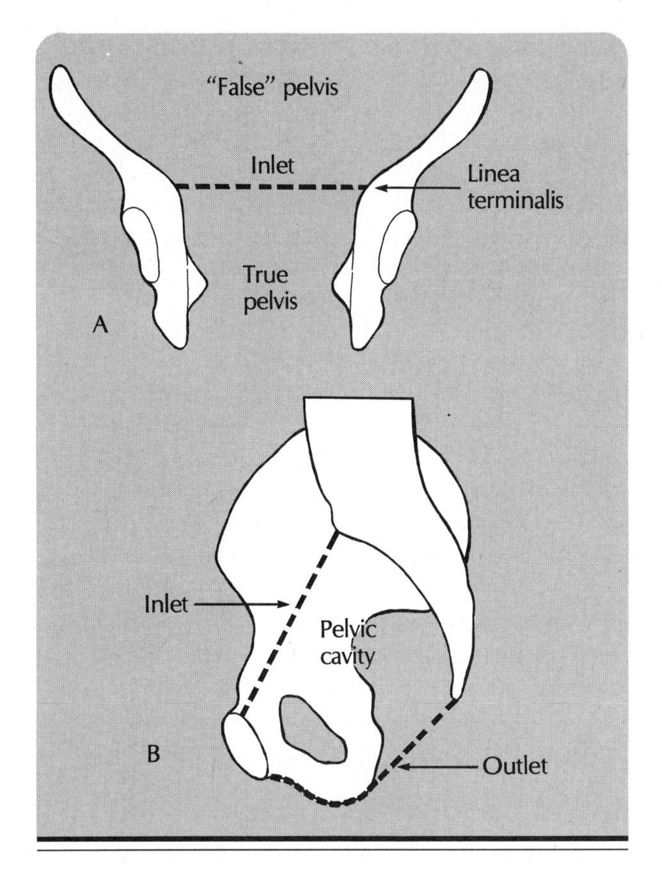

Figure 4–11. **A,** False and true pelves. **B,** Pelvic cavity.

Pelvic Division

The pelvic cavity is divided into the false pelvis and the true pelvis (Figure 4–11,*A*).

False Pelvis. The false pelvis, also known as the *major* or *greater pelvis,* is the portion above the pelvic brim, or linea terminalis, bounded by the lumbar vertebras posteriorly, the iliac fossae laterally, and the lower abdominal wall anteriorly. Its functions are to support the weight of the enlarged pregnant uterus and to direct the presenting fetal part into the true pelvis below.

True Pelvis. The true pelvis, also called the *minor* or *lesser pelvis,* lies below the pelvic brim and is bounded superiorly by the promontory and alae of the sacrum and the upper margins of the pubic bones and inferiorly by the pelvic outlet. The true pelvis represents the bony limits of the birth canal. It measures about 5 cm at its anterior wall at the symphysis pubis and about 10 cm at its posterior wall. When a woman is standing upright, the upper portion of the pelvic cavity or canal is directed downward and backward and its lower portion, downward and forward. This forms an axis or curved canal through which the presenting part of the baby must pass during birth (Figure 4–11,*B*). The inclination of the pelvis is the angle formed by two planes, a horizontal one through the tip of the coccyx and the superior border of the symphysis pubis and an inclined one through the sacral promontory and the superior border of the symphysis pubis. This pelvic angle of inclination usually measures 50°–60° (Figure 4–12).

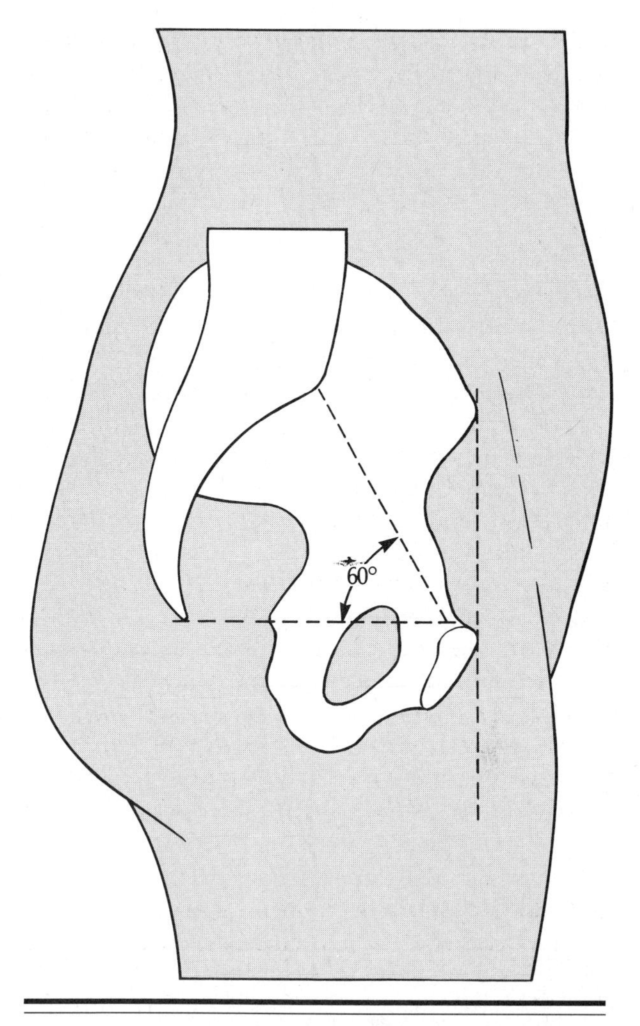

Figure 4–12. Pelvic angle of inclination while woman is standing.

The bony circumference of the true pelvis is made up of the sacrum, coccyx, and innominate bones below the linea terminalis. This area is of paramount importance in obstetrics, because its size and shape must be adequate for normal fetal passage during labor and at delivery. The rela-

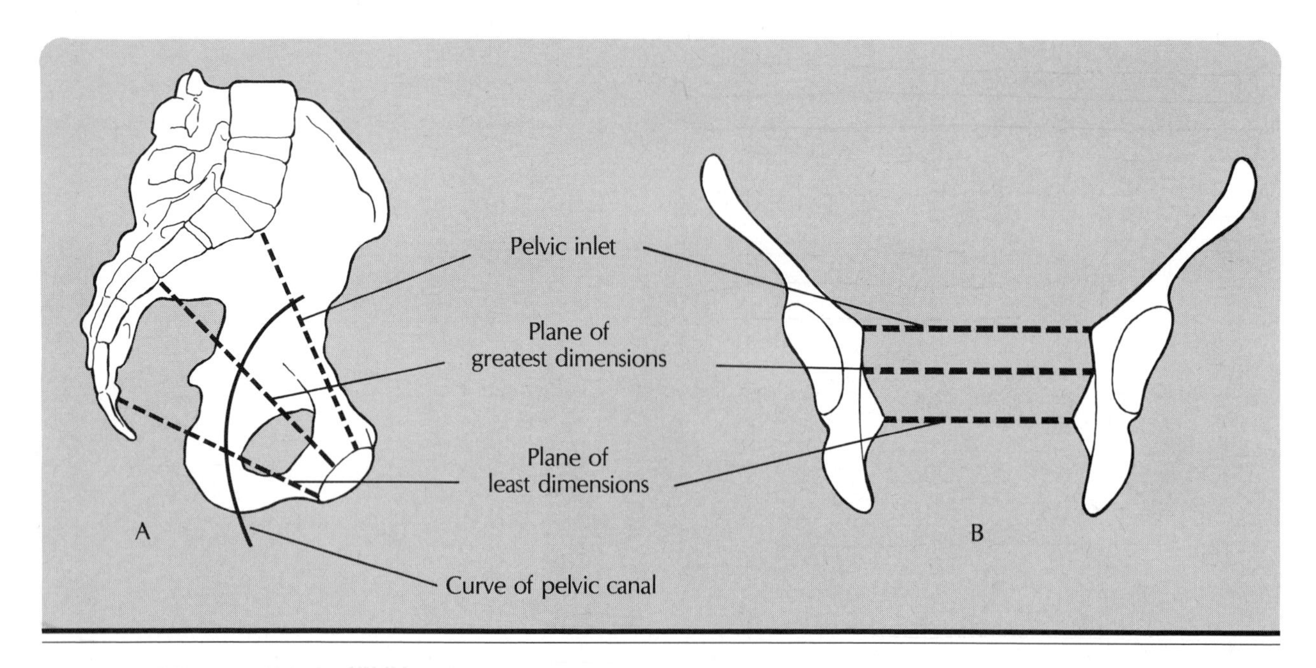

Figure 4–13. Pelvic planes. **A,** Sagittal section. **B,** Coronal section.

tionship of the fetal head to this cavity is of critical importance.

The true pelvis is considered to have three parts: the inlet, the pelvic cavity, and the outlet. The pelvic planes are imaginary flat surfaces drawn across the three parts of the true pelvis at strategic levels (Figure 4-13,*A*,*B*). Associated with each part are distinct obstetric measurements that aid in the evaluation of the adequacy of the pelvis for childbearing:

A. Pelvic inlet
    1. Anteroposterior diameters
        a. True conjugate
        b. Obstetric conjugate
        c. Diagonal conjugate
    2. Transverse diameter
    3. Right and left oblique diameters
B. Pelvic cavity
    1. Plane of greatest dimensions
    2. Plane of least dimensions
        a. Anteroposterior diameter
        b. Transverse (interspinous) diameter
        c. Posterior sagittal diameter
C. Pelvic outlet
    1. Anteroposterior diameters
        a. Anatomic
        b. Obstetric
    2. Transverse (intertuberous) diameter
    3. Anterior sagittal diameter
    4. Posterior sagittal diameter

The dimensions of the true pelvis and their obstetric implications are described here. Measurement techniques are discussed in Chapter 15. The effects of inadequate or abnormal pelvic diameters on labor and delivery are further considered in Chapter 19.

The *pelvic inlet,* also referred to as the *superior strait,* is the upper border of the true pelvis and is bounded posteriorly by the promontory and alae of the sacrum, laterally by the linea terminalis, and anteriorly by the upper margins of the pubic bones and symphysis pubis. The female pelvic inlet is typically round.

The anteroposterior, transverse, and right and left oblique diameters of the inlet are of obstetric importance (Figure 4-14). The anteroposterior diameter is the distance between the symphysis pubis and the sacrum. It is the shortest of the inlet diameters and therefore the most significant, because its inadequacy is the most common cause of inlet contraction. Three measures of this diameter may be made, depending on the specific point of the symphysis pubis used. The true (anatomic) conjugate, or conjugata vera, which has no obstetric significance, extends from the middle of the sacral promontory to the middle of the pubic crest (superior surface of the symphysis) and measures about 11.5 cm.

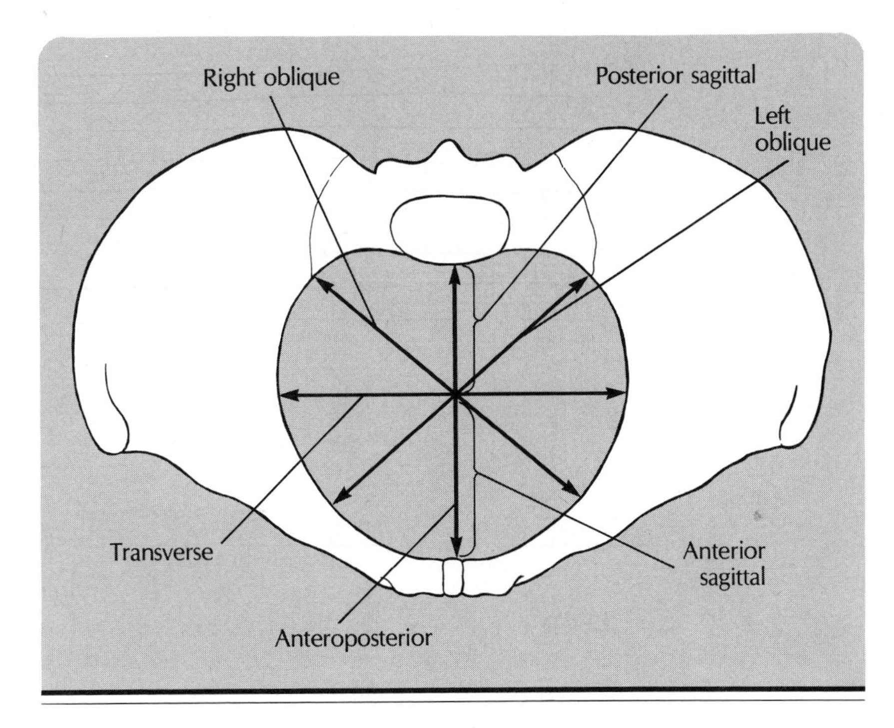

Figure 4–14. Diameters of pelvic inlet.

The obstetric conjugate extends from the middle of the sacral promontory to the posterosuperior margin of the symphysis, or about 1 cm below the pubic crest, and measures about 11 cm. Like the true conjugate, the obstetric conjugate is determined by radiographic measurement. In reality, it is through this diameter that the fetus must pass, and its size determines whether engagement of the fetal head will occur upon entering the superior strait.

The diagonal conjugate extends from the subpubic angle to the middle of the sacral promontory and measures about 12.5 cm. This measurement can be made manually (Chapter 16). By subtracting 1.5 cm from the diagonal conjugate, one can obtain an approximation of the vital obstetric conjugate.

The transverse diameter is the greatest measurement of the inlet and is measured from one side to the other using the lineae terminales as the points of reference. This diameter measures about 13.5 cm and assists in determining the shape of the inlet. It and the true conjugate lie at right angles to each other.

The suboccipitobregmatic diameter of the fetal head usually presents parallel to the transverse diameter because it is longer than the anteroposterior diameter. If the transverse or anteroposterior diameter is too short, the baby's head cannot enter the pelvis.

The right oblique diameter extends from the right sacroiliac joint to the left linea terminalis eminence and measures about 12.5 cm. The right and left oblique diameters have the same measurement.

Occasional mention is made of the posterior sagittal diameter, which extends from the intersection of the anteroposterior and transverse diameters to the middle of the sacral promontory and measures about 4.5 cm (Figure 4–14).

The *pelvic cavity* (canal) has varying diameters. The largest part of the pelvis is called the *plane of the greatest dimensions* (Figure 4–13,*A*,*B*). It is bounded by the junction of the second and third sacral vertebras posteriorly, the upper and middle thirds of the obturator foramen laterally, and the midpoint of the posterior surface of the pubis anteriorly. It is a curved canal with a longer posterior than anterior wall. A change in the lumbar curve can increase or decrease the pelvic inclination and can influence the progress of labor, because the fetus has to adjust itself to a curved path as well as to the different diameters of the true pelvis (Figure 4–11,*A*).

The smallest part of the pelvis is called the *plane of the least dimensions*, or the midpelvic plane (Figure 4–13). Arrest of labor occurs most frequently because of contracture in this plane, so its diameters are of great importance. The plane extends from the lower margin of the symphysis pubis, through the ischial spines, to the junction of the fourth and fifth sacral vertebras. Its anterior and posterior borders are bounded by the lower margin of the symphysis pubis, and fascia covering the obturator foramen, the ischial spines, the sacrospinous ligaments, and the sacrum. The anteroposterior diameter extends from the lower margin of the symphysis pubis to the junction of the fourth and fifth sacral vertebras and measures about 12 cm. The transverse (interspinous) diameter extends between the ischial spines and measures about 10.5 cm; it is the shortest pelvic diameter. The posterior sagittal diameter extends from the bispinous diameter to the junction of the fourth and fifth sacral vertebras and measures about 4.5–5 cm. At the midpelvic plane, the curve of the pelvic canal begins, and the axis of the birth canal changes. The fetal head, until it reaches the ischial spines, descends in a straight line. Then it curves forward toward the pelvic outlet.

The *pelvic outlet*, also called the *inferior strait*, is at the lower border of the true pelvis. It can be thought of as being composed of two triangles with a common base but in different planes. The common base as well as the most inferior part is the transverse diameter between the ischial tuberosities. The anterior triangle has as its apex the lower margin of the symphysis pubis, and the posterior triangle, the tip of the sacrum.

The anteroposterior diameter extends from the inferior margin of the symphysis to the tip of the coccyx and measures about 9.5 cm. This is the anatomic diameter. The obstetric anteroposterior diameter extends to the sacrococcygeal joint and measures about 11.5 cm (see Figure 16–7). The anteroposterior diameter increases during delivery to approximately 11.5 cm as the presenting part pushes the coccyx posteriorly at the mobile sacrococcygeal joint. As the infant's head emerges, the long diameter of the head (occipital frontal) parallels the long diameter of the outlet (anteroposterior).

The transverse diameter (bi-ischial or intertuberous) extends from the inner surface of one ischial tuberosity to the other and measures about 11 cm. It is the shortest diameter of the pelvic outlet and becomes shorter as the pubic arch narrows. The anterior sagittal diameter extends from the middle of the transverse diameter to the suprapubic angle and measures about 6 cm. The posterior sagittal diameter extends from the middle of the transverse diameter to the sacrococcygeal junction and measures about 9 cm. This is the most significant diameter of the outlet because it is the smallest diameter through which the infant must pass as it descends through the pelvic canal. The pubic arch has great importance, because the baby must pass under it. If it is narrow, the baby's head may be pushed backward toward the coccyx, making the extension of the head difficult. This situation is known as *outlet dystocia*, and forceps (outlet) delivery is required. Fetal head injury or deep maternal laceration may occur.

Types of Pelves

The Caldwell-Moloy classification of pelves is widely used to differentiate types of bony pelves (Caldwell and Moloy, 1933). Gynecoid, android, anthropoid, and platypelloid are the four basic types. However, variations in the female pelvis from plane to plane are so great that classic types are not usual. An imaginary line drawn through the greatest transverse diameter of the inlet divides it into anterior and posterior segments, and the pelvis type is always determined on the basis of the posterior segment of the inlet. With the posterior segment determining the type, the anterior segment of the inlet names variations. For example, an android pelvis with an anthropoid variation means that the posterior segment of the inlet is android and the anterior segment is anthropoid. These four types of pelvis are described further in Chapter 15. Each type has certain implications for labor and delivery, which are discussed in Chapter 19.

External Genitals

The female external genitals, referred to as the *vulva* or *pudendum*, include the following structures (Figure 4–15):

1. Mons pubis
2. Labia majora
3. Labia minora
4. Clitoris
5. Urethral meatus and paraurethral (Skene's) glands
6. Vaginal vestibule
   a. Vaginal orifice
   b. Vulvovaginal (Bartholin's) glands
   c. Hymen
   d. Fossa navicularis
7. Perineal body

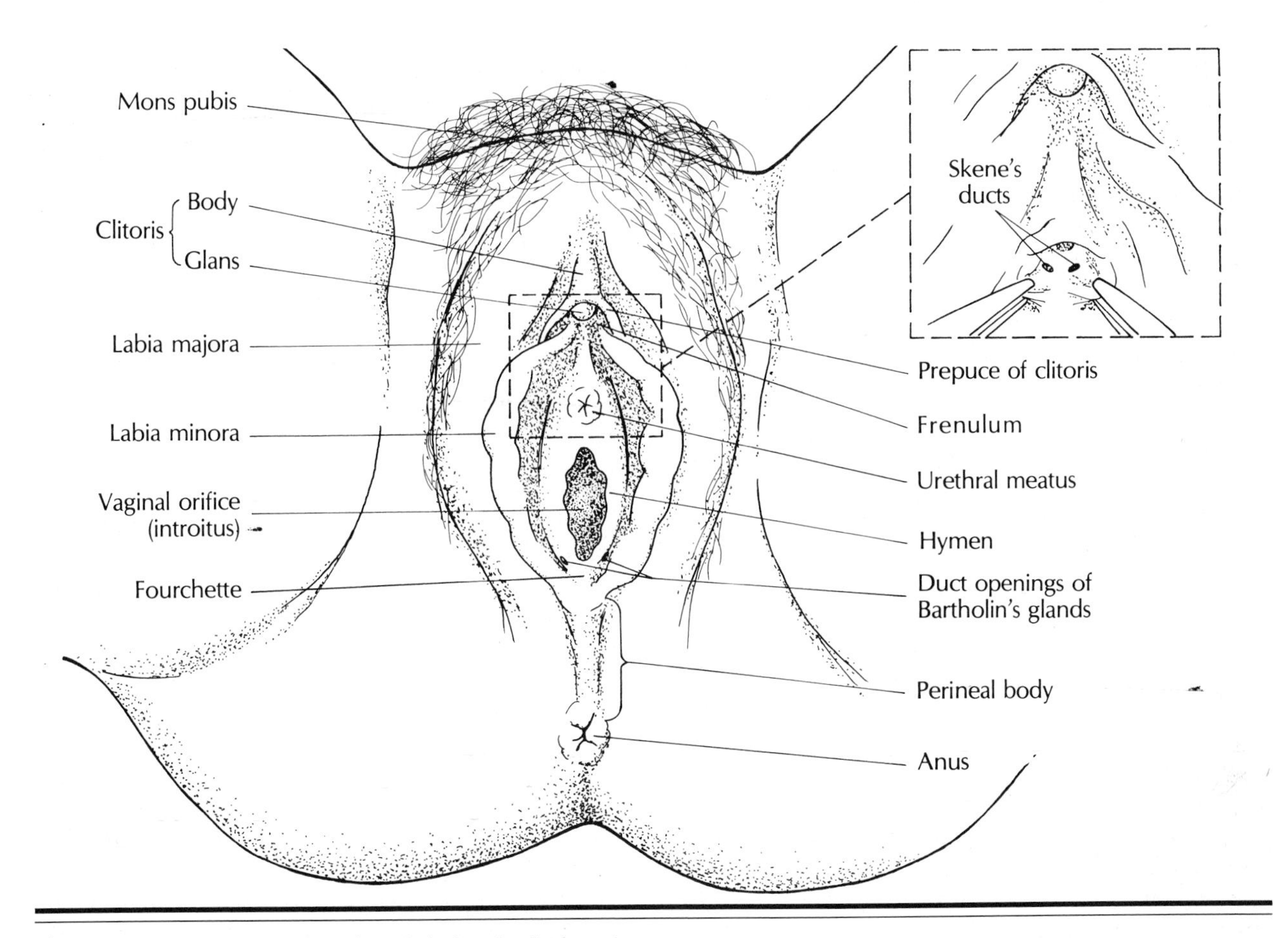

Figure 4–15. Female external genitals, longitudinal section.

Although not true parts of the female reproductive system, the urethral meatus and the perineal body will also be considered here because of their proximity and relationship to the vulva. All the external reproductive organs except the glandular structures can be directly inspected.

A composite structure, the vulva is a functional unit. Its organs, targets for estrogenic hormones throughout a woman's life (Beller et al., 1974), are endowed with a generous blood supply and complex innervation. With advancing age and decreased hormonal activity, these organs atrophy and are subject to a variety of lesions.

The size, color, and shape of these structures vary extensively among races and individuals. Racial characteristics, body size, and patterns of pigmentation all influence their appearance (Benson, 1976).

Mons Pubis

A softly rounded mound of subcutaneous fatty tissue beginning at the lowest portion of the anterior abdominal wall, the *mons pubis* (also known as the *mons veneris*) covers the anterior portion of the symphysis pubis (Figure 4–15). It is covered with hair in a typically female pubic pattern of distribution, with the hairline forming a transverse line across the lower abdomen. Approximately 75% of women display this pattern. The remaining 25% have hair extending toward the umbilicus along the linea alba. The hair is short and varies from sparse and fine in the Oriental woman to heavy, coarse, and curly in the black woman.

The function of the mons pubis is threefold. It helps protect the pelvic bones, especially during coitus. It contributes to the rounded contours of the feminine body. And finally, although it has no actual reproductive function, the mons appears to be sensually important (Masters and Johnson, 1966).

Because of the amount of loose connective tissue in the mons pubis, the incidence of edema is high relative to its occurrence in other parts of the body (Bloom and Van Dongen, 1972). During pregnancy, edema of the mons may accompany severe preeclampsia-eclampsia.

Labia Majora

The *labia majora* are longitudinal raised folds of deeply pigmented skin, one on either side of the vulval cleft (Figure 4–15). As the pair descend, they narrow, enclosing the vulval cleft, and merge posteriorly to form the posterior commissure of the perineal skin. The *vulval cleft* includes the clitoris, urethral meatus, vaginal vestibule, and vaginal orifice.

The labia majora are homologues of the unfused halves of the scrotum. With each pregnancy they become less prominent, so that in multiparous women they may be obliterated as distinct structures. The labia majora are covered by stratified squamous epithelium containing hair follicles and sebaceous glands with underlying adipose and muscle tissue. Immediately under the skin is a sheet of dartos muscle called the *dartos muliebris*, which is responsibile for the wrinkled appearance of the labia majora as well as for their sensitivity to heat and cold.

The subcutaneous tissues of the labia majora contain a great deal of loose connective tissue, which, as with the mons pubis, partially explains why edema occurs to a greater extent here than in any other part of the body, except the eyelids (Bloom and Van Dongen, 1972).

Arterial blood is supplied by the internal and external pudendal arteries, with numerous anastomoses. The venous drainage is composed of an extensive plexus in the area, in communication with the veins of the clitoris, labia minora, and perineum. Because of the extensive venous network in the labia majora, varicosities may occur during pregnancy, and obstetric or sexual trauma may cause hematomas of these structures.

The lymphatics of the labia majora are shared with other related structures of the vulva. They are extensive, diffuse, and a key to understanding malignancies of the female reproductive organs.

The labia majora are supplied with an extensive network of nerve endings that make them extremely sensitive to touch, pressure, pain, and temperature. The nerves supplying the area are mainly from the central nervous system: the anterior third is supplied primarily from the first lumbar segment of the spinal cord, and the posterior two-thirds are supplied mainly from the third sacral segment. Because of the central nervous system innervation of this area, certain regional anesthesia blocks will affect it.

The chief function of the labia majora is protection of the components of the vulvar cleft. Similar to the mons pubis, they have a potential erotic function.

Labia Minora

The *labia minora*, or nymphae, are soft folds of skin within the labia majora that converge both inferiorly and posteriorly (Figure 4–15). The labia minora are homologues of the unfused penile urethra of the male. Maldevelopment or fusion suggests anomalous sexual differentiation.

Toward their upper extremity each labium minus divides into two lamellas. The upper two merge to form the prepuce of the clitoris, and the lower pair fuse to form the frenulum of the clitoris. Inferiorly the labia minora unite to form the *fourchette*, a fold of skin below the vaginal orifice that is commonly torn or incised during childbirth.

Each labium minus has the appearance of shiny mucous membrane, moist and devoid of hair follicles. The labium minus is covered with stratified squamous epithelium, devoid of hair follicles but rich in sebaceous glands. The labia minora tissue is erectile, containing loose connective tissue, blood vessels, numerous large venous spaces, and involuntary muscle tissue. Because the sebaceous glands do not open into hair follicles but directly onto the surface of the skin, sebaceous cysts commonly occur in this area. Vulvovaginitis in this area is very irritating because of the many tactile nerve endings.

The functions of the labia minora are to lubricate and waterproof the vulvar skin, to provide bactericidal secretions, and to heighten sexual arousal and pleasure.

Clitoris

The *clitoris* is the most erotically sensitive part of the genital tract and is known to many females early in life as the site of masturbation. The term is derived from the Greek word *cleitoris*, meaning "key"; the ancients perceived it as the key to female sexuality. The clitoris is homologous to the male penis and is sometimes called the *penis muliebris*, or penis of woman (Bloom and Van Dongen, 1972). However, it contains no corpus spongiosum or urethral meatus.

The clitoris is at the anterior juncture of the labia minora (Figure 4–15), which form the prepuce anteriorly and the frenulum posteriorly.

The clitoris consists of the glans, the corpus or body, and two crura. The glans is partially covered by the prepuce at the distal end, and this area often appears as an opening to an orifice. Attempts to insert a catheter here produce extreme discomfort.

Visible between the folds of the labia minora, the clitoris is about 5–6 mm in length and 6–8 mm in diameter. Its tissue is essentially erectile, because of the large amounts of involuntary smooth muscle surrounding numerous venous channels. The clitoris has exceedingly rich blood and nerve supplies.

Clitoral innervation is through the terminal branch of the pudendal nerve, which lies next to the dorsal artery. Its branches terminate in the glans and prepuce. Heightened clitoral sensation may be dependent on an abundance of Dogiel, Krause, and Ruffini corpuscles (specialized genital receptor nerve endings). The incidence of free nerve endings is thought to be most prevalent in the prepuce of the clitoris (Benson, 1976). Overall, the clitoris is endowed with a nerve supply more plentiful than that of the male penis.

The clitoris exists primarily for female sexual enjoyment. In addition, it produces smegma. Along with other vulval secretions, smegma has a unique odor that may be erotically stimulating to the male.

Urethral Meatus and Paraurethral Glands

One to 2.5 cm beneath the clitoris in the midline of the vestibule is the *urethral meatus* (Figure 4–15). At times the meatus is difficult to see because of the presence of blind dimples, small mucosal folds, or wide variance in location. Its appearance is often puckered and slitlike.

The *paraurethral glands,* or *Skene's ducts,* open into the posterior wall of the female urethra close to its orifice (Figure 4–15). The paraurethral glands are homologous to the male prostate glands. Skene's ducts can become infected with gonococcus.

Vaginal Vestibule

The *vaginal vestibule* is a remnant of the urogenital sinus of the embryo. It is bordered anteriorly by the clitoris and urethra, laterally by the labia minora, and posteriorly by the fourchette (Figure 4–15). The vaginal vestibule is a boat-shaped fossa, visible when the labia majora are separated. Part of its contents, the vaginal introitus, has special significance, because it is the border between the external and internal genitals.

The junction of the vaginal orifice with the vestibule is limited by a thin, elastic membrane called the *hymen.* Its strength, shape, and size vary greatly among individuals and can change within the same individual as a result of age, coitus, and parity. The belief that the intact hymen is a sign of virginity and that it is perforated at first sexual intercourse with resultant bleeding is not valid. The hymen is essentially avascular. Intact hymens are found in heterosexually active and parous women, whereas virgins may possess broken hymens. The hymen may be broken through strenuous physical activity, masturbation, menstruation, or the use of tampons. Once it is broken, the irregular tags that remain are called *carunculae myrtiformes.*

External to the hymenal ring at the base of the vestibule are two small papular elevations containing the orifices of the ducts of the *vulvovaginal (Bartholin's) glands.* They lie under the constrictor muscle of the vagina. Generally, the vulvovaginal glands are not palpable upon examination, being placed deep in the perineal structures. Their ducts measure 1.5–2 cm in length and about 0.5 cm in diameter. These compound, lobulated glands secrete mucus to lubricate the vaginal orifice and canal during sexual arousal. The mucous secretion is clear and viscid, with an alkaline pH, all of which enhance the viability and motility of the sperm deposited in the vaginal vestibule.

The *fossa navicularis* is a slight depression or pitted area between the fourchette and the hymen. This area is subjected to laceration or incision by episiotomy during childbirth.

Innervation of the vestibular area is mainly by the perineal nerve from the sacral plexus. The area is not sensitive to touch generally, although the hymen contains numerous free nerve endings as receptors to pain.

Perineal Body

The *perineal body* is a wedge-shaped mass of fibromuscular tissue found between the lower part of the vagina and the anal canal (Figure 4–15). In obstetrics and gynecology, the perineal body is referred to as the *perineum.* (In other specialties, the perineum consists of all the muscles and fascia of the urogenital and pelvic diaphragms.)

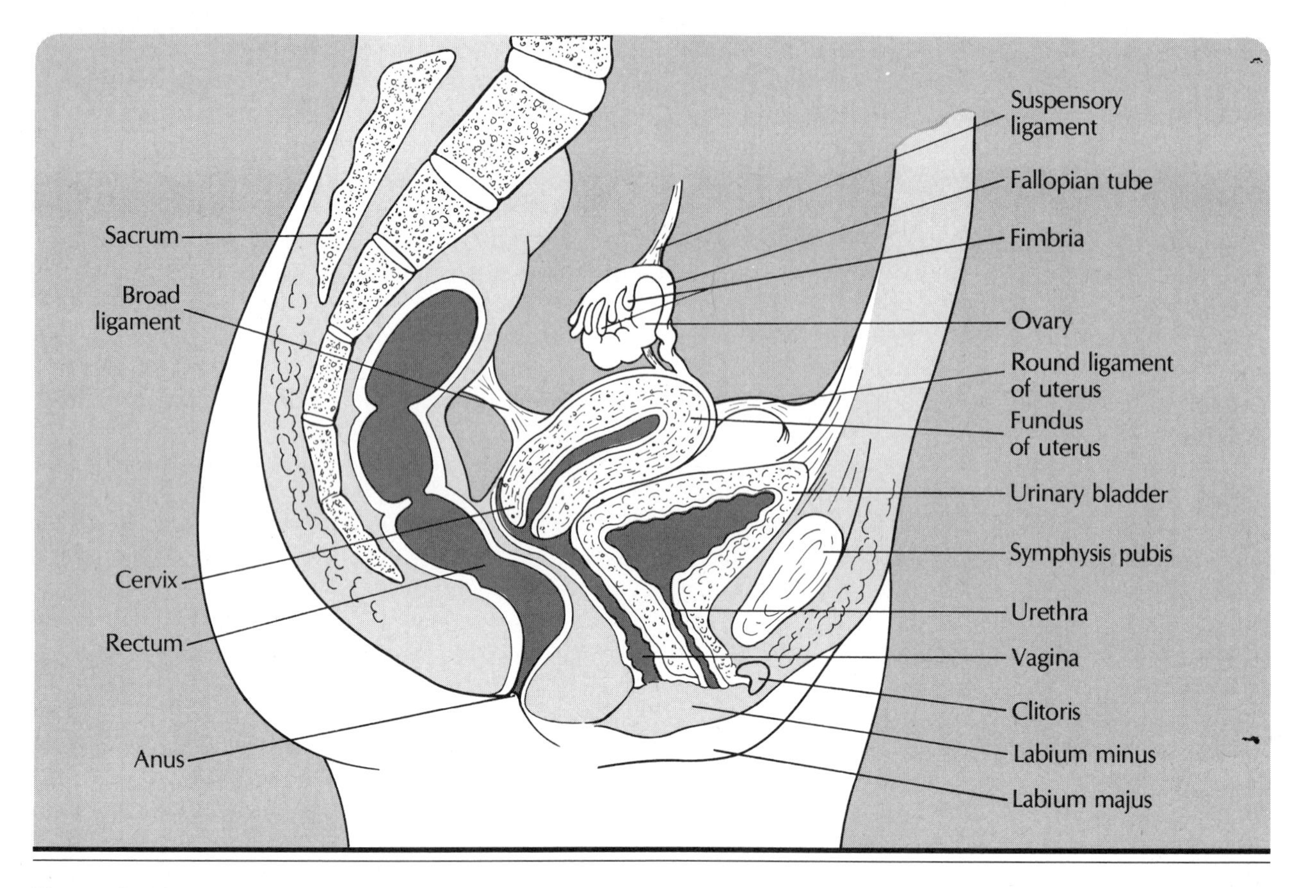

Figure 4–16. Female internal reproductive organs.

The muscles that meet at the central point of the perineum are the sphincter ani, both levator ani, the superficial and deep transverse perineal, and the bulbocavernosus. These muscles mingle with elastic fibers and connective tissue in an arrangement that allows a remarkable amount of stretching. The perineum is much larger in the female than in the male and is subject to laceration during chidbirth. Without proper repair, such damage may produce weakness of the pelvic floor.

Internal Genitals

The female internal reproductive organs are highly specialized in structure and function. The target organs for estrogenic hormones—the vagina, uterus, uterine or fallopian tubes, and ovaries—play a unique part in the reproductive cycle. They are shown in Figure 4-16. Each of these organs can be palpated manually or bimanually and can be observed through instrumentation with a speculum, laparoscope, or culdoscope. Radiography and sonography of these organs have contributed greatly to the study and diagnosis of the reproductive process and related functions. In addition, the recent techniques of transmission electron microscopy and scanning electron microscopy have yielded extremely detailed microphotographs of the cells and tissues of the reproductive organs (Ferenczy and Richart, 1974).

Vagina

The *vagina* is a musculomembranous tube that connects the external genitals with the center of the pelvis (Figure 4-16). Its passage superiorly and posteriorly from the vulva to the uterus is in a position nearly parallel to the plane of the pelvic brim. This direction is optimal for coitus. The vagina also forms the lower part of the axis through which the fetal head (or presenting part) must negotiate during its passage at birth.

Because the cervix of the uterus projects into the upper part of the anterior wall of the vagina, the anterior wall is approximately 2.5 cm shorter than the posterior wall. There is great individual variation in vaginal size. Measurements range from 6 to 8 cm for the anterior wall and from 7 to 10 cm for the posterior wall. The cervical projection (portio vaginalis cervicis) into the upper part of the vagina (vaginal vault) also creates a recess or hollow around the cervix, which for descriptive purposes is divided into four arches, referred to as the *vaginal fornices.* The anterior vaginal fornix is shallow, the two lateral fornices are deeper, and the posterior fornix is the deepest. These fornices are separated from surrounding organs by a single layer of connective tissue; the walls of the vaginal vault are very thin. Such structure enhances examination of the pelvic contents in a pelvic examination. Through the anterior fornix, the body of an anteverted uterus as well as the bladder, when distended with urine, can be palpated. Through the posterior fornix, the body of a retroverted uterus, rectouterine pouch (pouch of Douglas, or cul-de-sac) and any contents, uterosacral ligament, and rectum can be palpated. Through the lateral fornices, the ovaries, appendix, cecum, colon, and ureters can be palpated. Many examiners confuse the round ligament with the uterine tube, which usually cannot be palpated unless it is enlarged.

When a woman lies on her back, the space in the posterior fornix favors the pooling of semen after coitus. This space is called the *receptaculum seminis* and may enhance the chances of impregnation by the collection of large numbers of sperm close to a favorable cervical environment.

The vagina is divided into the lower, middle, and upper (vaginal vault) portions. Each portion is supported by ligaments and muscles attached to the vaginal wall by pelvic fascia. The upper vaginal portion is supported by the levator ani muscles and transverse cervical, pubocervical, and sacrocervical ligaments. The middle vaginal portion is supported by the urogenital diaphragm, and the lower vaginal portion, especially the posterior wall, is supported by the perineal body.

Generally, the anterior and posterior walls of the vagina are in approximation, so that the resting vagina has an H shape on transverse section. The embryologic development of the vaginal canal involves canalization and fusion of two separate halves of the paramesonephric ducts. Any interference with these processes can produce congenital malformations, frequently involving the presence of superfluous septa.

Extending into the lumen from the medial surface of the lower two-thirds of the vaginal anterior and posterior walls are prominent longitudinal ridges called *anterior* and *posterior vaginal columns.* Almost at right angles to these columns are the *rugae vaginales,* transverse ridges of the mucous membrane. Although these ridges are numerous at the midline, they almost disappear at the lateral walls. This patterned surface is present after menarche and is often obliterated with multiple pregnancies. These rugae allow for the profound vaginal stretching during the descent of the fetal head and may provide some additional friction or grasping effect for the erect penis during intercourse.

The noncornified, stratified, squamous epithelium lining of the vagina proliferates under the influence of estrogenic hormones and is an even more sensitive index of steroid hormonal effects than the uterine endometrium (Beller et al., 1974). Its structure parallels that of the skin, although there are no sweat glands, sebaceous glands, or hair follicles to weaken it. Immediately under the epithelial layer, the connective tissue is arranged to provide the epithelium with optimal nourishment by approximating a great number of mature basal cells with the underlying blood capillaries. The connective tissue layer has a profuse blood supply, occasional lymphoid nodules, and few somatic nerve endings. The rich blood supply is needed to maintain a high glycogen content in the epithelial cells as well as to nourish the underlying musculofascial layer, through which the vaginal vault gains strong attachments to the cervix. The two-layered smooth muscle component of the musculofascial layer is continuous with the superficial muscle fibers of the uterus. The outer layer is composed of longitudinal muscle fibers, and the inner layer is composed of circular muscle fibers. The outermost vaginal layer is a dense sheet of connective tissue, containing the larger vaginal arteries and venous plexus. A thin band of striated muscle, the sphincter vagina, is found at the lowest extremity of the vagina. However, the levator ani is the principle muscle that closes the vagina.

During a woman's mature reproductive life, a vaginal pH range of 4 to 5 is normal, with the lowest pH at midcycle and the highest premenstrually. Transudate of the vaginal epithelium provides a moist environment. The acidic pH is maintained by a symbiotic relationship beween the lactic acid–producing Döderlein bacillus

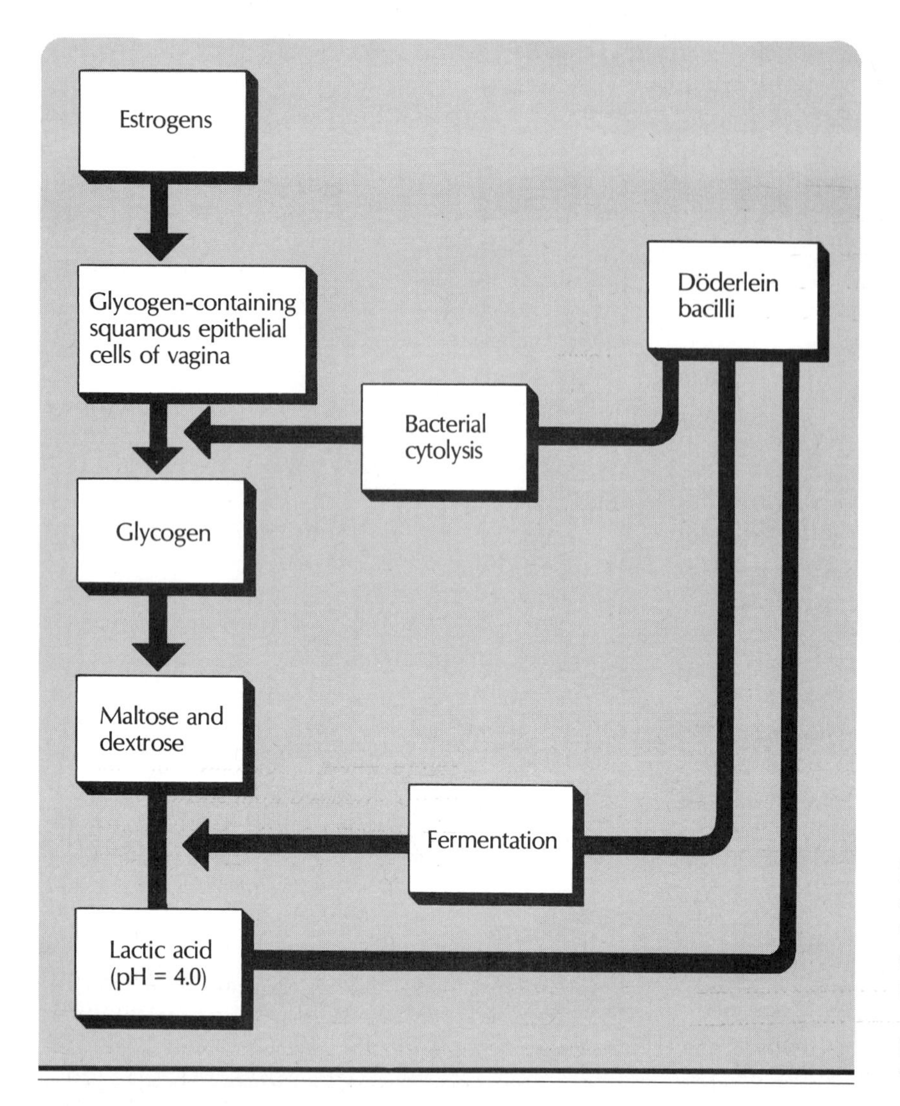

Figure 4–17. Scheme of biology of vagina: Reciprocal influence of the vaginal epithelium and Döderlein bacilli on maintenance of acidic vaginal milieu. (From Beller, F. K., et al. 1974. *Gynecology: a textbook for students.* New York: Springer Verlag New York, Inc., p. 220.)

(lactobacillus) and the vaginal contents. The bacilli depend on the desquamation of vaginal epithelial cells containing high levels of glycogen. Ovarian hormones regulate not only the glycogen content of these cells but their sloughing and renewal as well. The bacilli break down the glycogen enzymatically to simple sugars and finally to lactic acid. Figure 4–17 illustrates this process. Any interruption of this cycle can destroy the normal self-cleansing action of the vagina. Such interruption may be caused by antibiotic therapy, douching, or use of vaginal sprays or deodorants.

The acidic vaginal environment is normal only in the mature reproductive years and in the first days of life, when maternal hormones are operating in the infant. The relatively neutral pH of 7.5 is normal from infancy until puberty and after menopause.

Each third of the vagina is supplied by a distinct vascular pattern. Its upper third is supplied by the cervicovaginal branches of the uterine arteries; its middle third by the inferior vesical arteries (bladder arteries); its lower third by the internal pudendal and the middle hemorrhoidal arteries (rectal arteries). The venous drainage is accomplished by a closely interwoven, intercommunicating venous network. Because these venous plexus also anastomose with the vertebral venous plexus, it is possible for a pelvic embolism or carcinoma to bypass the heart and lungs and lodge in the brain, spine, or other remote part of the body (Bloom and Van Dongen, 1972).

Lymphatic drainage of the vagina follows a direct pattern. The upper third drains into the external and internal iliac nodes; the middle third, into the hypogastric nodes; and the lower third, into the inguinal glands. The posterior wall

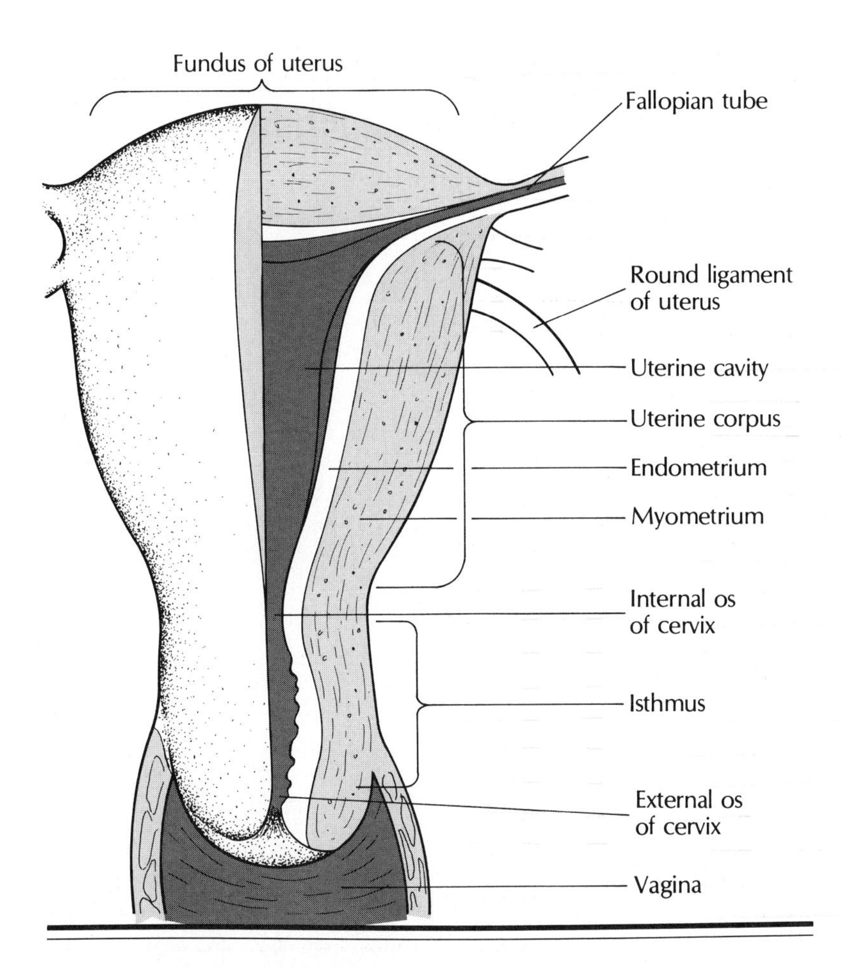

Figure 4–18. Anatomy of the uterus. (Modified from Spence, A. P., and Mason, E. B. 1979. *Human anatomy and physiology.* Menlo Park, Calif.: Benjamin/Cummings Publishing Co., p. 767.)

drains into nodes lying in the rectovaginal septum. Any vaginal infection follows these routes.

The vagina is a relatively insensitive organ, with meager somatic innervation to its lower third by the pudendal nerve and virtually no special nerve endings. Therefore sensation during sexual excitement and coitus is minimal and pain during the second stage of labor is less than if somatic innervation were greater. Nervous supply to the vagina is predominantly autonomic. Sensation arises in the vagina and terminates at the S2-3-4 level.

Serving as the copulatory and parturient passage, the vagina is frequently called the *birth canal.* It also functions to enable the discharge of menstrual products from the uterine endometrium to the outside of the body. Finally, the vagina protects against coital trauma and infection from pathogenic organisms.

Uterus

Throughout the ages, the *uterus,* or womb, has been endowed with a mystical aura. As the core of reproduction and hence continuation of the human race, the uterus and its bearer have received particular attention and treatment. Numerous customs, taboos, mores, and values have evolved about women and their reproductive function. Although scientific knowledge has replaced much of this folklore, remnants of old ideas and supersititions pervade the thinking of many persons who seek or provide maternal health care. The nurse must be able to recognize and deal with such attitudes and beliefs so that her application of the nursing process can be most effective.

The uterus is a hollow, muscular, thick-walled, pear-shaped organ lying central in the pelvic cavity between the base of the bladder and the rectum and above the vagina (Figure 4–18). It is at or slightly below the brim of the pelvis, with the external os about the level of the ischial spines. Its anterior and posterior surfaces are in opposition, making its cavity potential rather than actual. Although the anterior or vesical (bladder) surface is almost flat, the posterior surface is convex. Because the body of the uterus is flattened, the lateral diameter is greater than the anteroposterior diameter. Loops of the bowel are usually superior to the uterus. The mature organ weighs about 60 gm and is approximately 7.5 cm long, 5 cm wide, and 1–2.5 cm thick. Clinical approximation of size is inaccurate; a uterine sound is needed for a more exact measurement.

As Heinrich von Waldeyer, a Berlin anatomist, pointed out, "The uterus has one typical, but many normal positions" (Bloom and Van Dongen, 1972). Posture, parity, bladder and rectal fullness, and even normal respiratory patterns influence the position of the uterus; only the cervix is anchored laterally. The body of the uterus can move freely in the anteroposterior plane. The axis also varies. Generally, the uterus forms a sharp angle with the vagina. There is a bend in the area of the isthmus; from there the cervix faces downward. This is the so-called normal anteversion or angulation of the uterus.

The uterus is kept at its normal level in the pelvis by three sets of supports. The upper supports are the broad and round ligaments. The middle supports are suspensory and consist of the cardinal, pubocervical, and uterosacral ligaments. The lower supports are those structures considered to be the pelvic muscular floor (Bloom and Van Dongen, 1972).

Many uterine anomalies are thought to be congenital and can be understood more easily by reviewing the embryologic development of the uterus. Between the sixth and ninth week of embryonic development, the two paramesonephric ducts, which are adjacent to the mesonephric ducts, grow caudally. Their ultimate fusion gives rise to the fallopian tubes, uterine fundus, cervix, and upper vagina. A normal uterus therefore requires two symmetrical, parallel, equal-sized paramesonephric ducts to meet in the midline. Anomalies represent the absence of either one or both of the ducts, degrees of failure to fuse, or canalization defects. Figure 4–19 illustrates the normal uterus as contrasted with the common types of malformations (Jarcho, 1946). The bicornuate and didelphys uterine malformations are found most frequently.

In cases of habitual abortion, a hysterogram should be done to evaluate the normalcy of the uterus. Because both the urinary and reproductive systems develop from the common urogenital fold in the embryo, anomalies in one system are frequently accompanied by anomalies in the other. Problems of infertility and premature labor and delivery are common.

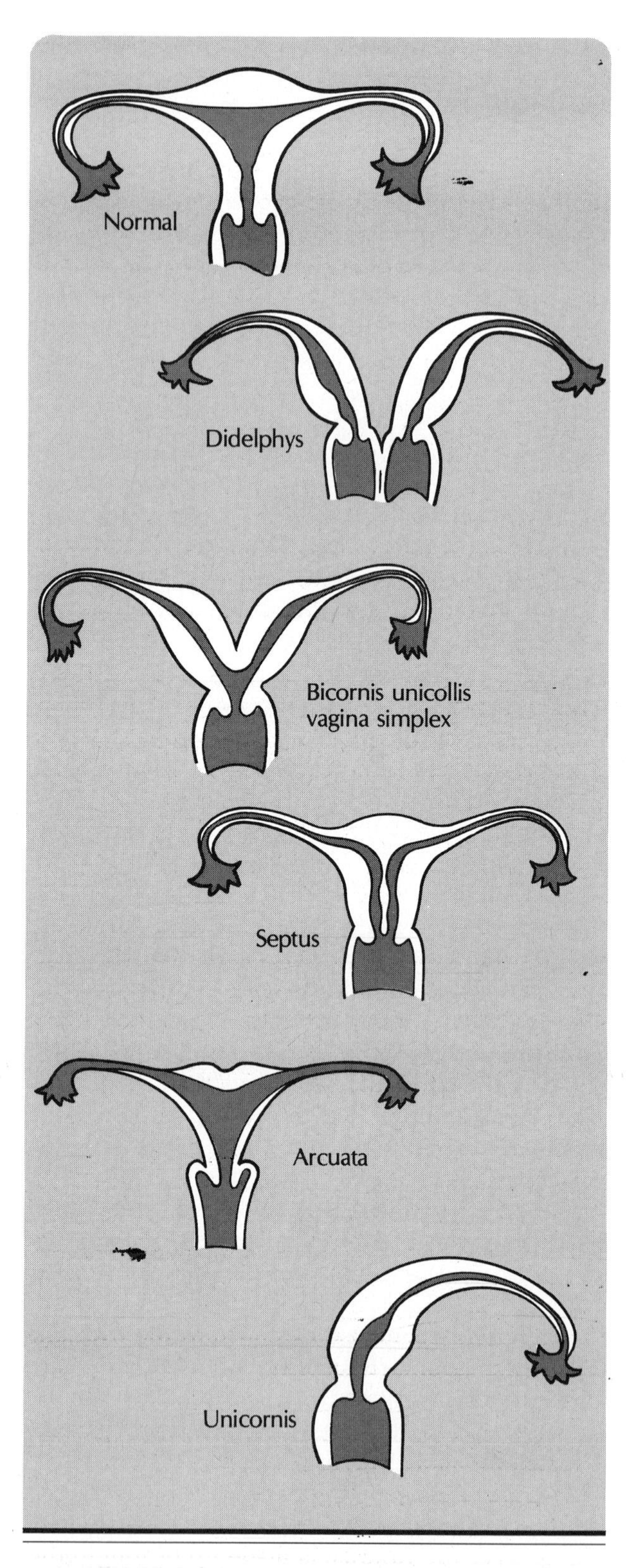

Figure 4–19. Congenital malformations of the uterus.

A slight constriction called the *isthmus* divides the uterus into two unequal parts. The upper two-thirds is the triangular body, or *corpus*, composed mainly of myometrium; the lower third is the neck, or *fusiform cervix*. The rounded uppermost portion of the corpus that extends above the points of attachment of the uterine tubes is called the *fundus*. The cervix, about 2.5 cm in both length and diameter, differs from the corpus both histologically and physiologically. It is canal-like, with its exit into the vagina called the *external os* and its entrance into the corpus, the *internal os* (Figure 4–18).

The isthmus is about 6 mm above the internal os, and it is in this area that the uterine endometrium changes into the mucous membrane of the cervix. The isthmus takes on significance in pregnancy, because it becomes the lower uterine segment. With the cervix, it is a passive segment and not part of the contractile uterus. At delivery, this thin lower segment, situated behind the bladder, is the site for lower-segment caesarean sections.

The corpus of the uterus is made up of three layers: outermost, or serosal (perimetrium); middle, or muscular (myometrium); and innermost, or mucosal (endometrium). Each layer is distinct in makeup and function.

The *serosal layer* is peritoneum, which passes down from the anterior abdominal wall onto the bladder surface, runs directly onto the anterior surface of the uterus at the level of the internal os, and continues over the fundus and down over the posterior surface of the corpus. As it covers the superior surface of the posterior vaginal fornix, it forms the anterior wall of the rectouterine pouch (pouch of Douglas). The two-layered folds of peritoneum, extending from the lateral uterine margins to the lateral pelvic walls, make up the broad ligament.

The *muscular uterine layer* has, in turn, three indistinct layers. It should be noted that myometrium is continuous with the muscle layer of the fallopian tubes as well as with that of the vagina. These muscle fibers also extend into the ovarian, round, and cardinal ligaments and minimally into the uterosacral ligaments, which helps explain the vague but disturbing pelvic "aches and pains" reported by many gravid patients.

Figure 4–20 shows these three layers of involuntary muscle. The outer layer, distributed mainly over the fundus, is made up of longitudinal muscles, especially suited for their expulsive function during the birth process. The middle layer is thick and made up of interlacing muscle fibers in figure-eight patterns. These fibers surround large blood vessels, and their contraction produces a hemostatic action. The inner muscle layer is made up of circular fibers, sparse over the fundus but concentrated to form sphincters at the uterine tube attachment sites (tubia ostia) and at the internal os. The internal os sphincter inhibits the explusion of the uterine contents during pregnancy. An incompetent cervical os can be caused by a torn, weak, or absent sphincter at the internal os. The sphincters at the tubia ostia prevent the regurgitation of menstrual blood into the uterine tubal lumen from the uterus.

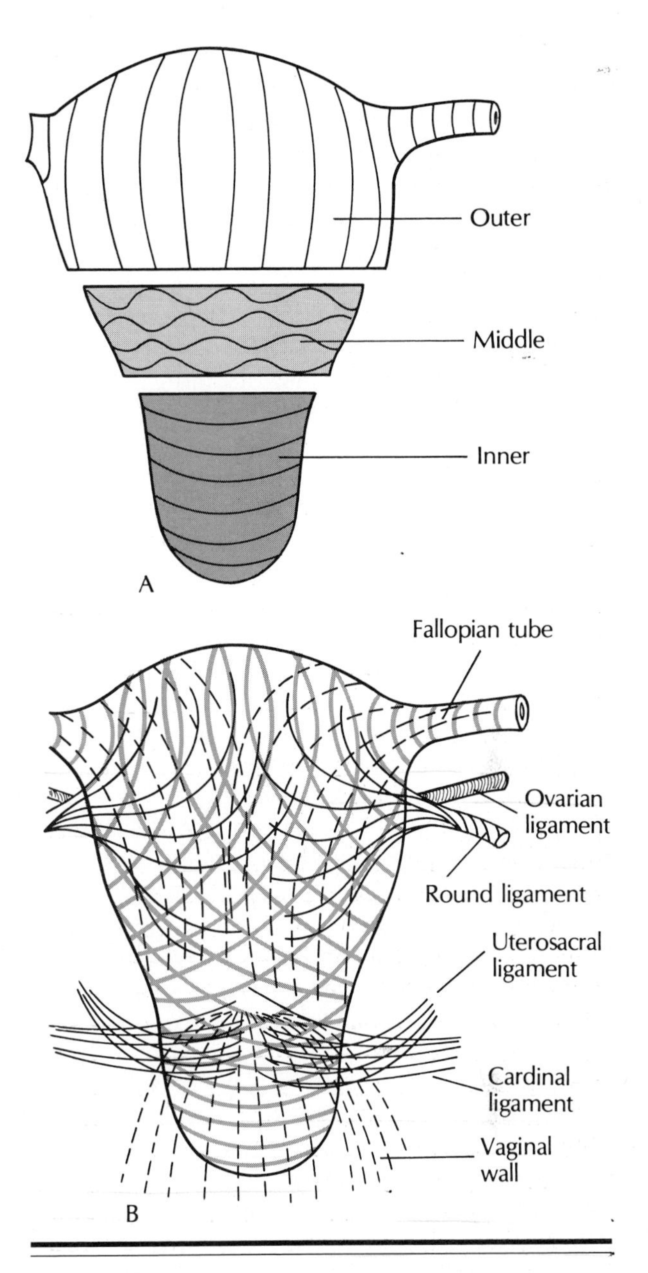

Figure 4–20. Uterine muscle layers. **A,** Muscle fiber placement. **B,** Interlacing of uterine muscle layers.

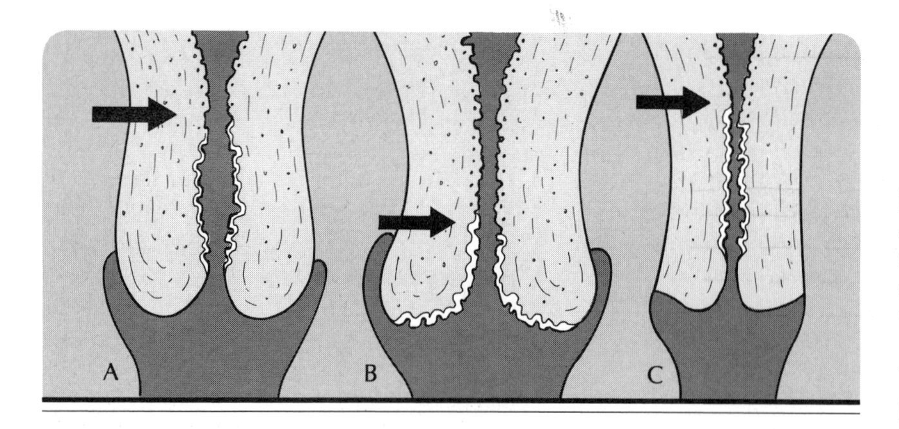

Figure 4–21. Changes in squamocolumnar junction (arrow) at various stages of life. **A,** Childhood. **B,** Reproductive years. **C,** Old age. (Modified from Beller, F. K., et al. 1974. *Gynecology: a textbook for students.* New York: Springer Verlag New York, Inc., p. 34.)

Although each layer of muscle has been discussed as having a unique function, it must be remembered that the uterine musculature works as a whole. The uterine contractions of labor are responsible for the dilatation of the cervix and provide the major impetus for the passage of the fetus through the pelvic axis and vaginal canal at birth.

The *mucosal* or *innermost layer* of the uterine corpus is the endometrium, a single layer of columnar epithelium, glands, and stroma. From menarche to menopause, the endometrium undergoes monthly degeneration and renewal in the absence of pregnancy. As it responds to a governing hormonal cycle, the endometrium varies in thickness from 0.5 to 5 mm.

Covering the endometrial surface are simple, tubular-type glands lined with columnar cells, which are continuous with those covering the surface of the endometrium. The glands produce a thin, watery, alkaline secretion that keeps the uterine cavity moist. Not only is this "endometrial milk" capable of assisting the sperm on their journey to the uterine tubes, but it provides nourishment to the blastocyst prior to implantation (Chapter 6).

There is no submucosa; the endometrium is directly over the myometrium, thereby facilitating the monthly regeneration of endometrium after menstruation. Some of the endometrial glands dip directly into the myometrium, and the new endometrium is derived from these irregular indentations of epithelium, called *endometrial seed.*

When pregnancy occurs and the endometrium is not shed, the reticular stromal cells surrounding the endometrial glands become the decidual cells of pregnancy. The stromal cells are highly vascular, channeling a rich blood supply to the endometrial surface.

The *cervix* is a protective portal for the body of the uterus as well as the connection between the vagina and the uterus. The cervix is divided by its line of attachment into the vaginal and supravaginal areas. The *vaginal cervix* includes about one-fourth of the anterior cervix and one-half of the posterior cervix. It projects into the vagina at an angle of 45°–90°. The *supravaginal cervix* is surrounded by the attachments that give the uterus its main support: the uterosacral ligaments posteriorly, the transverse ligaments of the cervix (ligaments of Mackenrodt) laterally, and the pubocervical ligaments anteriorly.

The vaginal cervix appears pink and is covered by pale squamous stratified epithelium, which is continuous with the vaginal lining. The vaginal cervix ends at the external os. The supravaginal cervix appears rosy red and is lined with tall columnar ciliated epithelium containing many branching mucus-secreting glands. Most cervical cancer begins at this squamocolumnar junction. Its exact location varies with age and parity. Figure 4–21 shows this junction at various stages of a woman's life.

Elasticity is a chief characteristic of the cervix. Its ability to stretch is made possible by the high fibrous and collagenous content of the supportive tissues and by the arrangement of vast numbers of folds and plications in the cervical lining. As in the vagina, anterior and posterior ridges with rugae branch off obliquely in the cervix. Thus the actual area is increased tremendously. About 10% of the cervix is composed of muscle cells.

The cervical mucosa has three functions: (a) to provide lubrication for the vaginal canal, (b) to act as a bacteristatic agent, and (c) to provide an alkaline environment to shelter deposited sperm from the acidic vagina. At ovulation, cervical mucus is clearer, more viscous, and higher in alkalinity.

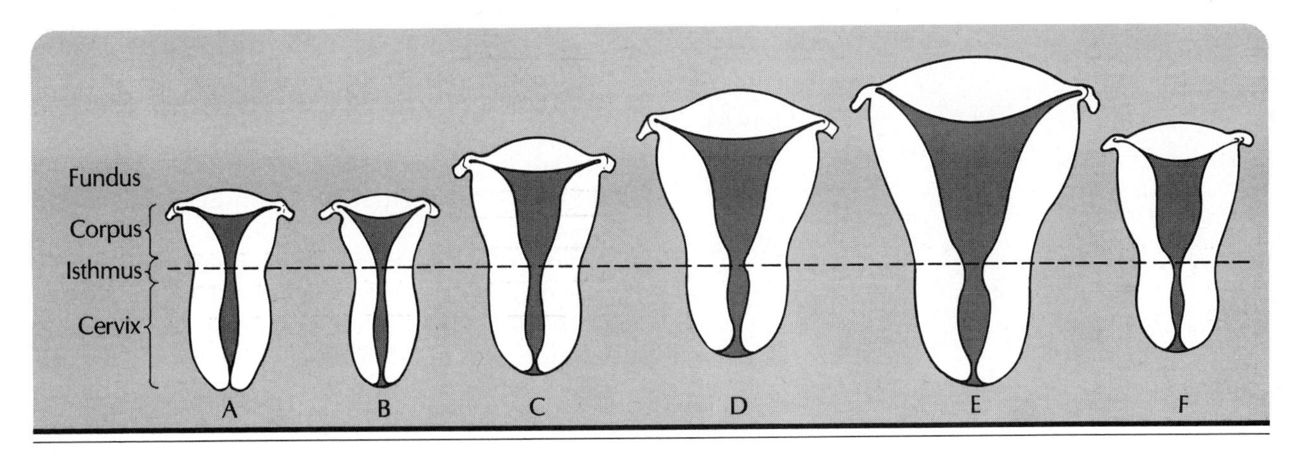

Figure 4–22. Changes in size of uterus and external os during a woman's life.

Both the body of the uterus and the cervix are changed permanently by pregnancy. The body never returns to its nulliparous size, and the external os changes from a circular opening of about 3 mm to a transverse slit with irregular edges. Figure 4–22 illustrates the changes in size of the uterus and the external os during the life span of a parous woman.

The ovarian artery arises from the abdominal aorta below the renal arteries and can supply the ovary, fallopian tube, and upper third of the uterus. The uterine artery arises from the internal iliac artery and supplies the lower two-thirds of the uterus. There are numerous anastomoses between the ovarian and uterine arteries and their branches. The uterine veins are arranged in a pattern similar to those of the uterine, ovarian, and tubal arteries (Figure 4–23).

Lymphatic drainage from the cervix moves in three areas: (a) external iliac nodes, (b) internal iliac nodes, and (c) sacral nodes. The body of the uterus is drained by a scant system for each of its three layers. One set of collecting vessels follows the broad ligament and ovarian vessels to end in the para-aortic nodes, another follows the round ligaments to terminate in the inguinal lymph glands, and the third set merges with lymphatics of the cervix into the external iliac nodes.

Innervation of the uterus is entirely by the autonomic nervous system and seems to be more regulatory than primary in nature. It is helpful to recall that generally sympathetic fibers stimulate muscle contraction and vasoconstriction; parasympathetic fibers inhibit contractions and stimulate vasodilatation. There is adequate contractility of the uterus without an intact nerve supply, as illustrated by the fact that hemiplegic patients have adequate uterine contractions (Beller et al., 1974).

Uterine parasympathetic fibers arise from the second, third, and fourth sacral nerves to form the pelvic nerves. Sympathetic fibers enter the pelvis through the hypogastric plexus. Although the sympathetic and parasympathetic fibers enter the pelvis separately, they become mixed in the uterovaginal plexus of Frankenhäuser (Figure 4–24).

Both the sympathetic and parasympathetic nerves contain motor fibers and a few sensory fibers. Pain of uterine contractions is carried to the central nervous system by the eleventh and twelfth thoracic nerve roots. Pain from the cervix and upper vagina passes through the ilioinguinal and pudendal nerves. The motor fibers to the uterus arise from the seventh and eighth thoracic vertebras. Because the sensory and motor levels are separated in this manner, caudal and spinal anesthesia can be utilized during labor and delivery.

The uterine functions are designed to provide a safe environment for fetal development. The uterine lining is cyclically prepared by steroid hormones for nidation (implantation of the embryo). Once implanted, the developing fetus is protected until it is expelled.

Uterine Ligaments

The uterine ligaments are shown in Figure 4–25.

Broad Ligament. The broad ligament, or *mesosalpinx,* is a double mesenteric layer continuous with the abdominal peritoneum. The peritoneum may be thought of as being draped over the blad-

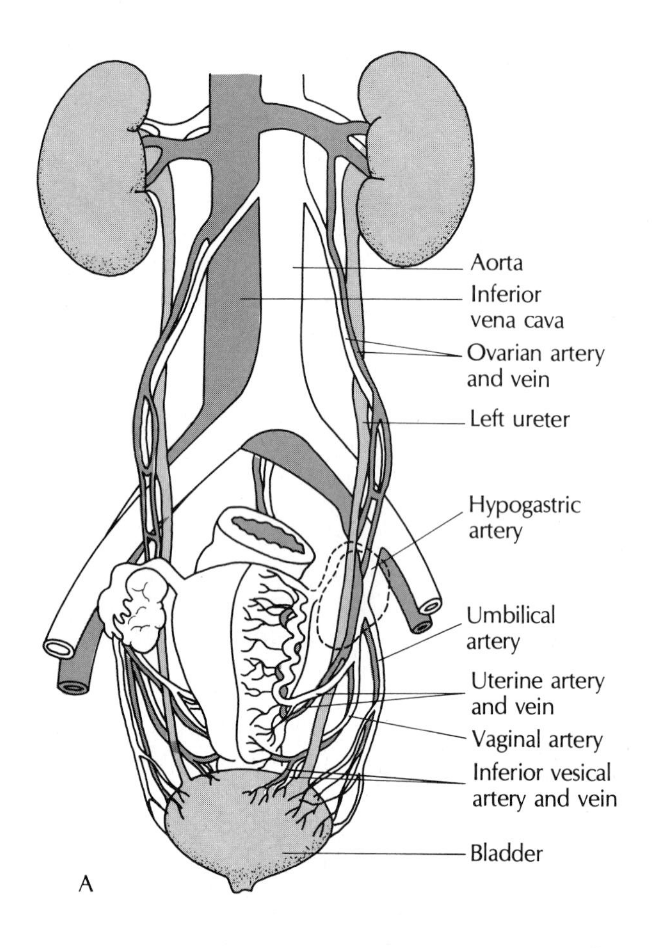

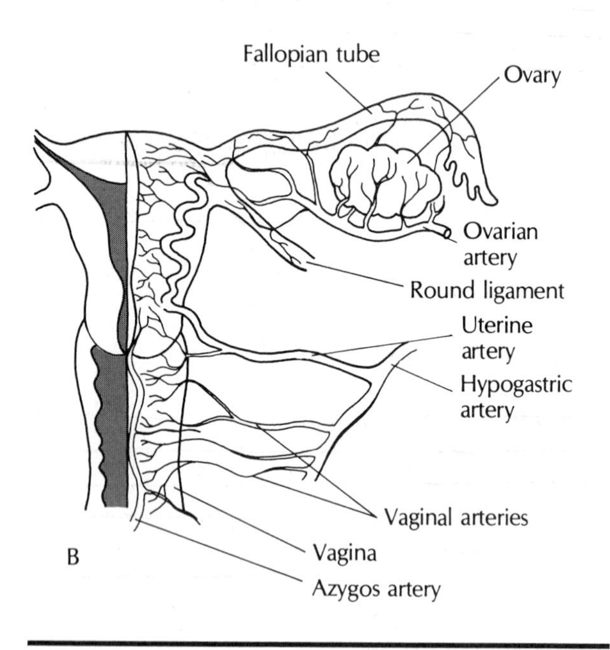

Figure 4–23. Blood supply to internal reproductive organs. **A,** Pelvic blood supply. **B,** Blood supply to vagina, ovary, uterus, and fallopian tubes.

der, over and around the uterus and extending uterine tubes, and down the posterior uterine border. Thus this double sheet of peritoneum, extending from the lateral margins of the uterus outward to the pelvic wall, enfolds the fallopian tubes and the round and ovarian ligaments at the upper border of the broad ligament. At its lower border, its fasciomuscular composition becomes more dense to form the cardinal ligaments. Laterally, beyond the uterine tubes, the broad ligament continues as the infundibulopelvic or suspensory ligament.

Between the folds of the broad ligament are large amounts of connective tissue, small amounts of involuntary muscle, blood vessels, lymph channels, and nerves. The broad ligament, with its specialized areas, keeps the uterus and tubes centrally placed within the pelvic cavity.

Between the tube and ovary in the mesosalpinx are vestigial tubules known as the *epoophoron* and *paroophoron*. They are homologous with the male structures of the epididymis and efferent ductules of the testicle. Parovarian or broad ligament cysts may arise in this area.

Round Ligaments. Each of the round ligaments arises below and anterior to the uterine tube insertion and courses outward between the folds of the broad ligament in a curved and tortuous manner, passing through the inguinal ring and canal, to fan out and fuse with the connective tissue of the labia majora. Made up of involuntary longitudinal muscle, which is continuous with that of the uterus, the round ligament hypertrophies during pregnancy. Although it shows signs of contractility and tonus, it probably does not contribute support to the uterus. However, during labor, the round ligaments steady the uterus, pulling downward and forward so that during the first stage the presenting part is forced into the cervix with encouragement to descend into the birth canal during the second stage (Bloom and Van Dongen, 1972).

Ovarian Ligaments. The ovarian ligaments are short, round fibromuscular cords that anchor the lower pole of the ovary to the cornu of the uterus. Structurally, the ovarian and round ligaments are the same and are homologous to the male gubernaculum testis. Although they begin as continuous structures in embryologic life, their continuity is interrupted by the developing uterus.

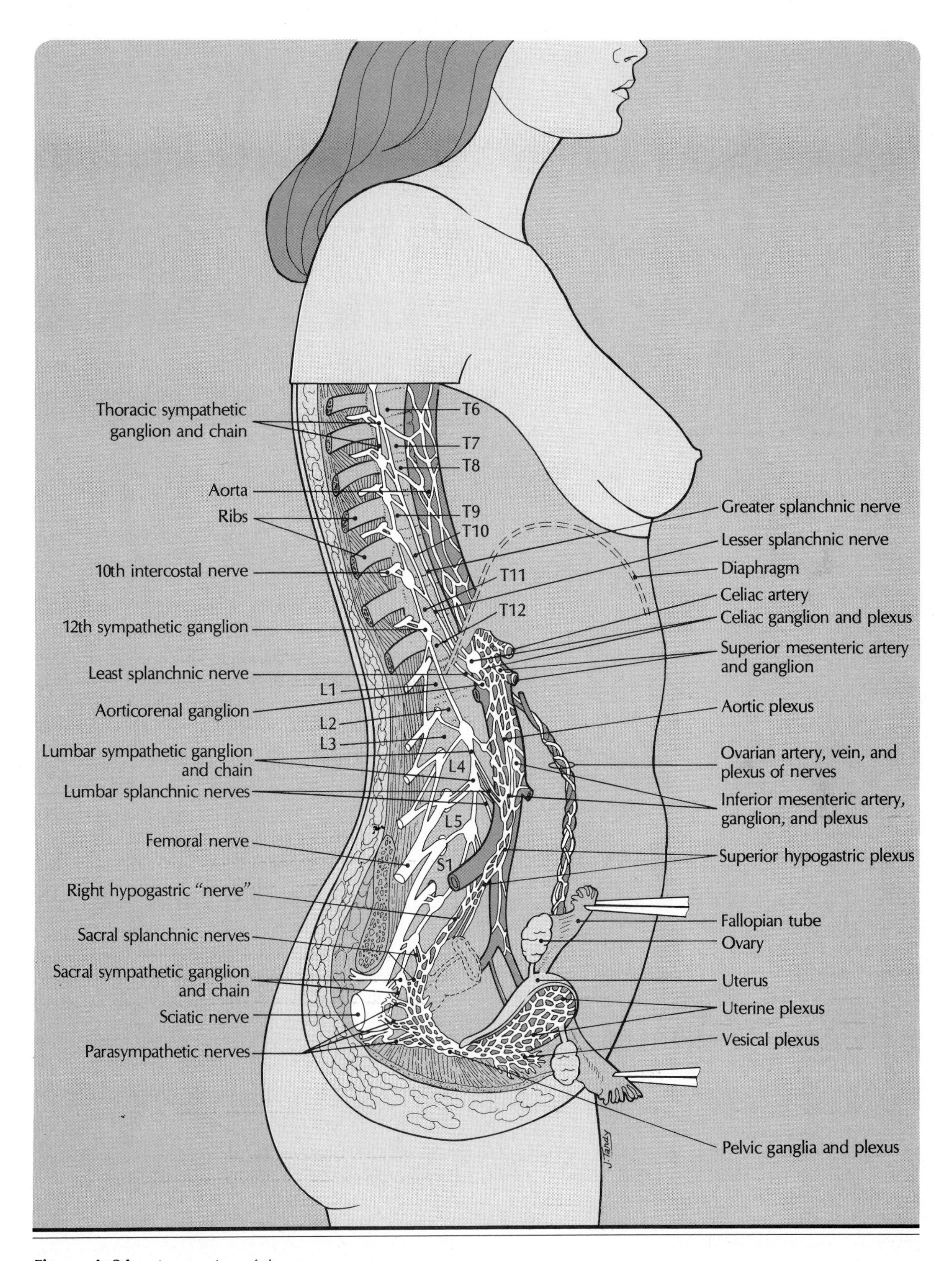

Figure 4–24. Innervation of the uterus.

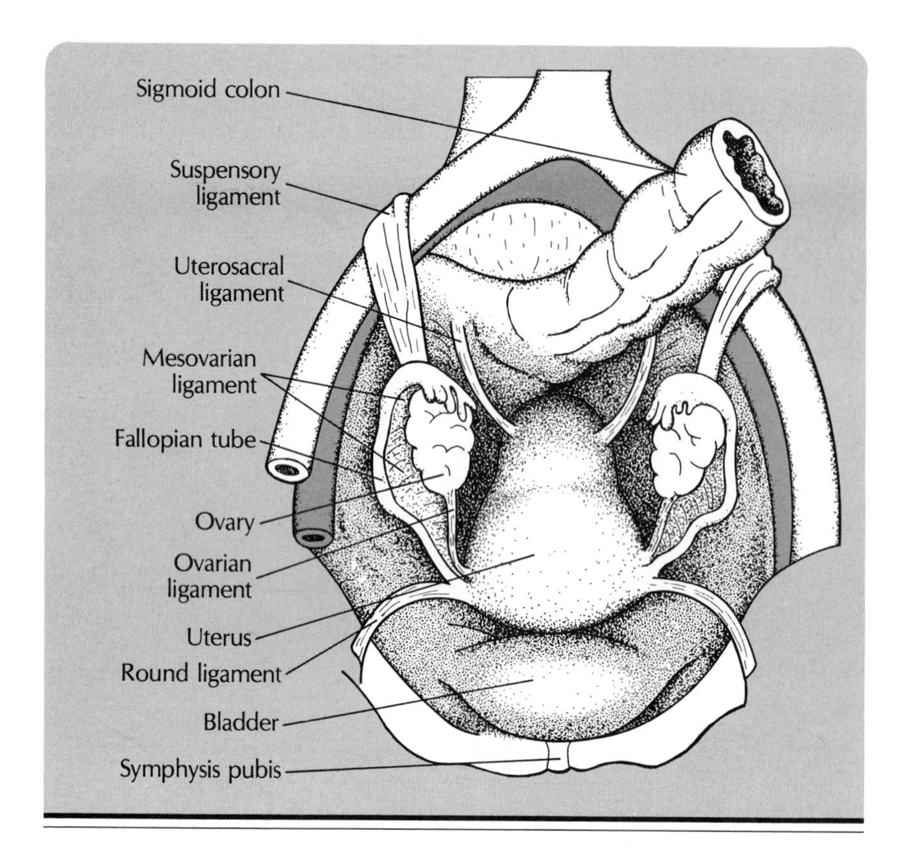

Figure 4–25. Uterine ligaments.

The contractile ability of the ovarian ligament allows it to influence the position of its ovary to some extent, thus assisting the fimbriae of the uterine tubes in "catching" the ovum each month as it is released.

Cardinal Ligaments. The cardinal ligaments, also known as *Mackenrodt's ligaments* or the *transverse cervical ligaments,* originate on the lateral pelvic walls and terminate in attachments to the lateral vaginal fornices and the supravaginal cervix. This thickened base of the broad ligament is continuous with the connective tissue of the pelvic floor and is made up of longitudinal smooth muscle fibers. It is the strongest band of the pelvic floor and the chief uterine support, suspending the uterus from the lateral walls of the true pelvis. It also supports the upper vagina.

Infundibulopelvic Ligament. The outer third of the broad ligament, extending from the fimbriated end of the uterine tube to the lateral pelvic wall, forms the infundibulopelvic, or suspensory, ligament. It contains the ovarian vessels and nerves and serves to suspend and support the ovaries.

Uterosacral Ligaments. The uterosacral ligaments arise on each side of the pelvis from the posterior wall of the uterus at the level of the internal os, sweep back around the lower third of the rectum, and insert on the lateral borders of the first and second sacral vertebras. These peritoneal folds make up the lateral boundaries of the pouch of Douglas. With the cardinal and pubovesical ligaments, the uterosacral ligaments make up a fibromuscular tissue support system extending from the pelvic wall to the uterus near the internal os.

The uterosacral ligaments contain smooth muscle fibers, connective tissue, blood and lymph vessels, and nerves. Providing support for the uterus and cervix at the level of the ischial spines, they also contain sensory nerve fibers that contribute to dysmenorrhea.

Fallopian (Uterine) Tubes

Derived embryologically from the paramesonephric ducts, the *fallopian* or *uterine tubes* (also known as the *oviducts*) arise laterally from the cornua of the uterus and progress almost to the side walls of the pelvis, where they turn posteri-

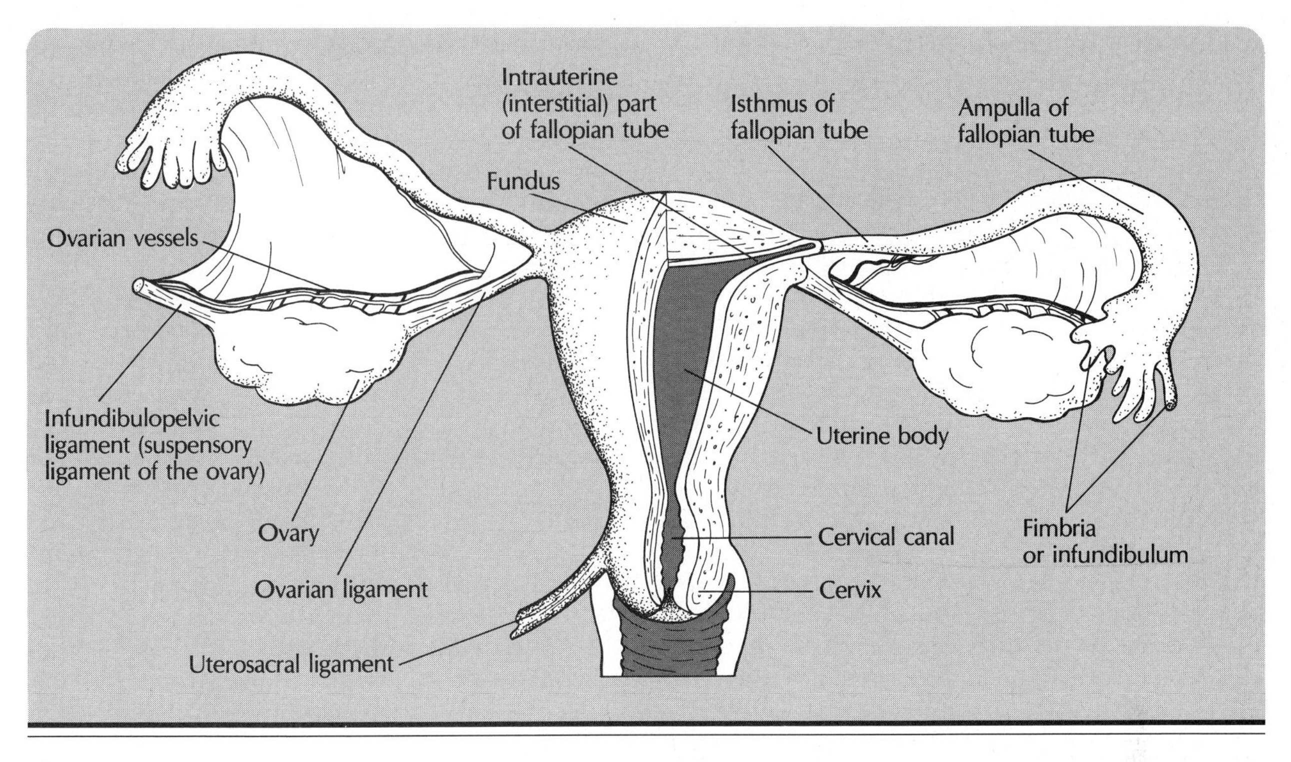

Figure 4–26. The fallopian tubes (oviducts or uterine tubes) and ovaries.

orly and medially toward the ovaries (Figure 4–26). Each tube is approximately 8–13.5 cm long, lying in the superior border of the broad ligament (mesosalpinx). These tubes are not inert, rigid structures; they are dynamic and restless, constantly seeking the ovum to be released from the ovary. The fallopian tubes link the peritoneal cavity with the external environment by way of the uterus and vagina, an arrangement that increases a woman's biologic vulnerability to disease processes.

A short section of each fallopian tube is intrauterine. Lying within the uterine muscular wall, its opening into the uterus (uterine ostium) is only 1 mm in diameter.

Each tube may be divided into three parts: the isthmus, the ampulla, and the infundibulum (fimbria). The isthmus is straight and narrow, with a thick muscular wall and a lumen 2–3 mm in diameter. It is the site of tubal ligation. Adjacent to the isthmus is the curved distal ampulla, comprising the outer two-thirds of the tube. Fertilization of the ovum by a spermatozoon usually occurs here. The ampulla has the widest lumen, and its muscular wall is thin and distensible. It terminates into the infundibulum, which is a funnellike enlargement with many moving fingerlike projections (fimbriae) reaching out to the ovary. The longest of these, the fimbria ovarica, is attached to the ovary to increase the chances of intercepting the ovum as it is released.

The wall of the fallopian tube is made up of four layers: peritoneal (serous), subserous (adventitial), muscular, and mucous tissues. The peritoneum of the broad ligament covers the tubes and becomes continuous with the mucous membrane lining the tube in the infundibular area. The subserous layer contains the blood and nerve supply, and the muscular layer is responsible for the peristaltic movement of the tube, created by the outer longitudinal and inner circular smooth involuntary muscle fibers. The mucosal layer, immediately adjacent to the muscular layer, is continuous with the uterine endometrium although less sensitive to hormonal cyclic changes. This layer is arranged in longitudinal folds, or plicae, which are few in number in the isthmus but increase in number and complexity in the ampulla to the extent that they extend beyond the ampulla as the fimbriae. The mucosal layer is composed of ciliated and nonciliated columnar epithelium, with the number of ciliated cells increasing at the fimbria. Nonciliated cells are goblet cells, which secrete a protein-rich, serous fluid that nourishes the ovum. The constantly roving tubal cilia create currents moving toward the uterus. Because the ovum is a large cell, this ciliary action is needed to augment the tubal peristalsis of the muscular layer. It is apparent that any malformation or malfunction of the tubes could result in infertility or even sterility.

In addition to physical problems, psychologic disturbances may influence fertility adversely. Bloom and Van Dongen (1972) report that a tense patient, with resultant autonomic nervous hyperactivity, may have spastic or tense fallopian tubes, causing reduced contractility and patency of the tubes. A well-functioning tubal transport system involves active fimbriae in close proximation to the ovary, peristalsis of the tube created by the muscular layer, and ciliated currents beating toward the uterus.

A double blood supply serves each oviduct. Branches of the uterine and ovarian arteries anastomose, creating a rich network in the mesosalpinx. Thus the uterine tubes have an unusual ability to recover from any inflammatory process. Venous drainage occurs through the pampiniform plexus and the ovarian and uterine veins. Lymphatic drainage occurs through the vessels close to the ureter into the lumbar nodes along the aorta.

Both parasympathetic and sympathetic motor and sensory nerves from the pelvic plexus and ovarian plexus supply the uterine tubes. The ampulla is supplied from ovarian branches, and the isthmus is supplied by the uterine branches. Pain arising from the tubes is referred to the area of the iliac fossae, because both areas are served by the same segmental skin innervation.

The functions of the uterine tubes are to provide transport for the egg from the ovary to the uterus; to act as a site for fertilization; and to serve as a warm, moist, nourishing environment for the egg or zygote (Chapter 6). The duration of the ovum's journey to the uterus is about five days.

Ovaries

The *ovaries* are two almond-shaped glandular structures lying on the posterior surface of the broad ligament, just below the pelvic brim and near the infundibulum (Figure 4-26). Their size varies among individuals and with the stage of the menstrual cycle. Right and left ovaries vary in size, weighing approximately 6–10 gm and measuring 1.5–3 cm in width, 2–5 cm in length, and 1–1.5 cm in thickness. During fetal life, they develop from the germinal epithelium of the urogenital ridge of the posterior abdominal wall and descend into the pelvis much as the testes do (Beller et al., 1974). The ovaries are small in childhood but increase in size after puberty. They also change in appearance: From a dull white, smooth-surfaced organ, the ovaries become a pitted gray because of scarring following ovulation.

The typical position of each ovary is in the upper part of the pelvic cavity at the lateral wall in a fossa created at the external iliac vein and ureteral junction. It is rare that both ovaries are at the same level. The ovary is connected to the uterus by the ovarian ligament, to the back of the broad ligament by the mesovarium, and to the lateral pelvic wall by the infundibulopelvic ligament (suspensory ligament of the ovary) (Figure 4-26). Blood vessels, nerves, and lymphatics enter the ovary through the hilum.

There is no peritoneal covering for the ovaries. Although this assists the mature ova to erupt, it also enhances the spread of malignant cells from cancer of the ovaries. A single layer of cuboidal epithelial cells, called the *germinal epithelium,* covers the ovaries. Three additional layers comprise the ovaries: the tunica albuginea, the cortex, and the medulla. The *tunica albuginea* is dense and dull white and serves as a protective layer. The *cortex* is the main functional part because it contains graafian follicles, corpora lutea, atretic follicles, and corpora albicantia held together by the ovarian stroma. The *medulla* is completely surrounded by the cortex and contains the nerves, blood and lymphatic vessels, and the rete ovarii (which develop into the testes in male embryos).

The ovary is a crucial component of reproduction. Even a small part of a functioning ovary will ovulate, providing an ovum for fertilization monthly. Every oocyte available for maturation within a woman's reproductive life is present at birth. No oogenesis occurs after fetal development. Close to a million oocytes are locked in the first meiotic division at birth. (See Chapter 6 for a discussion of meiosis and maturation of ova.) Because of follicular atretic processes, about 300,000 oocytes remain in a girl of 7 years, and about 30,000 are present at puberty (Bloom and Van Dongen, 1972). Almost 400 ova are actually extruded over the reproductive years. In spite of prepubescent bursts of pituitary activity that incite large numbers of follicles to attempt to ripen, they do not. The maturation of graafian follicles

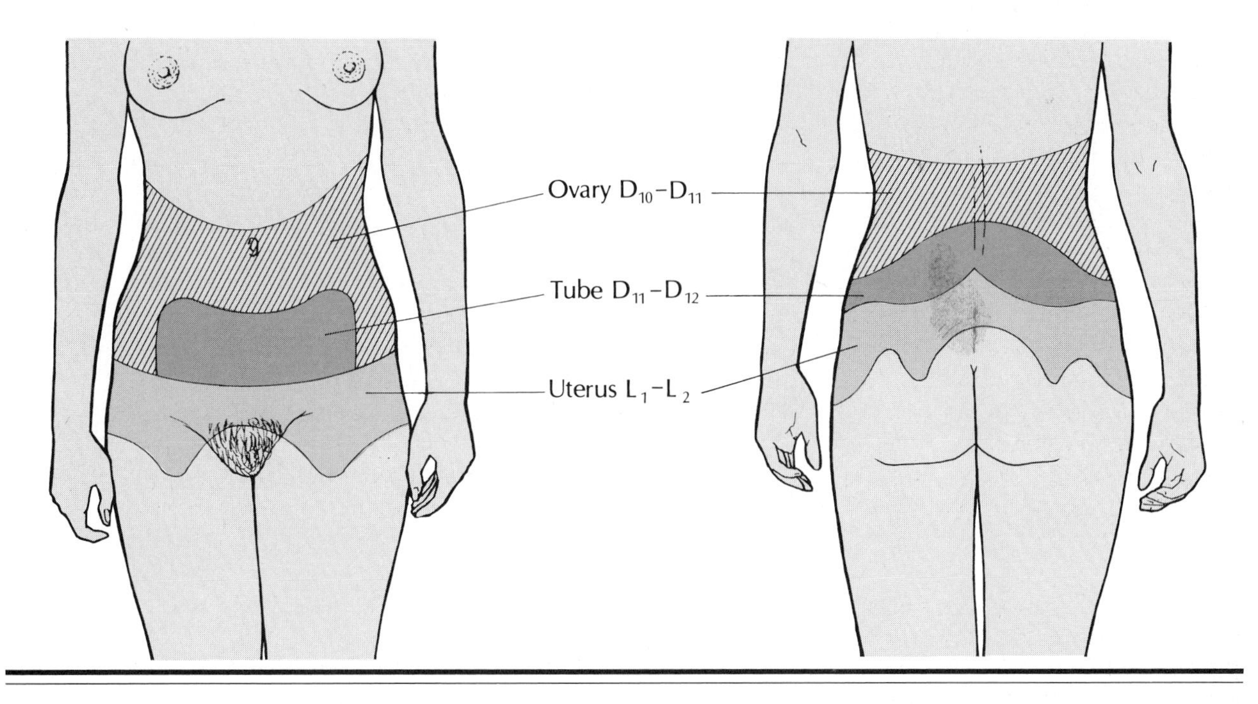

Figure 4–27. Location of referred ovarian pain. (Modified from Bloom, M. L., and Van Dongen, L. 1972. *Clinical gynaecology: integration of structure and function.* London: William Heinemann Medical Books Ltd., p. 175.)

and the release of a mature ovum are discussed in Chapter 5.

The motor and sensory parasympathetic and sympathetic nerves that accompany the ovarian artery from the abdomen transverse the infundibulopelvic ligament to reach the ovarian hilum. The ovaries are relatively insensitive unless they are squeezed or distended. Ovarian cancer usually originates in the germinal epithelium and is relatively painless (Bloom and Van Dongen, 1972). *Mittelschmerz,* or midcycle pain, is frequently noted and is due to irritation of the peritoneum caused by fluid or blood escaping along with the ovum. Pain can also be caused by follicular cysts. The location of referred ovarian pain is shown in Figure 4–27.

The singularly unique and vital function of the ovaries is to release a mature ovum monthly for fertilization (Chapter 6). When no more follicles remain in the ovary, resulting in the cessation of ovarian activity, usually in women in their mid-forties to early fifties, menopause occurs. Should this cessation occur in a woman in her thirties, it is called *premature menopause.* If sufficient viable follicles are not present in the twenties, gonadal or ovarian failure has occurred.

Breasts

Embryologically the breasts (mammae), which develop from ectoderm and mesoderm, appear about the sixth week of life along the mammary ridge. Although several mammary buds may appear on each ridge, only one develops. Solid cords evolve in the pectoral breast by the fifth month, and during the last trimester these cords become lumina, which ultimately are the chief ducts of the breast. Rudimentary acini are present at birth; the inverted nipple everts, and the areolar tissue is noticeable shortly after birth.

The breasts are considered accessories of the reproductive system and are specialized sebaceous glands known as *racemose* or *compound glands.* They appear in pairs and are symmetrically placed on the sides of the chest between the second and sixth ribs and the sternal edge and midaxillary line. Each breast, conical in shape, is separated from the underlying greater pectoral and anterior serratus muscles by a bed of connective tissue. The weight of each breast is about 150–200 gm (Goss, 1973). Occasionally a tag (tongue) of breast tissue extends into the axilla from the outer margin of normal breast tissue,

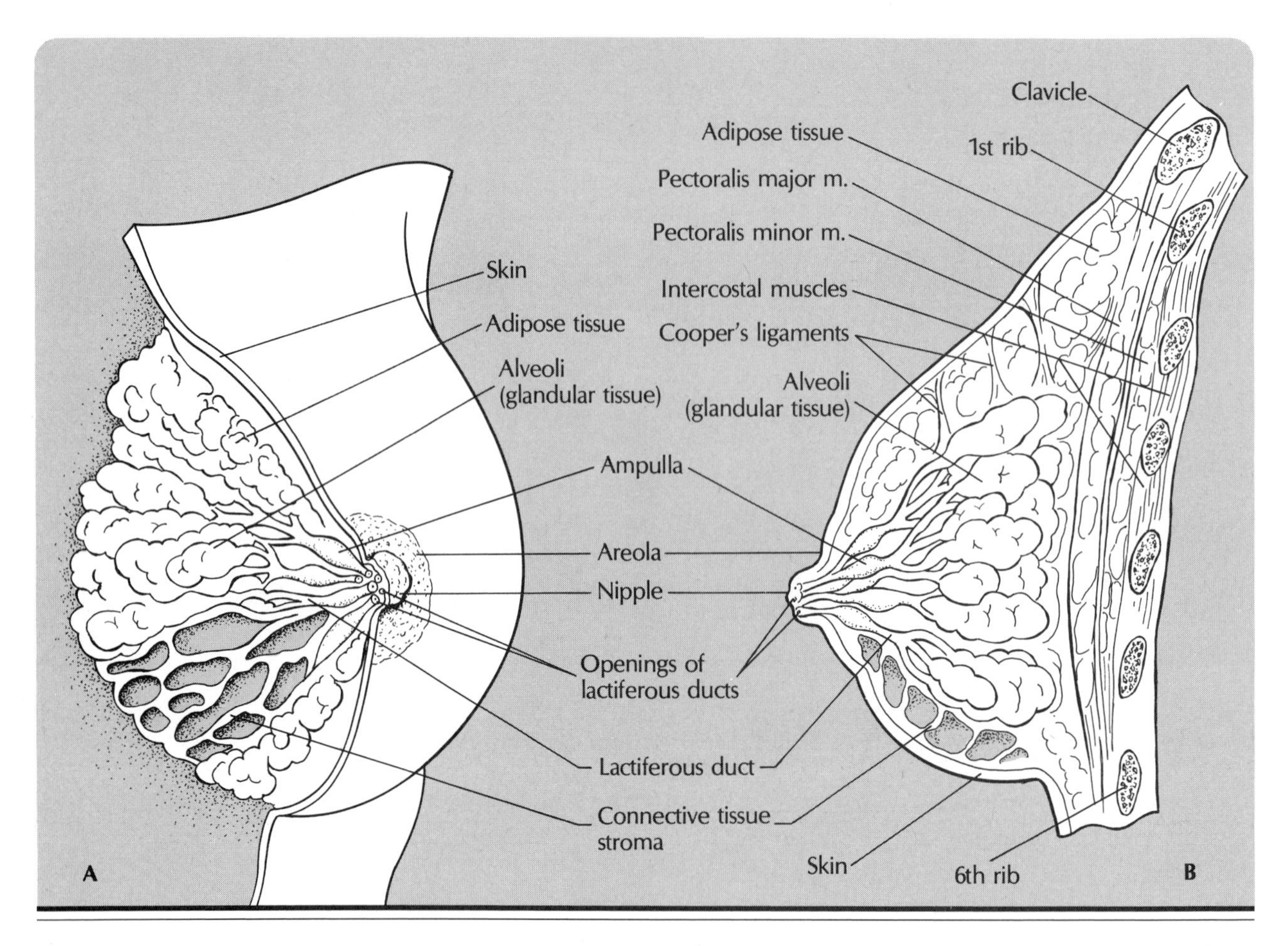

Figure 4–28. Anatomy of the breast. **A,** Anterior view of partially dissected left breast. **B,** Sagittal section. (Modified from Spence, A. P., and Mason, E. B. 1979. *Human anatomy and physiology.* Menlo Park, Calif.: Benjamin/Cummings Publishing Co., p. 774.)

called the *tail of Spence* (Donovan, 1977). Frequently, the left breast is larger than the right.

One or both breasts may be absent at birth (amastia), or one or both nipples may remain inverted or may be absent at birth (athelia). Supernumerary breasts may develop along the embryologic mammary ridges, which run in the midclavicular lines from the neck to the vulva. These extra breasts usually occur in pairs and are often small enough to be mistaken for moles but have distinct nipples. They also may occur in the axilla.

In the center of each mature breast is the nipple, a protrusion about 0.5 to 1.3 cm in diameter. The nipple is composed largely of erectile tissue and becomes more rigid and prominent during the menstrual cycle, sexual excitement, pregnancy, and lactation. The nipple is surrounded by the heavily pigmented areola, 2.5–10 cm in diameter. Both the nipple and areola are roughened by small papillae called *tubercles of Montgomery.* These tubercles are sebaceous glands that secrete a lipoid material during an infant's suckling that helps lubricate and protect the breasts.

The breasts are composed of glandular, fibrous, and adipose tissue. The glandular tissue consists of acini or alveoli (Figure 4–28), which are arranged in a series of 15 to 24 lobes. These lobes are in a radial pattern and are separated from one another by varying amounts of adipose and fibrous tissue. Fibrous tissues called *Cooper's ligaments* extend from the deep fascia overlying the chest wall muscles through the alveolar tissue and eventually fuse with the superficial fascial layer just under the skin. They suspend the breasts.

Each lobe of the breast is made up of several lobules, which in turn are made up of large numbers of alveoli in grapelike clusters around minute ducts. They are lined with a single layer of cuboidal epithelium, which secretes the various components of milk. The ducts from several lobules combine to form the larger lactiferous

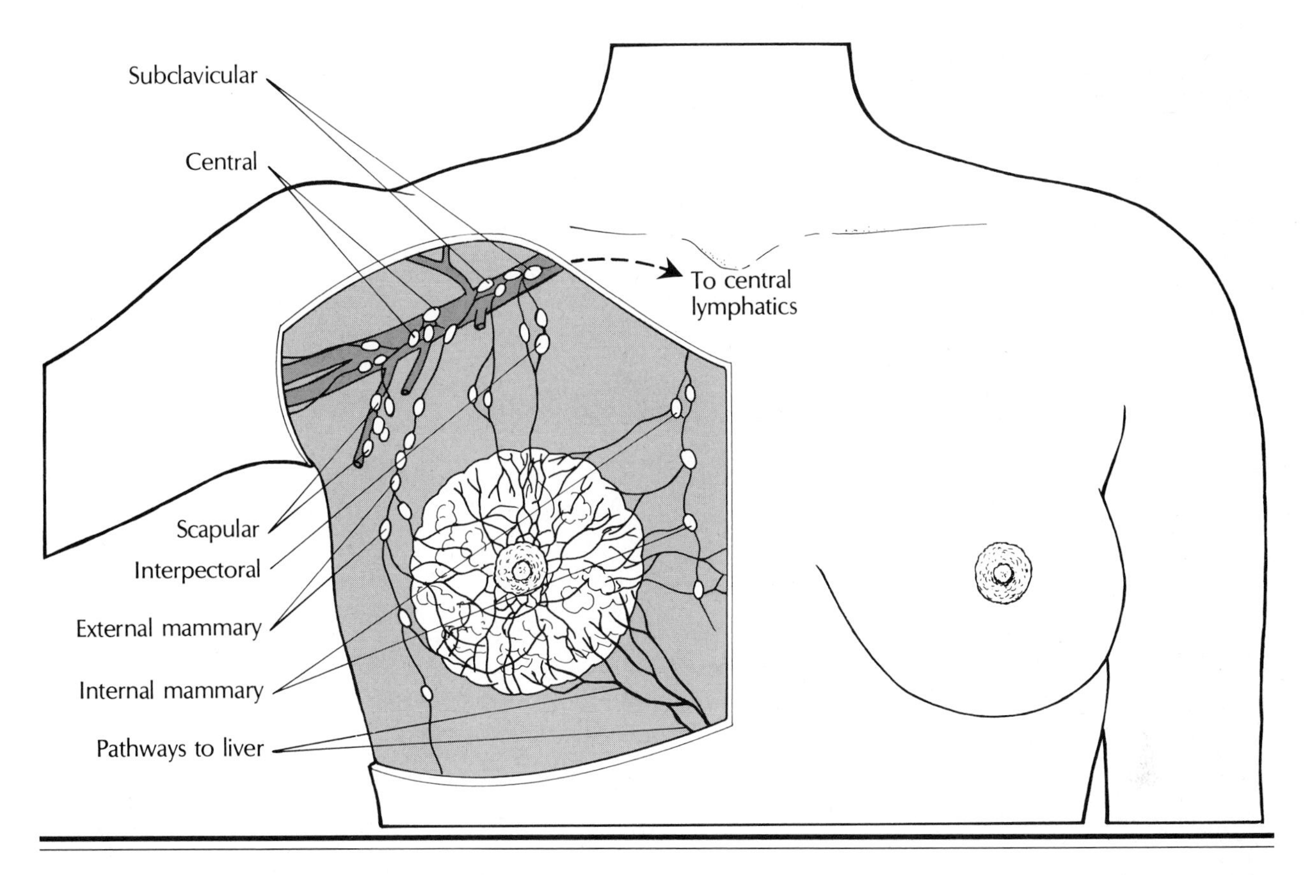

Figure 4–29. Lymphatic drainage of the breast.

ducts or sinuses. Each lactiferous duct opens separately on the surface of the nipple and may be seen as a tiny isolated orifice. The smooth muscle of the nipple causes erection of the nipple on contraction.

Cyclic hormonal control of the mature breast is complex. Essentially, estrogenic hormones stimulate the growth and development of the ductal epithelium. Progesterone, in association with estrogen, is responsible for the acinar and lobular development during the luteal phase of menstruation. In addition, adrenal corticosteroids, prolactin, somatotropin (growth hormone), and thyroxine are necessary for estrogen and progesterone to act.

The arterial, venous, and lymphatic systems communicate medially with the internal mammary vessels and laterally with the axillary vessels. Therefore, in cancer of the breast metastasis follows the vascular supply both medially and laterally (Figure 4–29).

The cutaneous nerve supply to the upper breast is from the third and fourth branches of the cervical plexus, whereas the supply to the lower breast is from the thoracic intercostal nerve.

The biologic function of the breasts is to provide nourishment and protective maternal antibodies to infants through the lactation process. Additionally, they are a source of much pleasurable sexual sensation. In the United States the breasts have become a sexual symbol; their size and sexual qualities receive more attention than their lactogenic functions.

SUMMARY

The miracle of life begins with the fusion of the egg and sperm in the woman's body and continues with the embryologic development of the zygote. This chapter has presented a discussion of the differences and similarities between the male and female reproductive organ development, blood supply, lymph supply, innervation, and functioning.

Many changes occur in the mother's body during the process of fetal growth. The foundation of knowledge necessary for understanding these numerous changes has been provided here through presentation of the embryologic development, anatomy, and physiology of the female and male reproductive systems.

SUGGESTED ACTIVITIES

1. In a small group discussion, explain the indifferent stage of embryologic development of the reproductive system.
2. During a classroom discussion, describe briefly the blood supply to the testes and the uterus.
3. During a postclinical conference, identify the muscles supporting the uterus and their importance during pregnancy, labor, and delivery.
4. Through a small group discussion, describe the different parts of the female pelvis and their implications for obstetric nursing.
5. During a clinical experience, determine the reason for low back pain with labor or cervical trauma.

REFERENCES

Beller, F. K., et al. 1974. *Gynecology: a textbook for students.* New York: Springer Verlag New York, Inc.

Benson, R. C. 1976. *Current obstetric and gynecologic diagnosis and treatment.* Los Altos, Calif.: Lange Medical Publications.

Bloom, M. L., and Van Dongen, L. 1972. *Clinical gynaecology: integration of structure and function.* London: William Heineman, Ltd.

Caldwell, W. E., and Moloy, H. C. 1933. Anatomical variations in the female pelvis and their effect on labor with a suggested classification. *Am. J. Obstet. Gynecol.* 26:479.

Donovan, A. J. 1977. The breast: anatomy, physiology and benign lesions. In *Rhoad's textbook of surgery: principles and practice.* 5th ed., ed. J. D. Hardy. Philadelphia: J. B. Lippincott Co.

Eliasson, R., and Lindholmer, C. 1976. Functions of male accessory glands. In *Human semen and fertility regulation in men,* ed. E. S. E. Hafez. St. Louis: The C. V. Mosby Co.

Ferenczy, A., and Richart, R. M. 1974. *Female reproductive system: dynamics of scan and transmission electron microscopy.* New York: John Wiley & Sons, Inc.

Goss, C. M., ed. 1973. *Gray's anatomy of the human body.* 29th ed. Philadelphia: Lea & Febiger.

Hafez, E. S. E., ed. 1976. *Human semen and fertility regulation in men.* St. Louis: The C. V. Mosby Co.

Jarcho, J. 1946. Malformations of the uterus. *Am. J. Surg.* 71:106.

Langley, L. L., et al. 1974. *Dynamic anatomy and physiology.* New York: McGraw-Hill Book Co.

Masters, W. H., and Johnson, V. E. 1966. *Human sexual response.* Boston: Little, Brown & Co.

Odell, W. D., and Moyer, D. L. 1971. *Physiology of reproduction.* St. Louis: The C. V. Mosby Co.

Oxorn, H., and Foote, W. R. 1975. *Human labor and birth.* 3rd ed. New York: Appleton-Century-Crofts.

Polakoski, K. L., et al. 1976. Biochemistry of human seminal plasma. In *Human semen and fertility regulation in men,* ed. E. S. E. Hafez. St. Louis: The C. V. Mosby Co.

Urban, J. A. 1977. Malignant lesions of the breast. In *Rhoad's textbook of surgery: principles and practice.* 5th ed., ed. J. D. Hardy. Philadelphia: J. B. Lippincott Co.

ADDITIONAL READINGS

Bailey, R. E. 1972. *Mayes' midwifery: a textbook for midwives.* 8th ed. London: Bailliere Tindall Publishers.

Bygdeman, M., and Wiquist, N. 1976. Prostaglandins in reproduction. In *Fertility and sterility,* eds. T. Hasegawa et al. New York: American Elsevier Publishing Co., Inc.

Crouch, J. E., and McClinitic, J. R. 1971. *Human anatomy and physiology.* New York: John Wiley & Sons, Inc.

Dawson, H. L. 1974. *Basic human anatomy.* 2nd ed. New York: Appleton-Century-Crofts.

Flechon, J. E., and Hafez, E. S. E. 1976. Scanning electron microscopy of human spermatozoa. In *Human semen and fertility regulation in men,* ed. E. S. E. Hafez. St. Louis: The C. V. Mosby Co.

Ganong, W. F. 1975. *Review of medical physiology.* 7th ed. Los Altos, Calif.: Lange Medical Publications.

Greisheimer, E. M., and Wiedeman, M. P. 1972. *Physiology and anatomy.* Philadelphia: J. B. Lippincott Co.

Guyton, A. C. 1977. *Basic human physiology: normal function and mechanisms of disease.* 2nd ed. Philadelphia: W. B. Saunders Co.

Hollander, M. M. July 1969. Hysterectomy and feelings of femininity. *Med. Asp. Hum. Sex.* 3:6.

Jensen, M. D., et al. 1977. *Maternity care: the nurse and the family.* St. Louis: The C. V. Mosby Co.

Kaufman, H. R., et al. 1975. Diseases of the vulva and vagina. In *Gynecology and obstetrics: the health care of women,* eds. S. L. Romney et al. New York: McGraw-Hill Book Co.

Novak, E. R., et al. 1975. *Novak's textbook of gynecology.* 9th ed. Baltimore: The Williams & Wilkins Co.

Pritchard, J. A. and MacDonald, P. C. 1976. *Williams obstetrics.* 15th ed. New York: Appleton-Century-Crofts.

Regenie, S., et al. Winter 1975. The self-instructional package: an educational resource, breast disease. *J. Nurse-Midwifery.* 20:8.

Reiffenstuhl, G., and Platzer, W. 1975. *Atlas of vaginal surgery.* Trans. E. J. Friedman and E. A. Friedman, ed. E. A. Friedman. Philadelphia: W. B. Saunders Co.

Romney, S. L., et al. 1975. Uterus. In *Gynecology and obstetrics: the health care of women,* eds. S. L. Romney et al. New York: McGraw-Hill Book Co.

Snell, R. W. 1973. *Clinical anatomy for medical students.* Boston: Little, Brown & Co.

Swanson, H. D. 1974. *Human reproduction: biology and social change.* New York: Oxford University Press.

Walker, J., et al., eds. 1976. *Combined textbook of obstetrics and gynaecology.* 9th ed. Edinburgh: Churchill Livingston.

Wynn, R. M., ed. 1977. *Biology of the uterus.* New York: Plenum Pub. Corp.

Ziegel, E., and Van Blarcom, C. C. 1972. *Obstetric nursing.* 6th ed. New York: The Macmillan Co.

CHAPTER 5

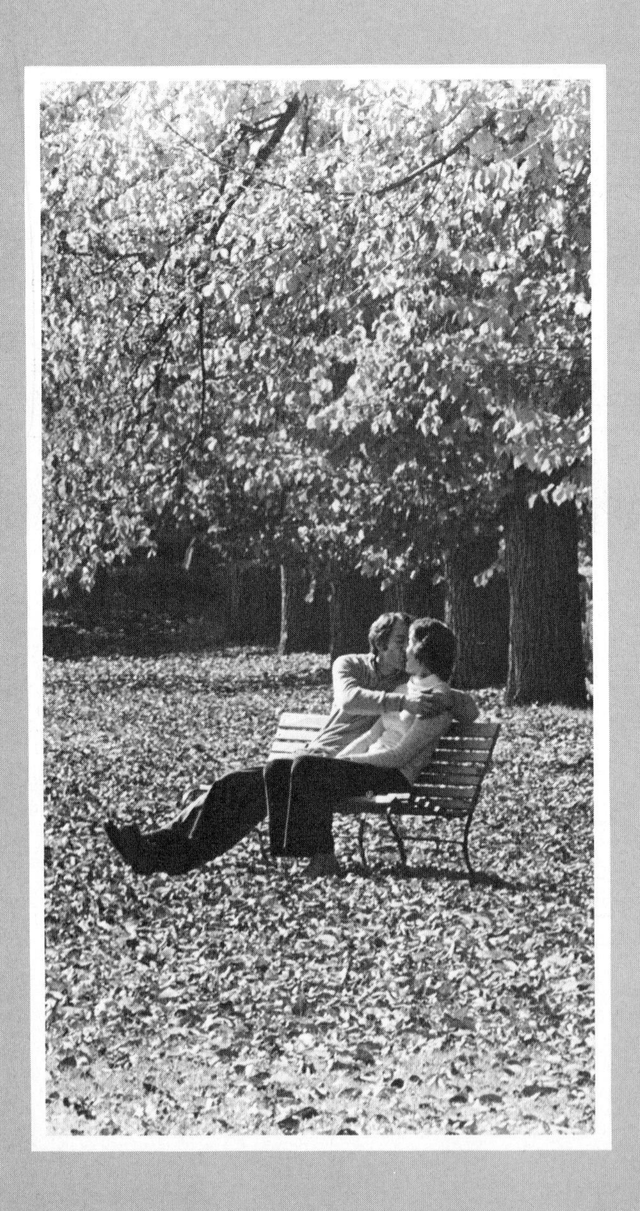

SEXUAL DEVELOPMENT AND SEXUALITY

OBJECTIVES

- Describe the components and development of sexuality.
- Describe puberty and the changes that the adolescent experiences.
- Explain the physical and psychologic aspects of the menstrual cycle.
- Identify the physical and emotional changes of the climacteric.
- Describe the physical and emotional aspects of coitus.

COMPONENTS OF HUMAN SEXUALITY

Sexuality is a dynamic force that is active throughout each person's life. And because its psychosocial and biologic components are intertwined and interdependent, sexuality is a forceful determinant of personality and behavior. Lief (1975) has developed a sexual system that emphasizes the pervasiveness of sexuality in our lives. The components of this sexual system are:

Biologic sex	Chromosomes; hormones; primary and secondary sex characteristics
Sexual identity (or core-gender identity)	Sense of maleness and femaleness
Gender identity	Sense of masculinity and femininity
Sexual role behavior	
Sex behavior	Behavior motivated by desire for sexual pleasure, ultimately orgasm (physical sex)
Gender behavior	Behavior with masculine and feminine connotations*

Biologic sex is determined at conception (this process is discussed in Chapter 6). A female embryo develops ovaries, and a male embryo develops testes. Generally, infants are born with clearly defined primary sex characteristics. Secondary sex characteristics develop at puberty. When primary sex characteristics are ambiguous at birth, the sex assigned to the child will be the determining factor in his ultimate concept of sexual identity.

Sexual identity (core-gender identity) is an individual's inner feeling of maleness or femaleness over a period of time. A child's sexual identity becomes firmly established by 3 years of age as a result of reinforcement of certain behaviors by parents and others (Lief, 1975). Sex-appropriate clothing (for example, pink-colored clothes for girls and blue for boys) and verbal reinforcers ("That's my big strong boy"; "That's my sweet baby girl") are among the most obvious methods parents use to assign sexual identity.

Gender identity refers to the broader, stereotypical ideas of masculinity and femininity. Traditionally, masculinity has been associated with courage, strength, stoicism, aggression, sexual assertiveness, rational thinking, stability, intelligence, and career achievement. Femininity has been associated with dependence, passivity, motherhood, tenderness, nurturance, and submission. Gender identity is learned over time through reinforcement. Self-doubts about gender identity are normal, especially during adolescence and middle age. Deviations in gender identity can lead to sexual behavior such as fetishism, homosexuality, promiscuity, or excessive competitiveness in nonsexual pursuits (Lief, 1975). Insecurity in one's gender identity may lead to poor adjustment with the opposite sex. Impotence may occur in the male; lack of arousal and response may occur in the female.

Sexual role behavior has two components: physical sex behavior and gender behavior. The act of coitus (sexual intercourse), physiologic responses, and sexual dysfunctions are all aspects of physical sex behavior; gender behavior is reflected in the sexual relationships between individuals. These two components of sexual role behavior do not stand isolated in life: they merge within the individual.

Many researchers are currently evaluating traditional sexual roles and relationships to determine what is biologically inherent and what is societally imposed. Some are questioning whether these sexual roles stifle rather than encourage an individual's quest for personal development and psychologic well-being. Many social critics promote the discarding of sterotyped roles; others encourage their modification. Unfortunately, the controversy about sexual role behavior has caused many individuals to become confused and disturbed about their sexuality and to experience feelings of inadequacy and lowered self-esteem.

*From Lief, H. I. 1975. Sexual counseling. In *Gynecology and obstetrics: the health care of women*, eds. S. L. Romney et al. New York: McGraw-Hill Book Co.

DEVELOPMENT OF SEXUALITY

The development of sexuality is modified and influenced by all life experiences—biologic, psychologic, sociocultural, and ethical. During the prenatal period, biologic sex is determined by the complex interaction of neurohormonal, genetic, and physiologic factors (Page et al., 1972). In addition, other senses and systems are developing that enable the infant at birth to react to sexual stimuli. For example, touch, which is fundamental in the development of sexuality, is highly developed by eight weeks' gestation (Berlin, 1976).

Tactile stimulation is essential for normal growth, development, and maternal-child bonding. Thus an infant responds positively to cuddling, holding, and touching. Adults demonstrate an identical need to be held, to be fondled, and to be physically close to a loved or cherished person. It should be noted that male and female children have traditionally been treated differently in our society with regard to physical affection. Males usually receive less tactile stimulation after infancy than do females, which certainly has implications for the development of sexual role behaviors.

Many sexual stereotypes are perpetuated by parents. Children's gender identity is established in part by the manner in which they are treated by parents and others, the toys they are given, the way they are disciplined, and the expectations others have for their behavior, education, and career. In addition, children are influenced by parental attitudes toward elimination, nakedness, and touching. A child senses parental embarrassment or reluctance to answer questions related to sexuality.

Sexual identity is also established by the functioning of the child's body. Male genitals are evident and responsive. Penile erections occur frequently, and masturbation begins early. Female genitals are less obvious, and the beginning of sexual feelings is more diffuse. For both sexes, the occurrence of puberty heightens sexual feelings and thoughts.

Adolescence finds sexually mature young persons trying to cope with new situations and sensations while they are still psychologically immature. Sexual experimentation begins in various ways. Masturbation accompanied by fantasy is prevalent. Homosexual experiences may occur in the form of exploratory erotic play, fondling, or bodily examination, and mutual masturbation for boys is not uncommon; but these activities are transient and do not signify a homosexual tendency. Heterosexual contacts range from initial kissing and fondling to mutual bodily exploration and masturbation to sexual intercourse. It is estimated that by 19 years of age, 45% of girls and 59% of boys in the United States have had coitus (Katchadourian and Lunde, 1975).

Adult sexuality has such wide individual variation that no average patterns can be formulated. New life-styles, changing morality, and effective contraceptive methods have separated sexual behavior from its reproductive function. Individuals engage in coitus for pleasure and do not necessarily remain with one partner. The new freedom is not without disadvantages. Unrealistic sexual expectations, exploitation of one partner by another, meaningless sexual contact, and overemphasis on sexual performance are some of the problems described by "sexually liberated" adults (Burt and Meeks, 1975). However, a majority of the people in the United States still equate love and sexual behavior and confine their sexual activities to one partner. For many, coitus within marriage remains the ideal (Burt and Meeks, 1975).

There is an unfounded belief that as men and women grow older they cease to be sexual beings. Perhaps this notion takes seed as young people observe the behavior of their parents and other adults, many of whom think that expression of sexual feelings in front of children is inappropriate. Children begin to believe that their parents and similar-age persons are incapable of experiencing passion and intense sexual urges and desires.

Many people view sexual activity among elderly persons as unseemly. Caretakers of the elderly in nursing homes discourage expression of sexuality among residents. The fact that sexual activity can and does continue well after the sixties (given an attentive partner and reasonable health) must receive recognition and planning. Positive attitudes toward the sexuality of the elderly as well as privacy for sexual expression should be encouraged.

PUBERTY

The term *puberty* refers to the transitional and developmental period that lies between childhood and the attainment of adult sexual characteristics and functioning. Its onset is never sudden, although it may appear so to parents or to the young person who is not prepared for the bodily and emotional changes of puberty. Generally, boys mature physically about two years later than girls. The average age of onset is 14 in boys and 12 in girls, although there is wide individual variation. The onset of puberty ranges in boys from 10 to 19 years of age and in girls, from 9 to 17 years of age. Puberty occurs over a period of time ranging from one and one-half years to four or five years and involves profound physical, psychologic, and emotional changes.

Closely associated with puberty is the period of *adolescence.* Adolescence is initiated by puberty and ends with the attainment of young adulthood. In our culture, it is equated with the teen years. Early adolescence begins one to two years before puberty occurs. Mid-adolescence is marked by behavioral as well as physical changes: Close identification with peer groups, rebellion against authority and parents, and increased interest in the opposite sex characterize this period. Late adolescence is associated with a more adult attitude toward oneself and one's life. This attitude may manifest itself in educational or career pursuits or in the search for a marriage partner and entrance into parenthood. The culmination of this stage is a unified sense of self (Schwartz and Schwartz, 1972). The ending of the adolescent period varies greatly and is influenced by the sociocultural and economic status of the family.

Major Physical Changes

In both boys and girls, puberty is preceded by a tremendous growth spurt. Widespread systemic changes occur, as well as maturation of the reproductive organs. One correlation between physical and sexual maturation can be seen: The broadening of the female hips and new distribution of adipose tissue and the broadening of the male shoulders and increasing muscularity of the body are associated with sexual maturation. These patterns occur prior to and during the maturation of the secondary sexual characteristics.

Although individual maturational patterns vary widely, usually males first note such changes as an increase in the size of the genitals; the appearance of pubic, axillary, and facial hair; the deepening of the voice; and nocturnal seminal emissions without sexual stimulation (mature sperm are usually not contained in the earliest emissions). Females experience a broadening of the hips, then budding of the breasts, the appearance of pubic and axillary hair, and the onset of menstruation. Table 5–1 summarizes the major developmental stages of puberty (Tanner, 1962). In Figure 5–1 the signs of puberty in females are correlated with age of onset.

Physiology of Onset

The specific cause of the onset of puberty is uncertain. However, it is known that onset is controlled by a neurohormonal regulatory system. The process is complex and sequential, involving several areas of the brain. The amygdala of the limbic system and the hypothalamus become involved after the individual reaches a certain level of maturation (Chinn, 1974). These centers are extremely sensitive to feedback information provided by levels of numerous circulating hormones, releasing factors, and inhibitory factors. The anterior pituitary and the ovaries or testes are part of this control mechanism, which initiates and sustains the hormones of mature reproductive functioning. The exact sequence of events is not yet known.

The hypothalamic nuclei synthesize and release *gonadotropin-releasing factor* (GnRF), which is transmitted by a portal system to the anterior pituitary. There it causes the synthesis and secretion of *follicle-stimulating hormone* (FSH) and *luteinizing hormone* (LH). Prior to puberty, the gonads do synthesize and secrete small amounts of androgens and estrogens, which are thought to inhibit production of GnRF. This inhibitory activity is decreased at puberty, and a new equilibrium is maintained whereby increased amounts of androgens and estrogens are required to inhibit the production of GnRF. Meanwhile, increased FSH and LH are released (Ticky and Malasanos, 1975). Figure 5–2 illustrates this feedback loop.

Other hormones are involved in the onset of puberty. Their action, although less direct, is essential. Abnormally high or low levels of adrenocorticotropic hormone (ACTH), thyroid hormone, or somatotropic (growth) hormone (STH) can cause disruptions in the occurrence of normal puberty.

Effects of Male Hormones

In addition to being essential for spermatogenesis, *testosterone* is responsible for the development of secondary male characteristics and for certain behavioral patterns. These androgenic effects include structural and functional development of the male genitals and accessory glands, emission and ejaculation of seminal fluid, distribution of bodily hair, and the hypertrophy of the vocal cords. The action of testosterone on the

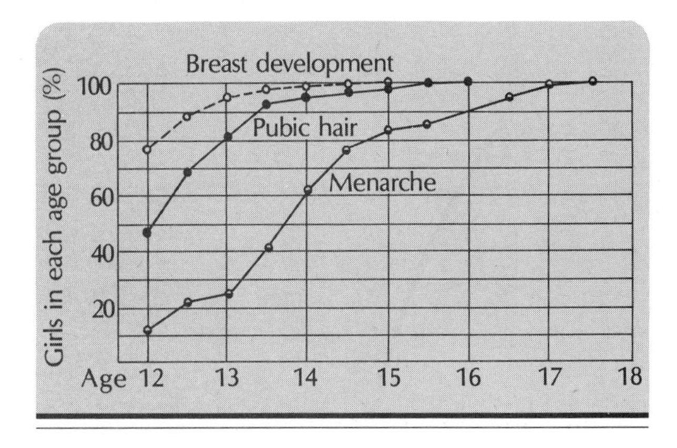

Figure 5–1. Signs of puberty in females according to age. (From Beller, F. K., et al. 1974. *Gynecology: a textbook for students*. New York: Springer Verlag New York, Inc., p. 69.)

Table 5–1. Pubertal Developmental Stages*

	Stage 1 (prepubertal)	Stage 2	Stage 3	Stage 4	Stage 5 (maturity)
Pubic hair (boys and girls)	No pubic hair	Sparse and fine at base of penis or along labia	Becoming darker, coarser, curlier, and more abundant	Adult in color and texture; small area covered	Normal adult male or female pattern; spread to medial aspect of thighs
Genital development (boys)	Penis, scrotum, and testes of childhood size and proportion	Testes enlarge; scrotum enlarges and becomes wrinkled and deeper in color	Penis enlarges in length; scrotum and testes enlarge	Penis increases in breadth; male glands begin to enlarge	Adult size, shape, color, function; no further growth; penis may decrease slightly in size
Breast development (girls)	Dormant breast tissue; everted nipple	Breast bud stage; increase in areolar size; small breast mound elevation	Continued enlargement of breast and areola	Projection of areola and nipple beyond countour of breast mound	Adult contour; only nipple projects
Menarche development (girls)	No menses; all primary oocytes dormant, locked in the first meiotic division	First menses occurs; usually scant and anovulatory; may be only spotting	Succeeding menses irregular in amount and interval; may involve dysmenorrhea, other physical complaints	Menses become increasingly regular in amount and interval; all internal genitals show cyclic changes	Adult cyclic ovulatory pattern established with consequent fertility

*From Tanner, J. M. 1962. *Growth in adolescence*. 2nd ed. Oxford: Blackwell Scientific Publications, Ltd.

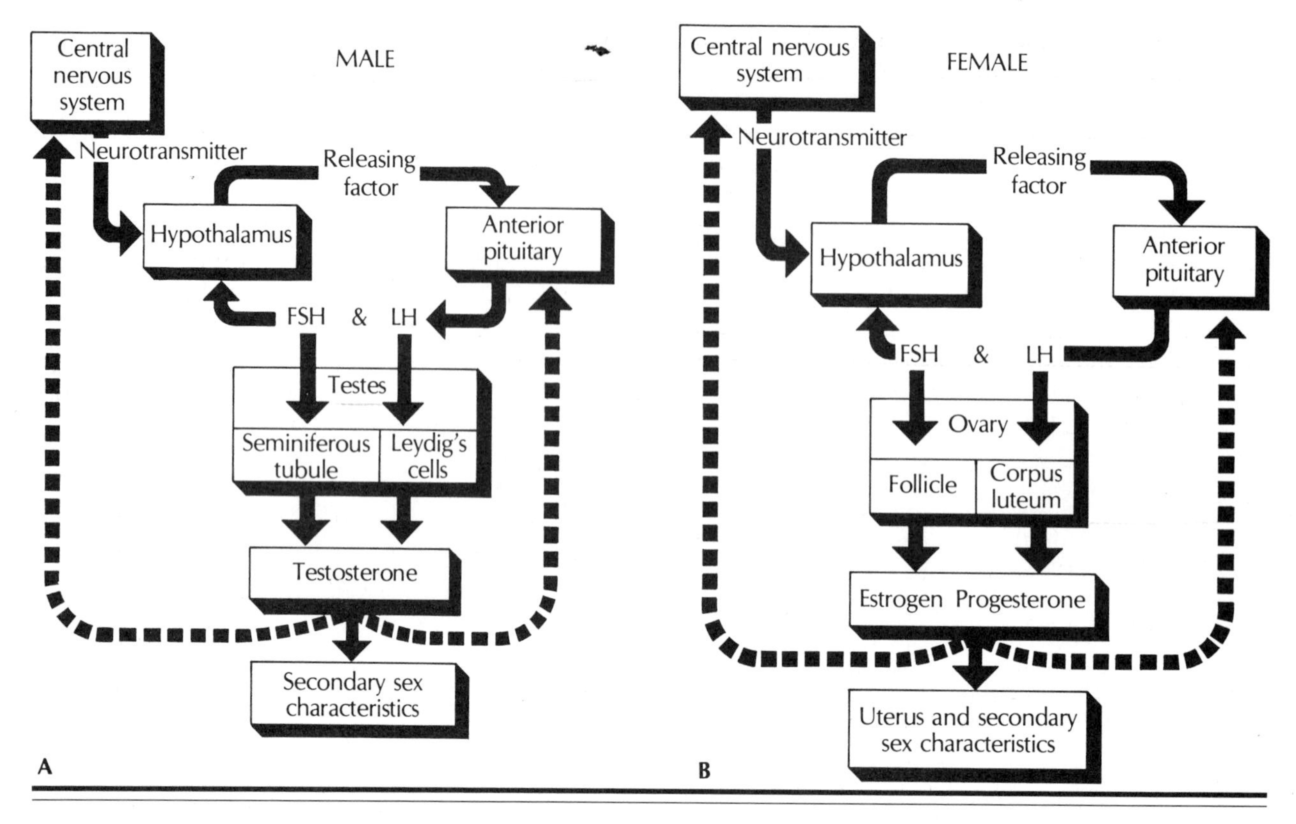

Figure 5–2. Positive feedback is illustrated with solid lines and negative feedback is illustrated with a broken line. Through a neurotransmitter, the central nervous system stimulates the hypothalmus, which in turn produces a releasing factor that causes the anterior pituitary to produce gonadotropins (FSH or LH). These hormones stimulate specific structures in the gonads to secrete steroid hormones (estrogen, progesterone, or testosterone). The increase in pituitary hormone production increases hypothalamus activity in a positive feedback relationship. The elevated steroid hormone levels stimulate the CNS and pituitary gland to inhibit hormone production in a negative feedback relationship.

central nervous system is thought to produce aggressiveness and sexual drive. Testosterone also stimulates the sebaceous glands' production of sebum, which contributes to the development of acne, and it assists in the lessening of subcutaneous fat deposits.

Anabolic activity of testosterone increases muscle mass, promotes growth and strength of the long bones, and enhances the rate of erythrocyte production. The resulting male characteristics of greater strength and stature, as well as a higher hematocrit than females, generally develop over a period of four or five years (Ticky and Malasanos, 1975). The action of testosterone is constant; it is not cyclic, nor is it limited to a certain number of years.

FSH, along with testosterone and the other androgens, maintains the spermatogenic function of the testes. LH supports the Leydig's cells of the testes as they synthesize testosterone from cholesterol. Testosterone in turn inhibits the secretion of LH by the anterior pituitary. Most of the circulating testosterone is converted in the liver to 17-ketosteroids, which are secreted in the urine. About one-third of these ketosteroids are metabolized from testicular testosterone; the rest is adrenal in origin (Sherman, 1971). See Figure 5-2,*A*.

In addition to the testes, the prostate and seminal vesicles are major target organs for testosterone.

Effects of Female Hormones

Having experienced menarche, a female undergoes a cyclic pattern of ovulation and menstruation (if pregnancy does not occur) for a period of 30 to 40 years. This cycle is an orderly process under neurohormonal control: Each month one ovum matures, ruptures, and presents itself for fertilization. The ovary, vagina, uterus, and fallopian tubes are target organs for female hormones.

Each organ undergoes changes indicative of the exact point in time of any menstrual cycle.

Like the testes, the ovaries produce mature gametes and secrete hormones. These activities are controlled by the continuous feedback system shown in Figure 5–2,*B*. Ovarian hormones include the estrogens (17-β-estradiol, estrone, and estriol), progesterone, and testosterone. The ovary is sensitive to FSH and LH. The uterus is sensitive to estrogen and progesterone. The relative proportion of these hormones to each other controls the events of both the ovarian and uterine (menstrual) cycles.

Pituitary Gonadotropic Hormones

The anterior pituitary produces FSH and LH. Generally, FSH determines the development of the primordial follicles through increased ovarian utilization of amino acids, electrolytes, and water. Thus the follicles mature—a prerequisite for the production of estrogens. Although FSH does not stimulate estrogen production directly, the event cannot occur without a mature follicle. It is LH that stimulates the follicle to synthesize estrogens.

There is a surge of LH prior to ovulation. The follicle changes into the corpus hemorrhagicum, which eventually becomes the corpus luteum. Under the control of LH and the anterior pituitary hormone luteotropin, or luteotropic hormone (LTH), the corpus luteum synthesizes progesterone. Thus both FSH and LH are necessary for the release of the mature ovum and for the ovarian synthesis of estrogen and progesterone (Ticky and Malasanos, 1975).

Estrogens

Estrogens control the development of the female secondary sex characteristics: breast development, the widening of the hips, and the adipose deposits in the buttocks and mons pubis. Certain characteristics, such as a high-pitched voice, occur because of low androgen levels, although the adrenal cortex supplies sufficient androgens to cause hair growth. The female pattern of hair growth is influenced by estrogens.

Estrogens assist in the maturation of the ovarian follicles and cause the endometrial mucosa to proliferate following menstruation. The amount of estrogens is greatest during the proliferative (follicular or estrogenic) phase of the menstrual cycle (p. 116). Estrogen also causes the uterus to increase in size and weight because of increased glycogen, amino acids, electrolytes, and water. Blood supply is augmented as well. Under the influence of estrogens, myometrial contractility increases in both the uterus and the fallopian tubes, and there is increased uterine sensitivity to oxytocin. The vaginal epithelium becomes thicker. More sodium and chloride are retained by the kidneys, causing mild edema and body weight increase. Estrogens inhibit FSH production and stimulate LH production. Clear cervical mucus is secreted.

Estrogens may increase libidinal feelings in humans. Estrogens decrease the excitability of the hypothalamus, which may cause an increase in sexual desire and contribute to so-called feminine behavior.

Although for many years estrogen has been considered a preventive factor for coronary artery disease in women, clear evidence for this seems to be lacking. Low estrogen levels do decrease serum cholesterol and β-lipoprotein and increase phospholipids and α-lipoprotein, but numerous other factors contribute to the development of coronary artery disease. Persistently high stress levels coupled with specific types of personality patterns seem influential in the current rising incidence of coronary artery disease in women (Friedrich, 1975).

Estrogens are metabolized in the liver to estriol and estrone, which are excreted in bile and urine.

Progestins

Progesterone is secreted by the corpus luteum and is found in greatest amounts during the secretory (luteal or progestational) phase of the menstrual cycle. It decreases the motility and contractility of the uterus caused by estrogens, thereby preparing the uterus for implantation after fertilization of the ovum. The endometrial mucosa is in a ready state as a result of estrogenic influence. Progesterone causes the uterine endometrium to further increase its supply of glycogen, arterial blood, secretory glands, amino acids, and water. This hormone is often called the *hormone of pregnancy*, because its effects on the uterus allow pregnancy to be maintained.

Under the influence of progesterone, the vaginal epithelium proliferates and the cervix secretes thick, viscous mucus. Breast glandular tissue increases in size and complexity.

The temperature rise of about 0.35C (0.5F) that accompanies ovulation and persists throughout the secretory phase of the menstrual cycle is probably due to progesterone. Traditionally, progesterone has been thought to cause passive behavior and to have a calming effect (Sherman, 1971).

MENSTRUAL CYCLE

Menarche—the onset of menstruation—occurs at approximately 12 to 13 years of age. A critical weight of 48 kg for menarche has been proposed (Chinn, 1974). Early cycles are often anovulatory and irregular in frequency, amount of flow, and duration. Within several months to two or three years, a regular cycle becomes established.

Menstrual parameters vary greatly among individuals. Generally, menses occur every 28 days, plus or minus 5 to 10 days. Approximately 60% of

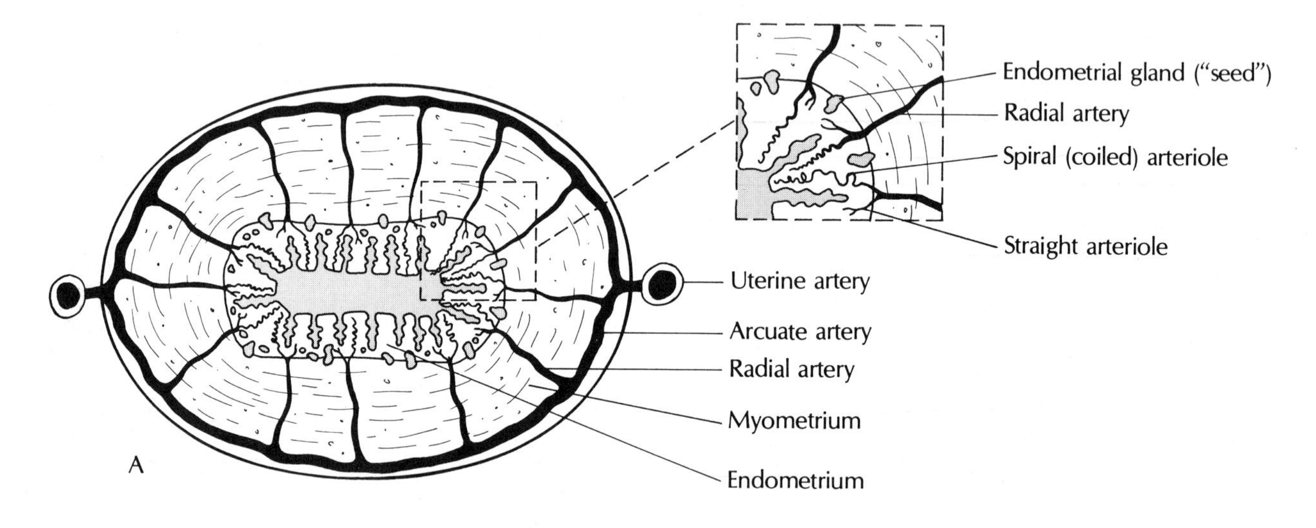

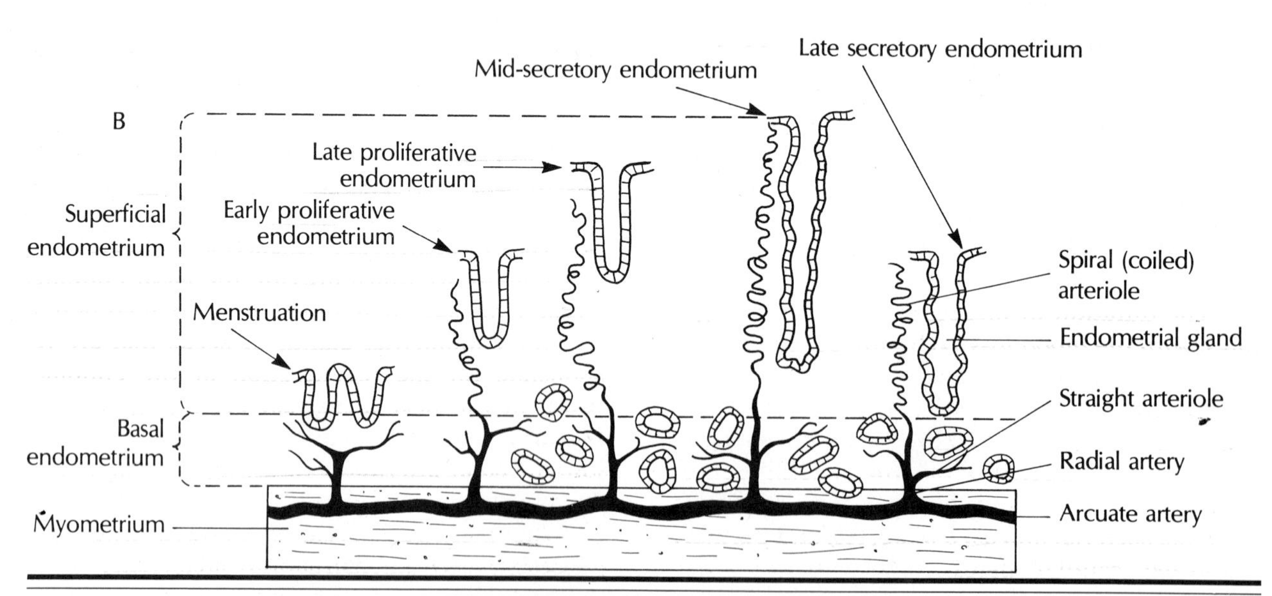

Figure 5–3. **A,** Blood supply to the endometrium (cross section view of the uterus). **B,** Schematic representation of blood supply during complete menstrual cycle. (Modified from Bloom, M. L., and Van Dongen, L. 1972. *Clinical gynaecology: integration of structure and function.* London: William Heinemann Medical Books Ltd., pp. 144–145.)

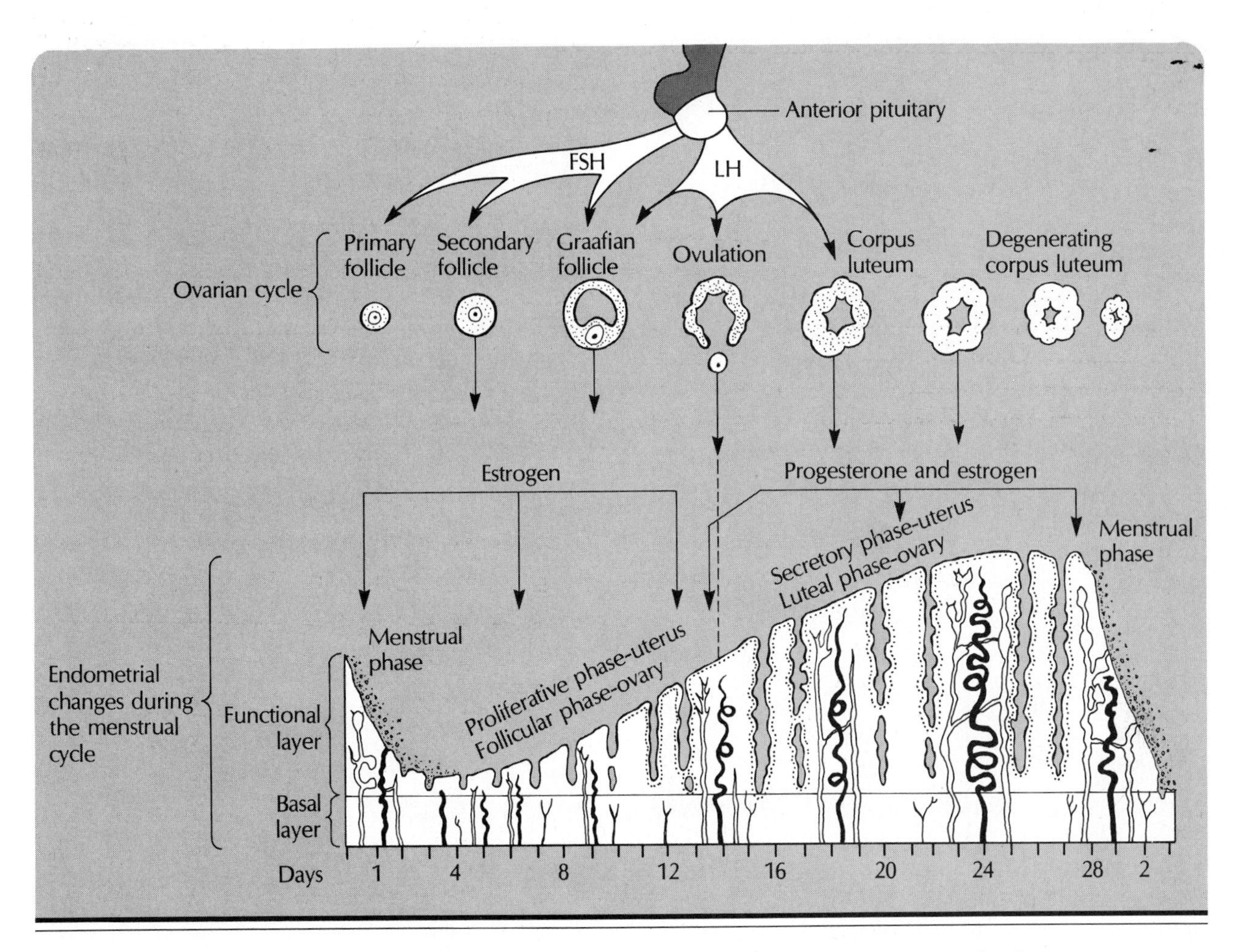

Figure 5-4. Changes in endometrium and ovary during menstrual cycle in response to hormone levels.

women experience menses every 25 to 30 days, but 1% menstruate as frequently as every 20 days or less and another 1% have periods 36 to 40 days apart. Emotional and physical factors such as illness, excessive fatigue, and high levels of stress or anxiety can alter the cycle interval. In addition, certain environmental factors such as temperature and altitude may influence the cycle.

The duration of menses is from two to eight days, with the blood loss averaging 30–100 ml and the loss of iron averaging 0.5–1 mg daily.

Menstruation may be defined as cyclic uterine bleeding in response to cyclic hormonal changes. The menstrual discharge or flow is composed of blood mixed with fluid, cervical and vaginal secretions, bacteria, mucus, leukocytes, and partially autolyzed cellular debris. The menstrual discharge is dark red and has a distinctive odor. It results from physiologic tissue necrosis caused by ischemia and anoxia of the endometrium. Menstruation occurs when the ovum is not fertilized.

A review of the endometrium and its arterial blood supply will provide further understanding of this process. Blood flow from the spiral arterioles in the superficial endometrium is reduced, with resultant ischemia and anoxia, which in turn produce necrosis and discharge of the superficial endometrium (menses). Concurrently, the straight arterioles provide the basal endometrium with sufficient blood flow to maintain it and the endometrial glands or seeds that are responsible for the regeneration of the endometrium in the next menstrual cycle (Figure 5-3). Bleeding is controlled by vasospasm of the straight basal arterioles, resulting in coagulative necrosis at the vessel tips.

The menstrual cycle is divided into four phases: *sloughing* (menstruation), *proliferative* (early and late), *secretory* (early and late), and *ischemic*. Days 1–5 are menstrual; days 6–13 are proliferative; day 14 is ovulatory; days 15–26 are secretory; and days 27 and 28 are ischemic. The proliferative

Know

Know

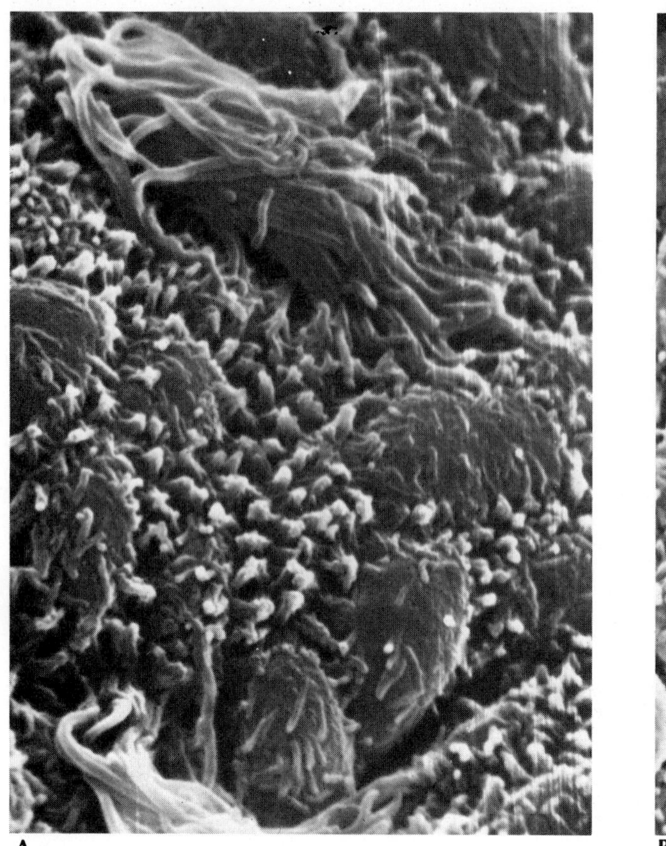

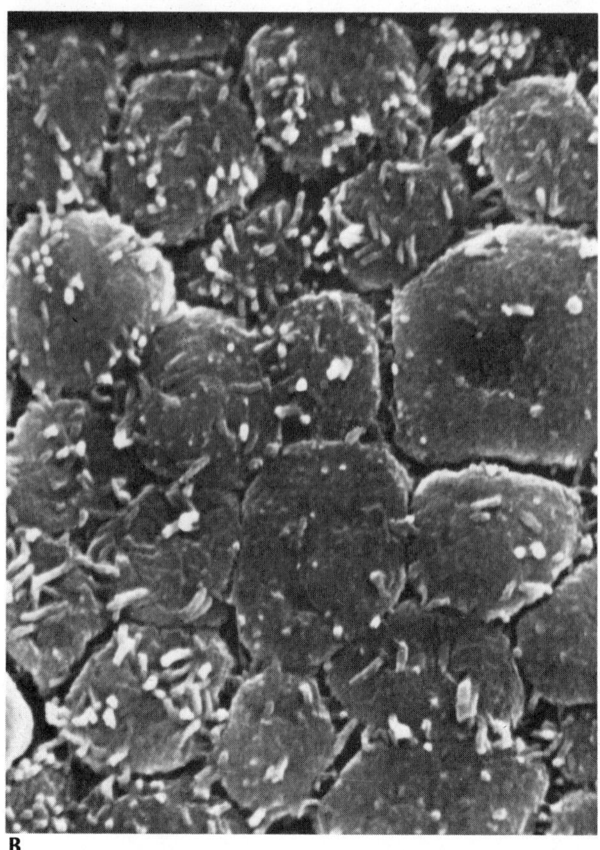

A B

Figure 5–5. Scanning electron micrographs of the lining of the uterus during different phases of the menstrual cycle. During the luteal phase **(A),** some of the cells have cilia and some are secreting droplets. The secreting cells are covered with microvilli. In the secretory phase **(B),** microvilli are still present on the surfaces of the secreting cells, but the general surface of the lining has a more lumpy appearance than during the proliferative phase, and the cilia appear shorter and less numerous. The named phases refer to the uterine condition at the time the photographs were taken. (Courtesy Dr. E. S. E. Hafez, Wayne State University, Detroit, Mich.)

phase is also known as the *estrogenic* or *follicular phase.* The secretory phase is frequently called the *progestational* or *luteal phase* (Figure 5-4).

Endometrial and Cervical Mucosal Changes

During menstruation and the sloughing of the functional endometrial layer, some of the remaining tips of the endometrial glands (seeds) begin to regenerate while other areas are being shed. Following menstruation, the endometrium is in a resting state. Its stromal cells are dense and compact, the epithelium is cuboidal, and the endometrial glands are short and straight. Estrogen levels are low. This earliest proliferative stage is a resting one. The endometrium is 1-2 mm deep. The cervical mucosa during this part of the cycle is scanty, viscous, and opaque.

In response to increasing amounts of estrogen, the glands hypertrophy, becoming tortuous and longer. The blood vessels become prominent and dilated and the endometrium increases sixfold to eightfold. This gradual process reaches its peak just before ovulation. Ovulation occurs in the presence of maximal amounts of estrogen. Subnuclear vacuoles have developed in the glandular endometrial epithelium. Under the influences of estrogen, the cervical mucosa becomes thin, clear, and watery, which is more favorable to spermatozoa. The cervical mucosal pH increases from slightly below 7.0 to 7.5 at the time of ovulation. The fernlike pattern of cervical mucus increases during the preovulatory phase, becoming full and complete and most pronounced at the time of ovulation. This fern pattern is a useful aid in assessment of ovulation time.

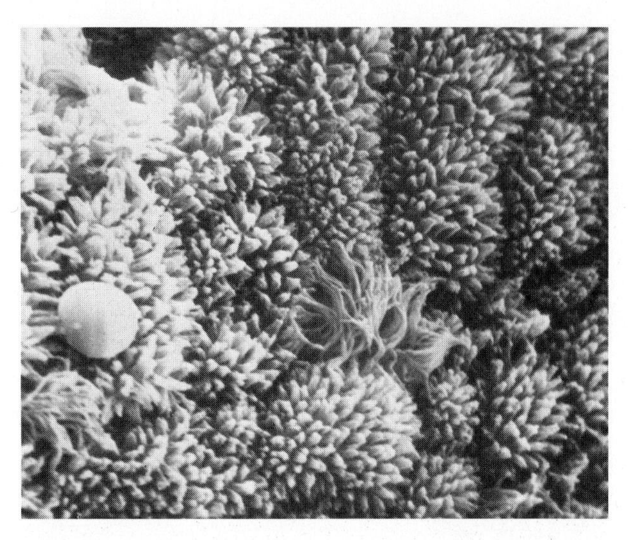

Figure 5–6. Scanning electron micrograph of the inner lining of the uterus at the time of implantation of the blastocyst. The blastocyst is an embryo at an early stage of development (see Chapter 6 for further discussion). (Courtesy Dr. E. S. E. Hafez, Wayne State University, Detroit, Mich.)

Following ovulation, the endometrium stops growing, and the glands begin to secrete (Figure 5–5). Endometrial growth is so pronounced that the epithelium is thrown into folds. This growth is in response to increasing amounts of progesterone produced by the corpus luteum. Increased amounts of tissue glycogen are present, and the glands begin to fill with cellular debris, become tortuous or like a corkscrew in appearance, and are increasingly dilated. During the secretory phase, the endometrium is prepared as for a fertilized ovum, providing optimal conditions for the protection and nurturance of the developing embryo. The vascularity of the entire uterus increases greatly, providing a succulent bed for implantation. Hypertrophy and hyperplasia of the myometrium occur. The postovulation cervical mucosa pattern is cellular, as progesterone appears. If implantation occurs, the endometrium, under the influence of progesterone, continues to develop and becomes even thicker (Figure 5–6).

If fertilization does not occur, the corpus luteum shows early signs of degeneration, resulting in withdrawal of both estrogen and progesterone. Small areas of necrosis appear under the epithelial lining. As the levels of progesterone fall, extensive vascular changes occur. Small blood vessels rupture and the spiral arteries constrict and retract, causing a deficiency of blood in the functional endometrial layer. The endometrium becomes pale. This ischemic phase is characterized by the extravasation of blood into the stromal cells and is followed by the menstrual flow. The basal layer remains, so that the tips of the glands can regenerate the new functional endometrial layer. These endometrial changes, as well as the ovarian follicular changes in response to hormone levels, are illustrated in Figure 5–4.

Ovarian Follicular Changes

At the beginning of the menstrual cycle, probably in response to the withdrawal of progesterone (and small amounts of estrogen), the hypothalamus produces GnRF. In response, the anterior pituitary produces FSH, which induces the growth and potential maturation of the primordial follicle. Within it, the oocyte grows. Follicular cells increase in number, and a fluid space (antrum) appears and increases in size. These changes occur during the proliferative phase in response to LH. LH increases gradually throughout this phase until just after the estrogen peak, when LH demonstrates a pulsating surge for about 24 hours. Under the dual control of FSH and LH, a mature *graafian follicle* appears about the fourteenth day. Figure 5–7 shows a mature graafian follicle in diagrammatic form.

In the mature graafian follicle, the cells surrounding the antral cavity are granulosa cells. The oocyte and follicular fluid are enclosed in the cumulus oophorus. The stromal elements of the ovary are condensed around the follicle in two layers: the *theca interna*, a vascular, hypertrophied layer; and the *theca externa*, an avascular layer of connective tissue. The theca interna cells resemble the luteal cells of the corpus luteum. The zona pellucida (oolemma), a thick elastic capsule, develops around the oocyte. The fully mature graafian follicle is a large structure, measuring about 5–10 mm. With maturity the follicle produces increasing amounts of estrogen.

Just before ovulation the mature oocyte completes its first meiotic division, in which the diploid number of 46 chromosomes found in somatic cells is reduced to the haploid number of 23. As another result of this division, the first polar body and the secondary oocyte are formed (see Chapter 6). This process is usually completed as ovulation is completed. It is not until after sperm penetration of the ovum that the second meiotic division occurs and the second polar body is formed.

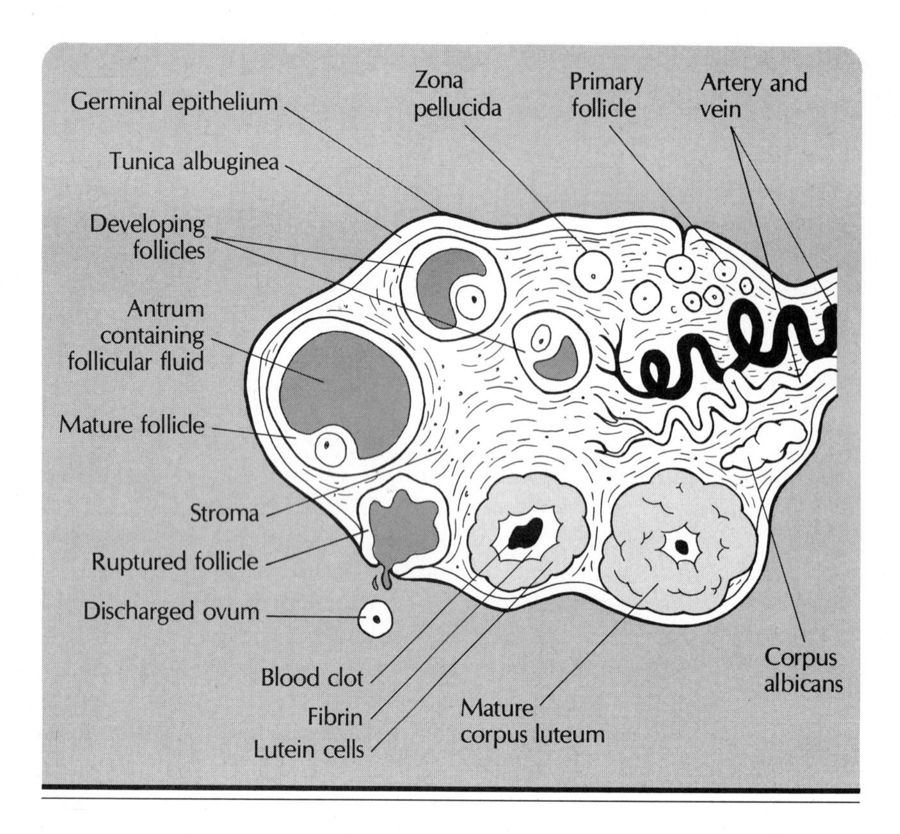

Figure 5–7. Various stages of development of the ovarian follicles.

Ovulation

As the graafian follicle matures and enlarges, it comes close to the surface of the ovary. The ovary surface has a blisterlike protrusion 10–15 mm in diameter, and the follicle's walls become so thin that its contents rupture out of the ovary. Thus the secondary oocyte, the polar bodies, and the follicular fluid are extruded. The egg carries with it the cumulus oophorus. Discharged near the fimbriated end of the fallopian tube, the egg is pulled into the tube and begins its journey through it. Occasionally ovulation is accompanied by midcycle pain, known as *mittelschmerz*, which may be caused by a thick ovarian tunica albuginea or by a local peritoneal reaction to the expelling of the follicular contents.

Vaginal secretion may increase during ovulation, and a small amount of blood (midcycle spotting) may be discharged as well. The body temperature increases around 0.5F at the time of ovulation or shortly thereafter and remains elevated throughout the secretory phase. There may be an accompanying sharp drop just before the increase. These temperature changes are useful clinically to determine the approximate time of ovulation (see Chapter 7). Ovulation is under complex hormonal control. Primarily, there is a marked surge of both LH and estrogen prior to ovulation.

Ovum transport is important to fertility. Because the ovum is thought to be fertile for only 6–24 hours, any delay in transport causes difficulty. Generally, it takes several minutes for the ovum to travel from the ruptured follicle to the fallopian tube opening. The contractions of the fallopian tube smooth muscle and ciliary epithelial action propel the egg through the tube. The ovum may remain in the ampulla so that it may be fertilized and cleavage can begin. It reaches the uterine lumen 72–96 hours after extrusion. By then, denudation of the cumulus mass is completed.

Under the effects of increasing amounts of LH, the corpus luteum develops from the ruptured follicle as a result of the luteinization of the granulosa cells. Following the disappearance of the antral cavity, the granulosa cells secrete steroids, primarily progesterone. Within two or three days the corpus luteum becomes yellowish and spherical and increases in vascularity. LTH governs the further changes of the corpus luteum. If the ovum is fertilized, followed by implantation of the resultant blastocyst in the endometrium, the blastocyst begins to secrete human chorionic gonadotropin (HCG), which is needed to maintain the corpus luteum. If fertilization does not occur within eight days after ovulation, the corpus luteum begins to degenerate and becomes the corpus albicans, which has a dull white appearance. Approximately 14 days after ovulation (in a 28-day cycle), in the absence of pregnancy, menstruation begins again.

Premenstrual Tension

In response to the sustained progesterone levels of the secretory phase, many women report a cluster of symptoms known as *premenstrual tension.* Symptoms include weight gain of 1-3 pounds, fatigue, backache, headache, a feeling of fullness in the pelvis, and enlarged and tender breasts. With these physical symptoms comes a predisposition toward irritability, loss of emotional equilibrium, and depression. Although this syndrome seems to be based more on empirical reports rather than on controlled physiologic studies, its management may include restriction of salt, increased rest balanced with increased exercise, and the prescription of mild diuretics or tranquilizers. An empathetic relationship with a health professional to freely discuss patient concerns is highly beneficial. With or without treatment, women report that the occurrence of menstruation removes all symptoms. It is likely that premenstrual tension is related to other personality and physical traits.

Bleeding Variations

Amenorrhea is the absence of menses. The most common cause is pregnancy, but other causes include emotional disturbances, lactation, debilitating disease, and malnutrition. Other causes of amenorrhea include congenital absence of the fallopian tubes, ovaries, uterus, or patent vagina, and a genetic abnormality causing hormonal imbalance.

An abnormally short menstrual cycle is termed *hypomenorrhea;* an abnormally long one is *hypermenorrhea.* Excessive, profuse flow is called *menorrhagia,* and bleeding between periods is known as *metrorrhagia.* Infrequent and too frequent menses are termed *oligomenorrhea* and *polymenorrhea,* respectively. Figure 5-8 graphically illustrates dysfunctional uterine bleeding. Such irregularities should be investigated to rule out any disease process.

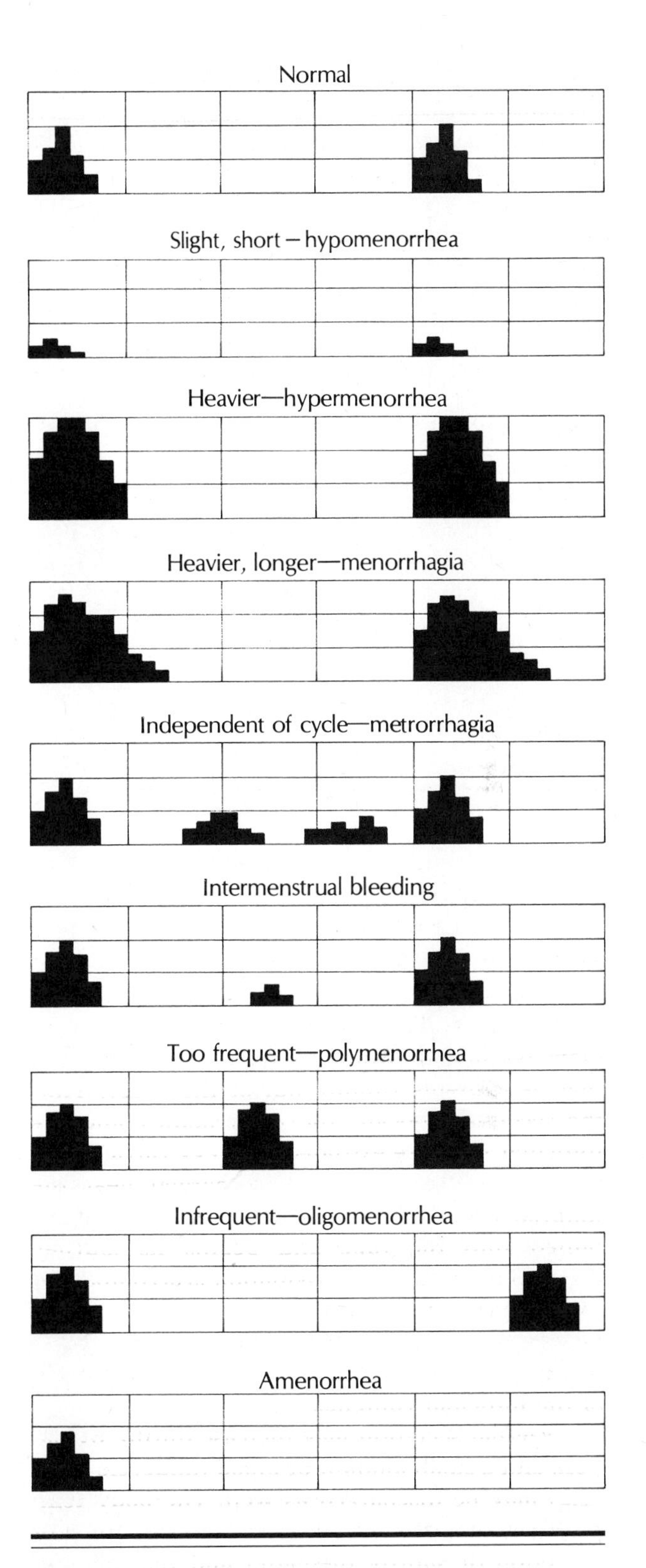

Figure 5-8. Dysfunctional uterine bleeding. (From Beller, F. K., et al. 1974. *Gynecology: a textbook for students.* New York: Springer Verlag New York, Inc., p. 142.)

Dysmenorrhea

Dysmenorrhea means painful menstruation. Primary dysmenorrhea usually appears two or three years after menarche, lasts for the first day of flow, and is absent when ovulation does not occur. This condition is most often physiologic in origin. Hypercontractility of the uterus (and the gastrointestinal tract as well) may be caused by excessive prostaglandin F_2. Treatment of physiologic primary dysmenorrhea includes hormonal therapy, dilatation of the cervix, and aspirin and codeine (Friedrich, 1975).

Dysmenorrhea may be psychologic in origin, resulting from an inability or unwillingness to cope with the sexual and reproductive meanings of the menses. Depending on the degree of conflict within the woman, some form of long-term counseling or psychotherapy may be needed to help uncover such feelings.

Secondary dysmenorrhea is caused by pelvic pathologic conditions such as congenital uterine anomalies or an imperforate hymen. Dysmenorrhea accompanies submucous myomas, intrauterine or intracervical polyps, endometriosis, and acute or chronic pelvic infection.

CLIMACTERIC

The *climacteric* is thought to occur in both men and women. It is commonly called the *change of life*. In women, it is associated with *menopause*, or cessation of menstruation, and with distinct hormonal changes leading to the inability to bear children. In men, there are no identifiable physical signs, and the vasomotor and psychologic disturbances reported in men age 45 to 52 may simply reflect a developmental crisis over the aging process. Therefore, the following discussion of the climacteric will be limited to the occurrence of menopause in women.

Psychologic Aspects of Menopause

Menopause is to the climacteric as menarche is to puberty—one indication of a larger, complex process. In addition to the normal physiologic cessation of ovarian function in women at about the age of 50, menopause can appear prematurely or can be surgically induced. Menopause is a turning point in any woman's life because it marks the end of her reproductive function—a meaningful event for a woman whether or not she has borne children.

More than at any other time, a woman's past, present, and future merge into one. She looks back on her life, with its accomplishments, disappointments, and limitations. She assesses her relationships with those she is close to, which may include a husband who is facing a developmental crisis; children who are leaving home and making life choices; and parents who are aged, ill, or facing death. Responsibilities may be heavy; conflicts between generations may be painful; satisfactions with oneself may be minimal. To this present, the uncertainty of the future is added: possible declining health, loss of physical beauty, and finally death. Clearly, adequate coping mechanisms and support systems are necessary for a woman to resolve this developmental crisis satisfactorily and to experience personal growth.

Physical Aspects of Menopause

The physical aspects of menopause are difficult to distinguish clearly, because subjective symptoms reported by women are much more extensive than those documented in the literature. However, certain physical findings are significant.

Menopause usually occurs between 45 and 52 years of age. The age of onset may be influenced by nutritional, cultural, or genetic factors. The physiologic mechanisms initiating its onset are not known.

Generally, ovulation ceases one or two years prior to menopause. However, individual variation does exist; as much as six to eight years of transition prior to menopause has been noted. There is some evidence of corpus luteal inadequacy as seen by changes in progesterone levels and basal body temperature (Friedrich, 1975). The change is usually gradual, and normal menstrual irregularities do not include menorrhagia or metrorrhagia. Atrophy of the ovaries occurs gradually; FSH levels rise permanently. The increased incidence of Down's syndrome in infants of mothers over 40 years of age is attributed to the lowered quality of the ova produced.

Contrary to popular thought, low levels of estrogen are maintained in about 40% of postmenopausal women. Estrone, produced by the adrenal glands, is the chief circulating estrogen.

The uterine endometrium and myometrium atrophy, as do the cervical glands. The uterine cavity becomes stenosed. The fallopian tubes atrophy extensively. The vaginal mucosa becomes smooth and thin and the rugae disappear, leading to loss of elasticity. As a result, painful intercourse, or dyspareunia, may occur. Dryness of the mucous membrane can lead to burning and itching. Vaginal pH increases as the number of Döderlein's bacilli decreases.

Vulval atrophy occurs late, and the pubic hair thins, turns gray or white, and may ultimately disappear. The labia shrivel and lose their heightened pigmentation. Pelvic fascia and muscles atrophy, resulting in decreased pelvic support. The breasts become pendulous and decrease in size and firmness.

These changes in the reproductive organs influence coital activity but in no way necessitate a decrease in its occurrence or enjoyment. In fact, sexual activity may increase at this time, as the need for contraception disappears and personal growth and awareness increase. The notion that sexual interest and activity decrease as a natural correlate of the aging process is a myth. Individual variations occur, but one's sexuality persists as long as one lives, although its expression may be limited by lack of a partner or of privacy.

In most menopausal women, certain vasomotor disturbances occur that are clearly related to the cessation of menstruation and to hormonal changes. Although the physiologic mechanism has not yet been clearly delineated, 75% of women report symptoms of heat arising on the chest and spreading to the neck and face, sweating (mild to drenching), and occasional chills. This cluster of symptoms is often referred to as *hot flashes.* There may be 20 to 30 of these a day, lasting three to five minutes. Dizzy spells, palpitations, and weakness are also reported.

Long-range physical changes may include osteoporosis, a decrease in the bony skeletal mass. The bones become more brittle and thus can more easily be broken. This change is thought to occur in association with lowered estrogen and androgen levels, lack of physical exercise, and a chronic low intake of calcium. The occurrence of diabetes mellitus increases at this age. Loss of protein from the skin and supportive tissues causes wrinkling. Frequently, postmenopausal women gain weight, which may be due to excessive caloric intake rather than to a change in adipose deposits.

Endocrine changes include a decrease in the steroid hormones produced by the ovary, and decreased estrogen levels cause the anterior pituitary to produce more FSH. The underlying causes of such endocrine changes are not clear.

Interventions

Until recently, menopausal symptoms were commonly treated with supplementary estrogen. However, estrogen therapy has been challenged in recent years. It has been determined that only vasomotor symptoms and vaginal atrophy are related to low estrogen levels. Also, sustained high-dosage estrogen therapy has been reported to predispose to malignancy of the reproductive tract. Currently the prescription of short-term, low-dose estrogenic therapy for extensive troublesome vasomotor disruptions and of intravaginal estrogenic creams for vaginal atrophy are preferred treatment measures.

Counseling of the menopausal woman to assist her in successfully overcoming this developmental crisis of life is receiving increased attention. Adjustment to this crisis is determined to a large extent by the kind of life the woman has lived, by the security she has in her feminine identity, and by her feelings of self-worth and self-esteem. The nurse or other health professionals can help such a patient to achieve high-level functioning at this time in her life.

A woman at menopause faces about 25 more years of life. If she can resolve the conflicts of the climacteric, work through the grieving process for the losses that occur, and affirm her worth and maintain her self-esteem, she is well on her way to leading a productive, fulfilling, sustaining mature period of her life.

COITUS (SEXUAL INTERCOURSE)

Among the numerous terms used to describe the sexual mating of a sexually mature female and male are coitus, coition, sexual intercourse, copulation, making love, and the sex act. *Coitus* may be defined as the insertion of the erect male penis into the female vagina. After repeated thrusting movements of the penis, the man experiences ejaculation of semen (seminal fluid) concurrent with orgasm. Ejaculation is the expulsion of semen from the genital tract to the exterior of the urethral meatus through the rhythmic contraction of the penile muscles. Orgasm is the involuntary climax or apex of the sexual experience, involving a series of muscular contractions, profound physiologic bodily response, and intense sensual pleasure. Orgasm may be achieved by other methods of sexual stimulation besides coitus, such as masturbation and oral stimulation. Orgasm in the absence of ejaculation can occur, usually in aged men.

Table 5-2. Summary of Female Sexual Response

Organ	Excitement (foreplay)	Plateau (entry and coital movements)	Orgasm (climax)	Resolution (relaxation)
Labia minora	Vasocongestion of erectile tissue occurs; color darkens; extension of tissue	Increases		Return to normal size and color
Labia majora	Vasocongestion and swelling occurs; nulliparous: flatten and widen; multiparous: widen by movement from vaginal introitus	Increases		Return to normal size and color
Clitoris	Size of glans increases; engorgement of dorsal vein occurs; shaft elongates	Glans retracts under hood after erection	Rhythmic muscular contractions occur, ranging from intense to mild	Returns to normal; no refractory period; multiple orgasms possible
Vagina	Vaginal lubrication appears; in 10-30 seconds, widens and lengthens 1 cm; walls become purplish; progressive distention occurs; upper portion "tents"; rugae become smooth	Engorgement occurs; outer third of vagina swells; interior lumen decreases to "grasp" penis	Outer third has spasm, then rhythmic contractions; perivaginal muscles contract	Outer third relaxes after clitoris returns to normal; remaining portion returns to normal
Cervix	Moves upward and backward posteriorly	Cervical os opens slightly		Returns to normal position; os closes in 20-30 minutes
Uterus	Moves upward and backward posteriorly	Increases in size	Rhythmic contractions from fundus to cervix occur	Returns to precoital size slowly
Breasts	Areolae increase in size; nipples become erect and size increases; sex flush may appear		Sex flush most pronounced	Slow return to normal; sex flush disappears

Although the basic events of coitus are the same for all couples, there is wide variation in sexual positions, technique, duration, intent, meaning, and reactions among individuals.

Psychosocial Aspects

Coitus is a personal act between two consenting adults. Its performance can signify a variety of feelings, beliefs, and attitudes.

The traditional purpose of coitus is procreation. However, with the availability of contraceptive methods and with changing social mores, sexual intercourse is also becoming accepted as a pleasurable and personally gratifying experience in itself. The sexual union of two individuals may reflect their mutual commitment and caring, or it may be a more immediate interaction, for the purpose of personal pleasure or merely temporary companionship. In our society, sexual intercourse ideally is the sharing of two persons' minds and bodies in a uniquely intimate way that represents the larger sharing of their lives together. Such sexual interactions are the result of mutual caring and love.

According to Fromm (1956), love has four essential components: labor, responsibility, respect, and understanding. If one person is willing to evaluate the consequences of his behavior as it affects the other and choose accordingly; if he does not exploit but enables the other to become; if he tries to understand the other's feelings, hopes, and desires—then he may be considered to love the other. Sexual interaction is an important

Table 5–3. Summary of Male Sexual Response

Organ	Excitement (foreplay)	Plateau (entry and coital movements)	Orgasm (climax)	Resolution (relaxation)
Scrotum	Skin thickens; scrotal sac elevates and flattens against body (spermatic cord contracts)			
Seminal vesicles			Semen is discharged into urethral bulb	
Urethra	Moistened with mucus	Mucus increases; becomes distended with semen just before orgasm	Semen ejected with force as bulb contracts	Minor contractions persist even after semen is ejected
Prostate			Contracts, expelling fluid into urethral bulb	
Testes	Elevate with scrotum	May increase in size by 50%		
Penis	Engorgement and erection is rapid; size increases; position changes: angle of protrusion created	Coronal ridge size increases; glans becomes purplish	Contracts	Becomes flaccid; refractory period: erection may not be experienced
Bulbourethral glands		Few drops of fluid may be discharged (contain sperm)		
Breasts	Nipple erections; sex flush may appear		Sex flush most pronounced	Slow return to normal; sex flush fades slowly

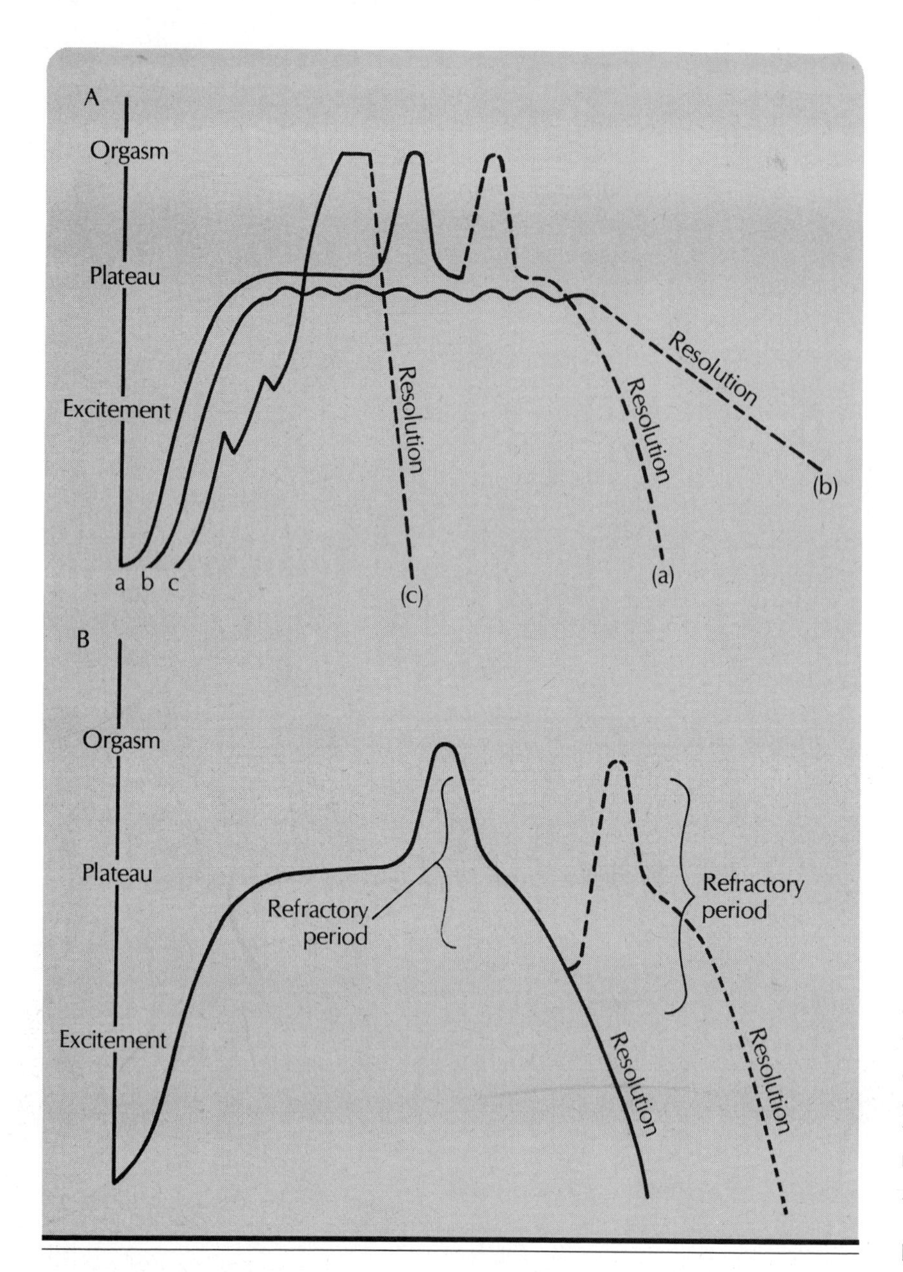

Figure 5–9. **A,** Cycle of female sexual response: *a,* reaction pattern with single or multiple orgasms; *b,* reaction pattern without orgasm; *c,* reaction pattern without distinct plateau. **B,** Cycle of male sexual response. (From Masters, W. H., and Johnson, V. E. 1966. *Human sexual response.* Boston: Little, Brown & Co., p. 55.)

way for individuals to express their love, and it is in this context that coitus can be most meaningful to the participants.

Physiology of Sexual Response

Masters and Johnson (1966) have identified and described the physiology of the sexual response in both males and females. Sexual response occurs in four phases: excitement, plateau, orgasm, and resolution. Essentially, the male and female sexual response is the same, involves the total body, and is a continuous process. Individual variation does occur.

All the responses can be classified as either vasocongestive or myotonic. *Vasocongestion* involves the congestion or engorgement of blood vessels and is the most common physiologic response to sexual arousal. *Myotonia,* a secondary physiologic response, is increased muscular tonus, which produces tension.

The sexual responses of female reproductive organs are given in Table 5–2; the male response is given in Table 5–3. Several responses are shared by both women and men. The *sex flush* consists of a maculopapular rash that may begin in the epigastric area and spread quickly to the breasts. Less than half of men experience this, whereas more than half of women do. Heart rate and blood pressure increase in proportion to the degree of sexual excitement. There may be tensing of the intercostal and abdominal muscles. This tension, beginning in the excitement phase, intensifies during the plateau phase and may involve the buttocks and anal sphincter. Hyperventilation occurs just before and during orgasm. At orgasm, muscle tension is extreme. The face may be contorted, while muscles of the neck, extremities, abdomen, and buttocks are tightly contracted. There may be uncontrollable groans, murmurings, or outcries. Grasping motions by each partner are not uncommon. There is a feeling of total surrender to bodily responses, and acute pleasure and relief are felt.

The male physical response is relatively constant, resulting in orgasm if erection and sexual stimulation are maintained. Female sexual response varies considerably. Not all women experience orgasm consistently; they are influenced by their subjective psychologic state, their health, their current sexual motivation, and environmental distractions. Therefore, a woman may not experience orgasm during a particular act of coitus, or she may experience one or multiple orgasms of varying intensity. Such variation is usual in a woman of "normal" sexual activity, interest, and response. Figure 5-9 illustrates the cycle of sexual response for the male and female.

Neurologic Control of Sexual Response

Cortical influences (limbic system and hypothalamus), peripheral nerves, autonomic pathways, spinal cord pathways, and reflex centers share the control of the sexual response.

In the male during the excitement phase, psychogenic or physical stimuli are transmitted by ascending sensory pathways or descending corticomotor pathways. Stimuli from pressure or tension in the pelvic organs or from touch of the external genitals create impulses carried by the pudendal and pelvic afferent fibers to the sacral cord. There they synapse with the parasympathetic efferent fibers to the pelvis. Reflex erection may result, as these fibers cause dilatation of the penile arteries and some constriction of the penile veins, with resultant vasoconstriction. Figure 5-10,*A*, shows the neural pathways involved in the male sexual response.

Heightened sexual arousal stimulates reflex centers of the spinal cord, which send out sympathetic impulses to the genital organs to initiate ejaculation. When the urethra is full of semen, impulses are transmitted to the sacral regions of the cord. The efferent fibers carry rhythmic impulses

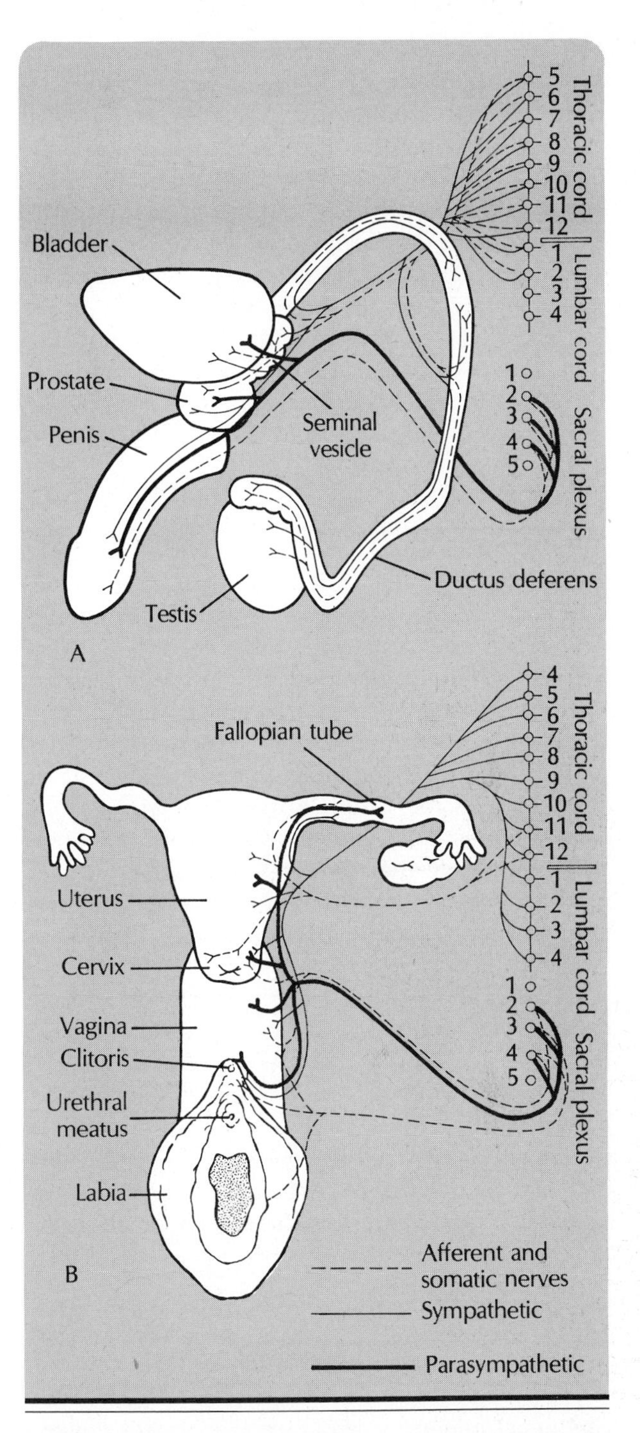

Figure 5-10. Neurologic basis of sexual response. **A,** Male neural pathways. **B,** Female neural pathways. (From Woods, N. F. 1975. *Human sexuality in health and illness.* St. Louis: The C. V. Mosby Co.)

from the cord to the skeletal muscles surrounding the erectile tissue, inducing rhythmic contractions. Sexual stimulation can arise from tubal fullness or irritation—the so-called morning erection is caused by fullness of the bladder.

A similar neurologic pattern is found in females. Tactile or psychogenic stimuli may cause sexual arousal. Local sexual sensations are carried to the spinal cord through the pudendal nerve and sacral plexus and are referred to cerebral centers. Reflexes associated with female orgasm seem to be associated with the lumbar and sacral regions of the cord. As in the male, erectile tissue is controlled by parasympathetic nerves. Figure 5–10,*B*, diagrams these neural pathways in the female.

Neural control of the female orgasm follows the same pathways as in the male.

To summarize, sympathetic innervation of sexual response causes vasoconstriction and orgasm in both sexes and ejaculation in the male. Parasympathetic innervation controls vasodilatation and erection of sex organs.

IMPLICATIONS FOR NURSES

Because sexuality is an intrinsic part of life from birth to death, people have many problems, needs, and questions concerning sex roles, sexual behaviors, family planning, sex education, sexual inhibitions, and other related areas. The nurse is frequently confronted with these concerns by her patients and thus may need to assume the role of sexual counselor. For the nurse to assume this role, she must be secure about her own sexuality. It is imperative that each patient's needs be met with appropriate knowledge, with lack of embarrassment and judgment, and with referral as required.

Rather than judging sexual behavior on predetermined standards of so-called normal behavior, the nurse should allow the couple to evaluate their own sexual activities. Each couple should determine their own patterns and preferences. If nurses are to satisfactorily meet the needs of their patients, they must accept these differences in sexual behaviors and provide support or information when requested.

SUMMARY

The development of sexuality is a function of societal, biologic, and physical factors. Society dictates many of the norms forming the framework for core-gender identity. Biologic factors are first established at conception and then are influenced by hormonal processes. Physical factors are influenced by hormonal levels and by an intricate feedback mechanism within the body.

The expression of sexuality is a learned process, and research has identified specific physiologic responses to sexual stimulation. Understanding the development and processes of sexuality will enable the nurse to interact with and counsel patients more appropriately.

SUGGESTED ACTIVITIES

1. In a classroom laboratory, describe the differences between sexual identity and gender identity.
2. During a postclinical conference, describe the hormonal aspects of the menstrual cycle.
3. Through independent study list the physical and psychologic aspects of menopause.
4. In a small group, discuss the similarities and differences between the female and male physiologic sexual responses.

REFERENCES

Berlin, H. July 1976. Effect of human sexuality on well-being from birth to aging. *Med. Asp. Hum. Sex.* 10:14.

Burt, J. J., and Meeks, L. B. 1975. *Education for sexuality: concepts and programs for teaching.* 2nd ed. Philadelphia: W. B. Saunders Co.

Chinn, P. L. 1974. *Child health maintenance: concepts in family-centered care.* St. Louis: The C. V. Mosby Co.

Friedrich, M. A. 1975. Psychophysiology of menstruation and the menopause. In *Gynecology and obstetrics: the health care of women,* eds. S. L. Romney et al. New York: McGraw-Hill Book Co.

Fromm, E. 1956. *The art of loving.* New York: Harper & Row Publishers, Inc.

Katchadourian, H. A., and Lunde, D. 1975. *Fundamentals of human sexuality.* New York: Holt, Rinehart & Winston, Inc.

Lief, H. I. 1975. Sexual counseling. In *Gynecology and obstetrics: the health care of women,* eds. S. L. Romney et al. New York: McGraw-Hill Book Co.

Masters, W. H., and Johnson, V. E. 1966. *Human sexual response.* Boston: Little, Brown & Co.

Page, E. W., et al. 1972. *Human reproduction: the core content of obstetrics, gynecology and perinatal medicine.* Philadelphia: W. B. Saunders Co.

Schwartz, L. H., and Schwartz, J. L. 1972. *The psychodynamics of patient care.* Englewood Cliffs, N.J.: Prentice-Hall, Inc.

Sherman, J. A. 1971. *On the psychology of women: a survey of empirical studies.* Springfield, Ill.: Charles C Thomas, Publisher.

Tanner, J. M. 1962. *Growth of adolescents.* 2nd ed. Oxford: Blackwell Scientific Publications, Ltd.

Ticky, A. M., and Malasanos, L. J. Nov.-Dec. 1975. The physiological role of hormones in puberty. *Am. J. Mat. Child Nurs.* 1:384.

ADDITIONAL READINGS

Abse, D. W., et al. 1974. *Marital and sexual counseling in medical practice.* New York: Harper & Row Publishers, Inc.

Adams, G. May-June 1976. Recognizing the range of human sexual needs and behavior. *MCN.* 1(3):166.

Adams, G. May-June 1976. The sexual history as an integral part of the patient history. *MCN.* 1(3):170.

Bardwick, J. M. 1971. *Psychology of women: a study of biocultural conflicts.* New York: Harper & Row Publishers, Inc.

Beach, F. A. 1977. *Human sexuality in four perspectives.* Baltimore: Johns Hopkins University Press.

Berezin, M. A. June 1972. Psychodynamic considerations of aging and the aged: an overview. *Am. J. Psychiatry.* 128:33.

Boettcher, J. H., and Boettcher, K. July-Aug. 1978. Sex education for fifth and sixth graders and their parents. *MCN.* 3(4):218.

Browning, M., and Lewis, E. 1973. *Human sexuality: nursing implications.* New York: The American Journal of Nursing Co.

Burgoyne, D. April 1974. Factors affecting coital frequency. *Med. Asp. Hum. Sex.* 8:143.

Chard, M. Jan.-Feb. 1976. An approach to examining the adolescent male. *MCN.* 1(1):41.

Cole, T. M. 1975. Sexuality and physical disabilities. *Arch. Sex. Behav.* 4:389.

Diamond, M. 1975. Sexual anatomy and physiology: clinical aspects. In *Human sexuality: a health practitioner's text,* ed. R. Green. Baltimore: The Williams & Wilkins Co.

Elder, M. S. Nov. 1970. Nurse counseling on sexuality—an unmet challenge. *Nurs. Outlook.* 18:38.

Grissum, M., and Spengler, C. 1976. *Womanpower and health care.* Boston: Little, Brown & Co.

Lennane, K. J., and Lennane, R. J. 1973. Alleged psychogenic disorders in women: a possible manifestation of sexual prejudice. *N. Engl. J. Med.* 288:288.

Maccoby, E. E., and Jacklin, C. 1974. *The psychology of sex differences.* Stanford, Calif.: Stanford University Press.

Moore, K. L. 1974. *Before we are born.* Philadelphia: W. B. Saunders Co.

Rybicki, L. L. May-June 1976. Preparing parents to teach their children about human sexuality. *MCN.* 1(3):182.

Vincent, C. E. 1973. *Sexual and marital health.* New York: McGraw-Hill Book Co.

Whitley, N. July-Aug. 1978. The first coital experience of one hundred women. *J. Obstet. Gynecol. Neonatal Nurs.* 7(4).

Woods, N. F. 1975. *Human sexuality in health and illness.* St. Louis: The C. V. Mosby Co.

Yorburg, B. 1974. *Sexual identity: sex roles and social change.* New York: John Wiley & Sons, Inc.

Zalar, M. K. May-June 1976. Sexual counseling for pregnant couples. *MCN.* 1(3):176.

CHAPTER 6

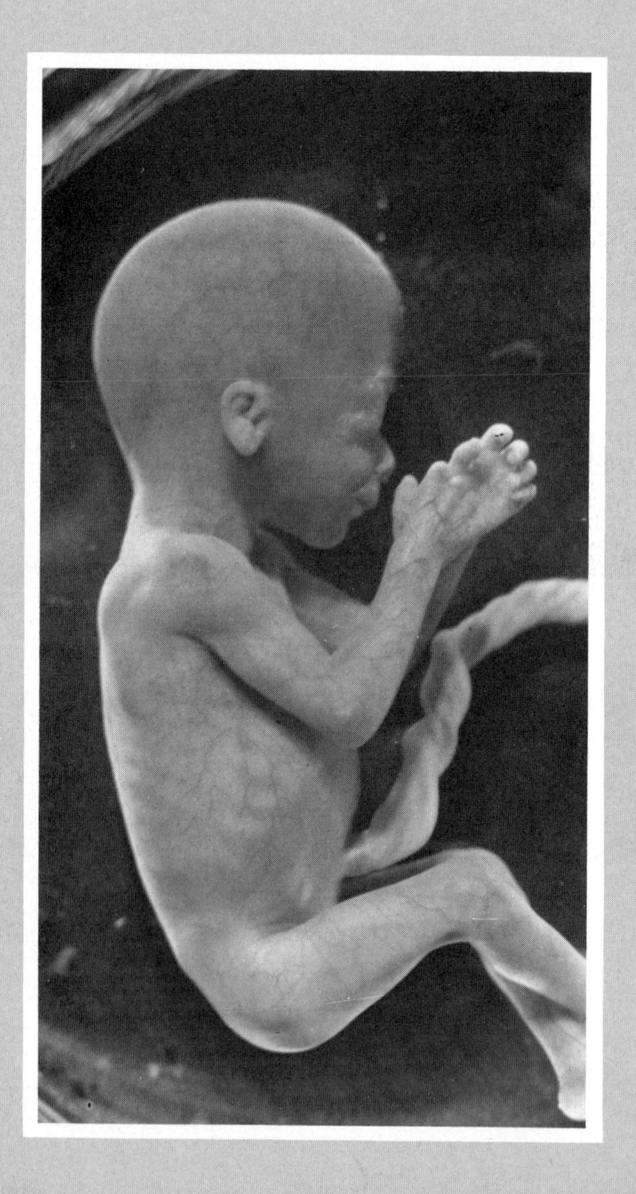

CONCEPTION AND FETAL DEVELOPMENT

OBJECTIVES

- Discuss meiotic cellular division and how it differs from mitotic cellular division.
- Describe the structure and functions of the umbilical cord and placenta during intrauterine life.
- Identify the significant changes in growth and development of the fetus in utero at 4, 8, 12, 16, 20, 24, 36, and 40 weeks' gestation.
- Identify the vulnerable periods in which malformations of various organ systems may occur and describe the resulting congenital malformations.

OVERVIEW OF GENETIC PROCESSES

Each person is unique. At the basis of this uniqueness are the physiologic mechanisms of heredity, which are reflected in the structure and function of cells and organ systems as determined by chromosomes and genes and the processes of cellular division.

Chromosomes and Genes

The somatic cells of each individual contain within their nuclei threadlike bodies known as *chromosomes,* which are composed of strands of deoxyribonucleic acid (DNA) and protein. *Genes* are regions in the DNA strands that contain coded information used to determine the unique characteristics of the individual; they are arranged in linear order on the chromosomes.

As the storage place for genetic information, DNA does not leave the cell nucleus. The DNA strand splits apart and forms the basis for a ribonucleic acid (RNA) molecule. The RNA passes out of the nucleus and carries coded information to the cytoplasm of the cell. A single error in the "reading" of the code can cause a change that may have serious effects on the functioning of the organism. For example, the alteration of one amino acid in the hemoglobin molecule produces abnormal hemoglobin, causing a disorder called sickle cell anemia. This type of genetic error is referred to as a *gene mutation.* Gene mutations can be induced by exposing cells to certain chemicals or to certain kinds of radiation (Winchester, 1966).

Each chromosome contains two longitudinal halves called *chromatids,* which are joined together at a point called the *centromere.* Each animal species tends to have a constant number of chromosomes. Human beings have 46 chromosomes divided into 23 pairs: 22 pairs of autosomes and one pair of sex chromosomes. Each member of a pair carries similar genes and is referred to as a *homologous chromosome* (Figure 6–1,*A*).

The chromosomes are classified according to their length and to the position of their centromere (Figure 6–1,*B*). When the centromere is centrally located, the longitudinal halves are divided into arms of approximately equal length, and the

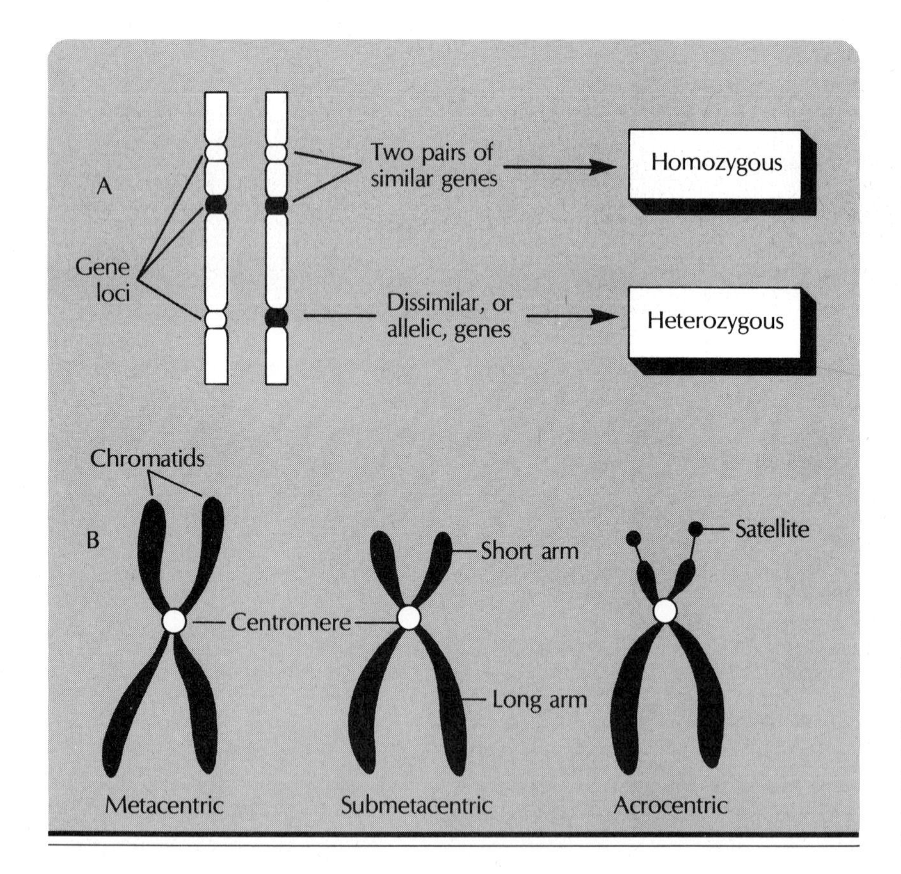

Figure 6–1. A, Pair of homologous chromosomes with similar (homozygous) and dissimilar (heterozygous) genes. **B,** Classification of chromosomal joining. (From Whaley, L. F. 1974. *Understanding inherited disorders.* St. Louis: The C. V. Mosby Co., pp. 6, 8.)

chromosome resembles an X. Such a chromosome is termed *metacentric.* If the centromere is located nearer one end of the chromosome than the other, the arms are of unequal length, and the chromosome resembles a Y. This configuration is termed *submetacentric.* A third type of chromosome (*acrocentric*) has a terminally located centromere at the distal end, where a second constriction occurs, referred to as a *satellite* (Figure 6–1,*B*). Satellites are often found in relation to abnormalities and can be induced by exposure to certain chemicals (Whaley, 1974).

Cellular Division

Although humans are multicellular animals, they begin life as a single cell. This cell reproduces itself, each of the new cells also reproduces, and so the process continues. The new cells must be basically similar to the cells from which they came.

Cells are reproduced by two different but related processes. The process of *mitosis* results in the production of additional body cells. Mitosis makes growth and development possible, and in mature individuals it is the process by which cells continue to divide and replace themselves. The other process of cell reproduction, *meiosis,* leads to the development of a new organism.

Mitosis

Although mitosis is a continuous process, it is generally divided into five stages: interphase, prophase, metaphase, anaphase, and telophase (Figure 6–2). During *interphase,* cell division is not taking place, but DNA is replicating itself within the chromosomes so that the genes will be doubled. Mitosis actually begins when the cell enters the *prophase.* The strands of chromatin shorten and thicken, and the chromosomes reproduce themselves by doubling the strands of chromatin. Next comes the appearance of a mitotic apparatus known as a *spindle,* in which fine threads extend from the top and bottom poles of the nucleus. At each pole of the spindle, a body known as the *centriole* is formed, so that the threads of the spindle extend from one centriole to the other. Next the nuclear membrane, which separates the nucleus from the cytoplasm, disappears; the nucleus thus disappears, and the cell enters metaphase. During *metaphase,* the chromosomes line up at the equator (midway between the poles) of the spindle. Metaphase is followed by *anaphase,* in which

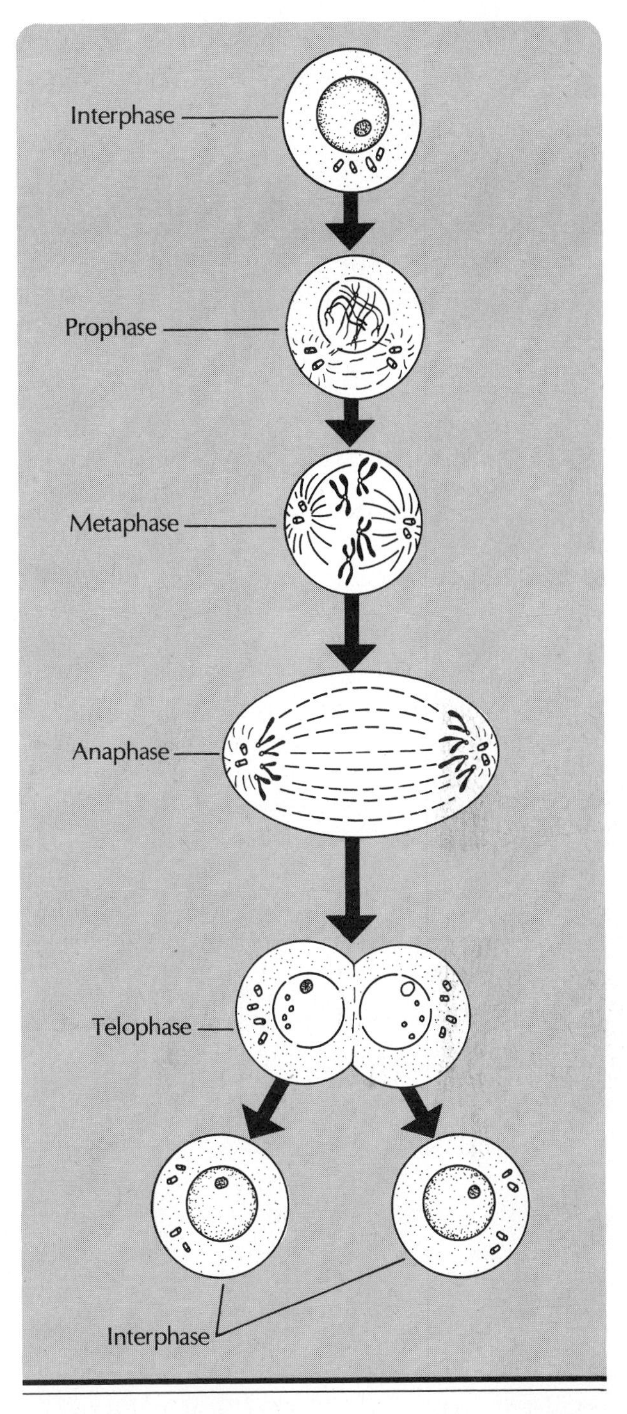

Figure 6–2. Somatic cell undergoing mitosis. Only four chromosomes are illustrated. (From Whaley, L. F. 1974. *Understanding inherited disorders.* St. Louis: The C. V. Mosby Co., p. 11.)

the two chromatids of each chromosome separate and move to opposite ends of the spindle, where they cluster in masses near the two poles of the cell. *Telophase* is essentially the reverse of pro-

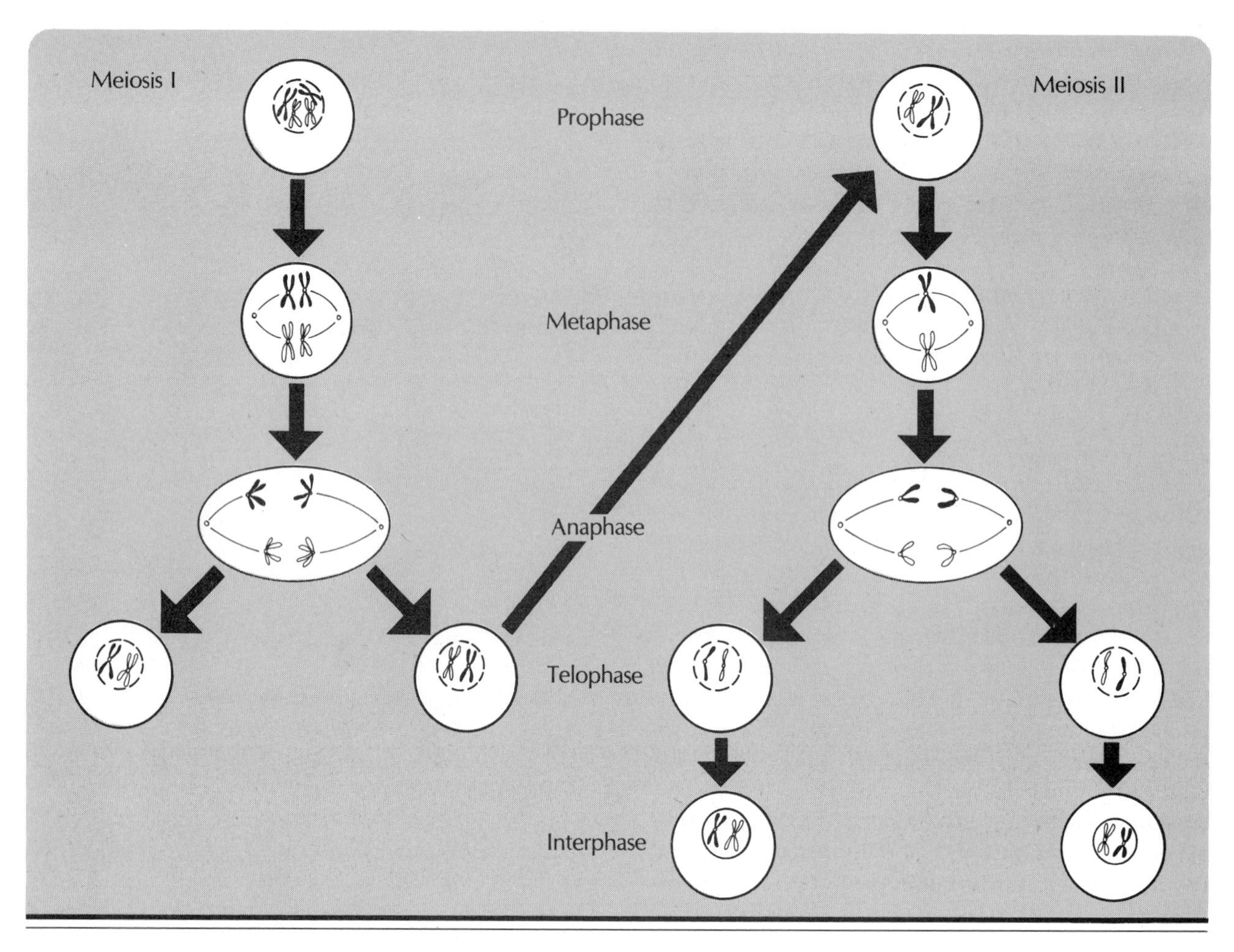

Figure 6–3. Meiosis in a germ cell. This illustration indicates the behavior of two pairs of homologous chromosomes. (From Whaley, L. F. 1974. *Understanding inherited disorders*. St. Louis: The C. V. Mosby Co., p. 13.)

phase. A nuclear membrane forms, separating each newly formed nucleus from the cytoplasm. The spindle disappears, and the centrioles relocate outside of each new nucleus. Within the nucleus the nucleolus again becomes visible, and the chromosomes lengthen and become threadlike. As telophase nears completion, a furrow develops in the cytoplasm at the midline of the cell and divides it into two *daughter cells*. Daughter cells have the same diploid number of chromosomes and the same genetic makeup as the cell from which they came (Winchester, 1966).

Meiosis

Meiosis occurs during *gametogenesis*, the process by which germ cells, or *gametes*, are produced. The male gamete (sperm) is produced in the seminiferous tubules of the testes by the process of spermatogenesis (Chapter 4 and p. 135). Oogenesis takes place in the graafian follicle of the ovary and results in the production of the female gamete (ovum) (p. 133). To maintain genetic balance, the chromosomes, through meiosis, are reduced by either reduction division or extrusion to form a gamete with 23 chromosomes, the haploid number.

Meiosis consists of two successive cell divisions, each of which includes the stages of interphase, prophase, metaphase, anaphase, and telophase (Figure 6–3). The chromosomes are replicated early in meiosis, although exactly when this occurs is not known, and the chromatids of each chromosome are joined together at the centromere. At this point, an essential difference between mitosis and meiosis becomes apparent.

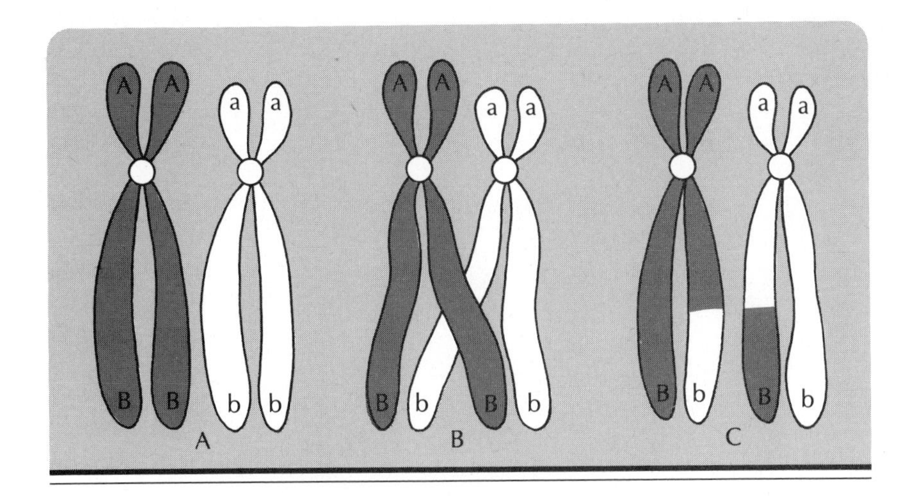

Figure 6–4. Phenomenon of crossing over. (From Spence, A. P., and Mason, E. B. 1979. *Human anatomy and physiology.* Menlo Park, Calif.: Benjamin/Cummings Publishing Co., p. 67.)

Whereas the replicated chromosomes function independently in mitosis, they become closely associated in meiosis. They often become entwined, forming a bundle of four chromatids referred to as a *tetrad.* At this stage an exchange of parts between chromatids, known as *crossing over,* often takes place (Figure 6–4). At each point of contact, there is physical exchange of genetic material between the chromatids. New combinations are provided by the newly formed chromosomes, accounting for the wide variation of traits seen in individuals. The replicated pairs of chromosomes line up at the equator of the spindle, and each member of a pair moves toward an opposite pole of the spindle. (In mitosis, the chromatids of each chromosome move together toward the poles.)

One of the members of each chromosome pair came originally from the father and the other, from the mother. At the end of the first meiotic division, the maternal and paternal chromosomes are randomly distributed between two separate daughter cells. Each of these cells contains half the usual number of chromosomes, but these chromosomes are still made up of two chromatids.

At the beginning of the second meiotic division, the chromosomes of each daughter cell line up along the equator of the spindle. The centromeres split, and the chromatids of each chromosome separate and move to opposite poles. The result of the second division is the formation of four cells, each containing the haploid number of chromosomes.

Occasionally during the second meiotic division, two of the chromatids may not move apart rapidly enough when the cell divides. The still-paired chromatids are carried into one of the daughter cells and eventually form an extra chromosome. This condition is referred to as an *autosomal nondisjunction* (chromosomal mutation) and is harmful to the offspring that may result should fertilization occur. The implications of nondisjunction are discussed in Chapter 8.

Another type of chromosomal mutation can occur if chromosomes break during meiosis. If the broken segment is lost, the result is a shorter chromosome; this situation is known as *deletion.* If the broken segment becomes attached to another chromosome, it is called *translocation,* which often results in harmful structural mutations (Whaley, 1974). The effects of translocation are described in Chapter 8.

Maturation of Gametes

Ovum

As discussed in Chapter 4, the ovaries begin development early in the fetal life of the female, and all the ova that an individual will produce are formed by about the sixth month of fetal life. The germinal epithelium of the outside of the ovary gives rise to oogonial cells, which develop into oocytes. Meiosis takes place within the oocytes, and meiotic division begins in all oocytes before the child is born. Meiosis stops just prior to the first meiotic metaphase in all oocytes and remains retarded until puberty. During puberty, the mature primary oocyte proceeds through the first

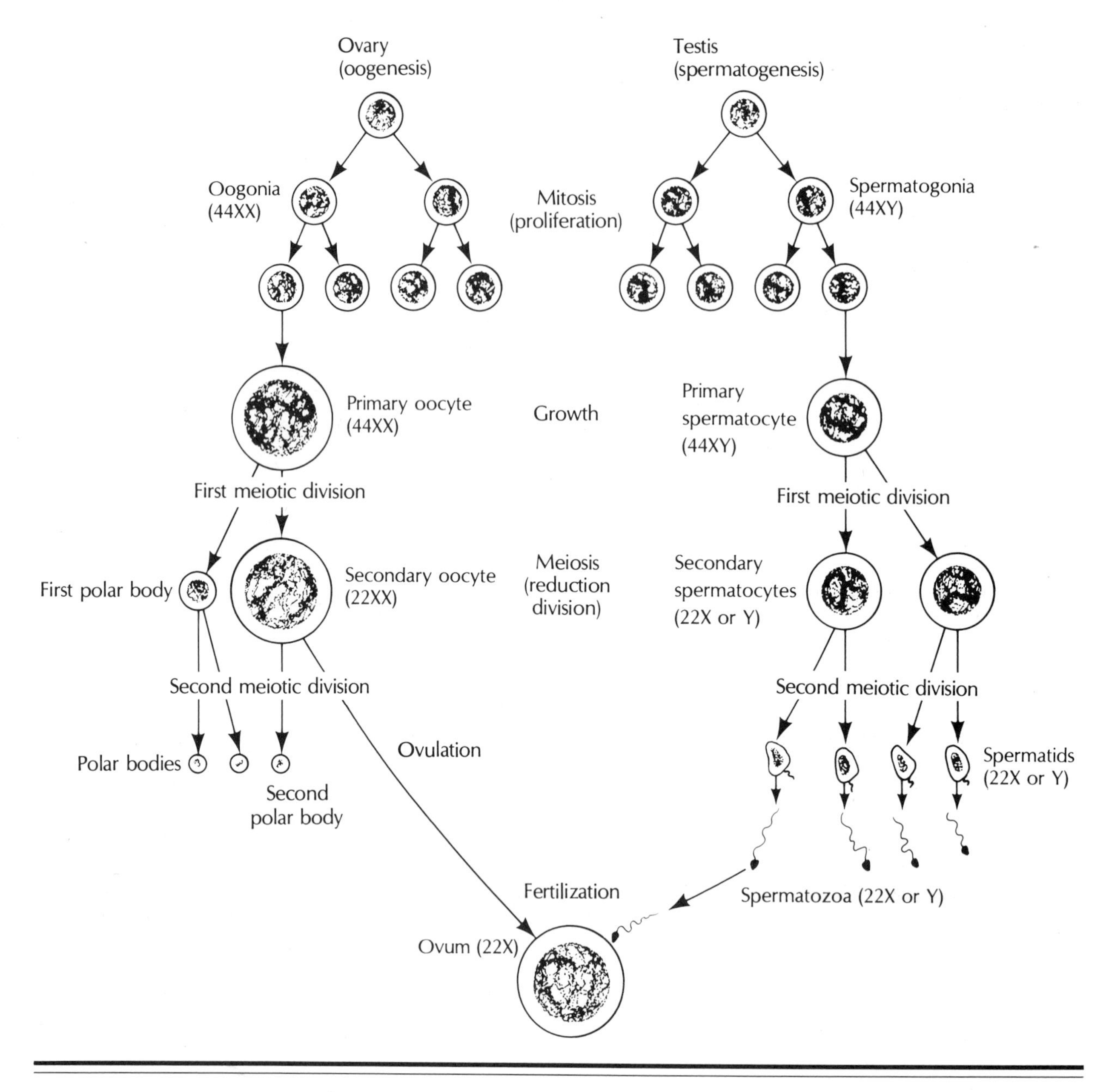

Figure 6–5. Gametogenesis involves meiosis within the ovary and testis. Note that during meiosis, each oogonium produces a single haploid ovum, whereas each spermatogonium produces four haploid spermatozoa. (From Spence, A. P., and Mason, E. B. 1979. *Human anatomy and physiology.* Menlo Park, Calif.: Benjamin/Cummings Publishing Co., p. 789.)

meiotic division through the process of oogenesis.

The first meiotic division gives rise to two cells of unequal size—a result of unequal division of the cytoplasm. These two cells are a secondary oocyte and a minute *polar body*—the end of the spindle and its pole with half of the chromosomes are actually extruded outside the cell membrane of the secondary oocyte. When fertilized by a sperm, both the secondary oocyte and the polar body proceed rapidly through the second meiotic division. The second meiotic division is similar to the first, except that the chromatids separate before migrating to opposite poles. Division is again not equal, producing an ovum with the haploid number of chromosomes and another extrusion of chromosomes into a second polar body. In the meantime, the first polar body has divided, and as a result of meiosis, four haploid cells have been produced: three small polar bodies, which eventually disintegrate, and one ovum, which will be functional (Figure 6-5).

Sperm

When a boy reaches puberty, at about 14 years of age, the germinal epithelium in the seminiferous tubules of the testes begins the continuous process of spermatogenesis, which will continue until senescence. As the diploid spermatogonium enters the first meiotic division, it is referred to as a *primary spermatocyte.* During the first meiotic division it forms two haploid cells, termed *secondary spermatocytes,* which will divide during the second meiotic division and form four *spermatids* with the haploid number of chromosomes. The spermatids undergo a series of changes during which they lose most of their cytoplasm. The nucleus becomes compacted into the head of the sperm, which is covered by a cap called an *acrosome,* and a long tail is produced from one of the centrioles (Figure 6-5).

Sex Determination

The two chromosomes of the 23rd pair are called *sex chromosomes.* The larger of the sex chromosomes has a centrally located centromere and is designated the *X chromosome.* The smaller sex chromosome has a terminally located centromere and is designated the *Y chromosome.* Females have two X chromosomes, and males have an X and a Y chromosome. Because male cells contain both an X and a Y chromosome, meiosis produces two gametes with an X chromosome and two gametes with a Y chromosome from each primary spermatocyte. The sex chromosomes in oocytes are both X, and thus the mature ovum can have only one type of sex chromosome, an X. For a child to be female, she must get an X chromosome from her mother and an X chromosome from her father. A male receives an X chromosome from his mother and a Y chromosome from his father. Maleness in humans thus depends on the father supplying the necessary Y chromosome.

When genes for two or more traits are situated on the same chromosome, the term *linkage* is used to describe their tendency to travel together during cell division. Y chromosomes contain mainly genes for maleness, but X chromosomes carry several genes other than those for sexual traits. These other traits are termed sex-linked because they are controlled by the genes on the sex chromosome. Hemophilia and color blindness are examples of sex-linked traits.

As discussed in Chapter 8, it is postulated that one X chromosome in every somatic cell of the female becomes genetically inactivated. This inactive X chromosome is pressed to the edge of the nucleus, where it remains as a tightly coiled small mass of material. Under laboratory conditions using certain dyes, this small mass of material, called the *sex chromatin* or *Barr body,* stains dark red in the cell. Female cells are sex chromatin-positive; their cell nuclei contain Barr bodies. Male cells are sex chromatin-negative; their cell nuclei do not contain Barr bodies. Sex chromatin is useful in determining the sex of an unborn fetus and in detecting the presence or absence of sex chromosomes in individuals (Whaley, 1974).

FERTILIZATION

The mature ovum and a spermatozoon must unite within a brief period of time, as their life span is limited. Ova are thought to be viable for only 24 hours, and the average life of spermatozoa in ejaculated semen at normal body temperature is thought to be 24-72 hours.

The process of *fertilization* takes place in the ampulla of the fallopian tube. The high estrogen level at the time of ovulation increases the contractility of the fallopian tube, propelling the ovum through its passageway. This high estrogen level also causes an increase in cervical mucus, which becomes less viscous and more readily penetrated by spermatozoa.

The ovum is surrounded by two layers of tissue. The layer closer to the cell membrane is called the *zona pellucida.* It is a clear, noncellular layer whose function is not known. Outside the zona pellucida is a ring of elongated cells, called the *corona radiata* because they radiate from the ovum like the gaseous corona around the sun. These cells are held together by hyaluronic acid.

A single ejaculation deposits about 2.5-4 ml of semen, containing approximately 200-400 million spermatozoa, in the vagina. The spermatozoa ascend the female tract by means of the whiplike action of their tails and with the assistance of uterine contractions (Danforth, 1977). The ovum has no power of movement.

The acrosome covering the head of the spermatozoon is believed to contain the enzyme hyaluronidase. Several million spermatozoa surround the ovum and deposit their minute amount of hyaluronidase, which breaks down enough hyaluronic acid for one spermatozoon to penetrate the ovum (DeCoursey, 1974). Only the head and neck of the spermatozoon enter the ovum; the tail becomes detached and remains in the ovum's outer membrane (Figure 6-6). Simultaneously with penetration, a cellular change occurs in the ovum that renders it impenetrable to other spermatozoa; thus, only one spermatozoon enters a single ovum.

At the moment of penetration the second meiotic division is completed in the nucleus of the ovum, and the second polar body is extruded. Each gamete contains a haploid number of chromosomes (23 chromosomes); at their union, the diploid number is restored, for a total of 46 chromosomes. At this moment the sex of the offspring is also established. As the male and female pronuclei approach each other, a mitotic spindle forms between them, their nuclear membranes disappear, and their chromosomes pair up along the equatorial zone of the newly formed spindle apparatus. Thus a new cell is formed from the union of a male and a female gamete. This cell, referred to as the *zygote*, contains a new combination of genetic material, resulting in an individual different from either parent and from anyone else in the world.

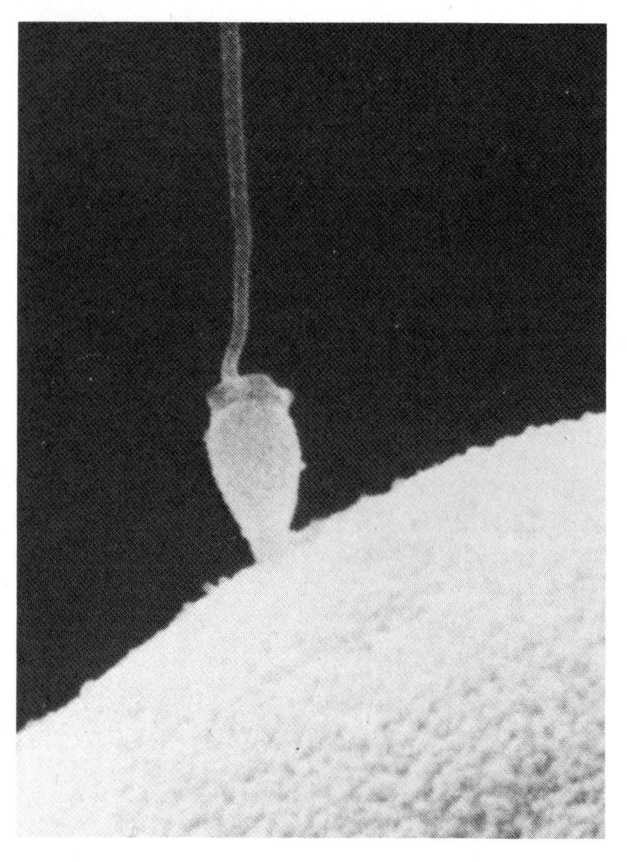

Figure 6-6. Electron micrograph of a sperm about to penetrate the surface of an ovum. (From Bloom, W., and Fawcett, D. W. 1975. *A textbook of histology.* 10th ed. Philadelphia: W. B. Saunders Co.)

Intrauterine human development after fertilization can be divided into three phases: cellular multiplication, cellular differentiation, and development of organ systems. These phases and the process of implantation will be discussed next.

CELLULAR MULTIPLICATION

Cellular multiplication begins as the recently fertilized ovum drifts down the fallopian tube to the uterus, a distance of 10-13 cm that takes about four or five days to accomplish. The zygote enters a period of rapid mitotic divisions called *cleavage,* in which it divides into two cells, four cells, eight cells, and so on. The cells that are produced during this period are called *blastomeres* and are so small that the developing mass is only slightly larger than the original zygote. The blastomeres are held together by the zona pellucida and eventually form a solid ball of cells referred to as the *morula.* After reaching the uterus, the morula floats freely for a few days, undergoing changes that result in the development of a cavity within the mass of cells. The inner, solid clump of cells is called the *blastocyst,* and the outer layer of cells forming the cavity and replacing the zona pellucida is referred to as the *trophoblast.* Eventually the trophoblast develops into one of the em-

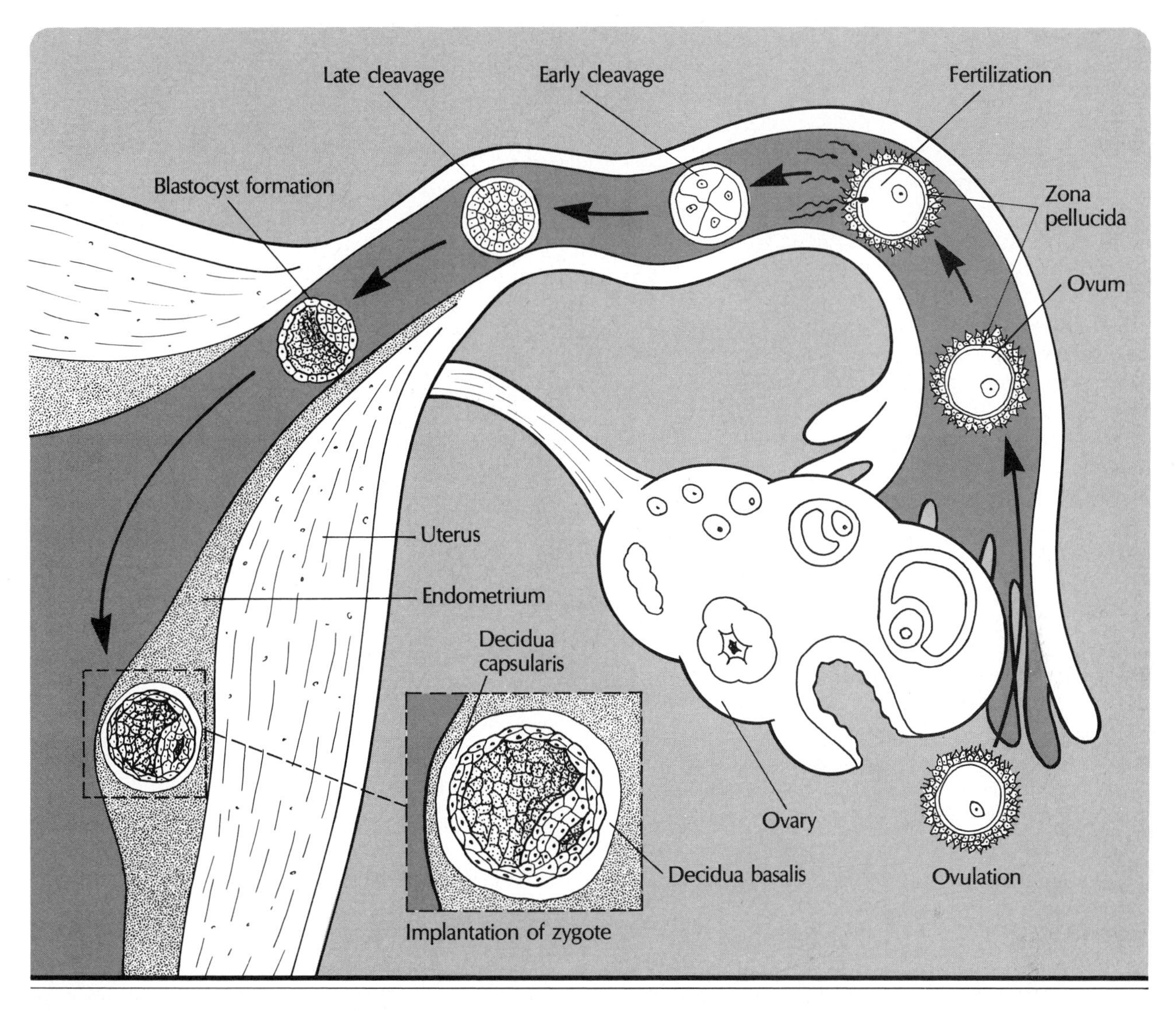

Figure 6–7. Fertilization generally occurs in the outer third of the fallopian tube. Illustrated is the cellular development of the ovum as it progresses to implantation in the uterus.

bryonic membranes, the chorion. The blastocyst develops into the embryo and the other embryonic membranes.

The journey of the fertilized ovum to its uterine destination is illustrated in Figure 6–7.

IMPLANTATION

While floating free in the uterine cavity, the blastocyst derives its nutrition from the uterine glands, which secrete a mixture of mucopolysaccharides, lipids, and glycogen. After the loss of the zona pellucida, the newly formed trophoblast must attach itself to the surface of the endometrium for further nourishment. The trophoblast most often selects a site for implantation in the upper part of the posterior uterine wall (Figure 6–7) and then burrows between the columnar epithelial cells, penetrating down toward the maternal capillaries. Between the seventh and ninth

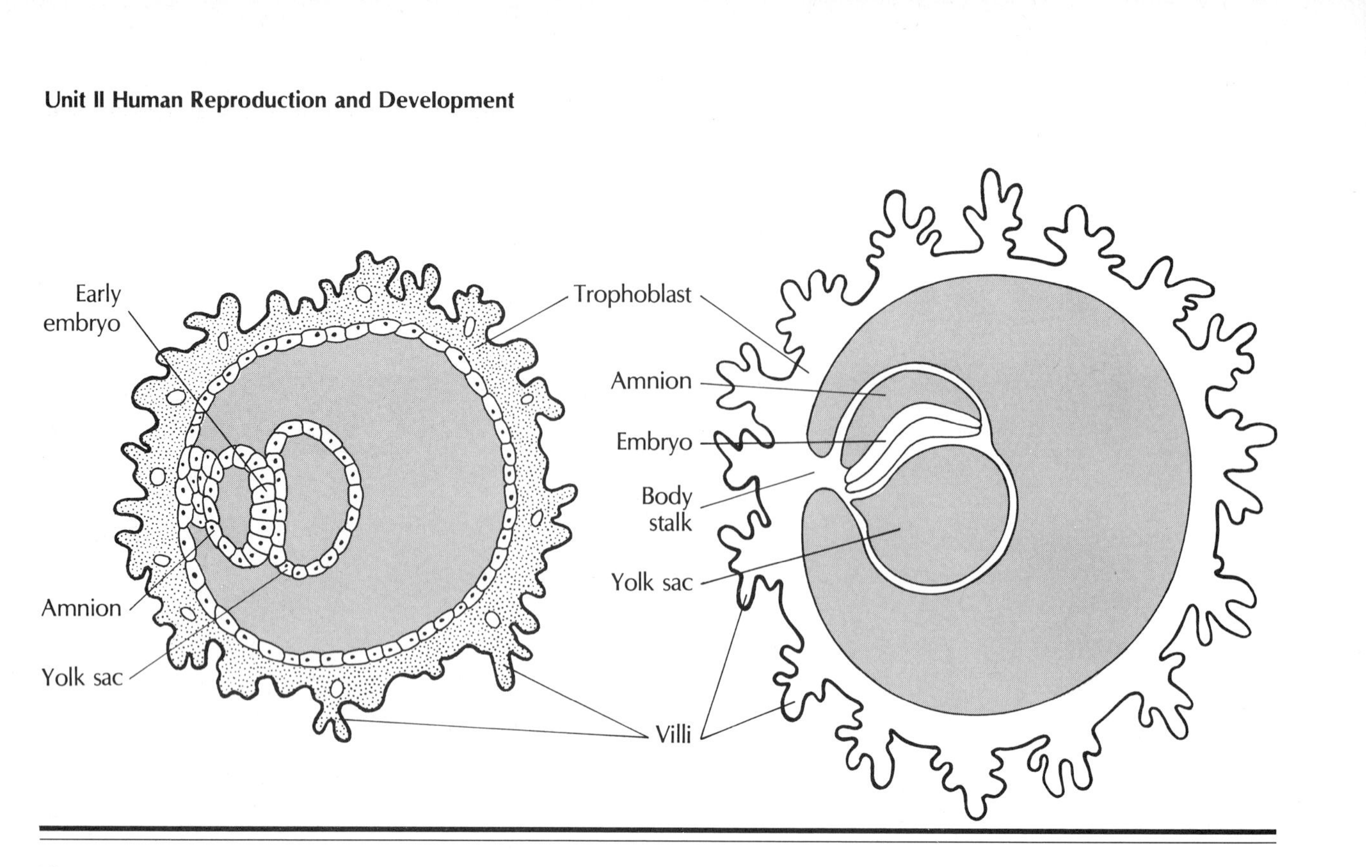

Figure 6–8. Formation of villi during implantation. (From Decoursey, R. M. *The human organism.* Copyright © 1968 by McGraw-Hill, Inc. Used with permission of McGraw-Hill Book Co.)

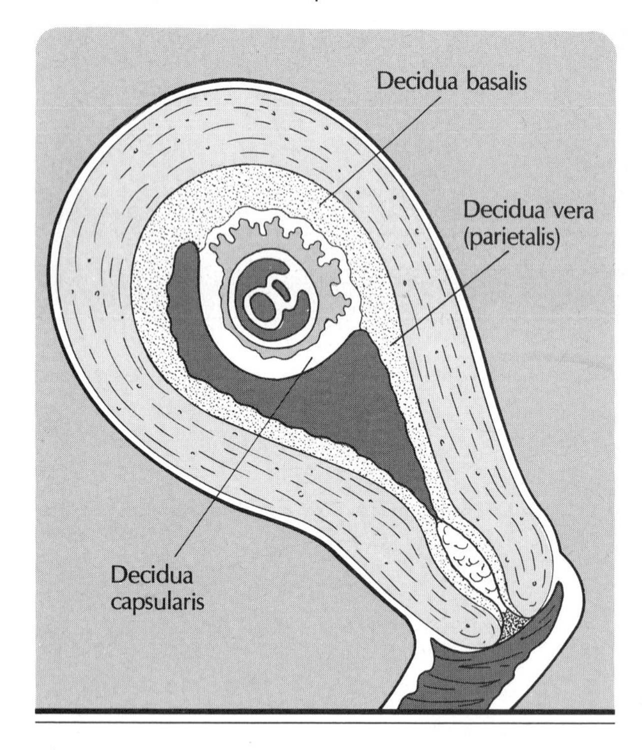

Figure 6–9. Layers of decidua early in pregnancy.

day after fertilization, the blastocyst implants itself in the uterus by sinking down into the uterine lining until it is completely covered. The lining of the uterus thickens below the implanted blastocyst and the cells of the trophoblast grow down into the thickened lining, forming processes called *villi* (Figure 6–8).

The endometrium, under the influence of progesterone, has undergone changes to prepare for implantation and nutrition of the ovum. Its vascularity and thickness are greatly increased. After implantation, the endometrium is referred to as the *decidua.* The portion of the decidua that overlies the blastocyst is called the *decidua capsularis;* the portion directly beneath the implanted blastocyst is the *decidua basalis;* and the portion that lines the rest of the uterine cavity is the *decidua vera* (parietalis) (Figure 6–9). The maternal portion of the placenta develops from the decidua basalis, which contains large numbers of blood vessels.

CELLULAR DIFFERENTIATION

At the time of implantation, the embryonic membranes begin to form (Figure 6–10). These membranes protect and support the embryo during its growth and development within the uterus.

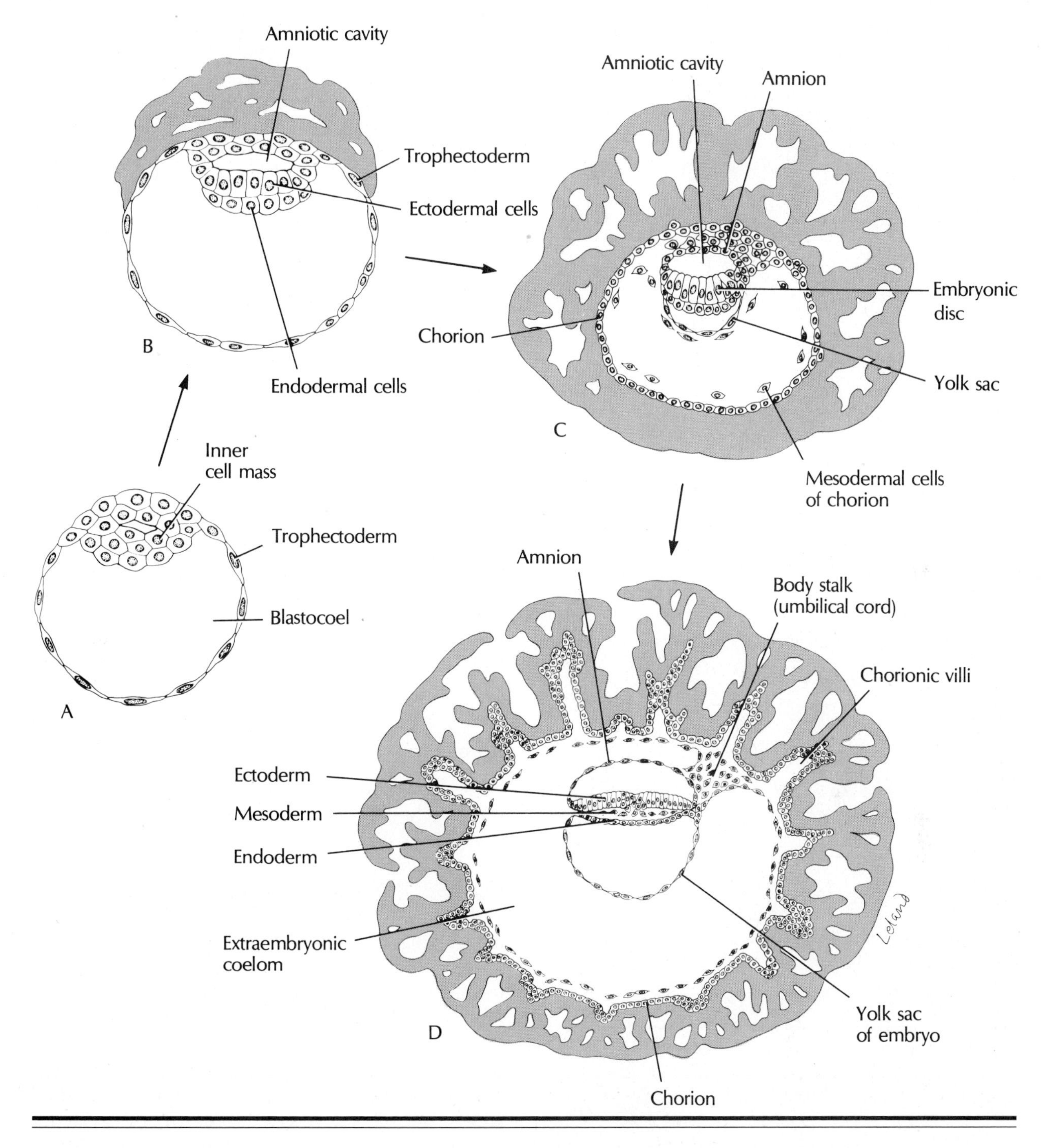

Figure 6-10. Early development of the embryonic membranes. (From Spence, A. P., and Mason, E. B. 1979. *Human anatomy and physiology.* Menlo Park, Calif.: Benjamin/Cummings Publishing Co., p. 800.)

The first membrane to form is the *chorion,* the outermost embryonic membrane, which encloses the amnion, embryo, and yolk sac. It is a thick membrane that develops from the trophoblast, with numerous fingerlike projections over its surface called *chorionic villi.* Soon after their development, the villi begin to degenerate, with the exception of those immediately beneath the embryo, which continue to grow and branch, fitting into depressions in the uterine wall and forming the embryonic portion of the placenta. By the fourth month of pregnancy, the surface of the

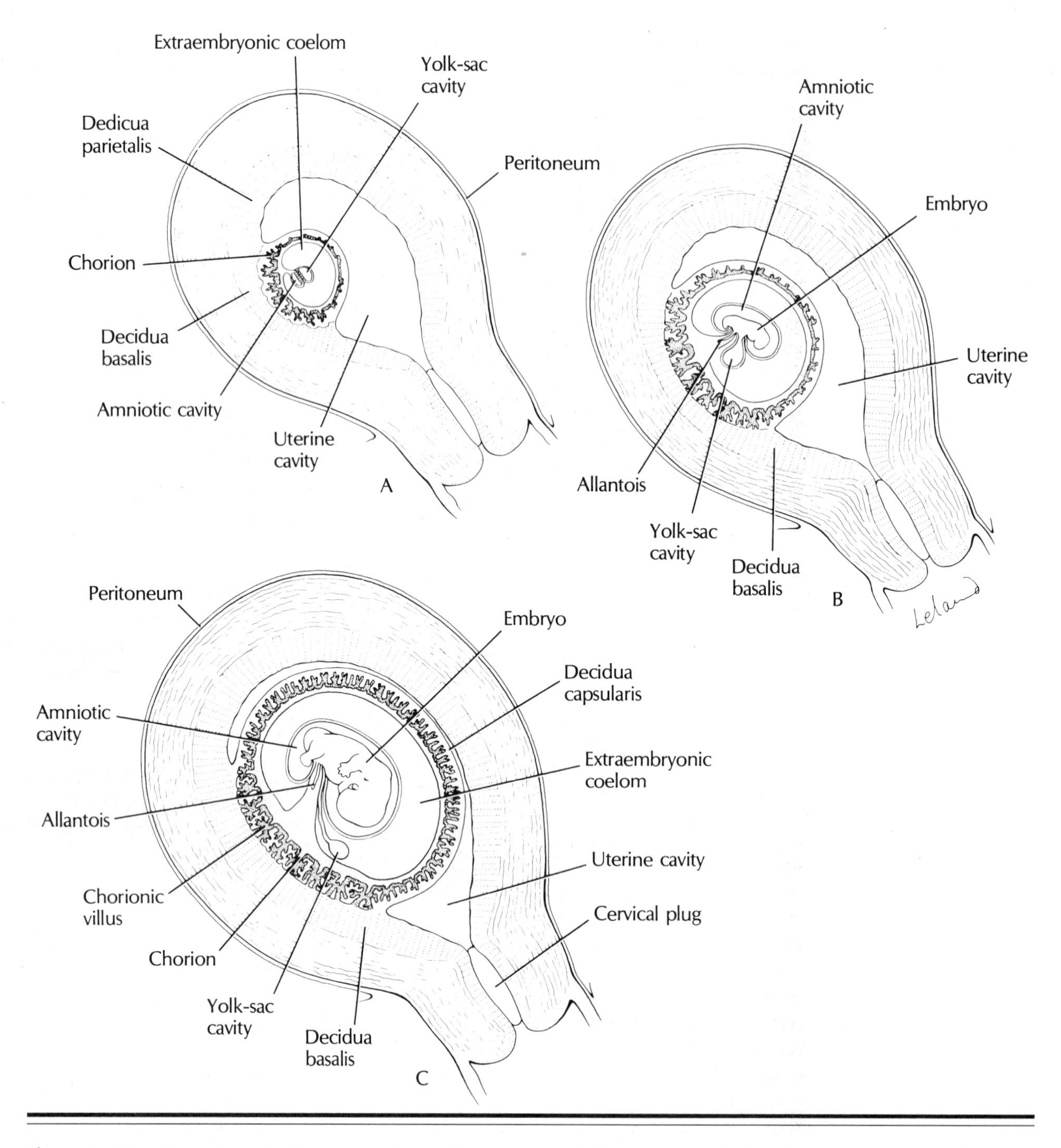

Figure 6–11. Formation of primary germ layers. (From Spence, A. P., and Mason, E. B. *Human anatomy and physiology.* Menlo Park, Calif.: Benjamin/Cummings Publishing Co., p. 802.)

chorion is smooth except at the place of attachment to the uterine wall.

The second membrane, the *amnion,* originates from the ectoderm during the early stages of embryonic development. It is a thin protective membrane that contains amniotic fluid. The space between the membrane and the embryo is the *amniotic cavity.* The amnion expands as the embryo grows, until it fills the extraembryonic cavity and comes into contact with the chorion. These two slightly adherent membranes form a fluid-filled sac, and the embryo literally floats within this protective envelope. The amniotic fluid acts as a cushion to protect against mechani-

Table 6–1. Derivation of Body Structures from Primary Cell Layers

Ectoderm	Mesoderm	Endoderm
Epidermis	Dermis	Respiratory tract
Sweat glands	Wall of digestive tract	Epithelium (except nasal), including pharynx, tongue, tonsils, thyroid, parathyroid, thymus, auditory tube
Sebaceous glands	Kidneys and ureter (suprarenal cortex)	Lining of digestive tract
Nails	Reproductive organs (gonads, genital ducts)	Primary tissue of liver and pancreas
Hair follicles	Connective tissue (cartilage, bone, joint cavities)	Urethra and associated glands
Lens of eye	Skeleton	Urinary bladder (except trigone)
Epithelium of internal and external ear, nasal cavity, sinuses, mouth, anal canal	Muscles (all types)	Vagina (parts)
Central and peripheral nervous systems	Cardiovascular system (blood, bone marrow)	
Nasal cavity	Pleura	
Oral glands and tooth enamel	Lymphatic tissue	

cal injury, helps control the embryo's body temperature, prevents adherence of the amnion, and allows freedom of movement so that the embryo can change position.

Initially, amniotic fluid is secreted by the amnion (Moore, 1977), but later most of it is derived from the maternal blood. The volume increases from about 30 ml at 10 weeks' gestation to 350 ml at 20 weeks' gestation. After 20 weeks, the volume ranges from 500 to 1000 ml. There is constant change in the amniotic fluid as a result of fluid movement in both directions through the placental membrane. Later in pregnancy the fetus contributes to the volume of amniotic fluid by excretion of urine, and it absorbs up to 400 ml/24 hr through its gastrointestinal tract by swallowing amniotic fluid. Amniotic fluid is slightly alkaline and contains albumin, urea, uric acid, creatinine, lecithin, sphingomyelin, bilirubin, fat, fructose, epithelial cells, leukocytes, enzymes, and lanugo hair.

About the eighth or ninth day, the yolk sac forms as a second cavity in the blastocyst. The yolk sac is small and functions only during early embryonic life. In animals other than mammals, the yolk sac is the source of nourishment. In humans, the yolk sac forms primitive red blood cells during the first six weeks of development until hematopoiesis begins in the liver of the embryo. As the embryo develops, the yolk sac is incorporated in the umbilical cord, where it can be identified as a degenerate structure.

About the tenth to fourteenth day, simultaneously with the development of the embryonic membranes, the once homogeneous mass of cells begins to differentiate. Three primary germ layers are formed: the ectoderm, mesoderm, and endoderm (Figure 6–11). From these three primary cell layers, all the tissues, organs, and organ systems will differentiate (Table 6–1).

How and why differentiation occurs are not clearly understood, although it is believed to be a gene-directed phenomenon that originates in the DNA of the zygote and that is carried out in the cytoplasm by an elaborate set of chemical reactions caused by the RNA-controlled synthesis of specific enzymes.

INTRAUTERINE ORGAN SYSTEMS

Placenta

The *placenta* is the means of metabolic exchange between embryonic and maternal circulation.

Development

Whereas the other embryonic membranes are formed during the time of implantation or shortly thereafter, true placental formation does not begin until the third week of development. The placenta forms at the place of attachment of the developing embryo to the uterine wall. The process begins with the chorionic villi.

Both the chorion and the uterus have extensive circulatory systems. The trophoblast cells of the chorionic villi form spaces in the tissue of the decidua basalis. These spaces fill with maternal blood, and it is into these spaces that the chorionic villi grow. As the chorionic villi proliferate, two distinct trophoblastic layers appear: an outer layer, called the *syncytium*, and an inner layer, known as the *cytotrophoblast*. Both layers are present during the first five months of pregnancy, but later the cells of the cytotrophoblast become fewer and eventually disappear, so that during the last half of pregnancy only a single layer of syncytium covers the chorionic villi.

Placental permeability is relatively slight during the early months of development because the villous membranes have not yet been reduced to their minimum thickness. Its permeability increases progressively until about the last month of pregnancy, when it begins to decrease again because of deterioration of the placenta with age. A third, inner layer of connective mesoderm develops in the chorionic villi and grows through the cell columns, forming anchoring villi. These anchoring villi eventually form the septa (partitions) of the placenta. The maturing placenta is divided by the well-developed septa into 15 to 20 segments called *cotyledons* (Figure 6–12,*B*). In each cotyledon the branching villi form highly complex vascular systems through which the exchange of gases and nutrients takes place.

Expansion of the placenta continues until about the 20th week, at which time it covers one-half of the internal surface of the uterus. After the 20th week, the placenta grows only in thickness, not in width. At 40 weeks' gestation, the placenta is a discoid organ about 15–20 cm in diameter and 2.5–3 cm in thickness and weighs about 400–600 gm.

The placenta is composed of two portions. The maternal portion is made up of the decidua basalis and its circulation. Its surface is red and fleshlike. The fetal portion consists of the chorionic villi and their circulation. The fetal surface is covered by the adherent amnion, which eventually gives it a shiny grayish appearance (Figure 6–12).

As the placenta is developing, the umbilical cord is also being formed. The developing embryo is connected to the yolk sac by an area of tissue known as the *body stalk*. A chain of vessels that communicate with the gut of the developing embryo develops in the body stalk. The chorion and the amnion are also attached at this structure. To obtain more nourishment, the chain of vessels in the body stalk extends into the chorionic villi. The body stalk then fuses with the embryonic

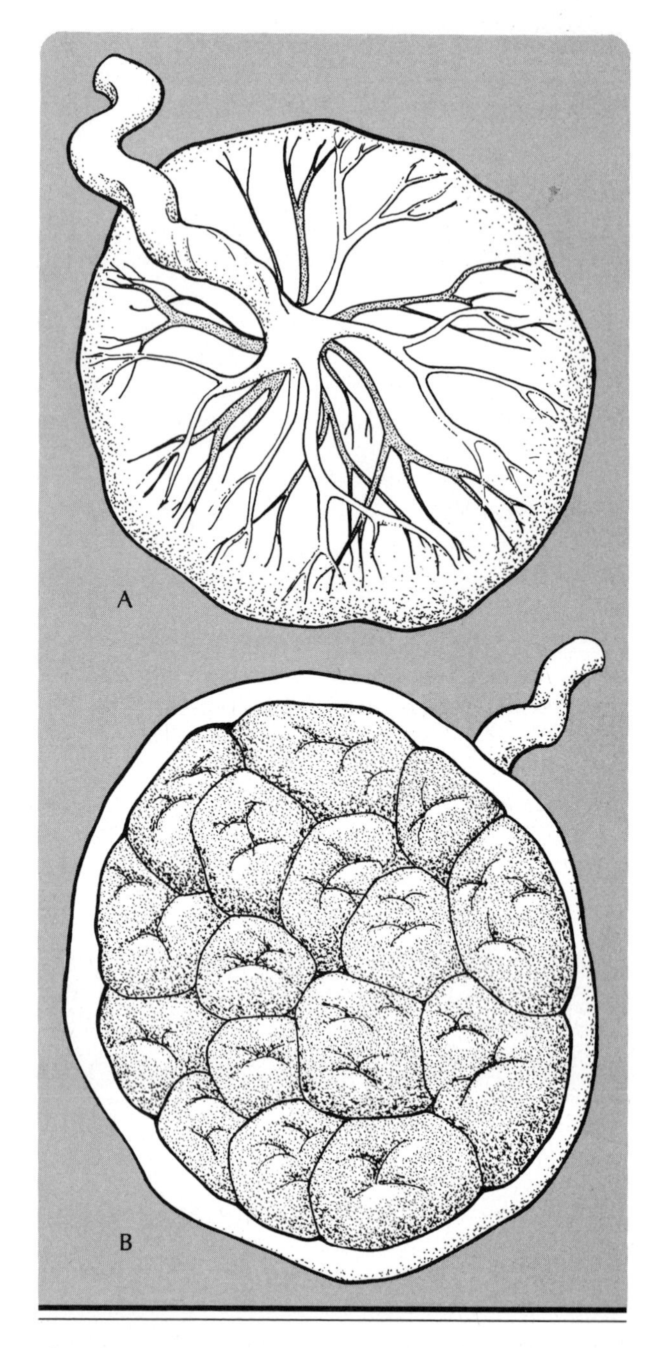

Figure 6–12. Fetal **(A)** and maternal **(B)** surfaces of the placenta.

portion of the developing placenta to provide circulatory pathways connecting the chorionic villi and the embryo. The body stalk elongates and becomes known as the *umbilical cord,* or *funis.* The vessels in the cord are reduced to one large vein and two smaller arteries. About 1% of umbilical cords have only two vessels, an artery and a vein; this condition is associated with congenital fetal malformations.

A specialized connective tissue known as *Wharton's jelly* surrounds the blood vessels. This tissue, plus the high blood volume pulsating through the vessels, prevents intrauterine compression of the umbilical cord.

At term, the cord averages 2 cm in diameter and is about 55 cm in length, extending from the umbilicus of the fetus to the fetal surface of the placenta. The attachment of the umbilical cord in the placenta is eccentric, having either a central or peripheral (battledore) insertion. In rare circumstances the cord inserts away from the placenta so that vessels run along the membranes from the site of cord insertion to the surface of the placenta. This configuration is called a *velamentous placenta.*

Circulation

After implantation of the blastocyst, the cells distinguish themselves into fetal cells and trophoblastic cells. The proliferating trophoblast successfully invades the decidua basalis of the endometrium, first opening uterine capillaries and later the larger uterine vessels. The placental villi are an outgrowth of the blastocystic tissue. As these villi continue to grow and divide, the fetal vessels begin to form. The intervillous spaces develop as the endometrial spiral arteries are opened.

By the fourth week, the placenta has begun to function as a means of metabolic exchange between embryo and mother. The completion of the maternal-placental-fetal circulation occurs about 22 days after conception when the embryonic heart begins functioning (Martin and Gingerich, 1976), and by the fourteenth week, it is a discrete organ.

Recall that the trophoblastic tissue of the villi is divided into the cytotrophoblast and the syncitium. The syncitium, an outgrowth of the cytotrophoblast and the functional layer of the placenta, is in direct contact with the maternal blood at the intervillous space. It also secretes the placental hormones of pregnancy.

The cotyledons of the maternal surface contain branches of a single placental mainstem villus, allowing for compartmentalization of the uteroplacental circulation (Martin and Gingerich, 1976).

In the fully developed placenta, fetal blood in the villi and maternal blood in the intervillous spaces are separated by three to four thin layers of tissue. The capillaries of the villi are lined with an extremely thin endothelium and are surrounded by a layer of mesenchymal (connective) tissue that is covered by chorionic epithelium (Figure 6–13). As previously discussed, one of the layers of the chorionic epithelium, the cytotrophoblast, thins out and disappears after the fifth month.

Fetal blood flows through two umbilical arteries, to the capillaries of the villi, and back through the umbilical vein into the fetus. Maternal blood, rich in oxygen and nutrients, flows from the uterine arteries into the intervillous spaces in spurts, which are produced by the maternal blood pressure. The spurt of blood is directed toward the chorionic plate, and as the flow loses pressure, it becomes lateral (or spreads out). Fresh blood continually enters and exerts pressure on the contents of the intervillous spaces, pushing blood toward the exits in the basal plate. Blood is then drained through the uterine and other pelvic veins (Figure 6–13).

Circulation within the intervillous spaces depends on maternal blood pressure, producing a gradient between arterial and venous channels. Braxton Hicks contractions are believed to facilitate placental circulation, although their role is not clearly understood. Maternal blood is forced into the intervillous spaces during contractions and drains out of the placental sinusoids back into maternal circulation with uterine relaxation (Jensen et al., 1977).

Functions

The placental functions, many of which begin soon after implantation, include fetal respiration, nutrition, and excretion. To carry out these functions, the placenta is involved in metabolic and transfer activities. In addition, it has endocrine functions and special immunologic properties.

Endocrine Functions. The placenta produces hormones that are vital to the survival of the preg-

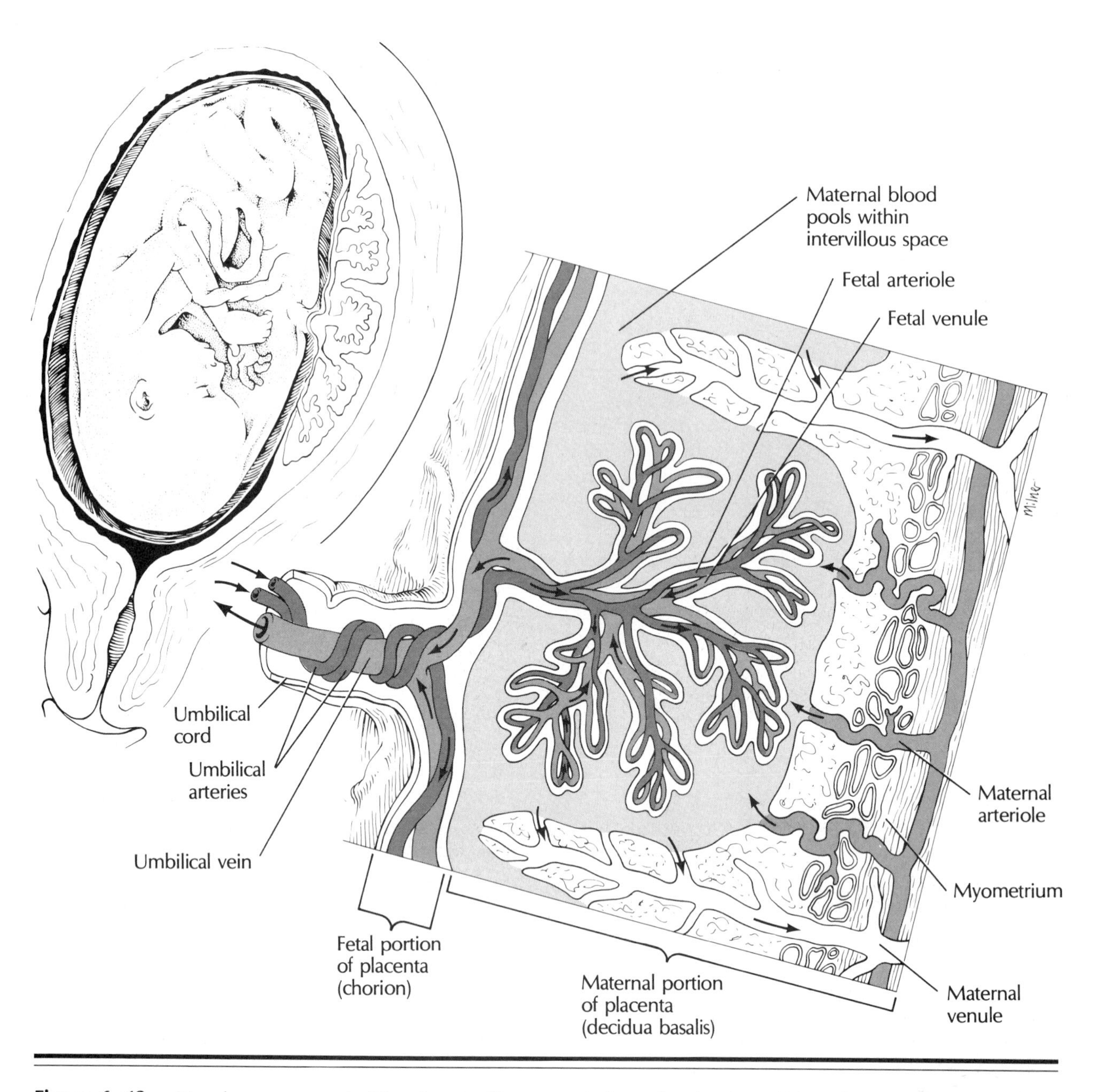

Figure 6–13. Vascular arrangement of the placenta. The arrows indicate the direction of blood flow. Maternal blood flows through the uterine arteries to the intervillous spaces of the placenta and returns through the uterine veins to maternal circulation. Fetal blood flows through the umbilical arteries into the villous capillaries of the placenta and returns through the umbilical vein to the fetal circulation. (From Spence, A. P., and Mason, E. B. 1979. *Human anatomy and physiology.* Menlo Park, Calif.: Benjamin/Cummings Publishing Co., p. 799.)

nancy. The syncytium is believed to be the site of hormone production. At the present time, four hormones are known to be produced by the placenta: two protein hormones, human chorionic gonadotropin (HCG) and human chorionic somatomammotropin (HCS) (also called human placental lactogen or HPL); and two steroid hormones, estrogen and progesterone.

Biochemically, *HCG* is similar to pituitary luteinizing hormone, and its most important function is to prevent the normal involution of the corpus luteum at the end of the menstrual cycle. HCG causes the corpus luteum to secrete increased quantities of estrogen and progesterone. If the corpus luteum ceases functioning before the eleventh week of pregnancy, spontaneous abortion occurs. After the eleventh week, the placenta produces enough progesterone and estrogen to maintain pregnancy. In the male fetus, HCG also exerts an interstitial cell-stimulating effect on the testes, resulting in the production of testosterone. This small secretion of testosterone during embryonic development is the factor that causes male sex organs to grow.

HCG is present in maternal blood serum 8 to 10 days after fertilization, just as soon as implantation has occurred, and is detectable in the maternal urine a few days after implantation by radioimmunoassay tests. Chorionic gonadotropin reaches its maximum level at 50–70 days' gestation and then begins to decrease as placental hormone production increases.

Progesterone is a hormone essential for pregnancy. It increases the secretions of the fallopian tubes and uterus to provide appropriate nutritive matter for the developing morula and blastocyst. Progesterone causes decidual cells to develop in the uterine endometrium, and it must be present in high levels for implantation to occur. It also decreases the contractility of the uterus, thus preventing uterine contractions from causing spontaneous abortion. The progesterone secreted during pregnancy also helps to prepare the breasts for lactation.

The production of progesterone by the corpus luteum prior to stimulation by HCG reaches a peak about 8 days after ovulation. Implantation occurs at about the same time as this peak. At 10 days after ovulation, progesterone reaches a level between 15 and 30 mg/ml of body plasma and continues to rise slowly in subsequent weeks (Vande Wiele et al., 1976). After the tenth week of pregnancy the placenta takes over the production of progesterone and secretes it in tremendous quantities, reaching levels of 188–560 mg/24 hr.

By the seventh week of pregnancy, more than 50% of the *estrogens* in the maternal circulation are produced by the placenta. Estrogens serve mainly a proliferative function, causing enlargement of the uterus, breasts, and breast glandular tissue. Estrogens also have a significant role in increasing vascularity and vasodilatation, particularly in the villous capillaries near the end of pregnancy. Placental estrogens increase markedly toward the end of pregnancy, to as much as 30 times the daily production in the middle of a normal monthly menstrual cycle. The primary estrogen secreted by the placenta is different from that secreted by the ovaries: the placenta secretes mainly estriol, whereas the ovaries secrete primarily estradiol. The placenta by itself cannot synthesize estriol. Essential precursors are provided by the adrenal glands of the fetus and are transported to the placenta for the final conversion to estriol. Therefore, measurement of the presence of estriol can be a test for both fetal well-being and placental functioning.

HCS is biochemically similar to human pituitary growth hormone. Secretion of this protein hormone begins about the fifth week of pregnancy. Placental lactogen stimulates key maternal metabolic adjustments and makes more protein and glucose available for the fetus. The lactogen also causes lipolysis, which increases the circulation of free fatty acids for maternal cellular metabolic usage and decreases maternal metabolism of glucose and amino acids. Because placental lactogen is a physiologic antagonist of insulin, it is considered to be the principal diabetogenic factor in pregnancy. Placental lactogen also promotes growth of the breasts and other maternal tissue during pregnancy.

A fifth hormone, *relaxin*, is also found in the blood of pregnant women. The placenta may be the site for relaxin production, or the ovaries may secrete relaxin in response to other placental hormones. Relaxin softens cartilage in the pelvic joints and symphysis pubis. It also promotes relaxation of pelvic ligaments and connective tissue elsewhere in the body. It serves to relax all smooth muscles—uterus, bladder, ureters, and gastrointestinal tract—and also promotes vasodilatation.

Immunologic Properties. The placenta is a transplant of living tissue within the same species and is therefore considered a homograft. Ordinarily, homografts are destroyed by the host within a week or two. The placenta and embryo, however, seem to be exempt from their host's immunologic reactivity. In fact, a totally unrelated embryo will grow after being transferred to a second uterus. The most accepted theory to explain this phenomenon is that trophoblastic tissue is immunologically inert. It may contain a cell coating that masks transplantation antigens and that repels sensitized lymphocytes (Beer and Billingham, 1974).

Metabolic Activities. The placenta is believed to have a metabolic rate comparable to that of an adult liver or kidney. Glycogen, cholesterol, and fatty acids are continuously synthesized by the placenta for fetal usage and hormone production. The placenta also produces the numerous enzymes necessary for fetoplacental transfer, and it breaks down certain substances such as epinephrine and histamine by enzymatic deamination. In addition, it functions as a storage unit for glycogen and iron.

Transport Mechanisms

The placenta is no longer considered to be an inert barrier with pores that prevent the transfer of large molecules and that permit the transfer of small molecules. It is a functional membrane that controls the transfer of a wide range of substances by four mechanisms:

1. *Simple diffusion.* This type of transport requires no energy output. Molecules move from an area of higher concentration to an area of lower concentration until an equilibrium is established. Substances that transfer across the placental membrane by simple diffusion are water, electrolytes, carbon dioxide, and drugs. Recent studies suggest that the rate of oxygen transfer across the placental membrane is greater than that allowed by simple diffusion, indicating that oxygen transfers by facilitated diffusion of some type (Martin and Gingerich, 1976).

2. *Facilitated transport.* This type of transport involves a carrier system to move molecules from an area of greater concentration to an area of lower concentration, thereby speeding up the transfer of certain substances through the placental membrane. Among molecules carried by facilitated placental transport are glucose, galactose, and some oxygen.

3. *Active transport.* This type of transport requires energy, involves an enzymatic pathway, and can work against a concentration gradient, with molecules moving from an area of lower concentration to an area of higher concentration. Amino acids, calcium, iron, iodine, and some vitamins transfer across the placental membrane by active transport.

4. *Pinocytosis.* In this type of transport, materials are engulfed by amebalike cells forming plasma droplets. This mechanism is important for transferring large molecules, such as albumin and gamma globulins, across the placental membrane.

Other modes of transfer exist. For example, fetal red blood cells pass into the maternal circulation through breaks in the placental membrane, particularly during labor and delivery. Certain cells, such as maternal leukocytes, and microorganisms, such as viruses and *Treponema pallidum* (which causes syphilis), can also cross the placental membrane, but the exact mechanism is not known. Some bacteria and protozoa infect the placenta by causing lesions, then enter the fetal blood system.

Parer (1974) has identified several factors that affect transfer rate: (a) molecular size, (b) electrical charge, (c) lipid solubility, (d) placental area, (e) diffusion distance, (f) maternal-fetal-placental blood flow, and (g) blood saturation with gases and nutrients. Substances that have a molecular weight of 1000 daltons or more have difficulty crossing the placenta by simple diffusion. Electrically charged molecules pass across the placenta more slowly. A lipid-soluble substance moves quickly across the placenta into the fetal circulation. Reduction of the placental surface area, as with abruptio placentae, will lessen the area that is functional for exchange. Placental diffusion distance also affects exchange; in conditions such as diabetes and placental infection, edema of the villi increases the diffusion distance, thus increasing the distance the substance has to be transferred.

The placental concentration gradient is altered by the concentration of substances in the maternal and fetal blood, by the placental blood flow from the fetus and the intervillous space blood flow from the mother, by the ratio of blood on each side of the placenta, and by the functioning of the carrier molecules in binding and dissociating. Decreased intervillous space blood flow is seen in labor and with certain maternal disease conditions such as hypertension. Mild hypoxia in the fetus increases the umbilical blood flow, and severe hypoxia results in decreased flow.

As the maternal blood picks up fetal waste products and carbon dioxide, it drains back into the maternal circulation through the veins in the basal plate (Parer, 1974). Fetal blood is hypoxic; it therefore attracts oxygen from the mother's blood. In addition, affinity for oxygen increases as the fetal blood gives up its carbon dioxide, which also decreases its acidity.

Fetal Circulation

Because the fetus must maintain the blood flow to the placenta to obtain oxygen and nutrients and to remove carbon dioxide and other waste products, the circulatory system of the fetus has several unique features.

The lungs of the fetus do not function in utero. Therefore, a special circulatory system is required to bypass the blood supply to the lungs. The placenta assumes the function of the lungs by allowing carbon dioxide to be excreted by the fetus and carried off by the maternal blood and by allowing oxygen as well as nourishing products to be acquired by the fetus. The blood from the placenta is carried through the umbilical vein, which penetrates the abdominal wall of the fetus. It divides into two branches, one of which circulates a small amount of blood through the liver and empties into the vena cava through the hepatic vein. The other larger branch, called the *ductus venosus*, empties directly into the vena cava. The blood then enters the right atrium, passes through the *foramen ovale* into the left atrium, and pours into the left ventricle, which pumps it into the aorta. Some blood returning from the head and upper extremities by way of the superior vena cava is emptied into the right atrium and passes through the triscupid valve into the right ventricle. This blood is pumped into the pulmonary artery, and a small amount passes to the lungs, to provide nourishment only. The larger portion of blood passes through the *ductus arteriosus* into the descending aorta, thus bypassing the lungs. Finally, blood returns to the placenta through the two umbilical arteries, and the process is repeated (Figure 6–14).

Fetal Heart

The heart of the fetus, as of the adult, is under the control of its own pacemaker. The sinoatrial (S-A) node sets the rate and is supplied by the vagus nerve. Bridging the atrium and the ventricle is the atrioventricular (A-V) node. It is also supplied by the vagus nerve. Baseline variability of the fetal heartbeat has been shown to be under the influence of this nerve. Atropine will block this effect.

Under the influence of the sympathetic nervous system, norepinephrine is released when the fetus is stressed, causing an increase in the fetal heart rate. To counteract the increase in blood pressure, baroreceptors, which respond to stretch, are present in the vessel walls at the junction of the internal and external carotid arteries. When stimulated, these receptors, under the influence of the vagus and glossopharyngeal nerves, cause the fetal heart rate to slow.

There are chemoreceptors in the fetal peripheral and central nervous systems that respond to decreased oxygen tensions and to increased carbon dioxide tensions, leading to fetal tachycardia and an increase in blood pressure. In studies conducted with the fetal lamb and monkey, it was concluded that the central nervous system also has control over heart rate. Increased activity of the lamb in a wakeful period was exhibited in an increase in the beat-to-beat variability of the fetal heart baseline. Sleep patterns demonstrated a decrease in the beat-to-beat baseline variability. In cases of severe hypoxia, increased levels of epinephrine and norepinephrine act on the fetal heart to produce a faster and stronger rate (Parer, 1974).

EMBRYO AND FETAL DEVELOPMENT AND ORGAN FORMATION

The basic events of organ development in the embryo and fetus are outlined in Table 6–2 on pp. 150–154.

Preembryonic Stage

The first 14 days of human development are referred to as the *preembryonic stage*, or the *stage of the ovum*. This period is characterized by extremely rapid growth, differentiation of tissues into essential organs, and development of main external features, as discussed in detail earlier in this chapter.

Embryonic Stage

The stage of the *embryo* begins with the third week and continues until approximately the end of the eighth week.

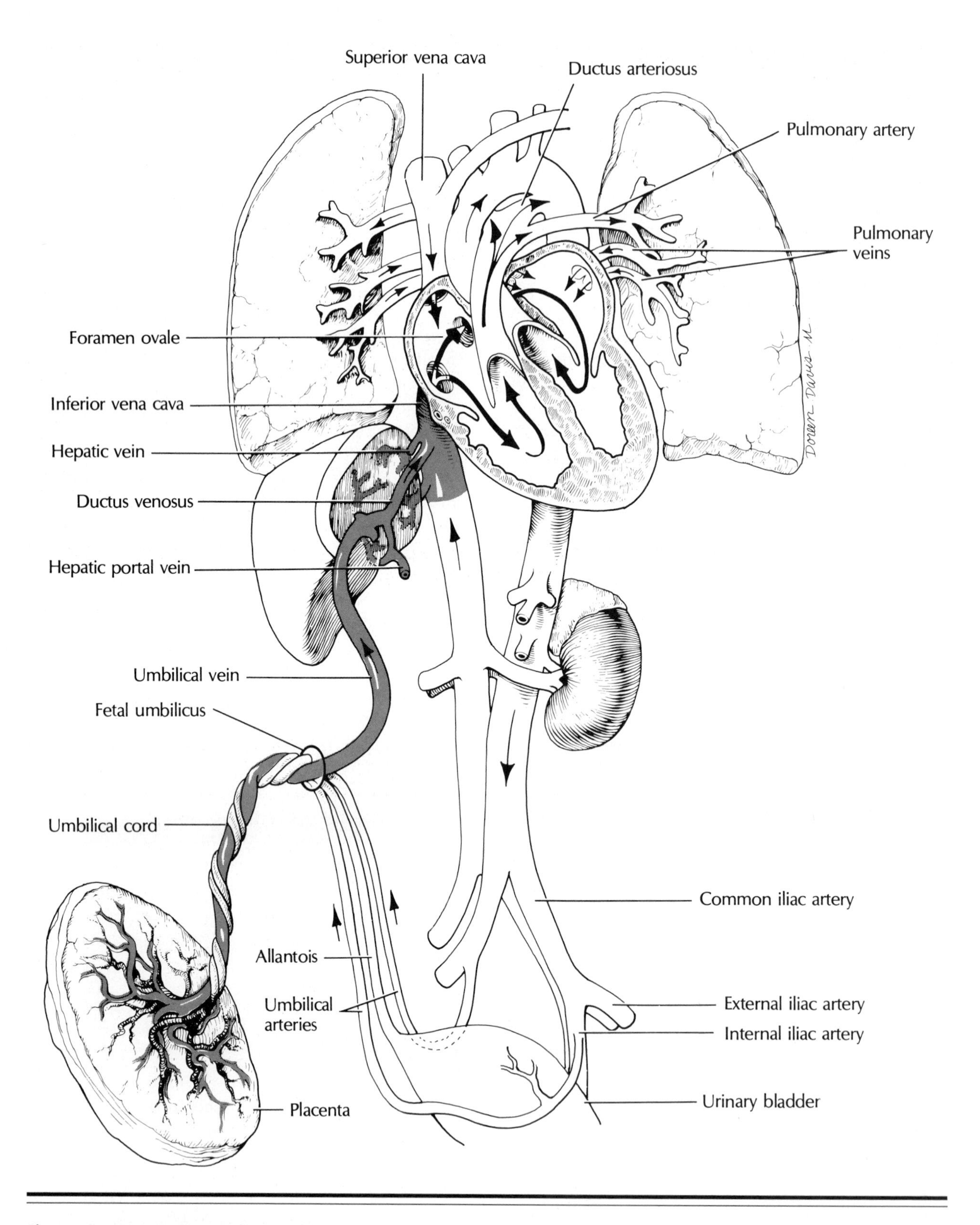

Figure 6–14. Fetal circulation. Blood leaves the placenta and enters the fetus through the umbilical vein. After circulating through the fetus, the blood returns to the placenta through the umbilical arteries. The ductus venosus, the foramen ovale, and the ductus arteriosus allow the blood to bypass the fetal liver and lungs. (From Spence, A. P., and Mason, E. B. 1979. *Human anatomy and physiology.* Menlo Park, Calif.: Benjamin/Cummings Publishing Co., p. 809.)

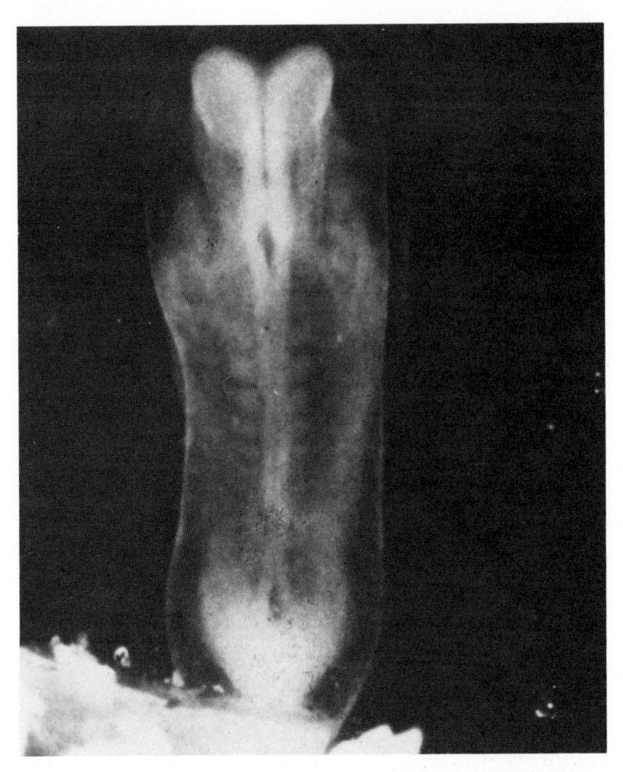

Figure 6–15. Third week. (Courtesy Dr. Roberts Rugh and Landrum B. Shettles.)

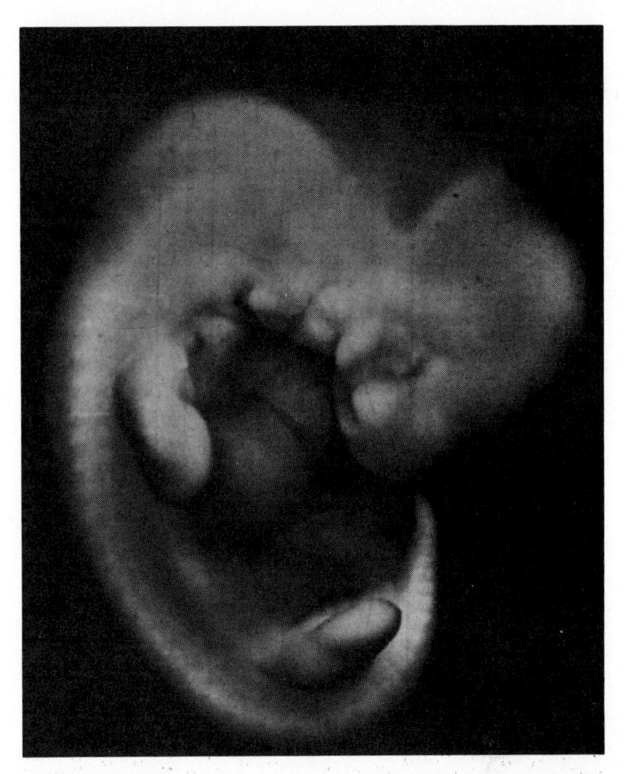

Figure 6–16. Fifth week. (Courtesy Dr. Roberts Rugh and Landrum B. Shettles.)

Third Week

In the third week the embryonic disk becomes elongated and pear-shaped, with a broad cephalic end and a narrow caudal end (Figure 6–15). The ectoderm has formed a long cylindrical tube for brain and spinal cord development. The gastrointestinal tract, created from the endoderm, appears as another tubelike structure communicating with the yolk sac. The most advanced organ is the heart. At three weeks, a single tubular heart forms just outside the body cavity of the embryo and by four weeks (28 days), it is beating at a regular rhythm and pushing its own primitive blood cells through the main blood vessels.

Fourth Week

The interval between the 21st and 32nd day is characterized by somite formation. Somites are a series of mesodermal blocks that form on each side of the midline of the embryo. By the 28th day, between 30 and 40 pairs of somites are present, appearing in a craniocaudal sequence. The vertebras that form the spinal column will develop from these somites. Arm and leg buds are not yet visible, but the tail bud is present. By this time four pairs of pharyngeal arches and five pairs of pharyngeal pouches have developed. The first arch will form the lower jaw (mandibular arch), the second arch will form the hyoid bone, and the third and fourth arches will form cartilage for the larynx. The first pouch, located just below the first arch, will form the eustachian tube and the cavity of the middle ear. The second pouch takes part in the formation of tonsils, and the third and fourth pouches contribute to the formation of the parathyroid and thymus glands. The fifth pouch is rudimentary and does not persist in the human embryo. The primordia of the eye and ear are also present. About the 30th day, the arm and leg buds become prominent and, by the 35th day, are well developed, with paddle-shaped hand and foot plates.

Fifth Week

During the fifth week, the optic cups and lens vesicles of the eye form and the nasal pits develop. Partitioning in the heart occurs with the dividing of the atrium. The embryo has a marked C-shaped body, accentuated by the rudimentary tail and the large head folded over a protuberant

Table 6–2. Classification of Organ System Development

Gestational age	Length*	Weight	Nervous system	Musculoskeletal system	Cardiovascular system	Gastrointestinal system
Conception						
2-3 weeks	2 mm C-R		Groove is formed along middle of back as cells thicken; neural tube formed from closure of neural groove		Beginning of blood circulation; heart begins to form during third week	
4 weeks	4 mm C-R	0.4 gm	Anterior portion of neural tube closes to form brain; closure of posterior end forms spinal cord	Noticeable limb buds	Tubular heart is beating at 24 days and primitive red blood cells are circulating through fetus and chorionic villi	Mouth: formation of oral cavity; primitive jaws present; esophagotracheal septum begins division of esophagus and trachea Digestive tract: stomach forms; esophagus and intestine become tubular; ducts of pancreas and liver forming
5 weeks	8 mm C-R	Only 0.5% of total body weight is fat (to 20 weeks)	Brain has differentiated and cranial nerves are present	Developing muscles have innervation	Atrial division has occurred	
6 weeks	12 mm C-R			Bone rudiments present; primitive skeletal shape forming; muscle mass begins to develop; ossification of skull and jaws begins	Chambers present in heart; groups of blood cells can be identified	Oral and nasal cavities and upper lip formed
7 weeks	18 mm C-R				Fetal heartbeats can be detected	Mouth: tongue separates; palate folds Digestive tract: stomach attains final form
8 weeks	2.5-3 cm C-R	2 gm		Digits formed; further differentiation of cells in primitive skeleton; cartilaginous bones show first signs of ossification; development of muscles in trunk, limbs, and head; some movement of fetus is now possible	Development of heart is essentially complete; fetal circulation follows two circuits—four extraembryonic and two intraembryonic	Mouth: completion of lip fusion Digestive tract: rotation in midgut; anal membrane has perforated
10 weeks			Neurons appear at caudal end of spinal cord; basic divisions of the brain present	Fingers and toes begin nail growth		Mouth: separation of lips from jaw; fusion of palate folds Digestive tract: developing intestines enclosed in abdomen
12 weeks	8 cm C-R, 11.5 cm C-H	45 gm		Clear outlining of miniature bones (12-20 weeks); process of ossification is established throughout fetal body; appearance of involuntary muscles in viscera		Mouth: completion of fusion of palate Digestive tract: appearance of muscles in gut; bile secretion begins; liver is major producer of red blood cells
16 weeks	13.5 cm C-R, 15 cm C-H	200 gm		Teeth: beginning formation of hard tissue that will become central incisors Mother can detect fetal movement		Mouth: differentiation of hard and soft palate Digestive tract: development of gastric and intestinal glands; intestines begin to collect meconium
18 weeks				Teeth: beginning formation of hard tissue (enamel and dentine) that will become lateral incisors	Fetal heart tones audible with fetoscope at 16-20 weeks	
20 weeks	18.5 cm C-R, 25 cm C-H	300 gm (6% of total body weight is fat)	Myelination of spinal cord begins	Teeth: beginning formation of hard tissue that will become canine and first molar Lower limbs are of final relative proportions		Fetus actively sucks and swallows amniotic fluid; peristaltic movements begin

*C-R = crown-rump; C-H = crown-heel

Genitourinary system	Respiratory system	Skin	Specific organ systems	Sexual development
				Determination of sex
Formation of kidneys beginning	Nasal pits forming		Endocrine system: thyroid tissue appears Eyes: optic cup and lens pit have formed; pigment in eyes Ear: auditory pit is now enclosed structure Liver function begins	
	Trachea, bronchi, and lung buds present		Ear: formation of external, middle, and inner ear continues Liver begins to form red blood cells	Embryonic sex glands appear
Separation of bladder and urethra from rectum	Diaphragm separates abdominal and thoracic cavities		Eyes: optic nerve formed; eyelids appear but are fused shut; thickening of lens Ear: external, middle, and inner ear assuming final structure forms	Differentiation of sex glands into ovaries and testes begins External genitals appear similar
Bladder sac formed Urine formed			Endocrine system: islets of Langerhans differentiated Eyes: development of lacrimal duct	
	Lungs acquire definitive shape	Skin pink, delicate	Endocrine system: hormonal secretion from thyroid Immunologic system: appearance of lymphoid tissue in fetal thymus gland	
Kidneys assume typical shape and organization		Appearance of scalp hair; lanugo present on body; transparent skin with visible blood vessels	Eye, ear, and nose formed Sweat glands developing	Sex determination possible; descent of testes into inguinal canal at 12–24 weeks
	Final cellular structure of alveoli	Lanugo covers entire body; brown fat begins to form; vernix caseosa begins to form	Immunologic system: detectable levels of fetal antibodies (IgG type normally) Blood formation: iron is stored and bone marrow is increasingly important	

trunk (Figure 6–16). The heart, circulatory system, and brain show the most advanced development. The brain has differentiated into five areas, and ten pairs of cranial nerves are recognizable.

Sixth Week

At six weeks, the head structures are more highly developed and the trunk is straighter than in earlier stages (Figure 6–17). The upper and lower jaws are recognizable, and the external nares are well formed. The trachea has developed, and its caudal end is bifurcated for beginning lung formation. The upper lip has formed, and the palate is developing. The ear is developing rapidly, as are the other postbranchial body parts. The arms have begun to extend ventrally across the chest, and both arms and legs have digits, although they may still be webbed. There is a slight elbow bend in the arm, and the arm is more advanced in development than the leg. The embryo at this time has a prominent tail, but beginning at this stage, the tail will regress. The heart now has most of its definitive characteristics, and fetal circulation begins to be established. The liver begins to produce blood cells.

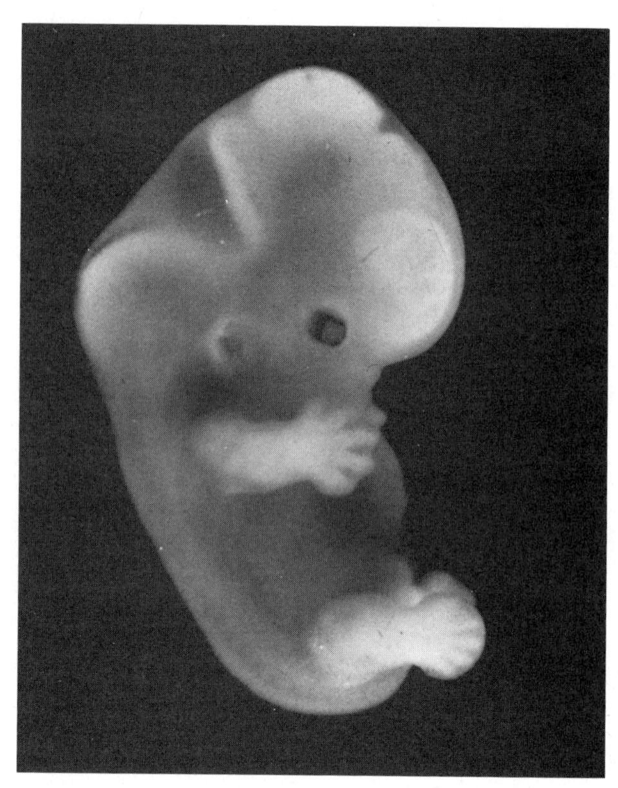

Figure 6–17. Sixth week. (Courtesy Dr. Roberts Rugh and Landrum B. Shettles.)

Table 6–2. Classification of Organ System Development

Gestational age	Length*	Weight	Nervous system	Musculoskeletal system	Cardiovascular system	Gastrointestinal system
24 weeks	23 cm C-R, 30 cm C-H	650 gm	Structure of brain; looks like mature brain	Teeth: beginning formation of hard tissue that will become second molar		
28 weeks	27 cm C-R, 35 cm C-H	1100 gm	Nervous system begins regulation of some body functions			
32 weeks	31 cm C-R, 40 cm C-H	1800 gm	More reflexes present			
36 weeks	35 cm C-R, 45 cm C-H	2200 gm		Distal femoral ossification centers present		
40 weeks	40 cm C-R, 50 cm C-H	3200+ gm (16% of total body weight is fat)				

*C-R = crown-rump; C-H = crown-heel

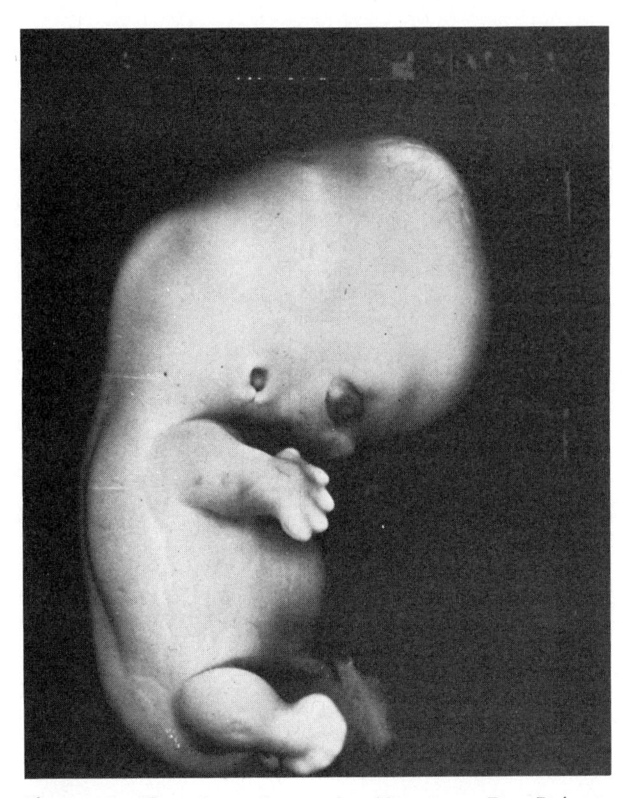

Figure 6–18. Seventh week. (Courtesy Dr. Roberts Rugh and Landrum B. Shettles.)

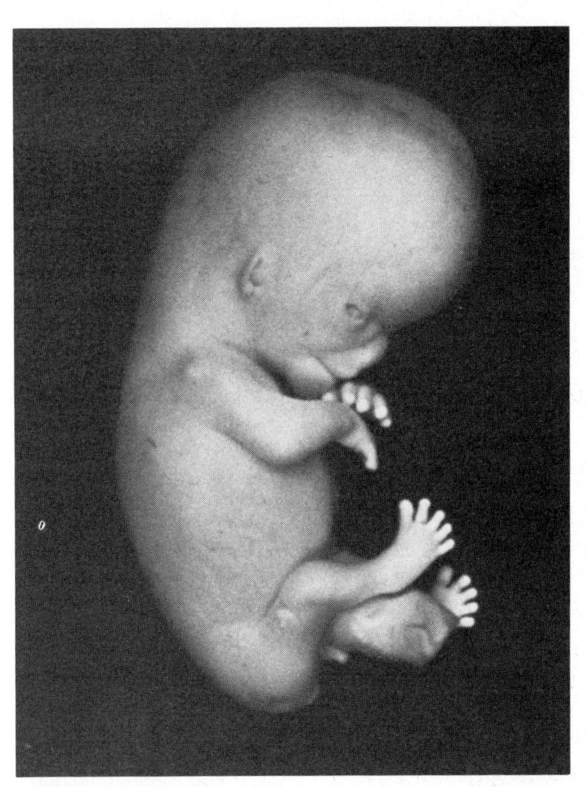

Figure 6–19. Eighth week. (Courtesy Dr. Roberts Rugh and Landrum B. Shettles.)

Genitourinary system	Respiratory system	Skin	Specific organ systems	Sexual development
	Respiratory movements may occur (24–40 weeks) Nostrils reopen Alveoli appear in lungs and begin production of surfactant; gas exchange possible	Skin reddish and wrinkled; vernix caseosa present	Immunologic system: IgG levels reach maternal levels Eyes structurally complete	
		Adipose tissue accumulates rapidly; nails appear; eyebrows and eyelashes present	Eyes: eyelids open (28–32 weeks)	Testes descend into scrotal sac
		Skin pale; body rounded; lanugo disappearing; hair fuzzy or woolly; few sole creases; sebaceous glands active and helping to produce vernix caseosa (36–40 weeks)	Ear lobes soft with little cartilage	Scrotum small and few rugae present; descent of testes into upper scrotum to stay (36–40 weeks)
	At 38 weeks, L/S ratio approaches 2:1	Skin smooth and pink; vernix present in skinfolds; moderate to profuse silky hair; lanugo hair on shoulders and upper back; nails extend over tips of digits; creases cover sole	Ear lobes stiffened by thick cartilage	Males: rugous scrotum Females: labia majora well developed

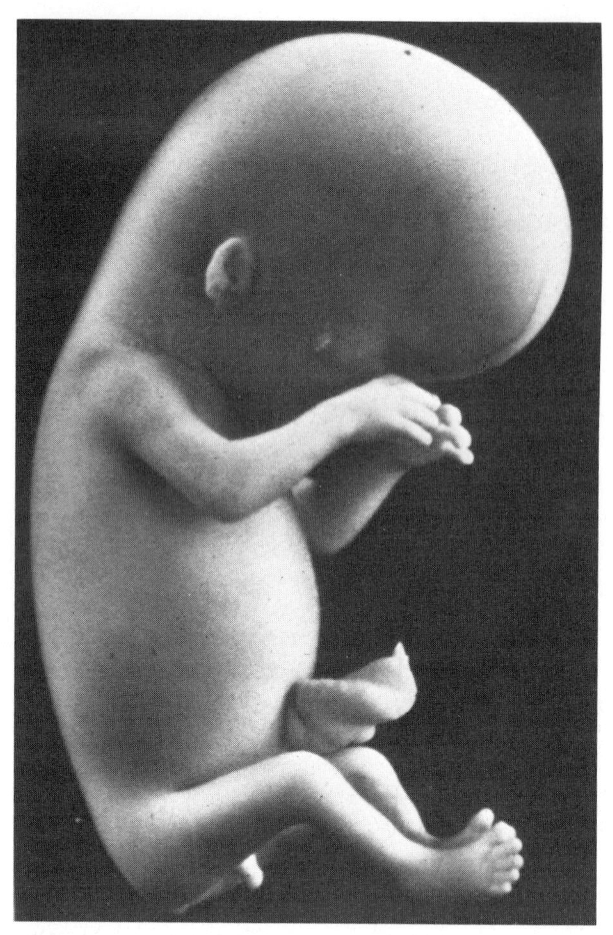

Figure 6–20. Ninth week. (Courtesy Dr. Roberts Rugh and Landrum B. Shettles.)

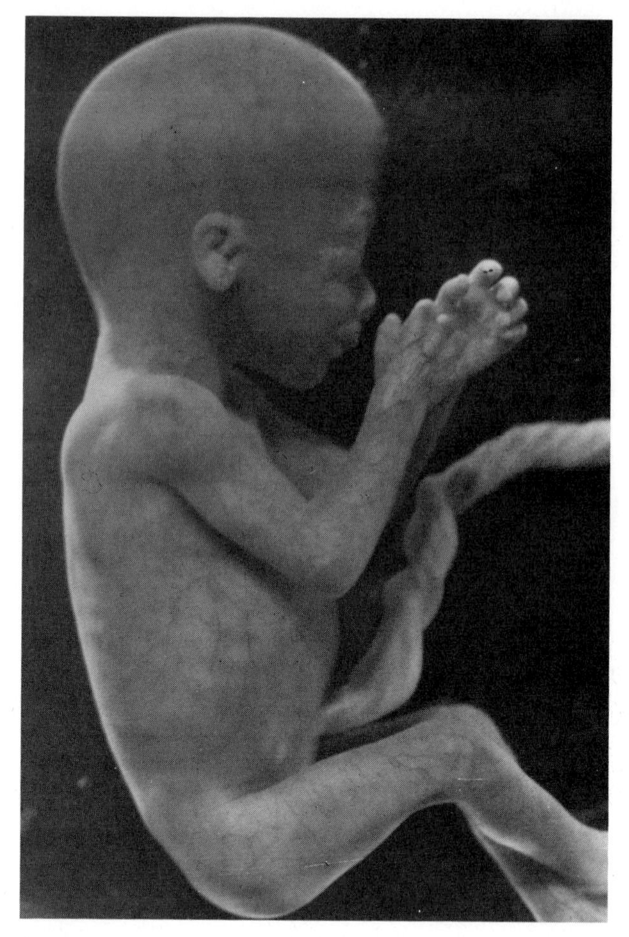

Figure 6–21. Twenty-eighth week. (Courtesy Dr. Roberts Rugh and Landrum B. Shettles.)

Seventh Week

At the seventh week the head of the embryo is rounded and nearly erect (Figure 6–18). The eyes have shifted from their original lateral position to a forward location, where they are closer together, and the eyelids are beginning to form. The palate is nearing completion, and the tongue also develops in the formed mouth. The gastrointestinal and genitourinary tracts undergo some significant changes during the seventh week. Prior to this time, the rectal and urogenital passages formed one tube that ended in a blind pouch; they now separate into two tubular structures. At this point, the beginnings of all essential external and internal structures are present.

Eighth Week

At the eighth week the embryo is approximately 2.5 cm long and clearly resembles a human being (Figure 6–19). Face and features continue their development. External genitals appear but are not discernible, and the rectal passage opens, with the anal membrane now perforated. The circulatory system through the umbilical cord is well established. Long bones are beginning to form, and the large muscles that have developed are capable of contracting. By the end of the embryonic period, all major organ systems have been started, if not become completely established, and the rest of the prenatal period is devoted to final refinements of structures and organization and practice of function.

Fetal Stage

By the end of the eighth week the embryo has become a *fetus*.

9–12 Weeks

The fetus has now reached a crown-to-heel length of 7–9 cm and probably weighs 5–20 gm. The head is large and comprises almost half of the fetus's entire size (Figure 6–20). The neck is distinct from the head and body, and both the head and neck are straighter than in previous stages of development. The face is well formed, with the nose protruding, the chin small and receding, and the ear acquiring a more adult shape. The eyelids close at about the 10th week and will not reopen until about 28 weeks. Some reflex movements of the lips suggestive of the sucking reflex have been observed at 3 months. Tooth buds now appear for all 20 of the child's first teeth (baby teeth). The limbs are long and slender, with well-formed digits. The fetus can curl the fingers toward the palm and make a tiny fist. The legs are still shorter and less developed than the arms. The urogenital tract completes its development, well-differentiated genitals appear, and the kidneys begin to form urine. Red blood cells are produced primarily by the liver. Spontaneous movements of the fetus now occur.

13–16 Weeks

At 13–16 weeks the fetus weighs from 55 to 120 gm and is about 10–17 cm in crown-to-heel length. Downy *lanugo hair* begins to develop, especially on the head. The fetal skin is so transparent that blood vessels are clearly visible beneath it. More muscle tissue and body skeleton have developed, which tend to hold the fetus more erect. Active movements are present—the fetus stretches and exercises its arms and legs. It makes sucking motions, swallows amniotic fluid, and forms meconium in the intestinal tract. Bronchial tubes are branching out in the primitive lungs, and sweat glands are developing. The liver and pancreas now begin production of their appropriate secretions.

17–20 Weeks

Growth is rapid in the fourth month. The fetus almost doubles its length and now measures about 25 cm. With this great increase in size, fetal weight increases to between 280 and 300 gm. Lanugo covers the entire body and is especially prominent on the shoulders. Subcutaneous deposits of brown fat have made the skin a little less transparent. Nipples now appear over the mammary glands. The head sports fine, "woolly" hair, and the eyebrows and eyelashes are beginning to form. The fetus has nails on both fingers and toes. Muscles are well developed, and the fetus is active. Fetal movement, known as *quickening*, is felt by the mother. The heartbeat is audible with the use of a stethoscope.

21–24 Weeks

The fetus has now reached a crown-to-heel length of 28–34 cm and weighs about 650 gm. The hair on the head is growing long, and eyebrows and eyelashes have formed. The eye is structurally complete and will soon open. The fetus has a reflex hand grip (grasp reflex), and by the end of the sixth month will have a startle reflex. Skin covering the body is reddish and wrinkled, with little subcutaneous fat. Skin on the hands and feet has thickened, with skin ridges on palms and soles forming distinct footprints and fingerprints. The skin over the entire body is covered with a protective cheeselike fatty substance secreted by the sebaceous glands called *vernix caseosa.* The alveoli in the lungs are just beginning to develop.

25–28 Weeks

At six months the fetus has the appearance of a little old man; the skin is still red, wrinkled, and covered with vernix caseosa (Figure 6–21). During this time the brain is developing rapidly, and the nervous system is complete enough to provide some regulation of body functions. The eyelids open and close under neural control. If the fetus is a male, the testes begin to descend into the scrotal sac. Respiratory and circulatory systems have developed sufficiently. The 28th week has traditionally been considered the earliest period of extrauterine viability. In some of the current literature, it has been suggested that extrauterine viability begins as early as 24 weeks' gestational age (Ziegel and Van Blarcom, 1978). However, very few infants survive at this gestational age, no matter how expert their care is. At 28 weeks' gestation the lungs are still immature, and the fetus requires specialized care to survive. The fetus at 28 weeks is about 35–38 cm long crown to heel and weighs about 1200 gm.

29–32 Weeks

The fetus is gaining weight from an increase in body muscle and fat and weighs about 2000 gm, with a length of about 38–43 cm. If born during this time, the infant has about a 60% chance of surviving with special care. Bones are now fully developed but are soft and flexible. The fetus begins storing minerals—iron, calcium, and phosphorus. Testicles may be located in the scrotal sac but are often still high in the inguinal canal.

33–36 Weeks

The body and extremities of the fetus are "filling out." The fetus is beginning to get plump, with less wrinkled skin covering the deposits of subcutaneous fat. Lanugo hair is beginning to disappear, and the nails have grown so they reach the edge of the fingertips. Weight is usually 1700–2600 gm, and the length of the fetus is about 42–48 cm crown to heel. If born at this time, the infant has a good chance of surviving but still requires some special care.

37–40 Weeks

The fetus is considered full-term at 38 weeks. Crown-to-heel length varies from 48 to 52 cm, with males being the longest. Males also weigh more. The weight at term is about 3000–3600 gm. The skin is pink and smooth with a polished look. The only lanugo hair remaining is on the upper arms and shoulders. On the head, the hair is no longer woolly but coarse and about an inch long. Vernix caseosa is still present but varies in amount, with heavier deposits remaining in creases and folds of the skin. The body and extremities are plump, with good skin turgor, and the fingernails extend beyond the fingertips. The chest is prominent but still a little smaller than the head, and mammary glands protrude in both sexes. The testes are in the scrotum or are palpable in the inguinal canals. As the fetus enlarges, amniotic fluid diminishes until there is about 500 ml or less, and the fetal body mass fills the uterine cavity. The fetus assumes what is referred to as its *position of comfort*, or *lie*. Generally, the head is down, because of the shape of the uterus and also possibly because the head is heavier than the feet. The extremities and often the head are well flexed. After the fifth month, feeding patterns, sleeping patterns, and activity patterns become established, so that at term the fetus has its own body rhythms and individual style of response.

Factors Influencing Embryonic and Fetal Development

Among factors that may affect embryonic development are the quality of the sperm or ovum from which the zygote was formed and the genetic code established at fertilization.

In addition, the adequacy of the intrauterine environment is important for optimal growth. If the environment is unsuitable before cellular differentiation occurs, all the cells of the zygote are affected. The cells may die, resulting in a spontaneous abortion, or growth may be slowed, depending on the severity of the situation. When differentiation is complete and the fetal membranes have formed, an injurious agent has the greatest effect on those cells undergoing the most rapid growth. Thus, the time of injury is critical in the development of anomalies.

Because organs are formed primarily during embryonic development, the growing organism is considered most vulnerable to noxious agents during the first months of pregnancy. Table 6-3 lists potential malformations related to the time of insult. Chapter 13 discusses the effects of specific teratogenic agents on the developing fetus.

The adequacy of the maternal environment is also extremely important to embryonic and fetal development. Those substances required for growth of a particular structure must be readily available at its time of development. In general, raw materials for development come from the mother's diet and not from her bodily reserves. Thus temporary deficiencies in the mother's diet, which may cause no manifest symptoms in her, may affect the developing embryo or fetus.

Research studies on animals have found that poor nutrition produces specific developmental anomalies (Moore, 1977). Such research has not been conducted on humans, so generalizations about the effects of diet on human development are of limited validity. Data concerning infants born to mothers with reportedly deficient diets during pregnancy indicate smaller intrauterine growth and more susceptibility to infections, particularly respiratory infections, during the first year of life. It is believed that barely adequate maternal nutritional intake may sustain growth and development during early pregnancy but may not meet the needs of the rapidly growing fetus during late pregnancy.

The period of maximum brain growth begins with the fifth lunar month before birth and con-

Table 6–3. Developmental Vulnerability Timetable

Weeks since ovulation	Potential malformation	Weeks since ovulation	Potential malformation
3	Ectopia cordis	6	Microphthalmia
	Omphalocele		Carpal or pedal ablation
	Ectromelia		Hairlip, agnathia
	Sympodia		Lenticular cataract
4	Omphalocele		Congenital heart disease
	Ectromelia		Gross septal or aortic abnormalities
	Tracheoesophageal fistula	7	Congenital heart disease
	Hemivertebra		Interventricular septal defects
5	Tracheoesophageal fistula		Pulmonary stenosis
	Hemivertebra		Digital ablation
	Nuclear cataract		Cleft palate, micrognathia
	Microphthalmia		Epicanthus
	Facial clefts		Brachycephaly
	Carpal or pedal ablation	8	Congenital heart disease
			Epicanthus
			Brachycephaly
			Persistent ostium primum
			Nasal bone ablation
			Digital stunting

tinues during the first six months after birth (Reeder, 1976). Amino acids, glucose, and fatty acids are considered to be the primary dietary factors in brain growth. A subtle type of damage that affects the associative capacity of the brain, possibly leading to learning disabilities, may be caused by nutritional deficiency at this stage and is the subject of current research.

Maternal nutrition during pregnancy is discussed in detail in Chapter 11.

TWINS

Twins may be either fraternal or identical. If they are fraternal, they are *dizygotic*, which means they arise from two separate ova fertilized by two separate spermatozoa. They have two placentas, two chorions, and two amnions; however, the placentas sometimes fuse together and look as if they are one. Despite their birth relationship, they are no more similar to each other than they would be to siblings born singly. They may be the same or different sex.

Identical, or *monozygotic*, twins develop from a single fertilized ovum. Consequently, they are of the same sex and have the same genotype. Division of the single fertilized ovum into two units does not occur at the first cleavage division, as was once believed, but only after the embryo consists of many thousands of cells. Complete separation of the cellular mass into two parts is necessary for twin formation. Identical twins have a common placenta and a single chorion but always two separate amnions (Figure 6–22).

Twins have been reported to occur more often among black than among white women and more often among white individuals than Orientals. Among all groups, as parity increases so does the chance for multiple births. In the United States, 2% of births are plural.

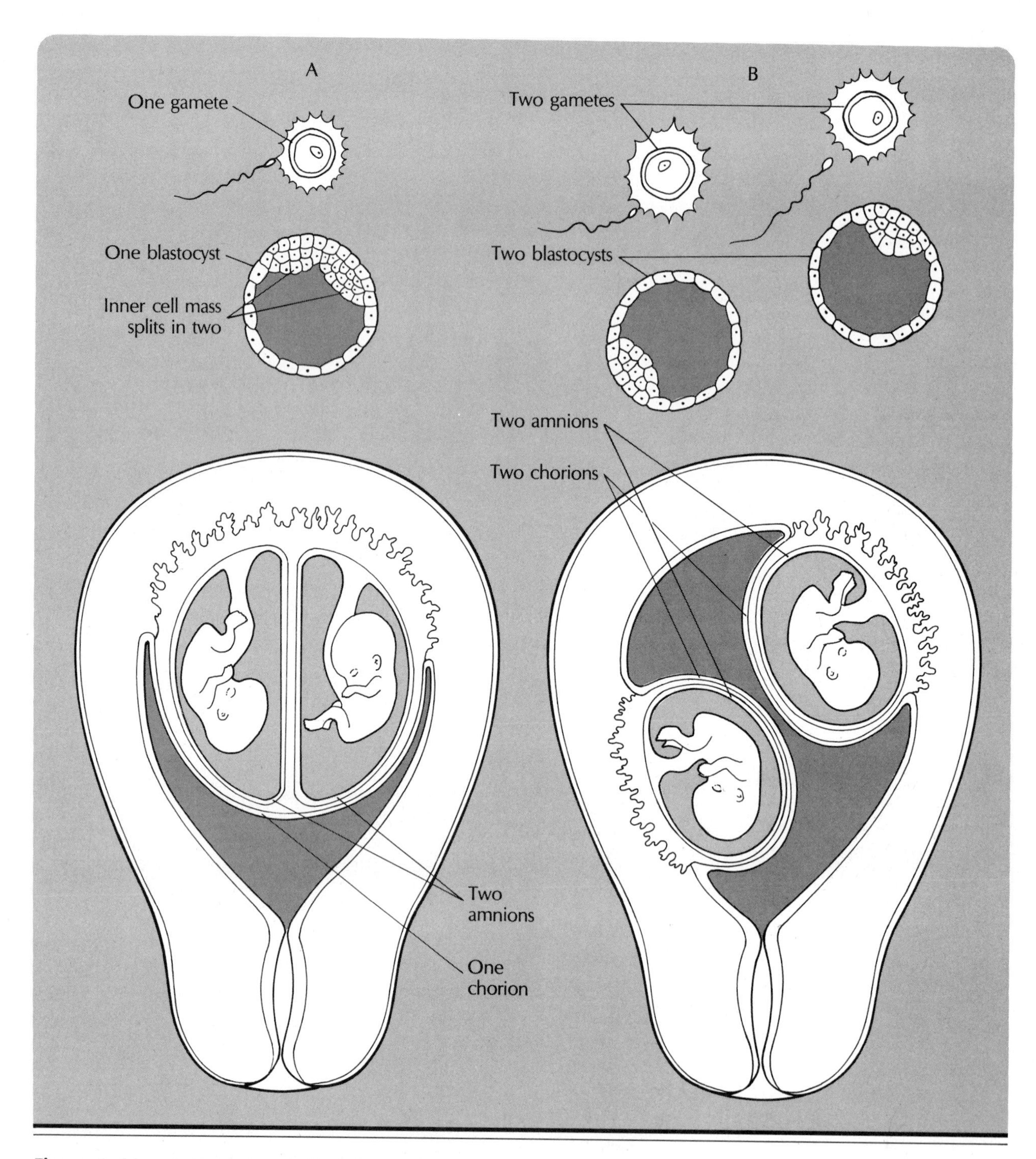

Figure 6–22. **A,** Formation of identical twins. **B,** Formation of fraternal twins.

SUMMARY

From a single fertilized cell, through an orderly series of events, a complex human being develops and begins his or her existence. This process is one of the most dynamic events in nature. The period of embryonic and fetal development is characterized by rapid cellular division, multiplication, and differentiation and by formation of the structures necessary for intrauterine development in the placenta, fetal membranes, and umbilical cord.

It is essential that the nurse comprehend the processes and mechanisms of embryonic, fetal, and placental development to understand the various critical influences that timing of cellular division and environment have on the successful completion of this complex process.

SUGGESTED ACTIVITIES

1. In the classroom laboratory, determine the weight and length of fetal specimens and note the significant growth and developmental changes associated with various gestational ages.
2. While assisting in a prenatal clinical setting or in prenatal classes, based on your knowledge of fetal development, answer parents' questions such as the following:
   When will the heartbeat be heard?
   How does my baby get its food?
   When will the fetus look like a baby?
   What determines if the fetus is a girl or a boy?

REFERENCES

Beer, A. E., and Billingham, R. E. April 1974. The embryo as a transplant. *Sci. Am.* 230:36.

Danforth, D. 1977. *Obstetrics and gynecology.* New York: Harper & Row Publishers, Inc.

DeCoursey, R. M. 1974. *The human organism.* 4th ed. New York: McGraw-Hill Book Co.

Jensen, M. D., et al. 1977. *Maternity care: the nurse and the family.* St. Louis: The C. V. Mosby Co.

Martin, C. B., and Gingerich, B. Sept.–Oct. 1976. Uteroplacental physiology. *J. Obstet. Gynecol. Neonatal Nurs.* 5 (supp.):16.

Moore, K. L. 1977. *The developing human: clinically oriented embryology.* 2nd ed. Philadelphia: W. B. Saunders Co.

Parer, J. T. 1974. Uteroplacental and fetal physiology. In *A clinical approach to fetal monitoring.* San Leandro, Calif.: Berkeley Bio Engineering, Inc.

Reeder, F. 1976. Fact or fantasy? Maternal and infant nutrition affect brain development and intellectual performance. In *Current practice in pediatric nursing,* vol. 1, eds. P. A. Brandt et al. St. Louis: The C. V. Mosby Co.

Vande Wiele, R. L., et al. 1976. Progesterones in pregnancy. In *Diabetes and other endocrine disorders during pregnancy and in the newborn,* eds. M. I. New and R. H. Fiser. New York: Alan R. Liss, Inc.

Whaley, L. F. 1974. *Understanding inherited disorders.* St. Louis: The C. V. Mosby Co.

Winchester, A. M. 1966. *Heredity: an introduction to genetics.* New York: Barnes & Noble, Inc.

Ziegel, E., and Van Blarcom, C. C. 1978. *Obstetric nursing.* 7th ed. New York: The Macmillan Co.

ADDITIONAL READINGS

Arey, L. 1965. *Developmental anatomy.* 7th ed. Philadelphia: W. B. Saunders Co.

Chinn, P. L. 1974. *Child health maintenance.* St. Louis: The C. V. Mosby Co.

Gordon, R., et al. 1978. The shaping of tissues in embryos. *Sci. Am.* 238:106.

Hong, S. K. 1976. Transport of essential elements in fetal-neonatal system. In *Childbearing: a nursing perspective,* eds. A. L. Clark and D. Affonso. Philadelphia: F. A. Davis Co.

McRedmond, A., et al. 1976. Placental development and circulation. *Ross Laboratories Clinical Education Aid,* no. 2, Teaching Reference. Columbus, Ohio: Ross Laboratories.

Nilsson, L., et al. 1975. *A child is born.* New York: Dell Publishing Co., Inc.

Pritchard, J. A., and MacDonald, P. C. 1976. *Williams obstetrics.* 15th ed. New York: Appleton-Century-Crofts.

Tanner, J. M., and Taylor, G. R., eds. 1968. *Growth.* New York: Time-Life Books.

Tuchmann, H. and Duplessis, G., et al. 1972. *Illustrated human embryology: embryologenesis,* vol. 1. New York: Springer Verlag New York, Inc.

Ville, C. A. 1970. Enzymatic development of the placenta in relation to fetal growth. In *Fetal growth and development,* eds. H. A. Waisman and G. R. Kerr. New York: McGraw-Hill Book Co.

Weingold, A. B. 1974. The fetus and fetal environment. In *Survey of clinical pediatrics,* eds. E. Wasserman and L. B. Slobody. New York: McGraw-Hill Book Co.

Whipple, D. V. 1966. *Dynamics of development: euthenic pediatrics.* New York: McGraw-Hill Book Co.

CHAPTER 7

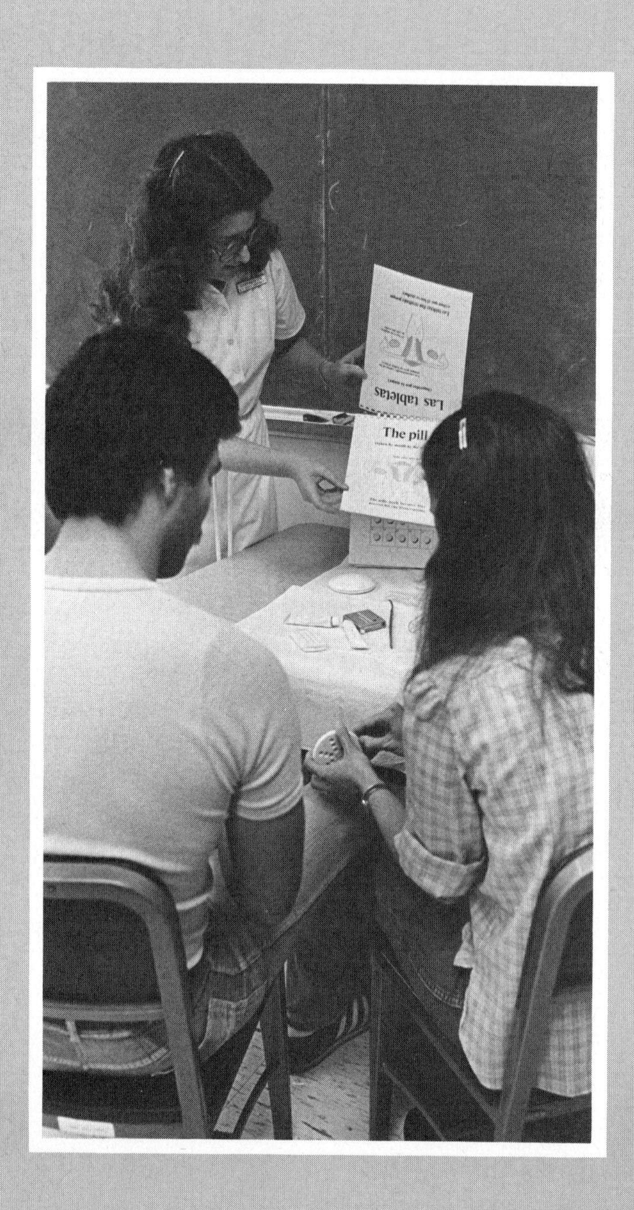

FAMILY PLANNING

CONTRACTION

Natural Family Planning

Mechanical Contraceptives

Ovulatory Suppressors

Spermaticides

Operative Sterilization

Induced Abortion

OBJECTIVES

- Identify the three main reasons for couples to seek family planning.
- Discuss infertility and its effect on couples.
- Compare various methods of contraception.
- Discuss the various types of abortions.

Control of reproduction has always been one of the foremost concerns of both men and women. Couples have eagerly sought fertility and sterility at appropriate times and under chosen circumstances. The man-woman relationship and the woman's self-concept have been greatly affected by the development of reliable methods for the control of reproductive functions. Motherhood has become a matter of choice, and birth control methods have reinforced the concepts of freedom of choice and the individual's right to self-determination.

Advances in medical-scientific knowledge and accompanying societal changes have expanded the processes and acceptance of family-planning techniques. Today competent nursing care requires an intellectual and emotional understanding of birth control techniques in order to adequately serve the growing numbers of people seeking or needing professional assistance for family planning.

The terms "family planning," "birth control," and "contraception" are used interchangeably. Usually, the term *family planning* is the broadest concept and includes voluntary interruption of pregnancy, seeking solutions to infertility, controlling the timing of pregnancies, and assessing the social, psychologic, economic, physical, and theologic concerns of couples making decisions about having children. *Contraception* and *birth control* generally refer to the methods employed to space or limit pregnancies.

Family planning is the responsibility of the involved couple. The health care professional can assist by providing clear, specific, and accurate information with which the couple may make informed decisions. Before they can reach a decision, the couple must evaluate sociocultural, economic, religious, physical, and psychologic factors in relation to their beliefs and values. After they reach a decision about which contraceptive method to use, the variables that contribute to acceptability of a method must be evaluated. Selection of a method of birth control requires information about cost, effectiveness, procedure for use, previous history of use or friends' use of a given method, personal objections and desires for use, and medical contraindications for a given couple. Health care professionals must be careful not to influence decision-making according to their preferences, because such persuasion is likely to reduce the effectiveness of the contraceptive method.

The reasons for a couple to engage in family planning are threefold: (1) to identify and correct causes of infertility; (2) to allow control over the number of children in the family; and (3) to predetermine the interval between desired children. Besides contributing to psychologic health by giving increased mastery over an important life event, family planning has physical benefits. It is well documented that the state of a woman's health is often negatively influenced by too frequent or too numerous pregnancies or by the absence of pregnancy. Given these facts, nursing personnel have a responsibility to provide information related to the various methods of family planning, in an objective and nonjudgmental manner.

INFERTILITY

Although the phrase "family planning" has come to imply planned limitation of pregnancies, an important aspect of family planning addresses itself to increasing the chances of conception, or to identifying couples for whom conception may be difficult or impossible.

Infertility can be defined as the inability of a couple to produce a living child as a result of failure to conceive or of failure to carry a conceptus to a viable state. There appears to be an increase in the incidence of infertility today, which may be related to the trend in delaying marriage and postponing childbearing until the couple has passed the age of optimal fertility (24 to 25 years). Other factors in infertility include increased risk of prolonged anovulation following the use of birth control pills, infections associated with use of intrauterine devices or following abortions, and obstructive diseases of the male and female reproductive systems caused by venereal disease.

Causes of Infertility

Understanding the elements essential for normal fertility can assist the professional nurse in identifying the many factors that may cause infertility.

The following conditions must be present for normal fertility:

Male partner:

1. The testes must produce spermatozoa of normal quality and quantity.
2. The male genital tract must not be obstructed.
3. The male genital tract secretions must be normal.
4. Ejaculated spermatozoa must be deposited in the female genital tract in such a manner that they reach the cervix.

Female partner:

1. The cervical mucus must be favorable for survival of spermatozoa.
2. There must be clear passage between the cervix and the fallopian tubes.
3. Fallopian tubes must be patent and have normal peristaltic movement to allow ascent of spermatozoa and descent of ovum.
4. Ovaries must produce and release normal ova.
5. There must not be obstruction between the ovaries and the fimbriae of the fallopian tubes.
6. The endometrium must be in a normal physiologic state to allow implantation of the blastocyst and to sustain normal growth.

In addition to these specific conditions, general physiologic and psychologic conditions must be such as to support conception.

With intricacies of timing and environment playing such a crucial role, it is an impressive natural phenomenon that approximately 85% of married couples in the United States are able to conceive. Of the remaining 15%, for every 100 couples about 40 will show a male deficiency, 20 a female hormonal defect, 30 a female tubal disorder, and 10 a cervical defect. In 35 of the couples multiple etiologies will be identified. Professional intervention can assist approximately 30% of infertile couples to achieve a pregnant state.

Couples present concerns about infertility following their inability to conceive after at least one year of attempting to achieve pregnancy. At the age of 25 years, which is identified as the couple's most fertile time, the average length of time needed to achieve conception is 5.3 months. For every 100 couples, 25 will achieve pregnancy after one month of unprotected intercourse, 63 by the end of six months, 75 by the end of nine months, and 80 by the end of twelve months (Shane, Schiff, and Wilson, 1976).

Preliminary Investigation

Evaluation and preliminary investigation should be made available for couples seeking help for infertility. Extensive testing should be avoided until data confirm that the timing of intercourse and the length of coital exposure have been adequate. Preliminary investigation should include a comprehensive history and physical examination for assessment of any obvious causes of infertility before a costly, time-consuming, and emotionally trying investigation is initiated. During the first visit for preliminary investigation, the requirements for a basic infertility investigation (the five basic tests) should be explained and a trusting relationship should be established between the health professionals and the infertile couple.

Health care interventions in cases of infertility are illustrated in Figure 7-1. Following the initial interview with the infertile couple, a complete history is taken and a comprehensive physical examination is conducted. The historical data base for the couple should include the following information:

Female:

1. Menstrual history
   a. Age of menarche; interval, duration, and quantity of menses
   b. Ovulation
      1. Symptoms, including molimina (premenstrual symptoms such as mood changes, breast tenderness, acne), mittelschmerz (midcycle ovulatory pain), intermenstrual spotting, increased midcycle discharge, and dysmenorrhea
   c. Date of last menstrual period
2. Previous pregnancies
   a. Number, and age at time of conception
   b. Interval of unprotected intercourse before conception
   c. Father of previous pregnancies
   d. Circumstances surrounding pregnancy loss
   e. Identification of any disease (such as pelvic inflammatory disease, intraabdominal operations, or endometriosis) that could

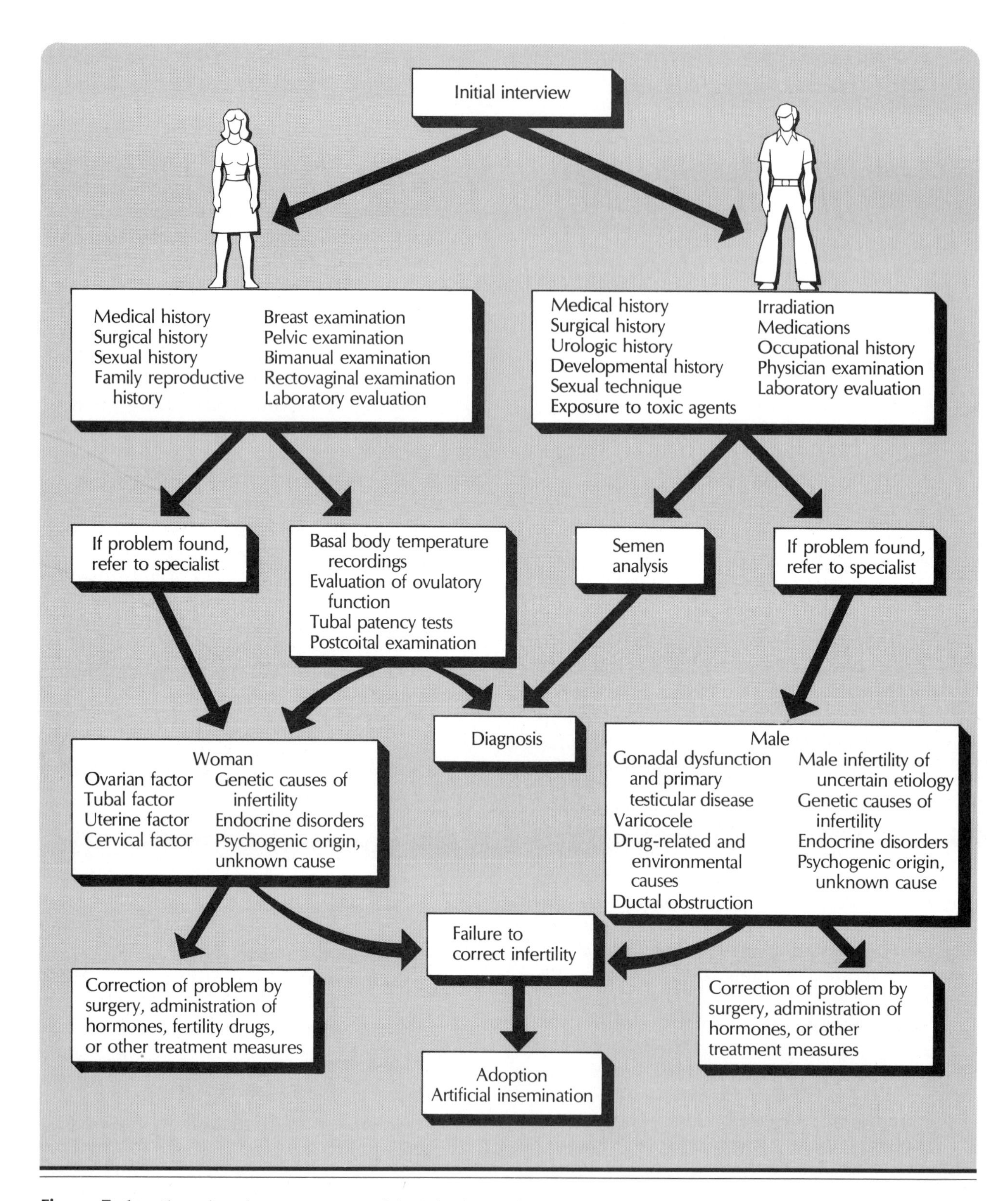

Figure 7–1. Flow chart for management of the infertile couple.

have adversely affected reproductive factors

3. Reproductive history
   a. Frequency of coitus
   b. Coital technique
   c. Family's reproductive history
   d. Past medical and surgical illnesses pertinent to reproductive potential (i.e., an appendicitis that might have caused tubal obstruction or adhesions)
   e. Medications (i.e., phenothiazines producing an amenorrhea-galactorrhea complex)

Male:

1. Age (sperm count decreases with age)
2. Occupation (some occupations expose the scrotum to excessive heat, which is harmful to spermatogenesis, e.g., cross-country truck-driving)
3. Medical history
   a. Mumps after adolescence
   b. Diabetes
   c. Tuberculosis
   d. Venereal disease, epididymitis, orchitis, or other medical conditions
4. Surgical history
   a. Accidental damage to testes
   b. Previous hernia repairs, cryptorchidism, circumcision, hypospadias, or other conditions requiring surgical intervention
5. Developmental history
   a. Endocrine diseases
   b. Age when growth spurt occurred; acne; appearance of facial hair
6. Sexual history
   a. Sexual technique
   b. Frequency of intercourse
   c. Presence of orgasm during coitus and ejaculation with orgasm
   d. Previous history of fathering other children with different sexual partner
7. Exposure to toxic substances or irradiation
   a. Toxic substance exposure (e.g., x-rays, lead, chemicals)
   b. Irradiation for genital cancer
8. Medications
   a. Drugs affecting potency (e.g., narcotics, alcohol, tranquilizers, monoamine oxidase inhibitors, and guanethidine and methyldopa, which interfere with the autonomic nervous system and cause retrograde ejaculation)
   b. Drugs affecting spermatogenesis (including amebicides, antimalarial drugs, nitrofurantoin, and methotrexate)
9. Personal habits
   a. Alcohol consumption
   b. Type of underwear worn (tight underwear may raise scrotal temperature)
   c. Bathing habits (hot baths and saunas may be harmful)

Following completion of the couple's histories, a complete physical examination of each partner is performed. At this time the following areas are evaluated:

Female:

1. Physical examination
   a. Endocrine evaluation of thyroid for exophthalmos, lid lag, tremor, or palpable gland
   b. Optic fundi evaluation for presence of increased intracranial pressure
   c. Reproductive features (including breast and external genital area)
   d. Physical ability to tolerate pregnancy
   e. General health
2. Pelvic examination
   a. Papanicolaou smear
   b. Culture for gonorrhea
   c. Shape of escutcheon (e.g., does pubic hair distribution resemble that of a male?)
   d. Size of clitoris
   e. Cervical mucus (evaluate for estrogen effect of spinnbarkeit and cervical ferning)
3. Bimanual examination
   a. Presence of congenital anomalies and tumors of corpus luteum
   b. Presence of endometriosis
   c. Ovarian size
4. Rectovaginal examination
   a. Presence of retroflexed or retroverted uterus

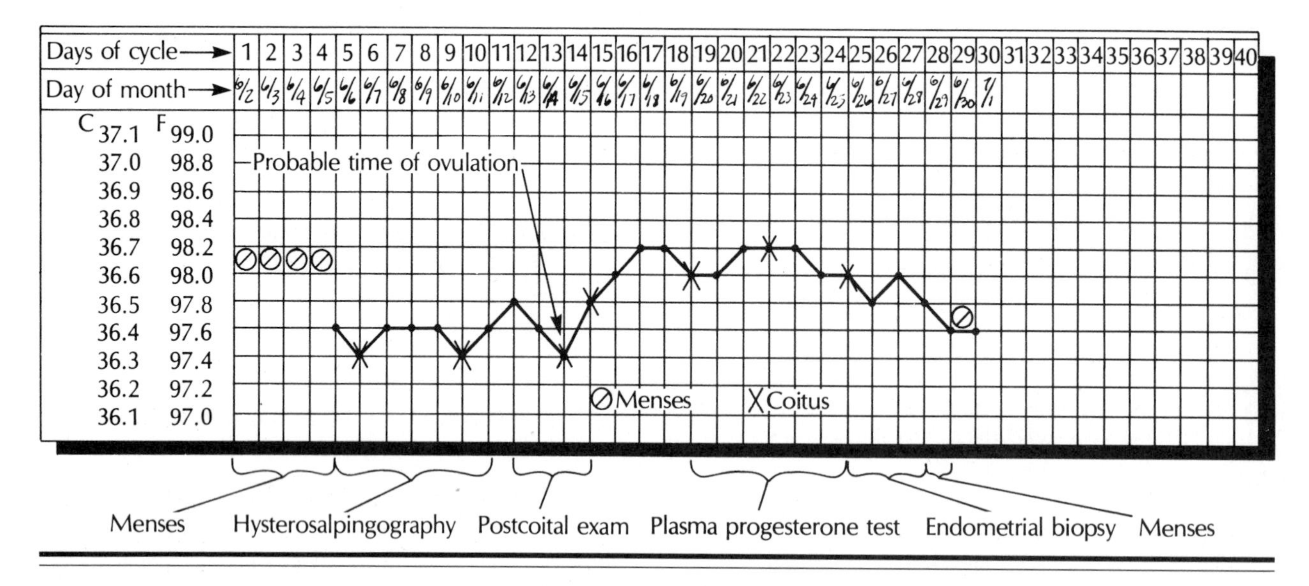

Figure 7–2. Basal body temperature chart with different types of testing and the time in the cycle that each would be performed.

   b. Presence of rectouterine pouch masses
   c. Presence of possible endometriosis

Male:

1. Physical examination
   a. General health (including blood pressure, height, arm span, weight, and so forth)
   b. Endocrine evaluation (e.g., presence of gynecomastia)
   c. Visual fields evaluation
   d. Abnormal hair patterns
   e. Urologic examination (includes notation of penis size; presence or absence of phimosis; location of urethral meatus; size and consistency of each testis, ductus deferens, and epididymis; presence of varicocele)
2. Rectal examination
   a. Size and consistency of the prostate, with microscopic evaluation of prostate fluid for signs of infection
   b. Size and consistency of the seminal vesicles

In addition to the physical examination, laboratory tests should be performed, including a complete blood count with sedimentation rate, urinalysis, diagnostic serology, and any other tests indicated from the history and physical examination.

Tests for Infertility

There are five basic tests that define the general areas in which fertility problems exist. These tests are designed to evaluate the anatomy, physiology, and sexual compatibility of the couple.

The first of the five basic tests is the *basal body temperature recording*. At the initial visit, the female is instructed in the technique of recording basal body temperatures, which may be taken with a basal body temperature thermometer. This special thermometer measures temperature between 96F and 100F and is calibrated by tenths of a degree, thereby enabling easier identification of slight temperature changes. The woman may choose the site to obtain the temperature. Possible sites include oral, axillary, rectal, or vaginal, and the same site should be used each time. For best results the thermometer should be kept beside the bed and the woman should take her temperature upon awakening, before any activity. After obtaining her temperature, she shakes the thermometer to prepare it for use the next day. This step is important, as even the activity of shaking the thermometer immediately before use can cause a small increase in the basal temperature. Other factors that may produce temperature variation are sleeplessness, digestive disturbances, illness, fever, and emotional upset. Daily variations should be recorded on the temperature graph. The temperature graph and the readings are used for detecting ovulation and for timing intercourse. The basal temperature for females in the preovulatory phase is usually below 98F (36.7C). As ovulation approaches, production of estrogen increases and may cause a drop in the basal temperature. When ovulation occurs, progesterone is produced, causing a 0.5 to 1F (0.3 to 0.6C) rise in basal temperature. Figure 7-2 shows a basal body temperature chart.

Further evaluation of ovulatory function is made by using a *biopsy of the endometrium,* which measures the effects of progesterone produced after ovulation by the corpus luteum. Progesterone concentrations can also be measured by plasma concentrations. A plasma progesterone concentration of 3 mg/ml suggests ovulation.

Tubal patency is confirmed with either tubal insufflation with carbon dioxide or hysterosalpingography. *Tubal insufflation* gives presumptive evidence of tubal patency, but its advantages are otherwise limited. The procedure does not tell whether one or both tubes are patent and gives no information about the contour of the uterine cavity, about uterine anomalies, or about distortion of one or both tubes as a result of pelvic adhesions.

Hysterosalpingography can reveal tubal patency and any distortions of the endometrial cavity. This procedure has also been known to have a therapeutic effect. Pregnancy is frequently achieved within the first three cycles following the test. This effect may be caused by the flushing of debris, by breaking of adhesions, or by induction of peristalsis by the media. Both procedures cause moderate discomfort, and thus the more informative of the two (hysterosalpingography) should be utilized. The hysterosalpingography should be performed in the proliferative phase of the cycle in order to avoid interrupting an early pregnancy and also to avoid the lush secretory changes in the endometrium that occur after ovulation and that may prevent the passage of the dye, presenting a false picture of cornual obstruction.

The *postcoital examination* is performed one to two days prior to the expected date of ovulation. The couple is asked to have intercourse two to four hours prior to being seen. The evaluation consists of examining the cervical mucus and the number and motility of sperm present at the endocervix.

The cervical mucus, which is produced by the mucus-secreting cells of the endocervix, consists predominantly of water. As ovulation approaches, increased secretion of estrogen by the ovary

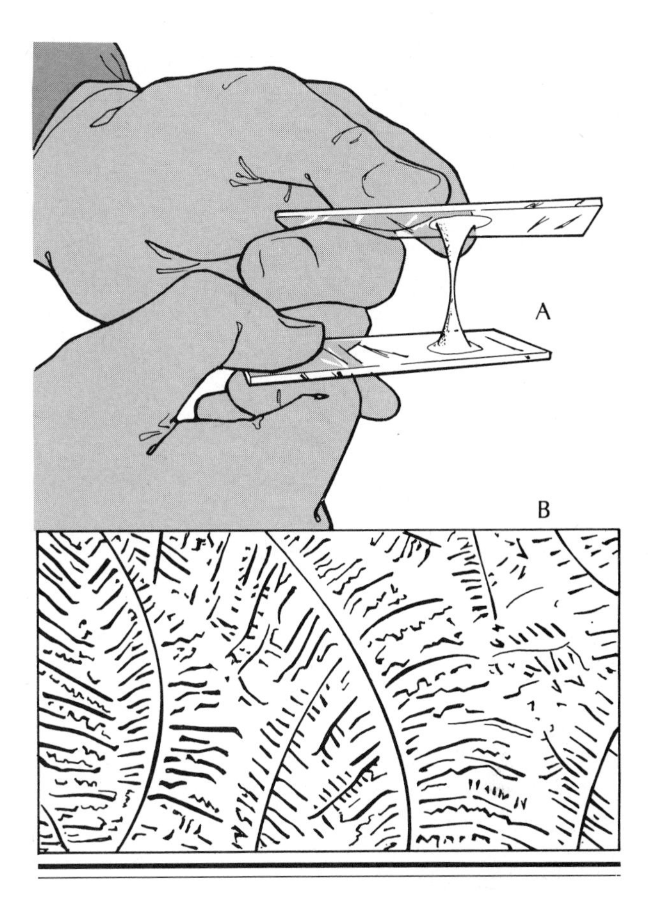

Figure 7-3. **A,** Spinnbarkeit (viscosity). **B,** Ferning.

causes a change in cervical mucus. The amount of mucus increases greatly, and the water content rises significantly. Elasticity (spinnbarkeit) increases, and viscosity decreases. The ferning capacity (Figure 7-3) of the cervical mucus also increases as ovulation approaches. Ferning, or crystallization, is caused by increased levels of salt and water interacting with the glycoproteins in the mucus during the ovulatory period and is thus an indirect indication of estrogen production. All of these factors increase the rate of sperm survival, which thus reaches its highest point at the time of ovulation.

Many physicians replace the postcoital examination with a *semen analysis,* which can be done anytime in the investigation and is the most important initial diagnostic study of the male. Optimum results are obtained after two days of abstinence. The sperm analysis (Figure 7-4) can provide information about sperm motility and morphology as well as a determination of the absolute number of spermatozoa present. A "normal" semen analysis may be defined as one that shows at least 20 million sperm per milliliter, a

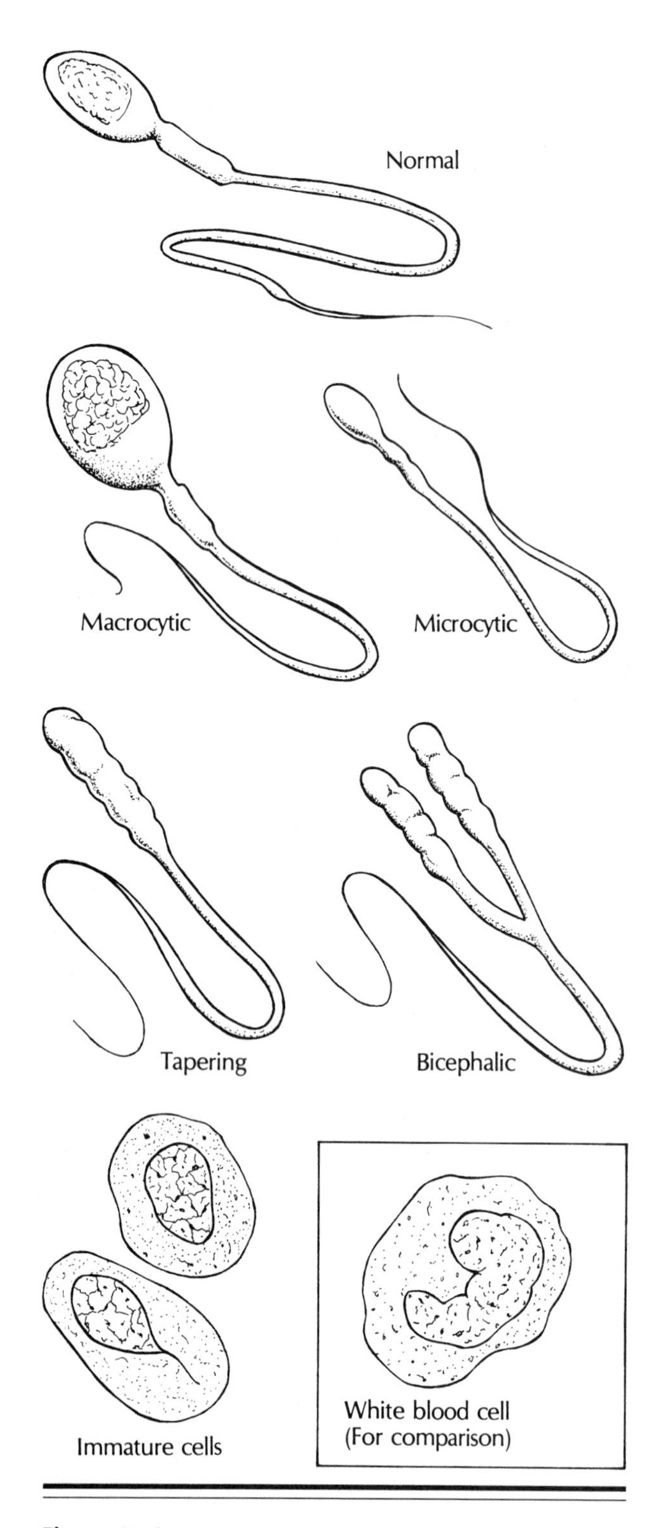

Figure 7–4. Semen analysis.

semen volume of 2 to 5 ml, sperm motility of greater than 60% (within two hours of collection) with normal progression, and at least 60% normal sperm forms. The chance to impregnate is remote if the semen analysis reveals less than 10 million sperm per ml, less than 50% active sperm, or less than 50% normal sperm forms.

Culdoscopy is another useful procedure in the treatment of infertility. The female client is given heavy analgesia and is placed in the knee-chest position. The posterior cul-de-sac is infiltrated with local anesthetic and entered with a metallic trocar (Figure 7–5). Culdoscopic examination of pelvic structures is accomplished by direct visual inspection. Indigo carmine or similar dyes can be injected through a cannula inserted into the cervix, and the patency of the fallopian tubes can thereby be evaluated.

Nursing Responsibility

Throughout the tests that one or both partners may undergo at this time, the nurse has a major responsibility for teaching and providing emotional support. The tests may heighten feelings of frustration or anger between the partners. In addition, the introduction of other parties to the problem in this intimate area of a relationship may precipitate feelings of guilt and shame.

Correction of the problem of infertility may require surgery, administration of hormones, or other treatment measures. The role of the nurse is to continue to provide information and emotional support to the infertile couple.

Infertility may be perceived as a loss by one or both partners, and like the loss of a loved one who dies, this situation is attended by feelings of grief and mourning. Nonjudgmental acceptance and a professional caring attitude on the nurse's part can go far to dissipate the negative effects the couple may experience while going through this process. This is also a time when the nurse may assess the quality of the couple's relationship—are they able and willing to verbally communicate and share feelings? Are they mutually supportive? The answers to such questions may help the nurse to identify areas of strength and weakness that will assist in the construction of an appropriate plan of care.

Tests for infertility may lead to a diagnosis of sterility, which is the absolute inability of the female to become pregnant or for the male to impregnate the female. At times, individual or group counseling with other couples may facilitate the couple's resolution of feelings brought about by this information.

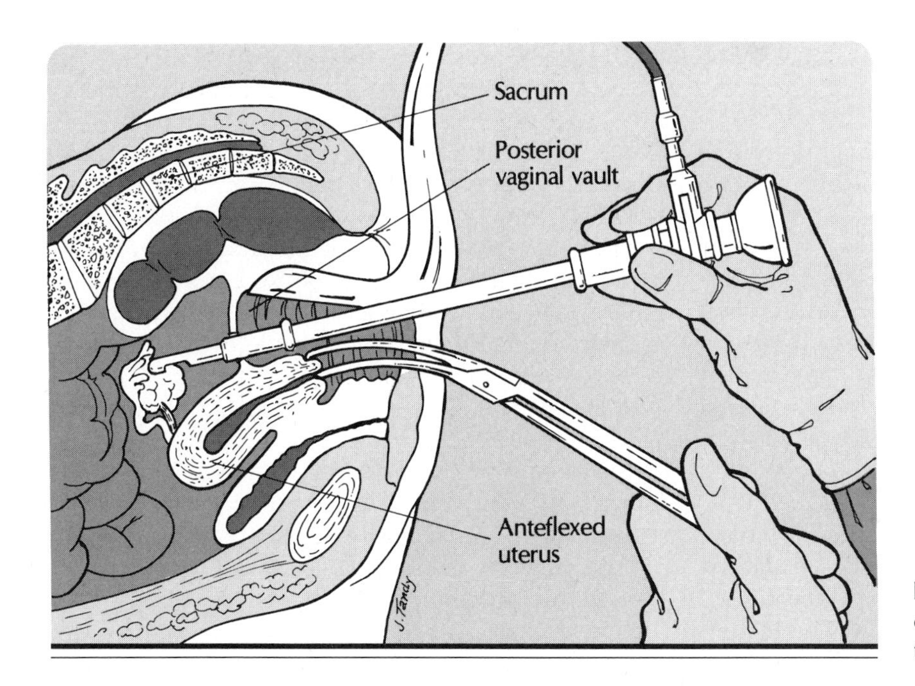

Figure 7-5. With woman in knee-chest position, culdoscope is inserted through the posterior vaginal vault.

HISTORY OF CONTRACEPTION

One of the most pressing problems of the twentieth century is human fertility. Population growth has decreased food supplies, resulting in poor nutrition for approximately 1 billion people. Rapid and increasing population growth can be devastating to mankind and has united health professionals, legislators, physiologists, chemists, researchers, and the general public in a common cause to slow or decrease the world's population.

The concerns of population control are not new. The Greek philosophers considered a stable population essential and suggested legally regulating reproduction and using abortion or infanticide as a population control method (Danforth, 1977).

Chemical means of contraception were identified in the Petrie medical papyrus, 1950 BC, with a recommended use of contraceptive pessaries of crocodile dung and honey or of vaginal fumigations with minnis, an ancient drug. Violent body movements to shake the semen free after intercourse were advocated by Lucretius, the Roman poet, whereas wearing an amulet of worms from the body of a hairy spider was proclaimed by Pliny the Elder to be the most effective birth control means. The *Kama-Sutra*, the Hindu love manual from the fourth century, listed the blossoms of the palash flower as an effective oral contraceptive.

During the Crusades, men supplied their wives and girlfriends with chastity belts, consisting of belts and girdles, to keep the women from accepting the advances of other men while they were gone to war. The continued use of chastity belts was suggested as recently as 1933 by the League of Awakened Magyars (Danforth, 1977).

The condom was invented in 1564 as a linen sheath worn for protection against veneral disease. Condoms made from animal's cecum in the eighteenth century were the first to become popular for contraception. Condoms evolved as a popular method for contraception in 1884, when they began to be inexpensively made from vulcanized rubber.

Between 1880 and 1965 many chemical agents and mechanical devices were available for contraception but were not widely distributed because of the moral issues surrounding their use. A Supreme Court ruling in 1965 was necessary before birth control clinics and dissemination of contraceptive advice became legal (Danforth, 1977).

By 1972 countries on every continent were being offered advice on contraceptives by the International Planned Parenthood Federation. During that year, 739,000 American women received contraceptive services from 700 Planned Parenthood-World Population clinics. Even with this impressive number of women receiving services, half of America's medically indigent women did not receive counseling about family planning.

CONTRACEPTION

Gaining control over the number of children they will conceive and spacing their children are two motivating factors in a couple's decision to use a contraceptive measure. In choosing a specific method, consistency of use outweighs the absolute reliability of a given method. Consideration of the risk factors and contraindications for use of a particular contraceptive method is important if the nurse is going to assist the couple in selecting a contraceptive method that has practical application and that is compatible with the couple's health and physical needs.

Women seeking contraception should have a history taken and a screening physical examination with minimal laboratory tests done before choosing a method of contraception. The history should include immediate family incidences of diabetes, bleeding or clotting problems, heart problems or high blood pressure, migraine headaches or seizure disorders, kidney or liver disease, anemia, tuberculosis, stroke, cancer, or mental problems. This information provides a baseline on risk factors that could influence or contraindicate the prescription of oral contraceptives. A past medical and surgical history is completed, as is a detailed menstrual and obstetric history. The data base should also include information on previous use of and experience with contraceptives, history of allergies, and social information.

A precontraception physical examination should include, as a minimum, a breast check, a pelvic examination and a Pap smear, and some type of health screen. Weight, age, and blood pressure can indicate risk factors that may preclude prescribing certain forms of birth control.

Minimal laboratory testing includes a hemoglobin/hematocrit; urinalysis for sugar and protein; Pap smear; endocervical culture for *Neisseria gonorrhoeae;* serologic test for syphilis; pregnancy test, if indicated; and any other test identified during the history or physical as being appropriate.

The couple's decisions about contraception should be made voluntarily, with full knowledge of options, advantages, disadvantages, effectiveness, side effects, and long-range effects; with access to alternatives; without pressure by health professionals; and with the strictest confidentiality. Many outside factors will influence a couple's choice, including cultural influences, religious beliefs, personality, cost, effectiveness, misinformation, practicability of method, and self-esteem. Different methods of contraception may be appropriate at different times in the couple's life.

Following is a review of the major contraceptive methods available, with an examination of their advantages and disadvantages.

Natural Family Planning

Increasing numbers of couples are becoming interested in natural methods of contraception because they are concerned about the use of artificial devices or substances. There are four methods of natural family planning based on the woman's menstrual cycle: basal body temperature, calendar rhythm, ovulation, and symptothermal. Periodic abstinence from sexual intercourse is a requirement of all four methods, as is the recording of certain events during the menstrual cycle. Advantages of the natural methods include an increased awareness of one's body and avoidance of artificial substances.

The *basal body temperature method* requires that the woman take her basal temperature every morning and record the readings on a temperature graph. The graph then provides data to identify the safe and unsafe periods of the menstrual cycle. Intercourse is avoided on the day of temperature rise and for the following three days.

The *calendar rhythm method* first requires the recording of each menstrual cycle for at least six months so that the shortest and longest cycles can be identified. The first day of menstruation is the first day of the cycle. The fertile phase "extends from and includes the 18th day before the end of the shortest likely cycle through the 11th day before the end of the longest likely cycle" (Britt, 1977). For example, if a woman's cycle lasts from 24 to 28 days, the fertile phase would be calculated as day 6 through day 17. Once this information is obtained, the woman can identify the fertile and infertile phases of the cycle and, for effective use of the method, she must abstain from intercourse during the fertile phase.

The *ovulation method* involves the assessment of cervical mucus changes that occur during the menstrual cycle. The amount and character of cervical mucus changes as a result of the influence of estrogen and progesterone. Type E mucus is predominant at the time of ovulation and is the result of the effect of estrogen on the 100 mucous secretory units present in the cervix. Type G mucus predominates during the luteal phase and is the result of the effects of progesterone.

As ovulation approaches, there is an increase in the amount of cervical mucus and it becomes clearer and more stretchable. This type E mucus consists of "96.7% water, 1% proteins, 0.8% NaCl, 1.5% mucin, and a few cells" (Britt, 1977). Type E mucus shows a fern pattern that becomes apparent when the mucus is placed on a glass slide and is allowed to dry (Figure 7-3).

The stretchability (spinnbarkeit) of the cervical mucus is greatest at the time of ovulation and may vary from 5 cm to 20 cm. Spinnbarkeit may be assessed by obtaining mucus from underwear, from the labia, or from the vagina and then placing the mucus between two glass slides or between two fingers.

Type E mucus allows increased permeability to sperm and enables sperm to pass through the cervix because of the presence of mucin fibers that lie parallel to each other. At ovulation, type E mucus is greatest in amount and stretchability. The woman notices a feeling of wetness around the vagina.

During the luteal phase, the characteristics of the cervical mucus change. It becomes thick and sticky and forms a network in the cervical canal that traps the sperm and makes their passage more difficult. This type G mucus consists of "90.2% water, 3% protein, 0.8% NaCl, 6% mucin, and an abundance of cells" (Britt, 1977).

To use the ovulation method, the woman should abstain from intercourse for the first menstrual cycle. Cervical mucus should be assessed for amount, ferning, and spinnbarkeit on a daily basis as the woman becomes more familiar with varying characteristics. After a pattern has been established, abstinence from intercourse is necessary when type E mucus predominates and for four days following ovulation.

The *symptothermal method* consists of various assessments that are made and recorded by the couple. They use a chart to record information regarding cycle days, coitus, basal body temperature, mucus and cervical changes, and secondary signs such as increased libido, abdominal bloating, and mittelschmerz. Through the various assessments, the couple learns to recognize signs that indicate ovulation.

Situational contraceptives also fall under the heading of natural family planning. These methods involve no prior preparation of the couple but involve motivation to abstain from intercourse or to interrupt the sexual act prior to the ejaculation of the sperm into the vagina. *Coitus interruptus,* or withdrawal, is the oldest method of contraception but has limited effectiveness as a birth preventative. This method depends on the male's ability to time his ejaculation. In the male partner experiencing premature ejaculation, withdrawal is an exceptional problem.

Douching after intercourse is another ineffective method of contraception. It may actually facilitate conception by helping to push the sperm farther up the birth canal.

Rhythm is the only method accepted by the Roman Catholic church and is a variation of the calendar rhythm method previously discussed. It is based on identification of the "unsafe period" of a menstrual cycle, which is a period of time immediately before and after ovulation. Theoretically, there are only three days in each cycle during which conception may occur, but women who have irregular cycles find it difficult to pinpoint the time of ovulation. (See Figure 7-2.) Basal body temperature has been used to determine ovulation, with an increased temperature persisting for three days indicating ovulation. Not all temperature curves are interpretable, however, so many people abstain from intercourse for an extended period of time, between days 12 and 18 in a cycle, to ensure safety. Those dedicated to the method may achieve success, but it requires continuous assessment.

Mechanical Contraceptives

These methods act either as a barrier preventing the transport of sperm to the ovum or increase the propulsion of the ovum/zygote, thereby preventing implantation. *Condoms,* although probably developed to protect against venereal disease, continue to offer a means of contraception when used consistently (Figure 7-6). They are applied to the erect penis, rolled from the tip to the end of the shaft. A small space must be left at the end of the condom to allow for collection of the ejaculate so that the condom will not break at the time of ejaculation. Care must be taken in removing the condom after intercourse. When the penis becomes flaccid following ejaculation, the man should hold the edge of the condom while withdrawing from the vagina to avoid spilling the se-

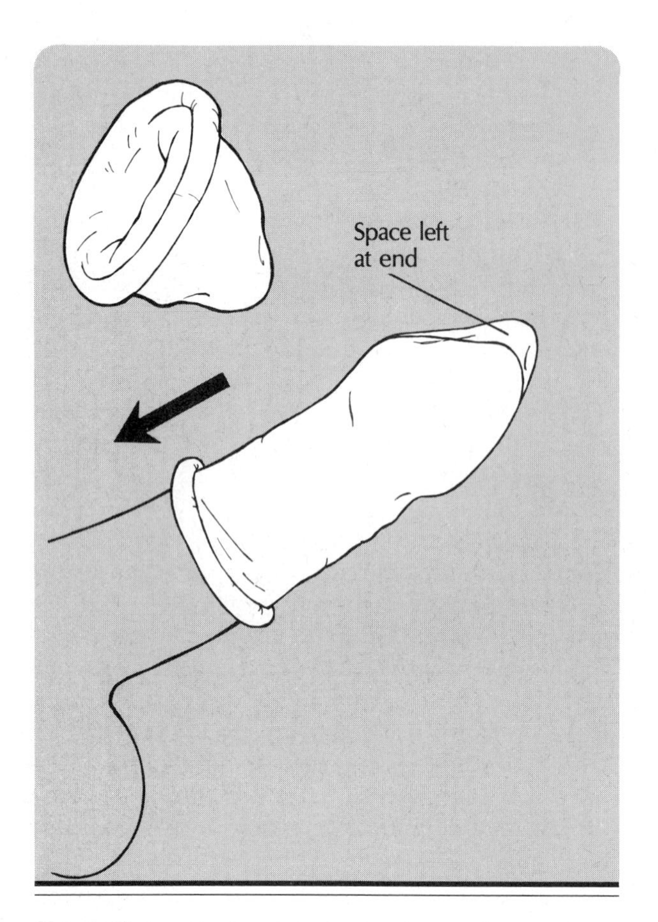

Figure 7–6. **A,** Condom. **B,** Condom applied to penis. Note space left at end to allow collection of ejaculate.

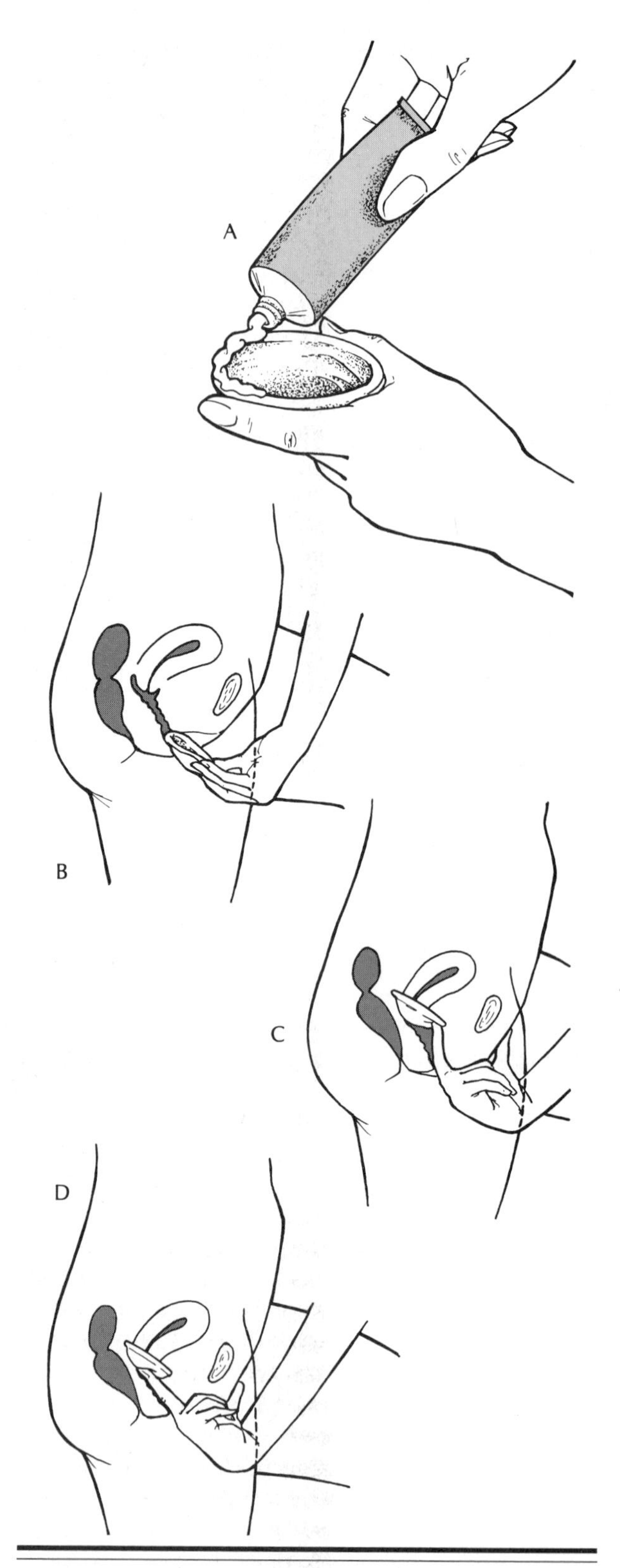

Figure 7–7. **A,** Diaphragm and gel. **B,** Insertion of diaphragm, **C,** Rim of diaphragm is pushed up under the symphysis pubis. **D,** Checking placement of diaphragm. Cervix should be felt through the diaphragm.

men and to prevent the condom from slipping off. Condoms are by no means foolproof, because they may split or become displaced during intercourse. Other disadvantages include possible perineal or vaginal irritation, and some couples feel the condom dulls sensation.

The *diaphragm* (Figure 7–7) offers greater protection from conception, especially when used with spermicidal creams. The client must be fitted with a diaphragm by trained personnel. The diaphragm should be rechecked for correct size after each delivery and if there is a weight gain or loss of 20 pounds. The diaphragm must be inserted prior to intercourse, with spermicidal jelly placed around its rim. It is inserted through the vagina and covers the cervix. The last step in insertion is to push the edge of the diaphragm under the symphysis pubis, which may result in a "popping" sensation. When correctly in place, the diaphragm should not cause discomfort to the wearer or her partner. Placement of the diaphragm can be checked by touching the cervix with a fingertip. The cervix feels like a small rounded structure and has a consistency similar to that of the tip of the nose. The center of the diaphragm should be over the cervix. Women who object to manipulation of the genitals for insertion, determination of correct placement, and removal may find this method offensive. If more than four hours elapses between insertion of the diaphragm and intercourse, additional spermicidal cream should be used. It is necessary to leave the diaphragm in for six hours after coitus. Some couples feel that the use of a diaphragm interferes with the spontaneity of intercourse. If intercourse is again desired within the next six hours, another type of contraception must be used.

The diaphragm should be periodically held up to a light and inspected for tears or holes.

Intrauterine devices (IUDs) come in many types and shapes, but all work by producing a local reaction in the endometrium. The mechanism of the action is not clear, although it is generally accepted that the IUD produces a local sterile inflammatory reaction. It is thought that the inflammatory reaction inhibits nidation if fertilization occurs (Danforth, 1977).

Possible side effects of the IUD include discomfort to the wearer, increased bleeding during menses, midcycle spotting, perforation of the uterus, and infection.

The IUD is inserted into the uterus with its string or tail protruding through the cervix into the vagina. There are four types currently in use: the loop, double coil, copper 7, and progesterone-releasing T. The copper 7 and the T-shaped IUD are smaller and have a lower incidence of pain after insertion, and therefore they are used more frequently in nulliparous women (Figure 7–8).

The copper 7 continuously releases a small amount of copper and has to be replaced every two to three years. Plastic IUDs may also have to be replaced on a regular basis. When they have been in place more than a year, calcium salts may become deposited on the plastic. This forms a rough surface that irritates the endometrium and can cause ulceration and bleeding. If these symptoms occur, the IUD should be removed and replaced.

The IUD may be inserted at the fourth-to-sixth-week postpartum check. After insertion, the woman should be instructed to check for the presence of the string once a week for the first month and then after each menses.

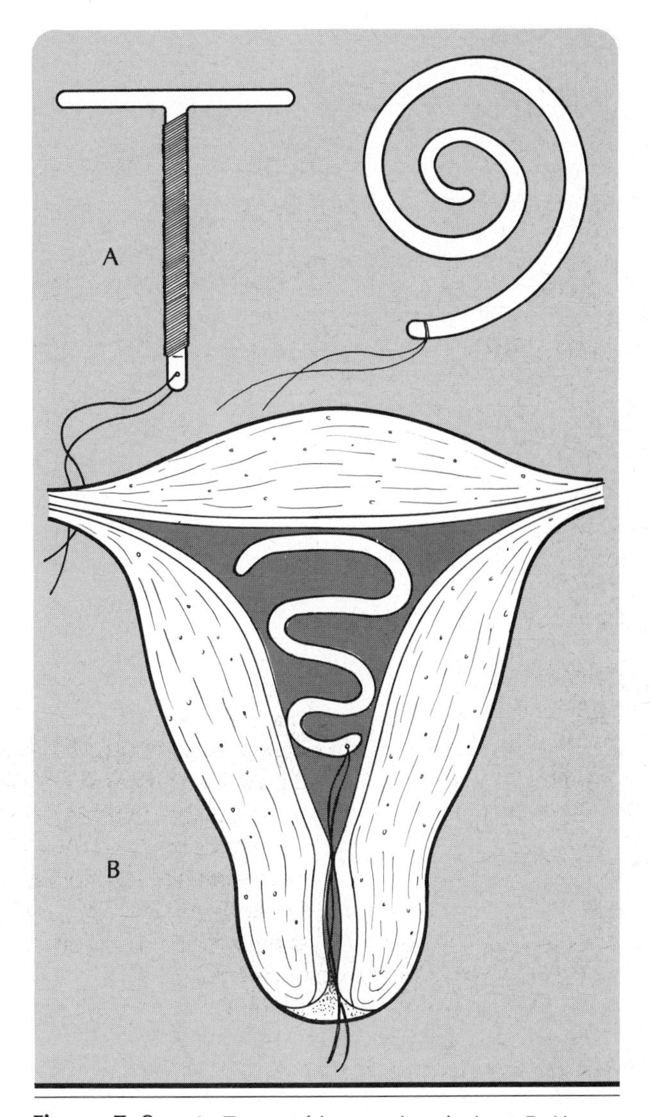

Figure 7–8. **A,** Types of intrauterine devices. **B,** Lippes loop in place within the uterus.

Ovulatory Suppressors

The use of hormones, specifically the combination of estrogen and progesterone, succeeds as a birth control method by inhibiting the release of an ovum and by maintaining type G mucus, which interferes with the passage of sperm through the cervix.

Numerous ovulatory suppressors are available. The dosage regimen consists of taking one tablet daily beginning on the 5th cycle day (the first day of menstruation is cycle day 1) and continuing for 20 to 21 days. In most cases, menstrual bleeding will occur one to four days after the last tablet.

Some pharmaceutical companies have added seven "blank" tablets so that the woman can continue to take one tablet daily and still maintain the monthly dosage regimen.

It is helpful if the woman establishes a routine in taking the tablets. For example, she may take a tablet daily with breakfast or may prefer to take it with supper. Establishment of a regular routine will reduce the chance of forgetting a day.

Although highly effective, ovulatory suppressors may produce side effects ranging from breakthrough bleeding to thrombus formation. Regulation of dosages has reduced many of the side effects, but the threat of potential risk is sufficient

CONTRACEPTIVE INFORMATION

Contraceptive Effectiveness*

Method	Theoretical effectiveness	Use effectiveness
Tubal ligation by laparotomy or laparoscopy	0	.04
Vasectomy	0	.15
Oral contraceptives (combined)	.1	3.0
Combination pill	.1	.2
Low-dose oral progestin	.1	.2
IUD	2	5
Condom	3	5
Diaphragm with spermicide	3	15
Foam or jelly only	3	20
Coitus interruptus	3	15–23
Rhythm (calendar)	14	35–40
Douche	—	35–40
Chance (sexually active)	80	80

Contraindications to Use of Oral Contraceptives†

1. Thrombophlebitis, thromboembolic disorders, cerebrovascular disease, or past history of any of these disorders.
2. Markedly impaired liver function of the cholestatic type.
3. Known or suspected breast cancer.
4. Known or suspected estrogen-dependent neoplasm.
5. Undiagnosed abnormal vaginal bleeding.
6. Known or suspected pregnancy.
7. Lack of regular menstrual cycles for at least 1 to 2 years (in adolescents).

Side Effects to Oral Contraceptives†

Estrogen component

Altered lipid metabolism
Altered convulsive threshold
Leukorrhea, cervical erosion, or polyposis
Headache
Excessive menstrual flow
Hypertension
Altered carbohydrate metabolism
Altered clotting factors—thrombophlebitis
Chloasma
Breast tenderness or engorgement
Venous or capillary engorgement (spider nevi)
Irritability, nervousness
Edema and cyclic weight gain
Nausea, bloating

Progestin component

Oligomenorrhea
Amenorrhea
Acne
Hirsutism
Breast regression
Anabolic weight gain
Increased appetite
Fatigue
Depression and altered libido
Moniliasis
Loss of hair

*Number of pregnancies per 100 woman-years of use. Adapted from Romney, S. L., et al. 1975. *Gynecology and obstetrics: the health care of women.* New York: McGraw-Hill, Blakiston, p. 552.

†Modified from Kreuther, A. K. K., and Hollingsworth, D. R. 1978. *Adolescent obstetrics and gynecology.* Chicago: Year Book Medical Publishers, Inc., pp. 369, 372.

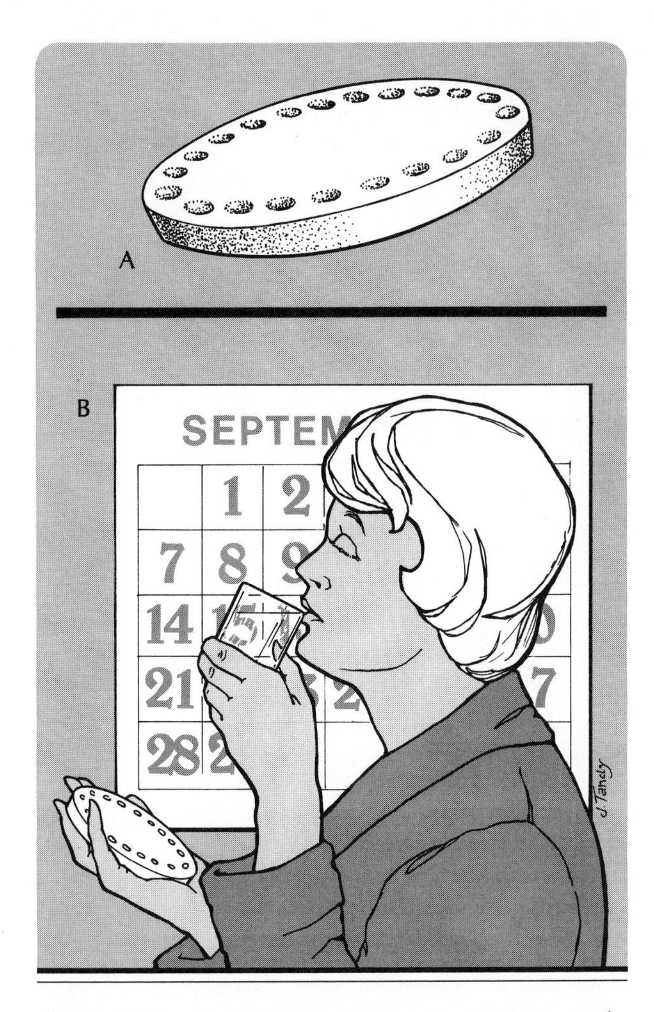

Figure 7–9. **A,** Ovulatory suppressors. **B,** Woman taking birth control pill.

to deter some women from using oral contraceptives (also known as birth control pills).

Contraindications to the use of oral contraceptives include pregnancy, previous history of thrombophlebitis or thrombolic disease, acute or chronic liver disease with abnormal function, presence of estrogen-dependent carcinomas, undiagnosed uterine bleeding, heavy cigarette smoking, hypertension, diabetes, toxemia, age over 40, and hyperlipoproteinemia. In addition, women with the following conditions who use oral contraceptives should be examined every three months: migraine headaches, epilepsy, depression, oligomenorrhea, and amenorrhea. Women who choose this method of contraception should be fully advised of potential side effects.

See Figure 7–9 for illustration of the oral contraceptives. See the accompanying boxed material for contraindications, side effects, and comparative effectiveness of oral contraceptives.

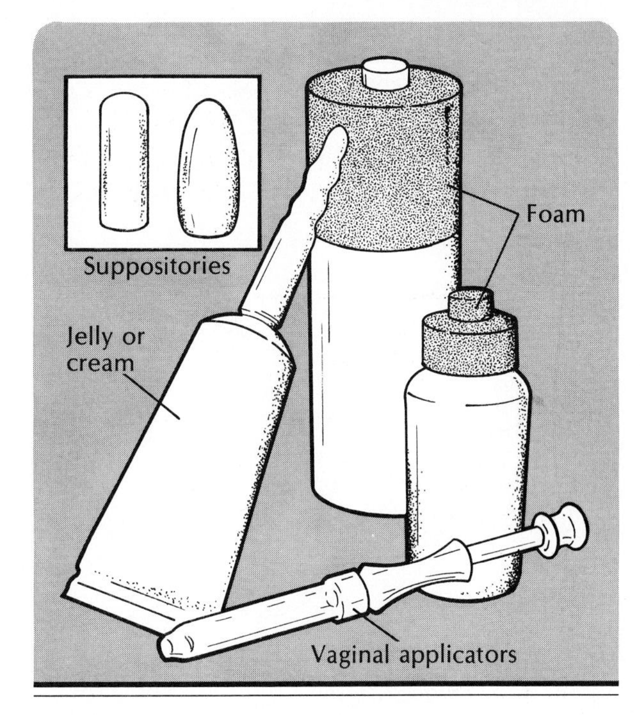

Figure 7–10. Types of spermaticides.

Spermaticides

A variety of creams, jellies, foams, and suppositories, inserted into the vagina prior to intercourse, destroy sperm or neutralize vaginal secretions and thereby immobilize sperm. Figure 7–10 illustrates the spermaticides. Spermaticides that effervesce in a moist environment offer a more immediate effect, and coitus may take place immediately after they are inserted. Suppositories, however, may require up to 30 minutes to dissolve and will not offer protection until they do so. Spermaticides are minimally effective when used alone, but in conjunction with a diaphragm or condom, their effectiveness increases.

Operative Sterilization

Male sterilization is achieved by a relatively minor procedure called a *vasectomy.* Under local anesthesia, a 2–3 cm incision is made over the ductus deferens on each side of the scrotum. The ducts are isolated; severed; and occluded by ligation of the ends, by coagulation of the lumen, by burial of the cut ends, or by use of clips or polyethylene tubing with a stopcock for potentially reversible procedures (see Figure 7–11). Absorbable sutures are used to close the skin, and the patient is instructed to apply ice when pain or swelling occurs and to use a scrotal support for a week. It takes

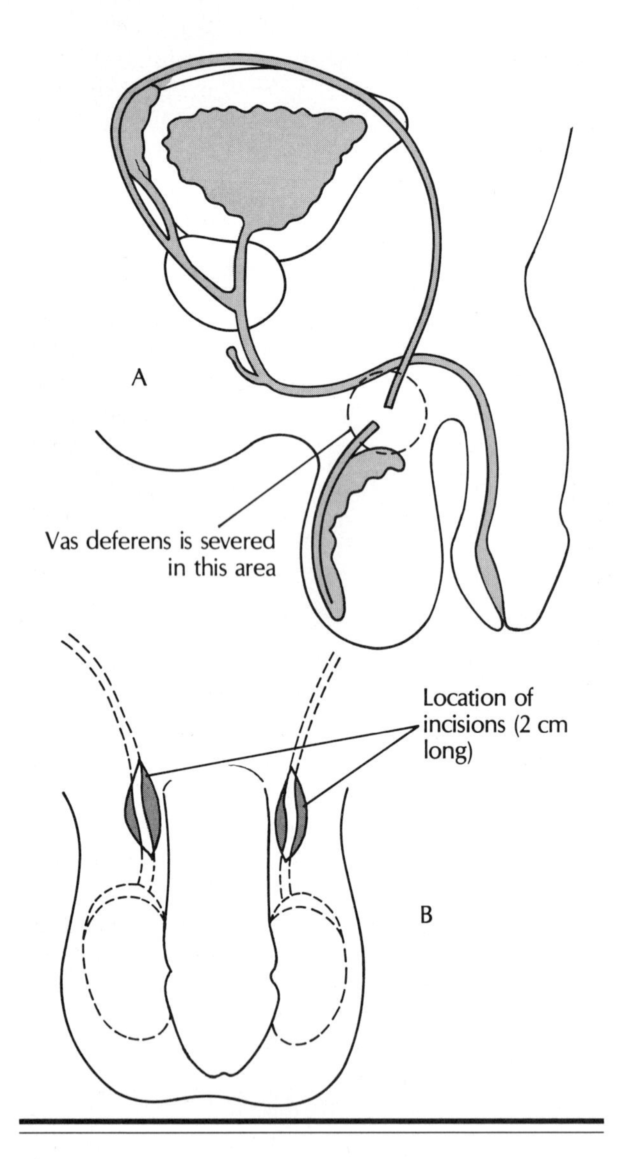

Figure 7–11. Vasectomy. **A,** Ligation of the ductus deferens. **B,** Location of incisions is at either side of the scrotum.

about 4–6 weeks and 6–36 ejaculations to clear sperm from the ductus. During that period, the couple is advised to use another method of birth control and to bring in two or three sperm samples for a sperm count. The man is rechecked at 6 and 12 months to insure that fertility has not been restored by recanalization.

Side effects of a vasectomy include hematoma, sperm granulomas, and spontaneous reanastomosis.

Female sterilization can be accomplished by many abdominal and vaginal procedures. In most cases the fallopian tubes are transected. Figure 7-12 shows the *tubal ligation*, which has been the

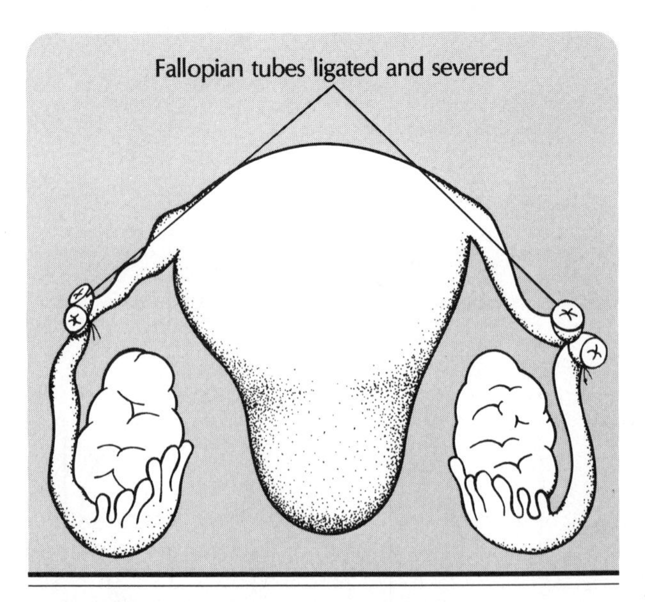

Figure 7–12. Tubal ligation. Both fallopian tubes are ligated and severed, which interrupts continuity of the tube.

most common method. The postpartal laparotomy is done one to three days after delivery, under general anesthesia and usually with a small subumbilical incision. The tubes are isolated and may then be crushed, ligated, or plugged (in the newer reversible procedures). The interval minilaparotomy uses a suprapubic incision with similar techniques for interrupting tubal patency and also requires about two days of hospitalization. Local anesthesia can be used for the minilaparotomy in certain cases. A newer method, laparoscopic sterilization, may be done at any time. A one incision (at the umbilicus) or two incision (between the umbilicus and pubic hairline) approach can be used. The abdomen is distended with carbon dioxide, the laparoscope introduced through a trocar, and the fallopian tube visualized. The isthmic portion of the tube is grasped and coagulated and may be transected. The procedure is repeated on the other fallopian tube.

Complications of female sterilization procedures include coagulation burns on the bowels, bowel perforation, infection, hemorrhage, and adverse anesthesia effects. Reversal of a tubal ligation results in an overall pregnancy rate of 15%. About three-quarters of these pregnancies result in live births, and 10% are tubal pregnancies.

Induced Abortion

Probably one of the most debated of all contraceptive measures is abortion by voluntary means.

For centuries, abortion was illegal according to church and public law. Nevertheless, many women still sought to terminate their pregnancies, and illegal abortions became the single highest cause of maternal death in this country. In 1973, as a result of action by the United States Supreme Court, induced abortion became a legal option. Under this ruling, an induced abortion may be performed legally during the first three months of pregnancy. All legal abortions must be performed by a licensed physician. It is left to individual states to determine what restrictions should be placed on abortions after the first trimester.

Although legalized abortion has been in effect for several years, the controversy over the moral and legal issues continues. This controversy is as readily apparent in the medical and nursing professions as among other groups. Not all physicians will perform the procedure. Some who appear to have decided to provide the service have not reached the decision on a moral level and therefore offer little, if any, psychosocial support to the woman.

Some nurses, too, have found the abortion issue threatening to their basic values. Ambivalence is often seen in nurses who perceive an incompatibility between their professional goal of helping to preserve life and the professional act of assisting clients who choose the option of abortion. Each nurse must decide for herself whether this type of nursing can be performed in view of her own moral code. In making such a decision, the nurse must consider the necessity of providing psychosocial support to clients who have had an abortion.

Many issues surrounding abortion still require clarification. Whether a minor can obtain an abortion without parental consent is under controversy in many states. The rights of the male partner in relation to the decision to terminate pregnancy are also being discussed. Another issue being debated is the "inappropriate" use of abortion as a contraceptive method. Continued education and counseling are needed to resolve these issues.

Factors Influencing the Decision to Seek Abortion

A number of factors influence a woman's decision to seek an abortion, most of them relating to interpersonal relationships. More specifically, the woman's self-concept and self-esteem and the couple's communication and relationship patterns enter into the decision. Many researchers have demonstrated that a breakdown in these areas can predispose to rejection of the pregnancy.

Counseling

Preabortion counseling is important and is most effective when it occurs before the evaluation exam. The initial health assessment includes biological data, such as medical history; laboratory tests of urine, blood type and cross-match, blood count, and Rh factor (for determination of RhoGAM use); and culture for gonorrhea. The nurse should also obtain psychosocial data about the woman's decision-making process in seeking an abortion.

Methods

Most induced abortions are performed in the hospital on a "same-day discharge" basis, although some states allow abortions on an outpatient basis. The decision about which method should be employed to terminate pregnancy is based primarily on the number of elapsed weeks of gestation. The gestational periods and the method of abortion specified for each period are shown in Table 7-1.

First Trimester

Several methods can be utilized at this time.

Morning-After Pill. This method requires the administration of relatively high doses of a synthetic estrogen during the first three days after possible conception. The drug causes the endometrial lining to be shed. The patient may experience nausea and vomiting following this procedure.

Vacuum Aspiration. Pregnancies of less than 10 weeks' gestation may be terminated by vacuum aspiration (menstrual extraction) using a cannula and suction (see Figure 7-13). Prior to suctioning, the cervix must be dilated. Dilatation to accommodate the cannula may be accomplished by one of two methods: use of a laminaria tent (the dried stem of a seaweed, fashioned in the shape of a cone, which swells and slowly dilates the cervical os, usually overnight) or introduction of increasingly larger sounds. In very early pregnancies, a

4–5 mm cannula can be used, and suction is accomplished with a closed-system 60 ml syringe. Later in pregnancy, a 6–10 mm cannula is necessary, and a small suction pump is used to remove the products of conception.

The patient, who may be premedicated, is

Table 7–1. Abortion Methods

Gestational age	Abortion method	Possible side effects	Facility required
Week 5 to 7	Menstrual extraction (endometrial aspiration, menstrual regulation, miniabortion, or EUE)	Allergic reactions, mild cramping, minimal vaginal bleeding, or incomplete removal of tissue	Physician's office or family planning clinic
Week 7 to 12	Vacuum aspiration (suction curettage) or dilatation and curettage (D&C)	Mild cramping and minimal bleeding after vacuum aspiration Uterine or cervic trauma, incomplete evacuation, or infection following D&C	Physician's office, family planning clinic, or hospital
Week 13 to 15	Prostaglandin suppository	Central nervous system reaction including vomiting, diarrhea, or temperature elevation	Hospital
Week 16 to 24	Prostaglandin intra-amniotic injection	Headache, vomiting, or diarrhea; retained placenta with hemorrhage; cervicovaginal fistula; allergic reaction to drug; hypotonic uterus	Hospital
	Urea intra-amniotic injection	Dehydration or alteration in coagulation factors	Hospital
	Saline injection	Hypernatremia resulting from infiltration into tissues Vascular system leakage may result in abdominal pain, severe headache, backache, tachycardia, drowsiness, confusion, seizures Ascending infection from vagina with external rupture of membranes When used with an oxytocin infusion: water intoxication, confusion, drowsiness, headache, cervical tear, uterine rupture	Hospital
	Hysterotomy	Future pregnancies may require repeat caesarean section	Hospital
After 24 weeks	Abortion is inadvisable; recommend other alternatives such as having baby and giving it up for adoption		

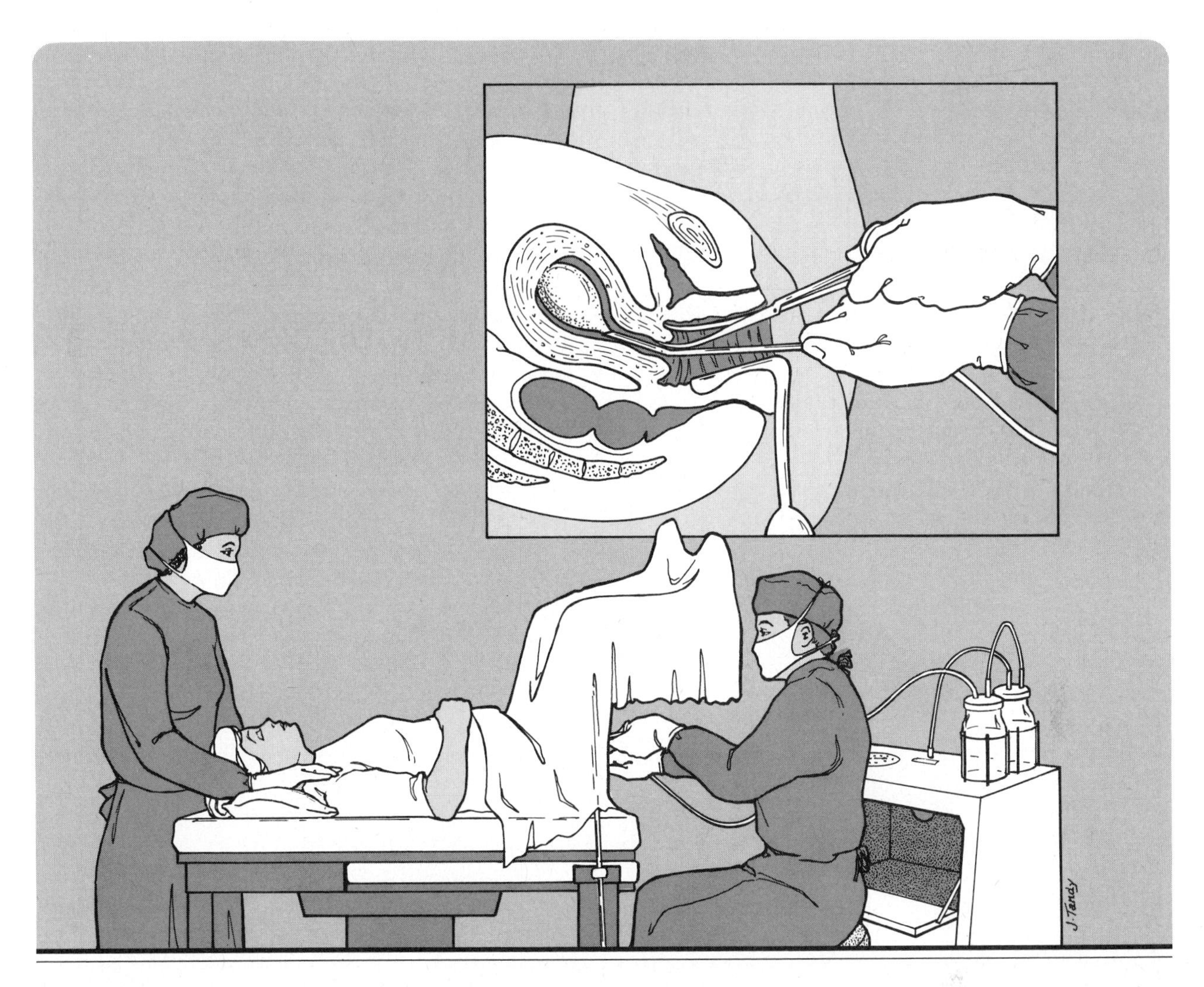

Figure 7–13. Vacuum aspiration. Suction catheter is attached to tube. The woman is in the lithotomy position. A speculum or retractor is inserted into the vagina so that the cervix can be observed. The suction catheter is attached to the suction machine by tubing and is inserted into the vagina and through the cervical os. The products of conception are then aspirated.

placed in a lithotomy position. A vulval and vaginal prep is performed using an antiseptic solution and sterile technique. The patient is draped. To facilitate control of the uterus, the cervix is stabilized with a tenaculum. A paracervical block may be administered using 1% Xylocaine or another anesthetic agent. "Supportive anesthesia" may be utilized in place of a blocking agent. In this case, the physician and nurse or another individual should provide emotional and physical support during the procedure. The abortion is usually performed in less than five minutes. Following suction, a curet may be introduced into the uterine cavity to assess completeness of the procedure.

During vacuum aspiration the patient may experience cramping or discomfort due to positioning. Following the procedure, she should experience little or no discomfort and only slight vaginal bleeding, which should stop prior to her discharge. The length of stay varies from setting to setting but is usually 1-4 hours. On discharge the patient is counseled to watch for signs of unusual bleeding or signs of infection, which include high temperature, foul-smelling discharge, or general malaise; and an appointment is set up for a postabortion checkup.

Prostaglandin. Today much research is being conducted on the use of prostaglandin. Its action is similar to oxytocin in that it causes smooth muscle tissue to contract and has a stimulating effect on the contractility of the myometrium. Side effects of prostaglandin are nausea and vomiting and marked constriction of bronchial musculature. Therefore, its use is contraindicated in the patient with asthma or other respiratory problems. Prostaglandin can be installed vaginally into the cul-de-sac or administered intraabdominally into the amniotic sac. The time required to expel the products of conception varies with the length of gestation. The mean time is approximately 24 hours.

Intraamniotic injection involves the injection of 20–40 mg of prostaglandin. A small test dose of 1 ml is injected slowly over 5 minutes. If no side effects occur, the remainder of the dose is given slowly. If side effects do occur, recovery takes about 30 minutes because of the short half-life of PG and the minimal test dose.

Following expulsion of the fetus, the placenta may be retained; a curet must be used to extract it. Additional side effects of this procedure include chills, vomiting, diarrhea, and tissue reaction at the site of injection.

Prostaglandin may be used for late first trimester or second trimester abortion.

Dilatation and Curettage. This procedure is performed prior to 12 weeks' gestation. It involves preparation of the patient similar to that mentioned for vacuum aspiration. The cervix is dilated with sounds and a curet is introduced into the uterus to scrape the products of conception from the uterine wall. A regional or general anesthetic may be used. Intravenous therapy may be utilized, and an oxytocic medication may be included to assist in the contraction of the uterus following the abortion. Following this method, the patient may experience some cramping with minimal vaginal bleeding. She may be discharged in one day with self-care instructions and an appointment to return for a postabortion checkup.

Second Trimester

In general, the more advanced the pregnancy, the greater the possibility of physiologic problems related to abortion. Thus the methods discussed in this section are considered a greater risk to the woman's health than first-trimester methods are.

Saline Induction. This abortion procedure is utilized only after 16 weeks' gestation, when the uterus is high enough and the amniotic fluid sufficient for safe amniocentesis. Hospitalization is required. The patient empties her bladder and is given an enema to decrease pressure when the fetus is expelled. The abdomen is shaved and cleansed and 1% Xylocaine is used to anesthetize the site of amniocentesis. A small amount of amniotic fluid is withdrawn and tested with nitrazine paper to be sure that the amniotic sac has been penetrated. Next, up to 250 ml of amniotic fluid is withdrawn, and a test dose of 10 ml of 20% hypertonic saline is injected. If severe side effects occur, such as tinnitus, tachycardia, dryness of the mouth, severe headache, or flushing, the procedure is terminated and 5% dextrose in water is administered intravenously to prevent cerebral dehydration. If no side effects are experienced, 30–40 gm of sodium chloride, diluted in 200–240 ml of fluid, is infused into the amniotic sac. This solution can be infused either in a short time or by the drop method. The needle is withdrawn carefully to avoid a spill of hypertonic solution into the peritoneal cavity. This could cause hypernatremia by drawing fluid from the serum and the extracellular tissues. Following the procedure, the patient may experience cramping and a feeling of fullness. Fetal death usually occurs within an hour of injection.

Some physicians may start an infusion of intravenous oxytocics about 6 hours after injection to speed up labor; others feel that this is unnecessary, because labor begins by itself in about 24 hours. Labor generally lasts about 22 hours, and may cause considerable discomfort to the patient. The placenta is usually spontaneously aborted 1–2 hours later. Occasionally the placenta is retained and curettage is necessary to remove it. Postabortion hemorrhage must be watched for carefully during the postpartum period.

Saline induction has many hazards, including hypernatremia and the inadvertent intravascular injection of the solution.

Hysterotomy. This method involves an incision into the uterus. It is primarily used when other methods are contraindicated or when the woman wants a tubal ligation for the purpose of sterilization.

Nursing Management

Perhaps the major contributing factor to quality nursing care for the abortion patient is the nurse's objective understanding and acceptance based on an adequate self-assessment. With this foundation a nurse can effectively assess the biologic and psychosocial needs of patients and plan to meet them. Important aspects of care include allowance for verbalization by the patient; support before, during, and after the procedure; monitoring of vital signs, intake, and output; providing for physical comfort and privacy throughout the procedure; and health teaching regarding self-care, the importance of the postabortion checkup, and contraception review. This type of involved, understanding nursing care can help the patient achieve an optimum level of health.

NURSING CARE PLAN

Saline Abortion

Patient Data Base

Nursing history

1. Previous pregnancies and outcome
2. Knowledge of procedure
3. Routine vital signs (temperature, pulse, respirations, blood pressure)
4. Weight
5. Patient questions

Physical examination

1. Confirmation of 16-20 weeks' gestation
2. Determination of optimum health level

Laboratory evaluation

1. Hematocrit
2. Papanicolaou smear
3. Gonococcal culture
4. Serum test for syphilis (STS) or VDRL
5. Urinalysis (routine)
6. Blood type and Rh

Nursing Priorities

1. Preparation of patient for procedure
   a. What will happen
   b. What to expect (contractions, feeling of fullness, expulsion of fetus)
   c. Psychologic support – presence of nurse
   d. Breathing techniques that can be used when contractions occur
2. Monitoring of contraction activity
3. Routine vital sign check every 4 hours, or every 15 minutes if intravenous oxytocin infusion is used
4. Completion of procedure – handling and disposal of fetal contents and assessment of patient status
5. Examination of patient, by physician, to assess complete explusion of uterine contents
6. Assessment of postpartal status
   a. Vital signs, per routine
   b. Fundal check, as ordered
   c. Pad check to assess blood loss
   d. Patient's emotional state

Problem	Nursing interventions and actions	Rationale
Patient preparation	Explain procedure: 1. What will happen. a. Injection of saline. b. Beginning of labor in approximately 12 hours.	To decrease fear and thus allow patient to maintain control.

NURSING CARE PLAN Cont'd

Saline Abortion

Problem	Nursing interventions and actions	Rationale
	2. Labor expectations. a. Contractions. b. Feeling of fullness. c. Expulsion of fetus. 3. Use of breathing and relaxation to minimize discomfort. 4. Use of analgesics. Physically prepare: 1. Empty bladder. 2. Enema if ordered.	
Vital signs and contractions	Assess vital signs every hour: 1. Temperature. 2. Pulse. 3. Respirations. 4. Blood pressure. 5. Contractions (if none, patient can be sent to unit and put on routine vital signs; once contractions begin, she is transferred to labor room and above procedure noted).	To assess for possible reaction to saline injection.
Retention of uterine contents	Check perineum for expulsion of uterine contents. Notify physician to assess expelled contents and patient. Place contents in container to be sent to laboratory for full evaluation. Assess size and firmness of uterine fundus. Assess amount of vaginal bleeding.	Incomplete expulsion of uterine contents causes infection and hemorrhage.
Postpartal status	Check every 15 minutes for 1 hour, then as ordered: 1. Fundus. 2. Perineum. 3. Perineal pads. 4. Blood pressure and pulse.	Postpartal complications following saline abortion can include infection at injection site; excessive bleeding, which may be due to length of labor (can be 36 hours, causing uterine relaxation); or retention of placental fragments or consumption coagulopathy.

Nursing Care Evaluation

1. Patient will briefly describe procedure.
2. Patient will exhibit no deviations in vital signs and will have regular uterine contractions.
3. Patient will expel all products of conception.
4. Patient's uterus will remain firm, bleeding controlled.
5. Patient will have received counseling as needed.

SUMMARY

Understanding a couple's desire to plan fertility for appropriate times and under chosen circumstances is important for the health care provider. Nurses can assist a couple in identifying and correcting causes of infertility or help them control the number and interval of children only when they disseminate contraceptive knowledge in an objective, nonjudgmental manner. Risk factors related to the woman's health, influences of culture and religion, psychosocial pressures, personal choices, and economic considerations are determining factors in the selection of a contraceptive method.

SUGGESTED ACTIVITIES

1. Ask four students or other women to complete a basal body temperature chart for one month. Compare the charts and identify the time of ovulation for each student.
2. Discuss four different methods of contraception and explain the advantages and disadvantages of each method.
3. Suppose that a 21-year-old woman appears in a health clinic and asks you for advice on an abortion. What would you tell her?
4. Explain what a woman should know about taking birth control pills.

REFERENCES

Britt, S. S. March–April 1977. Fertility awareness: four methods of natural family planning. *J. Obstet. Gynecol. Neonatal Nurs.* 6:9.

Danforth, D. H., ed. 1977. *Obstetrics and gynecology.* New York: Harper & Row Publishers, Inc.

Shane, J. M., Schiff, I., and Wilson, E. A. 1976. The infertile couple. *Clin. Symp.* 28(5).

ADDITIONAL READINGS

Boston Women's Health Book Collective. 1976. *Our bodies, ourselves.* New York: Simon & Schuster.

Dwyer, J. M. 1976. *Human reproduction: the female system and the neonate.* Philadelphia: F. A. Davis Co.

Eliot, J. W. 1973. Fertility control and coercion. *Family Planning Persp.* 5(3):132.

Hubbard, C. W. 1977. *Family planning education.* St. Louis: The C. V. Mosby Co.

Joel, C. A. 1971. *Fertility disturbances in men and women.* New York: Albert J. Phiebig.

Kessel, E., et al. 1975. Menstrual regulation in family planning services. *Am. J. Public Health.* 65(7):731.

Martin, L. 1978. *Health care of women.* Philadelphia: J. B. Lippincott Co.

Novak, E., et al. 1971. *Textbook of gynecology.* 8th ed. Baltimore: The Williams & Wilkins Co.

Robbie, M. O. July–Aug. 1978. Contraceptive counseling for the younger adolescent woman: a suggested solution to the problem. *J. Obstet. Gynecol. Neonatal Nurs.* 7(4):29.

Wiehe, V. 1976. Psychological reactions to infertility: implications for nursing in resolving feelings of disappointment and inadequacy. *J. Obstet. Gynecol. Neonatal Nurs.* 5:28.

CHAPTER 8

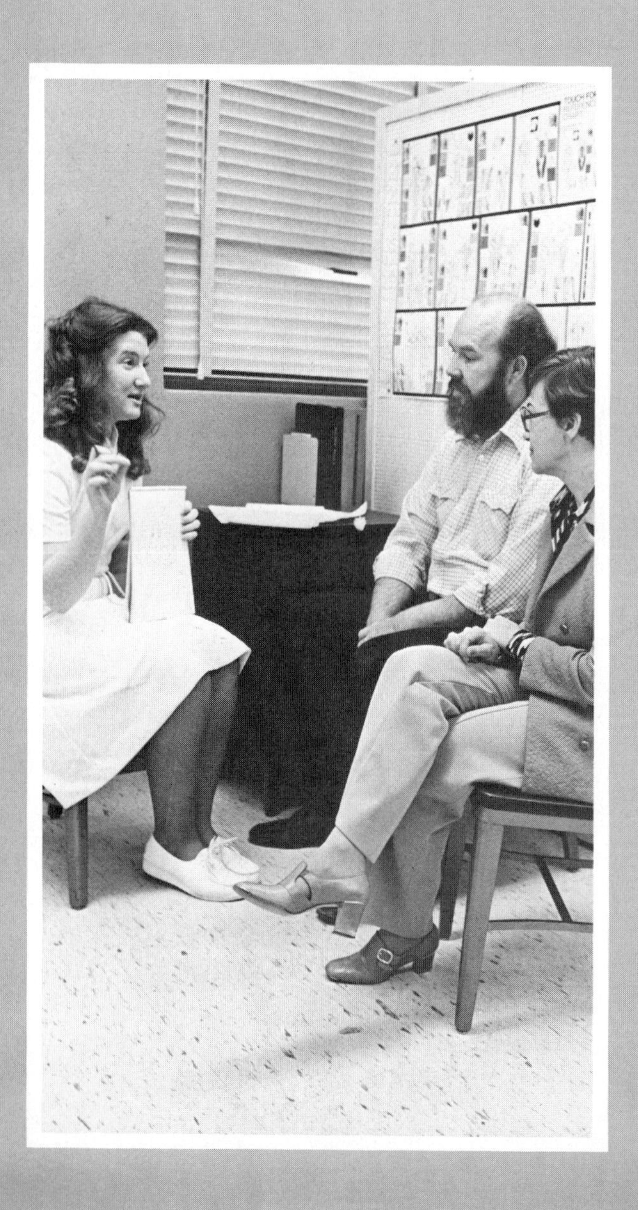

GENETIC COUNSELING

OBJECTIVES

- Identify indications for chromosomal analysis.
- Differentiate between Down's syndrome caused by trisomy 21 and Down's syndrome caused by a translocation.
- Discuss the significance of the Barr body in identifying sex chromosomal abnormalities.
- Identify general characteristics of an autosomal dominant disorder.
- Compare autosomal recessive disorders with X-linked (sex-linked) recessive disorders.
- Describe prenatal diagnostic procedures that may be utilized to determine the presence of genetic disease.
- Explain the nurse's responsibility in genetic counseling.
- Discuss the use of a family pedigree as a screening tool in genetic counseling.

The desired and expected outcome of any pregnancy is the birth of a healthy, "perfect" baby. In most cases, when parents gaze at their new son or daughter, they can sigh with relief at the ending of a nine-month period that was filled with hope, concern, and joyful anticipation. Unfortunately, a small but significant number of parents experience grief, fear, and anger at this moment, when they discover that their baby has been born with a defect or a genetic disease. Such an abnormality may be evident at birth or may not appear for some time. The child may have inherited the same genetic disease that one of his parents has, creating more guilt and strife within the family. The child may be mentally retarded and require institutional care.

Regardless of the type or scope of the problem, parents will have many questions: "What did I do?" "What caused it?" "Will it happen again?" The professional nurse must anticipate the parents' questions and concerns and be able to guide, direct, and support the family. To do so, the nurse must have a firm basic knowledge of genetics and genetic counseling. Many congenital malformations and diseases are genetic or have a strong genetic component. Others are not genetic at all. The genetic counselor attempts to categorize the problem and answer the patients' questions. Professional nurses can help expedite this process if they already have an understanding of the principles involved and are able to direct the family to the appropriate resources.

Is the magnitude of the problem great enough to warrant the nurse's time and effort? The problem of genetic disease can be likened to an iceberg—only the tip is immediately apparent. With the enormous strides and rapid increase in our understanding of heredity, more disease processes are now considered to be genetic, and their genetic components have been well—or reasonably well—established. Statistics indicate that:

1. Each couple has a 3%–5% risk of having a child with a major congenital abnormality.
2. Approximately 30%–50% of all spontaneous abortions are caused by gross chromosomal defects.
3. Approximately 0.5%–1% of all live newborns have a chromosomal abnormality.
4. Approximately one-third of all hospitalized pediatric patients have a genetic disease.
5. Of the 3% of the U.S. population who are mentally retarded, about four-fifths are believed to carry a genetic component.
6. There are over 2000 *known* inherited diseases (U.S. Department of Health, Education, and Welfare, 1976).

None of these statistics or estimations take into account the many diseases or conditions that have either been recently shown to have a genetic component or are strongly suspected to have one. Included among these are heart disease, cancer, and mental illness.

What of the cost of genetic disease? How do the costs of untreated genetic diseases compare with the costs of prevention and therapy? One can look at two well-known genetic problems—Down's syndrome and phenylketonuria (PKU). It has been estimated that the lifetime cost of maintaining a severely retarded individual who needs institutionalization is $250,000. The incidence of Down's syndrome is approximately 1 per 600 to 800 live births every year. If we take the mean, 1 per 700 live births, there are approximately 5000 children born with Down's syndrome each year. Thus, per year, the lifetime committed expenditure for Down's syndrome alone is approximately $1.25 billion.

However, with available technology, including prenatal diagnosis, it is possible to prevent the birth of a high proportion of such affected infants. It has been estimated that if fetuses of high-risk (older) pregnant women were screened in utero for Down's syndrome, approximately 1000 cases per year might be prevented—a savings of about $250 million in lifetime care. To detect 1000 cases, approximately 96,000 pregnancies would have to be monitored. The cost of such monitoring is estimated to be between $15 million and $25 million, less than a tenth of the cost of lifetime care.

Even the screening of fairly rare diseases such as PKU (1 per 14,000 births) appears to benefit society. The test to screen a newborn for PKU is about $1.25, or approximately $17,000 to detect each case. If an additional $8000–$16,000 is spent for dietary therapy, the cost of care to prevent severe mental retardation is approximately $33,000 per child. Compare this to the $365,000 it would cost to care for an untreated severely retarded child (50 years in an institution at $20 per day). Detection and prevention cost one-tenth that of lifetime care.

It would appear that the detection, treatment,

and prevention of genetic disease does indeed save a great deal of money. What cannot be accurately estimated in dollars and cents is the emotional and psychologic savings to the afflicted individual and his family when such genetic diseases are prevented or treated.

What is of most importance is that many genetic diseases can be either prevented or successfully treated to prevent irreversible damage. In some cases, to prevent the disease one must prevent the birth of an affected individual. This might be accomplished by a family deciding not to have any children, by using artificial insemination, or by prenatal diagnosis and elective termination of pregnancy. Some genetic diseases such as PKU and galactosemia are treatable with dietary modifications if detected early. Frequently, avoidance of substances that are toxic in certain genetic diseases is appropriate, such as the avoidance of copper in Wilson's disease.

Thus, even though more disease processes are being found to have a genetic basis, more methods of prevention and therapy are also being utilized. Nurses should find it imperative to be well informed so they can help families reach their maximum level of wellness and productivity. This chapter examines the principles of genetic counseling and the scientific data on which those principles are based.

CHROMOSOMES AND CHROMOSOMAL ABERRATIONS

As was discussed in Chapter 6, all hereditary material is carried on tightly coiled strands of DNA known as *chromosomes.* The chromosomes carry the genes, the smallest unit of inheritance. Although human chromosomes were described as early as the 1870s, it was not until 1956 that the normal human chromosome constitution was identified. All somatic cells contain 46 chromosomes, which is the *diploid* number, while the sperm and egg contain 23 chromosomes, or the *haploid* number. There are 23 pairs of *homologous* chromosomes (a matched pair of chromosomes, one inherited from each parent). Twenty-two pairs are known as *autosomes* (non-sex chromosomes), and one pair are the *sex chromosomes,* X and Y. A normal male, in standard notation, has a 46,XY chromosome constitution; the normal female is 46,XX (Figures 8-1 and 8-2).

The *karyotype,* or pictorial analysis of chromosomes, is usually performed on peripheral blood lymphocytes. These cells are stimulated to undergo mitosis and are arrested during metaphase. This preparation is stained, and the chromosomes can be seen (Figure 8-3). Although use of peripheral blood is an easy, convenient method for obtaining chromosomes, almost any tissue can be examined to get this information. Skin, bone marrow, and organ tissue can be used. In the case of a

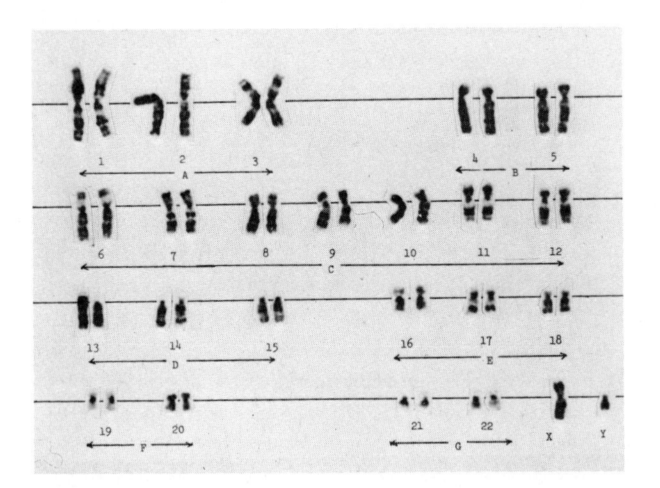

Figure 8-1. Normal male karyotype. (Courtesy Dr. Arthur Robinson, National Jewish Hospital and Research Center.)

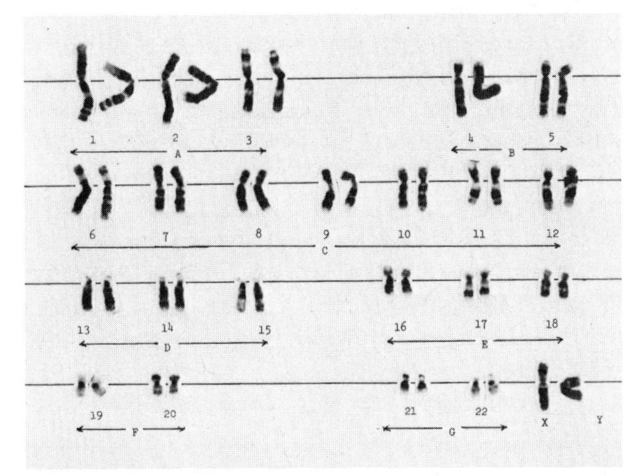

Figure 8-2. Normal female karyotype. (Courtesy Dr. Arthur Robinson, National Jewish Hospital and Research Center.)

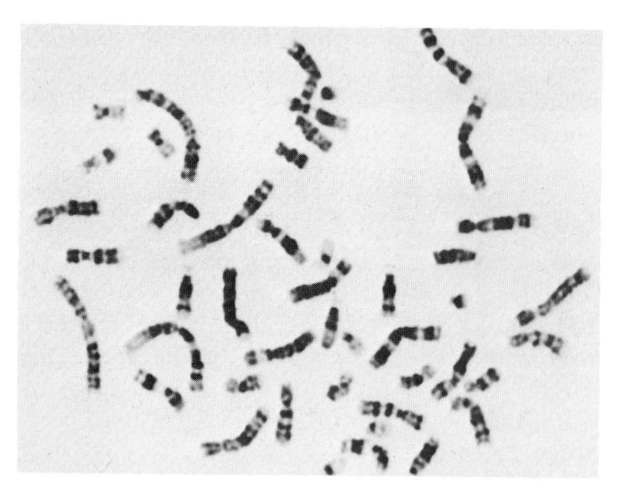

Figure 8–3. Chromosomes in metaphase spread. (Courtesy Dr. Arthur Robinson, National Jewish Hospital and Research Center.)

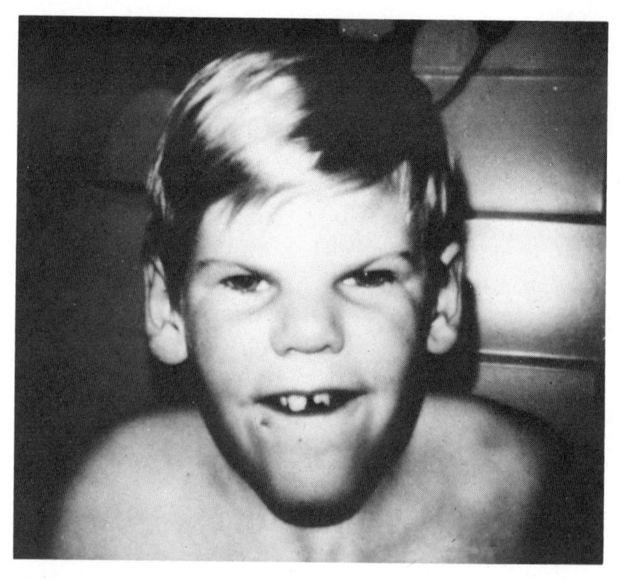

Figure 8–4. Ten-year-old boy who has a partial trisomy for the short arm of chromosome number 4; he is mentally retarded and has minor abnormalities.

stillbirth or perinatal death in which there are multiple congenital abnormalities and there is a question of diagnosis or cause, karyotypes of cells in the thymus can be examined if it has not been fixed in formalin.

Chromosome abnormalities can occur in either the autosomes or the sex chromosomes and can be divided into two categories: abnormalities of number and abnormalities of structure. With the advent of quinacrine mustard staining of chromosomes, begun by Caspersson in 1970, it has been possible to identify not only those cases in which an entire chromosome has been added or deleted but also those in which the addition or deletion of chromosomal material has been very small. Many children who received chromosomal analysis prior to this test were said to have normal chromosomes. But when examined with the new banding techniques, many were found to have additions or deletions of chromosomal material.

Even small aberrations in chromosomes can cause abnormalities, especially those associated with slow growth and development or with mental retardation. The child need not have obvious major malformations to be affected (Figure 8-4). In addition, some of these abnormalities can be passed on to other offspring. Thus, in some cases chromosomal analysis is appropriate even if clinical manifestations are mild. Whatever the case, too much or too little genetic material usually produces adverse effects on normal growth and development.

Indications for chromosomal analysis include:

1. Chromosome syndrome suspected (or patients with a clinical diagnosis of Down's syndrome).
2. Mental retardation and congenital malformations.
3. Abnormal sexual development (primary amenorrhea, lack of secondary sex characteristics).
4. Ambiguous genitals.
5. Multiple miscarriages.
6. Possible balanced translocation carrier.

Autosome Abnormalities

Abnormalities of Chromosome Number

In 1959 Lejeune described the presence of an extra chromosome 21 in children with *Down's syndrome,* also referred to as *mongolism.* The child with Down's syndrome has a chromosome constitution of 47,XX(or XY),+21; referred to as *trisomy 21* (Figure 8-5). This is by far the most common trisomy (Turpin and Lejeune, 1969).

Abnormalities of chromosome number are most commonly seen as trisomies or monosomies and as mosaicism. In all three cases, the abnormality is most often caused by *nondisjunction.* In

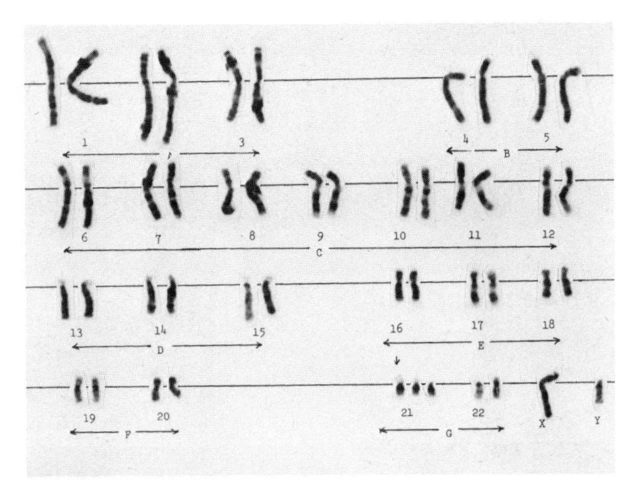

Figure 8–5. Karyotype of a male who has trisomy 21, Down's syndrome. (Courtesy Dr. Arthur Robinson, National Jewish Hospital and Research Center.)

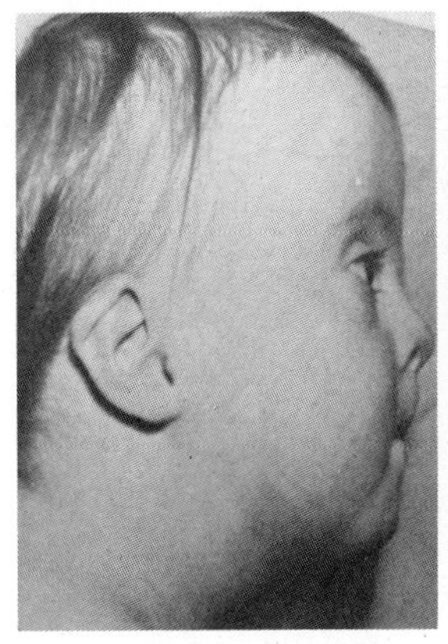

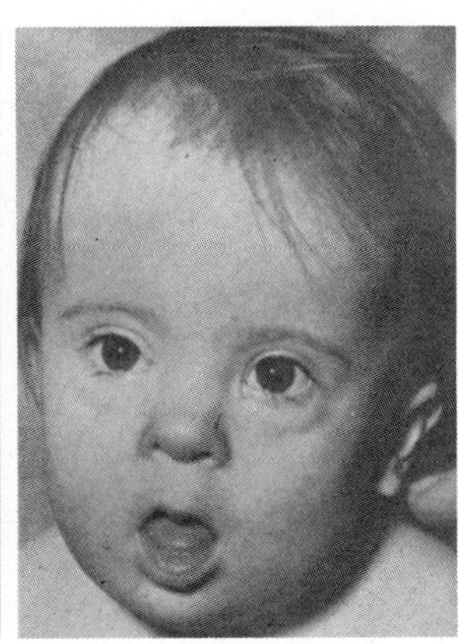

Figure 8–6. A child with Down's syndrome. (From Smith, D. W. *Recognizable patterns of human malformations.* © 1976 by the W. B. Saunders Company, Philadelphia, Pa.)

nondisjunction, a pair of chromosomes fails to separate during meiosis, resulting in the formation of one gamete (sperm or egg) that contains both members of the pair and one that contains neither. If the cell without the chromosome unites with a normal cell, the individual is said to be *monosomic.* Monosomy of an entire chromosome is incompatible with life. The only exception is the sex chromosomes. A female can survive with only one X chromosome; this condition is known as *Turner's syndrome.*

As already noted, Down's syndrome is the most common trisomy abnormality seen among children. The presence of the extra chromosome 21 produces distinct clinical features in the child (Figure 8–6). Those clinical features most commonly seen include:

CNS: Mental retardation
Hypotonia at birth
Head: Flattened occiput
Depressed nasal bridge
Mongoloid slant of eyes
Epicanthal folds
White speckling of the iris (Brushfield's spots)
Protrusion of the tongue
High arched palate
Low-set ears
Broad, short neck
Hands: Short fingers
Abnormalities of finger and foot dermal ridge patterns (dermatoglyphics)
Transverse palmar crease (simian line)
Other: Congenital heart disease

Congenital heart disease is seen in approximately one-half of those affected. With the advent of antibiotics and improved techniques in heart surgery, children with Down's syndrome are now living into adulthood. In fact, it is not uncommon for these individuals to survive into their fifth or sixth decade of life.

Trisomies can occur among other autosomes, the two most common being trisomy 18 and trisomy 13. Children with trisomy 18 have the following characteristics (Figure 8–7):

CNS: Mental retardation
Severe hypertonia
Head: Prominent occiput
Low-set ears
Corneal opacities
Ptosis (drooping of eyelids)
Hands: Third and fourth fingers overlapped by second and fifth fingers
Abnormal dermatoglyphics
Syndactyly (webbing of fingers)
Other: Congenital heart defects
Renal abnormalities
Single umbilical artery
Gastrointestinal tract abnormalities
Rocker-bottom feet
Cryptorchidism
Various malformations of other organs

A child born with trisomy 13 usually exhibits the following clinical characteristics (Figure 8–8):

CNS: Mental retardation

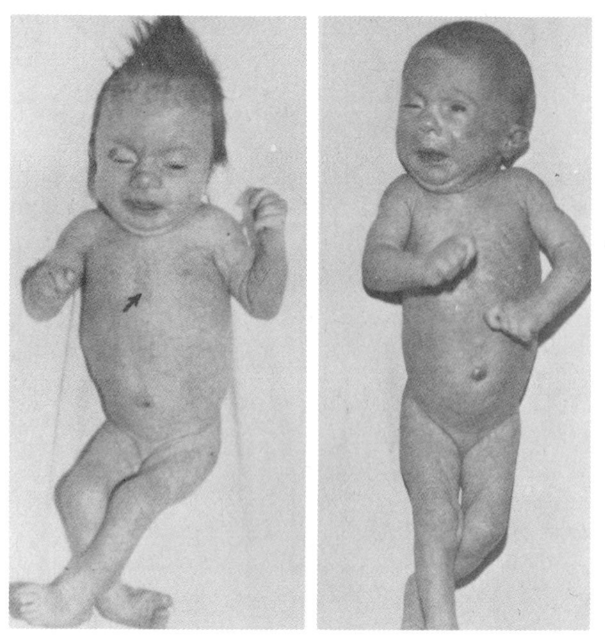

Figure 8–7. Infants with trisomy 18. In the child shown on the left, an arrow denotes the lower end of the sternum. (From Smith, D. W. *Recognizable patterns of human malformations.* © 1976 by the W. B. Saunders Company, Philadelphia, Pa.)

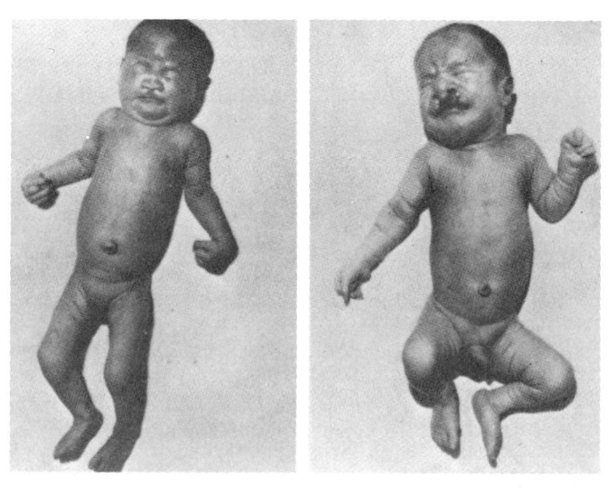

Figure 8–8. Infants with trisomy 13. (From Smith, D. W. *Recognizable patterns of human malformations.* © 1976 by the W. B. Saunders Company, Philadelphia, Pa.)

Severe hypertonia
Seizures

Head: Microcephaly
Microphthalmia and/or coloboma
Malformed ears
Aplasia of external auditory canal
Micrognathia
Cleft lip and palate

Hands: Polydactyly (extra digits)
Abnormal posturing of fingers
Abnormal dermatoglyphics

Other: Congenital heart defects
Hemangiomas
Gastrointestinal tract defects
Various malformations of other organs

The prognosis for both trisomy 13 and 18 syndromes is extremely poor. Most children (70%) die within the first three months of life. A very few children with trisomy 18 have survived into childhood, although this is rare. The major cause of death is usually secondary complications related to cardiac and respiratory abnormalities. The incidence of trisomy 18 is about 1 per 3000 live births. Trisomy 13 occurs less frequently, about 1 per 5000 live births.

Mosaicism, the other common abnormality caused by nondisjunction, occurs when an individual has two different cell lines, each with a different chromosomal number. Mosaicism tends to be more common in the sex chromosomes, but when it does occur in the autosomes, it is most common for Down's syndrome.

Nondisjunction before fertilization (meiotic nondisjunction) leads to an individual who has an abnormal chromosome constitution in all cells. Nondisjunction after fertilization (mitotic nondisjunction) results in cells with two or more different chromosome constitutions, evolving into two or more different cell lines. Depending on when mitotic nondisjunction occurs after fertilization, different tissues may have different chromosome constitutions. Or the tissue may have a mixture of cells and the ratio of normal to abnormal cells may vary from one tissue to the next. For instance, in Down's syndrome, one cell line may contain the normal 46 chromosomes while the other cell line contains 47 chromosomes, that is, an extra number 21. Or within a single tissue, some of the cells may be normal whereas others may contain the extra chromosome 21.

Clinical signs and symptoms may vary if mosaicism is present. In Down's syndrome, the clinical signs may be classic, minimal, or nonapparent, depending on the number and location of the abnormal cells. An individual with many classic signs of Down's syndrome but who has normal or near normal intelligence should be investigated for the possibility of mosaicism. More than one tissue may have to be examined to make the diagnosis. The peripheral blood may contain 46 chromosomes while the skin fibroblasts contain

47,+21. The frequency of mosaicism among children with Down's syndrome is approximately 1%.

Abnormalities of Chromosome Structure

Abnormalities of chromosome structure involving only parts of the chromosome generally occur in two forms: translocation and deletions and additions. Both types of structural abnormalities can produce distinct clinical signs and symptoms. Over 100 such abnormalities have been described in the literature. Again, Down's syndrome is one of the most common syndromes described.

Not all children born with Down's syndrome have trisomy 21. Instead, they may be the victims of an abnormal rearrangement of chromosomal material known as a *translocation.* Clinically, the two types of Down's syndrome are indistinguishable. What is of major importance to the family is that the two different types have different risks of recurrence. The only way to distinguish the two is to do a chromosome analysis.

The translocation occurs when the carrier parent has 45 chromosomes, usually with one of the number 21 chromosomes fused to one of the number 14 chromosomes (Figure 8-9). The parent has one normal 14, one normal 21, and one 14/21 chromosome. Since all the chromosomal material is present and functioning normally, the parent is clinically normal. This individual is known as a *balanced translocation carrier.* When this person mates with a person with a structually normal chromosome constitution, there are several possible outcomes (Figure 8-10). The offspring can receive the carrier parent's normal number 21 and normal number 14 chromosomes in combination with the noncarrier parent's normal chromosomes 21 and 14. In this case the offspring is chromosomally normal. Or the child may receive one of the balanced translocations, thus becoming a carrier like the carrier parent—chromosomally abnormal but clinically normal. If, however, the offspring receives the carrier parent's normal number 21 chromosome and the 14/21 chromosome and the noncarrier parent's normal chromosomes, the offspring receives two functioning number 14 chromosomes and three functioning number 21 chromosomes (Figure 8-11). Although the offspring has at first glance 46 chromosomes, on careful analysis he is discovered to have an extra chromosome 21. Thus he has an *unbalanced translocation* and has Down's syndrome.

In Down's syndrome, if the mother is a carrier of a 14/21 balanced translocation, there is a 10%-15% risk of having an affected offspring. If the father carries the balanced translocation, there is a 2%-5% risk. Other types of translocations can occur. But regardless of the chromosome involved, any person having a balanced chromosome rearrangement (translocation) has the potential of having a child with an unbalanced chromosome constitution. This usually means a substantial adverse effect on normal growth and development.

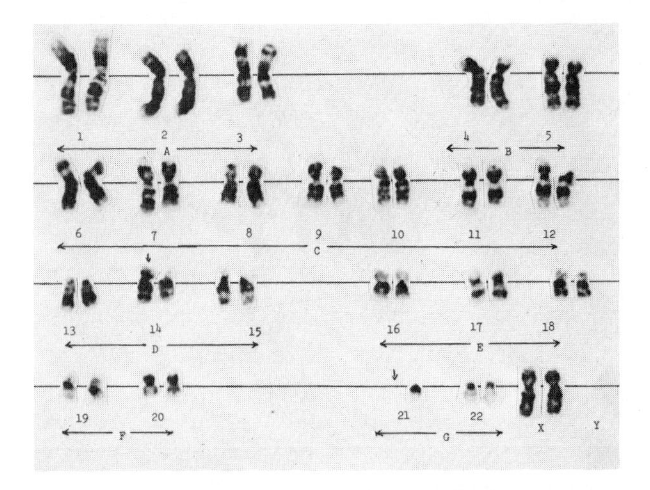

Figure 8-9. Karyotype of a female who is a balanced translocation carrier for chromosomes number 14 and 21. (Courtesy Dr. Arthur Robinson, National Jewish Hospital and Research Center.)

The other type of structural abnormality seen is caused by *additions and/or deletions* of chromosomal material. Any portion of a chromosome may be lost or added, generally leading to some adverse effect. Depending on how much chromosomal material is involved, the clinical effects may be mild or severe. Many types of additions and deletions have been described and new syndromes identified.

The cri du chat (cat cry) syndrome is associated with the deletion of one of the short arms of chromosome 5. Clinical features are severe mental retardation, a catlike cry in infancy, failure to thrive, microcephaly, hypertelorism, epicanthal folds, low-set ears, and various other organ malformations.

A deletion of the long arm of chromosome 18 usually results in severe psychomotor retardation, microcephaly, stenotic ear canals with conductive hearing loss, and various other organ malformations.

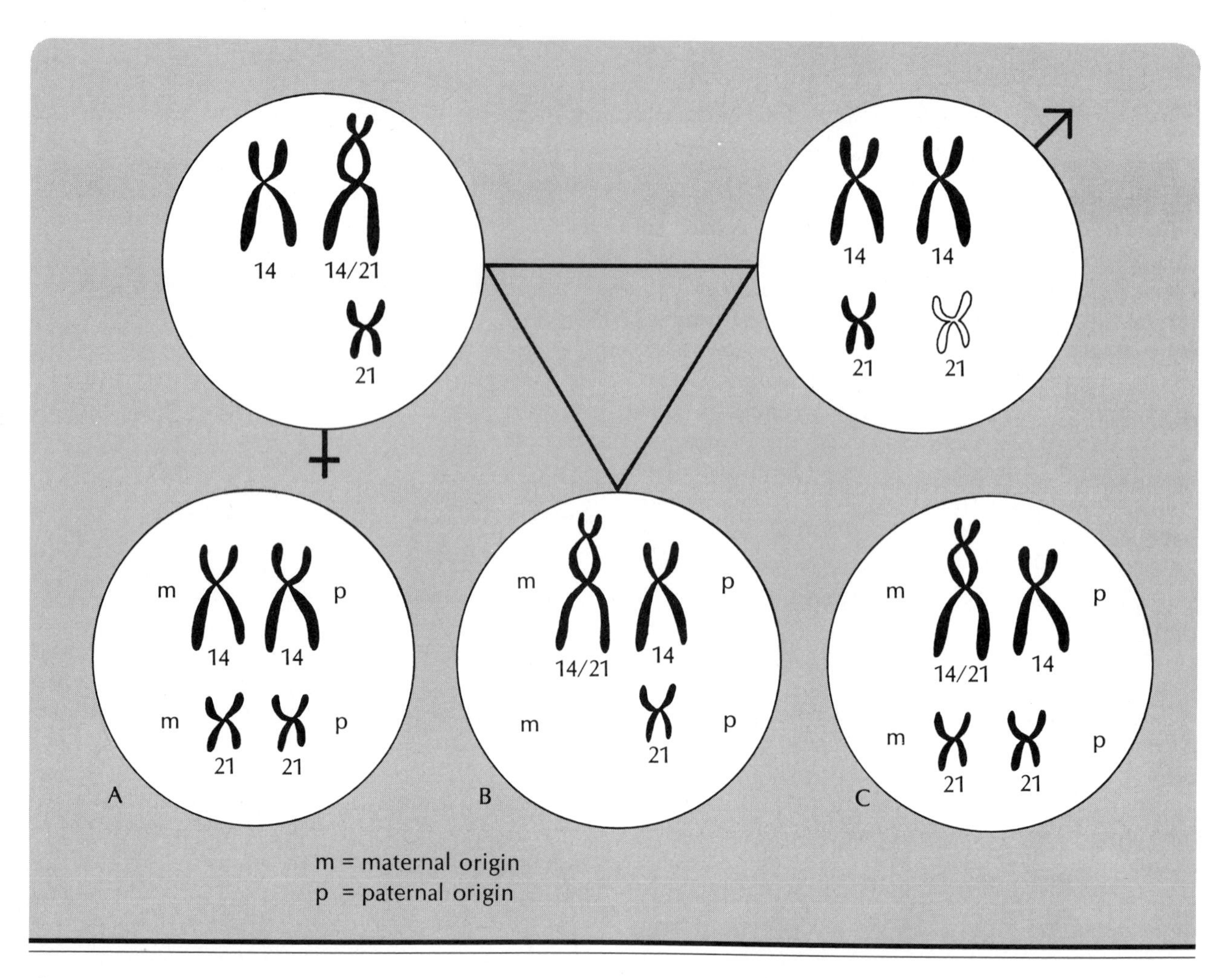

Figure 8–10. Diagram of various types of offspring when mother has a balanced translocation between chromosomes 14 and 21 and father has the normal arrangement of chromosomal material. **A,** Normal offspring. **B,** Balanced translocation carrier. **C,** Unbalanced translocation. Patient has Down's syndrome.

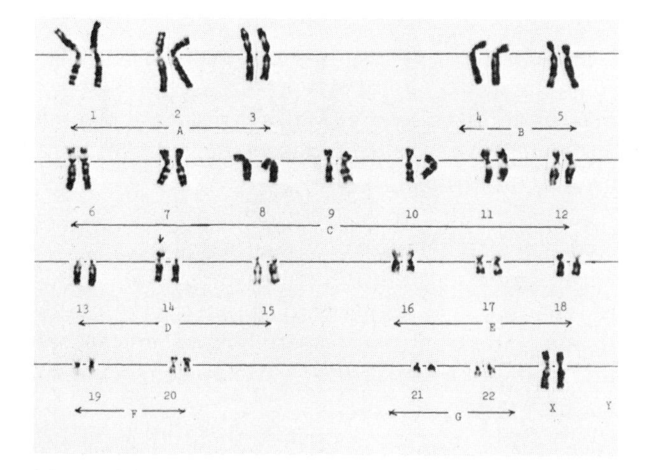

Figure 8–11. Karyotype of a female who has Down's syndrome as a result of an unbalanced translocation. (Courtesy Dr. Arthur Robinson, National Jewish Hospital and Research Center.)

Sex Chromosome Abnormalities

To better understand normal X chromosome function and thus abnormalities of the sex chromosomes, the nurse should have a basic understanding of the *Lyon hypothesis.* This well-established principle states that in females, at an early embryonic stage, one of the two normal X chromosomes becomes inactive, that all descendants of that cell will have the same X chromosome inactivated, and that inactivation is random and independent in each cell (Lyon, 1962). Thus, on an average, 50% of X chromosomes of maternal origin and 50% of X chromosomes of paternal origin become inactivated. The inactive X chromosome forms a dark staining area known as the *Barr body,* or *sex chromatin body* (Figure 8–12).

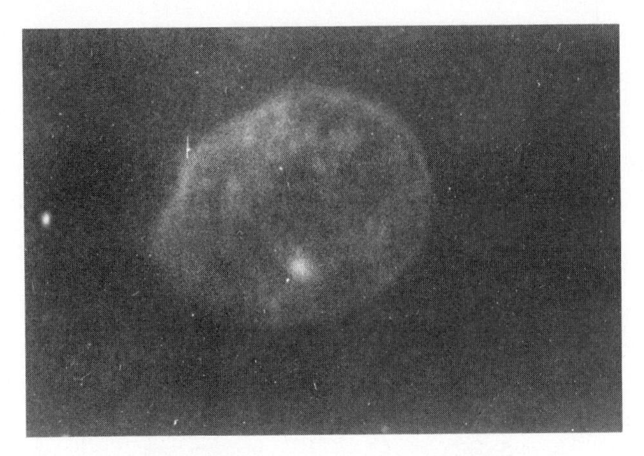

Figure 8–12. Nucleus with one Barr body; the patient is sex chromatin positive. (Courtesy Dr. Arthur Robinson, National Jewish Hospital and Research Center.)

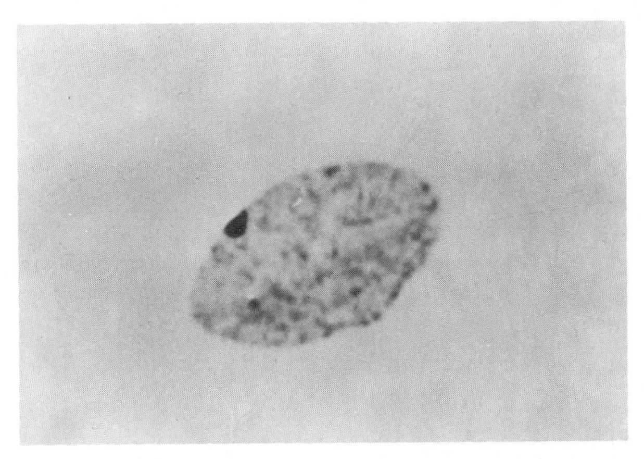

Figure 8–13. Nucleus with a Y body present. (Courtesy Dr. Arthur Robinson, National Jewish Hospital and Research Center.)

The Barr body may be observed by examining the cells scraped from the inside of a patient's mouth. This procedure, the *buccal smear,* will show the number of inactivated X chromosomes or Barr bodies present. In the normal female there is one Barr body, since one of her two X chromosomes has been inactivated. In the normal male, there are no Barr bodies, since he has only one X chromosome to begin with. The number of Barr bodies seen on the buccal smear is always one less than the number of X chromosomes present in the patient's cells.

This same technique may also be used to examine the Y chromosome. The cells are stained with a fluorescent stain, which under the fluorescent microscope shows the Y chromosome to be a bright body within the nucleus. The number of Y bodies present is equal to the number of Y chromosomes present. Males should have one Y body and females none (Figure 8–13).

The female with Turner's syndrome (Figure 8–14), on chromosomal analysis, is found to have only 45 chromosomes, with one X chromosome missing. There will be no Barr body present, since she is sex chromatin negative. During the newborn period, clinical signs and symptoms of Turner's syndrome are lymphedema of the dorsum of the hands and feet and excessive skin in the neck. Other features seen later in life are short stature, webbed neck, low hairline, cubitus valgus (increased carrying angle of arm), excessive nevi, broad shieldlike chest with widely spaced nipples, and underdeveloped secondary sex characteristics. The female external genitals and uterus are normal, but the ovaries are fibrous streaks. Primary amenorrhea is a striking symptom, and these patients are usually infertile. There are often renal anomalies, and the most common cardiac malformation is coarctation of the aorta. The patient with Turner's syndrome usually is not intellectually impaired, although she may have some perceptual difficulties. Turner's syndrome has an incidence of about 1 per 3000 to 7000 live female births.

When a female's cells contain two Barr bodies, this condition is known as *triple X.* She has a chromosome constitution consisting of 47,XXX. There are usually few physical features associated with this chromosomal abnormality, and recent studies have shown that intellectual impairment is inconsistent; that is, patients may or may not be impaired (Burns, 1976). The incidence of triple X is approximately 1 per 1000 to 1200 live female births.

Klinefelter's syndrome is one of the most common sex chromosome abnormalities among males (Figure 8–15). The patient has a chromosome constitution of 47,XXY and is chromatin positive (one Barr body present). Clinical signs associated with Klinefelter's syndrome include small, soft testes; eunuchoid body proportions; occasional gynecomastia (breast development); mild mental retardation; and underdeveloped secondary sex characteristics. These males are usually sterile. The incidence is approximately 1 per 1000 live male births. Approximately 1%–2% of institutionalized males have Klinefelter's syndrome.

Another sex chromosome abnormality among males is 47,XYY. In the past it was believed that these males were always very tall, aggressive or

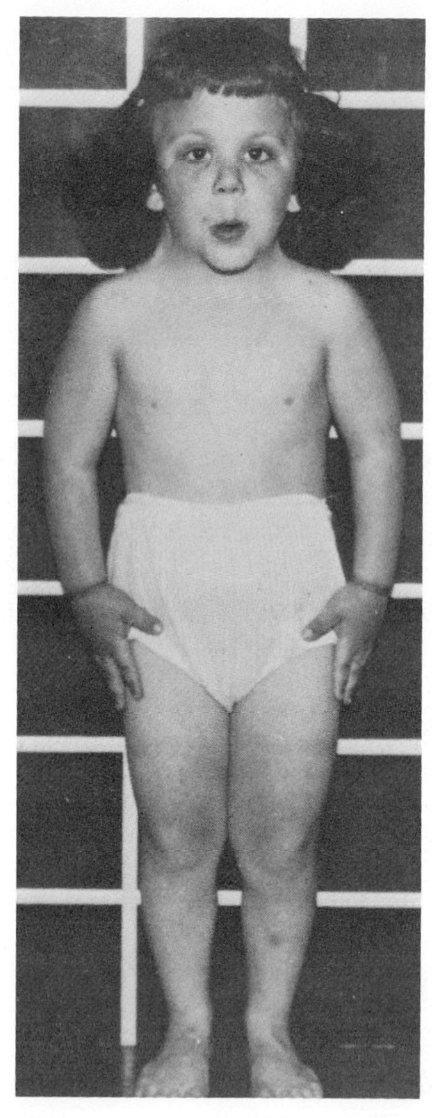

Figure 8–14. Patient with Turner's syndrome: 45,X karyotype. (From Smith, D. W. *Recognizable patterns of human malformations.* © 1976 W. B. Saunders Company, Philadelphia, Pa.)

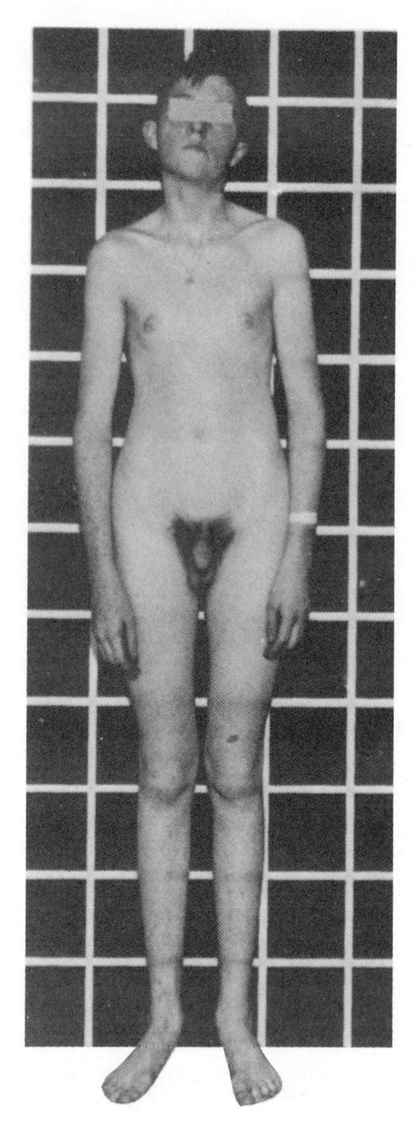

Figure 8–15. Patient with Klinefelter's syndrome: 47,XXY karyotype. (From Smith, D. W. *Recognizable patterns of human malformations.* © 1976 by the W. B. Saunders Company, Philadelphia, Pa.)

criminally inclined, and mentally retarded. Recent studies have not borne out this notion (Lubs and Lubs, 1975). However, the occurrence of mental retardation and psychiatric problems may be increased with this syndrome. There are no characteristic clinical findings.

Other sex chromosome abnormalities may occur. Whether there is an increased number of X chromosomes or Y chromosomes or both, the affected individual generally has an increased number of abnormalities and increased severity of mental retardation.

PATTERNS OF INHERITANCE

Not all genetic disorders are caused by abnormalities of the chromosomes. Many inherited diseases are produced by an abnormality in a single gene or pair of genes. In such instances the chromosomes are grossly normal, but the defect is at the gene level and cannot be detected by present lab-

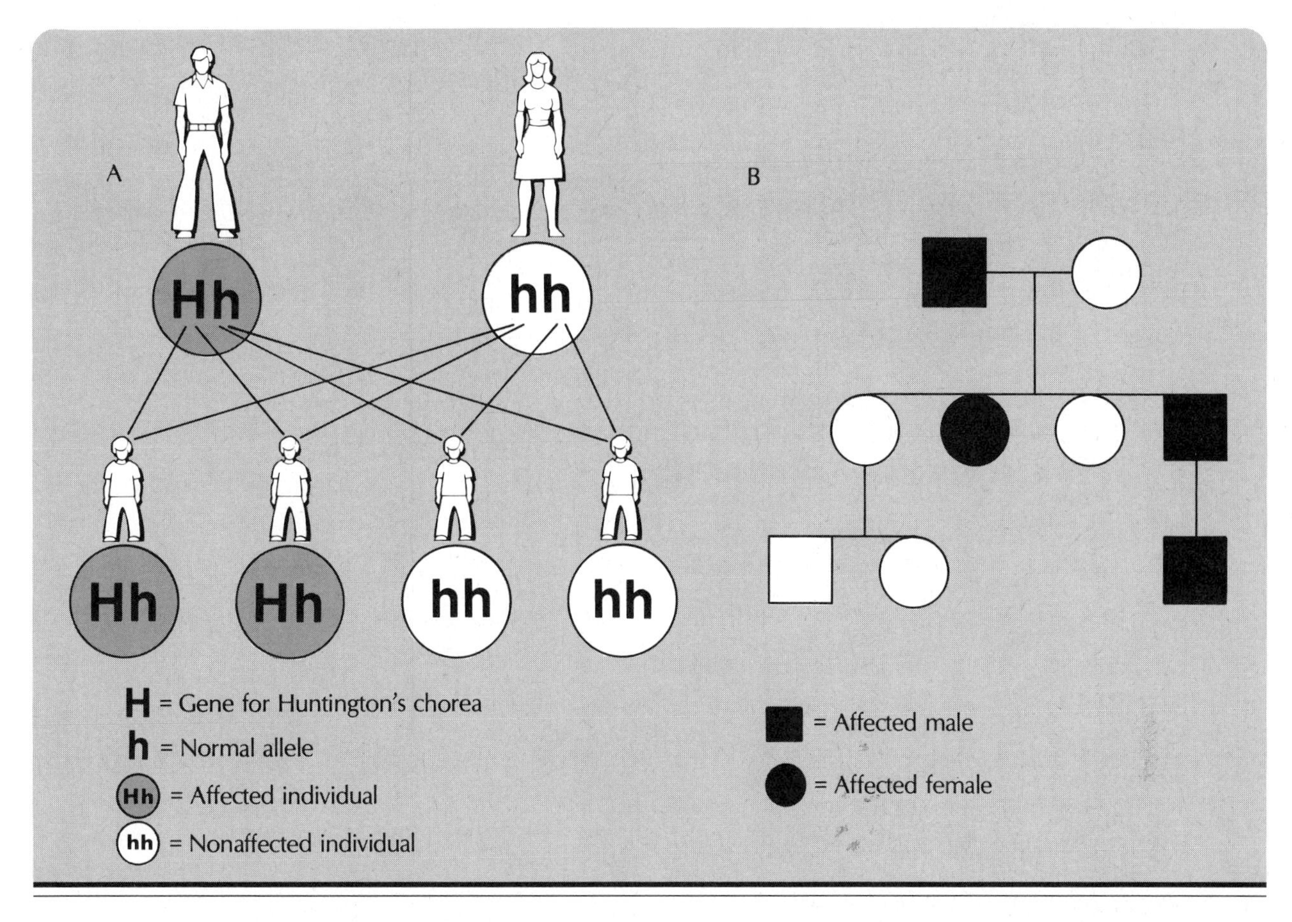

Figure 8–16. **A,** Autosomal dominant inheritance. One parent is affected. Statistically, 50% of offspring will be affected, regardless of sex. **B,** Autosomal dominant pedigree.

oratory techniques. The pattern of inheritance for a particular disease or defect is determined by two methods: (a) a close examination of the family in which the disease appears and (b) a knowledge of how the disease has been previously inherited as reported in the literature.

There are two major categories of inheritance: mendelian, or *single-gene, inheritance,* and nonmendelian, or *polygenic, inheritance.* Each single-gene trait is determined by a pair of genes working in concert. These genes are responsible for the observable expression of the trait, referred to as the *phenotype.* The total genetic endowment or constitution is referred to as the *genotype.* One of the genes for a trait is inherited from one's mother; the other, from one's father. The gene pairs are located on homologous (paired) chromosomes, and the place that each gene occupies is known as its *locus.* An individual who has two identical genes at a given locus is considered to be *homozygous* for that trait. An individual is considered to be *heterozygous* for a particular trait when he or she has two different *alleles* (alternate forms of the same gene) at a given locus on a pair of homologous chromosomes.

There are three well-known modes of single-gene inheritance: autosomal dominant, autosomal recessive, and X-linked (sex-linked) recessive. There is also an X-linked dominant mode of inheritance that is less common.

Autosomal Dominant Inheritance

An individual is said to have an autosomal dominantly inherited disorder if the disease trait is heterozygous. That is, the abnormal gene overshadows the normal gene of the pair, and the individual is thus affected. Autosomal dominant disorders have several distinctive characteristics:

1. An affected individual generally has an affected parent. Thus, the family pedigree usually shows multiple generations having the disorder (Figure 8–16).

2. The affected individual has a 50% chance of passing on the abnormal gene to each of his or her offspring, regardless of the genes of the other parent (Figure 8–16).
3. Both males and females are equally affected, and a father can pass the abnormal gene on to his son. This is an important principle when distinguishing autosomal dominant disorders from X-linked disorders.
4. There is a possibility of a mutation or a change of a normal gene into a dominant abnormal gene. In this case, this is the first time the disorder is seen in the family; an affected child is born to parents who are unaffected. In such instances, there is not an increased risk for future children of the same parents to be affected. The child, however, now has a 50% chance of passing the abnormal gene on to each of his or her offspring.
5. An unaffected individual in most cases cannot transmit the disorder to his or her children.
6. Dominant disorders may be clinically milder, since many affected individuals are able to reproduce and pass on the abnormal gene to their offspring.
7. Dominantly inherited disorders tend to have a variable pattern in their expression or observable characteristics. They may be more evident or more severe in one individual in the family than in others. This is an important factor when counseling families concerning autosomal dominant disorders. A parent may have a mild form of the disease, whereas his child may have a more severe form. Unfortunately, there is no method for predicting whether a child will be only mildly affected or more severely affected. The physician-geneticist must be thorough in the examination of family members to discern whether any of those individuals are indeed affected. They may express the disease in such a mild form that a cursory examination may miss clinical signs of the disease.

Some common autosomal dominantly inherited disorders are Huntington's chorea, polycystic kidney disease, neurofibromatosis (von Recklinghausen's disease), and achondroplastic dwarfism.

Autosomal Recessive Inheritance

An individual has an autosomal recessively inherited disorder if the disease manifests itself only as a homozygous trait. That is, because the normal gene overshadows the abnormal one, the individual must have two abnormal genes to be affected. The notion of a *carrier state* is appropriate here. An individual who is heterozygous for the abnormal gene is clinically normal. It is not until two individuals mate and pass on the same abnormal gene that affected offspring may appear. Characteristics of autosomal recessive disorders include:

1. An affected individual has clinically normal parents, but they are both carriers of the abnormal gene (Figure 8–17,*A*).
2. Parents who are both carriers for the same abnormal gene have a 25% chance of both passing the abnormal gene on to any of their offspring (Figure 8–17,*A*).
3. If the offspring of two carrier parents is clinically normal, there is a two-thirds chance that he or she is a carrier of the gene (Figure 8–17,*A*).
4. Both males and females are equally affected.
5. The family pedigree usually shows siblings affected in a horizontal fashion (Figure 8–17,*B*). Future generations are not affected unless both parents carry the same abnormal gene.
6. There is often an increased incidence of consanguineous matings. Parents who have a common ancestor are more likely to have the same genes in common than two parents who are unrelated.
7. Recessively inherited disorders tend to be more severe in their clinical manifestations. Clinically normal carrier parents pass on the disorder, and the affected offspring will often not reproduce. If an affected individual does reproduce, all the offspring will be carriers for that disorder.
8. For some autosomal recessively inherited disorders, the presence of the abnormal gene in a normal carrier parent can be detected. For instance, Tay-Sachs disease is caused by an inborn error of metabolism—that is, a deficiency of the enzyme hexosaminidase A. An affected individual has little or no enzyme activity present, whereas a carrier parent usually has 50% normal enzyme activity present.

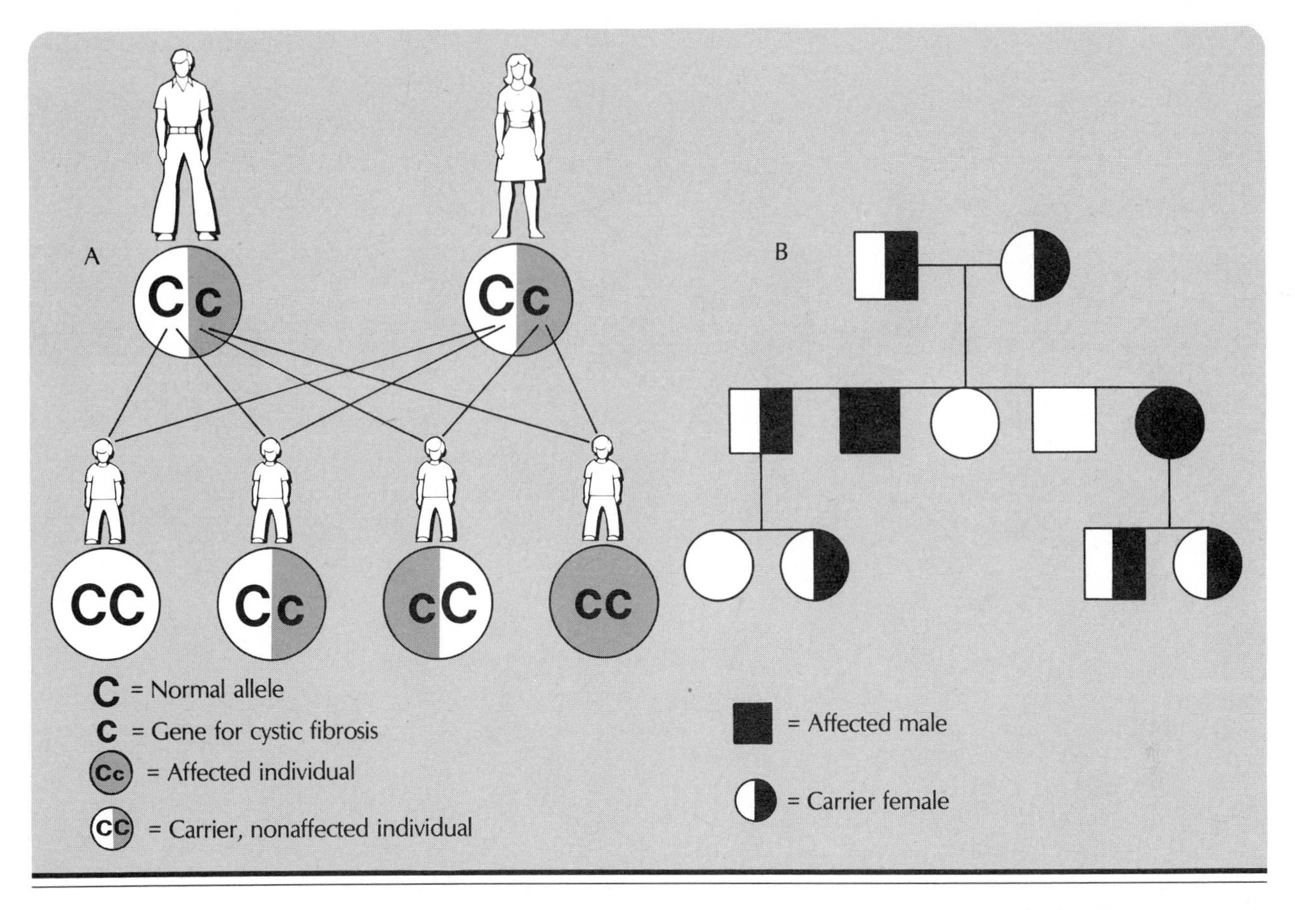

Figure 8–17. **A,** Autosomal recessive inheritance. Both parents are carriers. Statistically, 25% of offspring are affected, regardless of sex. **B,** Autosomal recessive pedigree.

Thus, biochemically the carrier is abnormal, and the heterozygous state can be detected, even though it is asymptomatic.

Some common autosomal recessive inherited disorders are cystic fibrosis, PKU, galactosemia, sickle cell anemia, Tay-Sachs disease, and most metabolic disorders.

X-Linked Recessive Inheritance

X-linked or sex-linked disorders are those for which the abnormal gene is carried on the X chromosome. A female may be heterozygous or homozygous for a trait carried on the X chromosome, since she has two X chromosomes. A male, however, has only one X chromosome, and there are some traits for which there are no comparable genes located on the Y chromosome. The male in this case is considered to be *hemizygous,* having only one allele instead of a pair for a given trait or disorder. Thus an X-linked disorder is manifested in a male who carries the abnormal gene on his X chromosome. His mother is considered to be a carrier when the normal gene on one X chromosome overshadows the abnormal gene on the other X chromosome.

The major distinguishing feature of X-linked disorders is that there is *no* male-to-male transmission. Males pass only their Y chromosomes to their sons and only their X chromosomes to their daughters. Thus a son always receives his X chromosome from his mother and his Y chromosome from his father. Daughters receive one of their mother's X chromosomes and their other X chromosome from their father.

Other characteristics seen in X-linked recessive disorders include the following:

1. The family pedigree is viewed in an oblique fashion (Figure 8–18). Affected males are related through the female line.
2. There is a 50% chance that a carrier mother will pass the abnormal gene on to each of her

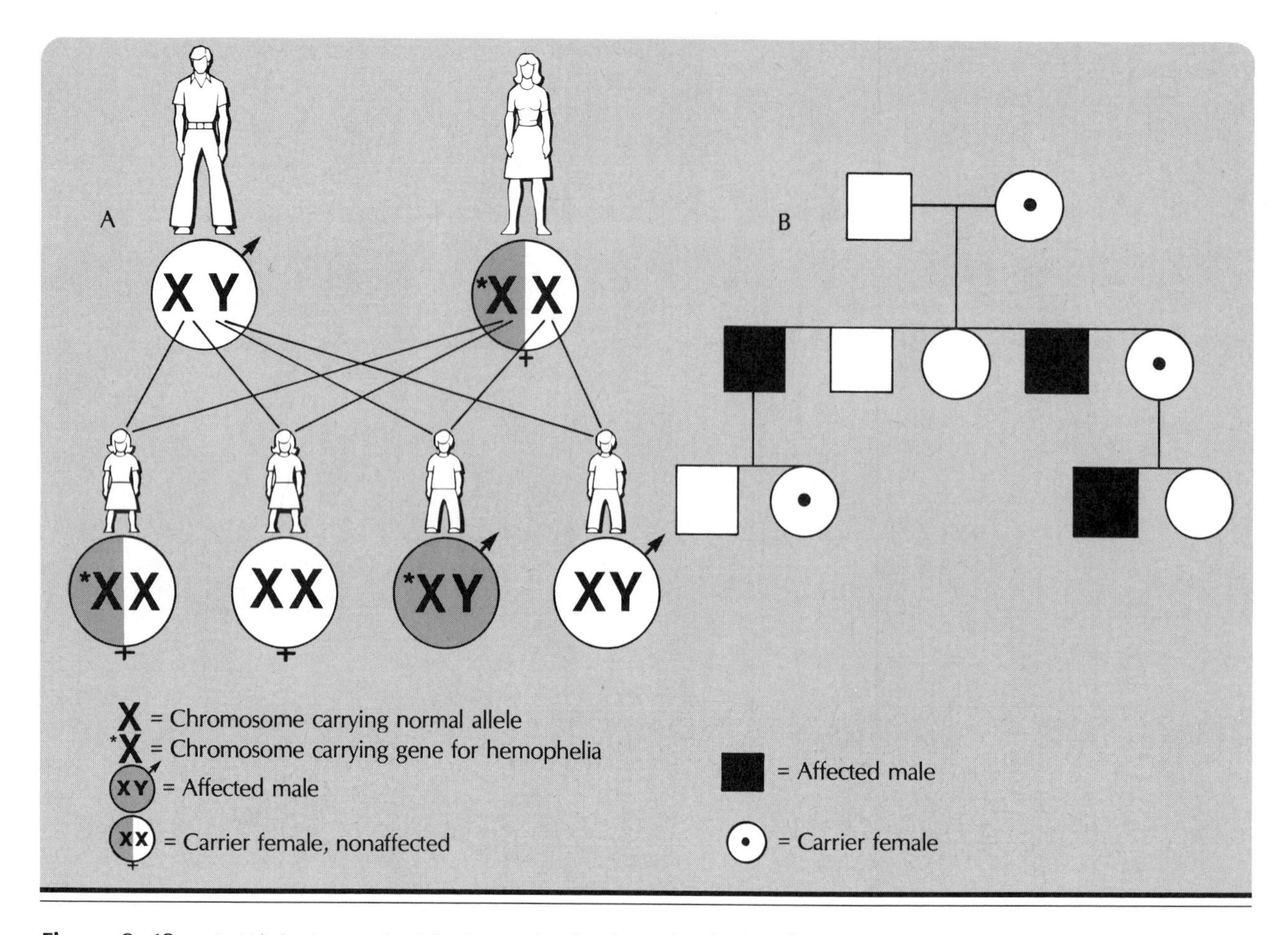

Figure 8–18. **A,** X-linked recessive inheritance. Mother is carrier. Statistically, 50% of male offspring are affected and 50% of female offspring are affected. **B,** X-linked recessive pedigree.

sons, who will thus be affected. There is a 50% chance that a carrier mother will pass the normal gene on to each of her sons, who will thus be unaffected. Finally, there is a 50% chance that a carrier mother will pass the abnormal gene on to each of her daughters; thus the daughters become carriers like their mother (Figure 8–18).

3. Fathers affected with an X-linked disorder cannot pass the disorder on to their sons. Conversely, *all* their daughters become carriers for the disorder.
4. Occasionally a female carrier may show some symptomatology of an X-linked disorder. This situation is probably due to random inactivation of the X chromosome carrying the normal allele (Lyon hypothesis). Thus, a heterozygous female may show some manifestation of an X-linked disorder.

Common X-linked recessive disorders are hemophilia, Duchenne type muscular dystrophy, and color blindness.

X-Linked Dominant Inheritance

X-linked dominant disorders are extremely rare, the most common being vitamin D–resistant rickets. When X-linked dominance does occur, the pattern is similar to X-linked recessive inheritance except that heterozygous females become affected. Since the abnormal gene is dominant, it overshadows the normal gene on the female's other X chromosome. Again, the major feature distinguishing this pattern from autosomal dominant inheritance is that there is no male-to-male transmission. An affected father will have affected daughters, but none of his sons will be affected.

Polygenic Inheritance

Many common congenital malformations, such as cleft palate, heart defects, spina bifida, dislocated hips, clubfoot, and pyloric stenosis, are not inherited in specific single-gene patterns but are caused by an interaction of many genes and an environmental influence on those genes. Instead of a single gene or a pair of genes being responsible for the manifestation of a disease or malformation, many genes appear to be coded to produce the defect. It is commonly hypothesized that each individual has a threshold above which such a defect will be manifested (Riccardi, 1977).

Several features are characteristic of polygenic inheritance:

1. The malformations are usually seen along a continuum from mild to severe. For example, spina bifida may range in severity from mild, as spina bifida occult; to more severe, as a myelomeningocele; to its most severe state, anencephaly. It is believed that the more severe the defect, the more genes are present for that defect.

2. There is often a bias of sex. Clubfoot is more commonly seen in males, whereas cleft palate is more common among females. Thus, when a member of the less commonly affected sex manifests this type of condition, a greater number of genes must be present to manifest the defect.

3. An environmental influence (such as weather, altitude, chemicals in the environment, or exposure to toxic substances) may be present. For example, suppose that it takes a certain number of genes to produce cleft lip and palate. If both parents pass on genes coded for cleft lip and palate and their offspring receives a particular number of genes above the threshold, he or she is affected. If, however, some environmental influence is present, it may take fewer genes to manifest the defect.

4. In contrast to single-gene disorders, there is an additive effect in polygenic inheritance. The more first-degree relatives affected with a malformation, the greater the risk for the next pregnancy to also be affected (Table 8–1).

Table 8–1. Risk of Recurrence of Spina Bifida or Anencephaly*

Family history of spina bifida and/or anencephaly	Estimated recurrence risk (percent)
One sibling affected	5
Parent and sibling affected	13
Two siblings affected	13
Three siblings affected	21
One sibling and 2nd-degree relative affected	9
One sibling and 3rd-degree relative affected	7
One sibling affected, no other family history	4

*From Smith, C. 1973. Implications of antenatal diagnosis. In *Antenatal diagnosis of genetic disease,* ed. A. Emery. Edinburgh: Churchill Livingstone, p. 137.

5. Risk figures are empirical. They are determined by the distribution of cases found in the general population as reported in the literature. Thus the risk of recurrence is usually 2%–5% for all first-degree relatives if one family member is affected; the recurrence figure continues to decrease with second-degree relatives and so forth.

Although most congenital malformations are polygenic traits, a careful family history should always be taken, since occasionally cleft lip and palate, certain congenital heart defects, and other malformations can be inherited as autosomal dominant or recessive traits. Other disorders thought to be within the polygenic inheritance group are diabetes, hypertension, some heart diseases, and mental illness.

PRENATAL DIAGNOSIS

Prenatal diagnosis of genetic disease has been one of the most exciting and significant advances made in preventive medicine in recent years. The ability to diagnose certain genetic diseases by various diagnostic tools, such as amniocentesis, carries with it enormous implications for the practice of preventive health care. Since parent-child and family-planning counseling have become a major responsibility of professional nurses, it has become imperative that nurses have the most current knowledge available concerning prenatal diagnosis.

Several methods are available for prenatal diagnosis, although some are still being used on an experimental basis. The use of *ultrasound,* a sonar-like procedure, involves directing sound waves over the abdomen. In areas of high density, such as bone, the sound waves are deflected and are picked up by the machine and projected on a screen. Information obtainable from the ultrasound includes the presence of a fetal head (from which fetal size and gestation can be approximated), localization of the placenta, the size of the uterus, the presence of twins, and structural abnormalities such as enlarged kidneys. There has been no evidence of harmful effects to either mother or fetus from exposure to ultrasound.

X-ray examination at approximately 20 weeks of pregnancy can be used to determine gross limb or generalized bone abnormalities. An x-ray film on an oblique axis can be used to rule out such inherited disorders as metatropic dwarfism and hypophosphatasia. Unfortunately, x-radiation may produce unwarranted effects on the fetus. However, if the risk and burden of a genetic disease are higher than the risk of problems due to x-ray exposure, then the use of x-rays should be considered.

Amniography (the instillation of dye into the amniotic cavity to outline the fetus) and *amnioscopy* (direct visual presentation of the fetus by a scope) are two methods of prenatal diagnosis that are not yet available for generalized clinical use. These methods are used primarily to observe the fetus for major structural abnormalities. Because the risks of these methods have not yet been determined, they remain experimental tools.

The major diagnostic method for prenatal diagnosis is *genetic amniocentesis.* This procedure, available for general clinical use since the early 1970s, differs from amniocentesis done late in pregnancy for Rh incompatibility in that it is performed early in pregnancy to diagnose a variety of genetic disorders. The 14th to 16th week of pregnancy (based on last menstrual period) appears to be the optimal time for the procedure, based on uterine size, volume of fluid, and the number of viable cells present in the fluid. After ultrasound is performed to localize the placenta and to estimate gestational size, a 22-gauge spinal needle is inserted through the abdomen (the puncture point is anesthetized) into the uterus. Approximately 20 ml of amniotic fluid is removed. This fluid contains fetal skin and mucous membrane cells, which can then be grown in culture or tested biochemically (Figure 8-19). The procedure is usually done on an outpatient basis, with no need for restriction of activities after the tap. (See Chapter 14 for an in-depth description of the procedure and specific nursing interventions.)

The indications for genetic amniocentesis include:

1. Previous child with a chromosomal abnormality.
2. Parent carrying a chromosomal abnormality (balanced translocation).
3. Increased maternal age (age 37 and over).
4. Mother carrying an X-linked disease.
5. Parents carrying an inborn error of metabolism that can be diagnosed in utero.
6. Family history of anencephaly or spina bifida.

Young couples who have had a child with trisomy 21 have approximately a 1%–2% risk of a future child having a chromosome abnormality. Although no statistics of recurrence risks for other chromosome abnormalities have been established, genetic amniocentesis is made available to any couple who has already had a child with a chromosome abnormality. In addition, any couple in which one of the partners is a carrier of a balanced translocation should be considered for prenatal diagnosis. Although the person with the chromosome rearrangement is clinically normal, he or she has the potential for conceiving a child with an unbalanced chromosome constitution, which usually has substantial adverse effects on normal development. For example, a woman who carries a balanced 14/21 translocation has a risk of approximately 10%–15% that her offspring will be affected with the unbalanced translocation of Down's syndrome; if the father is the carrier, there is a 2%–5% risk (Henry and Robinson, 1978).

One of the major indications for genetic amniocentesis is increased maternal age, since any woman age 37 or older is at greater risk for having children with chromosome abnormalities. This maternal age effect is most pronounced for trisomy 21. For women between 35 and 40 years of age, the risk for having children with Down's syndrome is 1%–3%; between 40 and 45 years, the risk is 4%–12%; after 45 years, it is 12% or greater.

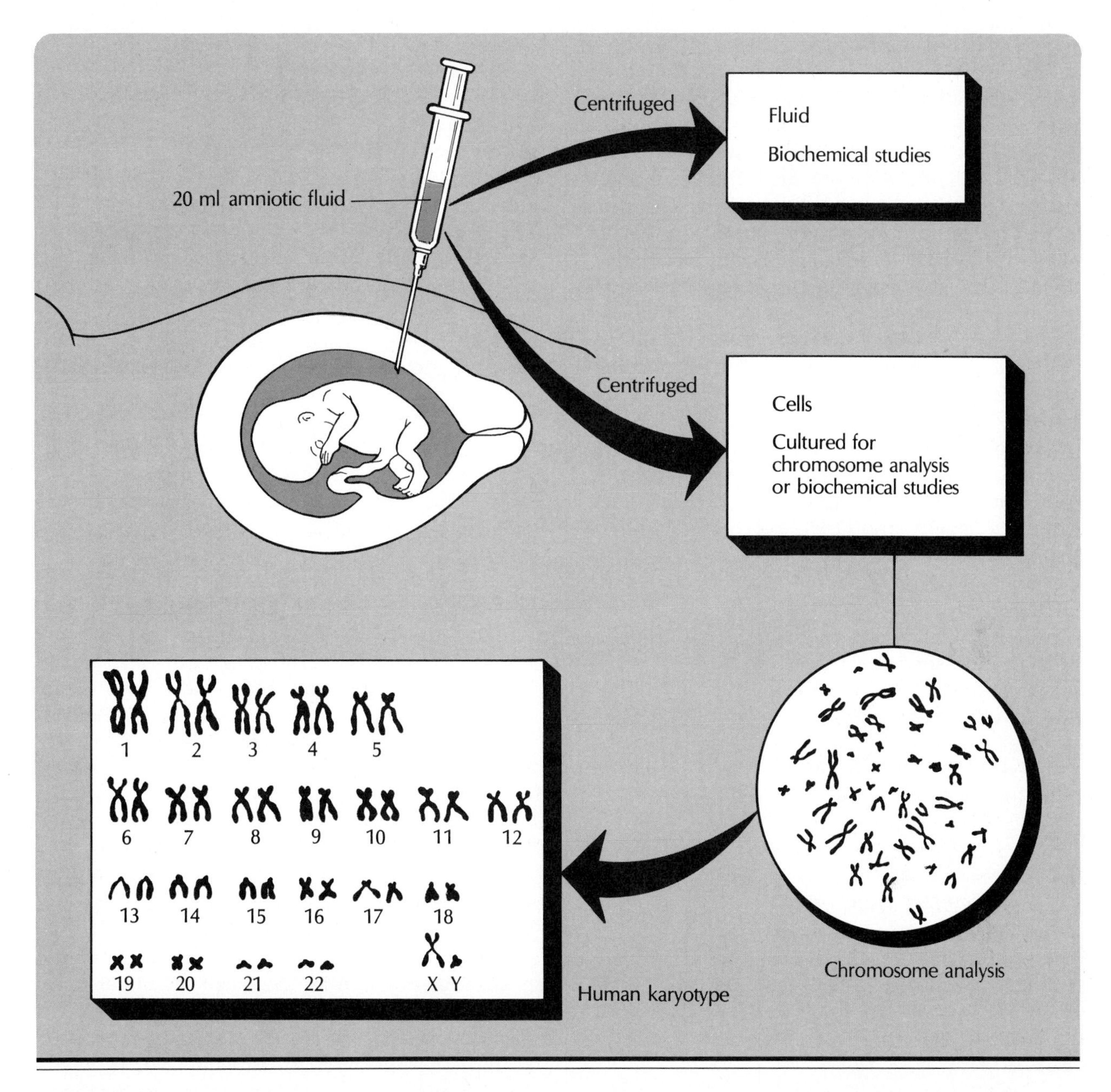

Figure 8–19. Genetic amniocentesis for prenatal diagnosis is done at about 15–16 weeks' gestation. (Modified from Ritchie, D. D., and Carola, R. 1979. *Biology.* Reading, Mass.: Addison-Wesley Publishing Co., p. 302.)

The occurrence of other autosomal trisomies (trisomy 13 and 18) also shows a correlation with increasing maternal age, although it is not as marked as in trisomy 21. The mechanism underlying the increased occurrence of nondisjunction (resulting in too many or too few chromosomes) is not known, but it is thought to be in some way related to the fact that women are born with their entire complement of eggs. The eggs are arrested in a stage of meiosis until ovulation and are subject to all the environmental factors that a given woman experiences.

In families in which the woman is a known or possible carrier of an X-linked disorder such as hemophilia or Duchenne type muscular dystrophy, genetic amniocentesis may be an appropriate option for the family. These disorders are not routinely diagnosable in utero. However, because they usually affect only males, the sex of the fetus can be determined and termination of pregnancy considered when it is found to be male. For a known female carrier, the risk of an affected male fetus is 50%. The decision to abort a possibly normal male fetus must be discussed and made within each family. Similarly, couples in which the father is affected with an X-linked disorder may elect to have only male children. The gene would not be continued in the family; all females (who would have to be carriers) could be aborted. To date, this has been an infrequent reason for genetic amniocentesis. However, since many males with X-linked disorders, especially hemophilia, are surviving to reproduce as greater advances in medical treatment become available, the situation may indeed become more common.

Another fairly common indication for genetic amniocentesis occurs when both parents carry a gene for the same autosomal recessive disorder, which is usually one of the biochemical inborn errors of metabolism.

Metabolic disorders detectable in utero include:

- Argininosuccinicaciduria
- Cystinosis
- Fabry's disease
- Galactosemia
- Gaucher's disease
- Homocystinuria
- Hunter's syndrome
- Hurler's disease
- Krabbe's disease
- Lesch-Nyhan syndrome
- Maple syrup urine disease
- Metachromatic leukodystrophy
- Methylmalonic aciduria
- Niemann-Pick disease
- Pompe's disease
- Sanfilippo's syndrome
- Tay-Sachs disease

When both parents are carriers of an autosomal recessive disease, there is a 25% risk for each pregnancy that the fetus will be affected. Diagnosis is made by testing the cultured amniotic fluid cells (either enzyme level, substrate level, or product level) or the fluid itself.

Most recently, genetic amniocentesis has been made available to those couples who have had a child with neural tube defects or who have a family history of these conditions, which include anencephaly, spina bifida, and myelomeningocele. Neural tube defects are usually polygenic traits. In cases in which there is an otherwise negative family history, an empiric recurrence risk is approximately 5% for the couple with a previously affected child (Table 8–1). Regardless of the numerical risk for a given family, whether for an isolated neural tube defect or a disorder in which a neural tube defect is a constant feature, the risk of recurrence can be reduced (possibly by as much as 90%) through α-fetoprotein (AFP) determination on the amniotic fluid. Normally α-fetoprotein is a substance found in high levels in a developing fetus and in low levels in maternal serum and in amniotic fluid. In pregnancies in which the fetus has an open neural tube defect, α-fetoprotein leaks into the amniotic fluid and levels are elevated. Elevation of α-fetoprotein may also occur in cases of fetal distress, imminent or actual fetal death, and several other disorders. Thus, genetic amniocentesis allows those families for whom the risk of a neural tube defect is increased the opportunity to choose whether to have a child affected with such a high-burden disorder.

With the advent of diagnostic techniques such as amniocentesis, couples who would not otherwise have additional children because of the risk or burden can decide to conceive without terminating pregnancy out of fear. Because the percentage of therapeutic abortions after amniocentesis is small, most couples find peace of mind throughout the remainder of the pregnancy.

Prenatal diagnosis offers an alternative to having children affected with certain genetic diseases. For many couples it is not an acceptable option, as the only method of preventing a genetic disease is preventing the birth of an affected child. This decision is an individual one to be made by the family. Most genetic centers do not require or even solicit an agreement or irrevocable decision regarding termination of pregnancy upon detection of an abnormal fetus. Genetic counselors do, however, discuss with the family those options available if an abnormal fetus is found.

Prenatal diagnosis cannot guarantee the birth of a normal child. It can only determine the presence or absence of specific disorders (within the limits of laboratory error). Nonspecific mental retardation, cleft lip and palate, cystic fibrosis, PKU, and sickle cell anemia are a few of the disorders that are not amenable to intrauterine diagnosis. A couple is at the same risk as the general population or at the risk calculated for their individual case based on their family history for any other disorder. It becomes imperative, then, that preamniocentesis counseling precede any procedure for prenatal diagnosis. There are many questions and points to consider if the family is to reach an appropriate decision.

In the future, if cure or treatment of diagnosable disorders is possible, prenatal diagnosis can allow for treatment to be initiated during the pregnancy, thus possibly preventing irreversible damage. For other disorders, effective postnatal treatment may make prenatal diagnosis unnecessary. The capability of diagnosis of many diseases in utero is realized every day. In light of the philosophy of preventive health care, this information should be made available to all couples who are expecting a child or who are contemplating pregnancy.

GENETIC COUNSELING: THE NURSE'S ROLE

Genetic counseling is a communication process in which the genetic counselor tries to provide a family with the most complete and accurate information on the occurrence or the risk of recurrence of a genetic disease in that family. The goals inherent in this definition are threefold. First, genetic counseling allows families to make informed decisions about reproduction. Second, it assists families in assessing the available treatments, examining appropriate alternatives to decrease the risk, learning about the usual course and outcome of the genetic disease or abnormality, and dealing with other psychologic and social implications that often accompany such problems. Finally, it is hoped that genetic counseling will help decrease the incidence and impact of genetic disease.

What Can Families Expect?

The process of genetic counseling usually begins after the birth of a child diagnosed as having a congenital abnormality or genetic disease. After the parents have been referred to the genetics clinic, they are sent a form requesting information on the health status of various family members. This type of previsit information form is used in many genetic centers throughout the country. At this time the nurse can be helpful to the family and the genetic counselor by discussing the form with the family or clarifying the information needed to complete it. It may be beneficial for the parents to write or telephone relatives to gather additional data. Perhaps someone in the extended family will recall pertinent events, such as the birth of a related child with spina bifida. In addition, medical records are requested for family members who may be similarly afflicted.

At the initial genetic counseling visit, an extensive family history is taken in the form of a pedigree. The counselor gathers additional information about the affected child, pregnancy, growth and development, and the family's understanding of the problem. Generally, a physical examination is performed on the affected individual. Other family members may also be examined. If any laboratory tests, such as chromosomal analysis, metabolic studies, or viral titers, are indicated, they are performed at this time. The genetic counselor may then give the family some preliminary information based on the data in hand.

When all the data have been carefully examined and analyzed, including any laboratory results, the family returns for a follow-up visit. At this time the parents are given all the information available, including the medical facts, diagnosis, probable course of the disorder, and any available management; the inheritance pattern for this particular family and their risk of recurrence; and the options or alternatives for dealing with the risk of recurrence. The remainder of the counseling session is spent discussing the course of action that seems appropriate to the family in view of their risk and family goals.

The family may return a number of times to allow ample time for airing their questions and concerns. It is most desirable for the nurse working with the family to attend many or all of these counseling sessions. Since the nurse has already established a rapport with the family, she can act as a liaison between the family and the genetic counselor. She hears directly what the genetic counselor has discussed with the family and can help the family members formulate their questions.

When the parents have completed the counseling sessions, a letter is sent to them and to their physician stating what was said during the sessions. This written document of the counseling session should be kept for the family to refer to as needed.

Appropriate Referrals

Genetic counseling is an appropriate course of action for any family who asks the question, "Will it happen again?" Referrals to the genetic counseling clinic may be made by anyone interested in helping the family answer this question. Occasionally families contact the clinic independently; most often their physician refers them. Increasingly, however, it is the nurse who makes the referral. If the nurse is aware of those families who are at an increased risk, she is in an ideal position to make the referral. The nursery nurse frequently has the first contact with the family of a child born with a congenital abnormality. The pediatric nurse, school nurse, or nurse practitioner often is the first to observe problems in growth and development or in perceptual and sensory functioning. The public health nurse has a rapport with the entire family and may be the only health professional to whom families will relate their questions and concerns. The family nurse practitioner or family-planning nurse is in an excellent position to reach at-risk families *before* the birth of an abnormal child.

Which families, then, are appropriate for the nurse to refer to genetic counseling? There are six major categories of indications that aid in determining referrals:

1. *Congenital abnormalities, including mental retardation.* Any couple who has had a child or a relative with a congenital malformation may be at an increased risk and should be informed as to what that risk is. Also, if mental retardation of unidentified cause has occurred in a family, they may be at an increased risk of recurrence. With the appropriate data, the genetic counselor will try to identify the risk.

In many cases the genetic counselor will identify the cause of a malformation as a teratogen (see Chapter 13). The family should be aware of what substances or exposures are teratogenic so they can be avoided with the next pregnancy.

2. *Familial disorders.* Families should be told that certain diseases may have a genetic component and that the risk of their occurrence within a particular family may be higher than that for the general population. Such disorders as diabetes, heart disease, cancer, and mental illness fall into this category.

3. *Known inherited diseases.* Families may know that a disease is inherited but not know the mechanism or the specific risk for them. A couple may be affected or may have a relative or child who is affected with an inherited disease and may wish to know the specific risk for passing the disorder on to other offspring. An important point to remember is that family members who are not at risk for passing on a disorder should be as well informed as those family members who *do* have an increased risk.

4. *Metabolic disorders.* Any families at risk for having a child with a metabolic disorder or biochemical defect should be referred. Because most inborn errors of metabolism are autosomal recessively inherited, a family may not be identified as at risk until the birth of an affected child. The three most common metabolic disorders for which families can be screened are PKU, sickle cell anemia, and Tay-Sachs disease. Infants are screened for PKU at birth, and an affected child can be treated by diet. However, no carrier test is available to identify parents before the birth of a PKU child.

Carriers of the sickle cell trait can be identified before pregnancy is begun, and the risk of having an affected child can be determined. Unfortunately, there is no method for identifying an affected fetus.

5. *Chromosomal abnormalities.* As discussed previously, any couple who have had a child with a chromosomal abnormality may be at an increased risk of having another child similarly affected. This group would include families in which there is concern for a possible translocation.

6. *Prenatal diagnosis.* Prenatal examination and diagnostic procedures can point out those families at risk, as discussed earlier in this chapter.

Alternatives to Increased Risks

During the genetic counseling session, an important area of discussion is the availability of alternatives for a family with an increased risk. Based on the family history, the inheritance pattern of the disease, and the disease process, none, one, or several alternatives may be appropriate for the family to consider. Among those options that may be considered are adoption, artificial insemination, delayed childbearing, prenatal diagnosis, and early detection and treatment.

If the risk of occurrence is high within the family or if the burden of the disease is high, a couple may choose not to have any of their own children but to *adopt*. In this case, the disease would not be passed on; the couple would not have the agonizing burden of caring for a chronically handicapped child. Their needs as parents would be fulfilled, and a parentless child would have a loving family. Unfortunately, the lack of available adoptive children makes this alternative less feasible than others.

The family may consider *artificial insemination by donor* (AID). This alternative is appropriate in several instances. For example, if the husband is affected with an autosomal dominant disease, AID would decrease the risk of having an affected child to zero, since the child would not inherit any genes from the affected parent. If the husband is affected with an X-linked disorder and does not wish to continue the gene in the family (all his daughters will be carriers), AID would be an alternative to terminating all pregnancies with a female fetus. If the husband is a carrier for a balanced translocation and if termination of pregnancy is against family ethics, AID is the most appropriate alternative. AID is also appropriate if both parents are carriers of an autosomal recessive disease. AID lowers the risk to a very low level or to zero if a carrier test is available. Finally, AID may be appropriate if the family is at high risk for a polygenic disorder.

Couples who are young may decide to delay childbearing for a few years. Medical science and medical genetics are continually making breakthroughs in early detection and treatment. Couples who are at risk may find in a few years that prenatal diagnosis will be available or that a disease can be detected and treated early to prevent irreversible damage.

Prerequisites of Counseling

Taking the family history and constructing the pedigree are the fundamental steps that must be taken before initiating any counseling session. The overall goal of eliciting a history is to identify those families for which the risk and burden is high enough that they may wish to alter their reproduction plans based on this information. Once a family has been identified as being at risk, the family history serves three additional purposes. First, even if a specific diagnosis cannot be made, the family history may indicate the mode of inheritance. If a family is afflicted with a neuromuscular degenerative disorder and the pedigree displays an autosomal dominant pattern of inheritance, a specific recurrence figure can be given to the family even if a specific name cannot be given to the disease. Second, the history and pedigree allow the genetic counselor to identify other areas that should be of concern to the family. Take the example of a pregnant woman, 45 years of age, who comes for preamniocentesis counseling and learns that she is at risk for having a child with a neural tube defect. This additional information may help to prevent a tragic situation. Finally, the pedigree and history allow the genetic counselor to identify other family members who might also be at risk for the same disorder. The family being counseled may wish to notify those relatives at risk so that they, too, can be given genetic counseling. When done correctly, the family history and pedigree become one of the most powerful and useful tools that the genetic counselor can use in determining a family's risk.

The pedigree is a fairly easy and productive method for screening families. The nurse can obtain the necessary information and draw a screening pedigree in approximately 15 minutes. Information that should be obtained when drawing the family pedigree includes names (maiden names if appropriate) and birth dates of members of the immediate family; names and ages of the remainder of the family (including deceased members), with a description of their health status; causes of death of family members; and any other information the family feels is significant. In discussing the affected individual, the nurse should obtain information on the pregnancy history of the mother (including miscarriages), medications and drugs taken during pregnancy, x-ray exposure, infections or illness during pregnancy, the type of birth control used prior to pregnancy, and the method used to diagnose the pregnancy. A complete delivery history should be taken, including a description of any complications. It is also appropriate for the nurse to ask the family when the problem was evident to them or was diagnosed.

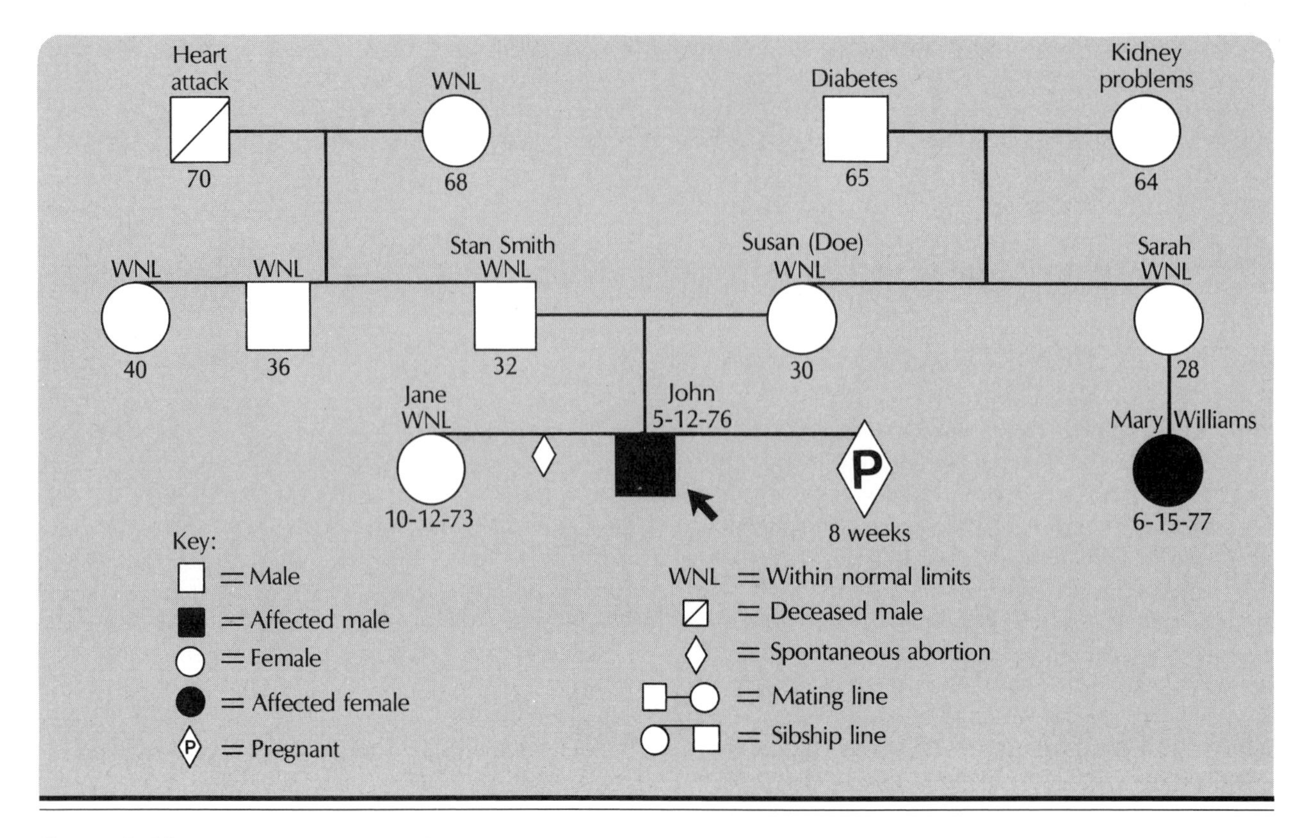

Figure 8–20. Screening pedigree. The arrow indicates the nearest family member affected with the disorder being investigated. Basic data have been recorded. Numbers refer to ages of the family members.

Finally, the nurse should inquire about the child's growth and development, including his developmental milestones, growth in comparison to siblings or other children his age, his symptoms of a problem, school records, and any previous testing.

A screening pedigree generally includes the affected individual, siblings, parents, aunts and uncles, and grandparents (Figure 8–20). If the family does not have all the necessary information at hand, the nurse can urge them to obtain the information in time for their first genetic counseling session, when a more extensive pedigree will be taken.

Principles in Counseling

For genetic counseling to be an effective avenue of health care, geneticists and health professionals must adhere to certain principles to guide them in their clinical practice. There are six major principles that govern genetic counseling: accurate diagnosis, nondirective counseling, confidentiality, truthfulness, timing, and follow-up counseling.

Accurate Diagnosis

Before any information can be given to a family, an accurate diagnosis must be established. The ability to provide information on the risk of recurrence, on the course of the disease process, on appropriate options, and on treatment modalities is based on an accurate diagnosis. Thus, special care and consideration must be given to establishing that diagnosis. When either confirming or establishing a diagnosis, the genetic counselor examines past medical records and the results of laboratory tests, requests photographs, reviews the literature, looks for minute details and subtleties on physical examination, and consults with colleagues. Only after the correct diagnosis has been confirmed or established does the genetic counseling process continue.

Unfortunately, a diagnosis is not always possible. Even more grave, the family may be given an inaccurate diagnosis. If there are insufficient data—if there are no medical records or if the syndrome has not been described previously—the genetic counselor may not be able to proceed with specific facts and figures. Instead, the counselor must speak in terms of "if" and must be acutely aware of the dilemma being created for the family. Fortunately, this situation is not common and affects only a small percentage of families.

Nondirective Counseling

Although it is impossible for the genetic counselor to be completely unbiased and unopinionated, he or she must strive to create a nonthreatening, noncoercive atmosphere in which families can make decisions for themselves. The counselor's role is to provide information and to assist and support families in their decisions, not to make the decision for them. What the counselor can and should provide to each couple is assistance in realizing what their personal priorities are and how their decisions may affect those priorities. Once they have decided on the course of action they wish to pursue, both the genetic counselor and the nurse should assist them as much as possible in accepting that decision.

Confidentiality

As with any client-professional relationship, confidentiality and trust are paramount to genetic counseling. Families should be assured that information they provide about their relatives' health status will not be loosely discussed or shared.

However, the issue of confidentiality is not clear-cut. What is the genetic counselor's moral obligation if an autosomal dominant disorder is diagnosed in a patient and the patient refuses to share this information with siblings, who are at 50% risk of being similarly affected? This situation is rare, and it is hoped that the geneticist can persuade the patient to share as much information with relatives as possible.

Truthfulness

Occasionally truthfulness in counseling becomes an issue. A counselor may be tempted to dilute or hide certain facts from a couple to protect them from undue anxiety or blame and guilt. While one does not have to dwell on all the "gruesome" facts concerning the disease process, the family does have a right to know what to expect. Similarly, the genetic counselor should discuss with the family members the problem of blaming someone in the family for passing on the disease and the ways the family can best deal with this problem.

On occasion, the genetic counselor may be privileged with potentially damaging information, such as laboratory results that clearly dispute paternity. In this case, the counselor must weigh truthfulness against family solidarity and survival. To divulge the truth in this instance may not be appropriate.

Timing

Timing is an important aspect of the counseling process. When should genetic counseling be initiated? Preferably, counseling should be *prospective*—before the birth of an affected child. Increasing numbers of young couples who are contemplating childbearing are seeking genetic counseling to discover their risk of having children with an abnormality or genetic disease. However, many genetic diseases do not present themselves until after an affected child is born. Genetic counseling in this case is *retrospective.*

In retrospective genetic counseling, time is a crucial factor. One cannot expect a family who has just learned that a child has a birth defect or has Down's syndrome to assimilate any information concerning future risks. However, neither should the couple be "put off" from counseling for too long a period, only to find that they have borne another affected child. Here the nurse can be instrumental in directing the parents into counseling at the appropriate time. At the birth of an affected child, the nurse can inform the parents that genetic counseling is available before they attempt having another child. Often, asking the genetic counselor to introduce himself to the family is enough to introduce the subject of genetic counseling. When the parents have begun to recover from the initial shock of bearing a child with an abnormality or when they begin to contemplate having more children, the nurse can persuade the couple to seek counseling.

Follow-up Counseling

Perhaps one of the most important and crucial aspects of genetic counseling in which the nurse can and should be involved is follow-up counseling. The nurse who has the appropriate knowledge in genetics is in an ideal position to help families review what has been discussed during the counseling sessions and to answer any additional questions they might have. As the family returns to the daily aspects of living, the nurse's extensive background in family dynamics will enable her to assist the family in making adjustments to living with and caring for a child with a handicap. The nurse can provide helpful information on the day-to-day aspects of caring for the child, can answer questions as they arise, can support the parents in their decisions, and can act as a resource for the family to other health and community agencies.

If the couple is considering having more children or if siblings want information concerning their affected brother or sister, the nurse should recommend that the family return for another follow-up visit with the genetic counselor. At this time, appropriate options can again be defined and discussed, and any new information available can be given to the family.

SUMMARY

Throughout the genetic counseling process, the nurse can provide the vital link between the genetic counseling team and those families at risk. With the appropriate knowledge base, the nurse can be involved in case finding, referral, and preparation of the family for counseling. She can serve as a liaison during the counseling sessions and as a resource person after the counseling sessions have been completed. Thus, it has become imperative that professional nurses have a sound background in the principles of genetics and genetic counseling to provide families with the benefits of this exciting aspect of preventive health care.

SUGGESTED ACTIVITIES

1. Obtain input from your family and develop a family pedigree.
2. Carry out a role-playing situation in which you must provide genetic counseling to a family whose only child was born with a bilateral cleft lip and palate.

REFERENCES

Burns, G. 1976. *The science of genetics: an introduction to heredity.* 2nd ed. New York: The Macmillan Co.

Henry, G. P., and Robinson, A. 1978. Prenatal genetic diagnosis. *Clin. Obstet. Gynecol.* 21:329.

Lubs, H. A., and Lubs, M. L. 1975. Genetic disorders. In *Medical complications during pregnancy,* eds. G. N. Burrow and T. S. Ferris. Philadelphia: W. B. Saunders Co.

Lyon, M. F. 1962. Sex chromatin and gene action in mammalian X-chromosome. *Am. J. Hum. Genet.* 14:135.

N.I.C.H.D. 1976. Amniocentesis Registry Symposium, 1975. *J.A.M.A.* 236:1471.

Riccardi, V. M. 1977. *The genetic approach to human disease.* New York: Oxford University Press.

Smith, C. 1973. Implications of antenatal diagnosis. In *Antenatal diagnosis of genetic disease,* ed. A. Emery. Edinburgh: Churchill Livingstone.

Turpin, R., and Lejeune, J. 1969. *Human afflictions and chromosomal aberrations.* (English translation of *Les chromosomes humaines,* 1965.) Elmsford, N.Y.: Pergamon Press, Inc.

U.S. Department of Health, Education, and Welfare. 1976. *What are the facts about genetic disease?* Publication No. (NIH) 76-370. Washington, D.C.: U.S. Government Printing Office.

ADDITIONAL READINGS

Carr, D. H. 1969. Chromosomal abnormalities in clinical medicine. In *Progress in medical genetics,* vol. 6, eds. A. G. Steinberg and A. G. Bearn. New York: Grune & Stratton, Inc.

Carr, D. H. 1971. Chromosomes and abortion. In *Advances in human genetics,* eds. H. Harris and R. Hirschhorn. New York: Plenum Press.

Carter, C. O. 1969. *An ABC of medical genetics.* Boston: Little, Brown & Co.

Carter, C. O. 1969. Genetics of common disorders. *Br. Medi. Bull.* 25:52.

Carter, C. O. 1973. Multifactorial genetic disease. In *Medical Genetics,* eds. V. McKusick and R. Claiborne. New York: H. P. Publishing Co., Inc.

Elber, E., et al. 1971. Prognosis in newborn infants with X-chromosomal abnormalities. *Pediatrics.* 47:681.

Erbe, R. W. 1976. Current concepts in genetics. *N. Engl. J. Med.* 294:381.

Gordon, H. 1971. Genetic counseling. *J.A.M.A.* 217:1215.

Jacobs, P., et al. 1974. A cytogenetic survey of 11,680 newborn infants. *Ann. Hum. Genet.* 37:359.

Leonard, M., et al. 1974. Early development of children with abnormalities of the sex chromosomes: a prospective study. *Pediatrics.* 54:208.

McKusick, V. A. 1969. *Human genetics.* 2nd ed. Englewood Cliffs, N.J.: Prentice-Hall, Inc.

McKusick, V. A. 1971. *Mendelian inheritance in man.* Baltimore: The Johns Hopkins University Press.

Milunsky, A. 1973. *The prenatal diagnosis of hereditary disorders.* Springfield, Ill.: Charles C Thomas, Publisher.

Milunsky, A., ed. 1975. *The prevention of genetic disease and mental retardation.* Philadelphia: W. B. Saunders Co.

Milunsky, A., and Atkins, L. 1974. Prenatal diagnosis of genetic disorders. *J.A.M.A.* 230:232.

Porter, I. H. 1968. *Heredity and disease.* New York: McGraw-Hill Book Co.

Smith, D. W. 1970. *Recognizable patterns of human malformations.* Philadelphia: W. B. Saunders Co.

Smith, D. W., and Wilson, A. A. 1973. *The child with Down's syndrome.* Philadelphia: W. B. Saunders Co.

Stanbury, J., et al. 1966. *The metabolic basis of inherited disease.* 2nd ed. New York: McGraw-Hill Book Co.

Stern, C. 1973. *Principles of human genetics.* 3rd ed. San Francisco: W. H. Freeman & Company, Publishers.

Stevenson, A. C., et al. 1970. *Genetic counseling.* Philadelphia: J. B. Lippincott Co.

Thompson, J. S., and Thompson, M. W. 1973. *Genetics in medicine.* 2nd ed. Philadelphia: W. B. Saunders Co.

Whaley, L. 1974. *Understanding inherited disorders.* St. Louis: The C. V. Mosby Co.

UNIT III

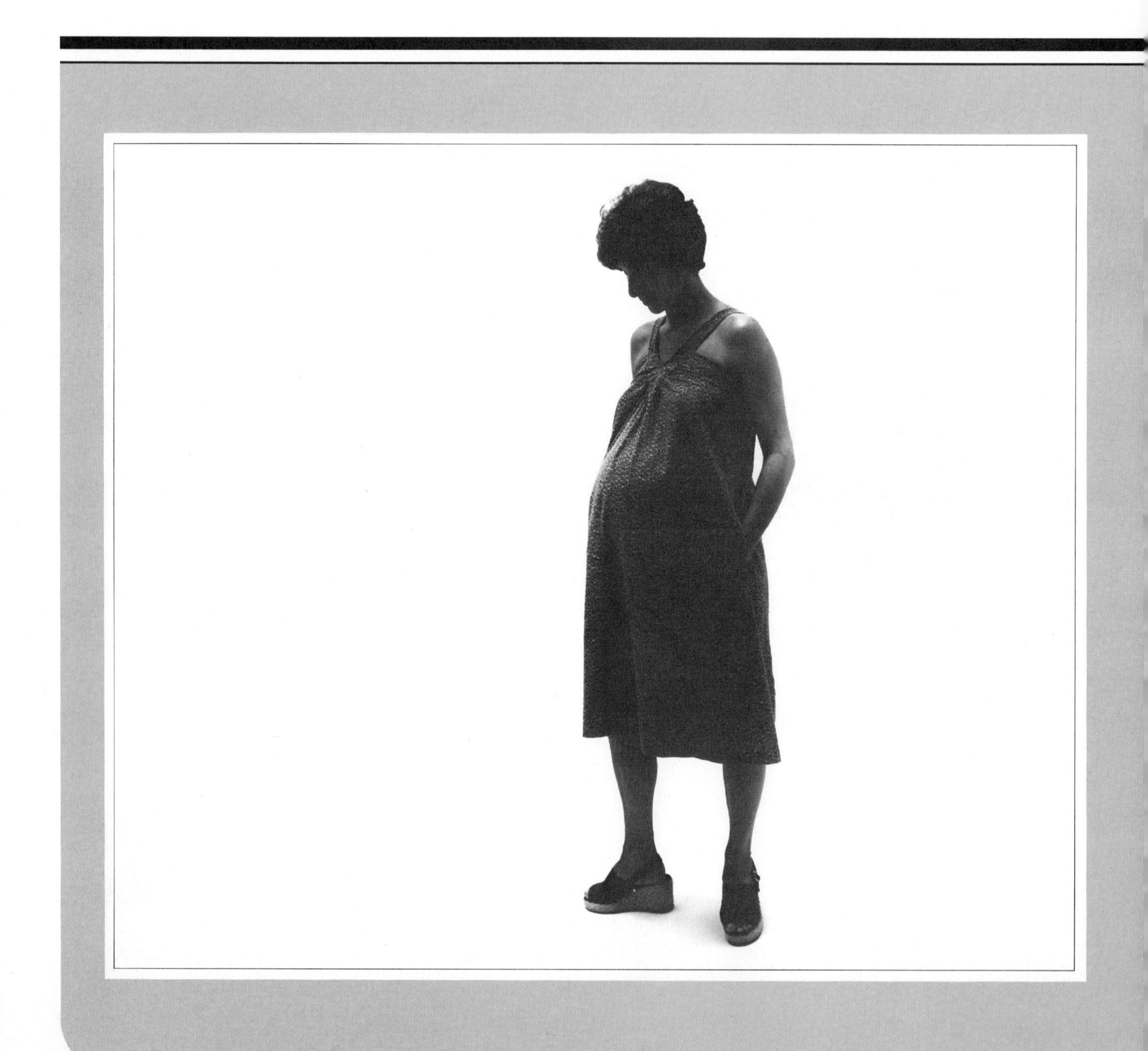

PREGNANCY

CHAPTER 9

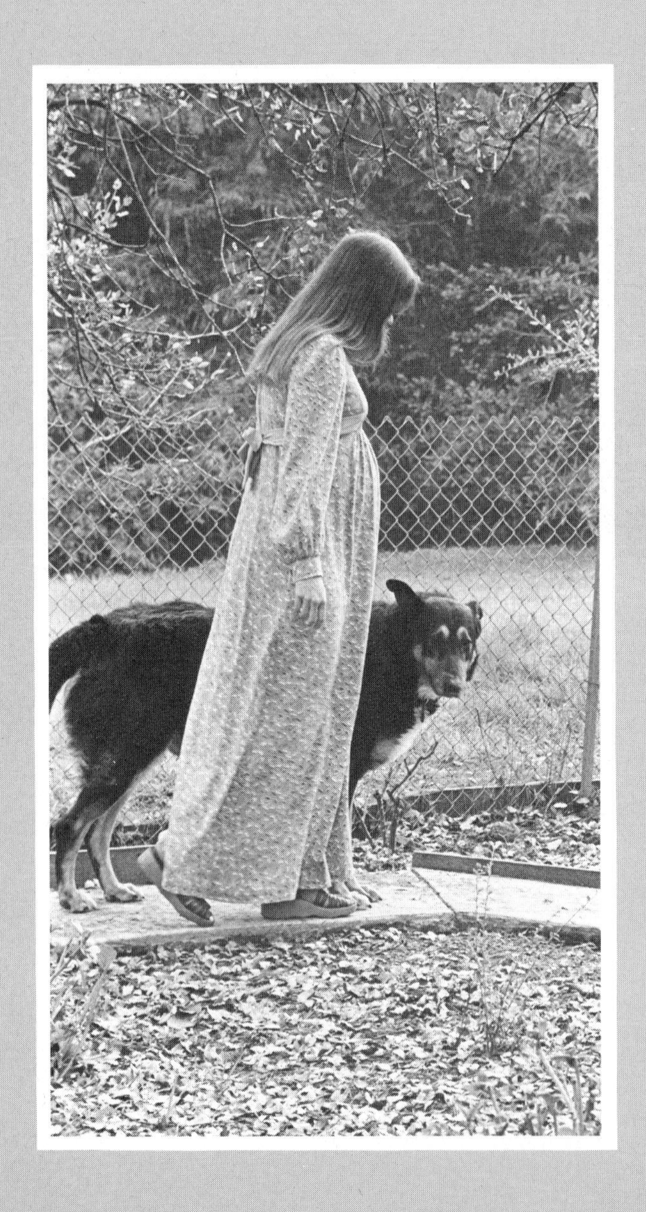

PHYSICAL AND PSYCHOLOGIC CHANGES OF PREGNANCY

OBJECTIVES

- Compare subjective (presumptive) and objective (probable) changes of pregnancy.
- Describe the various types of pregnancy tests that may be used to determine pregnancy.
- List the diagnostic (positive) changes of pregnancy.
- Relate the physiologic changes that occur in the body systems as a result of pregnancy to the signs and symptoms that develop.
- Discuss the emotional and psychologic changes that commonly occur in a woman during pregnancy.

The duration of human pregnancy is 9 calendar months, 10 lunar months, 40 weeks, or 280 days. The dating of a pregnancy is estimated from the first day of the last menstrual period (LMP), making the gestation period about 266 days, with considerable variation possible. Ovulation occurs approximately two weeks before the menstrual period begins. The last menses provides the most specific time for dating a pregnancy, since the times of ovulation and fertilization are usually unknown. The commonly used method for estimating the length of pregnancy is Nägele's rule. (This and other methods to determine the delivery date are discused in Chapter 10.)

Pregnancy is divided into three trimesters, each a three-month period. Each trimester has its own predictable developments, both fetally and maternally.

Generally, the diagnosis of pregnancy is not difficult for the physician. In most cases the woman is fairly certain of the diagnosis when she presents herself for the initial office visit. For a woman with regular menstrual periods, the absence of one or more menses usually confirms the diagnosis. The objective diagnosis is based on the subjective symptoms of the patient and on certain clinical signs, which can be noted on physical examination and through laboratory procedures. Pregnancy causes both obvious and subtle changes involving the psyche and every organ system of the body.

SUBJECTIVE (PRESUMPTIVE) CHANGES

The subjective changes of pregnancy can be caused by other conditions (Table 9–1) and therefore are inconclusive and not diagnostic of pregnancy. The following can be diagnostic clues when other signs and symptoms of pregnancy are also present.

Amenorrhea is the earliest symptom of pregnancy. In a healthy woman whose menstrual cycles are regular, one missed menstrual period leads to the consideration of pregnancy. The missing of successive menstrual periods increases the diagnostic value of this symptom.

Nausea and vomiting are experienced by almost half of all pregnant women during the first three months of pregnancy. The woman may feel merely a distaste for food or may suffer extreme vomiting. These symptoms frequently occur in the early part of the day and disappear within a few hours and hence are commonly referred to as *morning sickness.* Some women may complain of nausea or vomiting in late afternoon and evening, especially in association with fatigue. This gastrointestinal disturbance usually appears about the end of the first month of pregnancy and disappears spontaneously six to eight weeks later, although it may be prolonged in some instances.

Excessive fatigue may be noted within a few weeks after the first missed menstrual period and may persist throughout the first trimester.

Urinary frequency is experienced during the first trimester. In the early weeks of pregnancy, the enlarging uterus is still a pelvic organ and exerts pressure on the bladder, causing frequent micturition. This symptom decreases during the second trimester, when the uterus is an abdominal organ, but reappears during the third trimester when the presenting part descends into the pelvis.

Changes in the breasts are frequently noted in early pregnancy. Some women report significant breast changes prior to missing their first menses. Engorgement of the breasts due to growth of the secretory ductal system results in the subjective symptoms of tenderness and tingling, especially of the nipple area. Some women may report increased pigmentation of the areola and nipple and changes in Montgomery's glands.

Quickening, or the mother's perception of fetal movement, occurs about the 18th to 20th week after the last menstrual period. Quickening is a fluttering-type sensation in the abdomen that gradually increases in intensity and frequency. As with all the other symptoms of pregnancy, it can be simulated by other conditions.

OBJECTIVE (PROBABLE) CHANGES

The objective changes that occur in pregnancy are more diagnostic than the subjective symptoms. However, their presence does not offer a differential diagnosis of pregnancy.

Changes in the pelvic organs are the only physical signs detectable within the first three months of pregnancy and are caused by increased vascular congestion. These changes are noted on pelvic examination. There is a softening of the cervix, referred to as *Goodell's sign. Chadwick's sign* is the deep red to purple or bluish coloration of the mucous membranes of the cervix, vagina, and vulva due to increased vasocongestion of the pelvic vessels. (Some sources may consider Chadwick's sign a presumptive sign.) *Hegar's sign* is a softening of the isthmus of the uterus, the area between the cervix and the body of the uterus. This area may become so soft that on a bimanual exam there seems to be nothing between the cervix and the body of the uterus (Figure 9-1). *Ladin's sign* is a soft spot anteriorly in the middle of the uterus near the junction of the body of the uterus and cervix (Figure 9-2,*A*). *McDonald's sign* is an ease in flexing of the fundus on the cervix.

The uterus asumes an irregular globular shape during the early months of pregnancy. Irregular softening and enlargement at the site of implantation, known as *Braun von Fernwald's sign,* occurs about the 5th week (Figure 9-2,*B*). Occasionally an almost tumorlike, asymmetrical enlargement occurs, called *Piskacek's sign* (Figure 9-2,*C*). Generalized enlargement and softening of the body of the uterus are present after the 8th week of pregnancy. The fundus of the uterus is palpable just above the symphysis pubis at 8-10 weeks' gestation and at the level of the umbilicus at 20-22 weeks' gestation (Figure 9-3).

Enlargement of the abdomen during the childbearing years is usually regarded as evidence of pregnancy, especially if the enlargement is progressive and is accompanied by a continuing amenorrhea. However, since obesity or a pelvic tumor can also cause such an enlargement, this change cannot be relied on exclusively as a diagnostic sign.

Braxton Hicks contractions are painless contractions of the uterus occurring at irregular intervals throughout pregnancy but felt most commonly after the 28th week. They are not a positive sign of pregnancy, since they have been noted in pathologic states also, as in cases of hematometra and pedunculated myomas.

Uterine souffle may be heard when auscultating the abdomen over the uterus. It is a soft blowing sound at the same rate as the maternal pulse and is due to the blood pulsating through the placenta.

Changes in pigmentation of the skin and the *appearance of abdominal striae* are common cutaneous manifestations in pregnancy. The pigmentation of the nipple and areola may darken, especially in the primigravida and the dark-haired individual. The Montgomery tubercles, which are sebaceous glands of the areola, become enlarged. The skin in the midline of the abdomen may develop a

Table 9-1. Differential Diagnosis of Pregnancy

Subjective changes	Possible causes
Amenorrhea	Endocrine factors: early menopause; lactation; thyroid, pituitary, adrenal, ovarian dysfunction Metabolic factors: malnutrition, anemia, climatic changes, diabetes mellitus, degenerative disorders Psychologic factors: emotional shock, fear of pregnancy or venereal disease, intense desire for pregnancy (pseudocyesis) Obliteration of endometrial cavity by infection or curettage Systemic disease (acute or chronic), such as tuberculosis or malignancy
Nausea and vomiting	Gastrointestinal disorders Acute infections such as encephalitis Emotional disorders such as pseudocyesis or anorexia nervosa
Urinary frequency	Urinary tract infection Cystocele Pelvic tumors Urethral diverticula Emotional tension
Breast tenderness	Premenstrual tension Chronic cystic mastitis Pseudocyesis Hyperestrinism
Quickening	Increased peristalsis Flatus ("gas") Abdominal muscle contractions Shifting of abdominal contents

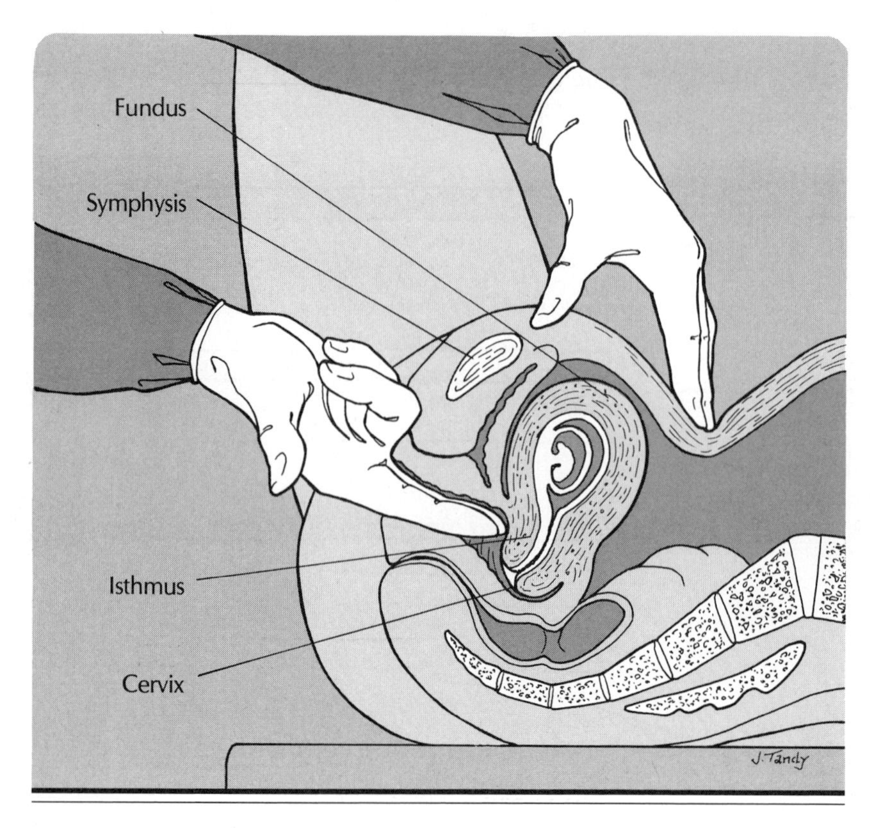

Figure 9–1. Hegar's sign.

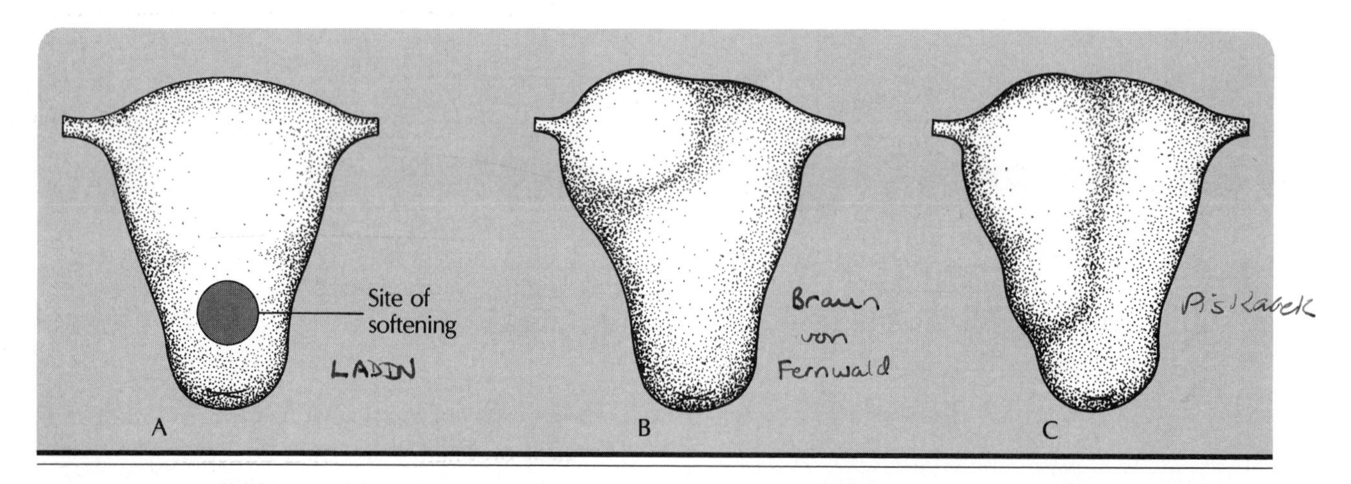

Figure 9–2. Early uterine changes in pregnancy. **A,** Ladin's sign. **B,** Braun von Fernwald's sign. **C,** Piskacek's sign.

pigmented line, known as the *linea nigra,* which may also include the umbilicus and surrounding area. As the uterus enlarges, reddish, irregular, wavy, depressed streaks (striae) appear on the abdomen and buttocks as the underlying connective tissue breaks down. These changes occur in about one-half of all pregnant women.

Facial chloasma (also referred to as "mask of pregnancy"), or darkening of the skin over the forehead and around the eyes, occurs in varying degrees in pregnant women after the 16th week. This condition is aggravated with exposure to the sun. It is hormonally induced and fades after pregnancy.

PREGNANCY TESTS

The endocrine pregnancy tests are divided into two types: the biologic and the immunologic. These tests are based on the presence of HCG in the urine of a pregnant woman (see Chapter 6). Due to the similarity of HCG and the pituitary-secreted luteinizing hormone, these tests cannot be absolute in diagnosing pregnancy. Most tests can be confused by a cross-reaction. Bioassays are subject to false results and require meticulous procedure and several days to obtain results. Consequently, with the development of more reliable immunoassay, HCG tests are being used less frequently.

Biologic Tests

The *Aschheim-Zondek test*, regarded as 98%–99% accurate, is the oldest and most reliable of the biologic tests. The urine of the presumably pregnant woman is injected into an immature female mouse. The mouse is then sacrificed and the ovaries inspected for significant follicular change, which would indicate a pregnancy.

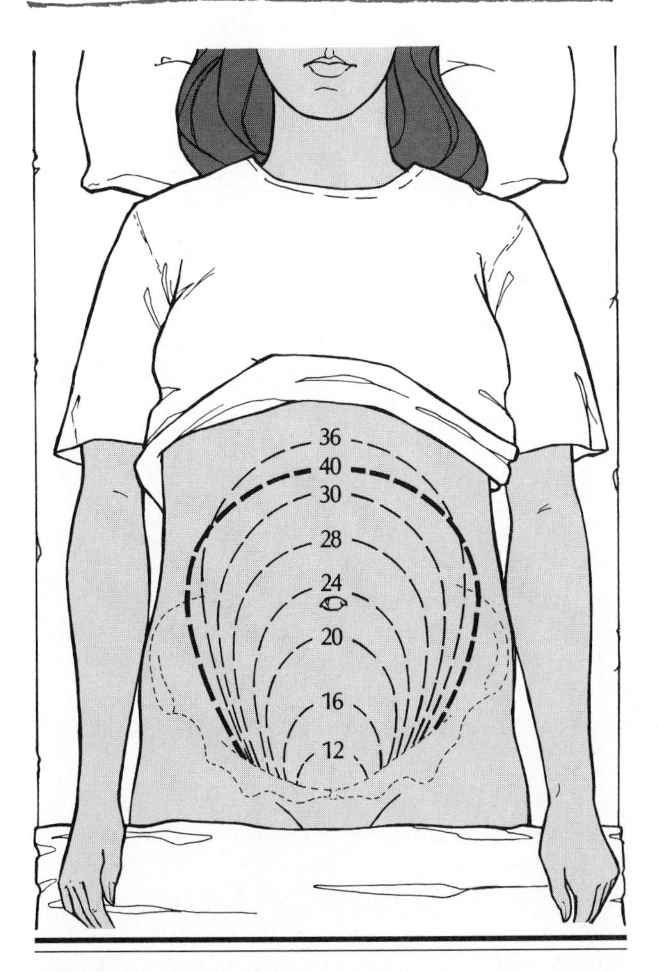

Figure 9–3. Approximate height of fundus at various weeks of pregnancy.

Friedman's test, a modification of the Aschheim-Zondek test, uses a virgin rabbit as the test animal. The test urine is injected into the animal on two successive days, with the animal being sacrificed on the third day. The ovaries are inspected for follicular changes. Friedman's test is approximately 97% accurate.

The *male frog test* is a simple, rapid test based on the ability to induce the emission of spermatozoa by the male frog through injection with the urine of a pregnant woman. The test is positive if spermatozoa are detected in the urine of the frog one-half to three hours after the injection. Hogben

In the *female frog test*, the animal is injected with the urine of the presumed pregnant woman. The test is positive if the frog extrudes ripe eggs within 18 hours of injection.

The *Kupperman* or *rat hyperemic test* is less reliable than other pregnancy tests. A female rat's ovaries are inspected for changes two hours after the injection of the woman's urine. The color changes, from pale pink to pink to dark red, are noted. Since the endpoint of color change is not sharp, a 10% rate of false negatives has been reported.

Immunologic Tests

The immunologic pregnancy tests are chemical urine tests that utilize the antigenic property of HCG. The tests are of two types:

1. *Hemagglutination-inhibition test (pregnosticon R).* No clumping of cells occurs when the urine of a pregnant woman is added to the HCG-sensitized red blood cells of sheep.
2. *Latex agglutination tests (Gravidex and pregnosticon slide test).* Latex particle agglutination is inhibited in the presence of urine containing HCG.

These tests have an accuracy of approximately 95% in the diagnosis of pregnancy and 98% in determining the absence of pregnancy. The tests become positive approximately 10–14 days after the first missed menstrual period. The specimen utilized for the tests is the first early morning midstream urine, free of extraneous protein material such as blood. This voiding is adequately concentrated for accuracy.

The newest development in the area of immunologic tests is the *solid-phase radioimmunoassay*, which utilizes an antiserum with specificity for the β subunit of serum HCG in blood plasma. This radioisotope procedure becomes positive a few days after presumed implantation. Another value of these tests is in diagnosis of ectopic pregnancy and spontaneous abortion and as a diagnostic tool prior to surgery, x-rays, or the administration of medication that may be harmful to the developing fetus.

False results may be obtained with any of the immunologic pregnancy tests if they are utilized too early in pregnancy, when the concentration of HCG is not sufficiently high to render the test positive.

Over-the-counter pregnancy test kits are available at the local pharmacy or grocery store. It is felt by some physicians and nurses that there is a problem (false negatives) with these tests due to lack of counseling and physical assessment that accompany pregnancy testing in the clinic setting.

DIAGNOSTIC (POSITIVE) CHANGES

The positive signs of pregnancy are completely objective, cannot be confused with pathologic states, and offer conclusive proof of pregnancy, but they are usually not present until after the fourth month of pregnancy (Table 9–2).

The *fetal heartbeat* can be detected and counted by approximately the 20th week of pregnancy. With the electronic Doppler device, it is possible to detect the fetal heartbeat as early as the 12th week of pregnancy. The fetal heart rate is between 120 and 160 beats/min and must be counted and compared with the maternal pulse for differentiation. Auscultation of the abdomen may reveal sounds other than that of the fetal heart. The maternal pulse, emanating from the abdominal aorta, may be unusually loud. The uterine souffle, a low blowing sound synchronous with the maternal pulse, is produced by the passage of blood through the dilated uterine vessels. The funic or umbilical souffle, a sharp whistling sound synchronous with the fetal heartbeat, is caused by blood pulsating through the umbilical arteries.

Fetal movements are actively palpable after about the 18th week of pregnancy. They vary from a faint flutter in the early months to more violent movements late in pregnancy.

The *fetal outline* may be identified by palpation in many pregnant women after the 24th week of gestation, becoming easier as term approaches. X-ray examination, which outlines the fetal skeleton, is not used to diagnose pregnancy because of the possibility of gonadal damage and genetic abnormalities. Identification of the fetal

Table 9–2. Occurrence of Signs and Symptoms of Pregnancy*

Signs and symptoms	Time of appearance (weeks of gestation)
Amenorrhea	2
Breast symptoms	3–4
Morning sickness	3–5
Immunologic pregnancy tests	1–6
Bladder symptoms	4–6
Biologic pregnancy tests	
Aschheim-Zondek	2
Friedman's	2–5
Rat hyperemia	5–6
Male frog	5–6
Female frog	6
Ladin's sign	6
Braxton Hicks contractions	6
Chadwick's sign	6
Braun von Fernwald's sign	6–8
Hegar's sign	8
Quickening	16
Abdominal enlargement	16
Palpation of fetal parts	16
X-ray demonstration of fetal parts	16
Fetal heart sounds	16
Palpation of active fetal movements	20–24

*Modified from Danforth, D.N., ed. 1971. *Textbook of obstetrics and gynecology.* 2nd ed. New York: Harper & Row Publishers, Inc., p. 275.

outline is usually not possible until after the fourth month of pregnancy and depends on a variety of factors, such as the thickness of the abdominal wall and the radiologic technique used. Foci of ossification have been demonstrated as early as the 14th week, but a true fetal skeletal outline is not visible until the 16th week of gestation (Pritchard and MacDonald, 1976). X-ray examinations are of special value in determining the death of a fetus or in differentiating a pregnant uterus from an abdominal tumor.

Fetal electrocardiographic evidence has been recorded as early as the 84th day of pregnancy and offers proof of a living fetus. The failure to detect fetal cardiac electrical activity does not exclude an early pregnancy, nor does it necessarily indicate the death of a fetus.

Ultrasonic echosound is a technique that can be utilized as early as the 6th week of pregnancy for a positive diagnosis. A sound wave is passed through the abdominal tissues, where it meets various densities. Each tissue returns a different echo depending on the energy reflected. This echo system is then converted into a two-dimensional picture of the area being examined. The gestational sac can be observed by 5–6 weeks and fetal parts can be seen as early as 10 weeks.

ANATOMY AND PHYSIOLOGY OF PREGNANCY

Reproductive System

The changes in the body during pregnancy are most obvious in the organs of the reproductive system.

Uterus

The changes in the uterus during pregnancy are phenomenal. Before pregnancy, the uterus is a small, semisolid pear-shaped organ measuring approximately 7.5 × 5 × 2.5 cm and weighing about 60 gm (2 oz). At the end of pregnancy the dimensions are approximately 28 × 24 × 21 cm, with an organ weight of approximately 1000 gm (2.2 lb). This growth represents an estimated 500- to 1000-fold increase in capacity.

The enlargement of the uterus is primarily a result of hypertrophy of the preexisting myometrial cells (Figure 9–4). Individual cells have been shown to increase 17 to 40 times their prepregnant size as a result of the stimulating influence of estrogen and the distention caused by the growing fetus. The amount of fibrous tissue between the muscle bands increases markedly, which adds to the strength and elasticity of the muscle wall.

The uterine walls are considerably thicker during the first few months of pregnancy than during the nonpregnant state. The myometrial hypertrophy ceases at about the fifth lunar month and the musculature begins to distend, resulting in a thinning of the muscle wall to a thickness of about 5 mm or less at term. The ease of palpating the fetus through the abdominal wall attests to this thinning.

The circulatory requirements of the uterus increase as the uterus enlarges and the fetus and placenta develop. By the end of pregnancy, one-sixth the total maternal blood volume is contained within the vascular system of the uterus.

The irregular, painless contractions of the uterus, which occur intermittently throughout the menstrual cycle, continue during pregnancy. They are stimulated by increasing amounts of estrogen and increasing distention of the uterus.

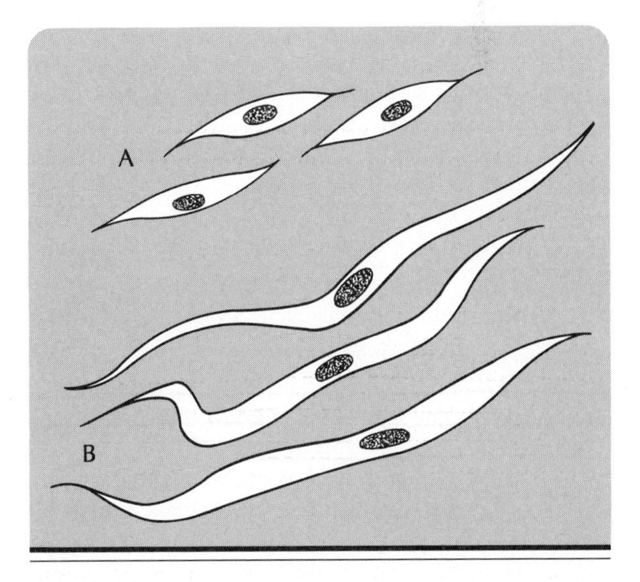

Figure 9–4. Hypertrophy of preexisting myometrial cells. **A,** Prepregnant state. **B,** Pregnant state.

These contractions occur despite the inhibiting effect of progesterone. They may be felt through the abdominal wall beginning about the fourth month of pregnancy. During a contraction, the previously relaxed uterus becomes firm or hard and then returns to its previously relaxed state. Braxton Hicks first called attention to this phenomenon, and the contractions bear his name. Some mothers report that Braxton Hicks contractions late in pregnancy are more uncomfortable than early labor contractions. Multigravidas tend to report greater incidence of Braxton Hicks than do primigravidas.

Cervix

The mucosa of the cervix undergoes marked changes during pregnancy. The glandular tissue becomes hyperactive and proliferates in number as well as in secretions. These increases are estrogen-induced. The endocervical glands occupy about half the mass of the cervix at term, as compared to a small fraction in the nonpregnant state (Figure 9-5). They secrete a thick, tenacious mucus, which accumulates and thickens to form the mucous plug that seals the endocervical canal and prevents the ascent of bacteria or other substances into the uterus. This plug is expelled when cervical dilatation begins. The hyperactive glandular tissue also causes an increase in the normal physiologic mucorrhea, at times resulting in extreme discharge. Increased vascularization causes both softening and the blue-purple discoloration of the cervix (Chadwick's sign). Increased vascularization is a result of hypertrophy and engorgement of the vessels below the growing uterus.

Ovaries

The ovaries cease ovum production during pregnancy. Many follicles temporarily develop but never to the point of maturity, because the appropriate hormonal stimulation is absent. The cells lining these follicles, the thecal cells, become active in hormone production and have been called the *interstitial glands of pregnancy*.

The corpus luteum persists and grows until about the 10th to 12th week of pregnancy. It engulfs approximately a third of the ovary at its peak of hypertrophy. By the middle of pregnancy, it has regressed to almost complete obliteration.

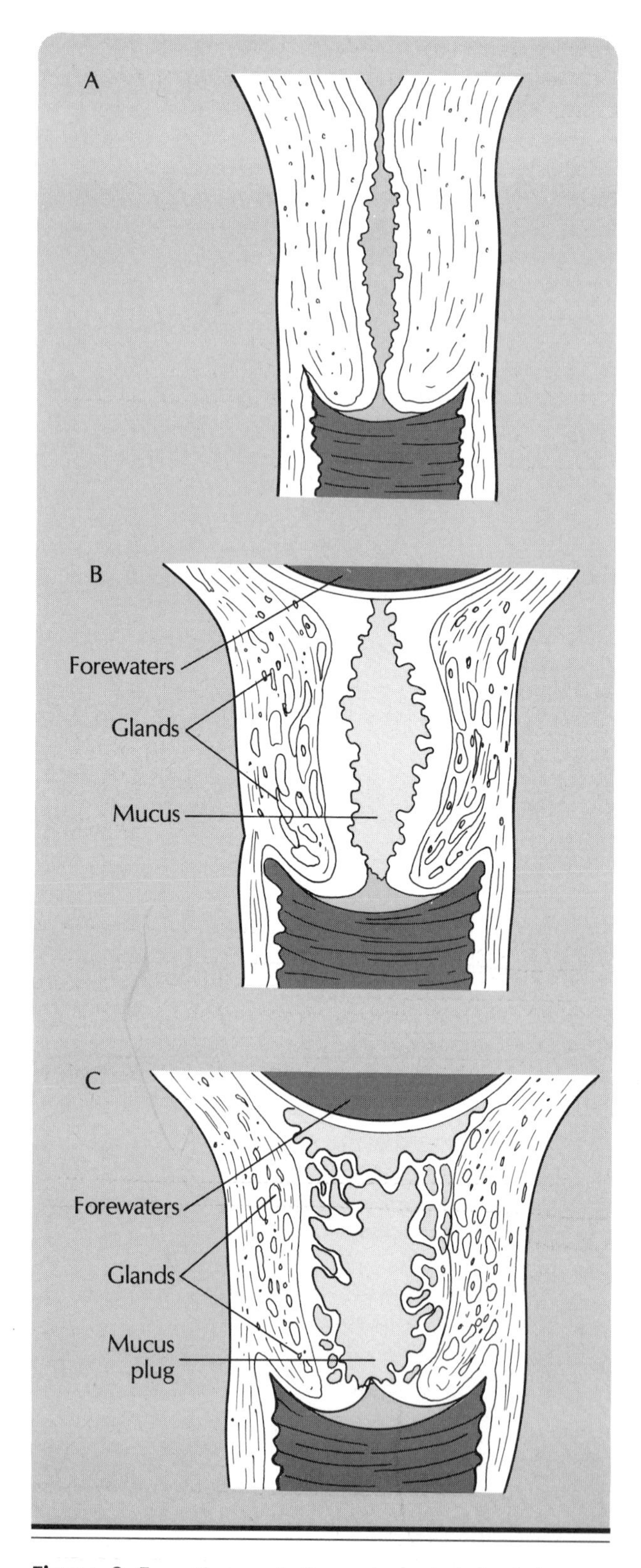

Figure 9-5. Changes in the endocervical glands in pregnancy. **A,** Normal prepregnant cervix. **B,** Cervix at third month of pregnancy. **C,** Cervix at term.

Progesterone secretion by the corpus luteum increases and decreases in relation to its size, maintaining the endometrial bed until adequate progesterone is produced by the placenta to maintain the pregnancy.

Vagina

The vaginal epithelium undergoes hypertrophy and hyperplasia during pregnancy. As with the cervical changes, these changes are estrogen-induced and result in a thickening of mucosa, a loosening of connective tissue, and an increase in vaginal secretions. The secretions are thick, white, and acidic (pH 3.5 to 6). The acid pH plays a significant role in preventing the invasion of pathogenic microorganisms. However, it also favors the growth of yeast organisms, resulting in moniliasis, a common vaginal infection during pregnancy.

As in the uterus, the smooth muscle cells of the vagina become hypertrophied, with an accompanying lessening of the supportive connective tissue. By the end of pregnancy, the vaginal wall and perineal body have become sufficiently relaxed to permit passage of the infant.

The increased vascularization of the uterus and cervix is also observed in the vagina. Within a short time after conception, the characteristic bluish purple color of Chadwick's sign is seen in the vaginal mucosa.

Breasts

Soon after the first menstrual period is missed, estrogen- and progesterone-induced changes are noted in the mammary glands. Increases in breast size and nodularity are the result of glandular hyperplasia and hypertrophy in preparation for lactation. By the end of the second month, superficial veins are prominent, nipples are more erectile, and pigmentation of the areola is more prominent. Hypertrophy of Montgomery's follicles is noted within the primary areola. Striae may develop as the pregnancy progresses. Breast changes are often most noticeable in the primigravida.

Colostrum, a yellow secretion, may be expressed or leaked from the breast during the last trimester of pregnancy. This substance has more protein and minerals but less sugar and fat than mature milk. The antibody-rich colostrum persists for about five to seven days after delivery, gradually undergoing conversion to milk.

Respiratory System

Pulmonary function is modified during pregnancy (Table 9–3). Pregnancy induces a small degree of hyperventilation as the respiratory rate and tidal volume (amount of air breathed with ordinary respiration) increase. There is a resulting 40% rise in the volume of air breathed each minute. Between the 16th and 40th week, oxygen consumption increases by approximately 14%. The vital capacity is not significantly altered with pregnancy. Total lung capacity remains relatively unchanged. Measurements of airway resistance show a decrease with pregnancy.

The diaphragm is elevated and the substernal angle is increased as a result of pressure from the enlarging uterus. This change causes the rib cage to flare, with a decrease in the vertical diameter and increases in the anteroposterior and transverse diameters. The circumference of the chest may increase by as much as 6 cm. There is a change from abdominal to thoracic breathing as pregnancy progresses, and descent of the diaphragm on inspiration becomes less possible.

Nasal "stuffiness" and epistaxis are not uncommon, because of estrogen-induced edema and vascular congestion of the nasal mucosa.

Cardiovascular System

As the growing uterus exerts pressure on the diaphragm, the heart becomes displaced upward and to the left and is lengthened in the longitudinal and transverse diameters. Blood volume progressively increases, beginning late in the first trimester, and peaks in the ninth lunar month at 30%–50% above the pregestational level. Because of this volume increase (hypervolemia), the pregnant woman is able to withstand moderate blood loss at delivery without problems. The pregnant woman also experiences a certain degree of cardiac dilatation because of increased blood volume and retained interstitial fluids. A rise in cardiac output has been demonstrated as early as the end of the first trimester (see Table 9–3).

Frequently, the pulse rate increases during pregnancy, although the amount varies from almost no increase to an increase approaching 20%, or 15 beats/min, at term. The blood pressure remains relatively unaltered, with the lowest levels occurring during the second trimester and the highest levels during the last week of pregnancy.

The femoral venous pressure slowly rises as the uterus exerts increasing pressure on return blood flow. There is an increased tendency toward stagnation of blood in the lower extremities,

Table 9–3. Measurable Pregnancy Changes*

Parameter	Increase (percent)	Decrease (percent)	Unchanged
Respiratory system			
Tidal volume	30–40		
Respiratory rate	X		
Resistance to tracheobronchial tree		36	
Expiratory reserve		40	
Residual volume		40	
Functional residual capacity		25	
Vital capacity			X
Respiratory minute volume	40		
Cardiovascular system			
Heart			
Rate	0–20		
Stroke volume	X		
Cardiac output	30–40		
Blood pressure			X
Peripheral blood flow	600		
Blood volume	48		
Blood constituents			
Leukocytes	70–100		
Fibrinogen	50		
Platelets	33		
Carbon dioxide		25	
Standard bicarbonate		10	
Proteins		15	
Lipids	33		
Phospholipids	30–40		
Cholesterol	100		
Gastrointestinal system			
Cardiac sphincter tone		X	
Acid secretion		X	
Motility		X	
Gallbladder emptying		X	
Urinary tract			
Renal plasma flow	25–50		
Glomerular filtration rate	50		
Ureter tone		X	
Ureteral motility			X
Metabolism			
Nitrogen stores	X		
Sodium stores	X		
Potassium stores	X		
Calcium stores	X		
Oxygen consumption	14		

*From Danforth, D. N., ed. 1971. *Textbook of obstetrics and gynecology.* Harper & Row Publishers, Inc., p. 244.

with a resulting dependent edema and tendency toward varicose vein formation in the legs, vulva, and rectum late in pregnancy. The pregnant woman is more prone to develop postural hypotension because of the increased blood volume in lower extremities.

The erythrocyte count undergoes a slight decline as a result of hemodilution. Although the concentration is lower, the total red blood cell volume actually increases about 33%. The hematocrit decreases by an average of about 7%, but the total amount of hemoglobin increases by an average of 12%–15% above prepregnancy levels. This increase is less than the plasma volume increase, so there is a decrease in hemoglobin concentration, which results in the physiologic anemia of pregnancy (pseudoanemia). Even though the gastrointestinal absorption of iron is moderately increased during pregnancy, it is usually necessary to add supplemental iron to the diet to meet the expanded red blood cell and fetal needs. The recommended daily allowance (RDA) of iron is 18 mg for the adolescent and adult female. This amount is difficult to obtain. In pregnancy the RDA is 18+ mg, and an iron supplement of 30–60 mg may be necessary to ensure adequate iron intake.

Leukocyte production equals or is slightly greater than the increase in blood volume. The average cell count is 10,000 to 11,000/mm^3, with an occasional woman developing a physiologic leukocytosis of 15,000/mm^3. The fibrin level in the blood is increased by as much as 40% at term, and the plasma fibrinogen has been known to increase by as much as 50%. The increased fibrinogen accounts for the nonpathologic rise of the sedimentation rate. The clotting time of the pregnant woman does not differ significantly from that of the nonpregnant woman. The body's physiologic response to reduce risks associated with pregnancy includes: (a) coagulation/fibrinolysis equilibrium, (b) increased blood volume, (c) increased red blood cells, and (d) increased oxygenation of tissues.

Gastrointestinal System

Many of the discomforts of pregnancy are attributed to the changes in the gastrointestinal system (see Table 9–3). Nausea and vomiting, so common during early pregnancy, are associated with the HCG secreted by the nidated ovum and with a change in carbohydrate metabolism that occurs in early pregnancy. Peculiarities of taste and smell are also common and can further aggravate gastrointestinal discomfort. Gum tissue may become softened and may bleed when only mildly traumatized. Oral and gastric secretions are altered with hypersalivation, or ptyalism, sometimes becoming excessive; decreased gastric acidity is the most noteworthy change.

In later months of pregnancy, numerous gastrointestinal symptoms are attributable to the pressure of the growing uterus. Anatomically, the intestines are displaced laterally and posteriorly and the stomach superiorly. Heartburn is caused by the reflux of acidic secretions from the stomach into the lower esophagus. Gastric emptying time and intestinal motility are decreased, leading to frequent complaints of bloating and constipation, which can be aggravated further by smooth muscle relaxation stimulated by the high level of placental progesterone. Hemorrhoids frequently develop in late pregnancy from the pressure on vessels below the level of the uterus.

Only minor liver changes occur with pregnancy. Because of the effects on the liver of high levels of circulating estrogen and progesterone, symptoms of cholestasis and pruritus gravidarum may occur, but they subside after delivery.

The emptying time of the gallbladder is decreased during pregnancy as a result of smooth muscle relaxation from progesterone. Hypercholesterolemia may follow, and it can predispose to gallstone formation.

Urinary Tract

The kidneys, ureters, and bladder undergo striking changes in both structure and function (see Table 9–3). The growing uterus puts pressure on the bladder and bladder irritation is present until the uterus rises out of the pelvis. Near term, when the presenting part engages in the pelvis, pressure is again exerted on the bladder. This pressure can impair the drainage of blood and lymph from the hyperemic bladder, rendering it more susceptible to infection and trauma. The bladder, normally a convex organ, is rendered concave from the external pressure, and its retention capacity is greatly reduced.

Dilatation of the kidney and ureter may occur, most frequently on the right side, above the pelvic brim, due to the lie of the uterus. This dilatation is accompanied by an elongation and curvature of the ureter. There appears to be no single factor accounting for this anatomic variation but rather a combination of ureteral atonia and hypoperistalsis, possibly caused by the placental hormones and by pressure from the enlarging fetus. The same type of hydroureter and bladder relaxation can be produced in the nonpregnant female with massive doses of progesterone.

The glomerular filtration rate and renal plasma flow increase early in pregnancy but return to normal within the month preceding delivery. An increased renal tubular reabsorption rate compensates for the increased glomerular activity. Glycosuria is not uncommon or necessarily pathogenic during pregnancy but is merely a reflection of the kidneys' inability to reabsorb all of the glucose filtered by the glomeruli. However, pregnancy can be diabetogenic, so the possibility of diabetes mellitus cannot be disregarded.

The increased renal function during pregnancy results in an increased clearance of urea and creatinine and in a lowering of the blood urea and nonprotein nitrogen values.

Skin

Changes in skin pigmentation commonly occur during pregnancy, in various areas of the body, stimulated by the hormones of pregnancy. In a fair-complexioned woman the nipple and areolar areas of the breasts darken. The abdominal wall frequently develops striae and the linea nigra. The cervix, vagina, and vulva become darker. Pigmentation of the cheeks, forehead, and nose may also occur. This facial pigmentation is termed *chloasma* and is also referred to as the *mask of pregnancy.* It is more prominent in dark-haired women and is occasionally disfiguring. Fortunately, it fades or at least regresses soon after delivery, when the hormonal influence of pregnancy has stopped. In addition, the sweat and sebaceous glands are frequently hyperactive during pregnancy.

Vascular spider nevi may develop on the chest, neck, face, arms, and legs. They are small bright-red elevations of the skin radiating from a central body. This condition frequently occurs in conjunction with palmar erythema and is of no clinical significance. Both usually disappear shortly after the termination of pregnancy, when there is a decrease in estrogen levels within the tissues.

Skeletal System

There are no demonstrable changes in the teeth of the pregnant woman. No demineralization takes place, and dental caries are the result solely of poor oral hygiene.

With a well-balanced diet, the pregnant woman's calcium and phosphorus requirements of 1.2 gm/day can be met. This is an increase of 0.4 gm over the needs of the nonpregnant body.

The fairly common occurrence of dental caries during pregnancy has led to the myth, "A tooth for every pregnancy." James' research showed that a dog maintained on a calcium-poor diet during pregnancy has a resultant decalcification of its bone but that its teeth show no change (Worthington et al., 1977). The dental caries that often accompany pregnancy are more often caused by a slight decrease in salivary pH and by inadequate oral hygiene and dental care.

The sacroiliac, sacrococcygeal, and pubic joints of the pelvis relax in the later part of the pregnancy. The result is often a waddling gait. A slight separation of the symphysis pubis, possibly the effect of the hormone relaxin, can often be demonstrated on x-ray examination.

As the pregnant woman's center of gravity gradually changes, there is an accentuation of the lumbodorsal spinal curve and a posture change (Figure 9-6). This posture change compensates for the increased weight of the uterus anteriorly and frequently results in low backache.

Metabolism

Most metabolic functions accelerate during pregnancy to support the additional demands of the growing fetus and its support system. The expectant mother must meet her own tissue replacement needs, those of the conceptus, and those preparatory for labor and lactation.

Weight Gain

The average weight gain during a normal pregnancy is 20–25 lb (9–11.25 kg). Weight may decrease slightly during the first trimester due to nausea, vomiting, and food intolerances of early pregnancy. But the lost weight is soon regained, and an average increase of 3, 11, and 11 lb occurs in the first, second, and third trimesters, respectively. The total weight gain may be accounted for

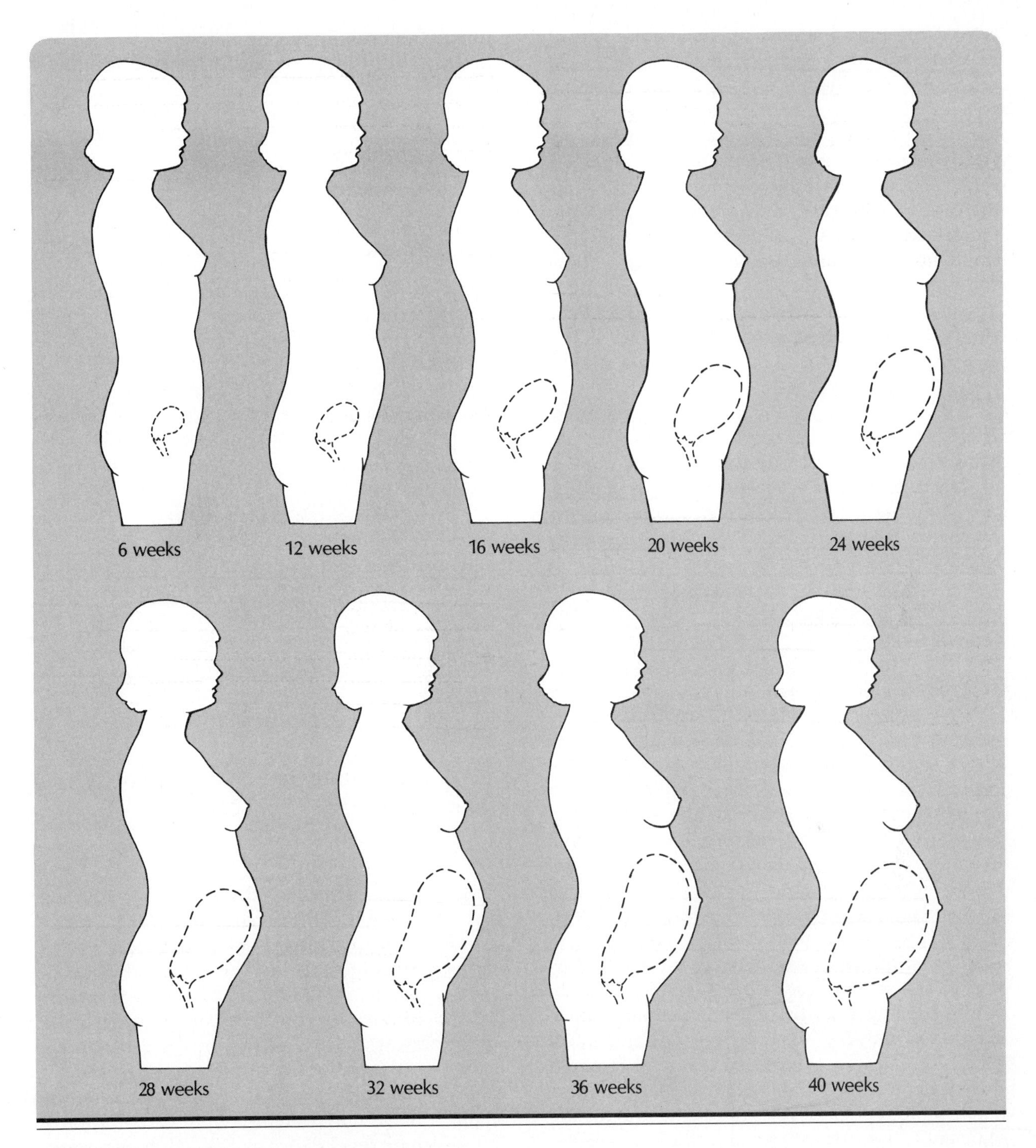

Figure 9-6. Postural changes during pregnancy.

as follows: fetus, 7½ lb; placenta, 1 lb; amniotic fluid, 2 lb; uterus, 2½ lb; breasts, 3 lb; and increased blood volume, 2-4 lb. The remaining 4-9 lb is extravascular fluid and fat.

Water Metabolism

Increased water retention is one of the basic chemical alterations of pregnancy. Several interrelated factors cause this phenomenon. The increased level of steroid sex hormones affects sodium and fluid retention. The lowered serum protein also influences the fluid balance, as does the increased intracapillary pressure and permeability. The products of conception—fetus, placenta, and amniotic fluid—account for an average increase of 3.5 liters of water. Another 3.5-liter increase is contained within the mother's hypertrophied organs and augmented blood volume and interstitial fluids. The extracellular fluid is distributed primarily below the uterus, the area of elevated venous pressure.

Nutrient Metabolism

The fetus makes its greatest protein and fat demands during the last half of gestation; it doubles in weight in the last 6–8 weeks. The increased nitrogen (protein) retention that begins in early pregnancy is initially utilized for hyperplasia and hypertrophy of maternal tissues, such as the uterus and breasts. Amino acid excretion accelerates during pregnancy largely because of the increased glomerular filtration rate. This accounts for the increased protein requirements of pregnancy.

Fats are more completely absorbed during pregnancy, resulting in a marked increase in the serum lipids and lipoproteins and decreased elimination through the bowel. Fat deposits in the fetus increase from about 2% at midpregnancy to almost 12% at term. The excess nitrogen and lipemia are considered to be a preparation for lactation. Nitrogen must be stored during pregnancy to maintain a constant level within the breast milk and to avoid depletion of maternal tissues.

Carbohydrate needs increase, especially during the last two trimesters. Ketosis can be a problem, especially with the diabetic patient, due to glycosuria, reduced alkaline reserves, and lipidemia. Intermittent glycosuria is not uncommon during pregnancy. When it is not accompanied by a rise in blood sugar levels, glycosuria is a physiologic entity secondary to the increased glomerular filtration rate. Fasting blood sugar levels tend to fall slightly to an average of 80–85 mg/100 ml, returning to more normal levels by the sixth postpartal month. The glucose tolerance test undergoes no change with pregnancy.

The possibility of diabetes must not be overlooked during pregnancy. Plasma levels of insulin are increased during pregnancy, and rapid destruction of insulin takes place within the placenta. Insulin production must be increased by the mother, and any marginal pancreatic function becomes apparent. The diabetic patient often experiences increased exogenous insulin demands during pregnancy.

Iron Metabolism

The demand for iron during pregnancy is accelerated, and the pregnant woman must guard against anemia. Iron is necessary for the increase in erythrocytes, hemoglobin, and blood volume, as well as for the increased tissue demands. The decrease in free hydrochloric acid in the stomach limits the amount of available iron from food, and the nausea and vomiting of early pregnancy may lower the ingestion of iron.

Iron transfer takes place at the placenta in only one direction: toward the fetus. It has been demonstrated that approximately five-sixths of the iron stored in the fetal liver has been assimilated during the last trimester of pregnancy. This stored iron in the fetal liver compensates in the first four months of neonatal life for the normal inadequate amounts of iron available in breast milk and non-iron-fortified formulas.

Endocrine System

Thyroid

Pregnancy influences the thyroid gland's size and activity. Often a palpable change is noted, which represents an increase in vascularity and hyperplasia of glandular tissue. The accompanying rise in the amount of iodine in the blood is in the form of thyroxine, with thyroxine-binding capacity increasing as early as the third week of pregnancy and continuing until term. Increased thyroxine-binding capacity is represented by the change in serum protein-bound iodine from a nonpregnant level of 4–8 μg/100 ml to a pregnant level of 6–11 μg/100 ml. The presumable cause is the increase in circulating estrogens; the same situation can be simulated by the exogenous administration of estrogens to the nonpregnant woman.

The basal metabolism rate (BMR) rises to a +25% level in late pregnancy. Blood studies and BMR indicate the existence of hyperthyroidism, but it is not present clinically. Within a few weeks after parturition, all thyroid function is within normal limits. It should be noted that, in the presence of hypothyroidism, spontaneous abortion often occurs.

Parathyroid

The concentration of the hormone secreted by the parathyroids and the size of the glands increase, paralleling the fetal calcium requirements. Parathyroid hormone concentration reaches its highest level between 15 and 35 weeks of gestation, returning to a normal or even subnormal level before parturition.

Pituitary

Enlargement of the pituitary gland is greatest during the last month of gestation, but it returns to normal size after delivery. There is no significant change in the posterior lobe of the gland, although the anterior lobe increases in weight with each successive pregnancy. On rare occasions the enlarged anterior lobe causes pressure on the optic chiasm, resulting in restriction of the visual field. Visual impairment subsides spontaneously postpartally as the gland recedes in size.

Pregnancy is made possible by the anterior pituitary hormones: FSH, which stimulates ova growth, and LH, which affects ovulation. Pituitary stimulation prolongs the corpus luteal phase of the ovary, which maintains the secretory endometrium for development of the pregnancy (see Chapter 6). Two additional pituitary hormones, thyrotropin and adrenotropin, alter maternal metabolism to support the pregnancy. Prolactin, also an anterior pituitary secretion, is responsible for initial lactation. (Continued lactation depends on the suckling of the infant.)

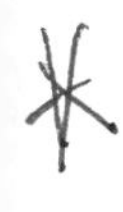

The posterior pituitary contains the mechanism for the release of oxytocin and vasopressin, which exert three physiologic effects: oxytocic, vasopressor, and antidiuretic. The main effects of oxytocin are the promotion of uterine contractility and the stimulation of milk ejection from the breasts. Vasopressin causes vasoconstriction, which results in increased blood pressure; it also has an antidiuretic effect and plays an important role in the regulation of water balance. Vasopressin secretion is controlled by changes in plasma osmolarity and blood volume.

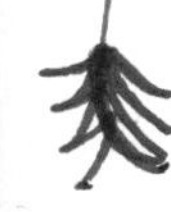

Adrenals

The adrenal cortex hypertrophies during pregnancy in response to the hyperestrogen state. There is an increase in the corticoid secretions, which regulate carbohydrate and protein metabolism. These substances are concentrated in the placenta but are not synthesized by the placenta. A normal level resumes 1–6 weeks postpartum.

Placental Hormones

Human Chorionic Gonadotropin. HCG, the "pregnancy hormone," was first described by Aschheim and Zondek in 1927 (Hellman and Pritchard, 1971). Its presence is the basis for the biologic and immunologic pregnancy tests.

The trophoblastic tissue of the placenta functions as an endocrine gland. Its secretion is detectable in the urine and, more recently, isolated in the serum of a pregnant woman. The detectable hormone levels in the serum and urine show a parallel increase shortly after the onset of pregnancy and a peak near the end of the second month. They then fall to a lower level, which is sustained until near the end of pregnancy. Frequently, no amount is detectable within an hour postpartum. Detectable amounts indicate retained placental tissue, a chorioadenoma, or a choriocarcinoma.

Estrogen. Because estrogen figures in the growth and development of the female reproductive system, it increases during pregnancy. The increase comes mainly from the placenta. As early as the 7th week of pregnancy, 50% of the circulating estrogens are generated by the placenta. Estrogens are not stored within the body; the unused portions are excreted in the urine in the form of estriol. This excretion increases as gestation progresses, being most marked after the 28th week of pregnancy. There is no fall in estrogen levels before labor ensues.

Estrogen levels can be used to determine and monitor fetal well-being, through analysis of a 24-hour urine specimen. The serum analysis is currently being standardized.

Progesterone. Progesterone is the hormone responsible for the preparation of the endometrium for pregnancy and for the maintenance of pregnancy. Progesterone production increases during pregnancy and does not decrease before labor begins.

After implantation, pregnanediol is excreted by the kidneys at a slightly higher rate than during the luteal phase of the menstrual cycle. The excretion rate begins to increase between the second and third months, when the placenta begins progesterone production. There is a progressive rise until the end of pregnancy. After labor and delivery of the placenta, blood and excretion levels of pregnanediol rapidly decline.

EMOTIONAL AND PSYCHOLOGIC CHANGES OF PREGNANCY

Pregnancy is a condition that causes alterations in the internal body milieu, hormonal balance, and external body image, necessitating a reordering of social relationships and changes in roles of family members. Any one of these situations produces stress. In pregnancy, they are present in concert. The way a particular woman meets the stresses of pregnancy is influenced by her emotional makeup, her sociologic and cultural background, and her acceptance or rejection of the pregnancy.

Ambivalence

Initially, even if the pregnancy is planned, there is an element of surprise that conception has indeed occurred. This feeling is generally coupled with a feeling that the timing is wrong, that pregnancy is desirable "some day" but "not now" (Rubin, 1970). The reasons women cite may vary widely—long-term plans, job commitments, financial stress, the needs of another child—but the feeling that one is not ready to have a child at this time remains. This feeling accounts for much of the ambivalence commonly experienced by women during early pregnancy. Ambivalence may also be related to the need to modify personal relationships or career plans, to fear coupled with excitement about assuming a new role, to unresolved emotional conflicts with one's own mother, and to fears about pregnancy, labor, and delivery themselves. Such fears may be even more pronounced in the event of an unplanned or unwanted pregnancy. Ambivalence may be verbalized by the woman or may be expressed as denial or rejection of the pregnancy, as depression, nausea, and vomiting, or in the form of somatic complaints.

During the early months the pregnant woman may seriously consider the possibility of an abortion if the pregnancy is unwanted. In the event of religious conflicts about induced abortion, the woman may experience guilt feelings about her thoughts or may tend to focus on the possibility of spontaneous abortion (miscarriage). Colman and Colman (1971) point out that even when the pregnancy is consciously planned and desired, thoughts of abortion and miscarriage arise. The idea that the baby might be lost has a certain emotional appeal because it represents the possible relief of fears and ambivalence.

Acceptance

During the first trimester, evidence of pregnancy is limited to amenorrhea and to the word of the caregiver that the pregnancy test was positive. In an effort to verify her condition, a woman may become minutely conscious of changes in her body that could validate the pregnancy. She closely watches for thickening of her waist, breast development, and weight increases. Morning sickness, though unpleasant, offers further corroboration. During the first trimester the woman's baby does not seem real to her and she focuses on herself and her pregnancy (Colman and Colman, 1971).

The second trimester is relatively tranquil. Morning sickness generally passes, the threat of spontaneous abortion diminishes, and the woman begins to accept the reality of her pregnancy. It is not unusual for excited primiparas to don maternity clothes at the beginning of this trimester even when it is not truly necessary. They serve as a verification of her pregnant state. During this time some women may seek to give substance to their baby by shopping for a crib or baby clothes, while other women may find they are not yet ready for that degree of preparation and involvement.

The highlight of the second trimester is quickening, which generally occurs about the 20th week—midway through the pregnancy. (With the increased use of the doppler to verify fetal heart tones during the last portion of the first trimester, the woman's acceptance of her baby's existence may occur earlier than it has in the past.) Actual perception of fetal movement frequently produces dramatic changes in the woman. She now perceives her baby as a real person and she generally becomes excited about the pregnancy even if she hasn't been prior to this time.

As quickening and her altered physical appearance confirm her pregnant state, the woman adjusts to the idea of change and begins to prepare for her new role and her new set of relationships—with her husband and family, with the child-to-be and with other children, with friends, and with loved ones. She also takes pleasure in the sensations of pregnancy and attempts to picture her baby in order to know him better. The mother may avidly delve into folklore regarding the child's sex and may carefully study photos of herself and her husband to gain some clues about her child's appearance. She may ask her friends about childbirth and seek out other women who are pregnant or who have recently given birth. She is eager to learn and to share. She feels well, is excited, and may exhibit the "glow" so often attributed to pregnant women.

The third trimester combines a sense of pride with anxiety about what is to come in order for the child to be born. During this time the special prerogatives of pregnancy may be most marked. As her protruding abdomen proclaims her advanced pregnancy, the woman may find that clerks become more solicitous, that a chair may be offered to her in a crowded room, that others may carry her parcels. The woman may actually need this help, she may simply enjoy it as a privilege of pregnancy, or she may reject it if she fears that such gestures indicate she is helpless.

During this final trimester physical discomforts again increase, and adequate rest becomes a necessity. The woman, eager for the pregnancy to end, wonders if her expected date of delivery is accurate. She makes final preparation for the baby and spends long periods selecting names for the child.

Rubin (1970) points out that during this time the woman feels very vulnerable to rejection, loss, or insult. She may worry about a variety of things and hesitate to go out unless accompanied by someone who cares about her. She withdraws into the security and quiet of her home. Toward the end of this period there is often a burst of energy as the woman prepares the "nest" for her expected infant. Many women report bursts of energy in which they vigorously clean and organize their home.

Introversion

Introversion, or turning in on one's self, is a common occurrence in pregnancy. An active, outgoing woman may become less interested in her previous activities and more concerned with her increased need for rest and time alone. This concentration of attention permits the woman to plan, adjust, adapt, build, and draw strength in preparation for her child's birth (Rubin, 1975). As she becomes more aware, she may appear overly sensitive to her husband, who may perceive her introversion and passivity as exclusion of him. He may in turn become unable to interact with his wife, either verbally or physically, and unable to provide the affection, support, and consideration she requires (Stickler et al., 1978). This may result in disequilibrium and stress for the entire family. It is essential that the couple work together to establish new, mutually acceptable patterns of response in order to overcome these blocks to communication (see Chapter 12).

Emotional Lability

Throughout pregnancy the emotions of the woman are characterized by mood swings, from great joy to deep despair. Frequently the woman will become tearful, with little apparent cause. When asked why she is crying, she may find it difficult or impossible to give a reason. This situation is extremely unsettling for the husband, causing him to feel confused and inadequate. Because the husband may feel unable to handle his wife's tears, he often reacts by withdrawing and ignoring the problem. Since the pregnant woman needs increased love and affection, she may perceive her husband as unloving and nonsupportive. Once the couple understand that this behavior is characteristic of pregnancy, it becomes easier for them to deal with it more effectively—although it will be a source of stress to some extent throughout pregnancy.

Body Image

Body image refers to "the picture of our own body which we form in our mind, that is to say, the way in which the body appears to ourselves" (Schilder, 1950). It involves personal attitudes, feelings, and perceptions and may be influenced by environmental, cultural, temporal, physiologic, psychologic, and interpersonal factors. Thus, it is dynamic and everchanging.

Pregnancy produces marked changes in a woman's body, resulting in major alterations in body configuration within a relatively short period of time (Fisher, 1972). These alterations result in a change in the pregnant woman's body image. The degree of this change is related to personality factors and attitudes toward pregnancy (Fawcett, 1978).

In the second trimester, the woman becomes aware that her body is widening and requires more body space. By the third trimester she is very aware of her increased size and may feel ambivalent about the changes that have occurred in her figure (Jessner et al., 1970).

Body boundary is another aspect of body image. It is the "perceived zone of separation between self and non-self" (Fawcett, 1978). When the body boundary is definite, the body is seen as firm, strong, and distinct from its environment. Body boundary vulnerability occurs when the body boundary is perceived as delicate, capable of being penetrated, and not readily distinguishable from its environment. Recent studies suggest that the pregnant woman feels increased body boundary definitions and body boundary vulnerability during pregnancy, which suggests that the woman may perceive her body as vulnerable and yet as a protective container (Fawcett, 1978).

Research has long shown that the husband experiences changed body image and sympathetic symptoms during his wife's pregnancy (see Chapter 12). Fawcett's (1978) findings suggest that "wives and husbands demonstrate statistically similar patterns of change in perceived body space from the eighth month of pregnancy through the twelfth postpartal month." Fawcett suggests that husbands may be more involved in the course of their wives' pregnancies than it appears and that identification plays a role in promoting these changes in body image for the husband.

Changes in body image are normal but can be a cause of real concern to the pregnant woman and may even contribute to the crisis aspect of both pregnancy and parenthood (Russell, 1974). Expectation of the physiologic changes, coupled with discussion of alterations in body image for both wife and husband, may help decrease the stress associated with this aspect of pregnancy.

Changes in a pregnant woman's sexuality also occur and are discussed in Chapter 11.

SUMMARY

Although each pregnancy is unique physiologically and emotionally, certain functional and structural changes are common to all normal pregnancies. Deviations from normal anatomic and physiologic alterations may indicate pathology, and the nurse must be able to detect these abnormalities during prenatal care of the patient so that the nurse can institute appropriate interventions. A basic understanding of physical and psychologic changes of pregnancy forms a foundation from which the nurse can more effectively assess (Chapter 10) and intervene in (Chapters 11 and 13) the health problems of the expectant woman.

SUGGESTED ACTIVITIES

1. Spend time with an obstetrician during prenatal visits at his or her office and observe patients for signs and symptoms of physiologic changes of pregnancy.
2. Ask three friends or relatives about the first indications they had that they were pregnant. If they have more than one child, determine whether the signs were consistent with each pregnancy.

REFERENCES

Colman, A., and Colman, L. 1971. *Pregnancy: the psychological experience.* New York: Herder and Herder, Inc.

Fawcett, J. July–Aug. 1978. Body image and the pregnant couple. *Am. J. Mat. Child Nurs.* 3:227.

Fisher, S. 1972. *The female orgasm: psychology, physiology, fantasy.* New York: Basic Books.

Hellman, L. M., and Pritchard, J. A. 1971. *Williams Obstetrics.* 14th ed. New York: Appleton-Century-Crofts.

Jessner, L., et al. 1970. The development of parental attitudes during pregnancy. In *Parenthood: its psychology and psychopathology,* ed. E. J. Anthony and T. Benedek. Boston: Little, Brown & Co.

Pritchard, J. A., and MacDonald, P. 1976. *Williams obstetrics.* 15th ed. New York: Appleton-Century-Crofts.

Rubin, R. Mar. 1970. Cognitive style in pregnancy. *Am. J. Nurs.* 70:502.

Rubin, R. Fall 1975. Maternal tasks in pregnancy. *MCN.* 4:143.

Russell, C. S. May 1974. Transition to parenthood: problems and gratifications. *J. Marriage Fam.* 36:294.

Schilder, P. 1950. *The image and appearance of the human body.* New York: International Universities Press.

Stickler, J., et al. May–June 1978. Pregnancy: a shared emotional experience. *Am. J. Mat. Child Nurs.* 3:153.

Worthington, B. S., et al. 1977. *Nutrition in pregnancy and lactation.* St. Louis: The C. V. Mosby Co.

ADDITIONAL READINGS

Ascher, B. May–June 1978. Maternal anxiety in pregnancy and fetal homeostasis. *J. Obstet. Gynecol. Neonatal Nurs.* 7:18.

Caplan, G. 1957. Normal emotions in pregnancy. *Briefs.* 21(3):35.

Caplan, G. 1975. Psychological aspects of maternity care. *Am. J. Public Health.* 47:25.

Davis, M. E., and Rubin, R. 1962. *De Lee's obstetrics for nurses.* 17th ed. Philadelphia: W. B. Saunders Co.

Griffith, S. Nov.–Dec. 1976. Pregnancy as an event with crisis potential for marital partners: summary of a study of interpersonal needs. *J. Obstet. Gynecol. Neonatal Nurs.* 5:35.

Kosasa, T. S., et al. 1974. Clinical use of a solid-phase radio-immunoassay specific for human chorionic gonadotropin. *Am. J. Obstet. Gynecol.* 19:6.

Littlefield, V. 1973. Emotional considerations for the pregnant family. In *Maternity nursing today,* ed. T. Clausen et al. New York: McGraw-Hill Book Co.

McLennan, C. E. 1943. Antecubital and femoral venous pressure in normal and toxic pregnancy. *Am. J. Obstet. Gynecol.* 45:568.

Reeder, S. R., et al. 1976. *Maternity nursing.* 13th ed. Philadelphia, J. B. Lippincott Co.

Reigquist, M. A. 1976. Psychologic stress in the last 3 months of pregnancy. In *Current practice in obstetrics and gynecologic nursing,* eds. L. K. McNall and J. T. Galeener. St. Louis: The C. V. Mosby Co.

Taylor, E. S. 1971. *Beck's obstetrical practice.* 9th ed. Baltimore: The Williams & Wilkins Co.

CHAPTER 10

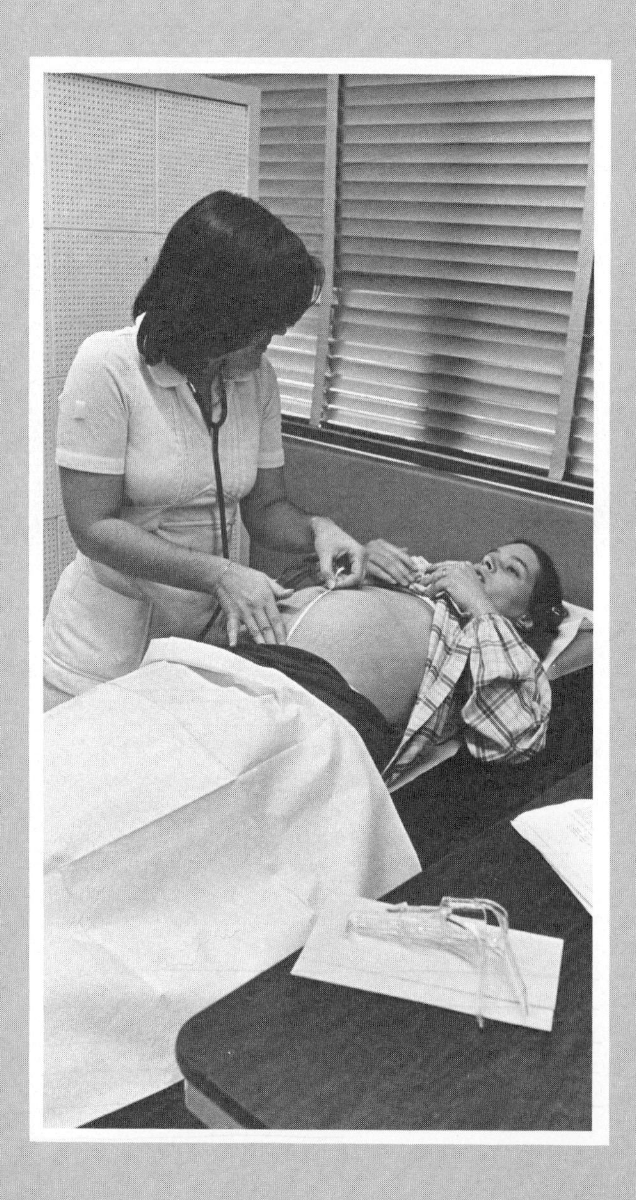

PRENATAL NURSING ASSESSMENT

DETERMINATION OF DELIVERY DATE

Nägele's Rule

Uterine Size

Quickening

Fetal Heartbeat

SUBSEQUENT PHYSICAL ASSESSMENT

SUBSEQUENT PSYCHOLOGIC ASSESSMENT

OBJECTIVES

- Identify the essential components of a prenatal history.
- Explain the common obstetric terminology found in the history of a maternity patient.
- Identify the factors of the father's health that should be recorded on the prenatal record.
- Describe the normal physiologic changes one would expect to find when performing a physical assessment on a pregnant woman.
- Explain how a mother's attitude toward childbearing can affect the course of her pregnancy.

The course of a pregnancy depends on a number of factors, including prepregnancy health of the mother, presence of disease states, emotional status, and past health care. Ideally, medical care before the advent of pregnancy has been adequate, and antenatal care will be a continuation of that established care.

If optimum maternal health is to be maintained, a thorough history and physical examination are essential to identify problem areas. The history and physical examination may be done by a nurse, by a physician, or by both.

PATIENT HISTORY

Definition of Terms

The following terms are used in the obstetric history of maternity patients:

Abortion: Loss of pregnancy before point of viability, usually less than 26 weeks' gestation or weight of 660 gms. As technology improves, the weeks of gestation determining viability become earlier.

Gravida: Any pregnancy, regardless of duration, including present pregnancy.

Multigravida: A woman who is in her second or any subsequent pregnancy.

Multipara: A woman who has given birth to two or more children, alive or dead, who had reached the age of viability.

Nullipara: A woman who has not carried a pregnancy to the point of viability.

Para: Past pregnancies that continued to the point of viability, regardless of whether the infant was dead or alive at birth.

Primigravida: A woman who is pregnant for the first time.

Primipara: A woman who has given birth to her first child, alive or dead, who had reached the age of viability.

The terms *gravida* and *para* refer to pregnancies, not to the fetus.

The following examples illustrate how these terms are applied in clinical situations:

1. Mrs. Smith has one child and is pregnant for the second time. At her initial prenatal visit, the nurse indicates her obstetric history as "gravida II para I ab 0." Mrs. Smith's present pregnancy terminates prematurely at 16 weeks' gestation. She is now "gravida II para I ab I."

2. Mrs. Alexander is pregnant for the fourth time. She has twins at home. She lost one pregnancy at 10 weeks' gestation and delivered another infant stillborn at term. At her prenatal assessment the nurse records Mrs. Alexander's obstetric history as "gravida IV para II ab I." Note that twins are considered as one pregnancy and delivery.

Patient Profile

The history is essentially a screening tool that identifies the factors that may detrimentally affect the course of a pregnancy. Thus, for optimal prenatal care, the following information should be obtained for each maternity patient at the first prenatal assessment:

1. Current pregnancy
   a. Date of last menstrual period
   b. Presence of cramping, bleeding, or spotting since last period
   c. Woman's attitude toward pregnancy (is this pregnancy planned?)
   d. Results of pregnancy tests, if they have been done
2. Past pregnancies
   a. Number of pregnancies
   b. Number of abortions, spontaneous or induced
   c. Number of living children
   d. History of preceding pregnancies—length of pregnancy, complications (antepartal, intrapartal, postpartal), length of labor
   e. Perinatal status of previous children—birth weights, general development, complications, feeding patterns
   f. Prenatal education classes

3. Gynecologic history
   a. Previous infections—vaginal, cervical, venereal
   b. Previous surgery
   c. Age of menarche
   d. Regularity, frequency, and duration of menstrual flow
   e. History of dysmenorrhea
   f. Contraceptive history (if birth control pills were used, did pregnancy immediately follow cessation of pills?)
4. Current medical history
   a. Weight
   b. Any medications presently being taken (including nonprescription medications) or taken since the onset of pregnancy
   c. Alcohol and tobacco intake
   d. Drug allergies
   e. Potential teratogenic insults to this pregnancy (e.g., viral infections, medications, x-ray examinations, surgery)
   f. Presence of disease conditions (e.g., diabetes, hypertension, cardiovascular disease, renal problems)
   g. Record of immunizations (especially rubella)
   h. Presence of any abnormal symptoms
5. Past medical history
   a. Childhood diseases
   b. Past treatment for any disease condition
   c. Surgical procedures
   d. Presence of bleeding disorders or tendencies (has she received blood transfusions?)
6. Family medical history
   a. Presence of diabetes, cardiovascular disease, hypertension, hematologic disorders, preeclampsia-eclampsia
   b. Occurrence of multiple births
   c. History of congenital diseases or deformities
7. Father's history
   a. Presence of genetic conditions or diseases
   b. Age
   c. Significant health problems
   d. Previous or present alcohol intake
   e. Blood type and Rh factor
8. Personal information
   a. Age
   b. Educational level
   c. Previous or present use of drugs, alcohol, and cigarettes
   d. Cultural patterns that could influence pregnancy (e.g., practice of pica)
   e. Acceptance of pregnancy
   f. Race or ethnic group (to identify need for prenatal genetic screening or counseling)
   g. Religion (e.g., Jehovah's Witnesses—refusal of blood transfusions)
   h. Stability of living conditions
   i. Economic level
   j. Housing
   k. Any history of emotional or physical deprivation (herself or children)
   l. History of emotional problems
   m. Support systems
   n. Over- or underutilization of health care system

Obtaining Data

A questionnaire like the one shown in Figure 10-1 is used in many instances to obtain information. The woman should be able to complete the questionnaire in a quiet place with a minimum of distractions.

Further information may be elicited by direct interview. A quiet setting where privacy is assured creates a comfortable environment for the interview process. During the interview, the pregnant woman can expand or clarify her responses to the questionnaire. In addition, the initial interview offers the nurse the opportunity to begin establishing rapport with the pregnant woman. This beginning dialogue sets the stage for a relationship in which the woman feels comfortable asking questions of and expressing concerns to the nurse about her pregnancy, and the nurse can be an active educator/counselor to facilitate the woman's understanding of her pregnancy, its influences on her, and how she influences her health care.

The expectant father should be encouraged to attend the initial and subsequent prenatal assessments. He may be able to contribute information to the history. In addition, the interview process

Name ______________________ Age __________

Address ______________________ Home Telephone __________

What was the last year of schooling completed? __________

How old were you when your menstrual periods started? ______

How many days does a normal period last? __________

How many days are there between periods? __________

Do you have cramping with your periods? yes__no__

Is the pain: minimal ____

moderate ____

severe ____

What was the date of your last normal menstrual period? ______

Have you had bleeding or spotting since your last menstrual period? yes__no__

Have you been on birth control pills? yes__no__

If yes, when did you stop taking them? __________

How many previous pregnancies have you had? __________

How many living children do you have? __________

Have you had any abortions or stillbirths? yes__no__

If yes, how many? __________

Were any of your previous babies born prematurely? yes__no__

List the birth weight of all previous children.

1. __________ 3. __________

2. __________ 4. __________

Did any of your children have problems immediately after birth? yes__no__

If yes, check the problems that occurred:

Respiratory ______ Feeding ______

Jaundice ______ Heart ______

Bleeding ______

Did you have any problems with:

previous pregnancies? yes__no__

If yes, what was the problem? __________

previous labors? yes__no__

If yes, what was the problem? __________

previous postpartal periods: yes__no__

If yes, what was the problem? __________

What is your present weight? __________

Are you presently taking any prescripton or nonprescription drugs? yes__no__

If yes, please list medications:

1. __________ 3. __________

2. __________ 4. __________

Do you smoke? yes__no__

If yes, how many cigarettes per day? __________

How much alcohol do you consume each day? __________

each week? __________

If you have had any of the following diseases, place a check beside it.

____ Chickenpox

____ Mumps

____ Measles (3 day)

____ Measles (2 week)

____ Asthma

____ High blood pressure

____ Heart disease

____ Respiratory disease

____ Kidney disease

____ Frequent bladder infections

If any of the following diseases is present in your family, place a check beside the item.

____ Diabetes

____ Cardiovascular disease

____ High blood pressure

____ Breast cancer

____ Preeclampsia-eclampsia

____ Multiple pregnancies

____ Congenital disorder

The following questions pertain to the father of this child.

What is the father's age? __________

Does he take prescription or nonprescription drugs? yes__no__

If yes, please list the medications:

1. __________ 3. __________

2. __________ 4. __________

What is his alcohol intake each day? __________

each week? __________

Figure 10–1. Sample prenatal questionnaire.

may provide him with the opportunity to ask questions and express concerns that may be of particular importance to him.

Prenatal High-Risk Screening

A valuable part of the prenatal assessment is the screening for high-risk factors. The following outline lists factors that have been associated with increased risk of complications for the mother, fetus, or newborn:

1. Personal factors
   a. Age—less than 16 or more than 35 years old
   b. Parity—primigravida or greater than gravida V
   c. Single parent
   d. Nutrition—weight under 100 or over 200 lb
   e. Use of habit-forming or addicting drugs or alcohol
   f. Smoking—one pack a day or more
   g. Environment—unstable living arrangements, financial instability
   h. Occupation of the mother and father
   i. History of abuse or neglect
   j. Over- or underutilization of medical care system
2. Preexisting medical disorders
   a. Hypertension
   b. Diabetes mellitus
   c. Cardiac disorders
   d. Respiratory conditions
   e. Renal disease
   f. Endocrine dysfunction
   g. Malignancy
   h. Anemia
   i. Positive serology for syphilis
   j. Psychiatric disorders
3. Obstetric factors
   a. Previous pregnancy
      (1) Abortion and/or stillbirth—neonatal morbidity
      (2) Premature labor
      (3) Cesarean section
      (4) Maternal complications—pregnancy, intrapartal (labor), postpartal
   b. Present pregnancy
      (1) Exposure to teratogens—chemical, environmental, radiation
      (2) Vaginal bleeding
      (3) Preeclampsia-eclampsia
      (4) Polyhydramnios or oligohydramnios
      (5) Abnormal presentation
      (6) Multiple gestation
      (7) Intrauterine growth retardation (IUGR)
      (8) Premature labor
      (9) Isoimmune disease
4. Genetic factors
   a. Previous infant with congenital anomalies
   b. Family history of inheritable disorder
   c. Parents who are known carriers of recessive disorders
   d. Consanguinity

Many of these factors can be identified during the initial prenatal assessment; other conditions predisposing to maternal or fetal compromise may be detected by subsequent examinations. The nurse must be aware of these high-risk factors and their implications for the successful termination of a pregnancy. It is important that high-risk pregnancies be identified early so that appropriate interventions can be instituted immediately.

All high-risk factors do not threaten the pregnancy to the same degree. To determine the possible effect of certain variables on the pregnancy, centers that provide prenatal care have devised various scoring tools. These scoring tools can be used to collect data and to identify the woman who needs to be observed more closely during the pregnancy course.

Table 10-1 illustrates one type of scoring tool. It is initiated at the first visit and then becomes a part of the patient's permanent record. Information may be updated throughout the pregnancy as necessary. Each of the listed factors is assessed, and the presence of a factor is assigned the appropriate score. A score of 4 or more points for several factors or 3 or more points for a single factor identifies the pregnancy as high risk.

In addition to scoring the factors listed in Table 10-1, the perinatal health team also needs to evaluate such psychosocial factors as ethnic back-

Table 10–1. Prenatal Assessment of Pregnancy Risk*

Factors			
1 point each	**2 points each**	**3 points each**	**4 points each**
Anemia: 8–10 gm/100 ml hemoglobin	Breech (present pregnancy)	Anemia: under 8 gm/100 ml hemoglobin (24% hematocrit)	Diabetes
Drug abuse and/or alcoholism	Hyperthyroidism	Breech position in primigravida	Hypertension
Height: <62 in.	Multiple births (present pregnancy)	Infertility	Symptomatic cardiac disease
Multiparity and over 40 years old	Three spontaneous abortions	Fetal death	Third trimester bleeding
Primiparity and under 16 years or over 35 years old	Previous abruptio placentae or placenta previa	Estriol deficit	
Parity: 4 or more	Prediabetic (abnormal glucose tolerance test)	Rh isoimmunization	
Previous stillborn or neonatal death		Previous cesarean section	
Previous prematurity		Hydramnios	
Previous toxemia		Liver dysfunction	
Pulmonary disease		Renal disease	
Smoking: 15 cigarettes/day or more		Preeclampsia	
Weight: under 100 lb (45 kg) or over 200 lb (90 kg)		Postmaturity (42 weeks' gestation or more)	

Prenatal assessment	Cumulative points	Noncumulative points (for single factor)
Normal pregnancy	0–2	0–1
Borderline (reassess)	3	2
High risk	4 or more	3 or more

*Modified from Antenatal Evaluation Risk Form. Antenatal Clinic, University of Maryland Hospital, Baltimore, Md.

ground; occupation; education; financial status; environment, including living arrangements and location; and the patient's concept of health and that of her family or significant others, which might influence her attitude toward seeking health care.

INITIAL PHYSICAL ASSESSMENT

After a complete history is obtained, the woman is prepared for a complete physical examination. The physical examination begins with assessment of vital signs, then proceeds to a complete examination of her body. The pelvic examination is performed last.

Before the examination, the woman should provide a clean voided urine specimen. After emptying her bladder, she is asked to disrobe and is given a sheet or some other protective covering. The woman who has emptied her bladder will be more comfortable during the pelvic examination, and the examiner will be able to palpate the abdominal organs more easily.

The physical examination is facilitated when the woman is at ease and comfortable.

Thoroughness and a systematic procedure are the most important considerations when performing a physical assessment. The accompanying Initial Prenatal Physical Assessment Guide may be used by the nurse who is performing the initial prenatal physical examination (see Chapter 9 for a discussion of the diagnosis of pregnancy). The assessment guide has been organized into four columns: the area that is to be assessed, normal findings, deviations and possible causes, and nursing actions for any deviations found. The nurse should be aware that certain organs and systems are assessed concurrently with other systems. Nursing interventions based on assessment of the normal physiologic and psychologic changes associated with pregnancy, and patient teaching and counseling needs that have been mutually agreed upon are discussed in more detail in Chapter 11.

INITIAL PRENATAL PHYSICAL ASSESSMENT GUIDE

Assess	Normal findings	Deviations and possible causes*	Nursing interventions[†]
Vital signs			
Blood pressure (BP)	90-140/60-90	High BP (essential hypertension, renal disease, pregestational hypertension, apprehension or anxiety associated with pregnancy diagnosis or other crises)	BP >150/90 requires immediate consideration. Establish patient's BP. Refer to physician if necessary. Assess patient's knowledge about high BP. Counsel on self and medical management.
Pulse	60-90/min Rate may increase 10 beats/min during pregnancy	Increased pulse rate (excitement or anxiety, cardiac disorders)	Count for one full minute. Note irregularities.
Respiration	16-24/min (or pulse rate divided by 4) Pregnancy may induce a degree of hyperventilation; thoracic breathing predominant	Marked tachypnea or abnormal patterns	Assess for respiratory disease.
Temperature	36.2-37.6C (98-99.6F)	Elevated temperature (infection)	Assess for infection process or disease state if temperature is elevated. Refer to physician.
Weight	Depends on body build	Weight <100 lb or >200 lb Rapid, sudden weight gain (toxemia)	Evaluate need for nutritional counseling. Obtain information on eating habits, cooking practices, foods regularly eaten, income limitations, need for food supplements, pica and other abnormal food habits. Note initial weight to establish baseline for weight gain throughout pregnancy.

*Possible causes of deviations are placed in parentheses.
[†]Nursing interventions are primarily directed toward identified deviations.

INITIAL PRENATAL PHYSICAL ASSESSMENT GUIDE Cont'd

Assess	Normal findings	Deviations and possible causes*	Nursing interventions†
Skin			
Color	Consistent with racial background; pink nail beds	Pallor (anemia) Bronze, yellow (hepatic disease, other causes of jaundice) Bluish, reddish, mottled Dusky appearance or pallor of palms and nail beds in dark-skinned patients (anemia)	Do following laboratory tests: CBC, bilirubin level, urinalysis, and BUN. If abnormal, refer to physician.
Condition	Absence of edema Slight edema of extremities normal during pregnancy	Edema (preeclampsia) Rashes, dermatitis (allergic response)	Refer to physician.
Lesions	Absence of lesions	Ulceration (varicose veins, decreased circulation)	Refer to physician.
	Spider nevi common in pregnancy	Petechiae, multiple bruises, ecchymosis (hemorrhagic disorders)	Evaluate for bleeding or clotting disorder.
	Moles	Change in size or color	Refer to physician.
Texture	Moderately smooth	Dryness, roughness (dry skin)	Evaluate thyroid function.
		Scaliness, broken skin (hypothyroidism, vitamin A deficiency)	Determine usual daily vitamin A intake. Counsel about sources and methods of obtaining necessary vitamin A. If necessary, refer to physician.
Turgor – pinch skin	Skin is elastic and returns to normal shape after pinching	Skin maintains pinched or "tent shape" (dehydration)	Assess for other symptoms of dehydration. Identify ways to control fluid loss and replace necessary fluids. Refer to physician.
Pigmentation	Café-au-lait spots	Six or more (neurologic disorders)	Refer to physician.
	Pigmentation changes of pregnancy include linea nigra, striae gravidarum, chloasma, spider nevi		Assure patient that these are normal manifestations of pregnancy and explain the physiologic basis for the changes.
Hair			
Distribution	Even over entire body	Hirsutism, alopecia (Cushing's syndrome, hypothyroidism)	Assess for presence of other symptoms of Cushing's syndrome and hypothyroidism. Refer to physician.

*Possible causes of deviations are placed in parentheses.
†Nursing interventions are primarily directed toward identified deviations.

INITIAL PRENATAL PHYSICAL ASSESSMENT GUIDE Cont'd

Assess	Normal findings	Deviations and possible causes*	Nursing interventions†
Texture	Consistent with racial background	Brittleness, dryness (hypothyroidism, nutritional deficiency)	Evaluate nutritional status. Initiate appropriate dietary education. Evaluate thyroid function.
Head			
Size, movement, general appearance	Size appropriate to body; symmetrical; easily supported and moves with smooth control; facial symmetry	Lesions (skin disorders); observable vascularity; drooping of musculature (muscle or nerve disorder); edema	Refer to physician. Urinalysis should be performed.
Temporal artery	Able to palpate to temporal artery without discomfort to patient	Bounding, hard nodules; sensitivity to pressure (high or low carotid pressure)	Refer to physician.
Scalp	Normal pattern	Scaliness, excess oiliness Nits or mites (head lice)	Evaluate hygiene. Institute programs to improve hygiene as needed and carry out medical treatment.
		Lumps or tenderness (infection)	Examine for local infection; if none found, refer to physician.
Neck			
Nodes	Small, mobile, nontender nodes	Tender, hard, fixed, or prominent nodes (infection, malignancy)	Examine for local infection. Refer to physician.
Trachea	Trachea should be in midline of neck; larynx, trachea, and thyroid rise with swallowing	Deviation to one side or the other; tension on one side or decreased expansion on one side	Do chest x-ray examination to identify normal or abnormal lung expansion. Refer to physician if deviation present.
Thyroid	Small, smooth lateral lobes palpable on either side of trachea; slight hyperplasia by third month of pregnancy	Enlargement or nodule tenderness (hyperthyroidism)	Listen over thyroid for bruits, which may indicate hyperthyroidism. Question patient about dietary habits (iodine intake), body composure. Ascertain history of thyroid problems. Refer to physician.
Major vessels	Easily palpable, good pulse in carotid	Absence or diminished pulses (cardiovascular disease)	Refer to physician.
	Jugular veins	Not distended, nonpulsable (low cardiac output)	Assess level of distention with patient at 45-degree angle. Refer to physician.

*Possible causes of deviations are placed in parentheses.
†Nursing interventions are primarily directed toward identified deviations.

INITIAL PRENATAL PHYSICAL ASSESSMENT GUIDE Cont'd

Assess	Normal findings	Deviations and possible causes*	Nursing interventions[†]
Eyes			
Near vision	Able to read print at about 18-in. distance	Any deviation from this standard	Refer to physician.
Conjunctiva	Salmon-colored	Pale or infected	Do following lab tests: CBC, bilirubin level.
Sclera	White with a few small blood vessels	Localized and/or general hemorrhage; lesions; jaundice; increased vascularity; excess tearing; thick, purulent discharge; opacity of lens; scars; thick pearllike covering over pupil	Refer to physician.
Eyelids	Smooth; move easily and close completely; when open, expose pupils equally; lashes full from inner to outer canthus; normal blinking	Exophthalmus (hypothyroidism), loss of elasticity, inflammation, purulent discharge, edema, ptosis, loss of lashes, accentuated or diminished blinking, nystagmus	Thyroid function tests (T_3-T_4) should be performed. Refer to physician.
Pupils	Round and equal; respond briskly to light	Constantly constricted or dilated, abnormal in shape, unresponsive to light	Evaluate for associated ptosis and facial muscle weakness. Refer to physician.
Ears			
External auricle	Size, position, and shape within normal limit for head size	Absence, deformity, lesions, swelling, discharge, foreign bodies	Evaluate for associated problems. Refer to physician.
Inner ear—pull pinna and tilt away; use otoscope to examine tympanic membrane; check hearing	Cerumen	Absence, bulging, inflammation, tears	
	Tympanic membrane flat, intact, pearly gray	Exaggerated sound; bulging membrane, reddened membrane (infection); poor perception of sound, no ability to hear	Refer to physician.
Jaw			
Temporomandibular	Smooth, voluntary opening and closing, full range of motion	Partial movement, pain or tenderness, crepitation, dislocation	Refer to physician.
Nose			
Patency and symmetry	Partial or fully open, normal contour	Closure or deformity (deviated septum), inflammation, bleeding, discharge, polyps, swelling, rhinitis, folliculitis	Refer to physician for deformities that are bothersome. Treat inflammation or bleeding.

*Possible causes of deviations are placed in parentheses.
[†]Nursing interventions are primarily directed toward identified deviations.

INITIAL PRENATAL PHYSICAL ASSESSMENT GUIDE Cont'd

Assess	Normal findings	Deviations and possible causes*	Nursing interventions†
Character of mucosa	Pale pink mucosa		
Olfactory ability – ask patient to identify familiar smell (food, perfume); tests adequacy of first cranial nerve	In pregnancy, nasal mucosa is edematous in response to increased estrogen, resulting in nasal stuffiness and nosebleeds		Refer to physician for olfactory loss.
Head movement			
Place hand on jaw and try to return head to midline while patient holds head firmly in lateral position	Able to move head from side to side Resists movement back to midline	Examiner able to return head to midline	Refer for neurologic evaluation.
Ask patient to shrug while examiner tries to prevent shoulders from rising	Equality of strength; able to raise shoulders	Unable to elevate shoulders under added pressure (weakness of sternocleidomastoid and trapezius muscles)	Refer for further neurologic evaluation.
Sinuses			
Palpate frontal and maxillary sinuses	Smooth; normal body temperature	Tenderness; increased temperature; swelling	Assess for other signs of allergy or infection.
Mouth			
Lips	Even border; pink mucous membrane, free of scaling, lesions; symmetrical shape and opening	Broken areas with mucocutaneous junction swelling, lesions	Refer to physician.
Tongue	Full mobility in mouth; pink color Moderate distribution of papillae over entire tongue Papillae moderately rough	Too large or thick; protruding from oral cavity; smooth; fissured, geographically "hairy"	Assess for signs of acromegaly, hypothyroidism, vitamin B_{12} deficiency. Reassure patient that some of these signs appear with age.
Buccal mucosa, palate, pharynx	Pink, unobstructed, moist mucosa; minimal or absent swelling in tonsillar area; hard palate	Canker sore; white, curdy patches Redness of pharynx; enlarged tonsil and uvula; white patches or gray membrane over throat	Refer if bony tumor not along midline. Culture for thrush and treat. Assess for infections. Counsel regarding seeking prompt health supervision for all infections or colds.
		Deviation of uvula plus soft palate fails to rise when patient says "ah" (tenth nerve paralysis)	Refer to physician for further neurologic evaluation.
Gums	May note hypertrophy of gingival papillae because of estrogen	Edema, inflammation (infection); pale (anemia)	Refer to physician.

*Possible causes of deviations are placed in parentheses.
†Nursing interventions are primarily directed toward identified deviations.

INITIAL PRENATAL PHYSICAL ASSESSMENT GUIDE Cont'd

Assess	Normal findings	Deviations and possible causes*	Nursing interventions†
Chest and lungs			
Chest	Symmetrical, elliptical, smaller anteroposterior (A-P) than transverse diameter	Increased A-P diameter, funnel chest, pigeon chest (emphysema; asthma, chronic obstructive pulmonary disease, COPD)	Evaluate for emphysema, asthma, pulmonary disease (COPD).
Ribs	Slope downward from nipple line	More horizontal (COPD) Angular bumps	Evaluate for COPD. Evaluate for fractures. Consult physician.
		Rachitic rosary (vitamin C deficiency)	Consult nutritionist.
	No retraction or bulging of intercostal spaces (ICS) during inspiration or expiration; symmetrical expansion	ICS retractions with inspiration, bulging with expiration; unequal expansion (respiratory disease)	Refer to physician.
	Tactile fremitus	Tachypnea, hyperpnea, Cheyne-Stokes respirations (respiratory disease)	Refer to physician.
Percussion of posterior lungs	Bilateral symmetry in tone	Flatness of percussion, which may be affected by chest wall thickness	Evaluate for pleural effusions, consolidations, or tumor.
	Low-pitched resonance of moderate intensity	High diaphragm (atelectasis or paralysis)	Refer to physician.
Auscultation (see Procedure 10-1)	Upper lobes: bronchovesicular sounds above sternum and scapulas; equal expiratory and inspiratory phases	Abnormal if heard over any other area of chest	Refer to physician.
	Remainder of chest: vesicular breath sounds heard; inspiratory phase longer (3:1)	Rales, rhonchi, wheezes; pleural friction rub; absence of breath sounds; bronchophony, egophony; whispered pectoriloquy	Refer to physician.
Breasts	Supple; symmetry in size and contour; darker pigmentation of nipple and areola; may have supernumerary nipples, usually 5-6 cm below normal nipple line	"Pigskin" or orange-peel appearance; nipple retractions; swelling, hardness (carcinoma); redness, heat, tenderness, cracked or fissured nipple (infection)	Refer to physician. Encourage monthly breast checks. Instruct patient how to examine own breasts (Procedure 10-2).
	Axillary nodes unpalpable or pellet size	Tenderness, enlargement, hard node; may be visible bump (infection)	Refer to physician for evidence of inflammation.

*Possible causes of deviations are placed in parentheses.
†Nursing interventions are primarily directed toward identified deviations.

INITIAL PRENATAL PHYSICAL ASSESSMENT GUIDE Cont'd

Assess	Normal findings	Deviations and possible causes*	Nursing interventions[†]
	Pregnancy changes: 1. Size increase noted primarily in first 20 weeks 2. Become nodular 3. Tingling sensation may be felt during first and third trimester; woman may report feeling of heaviness 4. Pigmentation of nipples and areolas darkens 5. Superficial veins dilate and become more prominent 6. Striae seen in multiparas 7. Tubercles of Montgomery enlarge 8. Colostrum may be present after 12th week 9. Secondary areola appears at 20 weeks, characterized by series of washed-out spots surrounding primary areola 10. Breasts less firm, old striae may be present in multiparas		Discuss normalcy of changes and their meaning with the mother. Teach and/or institute appropriate relief measures (see Chapter 11). Encourage use of supportive brassiere.
Heart (see Procedure 10-3)			
Size and placement	Lies in thoracic cavity within mediastinum; upper border lies behind upper portion of sternum; lower border lies at level of third left costal cartilage close to sternum	Enlargement (cardiac disease)	Refer to physician.
Point of maximal intensity (PMI) or apical pulse	PMI 1-2 cm in diameter and located 7-9 cm left of midsternal point in the fourth or fifth intercostal space	Diffuse PMI located farther than 9 cm left of midsternal point	Refer to physician.
	Thrills not present Palpitation may occur in pregnancy due to sympathetic nervous system disturbance	Thrills, palpable vibrations that resemble a cat's purr, are associated with cardiac defects; thrusting of chest wall felt	Refer to physician.

*Possible causes of deviations are placed in parentheses.
[†]Nursing interventions are primarily directed toward identified deviations.

INITIAL PRENATAL PHYSICAL ASSESSMENT GUIDE Cont'd

Assess	Normal findings	Deviations and possible causes*	Nursing interventions†
Rate and rhythm	Normal rate and rhythm	Gross irregularity or skipped beats	Refer to physician. Twelve lead EKG may be part of cardiac evaluation process to screen for abnormalities of rhythm or electrical conduction.
	Rhythm may vary slightly with respirations	Three heart sounds or gallop rhythm may signal presence of decompensation or carditis	
Sounds	Normal heart sounds	Extra or prolonged sounds may signify valvular disease	
	No murmurs present	Murmur (obstruction to cardiac blood flow)	
Abdomen			
General appearance	Skin clear with exception of whitish silver striae of multiparas	Purple striae (Cushing's syndrome)	Assess for presence of other symptoms of Cushing's syndrome.
	Fine venous network	Dilated veins (vena cava obstruction)	
	Peristalsis may be visible in very thin women	Increased peristaltic waves (intestinal obstruction)	Refer to physician.
	Aortic pulsation may be visible in epigastrium	Increased pulsation (aortic aneurysm)	
	Pubic hair limited to pubic area	Hair distribution extending to umbilicus (bilateral polycystic ovary, Cushing's ovary, ovarian tumor)	
	Umbilicus deeply indented early in pregnancy and more shallow as pregnancy progresses; at end of pregnancy, level with surface or may protrude slightly	Exudate or bleeding from umbilicus (infection, fistula)	Evaluate for infection.
Auscultation	Bowel sounds 5-34/min	Hyperactivity (hyperperistalsis)	Refer to physician.
Palpation	Abdomen nontender and relaxed, especially during expiration	Muscle guarding (anxiety, acute tenderness); tenderness, mass (inflammation, carcinoma)	Refer to physician.
	Diastasis of the rectus muscles late in pregnancy	Excessive separation of muscles	
	Liver nonpalpable	Rebound tenderness (peritoneal inflammation)	

*Possible causes of deviations are placed in parentheses.
†Nursing interventions are primarily directed toward identified deviations.

INITIAL PRENATAL PHYSICAL ASSESSMENT GUIDE Cont'd

Assess	Normal findings	Deviations and possible causes*	Nursing interventions[†]
		Liver palpable below right costal margin, tender and/or nodules (suggest malignancy) Costovertebral angle tenderness (kidney infection or disease)	
	Absence of pain	Pains in any abdominal quadrants; tenderness above inguinal ligaments (salpingitis)	Refer to physician for evaluation of specific cause.
Size	Flat or rotund abdomen Progressive increase in size of uterus due to pregnancy	Bulges (hernia, mass)	
	8-10 weeks: fundus slightly above symphysis pubis 16 weeks: fundus halfway between symphysis and umbilicus 20 weeks: fundus at umbilicus 28 weeks: fundus three finger-breadths above umbilicus 36 weeks: fundus just below ensiform cartilage	Size of uterus inconsistent with length of gestation	Evaluate increase in size using McDonald's method (p. 263). Use ultrasound to establish diagnosis.
Fetal heartbeats	120-160 beats/min May be heard with Doptone at 10-12 weeks' gestation May be heard with fetoscope at 16th week	Failure to hear fetal heartbeat after 16th week	Refer to physician. Administer pregnancy tests. Use ultrasound to establish diagnosis.
Fetal movement	Not felt prior to 20 weeks' gestation by examiner	Failure to feel fetal movements after 20 weeks' gestation	Refer to physician for evaluation of fetal status.
Ballottement	During fourth to fifth month, fetus rises and then rebounds to original position when uterus is tapped sharply	Failure to ascertain ballottement	Refer to physician for evaluation of fetal status.
Extremities			
Arms and hands	Hands warm, may be slightly moist; full range of motion; strong grip; good palpable pulses	Hands cold, stiff, tender; enlargement or deflation of phalanges; deviation of ulna or radius; presence of	Evaluate for other symptoms of vascular disease or arthritis. Refer to physician if these are found

*Possible causes of deviations are placed in parentheses.
[†]Nursing interventions are primarily directed toward identified deviations.

INITIAL PRENATAL PHYSICAL ASSESSMENT GUIDE Cont'd

Assess	Normal findings	Deviations and possible causes*	Nursing interventions†
	In late pregnancy, may have some edema of hands	nodules (arthritis) Marked edema (preeclampsia)	or if data are questionable. Initiate follow-up if patient mentions that her rings feel tight.
Nails	Pink nail beds, nail base angle 160°, nail base firm	Clubbing (hypoxia); spoon nails (iron-deficiency anemia)	Evaluate for anemia or heart disease.
Legs	Toes pink; popliteal, posterior tibial, and dorsalis pedis pulses palpable	Unpalpable or diminished pulses (arterial insufficiency); pallor on elevation, cool temperature, skin atrophic and shiny, ulcerations, brown pigmentation around ankles (venous insufficiency)	Refer to physician.
Musculoskeletal system	Full range of motion	Limitation or deviation of joints	Refer to physician.
		Swollen, tender, hot joints and subcutaneous nodules (rheumatoid arthritis)	Refer to physician.
		Bony enlargement of joints (osteoarthritis)	Refer to physician.
		Knock knees, bowlegs, painful swelling of metatarsophalangeal joint (gout)	Refer to physician.
Spine			
Curvature	Normal spinal curves: concave cervical, convex thoracic, concave lumbar	Abnormal spinal curves: flatness, kyphosis, lordosis	Refer to physician for assessment of cephalopelvic disproportion. May have implications for administration of spinal anesthesia.
	In pregnancy, dorsal and lumbar spinal curve may be accentuated	Backache	See p. 278 for relief measures.
	Shoulders and iliac crests should be even	Uneven shoulders and iliac crests (scoliosis)	Refer to physician.
Vertebras	In straight vertical line	Curvature (kyphosis, scoliosis)	Refer to physician.
	Absence of tenderness	Tenderness lateral to spine on flexion-extension or pressure	
	Able to do straight leg	Back pain (disc disease)	Refer to physician.

*Possible causes of deviations are placed in parentheses.
†Nursing interventions are primarily directed toward identified deviations.

INITIAL PRENATAL PHYSICAL ASSESSMENT GUIDE Cont'd

Assess	Normal findings	Deviations and possible causes*	Nursing interventions†
	raises without back pain		
	During advanced pregnancy, hypermotility of pelvic joints and accentuation of dorsal and lumbar curvature	Separation of symphysis, synchondrosis	
Reflexes	Reflexes normal and symmetrical	Hyperactivity, clonus (toxemia) Asymmetrical, diminished (cerebral or spinal nerve damage)	Evaluate for toxemia and cerebral or spinal nerve damage. (See Chapter 13 for specific nursing interventions.)
Pelvic area (see Procedure 10-4)			
External female genitals	Mons pubis covered with hair in shape of inverted triangle; labia majora symmetrical, not adherent or enlarged; vulva appears pink and moist	Lesions, hematomas, cellulitis, varicosities, urethral caruncle, inflammation of Bartholin's gland	Explain pelvic examination procedure (Procedure 10-4). Encourage patient to minimize her discomfort by relaxing her hips.
	Small clitoris not exceeding 2 cm in length and 1 cm in width	Clitoral hypertrophy (masculinization)	
	In multiparas, labia majora loose and pigmented		
Urinary meatus	Urinary and vaginal orifices visible and appropriately located	Single meatus for urethra and vagina (fistula)	Refer to physician.
		Fistulous opening	Refer to physician.
		Urethral irritation and/or discharge (urethritis, foreign body)	Obtain smear, urinalysis.
	No bulging into vagina when patient strains	Bulging into vagina from upper wall (cystocele)	Refer to physician.
		Bulging into vagina from posterior wall (rectocele)	Refer to physician.
Vagina	Pink or dark pink in color	Grayish white patches (carcinoma)	Refer to physician.
	Vaginal discharge odorless, nonirritating, thin or mucoid, clear or cloudy	Discharge associated with vaginal infections: 1. Monilial infection: thick, white, curdy 2. Trichomonal infection: profuse, watery, gray or green, frothy, with odor 3. Bacterial infection: with odor, gray	Obtain vaginal smear (Figure 10-2). See p. 371 for management of infections. Provide understandable verbal and written instructions to facilitate safe and effective treatment.

*Possible causes of deviations are placed in parentheses.
†Nursing interventions are primarily directed toward identified deviations.

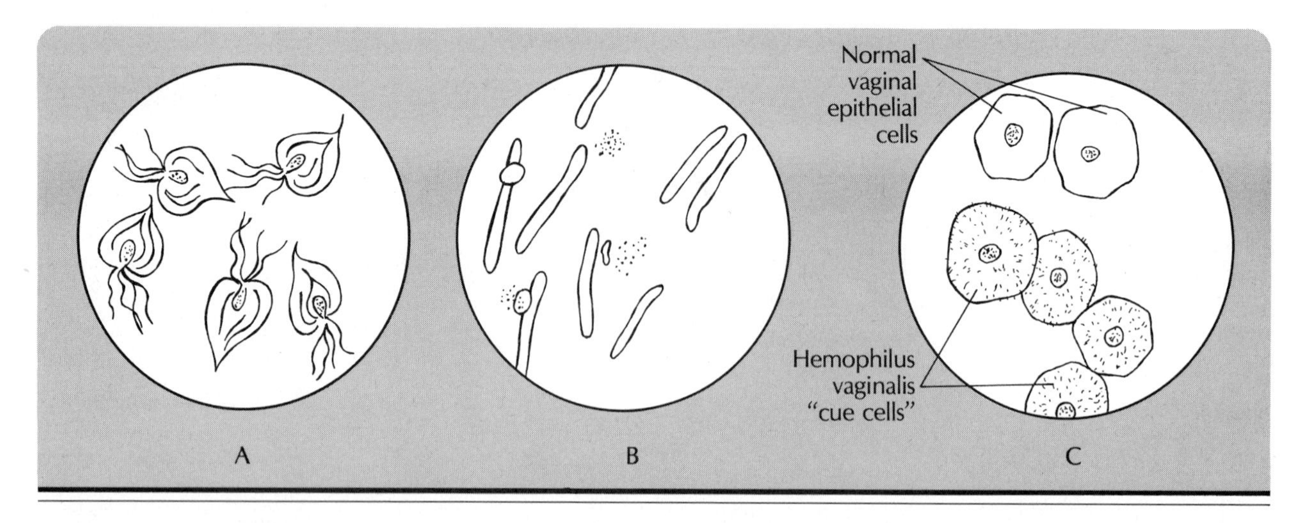

Figure 10–2. Microscopic appearance of microorganisms found in the vagina. **A,** *Trichomonas vaginalis.* **B,** Mycelia and spores seen in *Candida albicans.* **C,** Epithelial cells stippled by *Hemophilus vaginalis* bacteria.

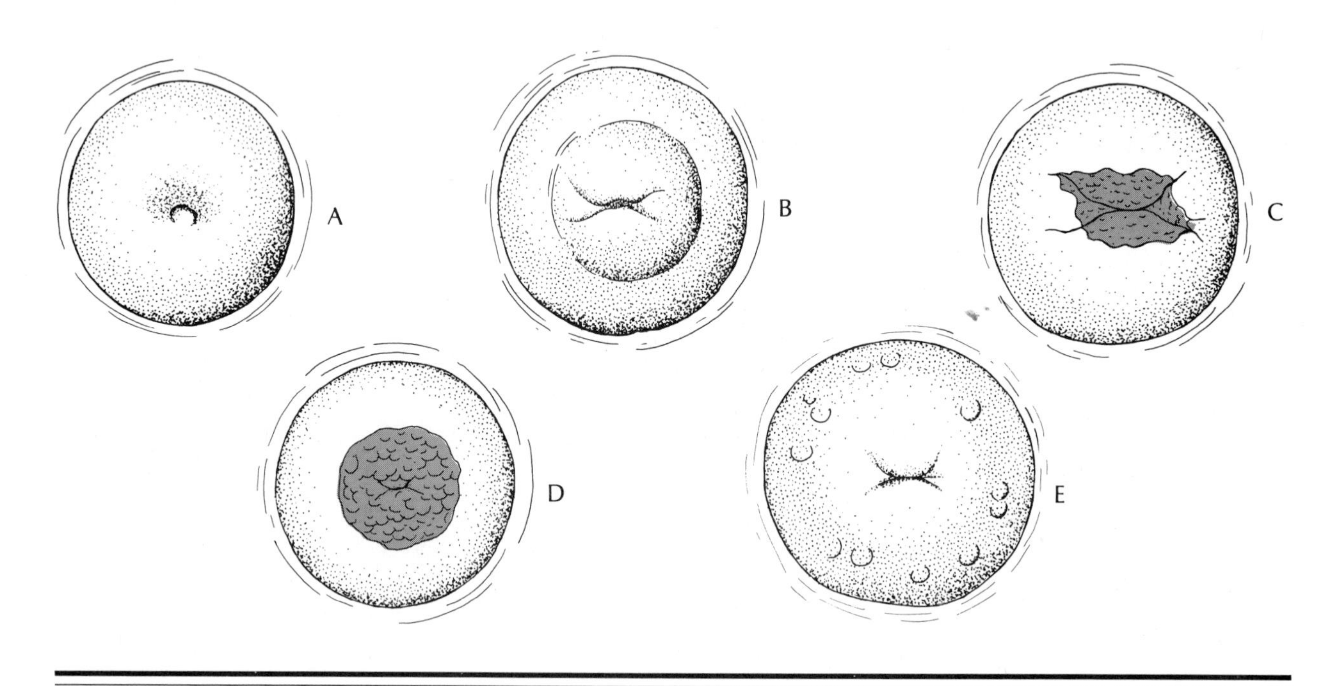

Figure 10–3. Common appearance of cervix on vaginal examination. **A,** Healthy nulliparous cervix. **B,** Lacerated multigravidous cervix. **C,** Everted cervix. **D,** Eroded cervix. **E,** Nabothian cysts.

INITIAL PRENATAL PHYSICAL ASSESSMENT GUIDE Cont'd

Assess	Normal findings	Deviations and possible causes*	Nursing interventions[†]
		4. Gonorrhea: green-yellow discharge, inflamed cervix and vulva	
	In multipara, vaginal folds smooth and flattened, entire vaginal canal widened; may have old episiotomy scar		
Cervix (Figure 10-3)	Pink color; os closed except in multiparas, in whom os admits fingertip	Eversion, reddish erosion, nabothian or retention cysts, cervical polyp, granular area that bleeds (carcinoma of cervix)	Refer to physician.
	Pregnancy changes: 1-4 weeks' gestation: enlargement in anteroposterior diameter 4-6 weeks' gestation: softening of cervix (Goodell's sign) and cervicouterine junction (Ladin's sign); softening of isthmus of uterus (Hegar's sign); cervix takes on bluish coloring (Chadwick's sign) 8 weeks' gestation: uterus globular in shape and anteflexed against bladder	Red spots on and around cervix (trichomonas vaginitis) Vulva inflamed, white patches present on mucosa and cervix (carcinoma) Inability to elicit Goodell's sign (inflammatory conditions and carcinomas)	Refer to physician.
	8-12 weeks' gestation: vagina and cervix appear bluish violet in color (Chadwick's sign)	Presence of string or plastic tip from cervix (IUD in uterus)	Refer to physician.
Uterus	Pear-shaped Located at upper end of vagina	Retroversion, retroflexion Prolapse	Refer to physician. Discuss appropriate individualized exercises and need for rest.
	Mobile within pelvis Smooth surface	Nodular surface (fibromas)	Refer to physician.
Ovaries	Small, walnut-shaped, nontender	Pain on movement of cervix (pelvic inflammatory	Refer to physician.

*Possible causes of deviations are placed in parentheses.
[†]Nursing interventions are primarily directed toward identified deviations.

INITIAL PRENATAL PHYSICAL ASSESSMENT GUIDE Cont'd

Assess	Normal findings	Deviations and possible causes*	Nursing interventions[†]
		disease) Enlarged or nodular ovaries (cyst, tumor, tubal pregnancy)	
Pelvic measurements	Internal measurements:		
	1. Diagonal conjugate 12.5 cm	Measurement below normal	Vaginal delivery may not be possible if deviations are present. Consider possibility of cesarean section. Determine CPD by radiological examination and ultrasound.
	2. Conjugata vera estimated by subtracting 1.5-2 cm from diagonal conjugate	Disproportion of pubic arch	
	3. Inclination of sacrum	Abnormal curvature of sacrum	
	4. Motility of coccyx	Fixed or malposition of coccyx	
	External measurements: intertuberosity diameter >8 cm		
Anus and rectum			
Inspect sacrococcygeal and perianal area	No lumps, rashes, excoriation, tenderness	Rectal prolapse	Refer to physician for further evaluation.
		Nodular lesion (carcinoma)	
	Cervix may be felt through rectal wall	Pilonidal cyst or sinus, anorectal fistula, anal fissure, rectal polyps, internal or external hemorrhoids	Counsel about appropriate relief measures (see Chapter 11).
	Stool negative for obvious or occult blood	Stool positive for blood (intestinal bleeding)	Refer to physician.
	Symmetrical buttocks		
Laboratory evaluation			
Hematologic tests			
Hemoglobin	12-16 gm/100 ml	<12 gm/100 ml (anemia)	Hemoglobin <12 gm/100 ml requires iron supplementation and nutritional counseling.
	Women residing in high altitude may have higher levels of hemoglobin		
ABO and Rh typing	Normal distribution of blood types (Table 10-2)	Rh negative	If Rh negative, check for presence of anti-Rh

*Possible causes of deviations are placed in parentheses.
[†]Nursing interventions are primarily directed toward identified deviations.

INITIAL PRENATAL PHYSICAL ASSESSMENT GUIDE Cont'd

Assess	Normal findings	Deviations and possible causes*	Nursing interventions†
			antibodies. Check partner's blood type. If partner is Rh positive, discuss with patient the need for antibody titers during pregnancy, management during the intrapartal period, and possible candidacy for Rhogam.
Complete blood count (CBC)			
Hematocrit	38%-47%	Anemia or blood dyscrasias	Perform WBC and Schilling differential cell count.
Red blood cells (RBC)	4.2-5.4 million/μl	Presence of infection	
White blood cells (WBC)	4500-11,000/μl		
Differential			
Neutrophils	56%		
Bands	3%		
Eosinophils	2.7%		
Basophils	0.3%		
Lymphocytes	34%		
Monocytes	4%		
Syphilis tests—STS (serologic test for syphilis); complement fixation test; VDRL	Nonreactive	Positive reaction STS tests may have 25%-45% incidence of biologic false positive	Positive results may be confirmed with the FTA-ABS tests (fluorescent treponemal antibody

*Possible causes of deviations are placed in parentheses.
†Nursing interventions are primarily directed toward identified deviations.

Table 10-2. Normal Distribution of Blood Types According to Race (in percent)*

Blood group	Whites	Blacks	American Indians	Orientals
O	45	49	79	40
A	40	27	16	28
B	11	20	4	27
AB	4	4	1	5
Rh-positive	60	72	86	95
Rh-negative	40	28	14	5

*From Miller, W. 1977. *Technical manual of American Association of Blood Banks.* Washington, D.C.: American Association of Blood Banks.

INITIAL PRENATAL PHYSICAL ASSESSMENT GUIDE Cont'd

Assess	Normal findings	Deviations and possible causes*	Nursing interventions†
(Venereal Disease Research Laboratory); flocculation test		results; false results may occur in individuals who have acute viral or bacterial infections, hypersensitivity reactions, recent vaccination, collagen disease, malaria, or tuberculosis	absorption tests). All tests for syphilis give positive results in the secondary stage of the disease; antibiotic tests may cause negative test results.
Gonorrhea culture	Negative	Positive	Refer for treatment.
Urinalysis			
Color	Pale golden yellow color	Orange, red, brown hues (porphyria, hemoglobinuria, urobilinuria, or bilirubinemia, treatment with phenazopyridine)	Assess for deviations. Porphyria may be indicated if urine becomes burgundy red on exposure to light.
Specific gravity	1.015-1.025	<1.015 (renal tubular dysfunction); >1.025 (ADH deficiency)	Refer to physician.
pH	4.6-8.0	Alkaline urine (metabolic alkalemia, *Proteus* infections, old specimen)	
Glucose	Negative (small amount of glycosuria may occur in pregnancy)	Glycosuria (low renal threshold for glucose, diabetes mellitus, Cushing's disease, pheochromocytoma)	Assess blood glucose. Test urine for ketones.
Protein	Negative	Proteinuria (urine specimen contaminated with vaginal secretions, strenuous physical exercise, fever, kidney disease, postrenal infection)	Repeat urinalysis. Instruct patient in collection technique.
Red blood cells	Negative	Blood in urine (calculi, cystitis, glomerulonephritis, neoplasm)	Refer to physician.
White blood cells	Negative	Presence of white blood cells (infection in genitourinary tract)	
Casts	Negative	Presence of casts (nephrotic syndrome)	
Rubella titer	Hemagglutination-inhibition test (HAI) >1:10 indicates patient is immune	HAI titer <1:10	Immunization will be given within six weeks after delivery. Instruct mother whose

*Possible causes of deviations are placed in parentheses.
†Nursing interventions are primarily directed toward identified deviations.

INITIAL PRENATAL PHYSICAL ASSESSMENT GUIDE Cont'd

Assess	Normal findings	Deviations and possible causes*	Nursing interventions†
			titers are <1:10 to avoid children who have rubella.
Antibody screen	Negative	Positive	For positive results, further testing should be done to identify specific antibodies. In addition, antibody titers may be done during pregnancy.
Sickle cell screen for black Americans	Negative	Positive; test results would include a description of cells	Refer to physician.
Papanicolaou (Pap) test	Negative‡	Test results that show atypical cells‡	Refer to physician. Discuss the meaning of the various classes with the woman and importance of follow-up.
Chest x-ray	Clear	Infiltrate (pulmonary lesions, tuberculosis)	Provide lead shield for abdomen while film is taken. Note: Current trend is to avoid x-ray exposure to growing fetus. Chest x-ray is not routinely done. If tuberculosis is suspected, tine test is performed. Chest x-ray examination would be indicated for positive tine test.

*Possible causes of deviations are placed in parentheses.
†Nursing interventions are primarily directed toward identified deviations.
‡The current trend is to report Pap test results as follows:
1. Negative
2. Atypical (this finding would describe the cells)
Some clinicians may still use Class I to Class V terminology, with Class I being negative and Class V cancer in situ.

Procedure 10–1. Auscultation of Chest

Objective	Nursing action	Rationale
Assess quality and intensity of breath sounds	Place diaphragm of the stethoscope on patient's chest and listen for breath sounds. Instruct patient to breathe in and out through her mouth. Note: Be observant for signs of hyperventilation. First listen to apexes or upper lobes of lungs, comparing one side with other.	Vesicular breath sounds can be heard over most of the lung area. Bronchovesicular breath sounds can be heard near main stem bronchi. Bronchial or tubular breath sounds can be heard over trachea.

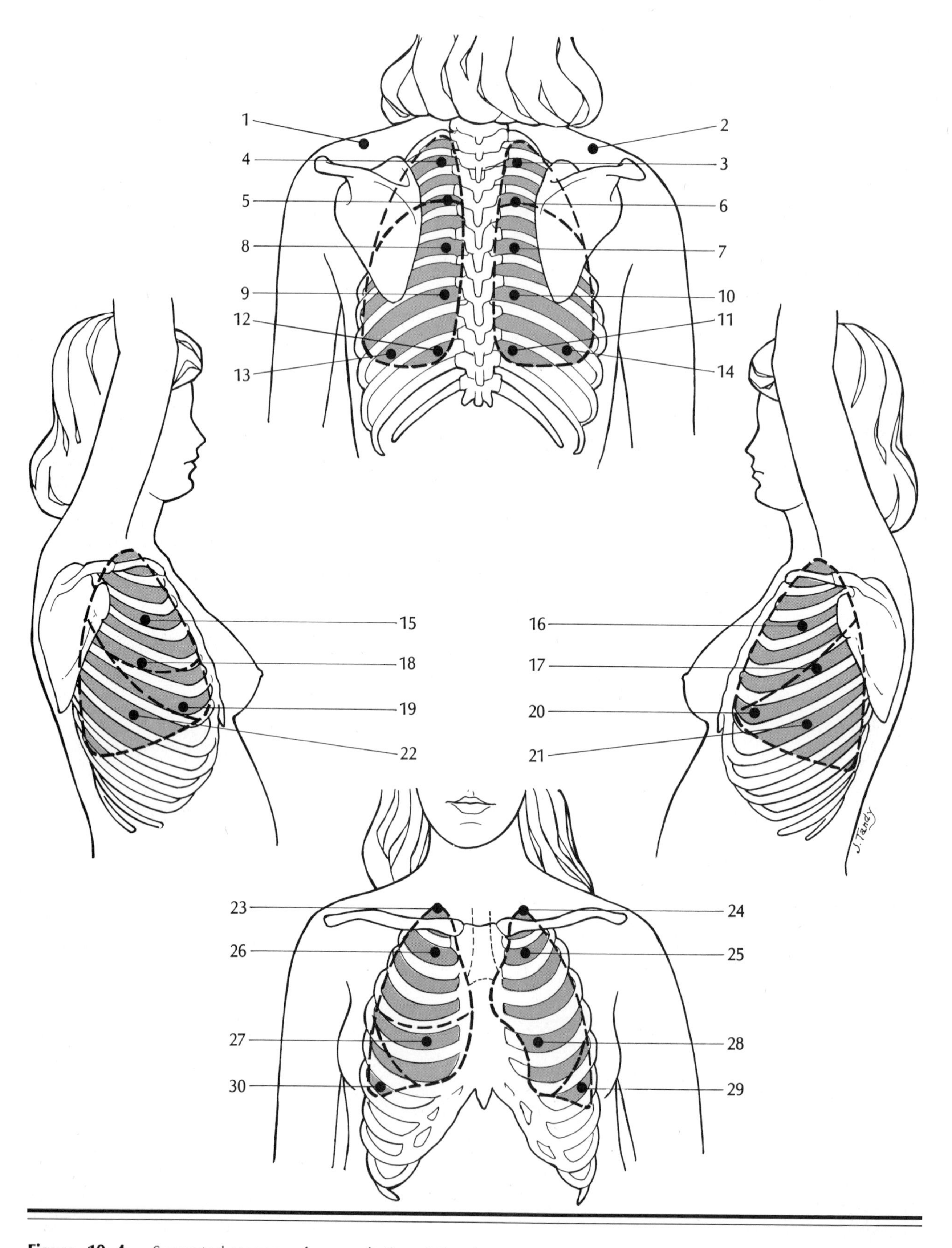

Figure 10–4. Suggested sequence for auscultation of the chest.

Procedure 10–1. Cont'd

Objective	Nursing action	Rationale
	Progress systematically downward from apexes to posterior, lateral, and anterior chest, always comparing both sides. Allow two to three breaths in each area (Figure 10–4).	
	Evaluate sounds as to pitch, intensity, quality, and relative duration of inspiratory and expiratory phases.	Absent or decreased breath sounds can occur in bronchial obstruction, emphysema, or shallow breathing. Increased breath sounds or change in pitch can occur in conditions causing lung tissue consolidation.
	Listen for adventitious or abnormal breath sounds.	Rales are noncontinuous sounds most frequently heard on inspiration. They are produced by moisture in tracheobronchial tree. Rhonchi and wheezes are continuous sounds and may be present on inspiration and expiration. They are produced when air flows across narrowed air passages. Friction rubs are grating or crackling sounds usually heard on inspiration and expiration. They are produced when pleura is inflamed.

Procedure 10–2. Breast Self-Examination

Objective	Nursing action	Rationale
Provide instruction	Instruct patient as follows: 1. Lie down. Put one hand behind your head. With the other hand, fingers flattened, gently feel your breast. Press ever so lightly (Figure 10–5,*A*). Now examine the other breast.	Over 74,000 American women develop breast cancer every year. About half die within five years. Experience shows that 95% of breast cancers are found by women themselves. When women discover lumps in their breasts at a very early stage, surgery can save 70%–80% of proven cancer cases.*
	2. Figure 10–5,*B* shows you how to check each breast. Begin where you see the A and follow the arrows, feeling gently for a lump or thickening. Remember to feel all parts of each breast.	

*From American Cancer Society. 1973. *Breast self-examination and the nurse.* No. 3408 PE.

Procedure 10–2. Breast Self-Examination

Objective	Nursing action	Rationale
	3. Now repeat the same procedure sitting up, with the hand still behind your head (Figure 10–5, *C*).	
	Instruct woman to perform breast self-examination on monthly basis.	Monthly assessment will increase opportunity to identify breast changes. Nonpregnant women should check breasts at end of menstrual period.

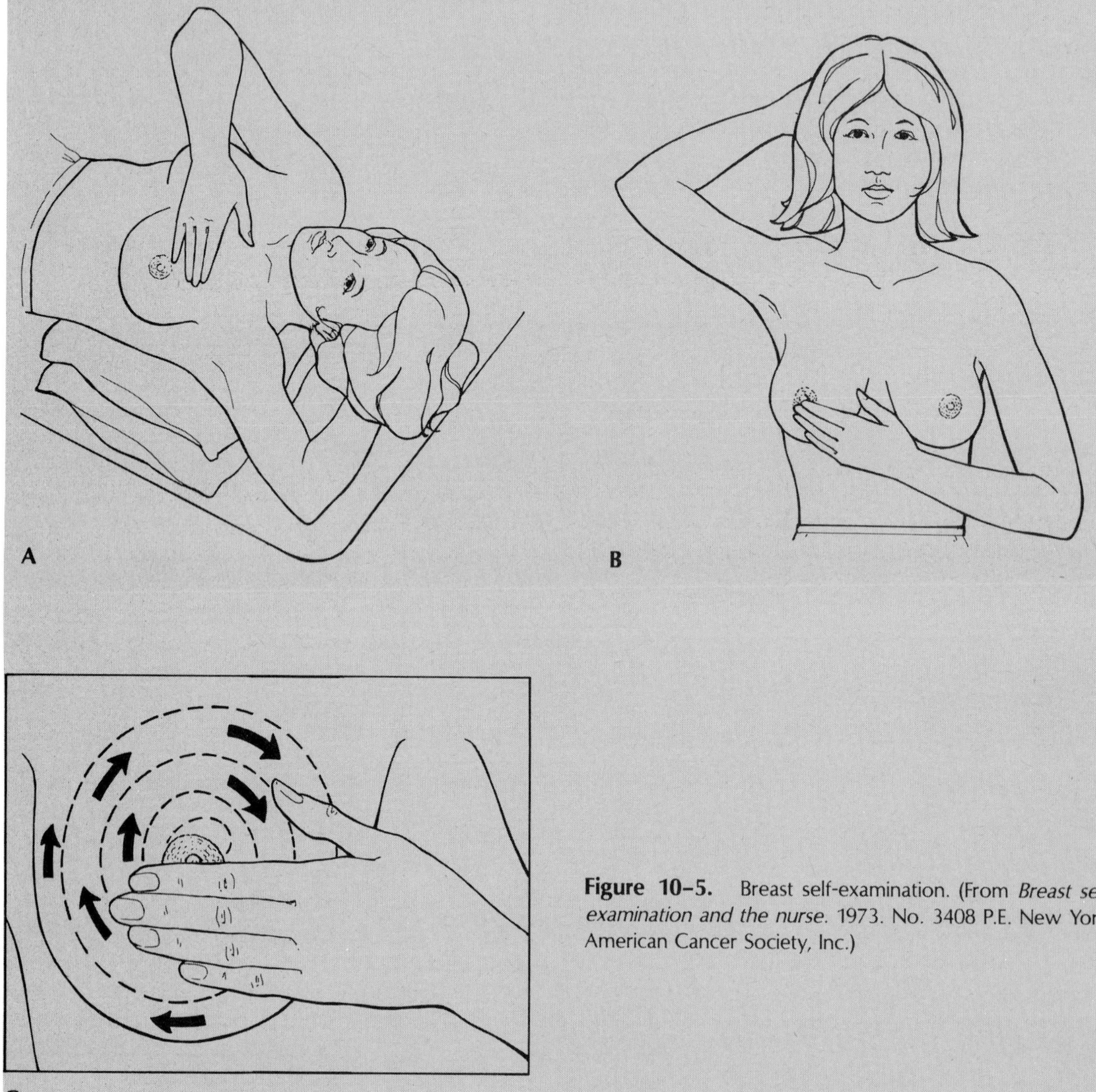

A

B

C

Figure 10–5. Breast self-examination. (From *Breast self-examination and the nurse*. 1973. No. 3408 P.E. New York: American Cancer Society, Inc.)

Procedure 10-3. Cardiac Examination

Objective	Nursing action	Rationale
Provide optimal positioning for assessment	In quiet, comfortably warm room, have patient remove all clothing from upper torso. Place patient in supine semi-Fowler's position with upper body elevated 30-40 degrees. Auscultate during normal respiration, in deep expiration, and when patient is holding her breath. Auscultate in same manner with patient on left side and then with patient sitting up and slightly forward.	Patient privacy is provided. Quiet warm room decreases shivering and subsequent muscular noises. Auscultation with patient in various positions allows detection of normal heart sound, low-frequency diastolic sounds, and high-pitched diastolic murmurs of aortic or pulmonic valve insufficiency.
Assess chest to ascertain heart size and position	Percuss chest.	Determine adequacy of cardiac and respiratory systems (enlargement or displacement of the heart).
Determine the apex beat or PMI	Standing to right of patient, use fingertips and palmar aspect of right hand to palpate first over apex toward axilla and lower rib margin. PMI is usually located at fifth intercostal space, 7-9 cm left of midsternal border, and is 1-2 cm in diameter. Optimal patient position is supine.	Malposition may indicate enlargement or abnormal placement of the heart.
Assess for presence of thrills	Palpate precordium at listening areas of heart.	Thrills are palpable vibrations that resemble cat's purr and are associated with cardiac defects.
Determine rate and rhythm	Auscultate with stethoscope (normal rate 60-100 beats/min). Palpate radial pulse; it should be simultaneous with the apical.	Rhythm may vary slightly with respirations. Deviations are gross irregularities or skipped beats.
Evaluate heart sounds	Auscultate with stethoscope for normal sounds, abnormal sounds, and extra sounds at the four listening areas* (Figure 10-6): 1. Apical or mitral area: midclavicular line at fifth ICS. 2. Tricuspid or xiphoid area: lower left sternal border at fourth ICS. 3. Aortic area: second right ICS at the sternal border. 4. Pulmonic area: second to third left interspace near sternal border. Lightly place bell of stethoscope on chest for low-frequency sounds; firmly place stethoscope diaphragm against chest for high sounds. Listen for frequency (pitch), intensity (loudness), duration, and timing during cardiac cycle.	
	Listen for first heart sound (S_1) at second right or left ICS. Use diaphragm of stethoscope.	S_1 is softer than S_2 in this area. S_1 may sound slightly split. Extra sound in right ICS may signify aortic valvular disease. Extra or prolonged sounds in left ICS space may indicate pulmonic valvular disease.
	Listen at heart apex in fifth left ICS.	S_1 louder than S_2; S_2 may sound split on inspiration.

*The student is referred to a physical examination book for practitioners for more in-depth information.

Procedure 10–3 Cont'd.

Objective	Nursing action	Rationale
	Use bell of stethoscope to listen for extra or abnormal heart sounds.	S_3 immediately follows S_2 and corresponds to syllable rhythm in "Kentucky." Physiologic third heart sound may be present in children. In older patient, third heart sound is pathologic. Fourth heart sound may immediately precede S_1, and heart rhythm is similar to syllable rhythm in "Tennessee."
	Listen for presence of murmurs. Determine location, timing, and duration.	Harsh blowing or rumbling sounds may radiate along flow of blood downstream from source and may be of continuous duration.

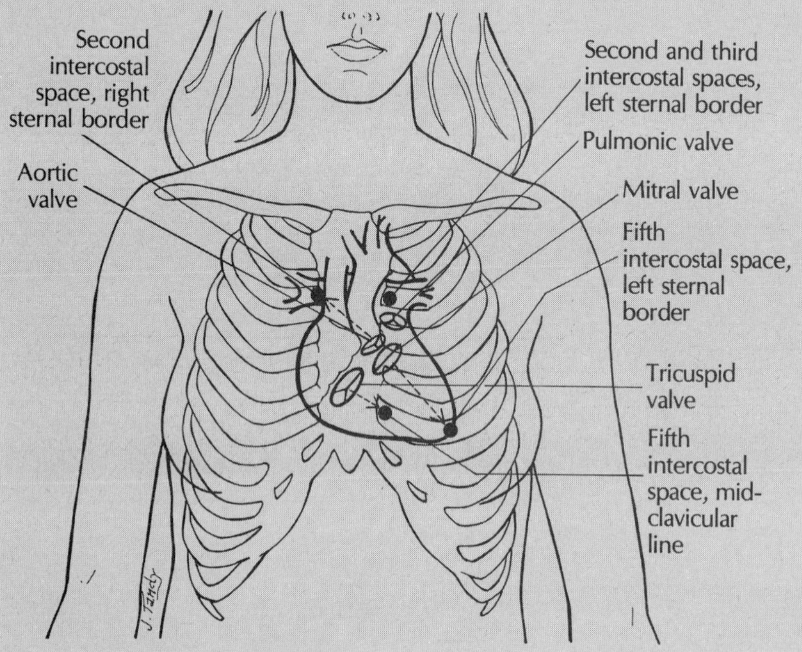

Figure 10–6. Auscultation of heart sounds.

Procedure 10–4. Assisting with Pelvic Examination

Objective	Nursing action	Rationale
Prepare patient	Explain procedure.	Explanation of procedure decreases anxiety.

Procedure 10–4 Cont'd.

Objective	Nursing action	Rationale
	Instruct patient to empty her bladder and to remove clothing below waist. She may be permitted to keep her shoes on.	Comfort is promoted during internal examination. Patient may feel more comfortable with shoes on rather than supporting her weight with bare heels against cold stirrups.
	Position patient in lithotomy position with thighs flexed and adducted. Place her feet in stirrups. Buttocks should extend slightly beyond end of examining table (Figure 10–7).	
	Drape patient with a sheet, leaving flap so perineum can be exposed.	

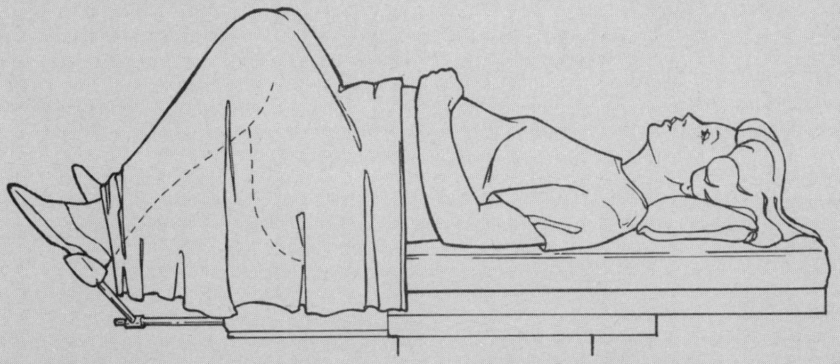

Figure 10–7. Patient in lithotomy position and draped for a pelvic examination.

Objective	Nursing action	Rationale
Ensure smooth accomplishment of procedure	Prepare and arrange following equipment so that they are easily accessible:	Examination is facilitated.
	1. Various-sized vaginal speculum, warmed prior to insertion.	Warmed speculum assists in lubrication and facilitates initial insertion when culture and smears are to be taken; many standard lubricants cannot be utilized.
	2. Glove.	
	3. Lubricant.	
	4. Pelvimeter.	
	5. Materials for Pap smear.	
	6. Good light source.	
Provide support to patient as physician or nurse practitioner carries out examination	Explain each part of examination as it is performed: inspection of external genitals, vagina, and cervix; bimanual examination of internal organs.	Relaxation of patient is promoted.
	Instruct patient to relax and breathe slowly.	
	Advise patient when speculum is to be inserted and ask her to bear down.	When speculum is inserted, woman may feel intravaginal pressure. Bearing down helps open vaginal orifice and relax perineal muscles.
	Lubricate examiner's finger well prior to bimanual examination.	
Provide patient comfort at end of examination	Assist patient to sitting position.	Supine position may create postural hypotension.
	Provide tissues to wipe lubricant from perineum.	Upon assuming sitting position, vaginal secretions along with lubricant may be discharged.
	Provide privacy for patient to dress.	Comfort and sense of privacy is promoted.

INITIAL PSYCHOLOGIC ASSESSMENT

At the initial visit the woman may be most concerned with the diagnosis of pregnancy. However, during this visit she (and her husband, if he is present) is also evaluating the health team that she has chosen. The establishment of the nurse-patient relationship will enable the woman to better evaluate the health team and also provides the nurse with a basis for an atmosphere that is conducive to interviewing, support, and education. A psychologic assessment is difficult to obtain if the patient does not feel free to talk.

Many patients are excited and anxious on the initial visit. Because of this, the initial psychologic assessment is general and the goal is to set the foundation for a trusting nurse-patient relationship.

INITIAL PSYCHOLOGIC ASSESSMENT GUIDE

Assess	Normal findings	Deviations and possible causes*	Nursing interventions†
Psychologic status	Excitement and/or apprehension; ambivalence	Marked anxiety (fear of pregnancy diagnosis, fear of medical facility)	Establish lines of communication. Active listening (see Chapter 12) is useful. Establish trusting relationship. Encourage woman to take active part in her care.
		Apathy	
		Display of anger with pregnancy diagnosis	Establish communication and begin counseling. Use active listening techniques.
Educational needs	May have questions about pregnancy or may need time to adjust to reality of pregnancy		Establish educational, supporting environment that can be expanded throughout pregnancy.
Support systems	Can identify at least two or three individuals with whom woman is emotionally intimate (husband, parent, sibling, friend, etc.)	Isolated (no telephone, unlisted number); cannot name a neighbor or friend whom she can call upon in an emergency; does not perceive parents as part of her support system	Institute support system through community groups. Develop trusting relationship with health care professionals.
Economic status	Source of income is stable and sufficient to meet basic needs of daily living and medical needs	Limited prenatal care Poor physical health Limited utilization of health care system	Discuss available resources for health maintenance and delivery. Institute appropriate referral for meeting expanding family's needs—WIC, food stamps, etc.
Stability of living conditions	Adequate, stable housing for expanding family's needs	Crowded living conditions Questionable supportive environment for newborn	Refer to appropriate community agency. Work with family on self-help ways to improve situation.

*Possible causes of deviations are placed in parentheses.
†Nursing interventions are primarily directed toward identified deviations.

DETERMINATION OF DELIVERY DATE

Nägele's Rule

The delivery date, or estimated date of confinement (EDC), can be determined in a number of different ways. The most common method is Nägele's rule. To utilize this method, take the first day of the last menstrual period (LMP), subtract three months, and add seven days. For example:

First day of LMP	November 21
Subtract three months	− 3 months
	August 21
Add 7 days	+ 7 days
EDC	August 28

A simpler method is to change the months to numerical terms:

November 21 becomes	11—21
Subtract 3 months	− 3
	8—21
Add 7 days	+ 7
EDC	August 28

If a woman with a history of menses every 28 days remembers her LMP and was not taking oral contraceptives prior to becoming pregnant, Nägele's rule may be a fairly accurate determiner of her predicted delivery date. However, if her cycle is irregular or 35–40 days in length, the time of ovulation may be delayed by several days. If she has been on oral contraceptives, ovulation may be delayed several weeks following her last menses. Ovulation usually occurs 14 days before the onset of the next menses, not 14 days after the previous menses.

Uterine Size

Physical Examination

When a woman is examined in the first 10–12 weeks of her pregnancy and the nurse practitioner or physician thinks that her uterine size is compatible with her menstrual history, uterine size may be the single most important clinical method for dating her pregnancy. In many cases, however, women do not seek obstetric attention until well into their second trimester, when it becomes much more difficult to evaluate specific uterine size. In the case of the obese woman, it is most difficult to determine uterine size early in a pregnancy.

Fundal Height

The physician may use fundal height as an indicator of uterine size, although this is at best only accurate within about four weeks and cannot be used late in pregnancy. A centimeter tape measure is used to measure the distance abdominally from the top of the symphysis pubis to the top of the uterine fundus. Fundal height usually correlates with gestational age until the third trimester, when fetal weights vary considerably. Thus at 26 weeks' gestation, fundal height is probably about 26 cm. At 20 weeks' gestation, the fundus is about 20 cm and at the level of the umbilicus in an average female.

McDonald's rule may also be used to measure fundal height in the second and third trimesters. Place the tape measure at the notch of the

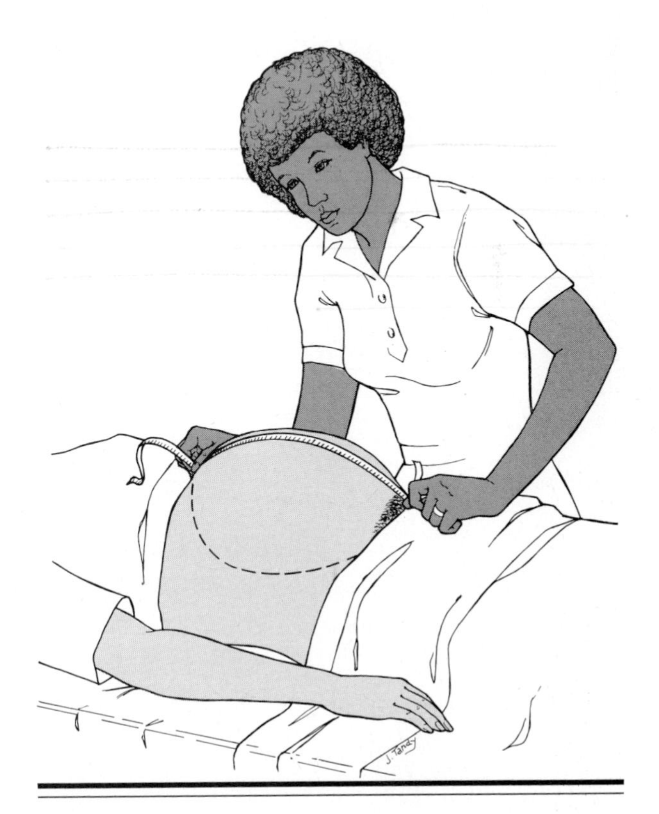

Figure 10–8. Use of McDonald's method to measure fundal height.

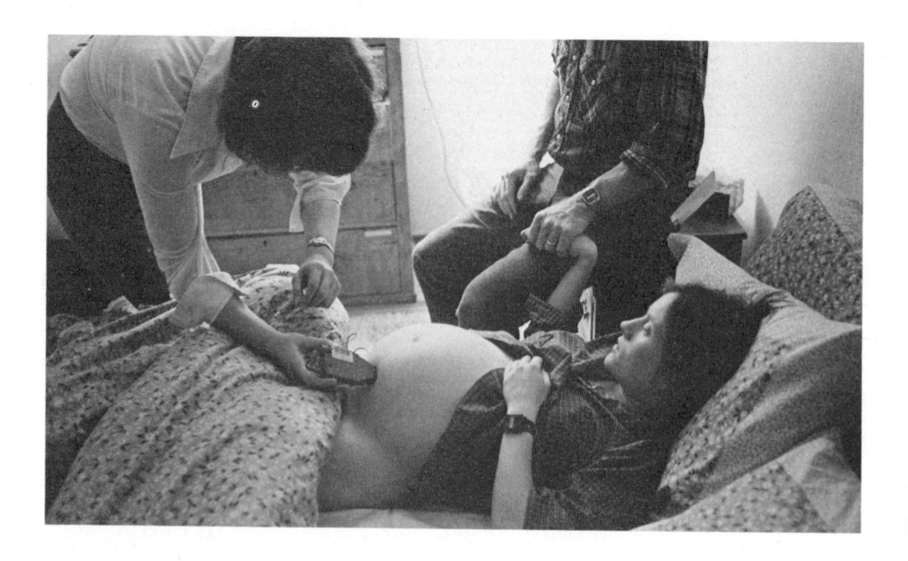

Figure 10–9. Listening to fetal heartbeat with Doppler device.

symphysis pubis and measure up over the fundus (Figure 10–8). Calculation is done as follows:

Height of fundus (in centimeters) × 2/7 = Duration of pregnancy in lunar months
Example: 28 cm × 2/7 = 8 lunar months

Height of fundus (in centimeters) × 8/7 = Duration of pregnancy in weeks
Example: 28 cm × 8/7 = 32 weeks

If the woman is very tall or very short, fundal height will differ.

Measurements of fundal height from month to month and week to week may give indications of intrauterine growth retardation (IUGR) if there is a lag in progression, or indications of the presence of twins or polyhydramnios if there is a sudden increase in height. Unfortunately, this method of dating a pregnancy can be quite inaccurate in obese women, in women with uterine fibroids, and in mothers who develop polyhydramnios.

Quickening

Fetal movements felt by the mother may give some indications that the fetus is nearing 20 weeks' gestation. However, quickening may be experienced between 16 and 22 weeks' gestation, so this is not a completely accurate method. One can begin to listen for a fetal heartbeat weekly after the mother experiences quickening and can use this indication as documentation for a delivery date.

Fetal Heartbeat

The fetal heartbeat can be detected as early as the 16th week and almost always by the 19th or 20th week of gestation with an ordinary fetoscope. In the case of twins or the obese patient, it may be later than this before the fetal heartbeat can be detected. Fetal heartbeat may be detected with the ultrasonic Doppler device (Figure 10–9) as early as the 8th week (Leopold and Asher, 1974).

SUBSEQUENT PHYSICAL ASSESSMENT

The recommended frequency of prenatal visits is as follows:

- Monthly for the first 32 weeks of gestation.
- Every two weeks to the 36th week.
- After the 36th week, every week until delivery.

The accompanying Subsequent Physical Assessment Guide provides a systematic approach to the regular physical examinations that the pregnant woman should undergo for optimal prenatal care.

SUBSEQUENT PHYSICAL ASSESSMENT GUIDE

Assess	Normal findings	Deviations and possible causes*	Nursing interventions†
Vital signs			
Temperature	36.2–37.6C (98–99.6F)	Elevated temperature (infection)	Evaluate for signs of infection. Refer to physician.
Pulse	60–90/min	Increased pulse rate (anxiety, cardiac disorders)	Note irregularities. Evaluate patient's anxiety and stress.
Respiration	16–24/min	Marked tachypnea or abnormal patterns (respiratory disease)	Refer to physician.
Blood pressure	90–140/60–90 (falls in second trimester)	>140/90 (preeclampsia)	Assess for edema, proteinuria. Refer to physician. Schedule appointments more frequently.
Weight gain	First trimester: 2–4 lb Second trimester: 11 lb Third trimester: 11 lb	Excessive weight gain (excessive caloric intake, edema, preeclampsia)	Discuss appropriate weight gain. Provide nutritional counseling. Assess for presence of edema.
Edema	Small amount of dependent edema, especially in last weeks of pregnancy	Edema in hands, face, legs, feet (preeclampsia)	Refer to physician. Identify any correlation between edema and activities and blood pressure.
Uterine size	See Initial Physical Assessment Guide for normal changes during pregnancy	Unusually rapid growth (multiple gestation, hydatidiform mole, polyhydramnios, miscalculation of EDC)	Evaluate fetal status. Determine height of fundus using McDonald's rule (p. 263). Use diagnostic ultrasound.
Fetal heartbeat	120–160/min Funic souffle	Absence of fetal heartbeat after 20th week of gestation (maternal obesity, fetal demise)	Evaluate fetal status.
Laboratory evaluation			
Hemoglobin	12–16 gm/100 ml Pseudoanemia of pregnancy	<12 gm/100 ml (anemia)	Provide nutritional counseling. Hemoglobin may be repeated at seven months' gestation. Women of Mediterranean heritage need a close check on hemoglobin because of possibility of thalassemia.
Antibody screen	Negative	Positive	Refer for further testing to identify specific antibodies. Titers may be indicated.
Urinalysis	See Initial Physical Assessment Guide (p. 254) for normal findings	See Initial Physical Assessment Guide (p. 254) for deviations	Repeat urinalysis at seven months' gestation.

*Possible causes of deviations are placed in parentheses.
†Nursing interventions are primarily directed toward identified deviations.

SUBSEQUENT PHYSICAL ASSESSMENT GUIDE Cont'd

Assess	Normal findings	Deviations and possible causes*	Nursing interventions†
Protein	Negative	Proteinuria, albuminuria (contamination by vaginal discharge, urinary tract infection, preeclampsia)	Obtain dipstick urine sample. Refer to physician if deviations are present.
Glucose	Negative Note: Glycosuria may be present due to physiologic alterations in glomerular filtration rate and renal threshold	Persistent glycosuria (diabetes mellitus)	

*Possible causes of deviations are placed in parentheses.
†Nursing interventions are primarily directed toward identified deviations.

SUBSEQUENT PSYCHOLOGIC ASSESSMENT

Periodic prenatal examinations offer the nurse an opportunity to assess the maternity patient's psychologic needs and emotional status. If the woman's partner attends the prenatal visits, his needs and concerns can also be identified.

The interchange between the nurse and patient will be facilitated if it takes place in a friendly, trusting environment. Provide time for the patient to ask questions and to air concerns. If the nurse provides the time and demonstrates genuine interest, the patient will feel more at ease bringing up questions that she may believe are silly or concerns that she has been afraid to verbalize.

During the subsequent psychologic assessments, a patient may manifest dysfunctional behavior patterns such as the following:

1. Increasing anxiety.
2. Inability to establish communication.
3. Inappropriate responses or actions.
4. Denial of pregnancy.
5. Inability to cope with stress.
6. Failure to acknowledge quickening.
7. Failure to plan and prepare for the baby (e.g., living arrangements, clothing, feeding methods, etc.).

If the patient appears to have these or other critical psychologic problems, the nurse should refer her to the appropriate professionals.

The accompanying Subsequent Psychologic Assessment Guide provides a model for the psychologic evaluation of both the pregnant patient and the expectant father.

SUBSEQUENT PSYCHOLOGIC ASSESSMENT GUIDE

Assess	Normal findings	Deviations and possible causes*	Nursing interventions†
Expectant mother			
Psychologic status	Pregnancy changes: First trimester: incorporates	Increasing stress and anxiety	Encourage mother to take an active part in her care.

*Possible causes of deviations are placed in parentheses.
†Nursing interventions are primarily directed toward identified deviations.

SUBSEQUENT PSYCHOLOGIC ASSESSMENT GUIDE Cont'd

Assess	Normal findings	Deviations and possible causes*	Nursing interventions†
	idea of pregnancy; may feel ambivalent, especially if she must give up desired role; usually looks for signs of verification of pregnancy, such as increase in adominal size, fetal movement, etc. Second trimester: baby becomes more real to woman as abdominal size increases and she feels movement; she begins to turn inward, becoming more introspective Third trimester: begins to think of baby as separate being; may feel restless and may feel that time of labor will never come; remains self-centered and concentrates on preparing place for baby	Inability to establish communication; inability to accept pregnancy; inappropriate response or actions; denial of pregnancy; inability to cope	Establish lines of communication. Establish a trusting relationship. Counsel as necessary. Refer to appropriate professional as needed.
Educational needs: self-care measures and knowledge	Knowledge about following: Breast care Hygiene Rest Exercise Nutrition	Inadequate information	Teach and/or institute appropriate relief measures (see Chapter 11).
	Relief measures for common discomforts of pregnancy	Inadequate information	
Sexual activity	Patient knows how pregnancy affects sexual activity	Lack of information about effects of pregnancy and/or alternate positions during sexual intercourse	Provide counseling.
Preparation for parenting	In last few weeks of pregnancy, parents have prepared equipment, clothing, and place for baby	Lack of preparation (denial, failure to adjust to baby, unwanted child)	Counsel. If lack of preparation is due to inadequacy of information, provide information (see Chapter 11).
Danger signs of pregnancy	Patient knows to report following danger signs immediately: 1. Sudden gush of fluid from vagina 2. Vaginal bleeding	Lack of information	Provide appropriate teaching. Encourage woman to report danger signs. Refer to physician immediately for evaluation.

*Possible causes of deviations are placed in parentheses.
†Nursing interventions are primarily directed toward identified deviations.

SUBSEQUENT PSYCHOLOGIC ASSESSMENT GUIDE Cont'd

Assess	Normal findings	Deviations and possible causes*	Nursing interventions†
	3. Abdominal pain 4. Temperature above 38.3C (101F) and chills 5. Dizziness, blurring of vision, double vision, spots before eyes 6. Persistent vomiting 7. Severe headache 8. Edema of hands, face, legs, and feet		
Preparation for childbirth	Patient aware of following: 1. Prepared childbirth techniques		If couple chooses particular technique, refer to classes (see Chapter 12 for description of childbirth preparation techniques).
	2. Normal processes and changes during childbirth		Encourage prenatal class attendance. Educate woman during visits based on current physical status. Provide reading list for more specific information.
	3. Problems that may occur as a result of drug and alcohol use and of smoking	Continued abuse of drugs and alcohol; denial of possible effect on self and baby	Review danger signs that were presented on initial visit.
	Woman has met other physician and/or nurse-midwife who may be attending her delivery in the absence of primary physician and/or nurse-midwife	Introduction of new individual at delivery may increase stress and anxiety for patient and partner	Introduce woman to all members of group practice.
Impending labor	Patient knows signs of impending labor: 1. Uterine contractions that increase in frequency, duration, intensity 2. Bloody show 3. Expulsion of mucous plug 4. Rupture of membranes	Lack of information	Provide appropriate teaching, stressing importance of seeking appropriate medical assistance.
Expectant father			
Psychologic status	First trimester: may express excitement over confirmation of pregnancy and of his virility; concerns move toward providing for financial needs; energetic; may identify with some	Increasing stress and anxiety Inability to establish communication Inability to accept pregnancy diagnosis Withdrawal of support	Encourage expectant father to come to prenatal visits. Establish lines of communication. Establish trusting

*Possible causes of deviations are placed in parentheses.
†Nursing interventions are primarily directed toward identified deviations.

Assess	Normal findings	Deviations and possible causes*	Nursing interventions†
	discomforts of pregnancy and may even exhibit symptoms	Abandonment of the mother	relationship.
	Second trimester: may feel more confident and be less concerned with financial matters; may have concerns about wife's changing size and shape, her increasing introspection		Counsel. Let expectant father know that it is normal for him to experience these feelings.
	Third trimester: may have feelings of rivalry with fetus, especially during sexual activity; may make changes in his physical appearance and exhibit more interest in himself; may become more energetic; fantasizes about child but usually imagines older child; fears of mutilation and death of mother and child arise		Include expectant father in pregnancy activities as he desires. Provide education, information, and support. Increasing number of expectant fathers are demonstrating desire to be involved in many or all aspects of prenatal care, education, and preparation.

*Possible causes of deviations are placed in parentheses.
†Nursing interventions are primarily directed toward identified deviations.

SUMMARY

Assessment of psychologic, social, cultural, and physical data forms the framework of specific medical and nursing interventions throughout a woman's pregnancy. The nurse must have a thorough understanding of the normal physical changes that occur during pregnancy so that deviations can be recognized and treated in an appropriate manner.

SUGGESTED ACTIVITIES

1. In the classroom laboratory, simulate an initial prenatal visit:
   a. Identify the essential components of the history and physical and psychologic assessments and identify needed laboratory tests.
   b. Outline the nursing and medical care needed on subsequent visits.
2. In a prenatal clinic or obstetrician's office, assist with a physical examination of a pregnant patient.

REFERENCES

Leopold, G. R., and Asher, W. M. 1974. Ultrasound in obstetrics and gynecology. *Radio. Clin. North Am.* 12:127.

Miller, W., ed. 1977. *Technical manual of American Association of Blood Banks.* Washington, D. C.: The Association.

University of Maryland. Antenatal evaluation risk form. Baltimore: Antenatal Clinic, University of Maryland Hospital.

ADDITIONAL READINGS

Bates, B. 1974. *A guide to physical assessment.* Philadelphia: J. B. Lippincott Co.

Danforth, D., ed. 1977. *Obstetrics and gynecology.* Hagerstown, Md.: Harper & Row Publishers, Inc.

Jensen, M., et al. 1977. *Maternity care: the nurse and the family.* St. Louis: The C. V. Mosby Co.

Malasnos, L., et al. 1977. *Health assessment.* St. Louis: The C. V. Mosby Co.

Ziegle, E., and Cranley, M. 1978. *Obstetric nursing.* New York: The Macmillan Co.

CHAPTER 11

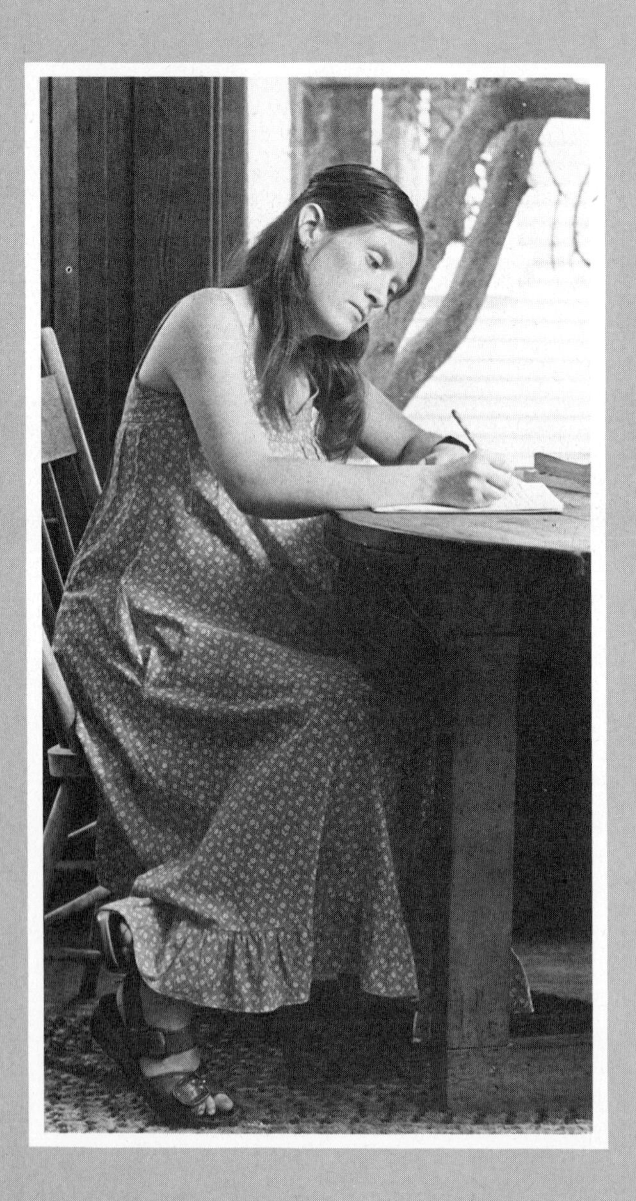

THE PREGNANT WOMAN: NEEDS AND CARE

OBJECTIVES

- Identify the common discomforts occurring during pregnancy, their possible causes, and appropriate nursing interventions to alleviate the discomforts.
- Discuss the main areas of prenatal care requiring nursing assessment and instruction.
- Identify some of the concerns that the expectant couple may have regarding sexual activity.
- Compare nutritional needs during pregnancy and lactation with normal requirements.
- Identify the special dietary needs of pregnant women of various ethnic backgrounds.
- Identify socioeconomic and cultural influences on pregnancy and prenatal practices.
- Explain how the general nutrition of the mother before pregnancy affects the development of the infant.

The body of the pregnant woman undergoes tremendous changes. These changes precipitate a number of physical discomforts that require intervention by the nurse who is managing the patient's prenatal care. Generally, the nurse will find it sufficient to educate the patient about self-care measures that promote relief of these annoying and possibly painful conditions. However, occasionally other nursing actions are required, depending on the severity of the problem or the ability of the patient to assume responsibility for her own care.

Pregnancy also precipitates a number of questions and concerns from the woman and her family regarding hygiene, possible changes in lifestyle, and nutrition. The nurse often assumes the roles of teacher and counselor for families who need information about pregnancy or who are having difficulty understanding how to adjust their lives to this event.

This chapter focuses on the common discomforts and concerns arising during pregnancy. In addition, it discusses hygiene and relief measures and examines the dynamics and significance of proper nutrition.

COMMON DISCOMFORTS OF PREGNANCY

Common discomforts of pregnancy are often referred to as minor discomforts by health care professionals. These discomforts, however, are not minor to the pregnant woman. A woman whose fourth pregnancy is aggravating her varicose veins and whose pendulous abdomen is creating severe backache will be quite uncomfortable. Varicose veins can even predispose her to complications if she does not use preventive methods that also promote relief. The primigravida who is unaware that the dizziness she is experiencing is common in pregnancy may suffer considerable anxiety.

The discomforts of pregnancy are a result of physiologic and anatomic changes. These changes are fairly specific to each of the three trimesters (Figure 11-1). Increased frequency of urination, for example, is most common in the first trimester, when the growing uterus creates pressure on the bladder; the problem is alleviated in the second trimester as the uterus rises out of the pelvis. Urinary frequency increases gradually during the third trimester when the enlarged uterus presses against the bladder as well as on all other internal organs.

Some preexisting problems, such as hemorrhoids and varicose veins, are aggravated during pregnancy. These discomforts worsen with enlargement of the gravid uterus; thus they may appear in the second trimester and become intensified in the third trimester. For women who do not have these preexisting conditions, the second trimester of pregnancy may be a relatively comfortable time. The discomforts caused by the enlarging uterus do not affect them until the last trimester or even until the last month.

First Trimester

Nausea and Vomiting

Nausea and vomiting are early symptoms in pregnancy, with some form of nausea occurring in the majority of pregnant women. This symptom appears sometime after the first missed menstrual period and usually ceases by the fourth missed menstrual period. Some women develop only an aversion to specific foods, many experience nausea upon arising in the morning, and others experience nausea throughout the day. Vomiting does not occur in the majority of these women.

Various theories attempt to explain the etiologic factors of nausea and vomiting in early pregnancy, but the specific cause is not known. A common theory attributes the nausea to hormonal changes related to HCG levels in the body. The initial presence of serum gonadotropin occurs at the same time that nausea and vomiting commence, and the gradual cessation of nausea and vomiting occurs as the reaction to serum gonadotropin subsides.

Another theory suggests that changes in carbohydrate metabolism may create a slight decrease in blood sugar levels in early pregnancy. Nausea may occur as the result of the sensations of intense hunger.

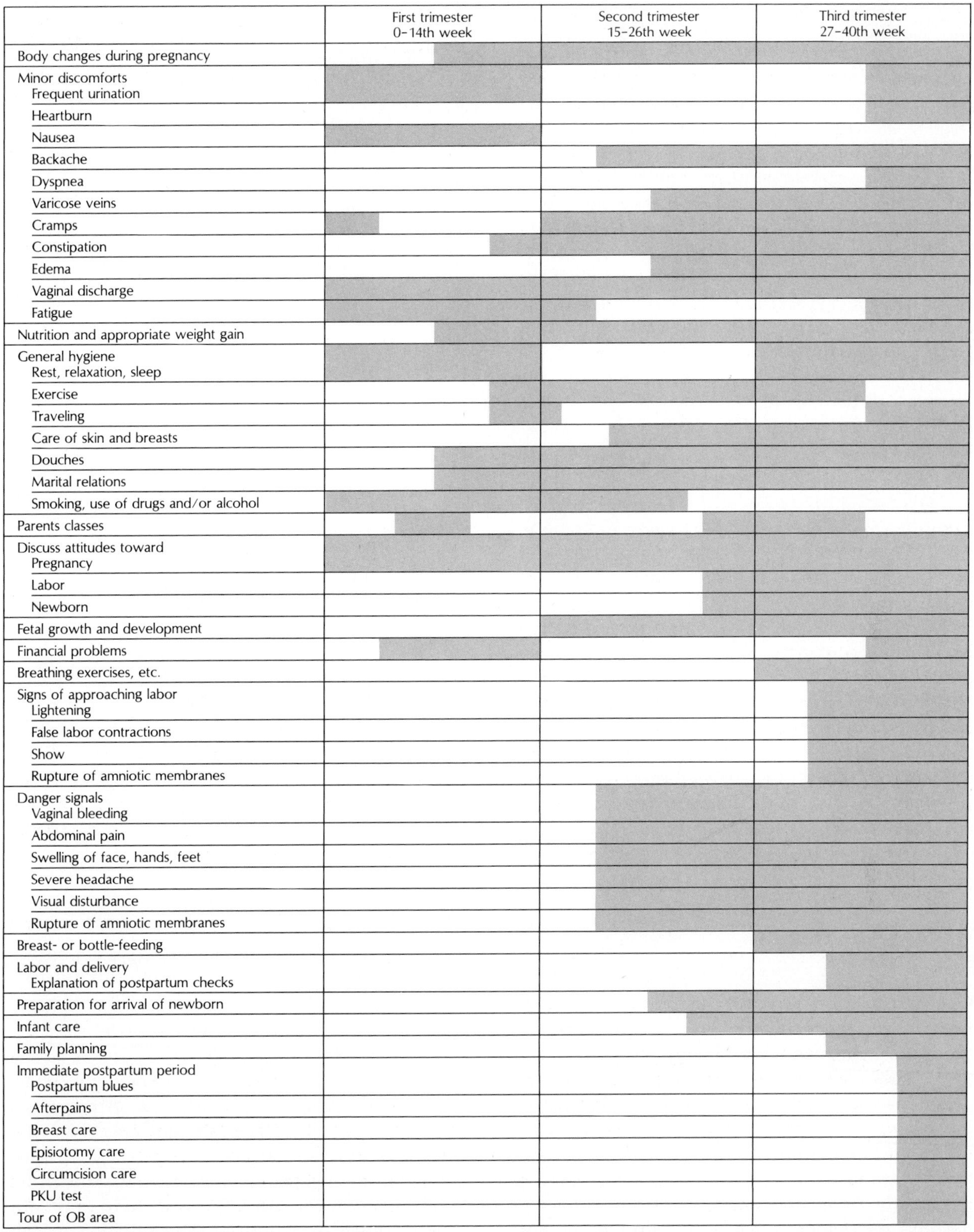

	First trimester 0–14th week	Second trimester 15–26th week	Third trimester 27–40th week
Body changes during pregnancy			
Minor discomforts Frequent urination			
Heartburn			
Nausea			
Backache			
Dyspnea			
Varicose veins			
Cramps			
Constipation			
Edema			
Vaginal discharge			
Fatigue			
Nutrition and appropriate weight gain			
General hygiene Rest, relaxation, sleep			
Exercise			
Traveling			
Care of skin and breasts			
Douches			
Marital relations			
Smoking, use of drugs and/or alcohol			
Parents classes			
Discuss attitudes toward Pregnancy			
Labor			
Newborn			
Fetal growth and development			
Financial problems			
Breathing exercises, etc.			
Signs of approaching labor Lightening			
False labor contractions			
Show			
Rupture of amniotic membranes			
Danger signals Vaginal bleeding			
Abdominal pain			
Swelling of face, hands, feet			
Severe headache			
Visual disturbance			
Rupture of amniotic membranes			
Breast- or bottle-feeding			
Labor and delivery Explanation of postpartum checks			
Preparation for arrival of newborn			
Infant care			
Family planning			
Immediate postpartum period Postpartum blues			
Afterpains			
Breast care			
Episiotomy care			
Circumcision care			
PKU test			
Tour of OB area			

Figure 11–1. Timetable for discomforts, concerns, and changes during pregnancy. This bar graph demonstrates the approximate times during pregnancy a woman will experience concerns or needs information in each category. From this data, a plan for teaching is made to present the information prior to her need, enabling the woman to better understand and be prepared for her experience. (From *Maternity Nursing Today* by Clausen, J. © 1977 McGraw-Hill, Inc. Used with permission of McGraw-Hill Book Company.)

Emotional factors and fatigue are considered by many authorities to have a role in the experience of nausea and vomiting (Pritchard and MacDonald, 1976).

Interventions. Treatment of nausea and vomiting is not always successful, but the symptoms can be reduced. It is important for the nurse to assess when the nausea and/or vomiting occurs to be helpful in suggesting methods of relief. For some women, nausea may be relieved simply by avoiding the odor of certain foods or other conditions that precipitate the problem. If nausea occurs most frequently during early morning, the woman can be encouraged to try various simple remedies, such as eating dry crackers or toast before slowly arising. In general, it is usually helpful to eat small but frequent meals and to avoid greasy and highly seasoned foods. Some women find unusual remedies that they claim to be helpful. If these remedies are not harmful to their pregnancy, they should be encouraged to continue using them.

Generally, nausea and vomiting cease by the fourth month of pregnancy. If they do not, hyperemesis gravidarum may develop, which is a complication of pregnancy discussed in Chapter 13. For women suffering extreme nausea and vomiting in the first trimester, antiemetics may be ordered by the physician, but they should be avoided if at all possible during this time because of possible teratogenic effects on the development of the embryo.

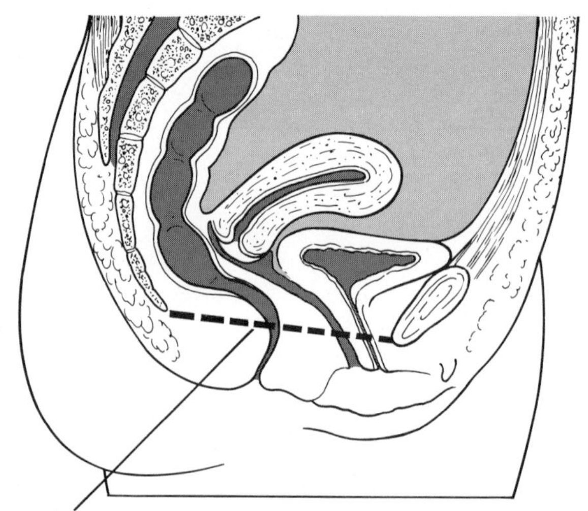

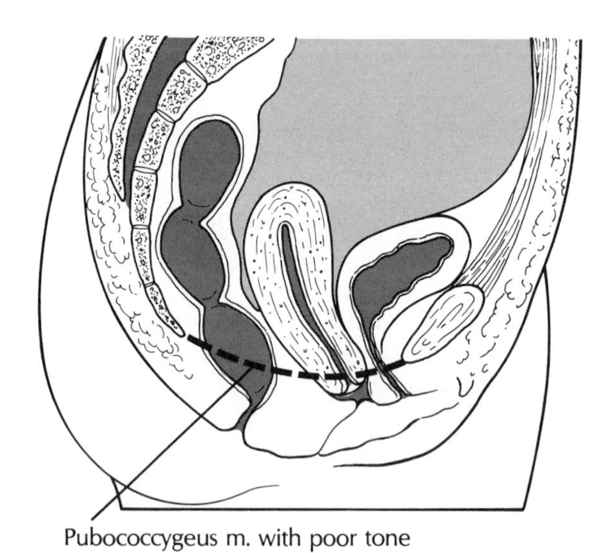

Figure 11–2. Kegel's exercises. The woman learns to tighten the pubococcygeus muscle, which improves support to pelvic organs.

Urinary Frequency and Urgency

One of the most common discomforts in pregnancy is frequency and urgency of urination. It occurs early in pregnancy because of the pressure of the enlarging uterus on the bladder. This condition subsides for a while when the uterus moves out of the pelvic area into the abdominal cavity, around the 12th week. Frequency recurs in the last trimester as the enlarging uterus begins to press on the bladder again. Coughing or sneezing in the last month may even cause leakage of urine.

As long as other symptoms of urinary tract infection do not appear, frequency and urgency of urination are considered normal during the first and third trimesters.

Interventions. There are no methods of decreasing the frequency and urgency of urination in pregnancy. Fluid intake should never be decreased in attempts to prevent frequency. Tightening of the pubococcygeus muscle, known as *Kegel's exercises* (Figure 11–2), can help maintain good perineal muscle tone. The function of the pubococcygeus muscle is to support internal organs and control voiding. The leaking of urine during pregnancy is usually limited only to pregnancy, unless there is excessive relaxation of the muscles. The muscle tone is believed to gradually weaken with each pregnancy, and bladder problems can occur when these women are older if perineal muscle tone is not maintained.

Breast Tenderness

Sensitivity of the breast occurs early and continues throughout the pregnancy. Increased levels of estrogen and progesterone play large roles in the soreness and tingling sensation felt in the breast and in the increased sensitivity of the nipples.

Interventions. A well-fitting supportive brassiere gives the most relief for this discomfort. The qualities of a proper supportive brassiere are discussed in the section on breast care (p. 282).

Increased Vaginal Discharge

Increased vaginal discharge (leukorrhea) is common in pregnancy. The discharge is usually whitish, consisting of mucus and exfoliated vaginal epithelial cells. It occurs as the result of hyperplasia of vaginal mucosa and increased production of mucus by the endocervical glands. In addition, an accompanying reduction in the acidity of the secretions allows organisms to grow more easily.

Interventions. Cleanliness is important in preventing excoriation and vaginal infections. Daily bathing should be adequate, and douching should not be necessary in pregnancy if vaginal infections do not occur. Nylon underpants and pantyhose retain heat and moisture in the genital area; thus absorbent cotton underpants should be worn to help prevent problems. Bath powder is also helpful in maintaining dryness and promoting comfort. The pregnant woman should be encouraged to report any change in vaginal discharge and any irritation in the perineal area. These changes frequently indicate vaginal infections (Chapter 13).

Second and Third Trimesters

It is more difficult to classify discomforts as specifically occurring in the second or third trimester, since many problems are due to individual variations in women, such as number of previously existing discomforts. The conditions discussed in this section usually do not appear until the third trimester in primigravidas but do occur earlier with each succeeding pregnancy.

Heartburn (Pyrosis)

Heartburn is the regurgitation of acidic gastric contents into the esophagus. It creates a burning or irritating sensation in the esophagus and radiates upward, sometimes leaving a bad taste in the mouth. It can occur anytime in pregnancy but is most common in the second half. Heartburn appears to be primarily a result of the displacement of the stomach by the enlarging uterus. Pregnancy is accompanied by a decrease in gastrointestinal motility and a relaxing of the cardiac sphincter, which also contribute to heartburn.

Interventions. Behaviors that aggravate heartburn are overeating, ingesting fatty and fried foods, and lying down soon after eating. These situations should therefore be avoided. The woman should be encouraged to eat smaller and more frequent meals to accommodate the decreased size of her stomach. Antacids such as aluminum hydroxide, magnesium trisilicate, and magnesium hydroxide (Amphojel, Gelusil, and Maalox) can be recommended. However, common household remedies containing sodium bicarbonate (baking soda) should never be used for heartburn during pregnancy because of potential electrolyte imbalance.

Ankle Edema

Most women experience ankle edema in the last part of their pregnancy because of the increasing difficulty of venous return from the lower extremities. Prolonged standing or sitting and warm weather increase the edema. It is also associated with varicose veins. Ankle edema becomes a concern only when accompanied by hypertension or proteinuria or when the edema is not postural in origin.

Interventions. The aggravating conditions just mentioned should be avoided. If the woman has to sit or stand for long periods, frequent dorsiflexion of her feet will help contract muscles, thereby squeezing the fluid back into circulation. Tight garters or other restrictive bands around the leg should not be worn. During rest periods, the woman should elevate her legs and hips as described in the following section on varicose veins.

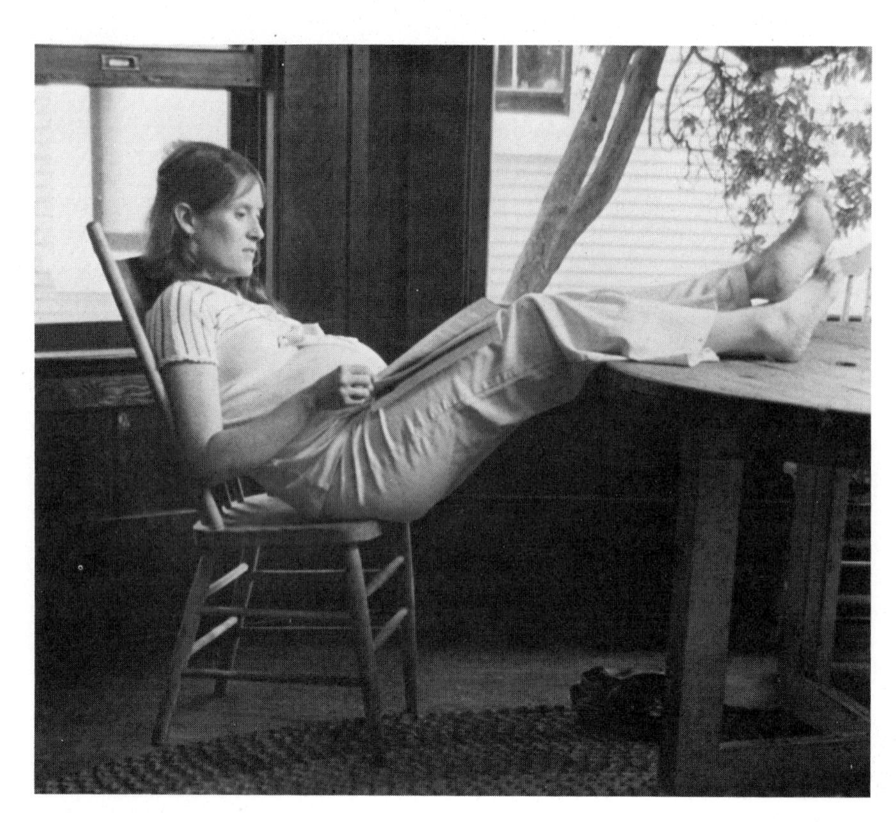

Figure 11–3. Sitting with her feet elevated helps to relieve the pregnant woman's discomfort and swelling of the lower extremities.

Varicose Veins

Varicose veins are a result of weakening of the walls of veins or faulty functioning of the valves. Some people have an inherited weakness in these walls. Poor circulation in the lower extremities predisposes to varicose veins in the legs and thighs. With poor circulation, the valves of the veins prevent the blood from going downward, and stasis of the blood exerts pressure, with gradual weakening of the walls, resulting in varicosities. In other instances, faulty functioning of the valves results in pooling of blood in the lower extremities with concomitant pressure on the vein walls. Occupations requiring prolonged standing or sitting contribute to congestion of blood in the lower extremities.

Pregnancy plays a significant role in creating conditions that cause varicose veins. The weight of the gravid uterus in the pelvis aggravates the development of varicosities in the legs and pelvic area by preventing good venous return. Most women who do not have other predisposing factors can avoid the development of varicose veins in pregnancy with good preventive measures. Some women, however, experience obvious changes in the veins of their legs. Increased maternal age, excessive weight gain, a large fetus, and multiple pregnancy can all contribute to the problem.

Women with varicosities in their legs experience aching and tiredness in the lower extremities, with the discomfort increasing throughout the day. They frequently become discouraged by the discoloration in the veins of their legs and by obvious blemishes. Prevention or relief of the discomfort occurs when good venous return from the lower extremities is restored.

Interventions. Preventive and relief measures include frequent elevation of the legs. One important habit that the pregnant woman can develop is always elevating her legs when she sits down (Figure 11–3). A more effective method the woman can use to promote venous return is to lie on her back on the floor or bed with her legs resting at a right angle against the wall (Figure 11–4).

A pregnant woman should not sit for long periods of time or cross her legs at the knees, because of the pressure on her veins. She should not wear garters or hosiery with constricting bands. She should also avoid standing for long periods of time. However, supportive hose or elastic stockings may be extremely helpful, depending on the amount of discomfort. Supportive hose should be put on upon rising in the morning and should be cleansed daily with soap and warm water to help retain their elasticity.

Treatment of varicose veins by the injection method or by surgery is not recommended during pregnancy. The woman should be aware that treatment may be needed after pregnancy because the problem will be aggravated by a succeeding pregnancy.

Phlebothrombosis and thrombophlebitis are possible complications of varicose veins, but they usually do not occur in a healthy pregnant woman. If these complications occur, the cause is often a local injury.

Vulval varicosities may also be a problem in pregnancy, although they are less common. Varicosities in the vulva and perineum cause aching and a sense of heaviness in these areas. Support in this area promotes relief. Elevation of only the legs aggravates vulval varicosities by creating stasis of blood in the pelvic area. Therefore, it is important that the pelvic area also be elevated to promote venous drainage into the trunk of the body. More than one firm pillow under the hips may be needed to accomplish this elevation. Near the end of pregnancy, this position may be extremely awkward; the woman may best relieve uterine pressure on the pelvic veins by resting on her side.

Hemorrhoids

Hemorrhoids are varicosities of the veins around the lower end of the rectum and anus. In the nonpregnant state, hemorrhoids are usually caused by the straining that occurs with constipation. When a woman becomes pregnant, the gravid uterus creates pressure on the veins and thus interferes with venous circulation. As the pregnancy progresses and the fetus grows, greater pressure on the veins and displacement of intestines occur, increasing the problem of constipation and often resulting in hemorrhoids.

Some women may not be aware of hemorrhoids in pregnancy until the second stage of labor, when the hemorrhoids appear as they push. Hemorrhoids that occur in pregnancy or at delivery usually subside, and they become asymptomatic after the early postpartal period.

Women who have hemorrhoids prior to pregnancy probably experience more difficulties with them during pregnancy because of the aggravating conditions just discussed.

Symptoms of hemorrhoids include itching, swelling, and pain, as well as hemorrhoidal bleeding. Internal hemorrhoids are located above

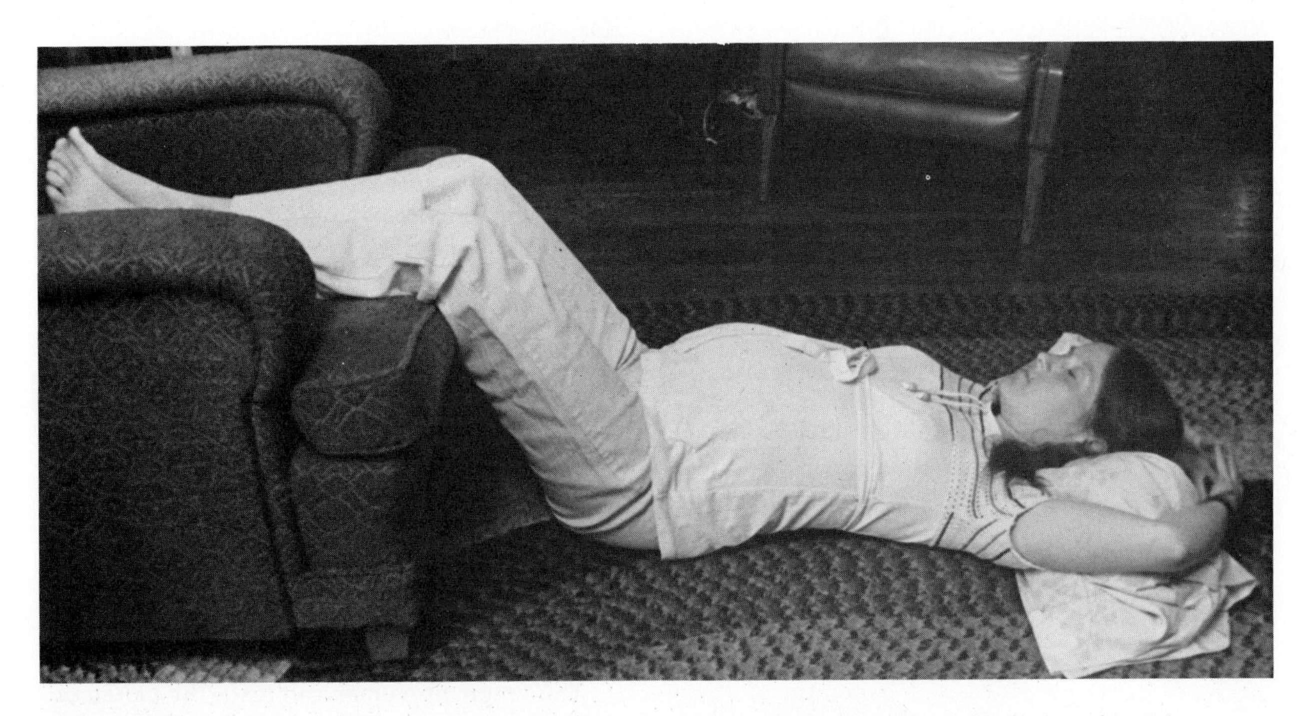

Figure 11–4. Swelling and discomfort from varicosities can be decreased by lying down with the legs elevated.

the anal sphincter and are responsible for bleeding, usually with defecation. They are not usually painful unless they protrude from the anus.

Interventions. Relief can be found by gently reinserting the hemorrhoids with the use of a lubricant. Reinsertion is aided by gravity; therefore, reinsertion is more successful if the woman lies on her side or in the knee-chest position. External hemorrhoids are located outside the anal sphincter. They are not usually the source of bleeding or pain; however, thrombosis of these hemorrhoids can occur, and in that case they become extremely painful. The thrombosis may resolve itself in 24 hours, or it can be treated in the physician's office by incising and evacuating the blood clot.

Avoidance of constipation is an important factor in preventing and/or relieving the discomfort of hemorrhoids. Relief measures for existing hemorrhoid symptoms include ice packs, use of topical ointments and anesthetic agents, and warm soaks.

Constipation

Conditions in pregnancy that predispose the woman to constipation include general bowel sluggishness caused by increased steroid metabolism; displacement of the intestines, which increases with the growth of the fetus; and oral iron supplements, which may be needed by the pregnant woman.

Interventions. Increased fluid intake, adequate roughage or bulk in the diet, daily bowel habits, and adequate daily exercise can often maintain good bowel function in women who have not had previous problems. Women who try to develop these daily habits during pregnancy will be prepared to maintain good bowel function after delivery; meanwhile, they may need to use mild laxatives, stool softeners, and suppositories as recommended by their physician. The nurse should help women with constipation to develop good daily bowel habits and to avoid becoming dependent on laxatives during pregnancy, a habit that may continue after delivery.

Backache

Many pregnant women experience backache. As the uterus enlarges, increased curvature of the lumbosacral vertebras occurs (Figure 11-5). The steroid hormones cause a softening and relaxation of pelvic joints; thus the growing uterus stretches the abdominal muscles, and the increasing weight creates a gradual tilt of the anterior portion of the pelvis. As the anterior portion of the pelvis tilts downward, the spinal curvature increases. If the woman does not learn how to correct this curvature, the strain on the muscles and ligaments will cause backache.

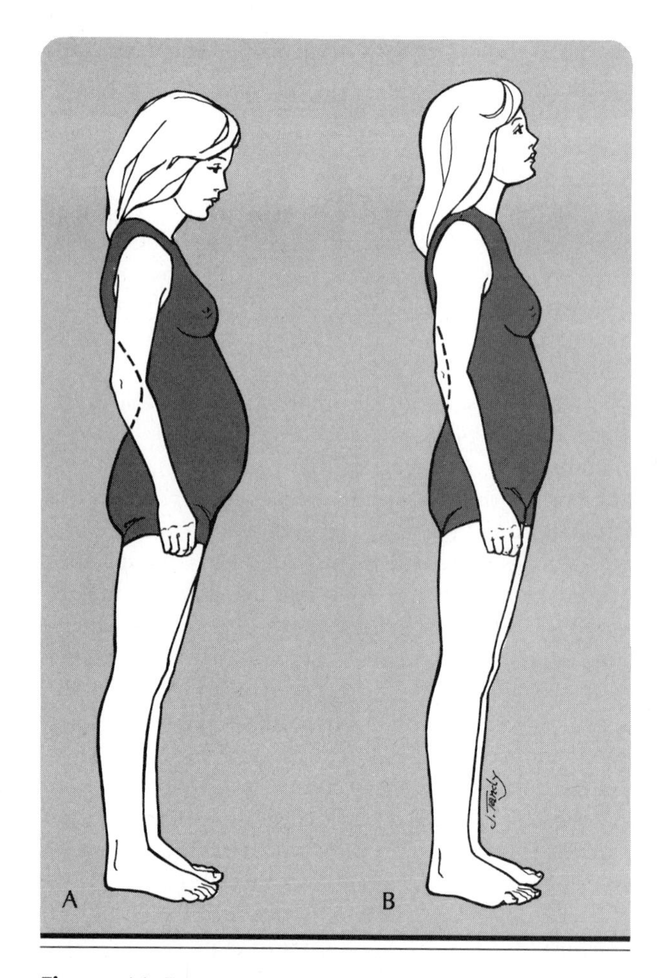

Figure 11-5. **A,** Increased curvature of lumbosacral vertebras. **B,** Approxpriate alignment with pelvic tilt.

Interventions. An exercise called the *pelvic tilt* can help restore proper body alignment. As the anterior pelvis is tilted upward, the curvature of the back is automatically decreased, relieving much of the discomfort. If proper body alignment is maintained throughout pregnancy, backaches can be relieved or even prevented.

The pregnant woman can learn the pelvic tilt in the following manner. While lying on her

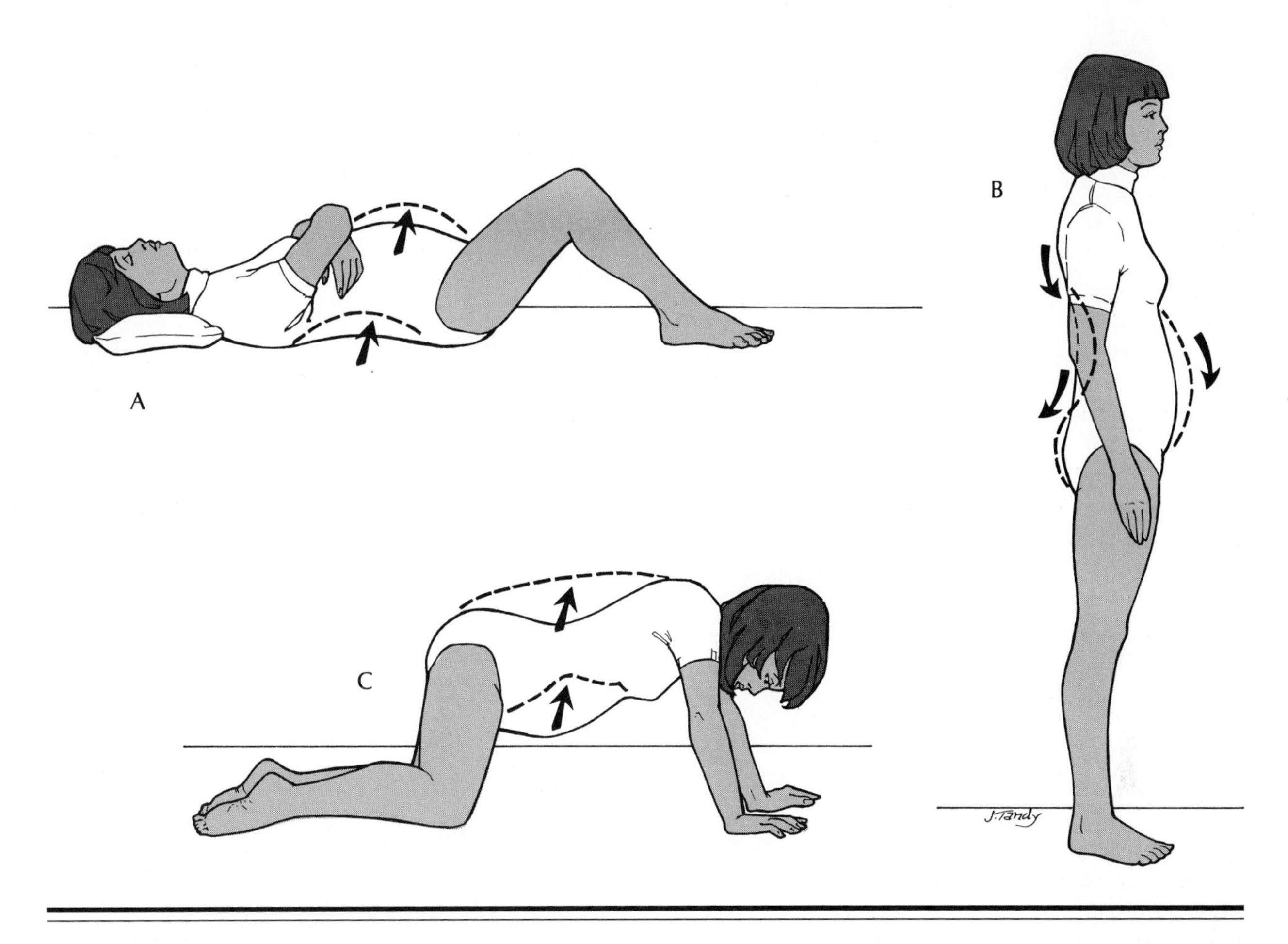

Figure 11–6. Pelvic tilt exercise relieves exaggerated lumbosacral curvature of pregnancy. The exercise may be done in three ways: **A,** lying supine; **B,** standing; **C,** on hands and knees.

back, she puts her feet flat on the floor with her knees in the air to help prevent further strain and discomfort (Figure 11–6). She relieves the curvature in her back by pushing the raised area toward the hard surface. She or her partner can place hands under her back to feel the change in body alignment. It is then easier to apply the pelvic tilt when she is standing with her back against a wall and to maintain this body alignment throughout the day. The pelvic tilt includes the simultaneous movements of tightening the buttocks and abdominal muscles and "tucking under" the buttocks. The exercise can be performed on hands and knees and used while sitting in a chair.

The application of proper body mechanics throughout pregnancy, in conjunction with proper posture, is also important. The pregnant woman should not curve her back by bending over to lift or pick up items from the floor. The strain is felt in the muscles of the back. Instead, leg muscles should be used to do the work. The woman can keep her back straight by bending her knees to lower her body into the squatting position (Figure 11–7). Her feet should be placed 12–18 in. apart to maintain body balance. When lifting heavy objects such as a child, she should place one foot slightly in front of the other, keeping it flat on the floor, and lower herself to the other knee. The object is held close to her body for lifting. This same principle of keeping the back straight and bending the knees applies when the woman sits down or gets out of a chair.

Work heights that require constant bending of the back can contribute to backache and therefore should be adjusted as necessary. Women who do not experience backache in pregnancy may become aware of it as they bend to change a newborn's diaper in the early puerperium.

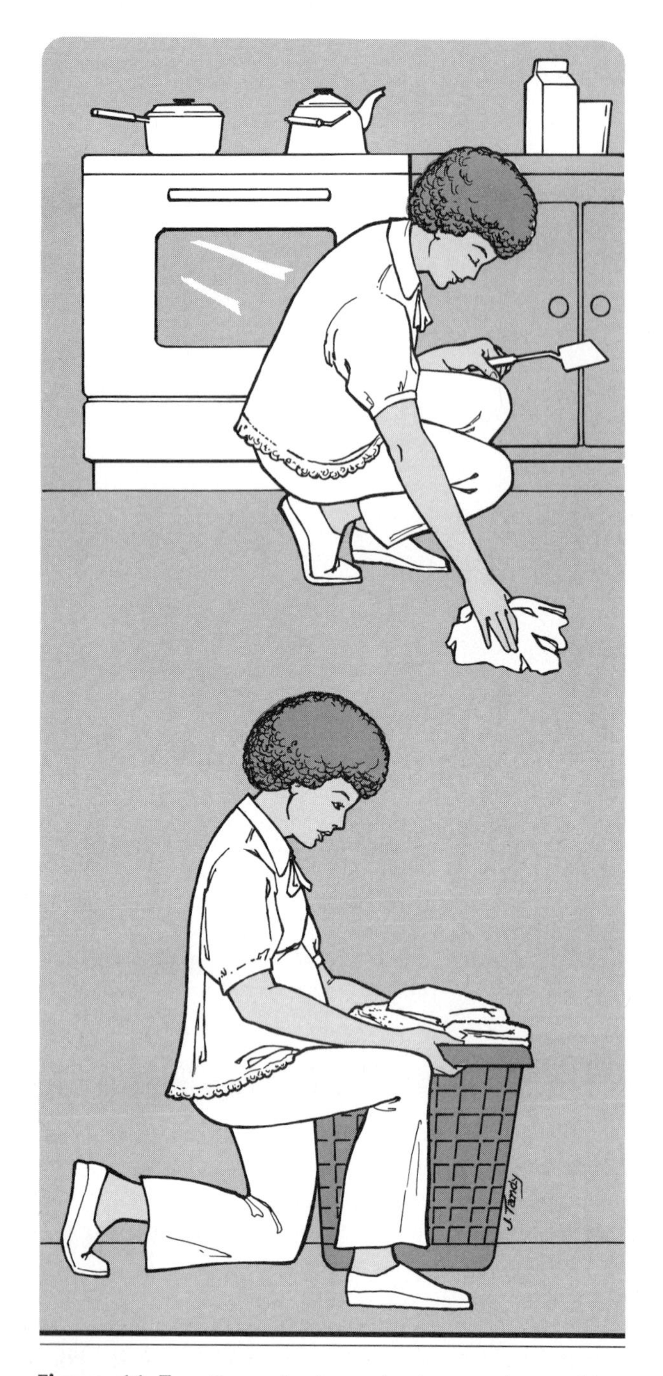

Figure 11–7. Proper body mechanics must be used by the pregnant woman when picking up objects from floor level or when lifting objects.

A pendulous abdomen contributes to backache by increasing the curvature of the back. The use of a good supportive maternity girdle is discussed in the section on clothing, as is the role of high-heeled shoes in increasing the lumbosacral curvature (p. 283).

Leg Cramps

Leg cramps are painful muscle spasms in the gastrocnemius muscles. They occur most frequently at night when the woman has gone to bed but may occur at other times. Extension of the foot can often cause leg cramps, so the pregnant woman should be warned not to do so while doing exercises for childbirth preparation or when she is resting.

It has been suggested that leg cramps are caused by an imbalance of the calcium/phosphorus ratio in the body (a high serum phosphorus content creates a hypocalcemic situation) (Williams, 1977), but this idea is controversial.

Leg cramps are more common in the third trimester because of increased weight of the uterus on the nerves supplying the lower extremities. Fatigue and poor circulation in the lower extremities contribute to this problem.

Interventions. Immediate relief of the muscle spasm is achieved by stretching the muscle. This is most effectively done with the woman lying on her back and another person pressing the woman's knee down to straighten her leg while pushing her foot toward her leg (Figure 11–8). Foot flexion techniques, massage, and warm packs can be used to alleviate discomfort from leg cramps.

Drinking large quantities of milk increases the calcium/phosphorus imbalance in the body because of the large quantities of phosphorus that milk provides. The high phosphorus levels depress the serum calcium. Therefore, the physician may recommend that the woman drink no more than a pint of milk daily and take calcium lactate, or the physician may allow a quart of milk daily and prescribe aluminum hydroxide gel. Aluminum hydroxide gel stops the action of phosphorus on calcium by absorbing the phosphorus and eliminating it directly through the intestinal tract. The treatment recommendations depend on the frequency of the leg cramps.

When planning a treatment regimen, one must be careful not to totally exclude milk from the woman's diet, because it is an excellent source of other essential nutrients.

Faintness

Faintness is experienced by many pregnant women, especially in warm, crowded areas. The cause of faintness is a combination of changes in

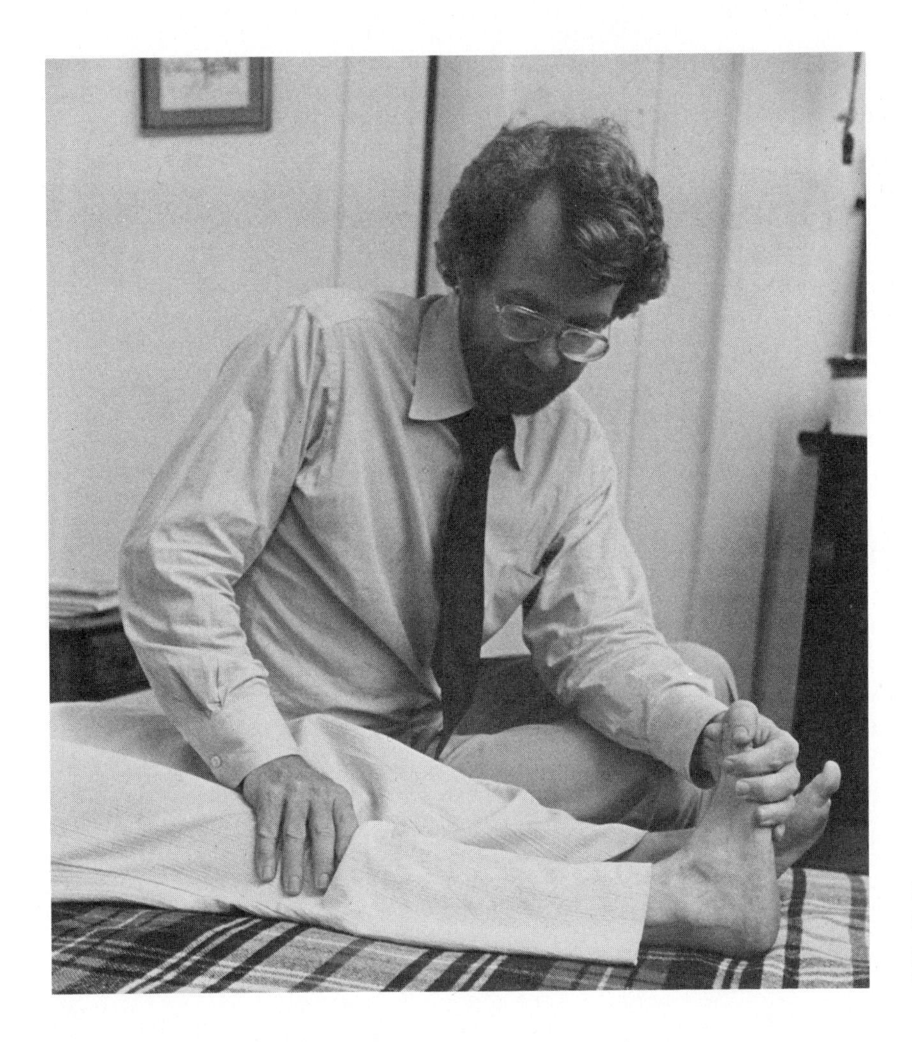

Figure 11–8. The expectant father can help relieve the woman's painful leg cramps by dorsiflexing the foot while holding her knee flat.

the blood volume and postural hypotension due to venous pooling of blood in the dependent veins. Sudden change of position or standing for prolonged periods can cause this sensation, and fainting can occur.

Interventions. If faintness is experienced from prolonged standing or from being in a warm, crowded room, the woman should lower her body to a sitting position, with her head lowered between her legs. If this procedure does not help, the woman should be assisted to an area where she can lie down and get fresh air. When arising from a resting position, she should move slowly.

Shortness of Breath

Shortness of breath occurs as the uterus rises into the abdomen and causes pressure on the diaphragm. This problem worsens in the last trimester as the enlarged uterus presses directly on the diaphragm, decreasing vital capacity. When lightening occurs in the last few weeks of pregnancy in the primigravida, she will experience considerable relief. Because the multigravida does not usually experience lightening until labor, shortness of breath will continue throughout her pregnancy.

Interventions. During the day, relief can be found by sitting straight in a chair and by using proper posture when standing. If distress is great at night, the woman can sleep propped up in bed, with several pillows behind her head and shoulders.

Nursing Actions

As described in this chapter, there is a fairly predictable pattern of concerns specific to the different trimesters of pregnancy. The health care of the maternity patient with these discomforts and concerns becomes more effective with the use of problem-oriented record-keeping. The PORK approach provides a system for obtaining a defined data base, a complete problem list, plans of care, and progress notes relating to the problem list. The plan of care for each identified problem includes diagnostic, therapeutic, and educational plans. The progress notes follow the SOAP format: subjective and objective information, assessment, and plans for each problem.

This format is designed to be used by all health care personnel when recording narrative notes and discharge notes. Flow sheets may be developed by the staff to aid in following the progress of specific problems. This system also provides an audit mechanism that can be used to correct deficiencies found in patient care. The expected outcome is improved patient care resulting from completeness, continuity, and consistency of care (Weed, 1969).

A basic responsibility of the nurse caring for the pregnant woman is to continually assess and anticipate the presence of discomforts. The nurse should be aware of appropriate interventions and should be able to evaluate the effectiveness of the relief measures used by the mother. If these methods are not effective, the nurse must determine why they are not helpful. Is it a result of inaccurate assessment of the source of discomfort or of incomplete patient education? The patient may not be using the self-care measures correctly, or the plan may include ineffective or inappropriate relief measures for this individual. After the situation is reevaluated, nursing interventions can be changed as necessary.

The major problem of prenatal care is maintenance of the intrauterine pregnancy. A related problem is the woman's reactions to the changes in her body and life-style she undergoes because of her pregnancy.

The following SOAP narrative note is an example of this nursing process. Mrs. B., gravida II para I, is 7 months pregnant. Her daughter is 18 months old.

Problem: Backache.
Subjective: "My back is really starting to bother me now. I can hardly pick up Sarah any more. I don't know what I'll do!"
Objective: Her posture exaggerates the curvature of her spine. She walks with her hand on the middle of her back as she enters the room.
Assessment: Back discomfort is causing increased distress for Mrs. B. She needs information about the relationship of her changing shape and body alignment and has to use good body mechanics when lifting her daughter.
Plan: Focus on educational needs in this area.

1. Explain causes of backache during pregnancy.
2. Teach use of leg muscles when lifting.
3. Discuss ways of limiting amount of lifting required.
4. Teach pelvic tilt exercises to be done twice a day.
5. If other measures do not provide enough comfort, discuss the helpfulness of a good supportive girdle.

COMMON CONCERNS DURING PREGNANCY

Breast Care

Whether the pregnant woman plans to bottle- or breast-feed her infant, proper support of the breasts is important to promote comfort, retain breast shape, and prevent back strain, particularly if the breasts become large and pendulous. The sensitivity of the breasts in pregnancy is also relieved by good support.

Because there is no voluntary muscle tissue in the breasts, loss of shape will occur if the woman does not wear a supportive brassiere. Many people falsely believe that sagging breasts are a result of breast-feeding. Breasts do become heavier when nursing, but it is the lack of proper support that causes tissues to sag.

A well-fitting supportive brassiere has the following basic qualities:

1. Straps are wide and do not stretch (elastic straps soon begin to lose their support with the weight of the breasts and constant washing).
2. All breast tissue fits comfortably into the bra cup.

3. The brassiere has tucks or other devices to expand its size with the enlarging chest circumference.
4. The nipple line is supported approximately midway between elbow and shoulder. At the same time, the brassiere is not pulled up in the back by the weight of the breasts.

Cleanliness of breasts is important, especially as the woman begins to produce colostrum. Colostrum, which can form crusts on the nipples, should be softened with the use of an ointment such as Massé cream and then removed with warm water. If a woman is planning to breast-feed, she should not use soap on the nipples because of its drying effect, which can lead to cracking of the skin.

Preparation of the breasts for breast-feeding is meant to help toughen the nipples and to prevent their dryness and cracking when the baby begins to nurse. After a daily bath, the woman should use a rough towel to dry the nipples, but the rubbing should not be allowed to cause soreness or irritation. The nipple can then be rolled by grasping it between thumb and forefinger and gently rolling it for a short time each day. Again, the nipple should not be irritated by this process. Women who have sensitive skin, such as those with red hair, can benefit considerably from this preparation.

Nipple-rolling is more difficult with fat or inverted nipples, but women with these kinds of nipples still find this measure helpful in preparing their breasts for breast-feeding. Inverted nipples are relatively uncommon but do make breast-feeding difficult and sometimes too frustrating. Breast shields designed specifically for correcting inverted nipples can be worn during pregnancy. The shields appear to be the only measure that really helps if nipples are inverted. The mother will need to be committed to breast-feeding to succeed if she has truly inverted nipples.

A woman can test for inverted nipples by gently pinching the areola at the base of the nipple with her forefinger and thumb. If the nipple comes out even a little, it is not truly inverted, and the preparation for breast-feeding previously described will be helpful. If it retreats, breast-feeding will be difficult because the baby cannot grasp the nipple and surrounding area.

Oral stimulation of the nipple by the woman's partner during sex play is also an excellent technique for toughening the nipple for breast-feeding. If a couple enjoys this, they should be encouraged to continue throughout the pregnancy.

Clothing

Clothing in pregnancy can be an important factor in how the woman feels about herself and her appearance. Maternity clothes, however, can be expensive, and are worn for a relatively short period of time. The maternity clothes that were worn during a first pregnancy may not be seasonally appropriate for the next pregnancy. Women who can afford the maternity clothes they want and those who can sew can dress stylishly. However, for women in lower socioeconomic levels, the expense may be a problem. Possible solutions include buying used clothing and trading or exchanging maternity clothes with friends or relatives.

Clothing affects a woman's general comfort in pregnancy. Clothing should be loose and nonconstricting for both general comfort and the prevention of some of the specific discomforts of pregnancy. For example, restricting bands around the waist can be uncomfortable; those around the lower extremities, such as garters, can interfere with venous circulation and predispose to varicose veins or aggravate existing ones.

Maternity girdles are not considered necessary for most pregnant women, but some women who are accustomed to wearing girdles may feel more comfortable in continuing this practice during pregnancy. It is important for them to be aware that the girdle is for support and not for constriction of the abdomen. Women who have large, pendulous abdomens benefit considerable from a well-fitting supportive girdle. Without this support, the pendulous abdomen increases the curvature of the back and is a source of backache and general discomfort. Tight leg bands on girdles should be avoided.

High-heeled shoes aggravate back discomfort by increasing the curvature of the back and should not be worn if the women experiences backache or problems with balance. Shoes should fit properly and should feel comfortable.

Bathing

With the increase of perspiration and mucoid vaginal discharge that occurs in pregnancy, daily bathing is important. Bathtub bathing was a controversial subject because of a concern about water entering the vagina and causing infection. This controversy no longer exists. The only time the pregnant woman is not allowed to bathe in a bathtub is in the presence of ruptured membranes or vaginal bleeding. However, caution is needed, since balance becomes a problem in pregnancy. Rubber mats in the tub and use of hand grips are important safety measures.

Some pregnant women have had difficulty getting out of the bathtub without assistance. This predicament seems to occur when extremely warm water is used or in hot weather in the latter part of pregnancy.

Employment

Fetotoxic hazards in the environment, overfatigue, excessive physical strain, and medical or obstetric complications are the major deterrents to employment during pregnancy. Employment involving balance should be terminated during the last half of pregnancy to protect the mother.

Fetotoxic hazards in the environment are always a concern to the expectant couple. If the pregnant woman or the woman contemplating pregnancy is working in industry, she should contact her company physician or nurse about possible hazards in her work environment. Some industrial products, such as turpentine and lead paint (which are also occasionally found in the home), are considered toxic substances during pregnancy.

Many women continue working during pregnancy because their income is necessary for the family or because their career is personally satisfying and important to them. Others may feel a need to work throughout pregnancy to help prevent boredom, which often occurs in the initial transition from being employed to being at home.

Travel

Pregnant women often have many questions about the effects of travel on them and on their fetus. If medical or obstetric complications are not present, there are no restrictions on travel. Travel does not harm the fetus or mother, although it can increase the discomforts of pregnancy and the possibility of accidents.

Travel by automobile can be especially fatiguing, aggravating many of the discomforts of pregnancy. The pregnant woman needs frequent opportunities to get out of the car and walk. A good pattern to follow is to stop every two hours and walk around for approximately ten minutes. Seat belts should be worn low, under the abdomen, and should not fit tight. Although these restraints can cause internal damage in the event of an accident, statistics demonstrate that within the general population, greater mortality occurs as a result of ejection from the car. Thus seat belts and shoulder straps are recommended for the pregnant woman (Crosby and Costiloe, 1971).

As pregnancy progresses, flying or travel by train is recommended for long-distance traveling. In the last month of pregnancy, airlines require a statement from the woman's physician before she is allowed to fly. The availability of medical care at one's destination also becomes an important factor for the near-term pregnant woman who is traveling.

Rest and Exercise

Adequate rest in pregnancy is important for both physical and emotional health. The pregnant woman experiences an increased need for sleep throughout her pregnancy, particularly in the first and last trimesters, when she tires easily. She will find that she has less resilience throughout pregnancy when she does not get adequate rest.

Eight hours of sleep is essential for many women, but individuals have varying needs. Time to rest during the day is also important. Finding this time may be difficult for mothers of small children and for women who work. The nurse can help the expectant mother examine her daily schedule and develop a realistic plan for short periods of rest and relaxation.

Sleeping becomes more difficult during the last trimester of pregnancy with the enlarging abdomen, increased micturition, and activity of the fetus. It becomes difficult for the pregnant woman to find a comfortable position. Figure 11–9 shows a position most pregnant women find helpful. Various methods of progressive relaxation of the mind and muscles similar to exercises taught in prepared childbirth classes can be helpful in preparing the woman for sleep. The most simple technique involves the gradual contraction and relaxation of muscle groups, beginning with flexion of the feet and moving upward to the top of the head.

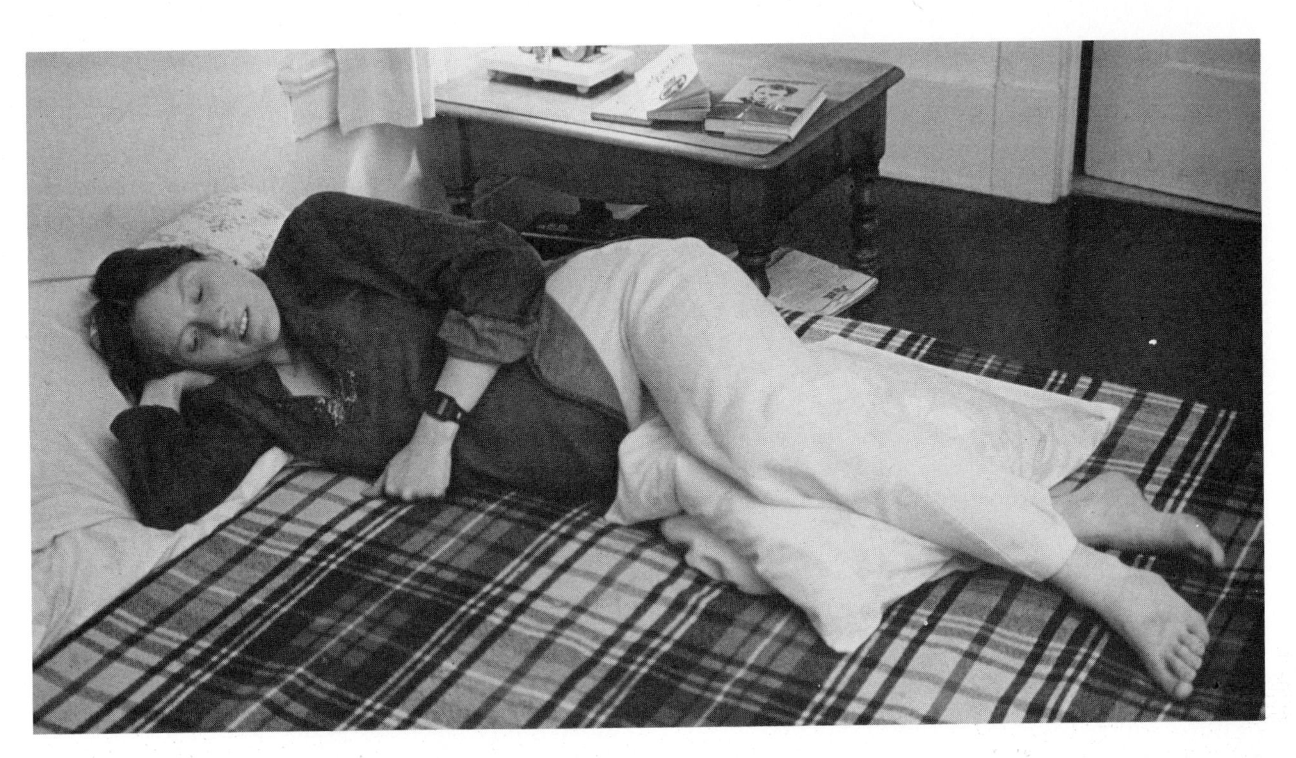

Figure 11–9. Position for relaxation and rest as pregnancy progresses.

Normal participation in exercise can continue throughout pregnancy. Pregnancy, however, is not the appropriate time to introduce new strenuous sports such as tennis. The woman should check with her physician about strenuous sports in which she is skilled, such as skiing, diving, and horseback riding. Walking is an excellent exercise for pregnant women and is recommended as a daily outdoor activity.

Exercise plays a role in prevention of constipation, in body conditioning, and in good mental hygiene. However, an important rule to follow, especially during pregnancy, is not to overdo.

Sexual Activity

As a result of the physiologic, anatomic, and emotional changes of pregnancy, the couple usually has many questions and concerns about sexual activity during pregnancy. These questions most commonly relate to concerns about injuring the baby or the mother and about changes in sexual desire of the couple.

In the past, only minimal information on this subject could be found in medical and nursing textbooks and in literature for expectant couples. Generally, couples were warned to refrain from intercourse in the last six to eight weeks of pregnancy and to continue their abstinence for another period of time after the baby was born. It was thought that abstaining from sexual activity would help prevent discomfort for the mother and, theoretically, prevent infection, premature rupture of the membranes, and premature labor. In practice, however, these fears seem to be unfounded. With the growing amount of research about sexual response in the general population, reliable information is being gathered concerning the sexual activity of expectant couples. Valid obstetric contraindications to coitus in pregnancy are limited only to pregnancies in which bleeding complications are present, membranes are ruptured, or there are other complications that may lead to premature delivery.

The expectant mother experiences many changes in sexual desire and response; they seem to be related to the various discomforts that occur during pregnancy. In the first trimester, many women experience loss of desire for sexual intercourse, which is probably related to the degree of fatigue or nausea and vomiting they are experiencing. For women who develop breast tenderness, any fondling of the breasts may no longer be desirable. To prevent discomfort, it may be necessary to use coital postions in which there is no direct pressure on the pregnant woman's breasts.

Probably the optimum time for sexual activity during pregnancy is in the second trimester. The excessive fatigue, nausea, and vomiting have subsided, and with the vascular congestion of the pelvis, the woman may experience greater sexual satisfaction than she experienced prior to pregnancy.

Interest in coitus usually begins to decrease again around the third trimester, as the woman's abdomen begins to protrude prominently. She is more uncomfortable in general, and fatigue occurs frequently. If they are not already being used, alternative coital positions other than the traditional male superior position will have to be considered. Other positions are side-by-side, female superior, and rear-entry. Alternatives to intercourse, such as mutual masturbation, can be considered. It is important, however, that the couple feel comfortable with their chosen alternatives.

The pregnant woman may be alarmed by the orgasmic changes that may occur in the last trimester. Instead of the rhythmic contractions of orgasm, she may experience a contraction lasting up to one minute, which may be followed by cramps and backache (Zalor, 1976). Masturbation creates a more intense contraction than occurs with intercourse (Masters and Johnson, 1966). There is no evidence, however, that these contractions cause premature labor in the large majority of pregnant women (Solberg et al., 1973).

There have been reports in the literature of maternal deaths from air embolism caused by forceful blowing of air into the vagina during orogenital sex play (Aronson and Nelson, 1967; Fatteh et al., 1973).

Sexual activity does not have to include intercourse. Many of the nurturing and sexual needs of the pregnant woman can be satisfied by cuddling, kissing, and being held by her partner. The warm, sensual feelings that are present during these activities can be an end in themselves. Increased use of masturbation, however, may be important for her partner.

The sexual needs of men during their partner's pregnancy have not been studied. Their sexual desires, however, are also affected by many factors in pregnancy, such as their previous relationship with their partner, acceptance of the pregnancy, attitudes toward their partner's change of appearance, and concern about hurting the expectant mother or baby.

It is important for the expectant couple to be aware of their changing sexual desires, the normality of these changes, and the importance of communicating these changes to each other so that they can make nurturing adaptations. The nurse has an important role in helping the expectant couple facilitate this process. Thus it is essential that the nurse feel comfortable about her sexuality and be well informed about the subject. In counseling expectant couples, an accepting and nonjudgmental attitude is important. The couple must feel free to express concerns about sexual activity, and the nurse must be able to respond and give anticipatory guidance in a comfortable manner.

Occasionally an expectant mother will initiate discussion about her sexual concerns, especially if she feels that she has good rapport with the nurse. More often the nurse must introduce the matter.

A statement such as "Many couples experience changes in sexual desire in pregnancy" can initiate the discussion. This generalization can be followed by an exploration of the couple's personal experience (Green, 1975). The nurse can ask a question such as "What kind of changes have you experienced?" rather than "Have you experienced any changes?"

The presence of both partners during sexual counseling is most effective in helping to facilitate communication between them.

Smoking

Many studies in the last several years have shown that infants of mothers who smoke have a lower birth weight than babies of mothers who do not smoke. The specific mechanism involved is not known, but various theories have been proposed.

Many authorities theorize that passage of carbon monoxide through the placenta produces intrauterine hypoxia. The carbon monoxide blood levels are increased in smoking mothers, and the carbon monoxide attaches to hemoglobin before oxygen does (Underwood et al., 1965). Others suggest that the nicotine in tobacco has a direct effect on the fetus through its vasoconstrictive actions.

A relatively recent study with a different orientation was conducted by Davies et al. (1976). They investigated the various effects of cigarette smoking in the latter half of pregnancy on maternal weight gain and fetal growth. They studied 1159 mother-infant pairs and found that pregnant women who did not smoke gained significantly more weight than women who were heavy smokers (15 cigarettes/day), with an intermediate weight gain by light-to-moderate smokers (1–14 cigarettes/day). The size of the infants varied similarly. Infants born to nonsmokers were larger than those born to heavy smokers. Drawing on their study, Davies et al. suggested that increasing weight gain in smoking mothers might help to prevent the harmful effects of smoking on fetal growth.

This study and others demonstrate that any decrease in smoking during pregnancy will result in better fetal outcome. Pregnancy may be a difficult time for a woman to stop smoking, but she should be encouraged to reduce the number of cigarettes she smokes daily.

Dental Care

Proper dental hygiene is important in pregnancy. In spite of such discomforts as nausea and vomiting, possible ptyalism (excessive salivation), and heartburn, regular oral hygiene must not be neglected. The hyperemia of pregnancy, however, may cause conditions that discourage the woman from taking proper care of her teeth. These conditions are hypertrophy and tenderness of the gums and susceptibility to pain associated with her teeth.

Many people believe that the fetus derives its calcium from the mother's teeth to aid in the development of its tooth and skeletal structure. This is not true. The calcium in the mother's teeth cannot be altered. The calcium and phosphorus required by the fetus are obtained from the mother's diet.

The pregnant woman is encouraged to have a dental checkup early in her pregnancy. Women who neglect to obtain dental care prior to pregnancy become aware of dental problems during this time and thus may associate these problems with pregnancy. General dental repair and extractions can be done during pregnancy, preferably under local anesthetic. Dental x-ray examinations and extensive dental work should be delayed when possible until after delivery. Dental care needed during pregnancy requires consultation between the dentist and the health care professional supervising the pregnancy.

Immunizations

All women of childbearing age need to be fully aware of the risks of receiving specific immunizations if pregnancy is possible. Expectant women, especially those who intend to travel throughout the world, should be aware of the immunizations that are contraindicated during pregnancy. In addition, it is important that expectant women clearly understand the recommendations that are made regarding immunizations at certain times, as when influenza epidemics occur.

Immunizations with attentuated live viruses should not be given in pregnancy because of the teratogenic effect of the live viruses on the developing embryo. Vaccinations using killed viruses can be used. Recommendations for immunizations during pregnancy are given in Table 11-1.

Table 11-1. Recommendations of American College of Obstetricians and Gynecologists for Specific Immunizations During Pregnancy*

Immunizations	Notes
Tetanus-diphtheria	May be given as needed
Poliomyelitis	Not recommended routinely for adults but mandatory in epidemics
Mumps	Contraindicated
Rubella	Contraindicated
Influenza	Recommended for those with serious underlying disease
Typhoid	Recommended if traveling in endemic region
Smallpox	Avoid in pregnancy unless there has been probable exposure
Yellow fever	Contraindicated except for unavoidable exposure
Cholera	Only to meet travel requirements
Rabies	Same as nonpregnant
Hepatitis-A	After exposure or before travel in developing countries

*From Pritchard, J. A., and MacDonald, P. 1976. *Williams obstetrics.* 15th ed. New York: Appleton-Century-Crofts, p. 258.

Medications

Factors that can cause malformations in the developing embryo are called *teratogenic agents*. Regardless of etiology, malformations in the embryo can develop from the time of fertilization until the end of the first trimester. Organogenesis occurs during this time. Medications should thus be avoided in the first trimester, since the teratogenicity of most drugs and combinations of drugs is not known. This is a difficult task, however, since development of vital structures such as the brain begins before most women are aware that they are pregnant.

The teratogenic effects of medications commonly prescribed in this country are being studied. A recent study has found that infants of mothers who took meprobamate (Equanil, Miltown) or chlordiazepoxide (Librium) during early pregnancy produced a higher than normal rate of birth defects (Rodman, 1976). Similar studies involve medications prescribed for specific medical problems, such as phenytoin (Dilantin), which is given to control epilepsy. In a few instances, infants of women taking phenytoin have been born with deformed palates and lips (Rodman, 1976).

Teratogenic effects do not usually occur after the first trimester, but medications still pass through the placenta to the fetus. Although the amount that reaches the fetus is usually small, the medication can affect the fetus in much the same way that an adult is affected by an overdosage. For example, the use of anticoagulants to treat thromboembolism in the mother can interfere with clotting factors in the fetus; however, this risk is lessened by frequent monitoring of prothrombin time in the mother, accompanied by appropriate changes in dosages of the anticoagulants. Heparin does not cross the placenta, so it is safer for the fetus than warfarin (Coumadin) and bishydroxycoumarin (Dicumerol) (Rodman, 1976). Table 13–3 (p. 375) lists selected drugs and their possible effects on the fetus.

Medications sold over the counter may be as dangerous as prescription drugs. Studies involving aspirin demonstrate that it induces a degree of platelet dysfunction in the fetus. Analgesic compounds containing salicylates in combination with caffeine or phenacetin are associated with increased incidence of anemia, hemorrhage, prolonged gestation, perinatal mortality, and low birth weight (Pritchard and MacDonald, 1976).

Caution should be the watchword when working with pregnant women who have been taking any of these medications. Although some studies demonstrate conclusive results, many cases are isolated, and the mother should not be unduly alarmed. When a pregnant woman asks about the harmful effects of medication in pregnancy, it is important to find out why she is asking before listing examples. It is essential that the pregnant woman check with her physician about medications that she was taking when pregnancy occurred and about any nonprescription drugs that she is contemplating using. A good rule to follow is that the advantage of using a particular medication must outweigh the risks. Any medication with possible teratogenic effects must be avoided in the first trimester.

Women who are addicted to heroin or other narcotics usually have addicted babies. These infants suffer from withdrawal symptoms after birth and must be observed closely for symptoms and treated appropriately. Studies show that the incidence of withdrawal symptoms in newborns of mothers maintained on methadone is similar to the withdrawal incidence when their mothers are untreated heroin addicts (Henderlich, 1977). Interestingly, the newborns do not seem to be depressed by the heroin at birth, as demonstrated by Apgar scores, because of the tolerance developed in utero. The effects of drug addiction on pregnancy are discussed further in Chapter 13 (p. 374).

The possible teratogenic effects of such drugs as lysergic acid diethylamide (LSD) have not been clearly delineated. Some women who conceived after taking the drug have given birth to babies with limb defects. However, proof that LSD can cause chromosomal damage is not available.

Alcohol

Alcohol taken in even minimal to moderate amounts during pregnancy may be harmful to the fetus. Small quantities of alcohol do reach the fetus when the pregnant woman has one or two drinks, but the significant factor is the resultant blood alcohol level. For some women 2 ounces of alcohol per day could produce a blood alcohol level with teratogenic effects upon the fetus.

Chronic alcoholism does become a problem because of the maternal malnutrition that usually occurs in conjunction with the drinking. Fetal underdevelopment occurs as a result of malnutrition. Infants of alcoholic women show the same kind of withdrawal symptoms at birth that occur with the infants of drug-addicted mothers. See Chapter 13 for additional discussion about the effects of alcoholism on the fetus and mother.

NUTRITION

Efficient childbearing is influenced by many factors, but the most important is health of the mother. Pregnancy is affected not only by the nutritional intake of the woman during pregnancy but also by her nutritional status prior to the pregnancy. Good nutrition is the result of proper eating for a lifetime, not just during pregnancy. The age of the mother is also an important factor. An expectant teenager has the additional needs of pregnancy superimposed on her needs for continued growth. This situation presents a double dilemma, since nutritional intake tends to be deficient during teenage years.

An additional factor is the parity of a woman. The mother's nutritional needs and pregnancy outcome are influenced by the number of pregnancies she has had and the interval between them.

The 1969 White House Conference on Nutrition recognized as its most pressing goal the setting of norms for pregnant women. The Conference's panel on National Goals and Objectives for pregnant women put forth the following statement:

> There must be a national affirmation that every woman has the right to high quality and high standard health care. This includes food that will prepare her for and carry her through childbirth and permit her infant to flourish. It affirms that the right to adequate nutrition is an inseparable part of the basic right to health care and that women require and are entitled to sufficient amounts of nutritious food.*

A widely known program is the Special Supplemental Food Program for Women, Infants and Children, or the WIC Program. It is sponsored by the Food and Nutrition Service of the U.S. Department of Agriculture. Supplemental foods for infants, young children (under 5 years of age), mothers with low incomes, and mothers in rural areas are supplied by the WIC Program. Under its provisions, persons judged to be at nutritional risk by medical or nutritional professionals, because of low income and patterns of inadequate nutrition, are eligible to receive free each month about $20 worth of high-protein, high-vitamin, and high-mineral foods. These supplements are coupled with dietary counseling. In order to qualify for such a program, participants must secure routine health care maintenance and physical examinations through facilities such as child health, family planning, or prenatal clinics.

The effects of the mother's nutritional status on the fetus have been demonstrated by animal studies. Such experiments have shown that nutritional deficiencies may cause smaller litters, increased malformations, and smaller offspring. Nutrition and many other factors are interrelated; more evidence points to the role of prenatal nutrition in infant well-being (Committee on Maternal Nutrition, 1970).

Conditions that occurred in several European countries during World War II, as well as experiments conducted during that period, led to informative conclusions as to the role of nutrition in pregnancy. The following dietary factors were recognized as affecting the outcome of pregnancy (Committee on Maternal Nutrition, 1970):

1. The nutritional status of the mother prior to pregnancy.
2. The severity of the deficiency and its duration.
3. The time of gestation during which the deficiency occurs.

As a result of the work of researchers such as Winick (1968, 1977) it is now possible to measure the effects of nutrient deficiency on cell and organ growth. Because the DNA content of mammalian cells remains a constant factor, the cell size and cell number of various organs can be estimated. Two formulas are used to obtain the information needed:

1. $\dfrac{\text{Amount of DNA in tissue}}{\text{Amount of DNA per cell (6.22 ng)}} = \text{Number of cells in organ or tissue}$

*From Jacobsen, H. N. Dec. 1974. Maternal nutrition since the 1969 White House Conference. *Nutrition News.* 37(4):13.

$$2.\ \frac{\text{Amount of protein in tissue sample}}{\text{Total DNA of sample}} = \text{Cell size}$$

Nutritional effects on growth during the prenatal period and early development have been measured using these formulas.

The result is the theory that growth occurs in three overlapping stages: (a) growth by increase in cell number, (b) growth by increases in cell number and cell size, and (c) growth by increase in cell size alone. It is now thought that nutritional problems that interfere with cell division may have permanent consequences; but if the nutritional insult occurs when cells are mainly enlarging, the changes are reversible when normal nutrition occurs. These concepts are of supreme importance when related to brain development. A deficiency of vital nutrients does interfere with neuronal division, and its effects may continue into the neonatal period for about 2½ years, until myelination and other aspects of brain development are complete.

Growth of fetal and maternal tissues requires increased quantities of essential dietary components. Table 11-2 compares the *recommended dietary allowances* (RDA) of the National Academy of Sciences for nonpregnant females with those for pregnant and lactating teenage and adult women.

Most of the recommended nutrients can be obtained by eating a well-balanced diet each day. The basic food groups and recommended amounts during pregnancy and lactation are presented in Table 11-3.

Maternal Weight Gain

It has been shown that a relationship exists between maternal weight gain and infant birth weight. A weight gain of 9-12 kg (20-30 lb) is recommended, with the average being 12 kg (25 lb). The weight gain should depend on the height and bone structure of the individual and also on the prepregnant nutritional state.

The patient whose weight gain during pregnancy is inadequate has an increased risk of delivering a low-birth-weight infant. This is par-

Table 11-2. Recommended Dietary Allowances for Women 15-35 Years of Age*

	Teenage allowance (15-18 years)			Adult female allowance (19-35 years)		
Nutrient	Nonpregnant	Pregnant	Lactating	Nonpregnant	Pregnant	Lactating
Energy, calories	2100	2400	2600	2000	2300	2500
Protein (gm)	48	78	68	46	76	66
Vitamin A (IU)	4000	5000	6000	4000	5000	6000
(Re)	800	1000	1200	800	1000	1200
Vitamin D (IU)	400	400	400	—	400	400
Vitamin E (IU)	12	15	15	12	15	15
Ascorbic acid (mg)	45	60	80	45	60	80
Folacin (mg)[†]	0.4	0.8	0.6	0.4	0.8	0.6
Niacin (mg)	14	16	18	13	15	17
Riboflavin (mg)	1.4	1.7	1.9	1.2	1.5	1.7
Thiamine (mg)	1.1	1.4	1.4	1.0	1.3	1.3
Vitamin B_6 (mg)	2.0	2.5	2.5	2.0	2.5	2.5
Vitamin B_{12} (μg)	3.0	4.0	4.0	3.0	4.0	4.0
Calcium (mg)	1200	1600	1600	800	1200	1200
Phosphorus (mg)	1200	1600	1600	800	1200	1200
Iodine (mμg)	115	140	165	100	125	150
Iron (mg)[‡]	18	18+	18+	18	18+	18
Magnesium (mg)	300	450	450	300	450	450
Zinc (mg)	15	20	25	15	20	25

*From Food and Nutrition Board. 1974. *Recommended dietary allowances.* 8th ed. Washington, D.C.: National Academy of Sciences, National Research Council.

[†]Folacin allowances refer to dietary sources as determined by lactobacillus casein assay. Pure forms of folacin may be effective in doses less than one-fourth of the recommended dietary allowance.

[‡]This iron requirement cannot be met by ordinary diets. Therefore the use of 30-60 mg supplemental iron is recommended.

Table 11-3. Daily Food Plan for Pregnancy and Lactation*

Food group	Nutrients provided	Food source	Recommended daily amount during pregnancy	Recommended daily amount during lactation
Dairy products	Protein; riboflavin; vitamins A, D, and others; calcium; phosphorus; zinc; magnesium	Milk – whole, 2%, skim, dry, buttermilk Cheeses – hard, semisoft, cottage Yogurt – plain, low-fat Soybean milk – canned, dry	3-4 eight-ounce cups; used plain or with flavoring, in shakes, soups, puddings, custards, cocoa Calcium in 1 c milk equivalent to 1½ c cottage cheese, 1½ oz hard or semisoft cheese, 1 c yogurt, 1½ c ice cream (high in fat and sugar)	4-5 eight-ounce cups; equivalent amount of cheeses, yogurts, etc.
Meat group	Protein; iron; thiamine, niacin, and other vitamins; minerals	Beef, pork, veal, lamb, poultry, animal organ meats, fish, eggs; legumes, nuts, seeds, peanut butter, grains in proper vegetarian combination (vitamin B_{12} supplement needed)	2 servings (1 serving = 3-4 oz) Combination in amounts necessary for same nutrient equivalent (varies greatly)	2½ servings
Grain products, whole grain or enriched	B vitamins; iron; whole grain also has zinc, magnesium, and other trace elements; provides fiber	Breads and bread products such as cornbread, muffins, waffles, hot cakes, biscuits, dumplings; cereals; pastas; rice	4-5 servings daily: 1 serving = 1 slice bread, ¾ c or 1 oz dry cereal, ½ c rice or pasta	5 servings
Fruits and fruit juices	Vitamins A and C; minerals; raw fruits for roughage	Citrus fruits and juices, melons, berries, all other fruits and juices	3-4 servings (1 serving for vitamin C): 1 serving = 1 medium fruit, ½-1 c fruit, 4 oz orange or grapefruit juice	Same as for pregnancy
Vegetables and vegetable juices	Vitamins A and C; minerals; provides roughage	Leafy green vegetables; deep yellow or orange vegetables such as carrots, sweet potatoes, squash,	3-4 servings (1 or 2 servings should be raw; 1 serving of dark green or deep yellow vegetable for vitamin A): 1 serving	Same as for pregnancy, except 1-2 servings of foods that provide vitamin A

*The pregnant woman should eat regularly, three meals a day, with nutritious snacks of fruits, cheese, milk, or other foods between meals if desired. (More frequent but smaller meals are also recommended.) One should diet only under the guidance of one's primary health care provider.

Four to six glasses (8 oz) of water and a total of eight to ten cups (8 oz) total fluid should be consumed daily. Water is an essential nutrient.

An occasional alcoholic drink is permissible, but the expectant woman should avoid frequent or heavy drinking.

Table 11-3 Cont'd.

Food group	Nutrients provided	Food source	Recommended daily amount during pregnancy	Recommended daily amount during lactation
		tomatoes; green vegetables such as peas, green beans, broccoli; other vegetables such as beets, cabbage, potatoes, corn, lima beans	= ½–1 c vegetable, 2 tomatoes, 1 medium potato	
Fats	Vitamins A and D; linoleic acid	Butter, cream cheese, fortified table spreads; cream, whipped cream, whipped toppings; avocado, mayonnaise, oil, nuts	As desired in moderation (high in calories): 1 serving = 1 tbsp butter or enriched margarine	Same as for pregnancy
Sugar and sweets		Sugar, brown sugar, honey, molasses	Occasionally, if desired, but not recommended	Same as for pregnancy
Desserts		Nutritious desserts such as puddings, custards, fruit whips, and crisps; other rich, sweet desserts and pastries	Occasionally, if desired (high in calories)	Same as for pregnancy
Beverages		Coffee, decaffeinated beverages, tea, bouillon, carbonated drinks	As desired, in moderation	Same as for pregnancy
Miscellaneous		Iodized salt, herbs, spices, condiments	As desired	Same as for pregnancy

*The pregnant woman should eat regularly, three meals a day, with nutritious snacks of fruits, cheese, milk, or other foods between meals if desired. (More frequent but smaller meals are also recommended.) One should diet only under the guidance of one's primary health care provider.

Four to six glasses (8 oz) of water and a total of eight to ten cups (8 oz) total fluid should be consumed daily. Water is an essential nutrient.

An occasional alcoholic drink is permissible, but the expectant woman should avoid frequent or heavy drinking.

ticularly true for the woman who is 10% or more below the recommended weight prior to conception. Although excessive weight gain has been thought to be an important factor in the development of preeclampsia-eclampsia, this belief is now being questioned; evidence fails to support a relationship between caloric intake and preeclampsia (Committee on Maternal Nutrition, 1970). However, energy intake above normal requirements does result in increased fat deposition and may contribute to obesity.

The optimum pattern of weight gain during pregnancy consists of a gain of 1–2 kg (2–4 lb) in the first trimester followed by a relatively linear rate of gain averaging 0.4 kg (slightly less than a pound) per week throughout the last two trimesters. The pattern of gain is more important than the total amount. Sudden sharp increases in weight after the 20th week of pregnancy may indicate excessive water retention and should be evaluated.

Nutritional Requirements

Calories

Calorie (cal) is a term used to designate that amount of heat required to raise the temperature of 1 gm of water 1 C. The *kilocalorie* (kcal) is equivalent to 1000 cal and is the unit used to express the energy value of food.

An extra daily caloric allowance of 200–300 cal above the individual requirement, or a total of 1800–2000 calories per day, throughout pregnancy is considered adequate for most women.

Protein

Protein supplies the amino acids (nitrogen) required for the growth and maintenance of tissue and other physiologic functions. Protein also contributes to the body's overall energy metabolism. In the absence of the preferred energy source, carbohydrate, about 58% of total dietary protein may become available as glucose and is oxidized as such to yield energy. The protein requirement for the pregnant woman is 70–80 gm/day.

An important source of protein is milk, which provides approximately half the protein in the diet. A quart of whole milk supplies 32 gm of protein, whereas the same quantity of skim or 2% low-fat milk yields 40 gm.

Milk can be incorporated into the diet in a variety of ways, including soups, puddings, custards, sauces, and yogurt. Beverages such as hot chocolate and milk-and-fruit drinks can also be included, but they are high in calories. Various kinds of hard and soft cheeses and cottage cheese are excellent protein sources, although cream cheese is categorized as a fat source only.

Protein equivalents for a cup of milk are 1 cup of yogurt, 1½ ounces of hard or semisoft cheese, ¼ cup (2 ounces) of cottage cheese, or 1½ cups of ice cream (which also contains more fat and calories).

In cases of allergy to milk or of those women who practice vegetarianism, dried or canned soy-base milk may be tolerated. It can be used in food preparation or as a beverage. Tofu, or soybean curd, may be used to replace cottage cheese. Goat's milk and goat's milk cheese sometimes may be tolerated by those who are allergic to cow's milk. Frequently, milk in cooked form is readily tolerated. Commercial coffee creamers have little or no nutritional value and must not replace milk in the diet.

Individuals who have difficulty drinking milk or who are vegetarians sometimes prepare a high-protein drink made from a mixture of ingredients. A quart of this drink prepared in the morning can be used between meals throughout the day and is an easy way to increase protein intake. Ingredients may vary but generally include 3 cups of milk (cow, goat, or soy), ½ cup dry nonfat milk powder (cow or soy), 2 tbsp wheat germ, 2 tbsp brewer's yeast or protein powders, fruit, and vanilla (eggs are optional). These ingredients are mixed together and stored in a covered container.

Meat, poultry, fish, eggs, and legumes are also good sources of protein. Small amounts of complete animal protein can be combined with partially complete plant protein for an excellent, well-utilized supply of protein. Several examples of complementary proteins are eggs and toast, tuna and rice, cereal and milk, spaghetti with meat sauce, macaroni and cheese, and a peanut butter sandwich.

Fats

Fats serve as valuable sources of energy for the body. The fat content of the maternal diet is associated with calorie level and linoleic acid intake. Linoleic acid is an essential nutrient found mainly in plant sources.

Research in the past decade has greatly increased our understanding of lipid and lipoprotein metabolism at all ages. This knowledge may eventually be used to normalize the cholesterol metabolism of the fetus and infant, thereby controlling these factors for a lifetime.

A high cholesterol level is the most common hyperlipidemia found in the perinatal state. It can be modified in the infant by changing dietary cholesterol and saturated fat. Commercial formulas with modified lipid content are now available for those concerned about dietary fat control in infant feeding (Tsang and Glueck, 1975).

It is difficult to determine the amount of maternal cholesterol being transferred to the fetus through the placenta. Fetal plasma levels do not correlate with maternal levels. The fetus does synthesize cholesterol, mainly in its liver and adrenals and in the placenta. The fetal brain synthesizes its own cholesterol, using primarily glucose, whereas the other sites use both glucose and acetate for cholesterol production.

Cholesterol content of cord blood is usually lower than adult levels. The lipoprotein content and composition may also be different (Tsang and Glueck, 1975).

Carbohydrates

Carbohydrates provide protective substances and bulk as well as energy. Carbohydrates contribute to the total need for calories. If the total caloric intake is not adequate, the body uses protein for energy. Protein then becomes unavailable for growth needs. In addition, protein breakdown leads to acidosis. Ketosis can be a problem, especially in diabetic patients, due to glycosuria, reduced alkaline reserves, and lipidemia. Intermittent glycosuria is not uncommon during pregnancy.

Carbohydrate needs increase, especially during the last two trimesters, as do the caloric needs for optimal weight gain and growth of the fetus, placenta, and other related maternal tissues. Productive carbohydrates can be found in milk, fruits, vegetables, and whole-grain cereals and breads.

Minerals

The absorption of minerals improves during pregnancy, and mineral allowances are increased to allow for the growth of new tissue.

Calcium and Phosphorus. Calcium and phosphorus are involved in energy and cell production and in acid-base buffering. Calcium is absorbed and utilized more efficiently during pregnancy, so the mother may store more than needed. Some calcium and phosphorus are required early in pregnancy, but most of the fetus's bone calcification occurs during the last two to three months. Teeth first begin to form at about the eighth week of gestation and are formed by birth. The six-year molars begin to calcify just before birth. This means that calcium is particularly important as a structural element. At term, the fetus contains about 28 gm of calcium.

If the mother's reserves of calcium are low, she should increase her calcium intake early in pregnancy. The minimum daily requirement of calcium for the pregnant adult woman is 1200 mg.

A diet that includes three to four cups of milk or an equivalent alternate and is nutritionally adequate for pregnancy will provide sufficient calcium and phosphorus. Frequently, the dietary intake of phosphorus exceeds the calcium intake. An excess of phosphorus can be avoided by limiting milk to one pint and meat to one serving daily and by ensuring that magnesium intake is adequate to effect proper utilization of calcium.

Table 11–4. Calcium Content of Some Common Foods*

Food	Amount	Calcium (mg)
Milk, whole	1 c (240 gm)	289
Turnip greens, raw	½ c	246
(cooked)	(½ c)	(58)
Cheese, American	1-inch cube (1 oz)	211
Salmon, pink, canned	3⅓ oz (100 gm)	196
White beans	½ c	144
Soybean curd, tofu	½ c (100 gm)	128
Almonds, shelled, dried	⅓ c	127
Cottage cheese	½ c (100 gm)	94
Broccoli, fresh, cooked	⅔ c (100 gm)	88
(frozen, cooked)	3½ oz (100 gm)	54
Soybean milk, fluid	1 c (240 gm)	50
Cabbage, raw	1 c	49
Blackberries, raw	1 c	46
Orange	1 small	41
Egg	1 large	29
Oatmeal, cooked	1 c	21
Bread, whole wheat, enriched	1 slice (23 gm)	20
Apricots	2–3 medium (100 gm)	17
Egg noodles, enriched	1 c	16
Artichoke, Jerusalem	4 small, 1½ in. in diameter	14
Banana	1 small, 6 in. long	8
Apple	1 small, 2 in. in diameter	7

*Modified from Bowes, A. D., and Church, C. F. 1975. *Food value of portions commonly used.* 11th ed. Rev. by Church, C. F., and Church, H. N. Philadelphia, J. B. Lippincott Co.

Sources of calcium are listed in Table 11–4. Phosphorus is readily supplied through calcium- and protein-rich foods, especially milk, eggs, and meat.

Iodine. Inorganic iodine is excreted in the urine during pregnancy. Enlargement of the thyroid gland may occur if iodine is not replaced by adequate dietary intake or additional supplement.

The iodine allowance of 125 μg/day can be met by using iodized salt. When sodium is restricted, the physician may prescribe an iodine supplement.

Sodium. The sodium ion is essential for proper metabolism. Sodium intake in the form of salt is never entirely curtailed during pregnancy, even when hypertension or preeclampsia-eclampsia is present. It is recommended that food be seasoned to taste during cooking. Salty foods such as potato chips, ham, sausages, and sodium-based seasonings can be eliminated to avoid excessive intake.

Zinc. Zinc was added to the National Academy of Sciences' list of recommended dietary allowances in 1974, when it was recognized as a nutrient factor affecting growth. The RDA in pregnancy is 20 mg. Sources include milk, liver, shellfish, and wheat bran.

Magnesium. Magnesium is essential for cellular metabolism and structural growth. The RDA for pregnancy is 450 mg. Sources include milk, whole grains, beet greens, nuts, legumes, and tea.

Iron. Normal red blood cell formation is dependent on adequate intake of several nutrients, including essential amino acids, vitamins B_6 and B_{12}, folic acid, ascorbic acid, and other vitamins and minerals, such as iron, copper, and zinc. If any one of these nutrients is missing from the diet, various types of anemia can result. Anemia is probably the most common problem in pregnancy, because nutritional anemia occurs frequently in nonpregnant women and the risk of anemia is increased by normal physiologic changes of pregnancy.

Anemia is generally defined as a decrease in the oxygen-carrying capacity of the blood. It results in a significant reduction in hemoglobin per 100 ml of blood, in the volume of packed red cells per 100 ml of blood (hematocrit), or in the number of erythrocytes per mililiter of blood.

The normal hematocrit in the nonpregnant woman is 38%–40%. In pregnancy the level may drop as low as 34%, even in the presence of adequate nutrition. This condition is called the *physiologic anemia of pregnancy* and is a result of increased plasma volume, which dilutes the hemoglobin and causes a drop in hemoglobin level between 24 and 32 weeks' gestation. After the 20th week, the fetus requires extra iron stores, which further contributes to the symptoms of anemia.

Thus anemia in pregnancy is caused by low iron stores, low nutrient intake, and increased needs. It is essential that the iron requirements balance the iron intake. This is a problem in nonpregnant women and even more so in pregnant ones. Total iron requirement for a single pregnancy varies from 750 to 900 mg, with the average being 800 mg (Kitay and Harbart, 1975). The iron cost of pregnancy is as follows:

Extra iron used in	
Products of conception	370 mg
Maternal blood increase	+290 mg
	660 mg
Less iron saved by cessation of menses	−120 mg
Total	540 mg

The Committee on Maternal Nutrition (1970) recommends that a simple iron salt such as ferrous gluconate, ferrous fumarate, or ferrous sulfate be given in amounts of 30–60 mg daily during the second and third trimesters of pregnancy. Supplements may not be given during the first trimester because of rapid changes that are occurring in the developing embryo. Ingesting more than 200 mg/day does not improve hematologic response significantly and may contribute to constipation.

By careful selection of foods high in iron, the daily iron intake can be increased considerably. Good sources of iron include liver and green leafy vegetables. Cereals are highly fortified with iron. Check the labels of various cereals to determine the approximate quantity of iron added. It should be noted that nonmeat sources of iron need an enhancing factor such as vitamin C to improve their absorption. Table 11–5 lists the iron content of certain foods.

Table 11–5. Iron Content of Selected Foods*

Food[†]	Weight or approximate measure	Iron (mg)	Food[†]	Weight or approximate measure	Iron (mg)
Prune juice	1 c	10.5	Sausage, bologna	2 slices	1.0
Beans, lima	1 c	5.6	Sweet potato	1 medium	1.0
Beans, red	1 c	4.6	Oatmeal, cooked	⅔ c	0.9
Peas, split	1 c	4.2	Banana, raw	1 medium	0.8
Barley	1 c	4.1	Cantaloupe	½ melon	0.8
Liver, beef	2 oz	4.0	Frankfurter	1 medium	0.8
Peas, blackeye	1 c	3.2	Squash, winter	½ c	0.8
Beef, pot roast	3 oz	2.9	Strawberries, raw	½ c	0.8
Beans, green	1 c	2.9	Lettuce leaves	2 large or 4 small	0.7
Pork chop	1 medium	2.2	Potato, white	1 medium	0.7
Spinach	½ c	2.0	Salmon, canned	½ c	0.7
Ham, boiled	2 oz	1.6	Bread, white, enriched	1 slice	0.6
Apricots, dried, stewed	½ c	1.5	Broccoli	½ c	0.6
Peas, green	½ c	1.5	Peanut butter	2 tbsp	0.6
Prunes, dried, cooked	5 with juice	1.5	Bacon, crisp	2 slices	0.5
Rice	1 c	1.5	Carrots, diced	½ c	0.5
Chicken, fried	½ breast	1.3	Corn, canned	½ c	0.5
Egg	1 medium	1.1	Grapefruit	½ medium	0.5
Rice, cooked, enriched	¾ c	1.1	Orange	1 medium	0.5
Tomato juice, canned	½ c, small glass	1.1	Apple, raw	1 medium	0.4
Haddock	1 filet	1.0	Beans, snap, green	½ c	0.4
Macaroni, enriched, cooked	¾ c	1.0	Peaches, canned	½ c with juice	0.4
			Pineapple juice, canned	½ c, small glass	0.4

*From Nielsen, I. *Childbirth education notebook.* Eugene, Ore.: Lucinia Birth Center, p. 35 (assisted by Eleanor Latterell, R. D.).

[†]All meats and vegetables are cooked unless otherwise indicated.

Vitamins

Many persons speak knowingly about the need for vitamins, but few have a thorough understanding of what they are and how they function in the body. Essentially, vitamins are organic substances that are necessary for life and growth. They are found in small amounts in specific foods and cannot be synthesized by the body.

Vitamins are grouped according to solubility. Those vitamins that dissolve in fat are A, D, E, and K; those soluble in water include vitamin C and the B complex. An adequate intake of all vitamins is essential during pregnancy; however, several are required in larger amounts to fulfill specific needs.

Fat-Soluble Vitamins

Vitamins A, D, E, and K are stored in the liver and thus are available should the dietary intake become inadequate. The major complication related to these vitamins is not deficiency but toxicity due to overdose. Toxic symptoms include nausea, gastrointestinal upset, dryness and cracking of skin, and loss of hair.

Vitamin A. Vitamin A is involved in the growth of epithelial cells, which line the entire gastrointestinal tract and which compose the skin. Vitamin A plays a role in the metabolism of carbohydrates and fats. In the absence of A, the body loses its ability to synthesize glycogen, and the manner in which the body handles cholesterol is also affected. The protective layer of tissue surrounding nerve fibers does not form properly if vitamin A is lacking.

Probably the best-known function of vitamin A is its effect on vision in dim light. The components of the light-sensitive color pigments in the eye recombine in the dark to form visual purple, which depends on a constant supply of vitamin A in its alcohol form, retinol. In this manner, vitamin A prevents night blindness. Thus vitamin A is associated with the formation and development of healthy eyes in the fetus.

If maternal stores of vitamin A are adequate, the overall effects of pregnancy are not very remarkable. The blood serum level of vitamin A decreases slightly in early pregnancy, rises in late pregnancy, and falls before onset of labor.

Both vitamin A (retinol) and its precursor, carotene, cross the placenta. Levels of vitamin A in the fetus are somewhat less than maternal values. The RDA for vitamin A during pregnancy is increased to 5000 IU (international units) from 4000 IU to allow for fetal storage of the vitamin.

Excessive intake of preformed vitamin A in large doses is toxic to both children and adults. Careful monitoring should be provided for those who regularly ingest more than 2000 retinol equivalents (6700 IU) of preformed vitamin A. The carotenes are not harmful if taken in excess but cause yellow skin; the discoloration disappears when intake is reduced. There are indications that excessive intake of vitamin A in the fetus can cause bone malformation, cleft palate, possible renal anomalies, jaundice, and skeletal pain.

Rich plant sources of vitamin A include deep green and yellow vegetables; animal sources include liver, liver oil, kidney, egg yolk, cream, butter, and fortified margarine.

Vitamin D. Vitamin D is best known for its role in the absorption and utilization of calcium and phosphorus in skeletal development. Calcium metabolism is a complex process involving ionized and protein-bound calcium, inorganic phosphorus, vitamin D, parathyroid hormone, and calcitonin. In the serum, calcium and phosphorus tend to have a reciprocal relationship. Approximately half of the total serum calcium is protein-bound and half is ionized. More than 98% of the calcium and 85% of the phosphorus exist as hydroxyapatite, a calcium phosphate salt, in bone. Calcium ions in the bone and serum are in a state of flux with each other, and this dynamic condition is regulated by parathyroid hormone and calcitonin. A form of vitamin D, D_3 (hydroxycholecalciferol), is responsible for intestinal transport of calcium and for parathyroid hormone–induced bone resorption.

To supply fetal needs for the development of skeletal tissue, the RDA for the second half of pregnancy is 400 IU of vitamin D. A deficiency of vitamin D results in rickets, a condition caused by improper calcification of the bones. It is treated with relatively large doses of vitamin D under a physician's direction.

Main food sources of vitamin D include fortified milk, margarine, butter, liver, and egg yolk. A quart of milk in the daily diet provides the 400 IU needed during pregnancy.

Excessive intake of vitamin D is not usually a result of food ingestion but of high-potency vitamin preparations. Overdoses during pregnancy can cause hypercalcemia or high blood calcium levels due to withdrawal of calcium from the skeletal tissue. Continued overdose can also cause hypercalcemia and eventually death, especially in young children. Symptoms of toxicity are excessive thirst, loss of appetite, vomiting, weight loss, high irritability, and high blood calcium levels.

Vitamin E. Tocopherol, or vitamin E, was first discovered in relation to reproduction. The term *tocopherol* is derived from the Greek words *tokos,* meaning childbirth; *phero,* meaning to bear or bring forth; and *ol,* to indicate alcohol. Its role during pregnancy has not been defined. The recommended intake is increased from 12 IU for nonpregnant females to 15 IU for pregnant women.

The major function of vitamin E in the body lies in its role as an antioxidant. This substance will take on oxygen, thus preventing another substance from undergoing chemical change. For example, vitamin E helps spare vitamin A by preventing its oxidation in the intestinal tract and in the tissues. It decreases the oxidation of polyunsaturated fats, thus helping to retain the flexibility and health of the cell membrane. In protecting the cell membrane, vitamin E affects the health of all cells in the body.

Vitamin E is also involved in certain enzymatic and metabolic reactions. It is an essential nutrient for the synthesis of nucleic acids required in the formation of red blood cells in the bone marrow. Vitamin E has also been found to be beneficial in treating certain types of muscular pain and intermittent claudication, in surface healing of wounds and burns, and in protecting lung tissue from the damaging effects of smog. Another well-established use for vitamin E is in the treatment of hemolytic anemia of infants. The newborn's need for vitamin E has been widely recognized, and human milk provides adequate vitamin E, whereas cow's milk is lower in E content. These functions may help explain the abundant claims and cures attributed to vitamin E, many of which have not been scientifically proved.

Deficiency symptoms of vitamin E are related to long-term inability to absorb fats. In humans, malabsorption problems exist in cases of cystic fibrosis, liver cirrhosis, postgastrectomy, obstructive jaundice, pancreatic problems, and sprue.

The vitamin E requirement varies with the polyunsaturated fat content of the diet. Vitamin E is widely distributed in foodstuffs, especially vegetable fats and oils, whole grains, greens, and eggs.

Vitamin E oil has been used by pregnant women externally on abdominal skin to facilitate stretching of the skin and possibly to alleviate permanent stretch marks. It is questionable whether taking high doses of vitamin E internally will accomplish this goal or will satisfy any other claims related to reproduction or virility.

Vitamin K. Vitamin K, or menadione as used synthetically in medicine, is an essential factor for the synthesis of prothrombin; its function is thus related to normal blood clotting. Synthesis occurs in the intestinal tract by the *Escherichia coli* bacteria normally inhabiting the large intestine. These organisms generally provide adequate vitamin K. Newborn infants, having a sterile intestinal tract and receiving sterile feeding, lack vitamin K. Thus a dose of menadione is often given the newborn as a protective measure.

Intake of vitamin K is usually adequate in a well-balanced prenatal diet; an increased requirement has not been identified. Secondary problems may arise if an illness is present that results in malabsorption of fats or if antibiotics are used for an extended period.

Water-Soluble Vitamins

Since water-soluble vitamins are excreted in the urine, only small amounts are stored, and so there is little protection from dietary inadequacies. It is therefore essential that adequate amounts be eaten daily. During pregnancy, the water-soluble vitamins are decreased in maternal serum levels, whereas high concentrations are found in the fetus.

Vitamin C. The requirement for ascorbic acid (vitamin C) is increased in pregnancy from 45 to 60 mg. The major function of vitamin C lies in the formation and development of connective tissue and the vascular system. Ascorbic acid is essential to the formation of collagen, an intercellular cementlike substance. Collagen may be thought of as the cement that holds cells together, just as mortar holds bricks together. If the collagen begins to disintegrate due to lack of ascorbic acid, cell functioning is disturbed and cell structure breaks down, resulting in muscular weakness, capillary hemorrhage, and eventual death. These are symptoms of scurvy, the disease related to vitamin C deficiency. Infants fed diets consisting mainly of cow's milk become deficient in vitamin C, and they constitute the main population group that develops scorbutic symptoms (Food and Nutrition Board, 1974).

Maternal plasma levels of vitamin C progressively decline throughout pregnancy, with values at term being about half those at midpregnancy. It appears that ascorbic acid concentrates in the placenta; thus levels in the fetus are 50% or more above maternal values.

There are no recognized effects of ascorbic acid deficiency on the outcome of pregnancy. However, the use of extremely high ascorbic acid supplements (up to 5 gm daily) in pregnancy is questionable. No specific complications of fetal hypervitaminosis C have been found, but the possibility exists that fetal metabolism could be adversely affected by an oxidizing agent such as ascorbic acid. The infant accustomed to a high maternal intake of ascorbic acid during the entire gestational period will suffer from an acute deficiency state that could be harmful when the maternal supply is stopped at birth.

A nutritious diet for pregnancy should meet the body's needs for vitamin C without additional supplementation. Common food sources of vitamin C include citrus fruit, tomatoes, canteloupe, strawberries, potatoes, broccoli, and other leafy greens. Ascorbic acid is readily destroyed by oxidation. Therefore, care must be taken in the storage and preparation of foods containing vitamin C.

B Vitamins. The B vitamins—which include thiamine (B_1), riboflavin (B_2), niacin, folic acid, pantothenic acid, vitamin B_6, and vitamin B_{12}—serve as vital coenzyme factors in many reactions, such as cell respiration, glucose oxidation, and energy metabolism. The quantities needed therefore invariably increase as caloric intake increases to meet the increased metabolic and growth needs of pregnancy.

The *thiamine* requirement for pregnancy increases during the last trimester to 0.6 mg/1000 kcal. Sources include pork, liver, milk, potatoes, enriched breads, and cereals.

Riboflavin allowances are possibly related to protein allowances, energy intake, and metabolic body size. Vitamin B_2 deficiency is manifested by cheilosis and other skin lesions. During pregnancy, women may excrete less riboflavin and still require more, because of increased energy and protein needs. An additional 0.3 mg/day is recommended. Sources include milk, liver, eggs, enriched breads, and cereals.

An increase of 2 mg daily in *niacin* intake is recommended during pregnancy and 4 mg during lactation, although there is no information on the niacin requirements of pregnant and nursing women. Sources of niacin include meat, fish, poultry, liver, whole grains, enriched breads, cereals, and peanuts.

Folic acid is directly related to the outcome of pregnancy and to maternal and fetal health. Folic acid deficiency is associated with several complications of pregnancy and can cause fetal damage. About 40 years ago, it was noted that pregnant women with macrocytic anemia often responded to treatment with autolyzed yeast or crude liver extract but failed to respond to the purified liver extract used in treatment of addisonian pernicious anemia. Later it was learned that these women were victims of folate deficiency and that the yeast and crude liver extracts contained folic acid (Committee on Maternal Nutrition, 1970).

Megaloblastic anemia due to folate deficiency is rarely found in the United States, but those caring for pregnant women must be aware that it does occur. When there is no iron deficiency, a series of changes characterizes overt megaloblastic anemia (Table 11-6). Note from the table that anemia and megaloblastic erythropoiesis do not develop until about the 20th week (Herbert, 1962).

Folate deficiency can occur in the absence of overt anemia. Any of the events identified in the table can occur late in pregnancy and are evidence of folate deficiency. Various studies have shown folate deficiency to be associated with abruptio placentae, abortion, fetal malformation, and other late bleeding conditions (Committee on Maternal Nutrition, 1970). It has been further pointed out that severe maternal folate deficiency may have other unrecognized effects on the fetus and newborn. Hemorrhagic anemia in the newborn infant is attributed to folate deficiency.

Hibbard suggests that folate deficiency causes irreversible damage to the products of conception—embryo and trophoblast—very early in pregnancy (Committee on Maternal Nutrition, 1970). He urges that folic acid supplementation begin no later than onset of pregnancy and preferably before.

Normal serum folic acid levels in pregnancy should range from 3 to 15 mg/ml; a value less than 3 mg/ml constitutes acute deficiency. Serum folate depends on absorption and ingestion of folic acid; thus, if the level is low in pregnancy, a folate deficiency may exist. The erythrocyte folate level is perhaps a better indicator of folate nutrition, but it is a late indicator of the anemia present (Kitay and Harbart, 1975). If no other complica-

Table 11-6. Morphologic and Biochemical Sequence of Events in Folic Acid Deficiency in Humans*

Events	Time of onset after folate deprivation (weeks)
Low concentration of serum folate (<3 mg/ml)	3
Hypersegmentation of neutrophils in peripheral blood	7
Elevated FIGLU excretion[†]	14
Low folate in erythrocytes (<20 mg/ml)	16
Macro-ovalocytosis	18
Megaloblastic marrow	19
Anemia	19

*From Herbert, V. 1962. Experimental nutritional folate deficiency in man. *Trans. Assoc. Am. Physicians.* 75:307.

[†]FIGLU = formiminoglutamic acid.

tions are present, folic acid therapy brings immediate response. The stage of pregnancy or puerperium is important in determining the dosage. Prenatally an intake of 400 μg (0.4 mg) daily by mouth may induce remission. Postnatally a routine nutritious diet generally provides adequate folate to alleviate symptoms; however, it is wise to give additional folate therapy to build up stores and promote rapid hematologic changes. Iron supplementation is also recommended, since iron is an essential factor in hemoglobin formation. The latest revision of the RDA recommends 800 μg (0.8 mg) for all dietary sources during pregnancy. Pure sources of folacin are effective in less than a fourth of this amount.

Folic acid and iron are the only nutritional supplements generally recommended during the course of pregnancy. The increased need for other vitamins and minerals can be met with an adequate diet.

The best food sources of folates are green leafy vegetables, kidney, liver, food yeasts, and peanuts. As indicated by the list of food sources in Table 11-7, many foods contain small amounts of folic acid. In a well-planned diet, folate intake should be adequate. Note that cow's milk contains a small amount of folic acid, but goat's milk contains none. Therefore, infants and children who are given goat's milk must receive a folate supplement to prevent a deficiency. Adults can generally receive adequate folate from other food sources.

Dietary intake of folic acid can be altered by preparation methods. Since folic acid is a water-soluble nutrient, care must be taken in the cooking process. Loss of the vitamin from vegetables and meats can be considerable when cooked in large amounts of water.

No allowance has been set for *pantothenic acid* in pregnancy. On the basis of some studies, it may

Table 11-7. Folic Acid Content of Selected Foods*

Food	Amount	Folic acid (μg)	Food	Amount	Folic acid (μg)
Yeast, torula	1 tbsp	240.0	Snap beans, green, fresh	3½ oz	27.5
Beef liver, cooked	2 oz	167.6	Peas, green, fresh	3½ oz	25.0
Yeast, brewer's	1 tbsp	161.8	Cauliflower buds, fresh	1 c	22.2
Cowpeas, cooked	½ c	140.5	Shredded wheat cereal	1 biscuit	16.5
Pork liver, cooked	2 oz	126.0	Wheat flakes cereal	1 c	16.4
Asparagus, fresh	3½ oz	109.0	Figs, fresh	3 small	16.0
Wheat germ	1 oz	91.5	Blackberries, fresh	⅔ c	13.7
Spinach	3½ oz	75.0	Sweet potatoes, fresh	½ medium	12.0
Soybeans, cooked	½ c	71.7	Walnut halves, raw	8-15	11.5
Wheat bran	1 oz	58.5	Oysters, canned	3½ oz	11.3
Kidney beans, cooked	½ c	57.6	Pork (ham)	3½ oz	10.6
Broccoli, fresh	⅔ c	53.5	Filberts, raw	10-12	10.0
Brussels sprouts, fresh	3½ oz	49.0	Banana, fresh	1 medium	9.7
Whole-wheat flour	1 c	45.6	Cantaloupe, diced, fresh	⅔ c	9.0
Garbanzos, cooked	½ c	40.0	Cottage cheese	1 oz	8.8
Wheat bran cereal	1 c	35.0	White flour	1 c	8.8
Beans, lima, fresh	3½ oz	34.0	Peanut butter	1 tbsp	8.5
Asparagus, green, fresh	3½ oz	32.4	Blueberries, fresh	⅔ c	8.0
Cabbage, fine shreds	1 c	32.3	Turkey	3½ oz	7.5
Chocolate	1 oz	28.1	Celery, diced, fresh	1 c	7.0
Corn, fresh	3½ oz	28.0	Potatoes, peeled	1 medium	6.8
			Raspberries, fresh	¾ c	5.0

*Modified from Hardinga, M. G., and Crooks, H. N. 1961. Lesser known vitamins in food. *J. Am. Diet. Assoc.* 38:240.

be advisable to supplement the diet with 5–10 mg of pantothenic acid daily. Sources include liver, egg yolk, yeast, and whole-grain cereals and breads.

Vitamin B_6 (pyridoxine) has long been associated biochemically with pregnancy. The classic test for B_6 nutrition is xanthinuric acid excretion following a tryptophan test load. The excretion of xanthinuric acid increases progressively throughout pregnancy until term, when levels may be 10 to 15 times those found in nonpregnant women. Also, blood levels of B_6 fall during gestation to about one-fourth the amounts found in nonpregnant women or during early pregnancy. The B_6 levels in the fetus are greater than those in the mother.

It is believed that these changes are due to metabolic adjustment during pregnancy rather than to B_6 deficiency. Rose and Braidman (1971) suggest that estrogenic stimulation of corticosteroid and the resultant increase in tryptophan oxygenase are responsible. Later in pregnancy, a true deficiency state may occur due to increased fetal uptake combined with the changes induced by hormones (Pitkin, 1975).

The RDA for vitamin B_6 during pregnancy is 2.5 mg, an increase of 0.5 mg over the allowance for nonpregnant women. Since pyridoxine is associated with amino acid metabolism, a higher-than-average protein intake requires increased pyridoxine intake. Generally, meeting the slightly increased need is possible from dietary sources, which include wheat germ, yeast, fish, liver, pork, potatoes, and lentils.

Vitamin B_{12}, or cobalamin, is the cobalt-containing vitamin and is found in animal sources only. Rarely is B_{12} deficiency found in women of reproductive age. Vegetarians are known to develop a deficiency, however, so it is essential that their dietary intake be supplemented with this vitamin. Occasionally vitamin B_{12} levels decrease during pregnancy but increase again after delivery. The RDA during pregnancy is 4 μg/day.

Vitamin B_{12} is absorbed either by simple diffusion or by a specific mechanism involving the intrinsic factor, which is a glycoprotein secreted by the parietal cells of the stomach. The intrinsic factor acts as a carrier for the vitamin in its passage to the ileum and ileal mucosal cells (Food and Nutrition Board, 1974).

A deficiency in vitamin B_{12} may occur when there is difficulty related to absorption. Pernicious anemia results when the body is unable to absorb cobalamin. Infertility is a complication when this type of anemia is present.

Vegetarianism

Vegetarianism is the dietetic choice of many persons. Some are vegetarians for religious reasons (Seventh-Day Adventists); others believe that this practice leads to a healthier body and mind.

There are several types of vegetarians. *Lacto-ovovegetarians* include milk, dairy products, and eggs in their diet. Occasionally fish, poultry, and liver are allowed. *Lactovegetarians* include dairy products but no eggs in their diets. *Vegans* are considered "pure" vegetarians; they will not eat any food from animal sources.

Persons who are concerned with the problem of preservatives and additives in food may be considering vegetarianism. The family with children or the couple expecting a child may alter their dietary habits in the belief that they are improving their nutritional status. Whether the family is currently practicing vegetarianism or is considering it as an alternative, during pregnancy it is vital that the expectant woman eat the proper combination of foods to obtain adequate nutrients.

An adequate pure vegetarian diet contains protein from unrefined grains (brown rice and whole wheat), legumes (beans, split peas, lentils), nuts in large quantities, and a variety of cooked and fresh vegetables and fruits. Complete protein may be obtained by eating any of the following food combinations at the same meal: legumes and whole-grain cereals, nuts and whole-grain cereals, or nuts and legumes. Seeds may be used in the vegetarian diet if the quantity is large enough. Because proteins are less concentrated in plant tissue than in animal tissue, it is necessary for vegetarians to eat larger quantities of food to meet body needs.

Sample vegetarian menus that meet the requirements of good prenatal nutrition are given on p. 302.

For those families interested in altering their dietary habits, Register and Sonnenberg (1973) provide practical suggestions in the use of the vegetarian diet. They recommend the following principles in changing from a nonvegetarian to a lacto-ovovegetarian diet:

1. Decrease all empty-calorie foods as much as possible.

Suggested Menus for Adequate Prenatal Vegetarian Diets—Day 1

Meal pattern	Mixed diet	Lacto-ovovegetarian	Lacto-vegetarian	Seventh-Day Adventist	Vegan
Breakfast					
Fruit	¾ c orange juice	Same as mixed diet	Same as mixed diet	Same as lacto-ovovegetarian	¾ c orange juice
Grains	½ c granola, 1 slice whole wheat toast				1 c granola, 1 slice whole grain toast
Meat group	1 scrambled egg with cheese		1 oz cheese melted over toast (no egg)		
Fat	1 tsp butter				1 tsp sesame butter
Milk	½ c milk				1 c soy milk
Midmorning					
Milk	1 c hot chocolate	Same	Same	Same	1 c protein drink*
Lunch					
Meat group/ vegetable	1 c lentil chowder† (made with ground beef)	1 c lentil chowder† (no ground beef)	1 c lentil chowder† (no ground beef)	1 c lentil chowder† (made with vegeburger)‡	1½ c lentil chowder† (1 tbsp torula yeast, wheat germ added)
Grains	1 corn muffin	Same	Same	Same	2 corn muffins**
Fat	1 tsp butter, honey				2 tsp margarine, honey
Fruit/dessert	½ peach, ½ c cottage cheese salad				½ peach, ½ c tofu salad
Tea	1 c tea				
Midafternoon					
Milk	¾ c vanilla pudding	Same	Same	Same	1 c pudding (soy milk)
Fruit	¼ c sliced banana				½ banana
Grain	1 graham cracker				1 graham cracker with peanut butter
Dinner					
Meat group/ vegetable	¾ c meat sauce (onion, celery,	¾ c tomato sauce (same	Same as lacto-ovovegetarian	Same as lacto-ovovegetarian	Same as lacto-ovovegetarian

*Protein drink recipe is given on p. 293. Use soy milk instead of cow or goat milk. Do not use eggs.

†Lentil chowder is made from lentils, celery, carrots, potatoes, onion, and tomatoes.

‡Vegeburger is made from meat analogs.

**Wheat germ and soy flour are added to corn muffin mixture.

Suggested Menus for Adequate Prenatal Vegetarian Diets—Day 1 Cont'd

Meal pattern	Mixed diet	Lacto-ovovegetarian	Lacto-vegetarian	Seventh-Day Adventist	Vegan
	carrot, tomato, mushroom in sauce), parmesan cheese	vegetables as in mixed diet), ¼ c cheese		(add vegeburger‡ to tomato sauce)	(use tofu instead of cheese)
Grains	¾ c spaghetti, bread	1 c whole wheat spaghetti, 1 slice French bread	Same as lacto-ovovegetarian		
Vegetable	Mixed vegetable salad	Mixed vegetable salad with ¼ c sprouts, ½ egg, ½ oz cheese, ¼ c kidney beans added	(No egg in salad)		(Add tofu; no egg in salad)
Fat	Oil-vinegar dressing, ½ tsp butter	Same as mixed diet			1 tsp margarine
Fruit	Fresh pear or baked pear half				
Tea	1 c tea				
Bedtime					
Milk	1 c milk	Same	Same	Same	
Meat group/ vegetable	2 tsp peanut butter in celery or on wheat crackers				1 c protein drink*
Grain					Corn muffin**

Suggested Menus for Adequate Prenatal Vegetarian Diets—Day 2

Meal pattern	Mixed diet	Lacto-ovovegetarian	Lacto-vegetarian	Seventh-Day Adventist	Vegan
Breakfast					
Fruit	½ c applesauce	Same	Same	Same	Same
Grains	¾ c oatmeal, 1 slice whole grain toast				

*Protein drink recipe is given on p. 293. Use soy milk instead of cow or goat milk. Do not use eggs.

†Lentil chowder is made from lentils, celery, carrots, potatoes, onion, and tomatoes.

‡Vegeburger is made from meat analogs.

**Wheat germ and soy flour are added to corn muffin mixture.

Suggested Menus for Adequate Prenatal Vegetarian Diets—Day 2 Cont'd

Meal pattern	Mixed diet	Lacto-ovovegetarian	Lacto-vegetarian	Seventh-Day Adventist	Vegan
Meat group	2 tbsp peanut butter, 1 tsp honey				
Milk	½ c milk				
Midmorning					
Fruit	1 medium orange	Same	Same	Same	Same
Lunch					
Meat group	Sandwich: ½ c tuna or egg salad, 2 tsp mayonnaise, 2 slices whole grain bread, ¼ c alfalfa sprouts, lettuce	(½ c egg salad)	(2 oz cheese)	(½ c egg salad)	½ c tofu in mixed vegetable scramble, 2 tbsp wheat germ, 2 slices whole grain bread, 2 tbsp sesame butter, honey
Fat		Same	Same	Same	
Grains					
Vegetables					
Fruit/dessert	Small banana				1 medium banana
Milk	1 c cream of tomato soup; ½ c milk				Cream of tomato soup; ½ c soy milk
Midafternoon					
Milk	½ c yogurt	Same	Same	Same	1 c soy yogurt
Fruit	½ c fruit				½ c fruit
Grain	2 tbsp wheat germ				2 tbsp wheat germ
Dinner					
Meat group	3 oz baked chicken	1 c bean and cheese enchilada casserole	Same as lacto-ovovegetarian	Same as lacto-ovovegetarian	1 c bean and tofu enchilada casserole
Grain	½ c brown rice pilaf, bran muffin	1 c brown rice pilaf, bran muffin			1 c brown rice pilaf, bran muffin
Vegetables	½ c broccoli, tossed green salad with tomato	¾ c broccoli, tossed green salad with tomato			¾ c broccoli, tossed green salad with tomato

*Protein drink recipe is given on p. 293. Use soy milk instead of cow or goat milk. Do not use eggs.

†Lentil chowder is made from lentils, celery, carrots, potatoes, onion, and tomatoes.

‡Vegeburger is made from meat analogs.

**Wheat germ and soy flour are added to corn muffin mixture.

Suggested Menus for Adequate Prenatal Vegetarian Diets—Day 2 Cont'd

Meal pattern	Mixed diet	Lacto-ovovegetarian	Lacto-vegetarian	Seventh-Day Adventist	Vegan
Fat	Russian dressing Butter	Cheese dressing Butter			French dressing Margarine
Fruit/dessert	Peach crisp	Peach crisp (with wheat germ and sunflower seeds)			Peach crisp (with wheat germ and sunflower seeds)
Milk	1 c milk	1 c milk			Soya hot chocolate
Bedtime					
Milk	1 c hot chocolate	Same	Same	Same	1 c hot soya/carob beverage
Meat group	1 oz cheese				Peanut butter (2 tbsp)
Grain	Rye-Krisp				Sesame crackers

*Protein drink recipe is given on p. 293. Use soy milk instead of cow or goat milk. Do not use eggs.

†Lentil chowder is made from lentils, celery, carrots, potatoes, onion, and tomatoes.

‡Vegeburger is made from meat analogs.

**Wheat germ and soy flour are added to corn muffin mixture.

2. Increase the intake of the basic food groups to provide sufficient calories.
3. Use an increased amount of legumes, nuts, and possibly meat analogs (food products derived from soy and wheat) to replace meat.
4. Increase the intake of whole-grain products that supply protein, B vitamins, and iron to the diet.
5. Increase the intake of dairy products, using nonfat and low-fat milk, cottage cheese, cheeses, and other foods, to provide additional protein and vitamin B_{12}.

For changing from a lacto-ovovegetarian diet to a pure vegetarian diet, Register and Sonnenberg (1973) have additional recommendations:

1. Maintain an adequate calorie intake so that the body will not burn protein for caloric needs.
2. Increase the intake of foods that contain nutrients such as calcium and riboflavin, which are supplied in significant amounts by the milk group. Other sources of these nutrients include fortified soybean milk preparations; leafy green vegetables; legumes, especially soybeans; nuts, particularly almonds; and dried fruits.
3. Supplement the diet with vitamin B_{12}, since there is no practical plant source.

Factors Influencing Nutrition

Armed with knowledge of nutritional needs and food sources for these nutrients, the nurse may educate the maternity patient so that nutritional adequacy can be maintained or instituted during pregnancy. In addition to the recommended diet, other factors need to be considered. What is the age, life-style, and culture of the pregnant woman? What food beliefs and habits does she have? What a person eats is determined by availability, economics, and symbolism. These factors and others will influence the expectant mother's acceptance of the nurse's intervention.

Pica

Pica is the eating of substances that are not ordinarily considered edible or to have nutritive value. Most women who practice pica in pregnancy eat such substances only during that time. The reasons given by many of these women are usually associated with relief of various discomforts of pregnancy or beliefs related to producing a beautiful baby (Curda, 1977).

Pica is most commonly found in poverty-stricken areas, where diets tend to be inadequate, but may also be found in other socioeconomic levels. The substances most commonly ingested in this country are dirt, clay, starch, and freezer frost. Iron-deficiency anemia is the most common concern. Studies indicate that ingestion of laundry starch contributes to iron deficiency not because of the number of calories it provides without the presence of iron but rather because of interference with iron absorption (Talkington et al., 1970). The same study reported that ingestion of large amounts of clay did not interfere with the absorption of iron. However, a study by Minich et al. (1969) reports significant impairment of iron absorption with clays from three specific regions. Other problems with pica have been reported, including severe hypokalemia and intestinal obstruction (Curda, 1977). The ingestion of starch may be associated with excessive weight gain.

It is important that nurses be aware of pica and its implications for the mother and fetus. Assessment for the practice of pica is an important part of a nutritional history. The nurse may detect this practice as she helps determine appropriate and effective relief measures for discomforts the woman is experiencing. Reeducation of the expectant woman is important in helping her to decrease or eliminate this practice.

Food Myths

The relationship of food to pregnancy is reflected in some common beliefs or sayings. Nurses frequently hear that the pregnant woman must eat for two or that the fetus takes from the mother all the nutrients it needs. The practice of pica, for example, has roots in myth. Common beliefs regarding pica include (a) that laundry starch will make the newborn lighter in color, and (b) that the baby will "slide out" more easily during delivery (Curda, 1977).

Cultural, Ethnic, and Religious Influences

Culture has been defined as the entire way of life of people, which includes all habits of daily living. The many facets of one's culture are learned gradually until they are internalized and become an intricate, unconscious part of each individual. The function of culture is twofold: (a) It helps people adapt to the environment, and (b) it helps them interpret common life experiences (Williams, 1977).

Cultural, ethnic, and occasionally religious background determines one's experiences with food and influences food preferences and habits. People of different nationalities are accustomed to eating different foods because of the kinds of foodstuffs available in their countries of origin. The way food is prepared varies, depending on the customs and traditions of the particular ethnic and cultural group. In addition, the laws of certain religions prescribe particular foods, prohibit others, and direct the preparation and serving of meals.

In each culture, certain foods have symbolic significance. Generally, these symbolic foods are related to major life experiences such as birth, death, or developmental milestones. (General food practices of different cultural and ethnic groups are presented in Table 11-8. Sample daily menus for differing cultural groups that meet minimal nutritional requirements during pregnancy are presented on p. 308.)

For example, Navajo Indian women believe that eating raisins will cause brown spots on the mother or baby. Many black Americans believe that craving one food excessively can cause the baby to be "marked"; in fact, they believe that a birthmark's shape can be correlated with the shape of the food the mother craved during pregnancy. This belief is also held by some Mexican-American women. Also, milk consumption is considered by some Mexican-Americans to make their babies too big, thereby creating difficult deliveries.

The traditional Chinese classify food as either hot or cold, and these classifications are related to the balance of forces for good health. Since childbirth is considered a cold condition, it must be treated with hot foods, such as chicken, squash, and broccoli. Vietnamese women believe that eating unclean foods such as beef, dog, and snake during pregnancy will cause the baby to be born an imbecile. Cabbage is also avoided because it is believed to produce flatulence that might bring on false labor (Clark, 1978).

Psychosocial Factors

Food is frequently considered a symbol of friendliness, warmth, and social acceptance. Sharing one's table with others has been practiced for centuries. Food has also been symbolic of motherliness; that is, taking care of the family and feeding them well is a part of the traditional mothering role. The mother influences her children's likes and dislikes by what she prepares and by her attitude about foods. Certain foods are assigned positive and negative values as reflected by such statements as "Milk helps one grow" and "Coffee stunts one's growth."

Some foods and food-related practices are associated with status. Some foods are prepared "just for company." Other foods are served only on specific occasions—for example, holidays such as Thanksgiving.

Table 11–8. Food Practices of Various Ethnic and Religious Groups

Cultural group	Staple foods	Prohibitions or foods not used	Food preparation
Jewish Orthodox	Meat: Forequarter of cattle, sheep, goat, deer Poultry: chicken, pheasant, turkey, goose, duck	No blood may be eaten in any form	Animal slaughter must follow certain rules, including minimal pain to animal and maximal blood drainage
	Dairy products	Combining milk and meat at meal not allowed; milk and cheese may be eaten before meal, but must not be eaten for six hours after meal containing meat	Two sets of dishes are used: one for meat, one for milk meals
	Fish with fins and scales No restrictions on cereals, fruits, or vegetables	No shellfish or eels	
Mexican-American	Main vegetables: corn (source of calcium) and chili peppers (source of vitamin C); pinto beans or calice beans; potatoes Coffee and eggs Grain products: corn is basic grain; tortillas from enriched flour made daily	Milk rarely used	Chief cooking fat is lard Usually beans are served with every meal
Chinese	Rice is staple grain and used at most meals Traditional beverage is green tea	Milk and cheese rarely used	Foods are kept short time and are cooked quickly at high temperature so that natural flavors are enhanced and texture and color are maintained
	Most meats are used, but in limited amounts Fruits are usually eaten fresh	Meat considered difficult to chew, so may be eliminated from child's diet	Chief cooking fat is lard or peanut oil
Japanese	Seafood (raw fish) eaten frequently Most meats; large variety of vegetables and fresh fruits Rice is staple grain, but corn and oats also used	Milk and cheese rarely used	Chief cooking fat is soybean oil

Suggested Menus for Adequate Prenatal Diet for Various Cultural Groups—Day 1*

Meal	Caucasian	Chicano†	Southern U.S.	Oriental†	Jewish	Italian†
Breakfast	Peaches Oatmeal/milk Toast with peanut butter Milk	Peaches Oatmeal/milk Corn tortilla Refried beans Milk	Peaches Oatmeal/milk Cornbread with molasses Milk	Peaches Steamed rice/milk (soy) Rice cracker Tea	Peaches Oatmeal/milk Bagel with unsalted butter Milk	Peaches Oatmeal/milk Bread with butter Cheese Coffee/milk
Midmorning	Fruit/juice	Fruit/juice	Fruit	Fruit	Fruit	Fruit/juice
Lunch	Cheese omelet and vegetables Whole grain muffin with butter Lettuce and tomato salad Raw apple Milk	1 fried egg Refried beans with cheese Corn tortilla Fresh tomato and chilis Banana Milk	1 fried egg Black-eyed peas and salt pork Cornbread with molasses Turnip greens Ice cream	Miso soup Chinese omelet (with bean sprouts, pepper, green onion, mushroom) and fried rice Spinach Tea	Cheese omelet Brown rice Lettuce and tomato salad Honey cookie Milk	Cheese omelet Zucchini, green salad Grapes/cheese Milk
Midafternoon	Fruit Cottage cheese	Fruit Cottage cheese	Fruit	Fruit Tofu	Fruit	Fruit Cheese
Dinner	Roast beef and gravy Whole grain roll with butter Parsley, carrots, cabbage slaw Banana cream pie Tea	Refried beans with cheese Fried macaroni Tortilla Carrots, steamed tomato, chilis Corn pudding Milk	Beef stew with vegetables (carrots, greens) Dumplings Steamed potato, cabbage slaw Corn pudding	Beef strips with pan-fried vegetables Brown rice, steamed Milk custard	Beef stew with vegetables Barley pilaf Cooked cabbage Unsalted butter Coffeecake Fruit/juice	Spaghetti and meatballs with tomato sauce Italian bread with butter Sauteed eggplant, cabbage, salad Fruit Coffee/milk
Bedtime	Milk Wheat crackers 1 oz cheese	Milk Tortilla with beans Cheese	Milk Corn pudding	Ice cream	Ice cream	Ice cream

Suggested Menus for Adequate Prenatal Diet for Various Cultural Groups—Day 2*

Meal	Caucasian	Chicano[†]	Southern U.S.	Oriental[†]	Jewish	Italian[†]
Breakfast	Orange juice Pancakes with butter/syrup Sausage Milk	Tortilla Scrambled egg with beans and cheese Milk	Melon or fruit in season Cornmeal grits with molasses Biscuit with cream gravy Milk	Steamed millet Rice cracker Tofu Tea	Orange juice Potato pancakes with unsalted butter Fried eggs Milk	Orange Farina/milk Whole grain bread with butter Coffee/milk
Midmorning	Fruit juice	Melon or orange	Fruit juice	Fruit Egg drop soup	Fruit/cheese Chicken noodle soup	Fruit/cheese
Lunch	Cheese on toasted whole wheat bread Vegetable soup Raw carrots, pickles Pineapple Milk	Bean and cheese enchilada Tomato, chilis Fruit Milk	Cheese on whole wheat bread Mustard greens, tomato wedges Buttermilk	Tofu with steamed brown rice and vegetables Cooked greens	Cottage cheese blintzes with fresh whipped butter Broccoli, tomatoes Milk	Cheese on whole wheat bread Minestrone soup Green salad Fruit Coffee/milk
Midafternoon	Milk and fruit shake	Apple or banana	Fruit	Ice cream	Ice cream	Ice cream
Dinner	Baked chicken Biscuit with butter Sweet potato Broccoli Fruit salad Sponge cake Beverage	Stewed chicken Tortilla Sweet potato Spinach, raw carrots Juice	Ham hocks with rice and tomato, onion, and okra Cornbread with molasses Sweet potato, collards Buttermilk	Pork with fried rice and vegetables Broccoli, raw green salad Rice custard pudding Tea	Green cabbage with ground lamb stuffing Rye bread with unsalted butter Sweet potato, broccoli, raw green pepper, cucumber, pickles Fruit juice	Chicken tettrazini (with pasta) Whole grain Italian bread with butter Broccoli, green salad Grapes/cheese Coffee/milk
Bedtime	Milk Crackers with peanut butter Banana	Milk Cheese Tortilla with beans	Biscuit with peanut butter Fruit	Rice crackers Cheese Fruit	Pumpernickel bread Cheese Fruit	Cheese Fruit

*Modified from American Dietetic Association. *Cultural food patterns in the U.S.A.*

[†]Encourage use of milk, since it is not ordinarily included in diets of members of these cultural groups.

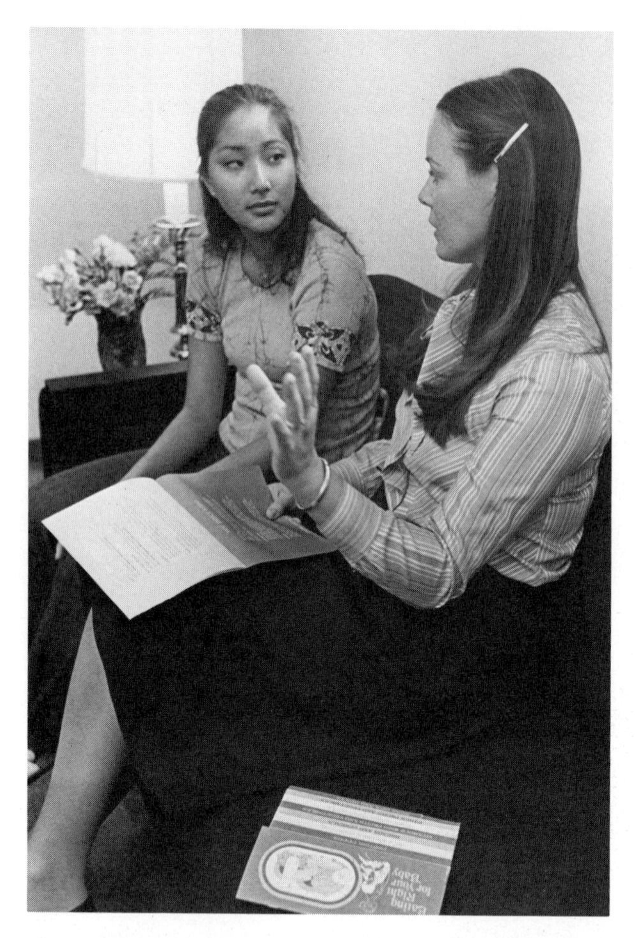

Figure 11–10. Evaluation of maternal nutritional status is part of a complete prenatal assessment.

Socioeconomic Factors. One's socioeconomic level may be a determinant of one's nutritional status. Poverty-level families are unable to afford the same types of food that higher-income families can. Thus, maternity patients with low incomes frequently are at risk for poor nutrition.

Education also plays a role in one's nutritional status, since one's educational level is frequently related to one's economic status.

Psychologic Factors. Nutritional well-being can be directly affected by a person's emotional state. For example, one psychologic disorder, anorexia nervosa, which occurs primarily in adolescent girls, is manifested chiefly by self-inflicted starvation, resulting in malnutrition and ultimately death if not treated. Loss of appetite is also a common symptom of serious depression.

The expectant woman's attitudes and feelings about her pregnancy will certainly have an influence on her nutritional status. The woman who is depressed or who regards this event as unwanted and unwelcome may manifest these feelings by loss of appetite or by improper food practices, such as overindulgence in sweets or alcohol.

Nursing Actions

The important components of and influences on a nutritionally balanced diet for the pregnant woman have been thoroughly discussed. Each person's view of nutrition and of its relationship to the pregnancy depends on previous teaching and dietary habits. A complete diet history and assessment of nutritional status must be made by the health care team to facilitate planning an optimal diet with each woman. During the data-gathering process, the nurse has an opportunity to discuss important aspects of nutrition in the context of the family's needs and life-style (Figure 11–10).

The nutritional questionnaire (Figure 11–11) can be used by the patient and nurse to record the data base from which the plan of nursing interventions can be developed to fit the patient's individual needs. The sample questionnaire has been filled in to demonstrate this problem-oriented process.

Assessment of nutritional status is begun by the nurse as the questionnaire is completed. According to the format of problem-oriented record-keeping, the formulation of a partial problem list and initial plans follow the assessment. Following is an example of the process of PORK:

Assessment:

- Weight gain of 10 pounds during first two months of pregnancy.
- Limited information about present nutritional needs.
- Limited budget, has obtained food stamps.

Problem list (partial):

1. Limited nutritional information.
2. Low intake of calcium and iron.
3. Excessive weight gain and empty calories.
4. Limited food budget.

Initial plans (partial):

Problem 1. Limited nutritional information.

a. Review basic food groups and requirements.

NUTRITIONAL QUESTIONNAIRE

Name Susan Longmont Date 2-20-80

Age 20

Ethnic group white middle class

Religion Protestant

Gravida 1 Para 0 EDC 10-7-80

Age of youngest child? NA

Birth weights of previous children? NA

Usual nonpregnant weight 115 Present weight 125

Weight gain during last pregnancy? NA

Vitamin supplements? none

Current medications? aspirin for headache

Do you smoke? yes How much per day? 1-1½ packs

Eating patterns:

1. How many meals per day? 2 when 12:30 pm 6:30 pm
2. How many snacks per day? 3 when 10:30 am 4:00 pm 10:00 pm
3. What other foods are important to your usual diet? chocolate and candy bars
4. Amount per day 4 bars/week
5. Do you have any different food preferences now? no
6. Do you eat nonfoods such as:

		Amount
laundry starch	no	NA
ice	yes	10 cubes/day
other (name)	no	NA

7. What foods do you dislike or do not eat? spinach and dried beans
8. For added information complete a typical daily intake (24 hour recall is suggested).

Do you have special problems in food preparation such as:

1. Physical disability yes ___ no ✓ Explain ___
2. Cooking appliances yes ___ no ✓ Explain ___
3. Refrigeration of food yes ___ no ✓ Explain ___

Who does the meal planning? I do. shopping? We both do.

cooking? I do most of the time but my husband likes to help.

Are there transportation problems? We have only one car but we go in the evening.

Financial situation: My husband is working and going to school.

I am not working. Foodstamps yes w/c no

Do you have any previous nutritional problems? No. I have never paid much attention to food before, but now I have a lot of questions.

Are there any problems with this pregnancy? Nausea Yes, in the morning.

Constipation No Other NA

Assessment by the nurse following the completion of the questionnaire.

Basic estimated nutrient and caloric value of typical daily intake.

Please circle one of the following:

Protein intake was	low	(adequate)	high
Caloric intake was	low	adequate	(high)
Calcium intake was	(low)	adequate	high
Iron intake was	(low)	adequate	high
Vitamin C intake was	low	(adequate)	high

Figure 11–11. Sample nutritional questionnaire used in nursing management of a pregnant patient.

b. Compare present intake with recommended diet for the pregnant young adult.

c. Recommend in-depth diet counseling if required.

Problem 2. Low intake of calcium and iron.

a. Plan additional 3–4 cups of milk in daily intake.

b. Encourage use of foods high in iron. If this is not realistic (dislikes liver and spinach), investigate use of iron supplement.

SUMMARY

Comprehensive knowledge of the physiologic and psychologic aspects of pregnancy is needed by the nurse so that she can counsel the pregnant woman and her family about hygiene, possible changes in life-style, acceptable relief measures for discomfort of pregnancy, and nutrition.

Each woman, family, and pregnancy is unique. But one must acknowledge that each pregnancy builds on what went before, such as the physical and psychologic status of the mother and family. Consideration must be given to these diverse and complex factors when identifying prenatal needs and nursing interventions.

SUGGESTED ACTIVITIES

1. Formulate an antepartal teaching plan that includes the following concepts: hygiene, rest, exercise, clothing, care of the breasts, and other common concerns of pregnancy.
2. Write nutritionally adequate menus for three days for the pregnant woman. Modify the same menu to supply the nutrient needs of the pregnant teenager and the lactating woman.
3. Following the dietary pattern for pregnancy, plan a week's menu for a woman of a specific cultural background in your community.
4. In a prenatal clinic, become involved in counseling patients about identified discomforts of pregnancy.
5. Check with the local health department and other agencies or groups who deal with childbirth to ascertain the amount of general prenatal education and nutritional information included in their educational programs.

REFERENCES

Aronson, M. E., and Nelson, P. K. 1967. Fatal air embolism in pregnancy resulting from an unusual sex act. *Obstet. Gynecol.* 30:127.

Bowes, A. D., and Church, C. F. 1975. *Food value of portions commonly used.* 11th ed. Rev. by C. F. Church and H. N. Church. Philadelphia: J. B. Lippincott Co.

Clark, A. L., ed. 1978. *Culture, childbearing, health professionals.* Philadelphia: F. A. Davis Co.

Committee on Maternal Nutrition. 1970. *Maternal nutrition and the course of pregnancy: summary report.* Washington, D.C.: Food and Nutrition Board, National Academy of Sciences, National Research Council.

Crosby, W. M., and Costiloe, P. J. 1971. Safety of lap-belt restraint for pregnant victims of automobile collisions. *N. Engl. J. Med.* 284:632.

Curda, L. R. Spring 1977. What about pica. *J. Nurse-Midwifery.* 23:8.

Davies, D. P., et al. 1976. Cigarette smoking in pregnancy associated with weight gain and fetal growth. *Lancet.* 1:385.

Fatteh, A., et al. May 1973. Fatal air embolism in pregnancy resulting from orogenital sex play. *Forensic Sci.* 2:247.

Food and Nutrition Board. 1974. *Recommended dietary allowances.* 8th ed. Washington, D.C.: National Academy of Sciences, National Research Council.

Green, R., ed. 1975. *Human sexuality: health practitioner's text.* Baltimore: The Williams & Wilkins Co.

Hardinga, M. G., and Crooks, H. N. 1961. Lesser known vitamins in food. *J. Am. Diet. Assn.* 38:240.

Henderlich, J. 1977. Health care of the heroin-dependent woman. In *Nursing of women in the age of liberation,* ed. N. Lytle. Dubuque, Iowa: William C. Brown Co.

Herbert, V. 1962. Experimental nutritional folate deficiency in man. *Trans. Assoc. Am. Physicians.* 70:307.

Jacobsen, H. N. Dec. 1974. Maternal nutrition since the 1969 White House Conference. *Nutrition News.* 37(4):13.

Kitay, D. Z., and Harbart, R. A. Sept. 1975. Iron and folic acid deficiency in pregnancy. *Clin. Perinatol.* 2:255.

Masters, W. H., and Johnson, V. E. 1966. *Human sexual response.* Boston: Little, Brown & Co.

Minich, V., et al. 1969. Pica in Turkey: effect of clay upon iron absorption. *Am. J. Clin. Nutr.* 21:73.

Nielsen, I. *Childbirth education notebook.* Eugene, Ore.: Lucinia Birth Center.

Pitkin, R. M., Sept. 1975. Vitamins and minerals in pregnancy. *Clin. Perinatol.* 2:221.

Pritchard, J. A., and MacDonald, P. 1976. *Williams obstetrics.* 15th ed. New York: Appleton-Century-Crofts.

Register, U. D., and Sonnenberg, L. M. 1973. The vegetarian diet. *J. Am. Diet. Assoc.* 62:253.

Rodman, J. J. 1976. The pregnant patient: treating her without harming the baby. In *Drugs used with neonates and during pregnancy,* eds. A. M. Overback and M. J. Rodman. Oradell, N. J.: Medical Economics Co.

Rose, D. P., and Braidman, I. P. 1971. Excretion of tryptophan metabolites as affected by pregnancy, contraceptive steroids and steroid hormones. *Am. J. Clin. Nutr.* 24:673.

Solberg, D. A., et al. 1973. Sexual behavior in pregnancy. *N. Engl. J. Med.* 288:1098.

Talkington, K., et al. 1970. Effect of ingestion of starch and some clays on iron absorption. *Am. J. Obstet. Gynecol.* 108:267.

Tsang, R. C., and Glueck, C. J. Sept. 1975. Perinatal cholesterol metabolism. *Clin. Perinatol.* 2:275.

Underwood, P., et al. 1965. The relationship of smoking to the outcome of pregnancy. *Am. J. Obstet. Gynecol.* 91:270.

Weed, L. L. 1969. *Medical records, medical education and patient care.* Cleveland: Cleveland Press, Case Western Reserve University.

Williams, S. 1977. *Nutrition and diet therapy.* 3rd ed. St. Louis: The C. V. Mosby Co.

Winick, M. 1968. Changes in nucleic acid and protein content of the human brain growth. *Pediatr. Res.* 2:352.

Winick, M. April 12, 1977. *Maternal and infant nutrition seminar.* Portland, Ore.

Zalor, M. K. May–June 1976. Sexual counseling for pregnant couples. *MCN.* 1:176.

ADDITIONAL READINGS

Brandl, E. Feb. 1965. Cigarette smoking and pregnancy. *Nurs. Sci.* 3:71.

Browne, J. C., and Dixon, G. 1970. *Browne's antenatal care.* 10th ed. Baltimore: The Williams & Wilkins Co.

Bruhn, C. M., and Panghorn, R. M. May 1971. Incidence of pica among migrant families. *J. Am. Diet. Assoc.* 58:417.

Butler, J., and Wagner, M. M. 1975. Sexuality during pregnancy and post partum. In *Human sexuality,* ed. R. Green. Baltimore: The Williams & Wilkins Co.

Caplan, G. 1957. Normal emotions in pregnancy. *Briefs.* 21(3):35.

Caplan, G. 1975. Psychological aspects of maternity care. *Am. J. Public Health.* 47:25.

Cardenas, J., et al. Sept. 1976. Nutritional beliefs and practices in primigravida Mexican-American women. *J. Am. Diet. Assoc.* 69:262.

Christakis, G. 1973. *Nutritional assessment in health programs.* Washington, D. C.: American Public Health Association, Inc.

Clark, A. L., and Affonso, D. D. 1976. *Childbearing: a nursing perspective.* Philadelphia: F. A. Davis Co.

Clark, A. L., and Hale, R. W. 1974. Sex during and after pregnancy. *Am. J. Nurs.* 3:1430.

Danforth, D. N. 1977. *Textbook of obstetrics and gynecology.* New York: Harper & Row Publishers, Inc.

Davis, M. E., and Rubin, R. 1962. *De Lee's obstetrics for nurses.* 17th ed. Philadelphia: W. B. Saunders Co.

Drugs and Therapeutic Information, Inc. March 1970. Safety of immunizing agents in pregnancy. *Med. Letters Drugs Therap.* 12:5.

Edwards, C. H., et al. Feb. 1964. Effects of clay and cornstarch intake on women and their infants. *J. Am. Diet. Assoc.* 44:109.

Emerson, K., et al. 1972. Caloric cost of normal pregnancy. *Obstet. Gynecol.* 40:786.

Falicov, C. J. 1973. Sexual adjustment during first pregnancy and post partum. *Am. J. Obstet. Gynecol.* 117:991.

Goodhardt, R. S., and Shils, M. E. 1973. *Modern nutrition in health and disease.* 5th ed. Philadelphia: Lea & Febiger.

Goodlin, R. C. 1976. Can sex in pregnancy harm the fetus? *Contemp. OB/Gyn.* 8:21.

Hunt, I., et al. 1976. Effect of nutrition education on the nutritional status of low-income pregnant women of Mexican descent. *Am. J. Clin. Nutr.* 29:675.

Huyck, N. July 1976. Nutrition services for pregnant teenagers. *J. Am. Diet. Assoc.* 69:60.

Jacob, M., et al. 1976. Biochemical assessment of the nutritional status of low-income pregnant women of Mexican descent. *Am. J. Clin. Nutr.* 29:650.

Jelliffe, D. 1976. World trends in infant feeding. *Am. J. Clin. Nutr.* 29:1227.

King, J. Spring 1977. Nutrition during oral contraceptive treatment. *J. Nurse-Midwifery.* 22:31.

Kosasa, T. S., et al. 1974. Clinical use of a solid-phase radioimmunoassay specific for human chorionic gonadotropin. *Am. J. Obstet. Gynecol.* 19:6.

Levine, M., et al. 1974. Live virus vaccines in pregnancy, risks and recommendations. *Lancet.* 2:34.

Luke, B. March–April 1977. Lactose intolerance during pregnancy: significance and solutions. *MCN.* 2:92.

Luke, B. March–April 1977. Understanding pica in pregnant women. *MCN.* 2:97.

McLennon, C. E. 1943. Antecubital and femoral venous pressure in normal and toxic pregnancy. *Am. J. Obstet. Gynecol.* 45:568.

Mason, M., and Rivers, J. April 1970. Factors influencing plasma ascorbic acid levels of pregnant women. *J. Am. Diet. Assoc.* 56:313.

Modlin, J. F., et al. 1976. Risk of congenital abnormality after inadvertent rubella vaccination of pregnant women. *N. Engl. J. Med.* 294:172.

Molony, C. H. 1975. Systematic valence coding of Mexican "hot"-"cold" food. *Ecol. Food Nutr.* 4:67.

Nabatoff, R. A., and Pencus, J. A. Dec. 1970. Management of varicose veins during pregnancy. *Obstet. Gynecol.* 36:928.

Osofsky, H. 1975. Relationships between prenatal medical and nutritional measures, pregnancy outcome, and early infant development in an urban poverty setting. I. The role of nutritional intake. *Am. J. Obstet. Gynecol.* 123:682.

Parker, L. Winter 1974. Coitus during pregnancy. *J. Nurse-Midwifery.* 9:4.

Parker, S., and Bowering, J. April–June 1976. Folacin in diets of Puerto Rican and black women in relation to food practices. *J. Nutri. Educ.* 8:73.

Pike, R. L. 1964. Sodium intake during pregnancy. *J. Am. Diet. Assoc.* 44:176.

Pitkin, R., et al. 1972. Maternal nutrition—a selective review of clinical topics. *Obstet. Gynecol.* 40:773.

Rajegowda, B. K., et al. 1972. Methadone withdrawal in the newborn infant. *J. Pediatr.* 81:532.

Robinson, C. 1972. *Normal and therapeutic nutrition.* 14th ed. New York: The Macmillan Co.

Rubovits, F. E. 1964. Traumatic rupture of the pregnant uterus from "seat belt" injury. *Am. J. Obstet. Gynecol.* 90:828.

Schneider, H., et al. 1977. *Nutritional support of medical practice.* New York: Harper & Row Publishers, Inc.

Schreier, A. C. Winter 1976. The nurse-midwifery management of physiological edema in pregnancy. *J. Nurse-Midwifery.* 21:4.

Shapiro, S., et al. 1976. Perinatal mortality and birthweight in relation to aspirin taken during pregnancy. *Lancet.* 1:1375.

Slone, D., et al. 1976. Aspirin and congenital malformations. *Lancet.* 1:1373.

Stevens, H. A., and Ohlson, M. A. April 1967. Nutritive value of the diets of medically indigent pregnant women. *J. Am. Diet. Assoc.* 50:290.

Streissguth, A. P. July 1977. Maternal drinking and the outcome of pregnancy: implications for child mental health. *Am. J. Orthopsych.* 47:422.

Taylor, E. S. 1971. *Beck's obstetrical practice.* 9th ed. Baltimore: The Williams & Wilkins Co.

Warshaw, J. B., and Uauy, R. Sept. 1975. Identification of nutritional deficiency and failure to thrive in the newborn. *Clin. Perinatol.* 2:327.

Winick, M., and Noble, A. 1967. Cellular growth in human placenta. I. Normal placenta growth. *Pediatrics.* 39:248.

Zelson, C., et al. 1971. Neonatal narcotic addiction: 10 year observation. *Pediatrics.* 48:178.

CHAPTER 12

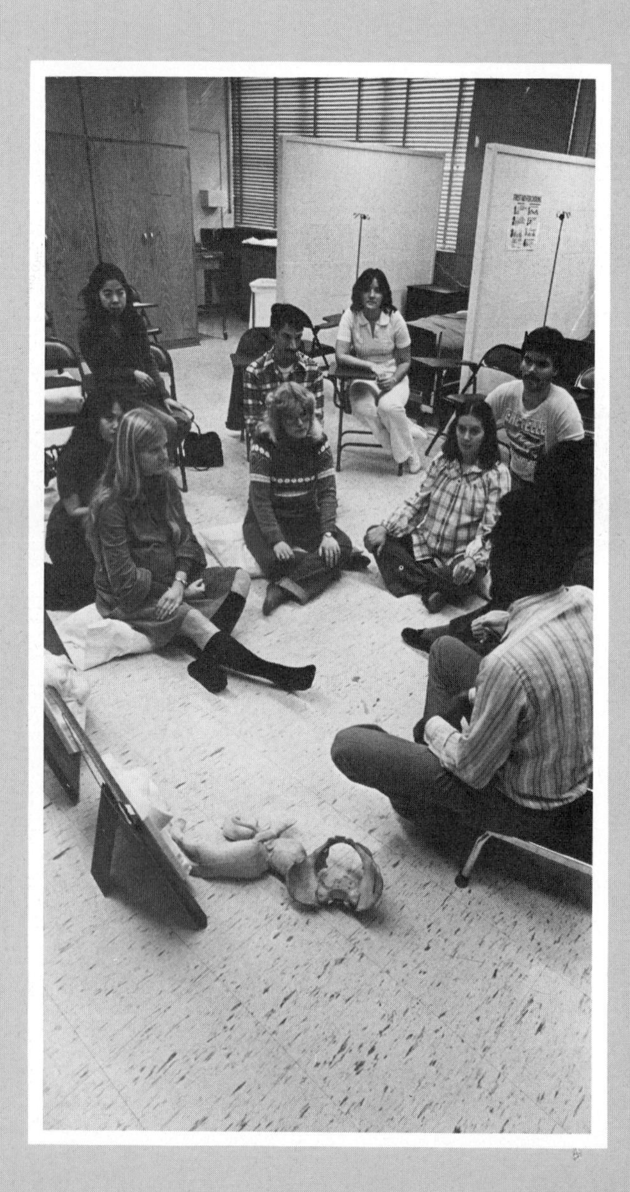

PREPARATION FOR PARENTHOOD

OBJECTIVES

- Identify a family's responses to pregnancy and the appropriate nursing interventions.
- Describe the areas of assessment utilized in establishing a data base for the expectant family.
- Discuss nursing interventions for the family during pregnancy.
- Describe communication skills that parents may use to enhance family well-being.
- Compare and contrast methods of childbirth preparation.
- Determine differences between nursing management for adolescent childbirth and adult childbirth.

PREGNANCY AND THE EXPECTANT FAMILY

Pregnancy as Crisis

Pregnancy is a crisis in a family's life and therefore is accompanied by stress and anxiety, whether or not the pregnancy is desired. *Crisis* can be defined as any naturally occurring turning point (courtship, pregnancy, parenthood, death, or loss of a loved one) that necessitates intrapersonal and interpersonal changes and reorganization. *Stress* is any stimulus that evokes the affective responses of anxiety. Stress disrupts the individual's usual behavior, affect, and attitude and results in anxiety. *Anxiety* is a free-floating, poorly defined apprehensiveness about a vague threat of loss. The loss or threat of loss may be physical (body integrity), psychosocial (established relationships), or economic.

During a crisis, the individual or family is in disequilibrium. Egos weaken, usual defense mechanisms lose their effectiveness, unresolved material from the past reappears, and intrapersonal and interpersonal relationships shift. The period of disequilibrium and disorganization is characterized by abortive attempts to solve the perceived problems.

Crisis and its potential for successful resolution are affected by the individual or family's (a) present level of organization or disorganization; (b) past experiences of success or failure with crisis, stress, and anxiety; (c) established coping patterns, productive or unproductive; and (d) availability and effectiveness of resources.

Pregnancy, whether it terminates in elective or spontaneous abortion or in a term infant, is a turning point in a couple's life. Pregnancy confirms one's biologic capabilities to reproduce, and it is evidence of one's participation in sexual activity and as such is an affirmation of one's sexuality. Pregnancy is the couple's transition period from childlessness to parenthood. If the pregnancy terminates in the birth of a child, the couple enters a new stage of their life together, one characterized by irreversibility and awesome responsibilities.

The expectant couple may be unaware of the physical, emotional, and cognitive state peculiar to pregnancy. The couple may anticipate no problem from such a normal event as pregnancy and therefore may be confused and distressed by the feelings and behaviors commonly associated with childbearing.

If the expectant woman is married or has a stable partner, she no longer is only a wife but also must assume the role of mother. Her partner will soon be a father. Career goals and mobility may be thwarted for one or both partners. Each partner begins to see the other in a different light. Their relationship takes on a different meaning to them and within the larger family and community. Their life-style changes. Role reorientation and reidentification are inevitable with each additional pregnancy and child. The set routines, family dynamics, and interactions are altered again with each pregnancy and require readjustment and realignment.

Even if a pregnant woman, by design or circumstance, is without a stable partner but plans to keep the baby or place it for adoption, her need for changes in role identity, for psychobiologic maturation, and for self-actualization still remains. The woman is no longer a separate individual. She must now consider the needs of another being who is totally dependent on her, at least during the pregnancy.

Decisions regarding financial matters also need to be made at this time. Will the wife work during the pregnancy and return to work after the baby is born? If she chooses to return to work, how soon after the birth of the child will she return? Many men have strong feelings about being the provider and caretaker of the family. Decisions may also need to be made about the division of tasks within the home. If the woman expects to share household and child-care tasks with the man but he believes that women take care of home and children and men provide the income, conflicts will inevitably arise. When these differences are discussed openly, needs are identified, and solutions are agreed upon, the newly forming family moves toward meeting the needs of its members.

Colman and Colman (1972) have done a comprehensive study of parents' reactions to pregnancy and find that, although it is a time of crisis, pregnancy can be a rewarding experience, especially if the couple has formed a trusting alliance and are sincere in their desire to share in every aspect of the experience. However, a weak relationship is often in greater jeopardy during pregnancy, especially if the husband is forced to become involved in childbirth education classes and to be the wife's coach during labor and her supporter in the delivery room.

The couple must face the realities of labor and delivery before parenthood can be realized. Many nonparents have little idea what labor entails. Frequently, their information is based on experiences related to them by family members or friends, and these tales are often fraught with myths and exaggerations. Classes in prepared childbirth can help them overcome much of this lack of information or misinformation (see the discussion on specific methods of childbirth preparation later in this chapter).

Labor is threatening in many respects. Pain, disfigurement, disruption of bodily function, and even death are potential threats for the woman. The man faces the potential disfigurement of his wife, impairment of her health, or her death. Both fear that the baby may be ill or disfigured. The expectant couple is subject to anxiety during this period, and no one can reassure them about the outcome.

Colman and Colman (1972) have described a wide range of expected and normal reactions during pregnancy. Some are physical, others are basically emotional, and they often overlap. Colman and Colman have observed that couples go through similar feelings and reactions during pregnancy whether it is their first, second, or third pregnancy, with a wide range of possible reactions. These reactions parallel the developmental tasks discussed in the next section, and the extremes of reactions may indicate the degree to which the task is accomplished. Both partners' possible reactions to the pregnancy are given in Table 12-1.

Pregnancy as a Developmental Stage

As discussed in Chapter 3, Duvall (1971) views the period of pregnancy and childbirth as a developmental stage in the expanding family that parallels the individual's psychosocial developmental tasks (Table 3-2). Pregnancy can be a period of support or conflict for the couple, depending on the amount of adjustment each is willing to assume to maintain the family's equilibrium.

Three tasks are likely to be complementary and are not likely to cause conflict:

1. The couple plans for the first child's arrival together, collecting information on how to be a mother and a father.
2. Each continues to participate in some separate activities with friends or family members. This may cause some conflict if the partners become too divergent in their activities unless an effort is made to limit these types of associations.
3. As time passes the husband assumes the role of breadwinner and the wife assumes the role of homemaker. She prepares for the birth with layette and nursery organization, and the husband becomes more overtly concerned with the financial responsibilities.

Each member of the expectant family must adjust to the experience of pregnancy and its implications. The psychologic integrity and growth of the family depends on the resolution of certain conflicts and acceptance of changes within the family structure as well as within each individual.

THE EXPECTANT FAMILY'S RESPONSES TO PREGNANCY

The Mother

The pregnant woman undertakes several psychologic tasks during pregnancy to establish a foundation for a healthy, mutually gratifying relationship with her infant:

1. *Acceptance of pregnancy.* She must resolve any ambivalence about pregnancy and eventually accept the embryo-fetus as part of herself; that is, she must establish bonds of attachment. Failure in this task may result in lack of responsivenesss or in a sense of detachment or estrangement after giving birth.

2. *Acceptance of termination of pregnancy.* Toward the end of pregnancy, the mother prepares herself psychologically for physical separation from the fetus. Quickening during the second trimester serves a dual purpose; it helps the mother form bonds of attachment and helps her perceive the fetus as a separate individual. The discomforts of late pregnancy, mounting tension over impending labor, and eagerness to know the sex and appearance of the baby assist her in relinquish-

Table 12–1. Parental Reactions to Pregnancy

Mother's reactions	Father's reactions
First trimester	
Informs father secretively or openly	Differ according to age, parity, desire for child, economic stability
Feels ambivalent toward pregnancy; anxious about labor and responsibility of child	Acceptance of wife's mothering attitude or complete rejection and lack of communication
Is aware of physical changes; daydreams of possible miscarriage	Is aware of his own sexual feelings; may develop more or less sexual arousal
Develops special feelings for, renewed interest in mother, with formation of own mother identity	Accepts, rejects, or resents mother-in-law May develop new hobby outside of family as sign of stress
Second trimester	
Feels movement and is aware of fetus and incorporates it into herself	Feels for movement of baby, listens to heartbeat, or remains aloof, with no physical contact
Dreams that husband will be killed, telephones him often for reassurance	May have fears and fantasies about himself being pregnant; may become uneasy with this feminine aspect to himself
Experiences more distinct physical changes; sexual desires may increase or decrease	May react negatively if wife is too demanding; may become jealous of physician and of his/her importance to wife and her pregnancy
Second trimester Cont'd	
Remains regressive and introspective; all problems with authority figures projected onto husband; may become angry as if lack of interest is sign of weakness in him	If he can cope, will give her extra attention she needs; if he cannot cope, will develop a new time-consuming interest outside of home
Continues to deal with feelings as a mother and looks for furniture as something concrete	May develop a creative feeling and a "closeness to nature"
May have other extreme of anxiety and wait until ninth month to look for furniture and clothes for baby	May become involved in pregnancy and buy or make furniture
Third trimester	
Experiences more anxiety and tension, with physical awkwardness	Adapts to alternative methods of sexual contact
Feels much discomfort and insomnia from physical condition	Becomes concerned over financial responsibility
Prepares for delivery, assembles layette, picks out names	May show new sense of tenderness and concern; treats wife like doll
Dreams often about misplacing baby or not being able to deliver it; fears birth of deformed baby	Daydreams about child as if older and not newborn; dreams of losing wife
Feels ecstasy and excitement; has spurt of energy during last month	Renewed sexual attraction to wife Feels he is ultimately responsible for whatever happens

ing intimacy with the fetus. Baby showers and gifts of baby clothes and equipment also help her identify the separateness (and smallness) of the coming baby.

3. *Acceptance of mother role.* Rubin (1967) describes three phases of establishing one's identity with the mother role: (a) rejection, (b) fantasizing oneself in the role, and (c) actively seeking information and role models. This self-concept as mother begins with the first pregnancy for most women. The self-concept expands with actual experience as a mother and continues to grow throughout subsequent childbearing and childrearing. Occasionally a woman never identifies with the mother role but instead plays the role of babysitter or older sister. For many women, the nurse is a role model. The way the nurse interacts with the baby and nurtures the mother's self-esteem and self-confidence can influence the mother's responsiveness to the baby and her view of herself.

4. *Resolution of fears about childbirth.* During pregnancy, primitive emotional material reemerges, including fantasies about childbirth. Some women do not resolve their fantasies; instead, they suppress their fears and refrain from preparing for labor. These women want to "leave it all up to the doctor" and often request "something to put me out completely." For these women, childbirth may be psychologically traumatic. Other women attempt to master their fears through various methods: psychoprophylactic preparation, reading, or classes.

5. *Bonding.* The attachment of a woman to her child and her binding commitment to nurture the child begin during pregnancy. Thus the maternal response may be influenced to some extent by the positiveness or negativeness of a woman's pregnancy. The maternal response and attachment are discussed in greater detail in Chapter 28.

The Father

For the expectant father, pregnancy is a psychologically stressful time because he, too, is facing the transition from nonparent to parent or from parent of one or more to parent of two or more. Although many fathers say that the event is "not real until I hold the baby in my arms," most undoubtedly experience many changes in their self-concept as a person, a man, and a husband-partner. The man is often confused by his wife's mood changes and perhaps bewildered by his responses to her changing body. He reevaluates himself in terms of his concept of a father, becoming the sole breadwinner (if his wife has worked) and assuming the responsibility for a totally dependent newborn. He may resent the attention given to his wife and the need to change their existing life-style and relationship. He may feel that he wants to be a father someday but that he is just not ready for it now.

For centuries, primitive societies recognized the crisis potential of childbearing and prescribed behaviors and imposed taboos related to pregnancy, birth, and new parenthood. The term *couvade* refers to the observance of certain rituals and taboos by the male to signify the transition to fatherhood. Acting out these socially acceptable and patterned behaviors establishes the man's new identity for himself and others. Some taboos restrict his actions. For example, he may be forbidden to eat certain foods, to kill certain animals, or to carry certain weapons prior to and immediately after the birth. Perhaps these societies recognized a potential threat to the wife and unborn child if the energy from some of his aroused feelings was not rechanneled.

With couvade, the father plays an active and vital role during his wife's labor. In one culture, the father is expected to cry out and writhe in apparent agony while he is attended by several people and ceremoniously "delivered" of a pile of stones between his legs. His cries draw the attention of any lurking harmful spirits. Meanwhile his wife delivers quietly, alone or with one attendant, some distance away and safe from the harmful spirits.

The husband's participation in the couvade affirms his psychosocial and biophysical relationship to the woman and child. Recent trends in this country toward a more active role of the father during pregnancy and childbirth may be a couvade in its embryonic stage.

Some expectant fathers experience *mitleiden* and develop symptoms similar to those of the pregnant wife: weight gain, nausea, and various aches and pains. Many men are unfamiliar with this phenomenon, but the nurse's matter-of-fact inquiry about these psychosomatic symptoms puts the father's experience into the realm of "normal." The exact significance of this phenomenon is unknown. It may be a means for the husband to identify with his wife and the pregnancy, thereby

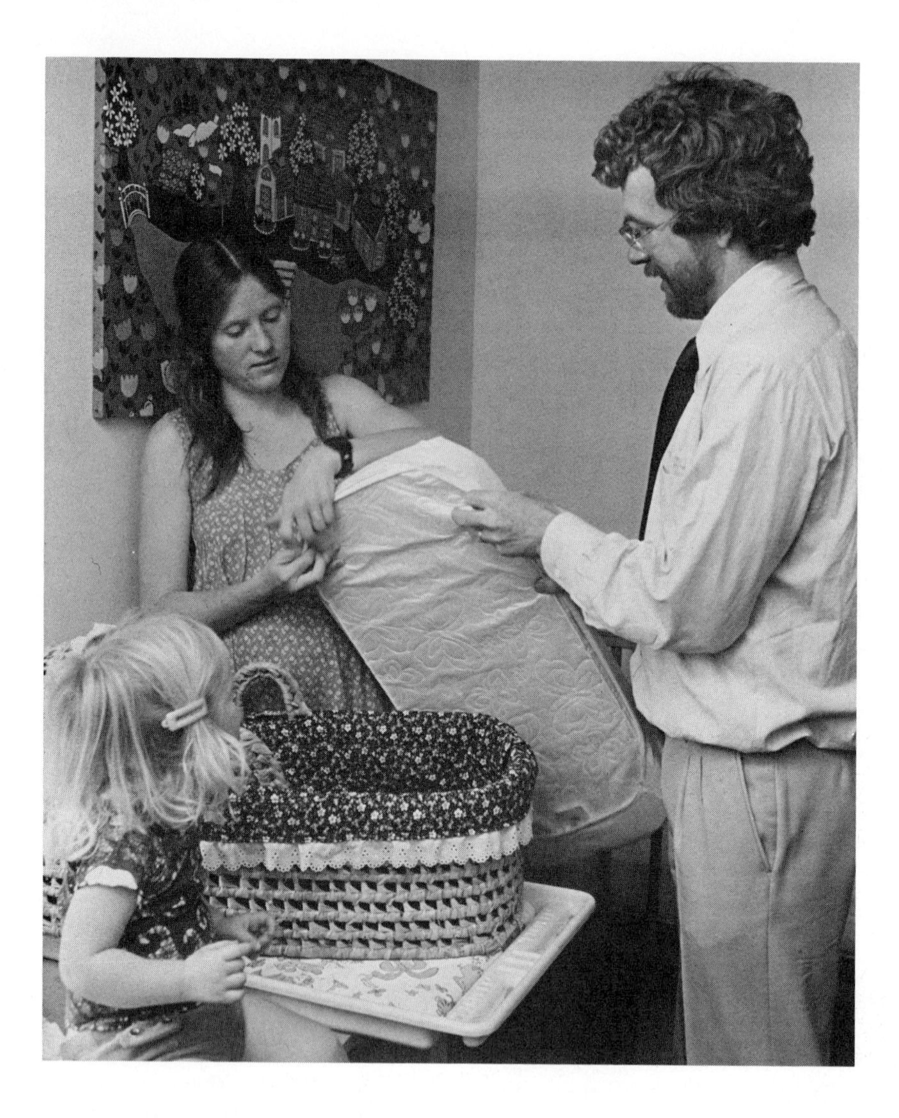

Figure 12–1. Expectant parents and their other children can prepare together for the advent of the new baby.

increasing his sensitivity to his wife's and child's needs.

Siblings

It is commonly recognized that the introduction of a new sibling into a family unit may cause an upheaval among the other children. This upheaval may be major or minor and may be temporary or longlasting. Older siblings may feel their parent-child relationship threatened and may undergo regressive behavior in an attempt to compete with the newly introduced sibling. Regressive behavior such as thumb-sucking, bedwetting, or soiling of underclothing is not uncommon, and its objective appears to be to regain the attentions and affection of one or both parents. This behavior is especially common if the older sibling has not been prepared for the introduction of a new sibling.

Thus for many expectant parents, concern for the newborn is coupled with concern for the needs of any older children at home. Many parents begin to prepare for introducing the new baby before its birth (Figure 12–1).

Preparation begins several weeks prior to the anticipated birth and is designed according to the age and experience of the child. Because they do not have a clear concept of time, young children should not be told too early about the pregnancy. The mother may let the child feel the baby moving in her uterus, explaining that this is "a special place where babies grow." (Many parents need to be reminded to use the word *uterus* versus *stomach*, because *stomach* connotes something being eaten and something that can be vomited. Thus some children develop a dread of eating or defecating or become afraid when they see their mother vomiting.) The child can assist in unpack-

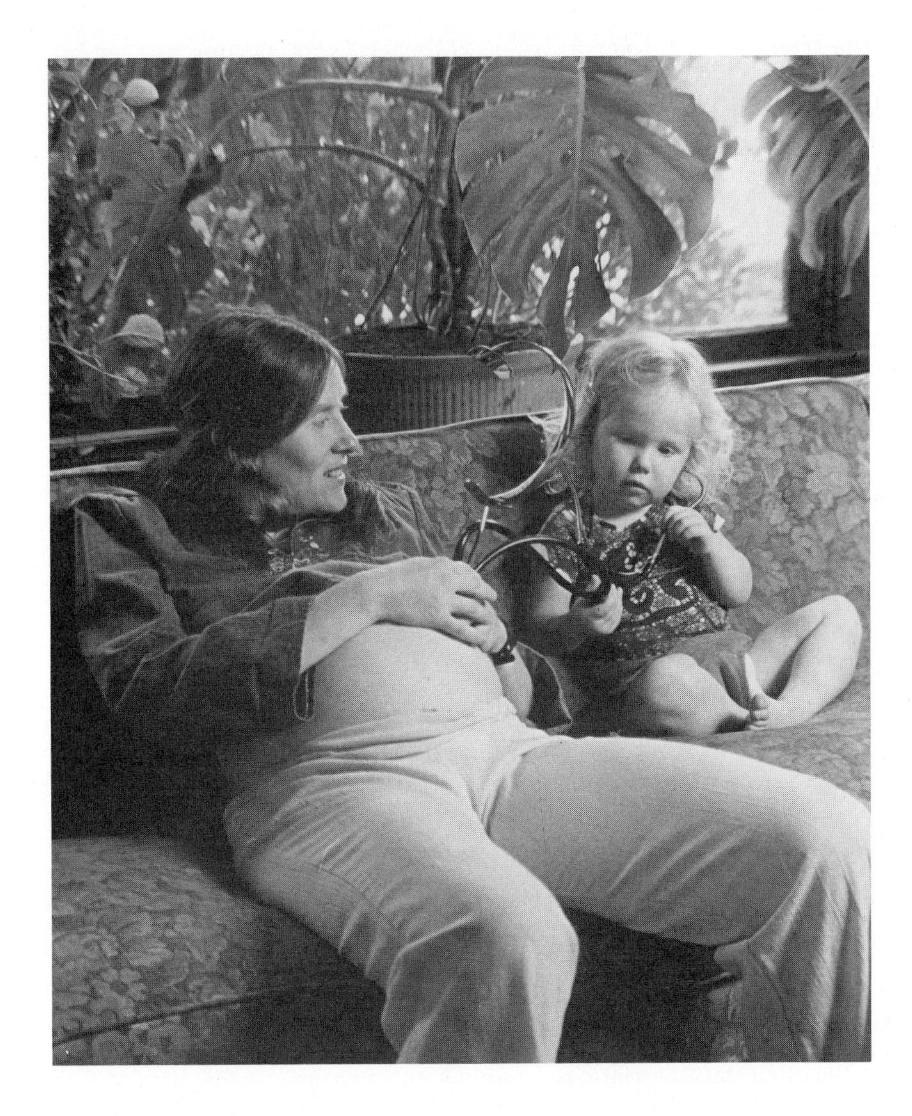

Figure 12-2. Children respond positively when they hear the heartbeat of their sibling-to-be.

ing clothes and putting them in drawers or in preparing the nursery room or area. The child will probably be interested in trying on the clothes, lying in the crib, and trying out other baby items.

If the child is ready for toilet training, it is most effectively done several months before or after the baby's arrival. Parents should know that the older, toilet-trained child may regress to wetting or soiling because he sees the new baby getting attention for such behavior. Any move from crib to bed or from one room to another should precede the baby's birth. The older, weaned child may want to drink from a bottle again after the new baby comes. Lack of knowledge of these common occurrences can be frustrating to the new mother and can compound the stress that she feels during the early days postpartum.

During the pregnancy, if possible, the older child should be introduced to a new baby for short periods to get an idea of what a new baby is like. This introduction dispels fantasies that the new arrival will be big enough to be a playmate.

A preliminary study is being undertaken by Ford* to see whether the inclusion of older siblings in family-oriented obstetrics and prenatal care will facilitate sibling bonding and the integration of the new baby into the family unit and will reduce the degree of regressive behavior in older siblings. For approximately two years, pregnant patients with preschool children (age 2–6) have been encouraged to bring these children to their prenatal visits. Usually parents have made their children aware of the fact that a new sibling is expected. When the children come, they are encouraged to actively participate in prenatal care. The children are encouraged to ask any questions

*From Ford, J. Personal communication, 1978.

they might have and to listen to the fetal heart tones (see Figure 12-2).

These children have shown a keen interest in prenatal activities. Upon hearing the FHTs, small children appear to be totally absorbed in listening to the heart sounds. They frequently stroke the earpieces and tubing of the fetoscope as they are listening. It has been theorized that the child in utero hears the sounds generated by the maternal circulatory system and that these sounds have a soothing effect on the fetus in utero. Perhaps it is a recognition of this type of sound that accounts for the behavior of the small child listening to FHTs.

Whatever the explanation, the results of the study appear to be very positive. Almost without exception, these children become excited participants in the prenatal visits. Frequently mothers report that the children come to look forward to the prenatal visits and comment excitedly about hearing the fetal heart sounds. A few mothers have commented that their children have demonstrated little enthusiasm for listening to music or sound through stereo headsets but have been eager to listen to the FHTs for as long as they are allowed to hold the fetoscope.

Two other interesting aspects of the sibling bonding process are observed when the mothers return for postpartal visits. Almost uniformly, parents report that the new sibling has been smoothly integrated into the family unit, with no apparent regressive behavior on the part of the older siblings who have been permitted to participate in the prenatal care. When older children have returned with the mother and the new baby for postpartal visits, extremely positive interactions between the older children and the new child are frequently observed. On a few occasions the mother has delegated care of the new baby to the older child while she gets her postpartal examination. Typically the older child cares for the new baby in a surprisingly mature and competent manner. Rarely if ever does the baby display any discomfort or disapproval. Parents often comment spontaneously that the siblings like each other or that the sibling relationship seems much better and more positive than previous sibling interactions.

NURSING MANAGEMENT

Assessment: Establishing the Data Base

During the initial contact with the expectant mother or couple, the nurse elicits an explicit patient profile (p. 234): the family's environment, life-style, habits, and relationships; sources and adequacy of income; race and/or culture; patient's temperament and usual way of coping with stressful situations; an average day; and impact of the pregnancy on self, family, and significant others. At subsequent visits the nurse may ask her what *mother* means to her, what she thinks an average day with the baby will be like, and what she expects from the father. The father can be asked similar questions about his expectations for fatherhood and for his wife as a mother.

Many nonparents are not prepared for the sleep and feeding patterns of newborns. They have not thought about their feelings about the inevitable crying of the newborn and what they will do when the baby cries. Many couples are surprised to discover the sometimes extreme discrepancy between the spouse's view of parenthood and expectation of the other. Guided discussion of these topics allows parents-to-be to attack problems, to arrive at compromises, and to appreciate each other's uniqueness.

Personal habits relevant to pregnancy include patterns of diet, sleep, and sexual activity; exercise; hobbies; and use of drugs (alcohol, tobacco, caffeine, and others). A past health history, describing the type and kind of therapies and responses to illness, adds significantly to the data base. The family history reveals the woman's placement within a family tree and her social relationship to its members. While taking the family history, the nurse can inquire about the geographic and social distance from family members, the frequency of visits, and the expected assistance from family members during pregnancy and after delivery.

The data base is completed with a description of body functioning, a complete physical examination, and laboratory values (see Chapter 10).

From the health assessment, the nurse develops an initial plan for interventions during the couple's preparation for childbearing and childrearing. The plan anticipates the need for information, guidance, and physical care. Interventions are timed to coincide with the woman's (couple's) readiness and needs.

Interventions

Any crisis situation makes the involved parties more vulnerable but also more amenable to intervention. Through physical and psychosocial closeness to the woman or couple and with a detailed health assessment, the nurse is in a good position to intervene therapeutically. Well-paced interventions reassure prospective parents and validate their feelings and thoughts.

Two primary functions of the nurse caring for the pregnant family are (a) to support the family unit and (b) to provide prenatal education. If these tasks are performed well, family members may gain greater problem-solving ability, self-esteem, self-confidence, feelings of self-worth, and ability to participate in health care. In addition, parents who feel good about themselves have a sounder foundation on which to build meaningful relationships with their children.

Support of Family Unit

Chapter 11 focuses on the problems and concerns of the pregnant woman, the relief of her discomforts, and maintenance of her physical health. However, her well-being also depends on the well-being of those she is closest to. Thus it is important that the nurse meet the needs of the woman's family in order to maintain the integrity of the family unit.

Husbands

Anticipatory guidance of the expectant father is a necessary part of any plan of care. He may need information about the anatomic, physiologic, and emotional changes that occur during pregnancy and postpartum, the couple's sexuality and sexual response, and possible reactions that he may experience. He may wish to express his feelings about breast- versus bottle-feeding, the sex of the child, and other topics. If it is culturally and personally acceptable to him, the nurse refers the couple to expectant parents' classes for further information and support from other couples.

The nurse ascertains the father's intended degree of participation during labor and delivery and assesses his knowledge of coaching and comfort measures and his preparation for the sights, sounds, and smells he may experience. If the couple prefers that his participation be minimal or restricted, the nurse supports their decision. With this type of consideration and collaboration, the father is less apt to develop feelings of alienation, helplessness, and guilt during the intrapartal period. Thus the relationship between the couple may be strengthened and his self-esteem raised. He is then better able to provide physical and emotional support to his wife during the birthing process.

Siblings

The nurse incorporates in her plan for prenatal care a discussion about the negative feelings that older children may have. It may distress parents to see an older child become aggressive toward the newborn. Parents who are unprepared for the older child's feelings of anger, jealousy, and rejection may respond inappropriately in their confusion and surprise. The nurse stresses that open communication between parents and children (or acting out feelings with a doll if the child is too young to verbalize) helps the children to master their feelings and may prevent them from hurting the newest sibling when they are unsupervised. Children may feel less neglected and more secure if they know that their parents are willing to help with their anger and aggressiveness.

Teaching Communication Skills

The nurse's role may be expanded to teaching parents specific communication skills that enhance family well-being. Whether this is the first child or not, learning and using these skills will strengthen family relationships. In addition, these communication skills directly benefit the nurse-patient relationship.

The communication skills described in this section are based on the work of Gordon (1970), who formulated an easily understood and practical adaptation of well-established psychotherapeutic techniques. The skills he described that facilitate growth are active listening, sending I-messages, resolving conflicts through the "no-lose" method, and handling values collisions.

Active Listening

Active listening is a well-tested technique for helping a person with a problem. The listener simply feeds back to the sender his understanding of the meaning and of the feelings underlying the sender's statement.

Active listening requires certain underlying attitudes, including (a) wanting to be helpful to the other person, (b) genuinely being able to accept his feelings, and (c) having a deep feeling of trust in the person's capacity to handle his feelings and to work through them to find solutions to his problems. Active listening is a profound but conceptually simple way to help another person in the sometimes frightening experience of being himself.

One important application of active listening in the maternity clinical setting is in deescalation of the patient's concern about her health or the couple's worries about the well-being of the fetus. Active listening can give the worried couple relief about the concern as well as a sense that the concern is being taken seriously. Active listening can also help the worried person arrive at the kind of emotional quiescence necessary to be able to hear, understand, and follow through on the nurse's professional recommendations.

Another use of active listening is in facilitating the sharing of information. Because active listening helps the other person feel comfortable sharing thoughts as well as feelings, the nurse's use of active listening enables her to obtain more data about the maternity patient upon which to base the nursing diagnosis. A further benefit is the feeling of collaboration in the effort to restore and maintain the health of family members. This way of building a relationship between nurse and patient also serves as a model for the expectant parent to emulate in responding to feelings, needs, and concerns expressed by the partner and eventually by their child.

Sending I-Messages

The second communication skill described by Gordon is the ability to send I-messages. An I-message lets the sender tell another person how he feels about behavior that he finds unacceptable. An I-message has three components: (a) a nonblameful description of the behavior of the other person, (b) a statement of the concrete and tangible effect of that behavior on the sender, and (c) a statement of the sender's feelings about the behavior.

Nurses have many opportunities for using I-messages to communicate their needs to patients. I-messages allow nurses to express their feelings yet cause patients minimal embarrassment, guilt, or shame. This type of communication enlists the patient's willingness to initiate behavior out of consideration for the nurse's needs. I-messages such as the following may be sent from nurses to patients: "I am concerned when you don't take your medication. It makes me afraid you'll have a relapse and the work done so far will be wasted." This nonblameful yet clear way for nurses to identify their needs generates minimal resistance, so that the patient remains willing to modify his behavior.

No-Lose Problem-solving

Many solutions to conflicts involve the imposition of one party's will on the other. For example, the parent "wins" at the expense of the child's needs, or the child "wins" at the expense of the parent's needs. In either case, the loser inevitably feels resentful of the winner, and there is damage to the relationship. The no-lose method of problem-solving is designed to make both parties "winners."

The first step is to identify the needs of each person, with full use of active listening and I-messages. Both persons then search for a solution that is acceptable to each. They offer possible solutions, evaluate them, and eventually make a decision on a final solution that satisfies both. No compromise is required after the solution has been selected, because both parties have already accepted it. No power is required to force compliance, because neither is resisting the decision.

Conflicts between nurses and their patients are inevitable, as they are in all human relationships. Authoritarian nurses who impose their solutions on patients without reference to the patients' needs will find that they have resentful and resistant patients who are less likely to adhere to the professional advice. Permissive nurses who yield to their patients often suffer through missed appointments, late payment for services, or incomplete medical histories; as a result, they feel abused and resentful of the time and energy spent with that patient. The no-lose problem-solving process gives nurses, couples, and parents the tools they need to avoid authoritarian or permissive responses to conflict and ensures that everyone's needs are met.

Handling Values Collisions

In values collision one person's behavior may cause consternation to the other without affecting the other's physical well-being. Both marriage partners hold values, and often they would like to influence each other to behave in ways consonant with those values. Nurses have values, too. In the clinical situation, for example, a nurse may want the expectant woman to adhere to a particular nutritional program, may feel that it is important that the couple talk more openly with each other about sex, or may want the couple to be less anxious about the dangers of childbirth. Although the nurse's well-being is not affected if the patients do not follow her advice, she nevertheless wants to influence the patients' behavior.

Gordon identifies three ways to influence the behavior of other people that have application to personal relationships as well as to the clinical setting:

1. Modeling by living congruently with professed values.
2. Acting as a consultant by sharing pertinent information with the other person on a one-time basis.
3. Modifying one's own values.

Modeling can be a potent influence on the behavior of another person. In the clinical situation, the patient often looks to the nurse for guidance. For this reason it is desirable that the nurse examine the values she is modeling; her credibility will be undermined if her behavior is not congruent with her professed values. Is the nurse negating the values she purports by being overweight and rundown and by smoking heavily? Is the nurse modeling a respect for her patients' concerns or merely offering treatment for the physical complaint and ignoring the emotional needs associated with illness? Are there ways that the nurse can enhance her commitment to modeling values that she considers important?

A second way to influence an individual's values is to act as a consultant. This role is not foreign to the nurse nor unexpected of a parent or a marriage partner. An important consideration, however, is the timing of such information-sharing; one person must want to hear the other person's advice. Before offering professional or personal advice, it is often necessary to use active listening to defuse the person's intense feeling and to restore the person's emotional equilibrium. Then it is advisable to determine whether the person would like advice, preferably by asking directly. The answer to that question will indicate whether the person is open to consultation and is willing to consider it carefully.

As in any consulting relationship, the nurse must allow the patient to decide about the usefulness of the advice—that is, whether to "buy" the consultation. Also, the nurse must realize that repeated attempts to convert the patient to her viewpoint, once it has been fully explained, only increase the patient's defensiveness and the likelihood that he or she will ignore the advice. These considerations are also applicable to advice-giving within the family situation.

Another way to lessen values collisions is to modify values through identifying them, examining them, learning why other people's values are different, and changing values when change seems appropriate and desirable.

In the clinical setting, the nurse's willingness to express values and attitudes but to remain open to examining other approaches can be a refreshing model for expectant parents, who sometimes feel that they must be consistent and must know all the answers about their relationship, about childbearing, and about childrearing. It can be helpful for them to realize that they have the freedom to change, that they need not be straitjacketed to traditional approaches to be effective within their marital relationship and with their children. This attitude also helps their children realize that they have the freedom to change and to redefine their values and attitudes.

Using these communication skills in the clinical setting and teaching them to the expectant couple have three primary benefits. First, the antepartal care will be more effective because the patient is more likely to discuss her concerns with the nurse and is also more likely to adhere to the treatment regimen. Second, these skills provide the expectant couple with tools for openly dealing with conflict, decision-making, and problems. Finally, the couple can use these skills in dealing with their children.

The maternity encounter is not the only or even necessarily the best place to teach and acquire effective communication. Courses for parents that focus on these skills are probably more

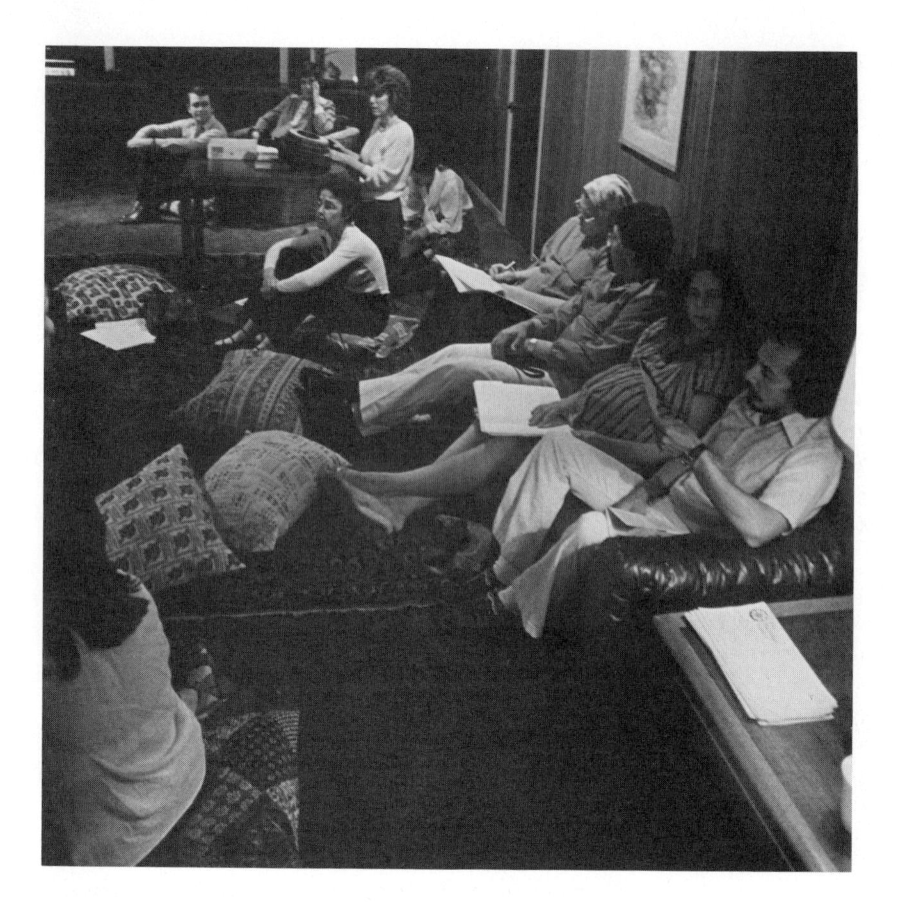

Figure 12–3. Childbirth preparation classes provide an opportunity for parents to learn together and exchange ideas.

effective educational vehicles. However, because support for parents is often scarce, the maternity setting may provide an opportunity to reinforce the learning of these skills.

Prenatal Education

Antepartal educational programs vary in their goals, content, leadership techniques, and method of teaching. Content of the classes is generally dictated by the goals. For example, the goals of some classes are to prepare the couple for childbirth, and therefore discomforts of pregnancy and care of the newborn may not be included. Other classes may be oriented only to pregnancy and not prepare the woman for labor and delivery. Nurses should be aware of these variations and the goals of the couple before directing couples to specific classes (Figure 12–3).

One-to-One Teaching

Teaching on an individual basis occurs when the patient needs it. Anticipatory guidance is also an important part of teaching, and its effective use is based on the nurse's knowledge of the maternity cycle, her assessment of its effect on the mother and other family members, and her judgment of how this knowledge should be applied to probable or existing needs. Anticipatory guidance is frequently used in discussion of such topics as care of breasts in pregnancy, sexual activity, and preparation for labor and delivery.

A nurse's teaching skills improve as she becomes more aware of the needs of expectant families and as she broadens her base of knowledge. A continuous evaluation of the effectiveness of her teaching is essential in developing these skills.

Group Teaching

Group discussion is an appropriate and effective teaching method, and it allows for optimum use of the nursing process. The nursing process basically involves the continuous assessment of patient needs through various methods of data collection, intervention determined by the nurse's interpretation of the needs and by her knowledge and skills, and evaluation of how well the nursing intervention has met the patient's needs. In group teaching, however, the nurse assesses the needs of the group instead of the needs of an individual. Her knowledge of group skills thus becomes essential.

Auerbach (1968) a leader in the field of parent education, has listed nine basic assumptions about parent group education:

1. Parents can learn.
2. Parents want to learn.
3. Parents learn best what they are interested in learning.
4. Learning is most significant when the subject matter is closely related to the parents' own immediate experience.
5. Parents can learn best when they are free to create their own response to a situation.
6. Parent group education is as much an emotional experience as it is an intellectual one.
7. Parents can learn from one another.
8. Parent group education provides the basis for a remaking of experience.
9. Each parent learns in his own way.*

Other factors are important in facilitating group teaching. Groups should contain no more than 20 members when couples are involved (many fewer if only mothers are in the group). An informal and friendly environment must be maintained. The members must attend consistently, and other activities should be encouraged in order to increase cohesiveness of the group. Large classes whose members sit in rows listening to didactic presentations by the nurse lose their effectiveness. Even when a short period is allowed for questions at the end of the lecture, only a few group members are able to participate. This traditional approach cannot provide for continuous identification of members' learning needs.

Helping the group to set an agenda at the initial session of a series of classes is one way of assessing members' needs. The individuals in the group must first become comfortable with each other so that there is a general sharing of concerns, questions, and information. Various techniques can be used to help the group members become familiar with one another. For example, the group can be divided into subgroups of two or three couples. Each subgroup is asked to list specific questions or concerns they would like discussed in the series of classes and to rank them in the order of interest. The subgroups are given a limited amount of time in which to accomplish their task. This method also stimulates much exchange of personal information.

Various methods can be used to compile the subgroups' lists. For example, a spokesperson for each group can submit a topic. As she clarifies what is meant, the individual who mentioned the topic elaborates, and often other members contribute their concerns on the subject. Eventually the group leader has an agenda set by the group. Anticipatory guidance is necessary if discussion of important areas of content is not requested by group members; the leader can check with the group to determine whether it is an area of interest to them. Time must also be allotted for helping the group to plan how the agenda will be utilized, say by grouping topics into general areas of focus, and letting the group determine the sequence in which these areas will be discussed.

Nursing intervention takes many forms in group discussion and frequently overlaps with assessment and evaluation as specific interests and concerns are clarified. The nurse may need to draw other members into the discussion or to clarify information. However, most prenatal classes are not purely discussion groups but include films, tours of maternity wards, demonstrations, and lengthy explanations. In classes concerned with selected methods of childbirth preparation, many group members have read extensively on the subject and can contribute considerably to the discussion, whereas other members may know nothing about it and thus require more explanations and demonstrations by the nurse. In situations where group members know little about the method, a more structured approach to discussion and exercises may be useful.

Evaluation of the effectiveness of the teaching-learning process is also continuous, but it is the most nebulous aspect. Checking each individual on a return demonstration of an exercise is the most concrete way to evaluate learning. Evaluating members' changes in attitude or misconceptions is more difficult. A general evaluation of the series may be conducted in the last class, or evaluation forms can be given to members to return by mail at a later date.

*From Auerbach, A. 1968. *Parents learn through discussion: principles and practice of parent group education.* New York: John Wiley & Sons, Inc.

Some excellent books have been written to give the beginning practitioner specific directions on how to establish classes and how to be an effective group leader. Initially the traditional didactic method is easiest to use; however, as she utilizes the nursing process in practice, the nurse will become dissatisfied with didactic presentations and find herself gradually developing skills as an effective leader in group discussion.

SELECTED METHODS OF CHILDBIRTH PREPARATION

Various methods of childbirth preparation are taught in North America. General antepartal classes cover various aspects of the maternity cycle and care of the newborn. Some classes, however, are more specifically oriented to preparation for labor and delivery, are labeled with a name indicating a theory of reduction of pain in childbirth, and are accompanied by specific exercises to accomplish this task. The three most common methods of this type are the Read (natural childbirth), the Lamaze (psychoprophylactic), and the Bradley (husband-coached childbirth). Hypnosis is also discussed here becaue it is sometimes used to help the expectant mother reduce or even eliminate pain in labor and delivery.

The programs in prepared childbirth have some similarities. All have an educational component to help eliminate fear. The classes vary in the breadth and depth of their coverage of various subjects related to the maternity cycle, but all prepare the participants in what to expect during labor and delivery and in methods of relaxation. Except for hypnosis, these methods also teach exercises to condition muscles and breathing patterns used in labor. The greatest differences among the methods are in the theories of why they work and in the relaxation techniques and breathing patterns that are taught (Figures 12-4 and 12-5).

The advantages of these methods of childbirth preparation are several. The most important is that a healthier baby may be produced because of the reduced need for analgesics and anesthetics. Another advantage is the satisfaction of the couples for whom childbirth has become a shared and profound emotional experience. In addition, proponents of each method claim that it shortens the labor process, which has been clinically validated.

All maternity nurses must know how these methods differ, so that they will be able to support the couple in their chosen method. It is important that the nurse assess the couple's emotional resources and their expectations for the birth experience, so that she can more effectively help them to achieve their goals.

Read Method

Dr. Grantly Dick-Read (1959) was an English physician and a pioneer in the childbirth preparation movement, as discussed in Chapter 1. After observing many women in labor and assisting them in delivery, he developed a theory of preparation for childbirth. In 1933 his first book was published, entitled *Natural Childbirth.* It created considerable furor among physicians in his country.

Dick-Read called his method *natural childbirth* because he felt the process of labor and delivery was originally a natural process. He believed that pain experienced during this time was mental in origin, stating that "theoretically nature made no provision for parturition to be painful." Most women experience pain because of the culturally induced fear that they associate with childbirth. Thus his preparation method is centered around the fear-tension-pain syndrome: If the fear of childbirth is removed, tension will be reduced and pain will minimized. Dick-Read believed that fear of childbirth could be removed by education. In his classes, mothers were taught what to expect in labor and delivery and to understand the process. Achievement of relaxation was also important. Additional exercises included conditioning of muscles that would be used in childbirth and others directed to the control of respiration during contractions. His program of physical preparation was developed with the assistance of Helen Heardman (1961), a physiotherapist who was a proponent of this method.

Classes teaching the Read method follow a basic pattern. Part of the class time is devoted to the educational component and the other part to demonstration and practice of exercises.

Relaxation is an important part of the Read method. The woman is taught to use passive re-

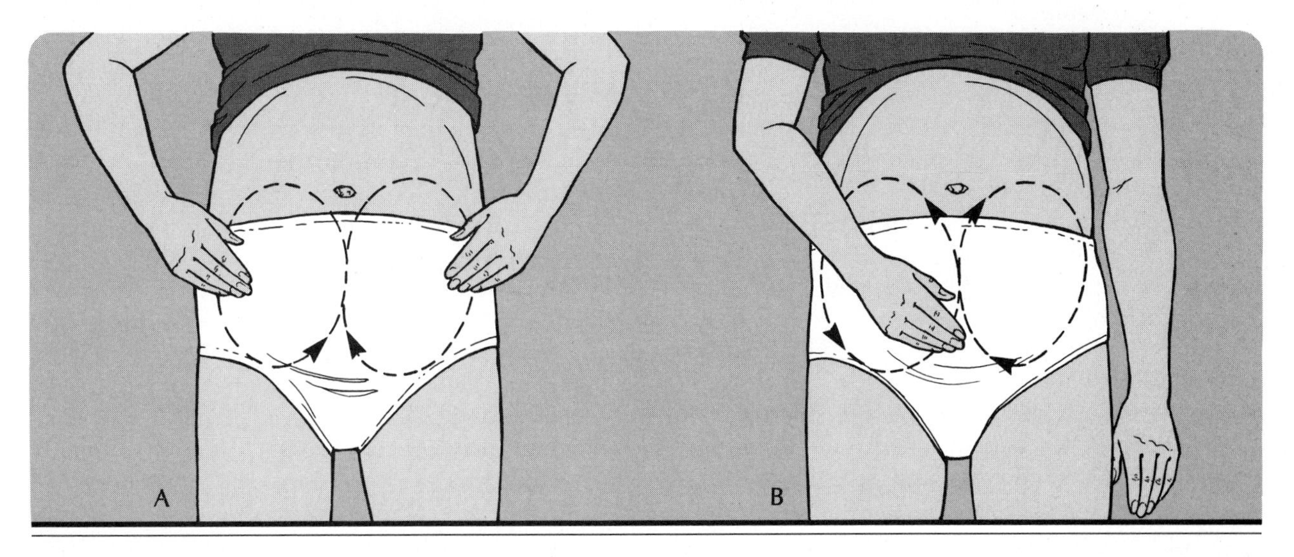

Figure 12–4. Effleurage is light stroking of the abdomen with the fingertips. **A,** Starting at the symphysis the patient lightly moves her fingertips up and around in a circular pattern. **B,** An alternate approach involves the use of one hand in a figure-eight pattern. This technique is used primarily during labor.

laxation methods, such as progressive contraction and relaxation of muscle groups from her head to her toes, which may result in her falling asleep. She is encouraged to use this technique in labor to help her sleep or nap between contractions. If she is not able to sleep, at least she can relax her muscles.

The pattern of respiration utilized in labor is basically abdominal breathing. The woman concentrates on forcing the abdominal muscles to rise. When she begins the class, she probably takes several breaths per minute, but she is gradually taught to take one breath per minute, with a 30-second inhalation and 30-second exhalation. This pattern of breathing lifts the abdominal muscles as the uterus rises forward with a contraction. Proponents of this method suggest that the pressure of the abdominal muscles on the contracting uterus increases pain. The woman is encouraged to practice her breathing in various positions and while involved in various activities. She begins the breathing technique with the first contraction in labor. Women utilizing the Read method should not be interrupted in the middle of a contraction while doing their breathing.

An effective "pushing" position is also taught, but pushing is not done until the second stage of labor when it is needed. Body conditioning exercises condition the appropriate muscles. Panting is also taught to prevent pushing when it is not necessary.

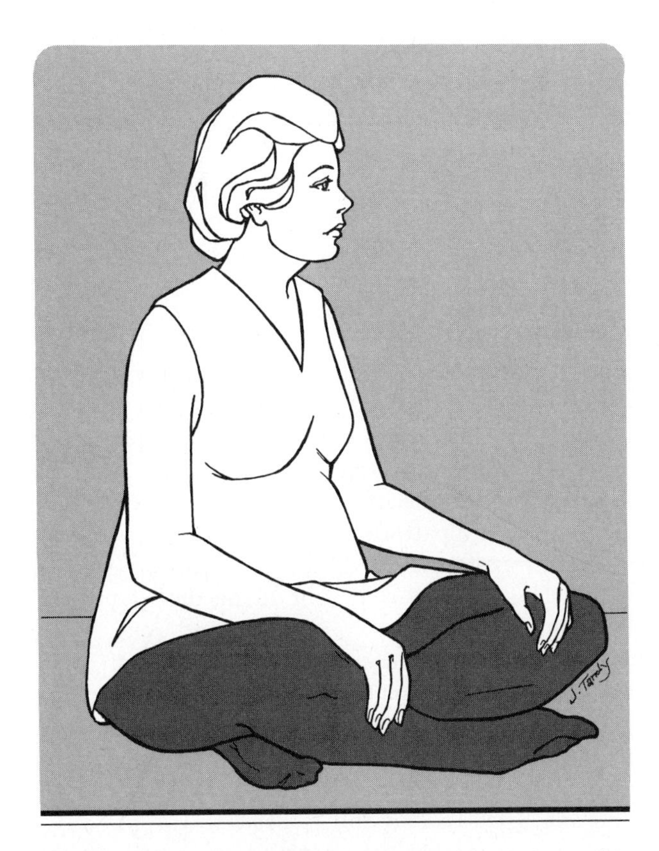

Figure 12–5. Tailor sit. The pregnant woman sits on the floor in cross-legged style. This exercise aids in stretching the adductor muscles of the legs.

Dick-Read emphasized the importance of a supportive environment throughout labor and delivery. He believed that a major source of discomfort for a woman during labor was the suggestion of pain, which "emanates from doctors, nurses, and relatives who believe in pain" (Dick-Read, 1959). Proponents of all prepared childbirth methods believe that this type of environment still exists in many institutions and is a major source of discomfort.

Dick-Read believed husbands should be educated because of their influence on their wives but that husbands should not be with their wives during labor if they were not helpful to them. He emphasized that analgesia and anesthesia were available for women using his method of natural childbirth but implied throughout his book that a woman is either improperly prepared or remiss in her duty as a mother if she requests them.

Abdominal breathing can be effectively utilized to reduce labor pain by women who have had no preparation of any kind, although it will not be as effective as for the woman who has practiced this method throughout the latter part of her pregnancy. The unprepared woman requires continuous support throughout labor to maintain any semblance of this pattern of slow, deep breathing.

Psychoprophylactic (Lamaze) Method

The terms *psychoprophylactic* and *Lamaze* are used interchangeably. *Psychoprophylactic* means "mind prevention," and Dr. Fernand Lamaze, a French obstetrician, was the first person to introduce this method of childbirth preparation to the Western world. Psychoprophylaxis actually originated in Russia and is based on Pavlov's research with conditioned reflexes. Pavlov found that the cortical centers of the brain can respond to only one set of signals at a time and that they accept only the strongest signal; the weaker signals are inhibited. Pavlov's research also demonstrated that verbal representation of a stimulus can create a response. When the real stimulus is substituted, the conditioned response continues to be produced. This theory was successfully applied to preparation for childbirth by Russian physicians.

Lamaze first became familiar with the psychoprophylaxis method when attending a conference in Russia. He introduced the method in France in 1951, adding innovations of his own. It was popularized soon after in this country through Marjorie Karmel's book *Thank You, Dr. Lamaze* (1965). The method was called "painless childbirth" and thus received much resistance from the medical profession in this country because it was believed that women inevitably experience pain in childbirth. Furthermore, with the growing development of many analgesic and anesthetizing agents, it did not seem necessary to condition women for childbirth.

Proponents of the method gradually organized and in 1960 formed a nonprofit group called the American Society for Prophylaxis in Obstetrics. Two of the founders were Marjorie Karmel and Elizabeth Bing, a physical therapist who had also written about childbirth preparation using this method (Bing, 1967). This organization helped establish many programs throughout the country and has become one of the most popular methods of childbirth education.

The two components of the class involve education and training. Couples are taught about childbirth and are trained to do specific exercises. Instructors teaching the method in this country have modified many of the original exercises, but the basic theory of conditioned reflex remains the same. Women are taught to substitute favorable conditioned responses for unfavorable ones. Rather than restlessness and loss of control in labor, the woman learns to respond to contractions with conditioned relaxation of the uninvolved muscles and a learned respiratory pattern. Exercises taught in these classes include proper body mechanics and body conditioning, breathing techniques for labor, and relaxation.

Some of the body conditioning exercises are similar to those taught in other childbirth preparation classes, such as the pelvic tilt, pelvic rock, and Kegel exercise. Other exercises strengthen the abdominal muscles for the expulsive phase of labor. The method of relaxing uninvolved muscle groups (neuromuscular control), however, is unique and is a pattern of active relaxation, which is in contrast to the Read method of passive relaxation. The woman is taught to become familiar with the sensation of contraction and relaxation of the voluntary muscle groups throughout her body. She then learns to contract a specific muscle group and relax the rest of her body. This process of isolating the action of one group of voluntary muscles from the rest of the body is called *neuromuscular disassociation* and is basic to the psychoprophylaxis method of prepared childbirth. This exercise conditions the woman to separate the voluntary muscles of her body from uterine activ-

Psychoprophylactic Method: Breathing Patterns*

Level 1 Woman breathes in through nose, out through mouth in a smooth rhythm. Her breathing is relaxed and at her own speed.

Level 2 Woman keeps mouth closed and quickly breathes in through nose as if sniffing and breathes out through mouth as she says the word "ah" ("sniff-ah"). The "sniff" is quick and short, and the expiration is slow and lazy.

Level 3 Woman breathes in and out through mouth. As she expires, she says the word "house" as if she has a lisp ("howth").

Level 4 Woman breathes in and out through her mouth. She breathes in and says "ah." She blows out through pursed lips and says "whew."

*From Childbirth Education Association of the Pikes Peak Region. *Levels of breathing.* Colorado Springs: The Association.

ity by relaxation of uninvolved muscles while the uterus contracts.

The breathing patterns utilized in the Lamaze method are also different from other methods. Chest breathing patterns vary according to the phase of labor; breathing becomes progressively more shallow. The breathing patterns most commonly utilized are slow, deep chest breathing; shallow, accelerated-decelerated breathing; and a "pant-blow" pattern utilizing shallow chest breathing. (See above for the various levels of breathing.) Proponents of this method believe that the variety of chest breathing patterns helps keep the pressure of the diaphragm off the contracting uterus. The patterns of breathing do vary across the country. Occasionally the woman is taught to use one pattern until it is no longer effective rather than in conjunction with the phases of labor.

Another major modification in the Lamaze method involves the goals of expectant couples. Lamaze and his supporters implied that, if the childbirth experience was to be successful (painless with no anesthetic), specific criteria must be adhered to. Couples using this method are now encouraged to set their own goals for success. Lamaze childbirth education in this country supplies them with the tools to assist them in accomplishing these goals.* The couple is encouraged to discuss their goals with the obstetrician and maternity nursing personnel in labor and delivery. When the nursing staff are aware of what the couple hopes to accomplish and of the resources they have available, they will be able to support them more effectively in their endeavors.

*Nurses who are interested in further information about the psychoprophylactic method of childbirth or are interested in becoming certified teachers can write to the American Society for Psychoprophylaxis in Obstetrics, 1523 L Street, NW, Washington, DC 20005. Individuals in other professional fields are also trained and certified to teach this method.

In France, *monitrices* are specially trained to assist the woman in labor and delivery. In this country, the husband has become the specially trained individual. In the United States, the Lamaze method no longer means childbirth without anesthetics or pain. The couple's training, however, helps the woman to reduce pain and even to eliminate the need for anesthetics. More important, the woman is prepared to be an active participant and to be in control of her experience.

Of concern when using this method is the hyperventilation that sometimes occurs in laboring women doing the rapid chest breathing. Couples are prepared to recognize and relieve the hyperventilation immediately, but it is still a concern to medical and nursing personnel. However, this condition can occur in any labor if the patient is not breathing properly. If prolonged, hyperventilation can cause maternal respiratory alkalosis and fetal acidosis. When the woman in labor is hyperventilating, the nurse needs to assess what can be changed in the woman's breathing technique and to help her correct the problem.

Bradley Method

The Bradley method, frequently referred to as husband-coached natural childbirth, is not as well known in this country as the childbirth preparation methods previously discussed. It is basically

Read's method with the important introduction of the husband, who plays a vital role in coaching the wife throughout pregnancy in preparation for labor and delivery.

In his writings and talks, Bradley compares his method of natural childbirth to the natural insticts in animals. He has observed that animals do not suffer pain during the birthing process. He suggests that their birthing behaviors can be adapted by women to alleviate their suffering. He lists environmental characteristics sought by birthing animals and their natural habits that he feels are necessary to achieve natural childbirth: darkness, solitude, quiet, physical comfort, physical relaxation, controlled breathing, and the appearance of sleep (Bradley, 1974). The exercises used to accomplish the relaxation and controlled breathing are basically those used in the Read method. A book titled *Exercises for True Natural Childbirth* (1975) gives more explicit instructions on how to do these exercises. The book was written by Rhonda Hartman, a nurse who was an early advocate of this method and who worked with Bradley in teaching and promoting it.

Bradley's goal is to help women achieve an unmedicated pregnancy, labor, and delivery. Proponents of his method have recently established the American Academy of Husband-Coached Childbirth for certifying teachers in his method. The teachers are usually individuals who have used the method successfully.*

Hypnosis

The use of hypnosis in childbirth is not as common as the other methods of preparation just discussed. It does not include active exercising and is not usually taught in a group situation. However, hypnosis is similar to the other methods in that it reduces fear of childbirth by telling the woman what to expect, produces relaxation, and reduces or eliminates pain. The success of this method depends on self-suggestibility and on rapport between the hypnotist and the woman.

The routine use of hypnosis is discouraged because many women are drawn to it out of curiosity and not many obstetricians are trained in this method. It is time-consuming because it is done on a one-to-one basis in most situations. The obstetrician is frequently the hypnotist and begins preparation of the woman around the fifth or sixth month of pregnancy. Most commonly, the first session is spent discussing the woman's motivation for using this method and clarifying what it is. Six to eight sessions may be incorporated as part of the woman's prenatal visits.

After clarification about the use of hypnosis, the woman is introduced to a method of achieving relaxation that works most effectively for her. When in the trancelike state associated with hypnosis, the woman is deeply relaxed but awake and has heightened awareness to suggestions by the hypnotist. All other external stimuli are blocked from her awareness, and her concentration is focused on the hypnotist's suggestions.

When the hypnotist feels that his patient is able to reach a medium or complete trance, he introduces "glove anesthesia" into the sessions. The hypnotist describes the process of anesthetizing the woman's hand from the wrist to her fingertips. He describes the tingling sensations she will experience and the eventual numbness of her hand. When the subject is able to achieve the numbness in her hand, she can transfer this anesthesia to other parts of her body by suggestion and touch. Throughout these sessions, the woman's experience in labor and delivery is described in a positive manner, and the hypnotist attempts to prepare her for her experience on a step-by-step basis to prevent any element of surprise. By the last session autohypnosis may be accomplished by the patient (Tinterow, 1972).

Cues—posthypnotic suggestions given while the woman is in stages of deep relaxation—are important during the woman's childbirth experience. An example of a cue is the suggestion that she enter deep relaxation; the hypnotist need not go through the lengthy hypnotic induction technique he uses initially to help her relax. Posthypnotic suggestions are utilized automatically in labor, with the numbness from the abdominal area to the knees being achieved rapidly, inside and out. During labor, the woman is never unconscious and can carry out such activities as voiding. She should be disturbed as infrequently as possible and spoken to softly; discomfort should never be suggested.

Immediately after delivery, the woman is brought out of her trance to see her baby. If an episiotomy repair is needed, she can achieve anesthesia of the perineum by the cue method. Her

*For further information on teacher preparation by this method write to the American Academy of Husband-Coached Childbirth, P.O. Box 5224, Sherman Oaks, Calif. 91403.

postpartal experience and even lactation have been found to be influenced by posthypnotic suggestions.

Even in cases in which the full effect of hypnotic anesthesia is not achieved, most women who try this method still report that the discomforts of labor are reduced immensely and are tolerated without difficulty (Tinterow, 1972). Minimal amounts of analgesia or anesthetic may be needed in these situations.

Much controversy has surrounded the use of hypnosis, perhaps because the mechanism of hypnosis is only vaguely understood. Trance also seems to connote mysticism and lack of control. Proponents of hypnosis, however, say that the subject does not follow through on suggestions that she ordinarily would not do anyway. The subject has a heightened awareness of what she is doing. In labor she is aware of contractions, but she experiences no pain when numbness of her abdominal area is achieved and feels tolerable discomfort when only deep relaxation is accomplished. There is no physical danger to the mother and baby, especially with the reduction or elimination of medications in labor and delivery.

The greatest disadvantage to the couple is that the husband is usually not involved. In addition, some authorities are concerned about the risk of producing psychosis in a woman who has emotional disorder. Others feel that this would be impossible (Tinterow, 1972).

PREPARING THE ADOLESCENT FOR CHILDBIRTH AND CHILDREARING

Pregnancy for the adolescent is a crisis situation, as it is for an adult. However, adolescent pregnancy is complicated by several factors: interrupted developmental tasks, immature physical development, change in educational or career pursuits, lack of family acceptance or paternal support, increased medical risks during pregnancy, and premature assumption of adult responsibilities. An acute emotional crisis may ensue for both male and female adolescents involved in an out-of-wedlock pregnancy.

Interruption of developmental tasks of adolescence affects teenagers' ability to delineate and confirm their sense of identity and synthesize their personality. During adolescence, struggles for independence and emancipation from family compete with a need for dependence. Oedipal conflicts are reviewed and resolved. The adolescent must come to terms with bodily changes, sexual development, and psychosexual drives while learning more about the sexual role. Exploration and experimentation within one's personal world and environment are characteristic of adolescent behavior. The adolescent strives to achieve peer approval and relationships. Resolution of these tasks is critical for the continued psychosocial development of the individual.

Pregnancy superimposes a second maturational crisis onto the existing maturational crisis of adolescence. Adolescence is a transitional period between childhood and adulthood. Childhood is characterized by dependency; during adolescence, one strives for independence; and an adult is one who realizes his interdependency. Ideally, the adult is able to cope with the responsibilities of childbirth and childrearing. Adolescent pregnancy forces the teenager to skip a step. Unwed expectant teenagers are now responsible for meeting the needs of another person while still learning how to be responsible for themselves.

Young persons may engage in sexual activities for a number of reasons. For example, some youths feel that this is a way to gain peer acceptance. Others may be rebelling against parental authority. For some young people, sex may be a way of meeting needs for physical affection. Usually childbearing and childrearing are not the goal. The teenager may not be willing or ready to assume a responsible position in life and to care for or support a family. His or her psychosocial maturation is incomplete.

The Pregnant Teenage Girl

Although the teenage girl may appear physically mature, her body is still developing. The younger the girl, the greater the medical risks imposed by pregnancy. The uterus does not reach maturity until the age of 18 or 19. Pregnancy before the uterus is mature may result in difficulties in later life, such as prolapsed uterus as a result of the strain on immature pelvic muscles. The increased nutrient demands of pregnancy may compromise the adolescent's growth potential as well as that of the fetus. Incomplete maturation of bones may be one reason for the increased incidence of cephalopelvic disproportion in the young adolescent.

The unwed pregnant adolescent is faced with an acute emotional crisis. She may experience feelings of guilt or of being trapped. At a time when she is trying to become independent from her family, she may need to seek her family's help and support. Her sexual partner may reject her or refuse to acknowledge his paternity, which reinforces a sense of unworthiness in the adolescent. Emotional upsets may result in behaviors reflecting hostility, rebellion, and anger. She may have frequent psychosomatic complaints related to the pregnancy. Panic behavior may be exhibited when the adolescent approaches labor and delivery.

During the first trimester, the unwed pregnant teenager must deal with the important issue of whether to seek an abortion or to carry the fetus to term. If she decides to obtain an abortion, the pregnant adolescent may experience another period of emotional upset. She may have feelings of ambivalence, guilt, denial, anger, disappointment, or sadness. Underlying conflicts may surface for the adolescent concerning her femininity, motherhood, and moral conduct. The girl may experience exaggerated fears and anxieties about dying, disgrace, physical punishment, possibilities of a deformed child in the future, withdrawal of love, isolation, and separation. The adolescent needs to consider her feelings about destroying living tissue.

If the adolescent decides to have an abortion, her reasons should be explored to ensure that she is not being forced by parents or the unwed father. The immaturity of the adolescent may contribute to ambivalence about the decision to seek an abortion. She may have distorted perceptions about the procedure, believing it to be dangerous, frightening, punitive, or violent. Regardless of the individual's coping mechanisms during this crisis, the adolescent undergoing an abortion will experience a period of mourning over the loss of the fetus.

The decision to carry the fetus is also fraught with crisis and emotional upset. The following issues related to the unborn child require careful consideration and must be resolved by the unwed mother:

- Will the baby be kept by the unwed mother or placed for adoption?
- Will the family be supportive during the pregnancy or will the unwed mother need placement in a home for unwed mothers?
- What adoption services are available?
- Will financial assistance be available from state programs or from the family?
- Will prenatal childbirth classes be available and geared to the unwed adolescent mother-to-be?
- Will support persons be available? Who are they?
- Will the unwed mother be able to develop nurturing behaviors toward the child, even though she may not have completed her own developmental tasks?
- Will her relationship with the child's father be strengthened or broken?

The Unwed Father

The unwed adolescent father is characterized in many different ways. He may be someone who has taken advantage of the girl and then refuses to stand by her, or he may be a supportive person who cares. He may be a casual sexual partner who is not informed about the pregnancy, he may refuse to acknowledge his paternity, or he may be forced to marry the pregnant girl.

The unwed father may experience many of the same feelings that the mother-to-be exhibits. He may be surprised that the relationship resulted in pregnancy, believing himself immune to such an occurrence. He may be extremely frightened. This pregnancy may mean an interruption of developmental tasks and withdrawal from the formal educational system. Many unwed fathers feel a deep sense of responsibility for the young woman and unborn child, which may result in despair and depression.

When it is appropriate, the unwed father should be included in programs to help the adolescent parents-to-be. Counseling sessions may be especially helpful to the unwed father, providing him with an arena wherein he can receive attention for his needs, particularly those related to sexuality. The young man may exhibit feelings of guilt or anxiety related to unsatisfactory sexual relationships. He may lack knowledge about the implications of the pregnancy. Legal issues may be in question because in some states the boy can be prosecuted for statutory rape. He may have strong feelings about being involved in decisions related to the unborn child and the mother-to-be. Involvement in decision-making and participation in crisis intervention counseling during the prenatal, intranatal, and postnatal periods are maturing experiences for the unwed father.

Nursing Management

Assessment: Establishing the Data Base

Within any one age group, the maturational level varies from one individual to another. Adolescent life-styles and support systems vary tremendously. It is imperative that the interdisciplinary health team have information regarding the expectant adolescents' feelings and perceptions about themselves, their sexuality, and the coming baby; their knowledge of, attitude toward, and anticipated ability to physically care for and financially support the infant; and their maturational level and needs.

The nurse must establish a data base to plan her interventions for the adolescent mother-to-be. The following information is necessary:

1. *Family and personal history.* Family diseases such as diabetes, cardiovascular diseases, epilepsy, blood dyscrasia, hereditary diseases, congenital anomalies, tuberculosis, mental illness; multiple pregnancies; cultural influences; relationship within family and with significant others; previous sexual experience and sex education; self-concept and family support; and coping methods.

2. *Medical history.* The adolescent's general health; past or current heart disease, diabetes mellitus, epilepsy, rheumatic fever, childhood diseases, blood dyscrasia, tuberculosis, urinary tract disease, drug sensitivity, allergies; immunization; recent viral diseases; and exposure to drugs or pollutants.

3. *Menstrual history.* Onset of menses, regularity and duration of menses, and any problems with menses.

4. *Obstetric history.* Number of pregnancies, interrupted pregnancies, abortions, premature deliveries, viable births; health status of any living children; neonatal complications and/or stillbirths; previous pregnancy complications; problems of infertility; experience with contraceptive methods.

During the assessment phase the nurse must obtain information while supporting the adolescent's feelings and encouraging problem-solving. Assessment questions may be prefaced with provocative statements such as the following (Poole, 1976): "Becoming a mother will change your life" (for example, plans for attending school, getting a job, dreams for self), and "The full-time demands of school or job and baby care will leave little time for you." Provocative statements like these will facilitate discussion and expression of feelings by the adolescent mother-to-be.

The adolescent will experience stress, so an assessment of her coping behaviors is necessary before crisis intervention techniques can be implemented. Failure of coping mechanisms frequently occurs in the face of the following: discovery of pregnancy, negative response from mate, withdrawal from educational system, decision to carry fetus or abort, labor and delivery, decision to keep child or place for adoption, and attempting to plan for the future. Resolution of the crisis can be facilitated with caring involvement of health team members.

Interventions

Nursing actions should focus on several problems areas:

- *Nutritional status:* The adolescent usually has poor nutrition and is a higher risk for anemia.
- *Medical status:* Preeclampsia and prematurity occur more frequently in adolescent pregnancies.
- *Psychosocial status:* Poor adaptation, ambivalence, and lack of family support present problems for the pregnant adolescent.
- *Developmental status:* Adolescent developmental tasks are interrupted and new developmental tasks of pregnancy must be completed.

The pregnant teenager should be taught the importance of adequate nutrition and ways to obtain the appropriate nutrients. The nurse can supply information, assist in menu planning, and encourage the mother-to-be to eat properly. Table 11–2 lists the recommended daily requirements for adolescents.

Periodic physical assessments (see Chapter 10) provide the nurse with a basis for identifying medical complications that may threaten the outcome of the pregnancy. Similarly, periodic psychologic evaluation will indicate any emotional problems or psychosocial difficulties.

The nurse can help the adolescent cope with the stress of this crisis. Problem-solving techniques can be taught to the adolescent mother-to-be for use not only during the pregnancy but for situations related to childrearing. Many adolescents view the pregnancy as overwhelming and need assistance in breaking the situation down into manageable "parts" or decisions. Not all decisions made by the pregnant adolescent will be correct, but with guidance many positive decision-making experiences can be acquired and utilized as a basis for handling adult responsibilities.

Regardless of the adolescent's age, level of maturity, support system, self-concept, and readiness for parenthood (or decision to abort or release for adoption), the nurse becomes her personal advocate, interpreting antepartal management to her and interpreting her needs to the involved members of the interdisciplinary health care team. Information is offered in a matter-of-fact manner; adolescents are often hesitant to ask for clarification for fear of being labeled "stupid."

One widely held but erroneous assumption is that the increase of sexual activity among adolescents in this country has been accompanied by increased sophistication about sex and reproduction, contraception, abortion, health care, and techniques related to sexuality. This is not always the case. Vaginal and bimanual examinations may be refused or poorly accepted if a girl's sexual experiences have been traumatic.

The option of abortion may be nonexistent if the adolescent's religion, culture, or personal philosophy proscribes the procedure.

Discussion of fetal development and expected physiologic changes prenatally, during labor and delivery, and postnatally counters misinformation and ameliorates fear based on myths and folklore to which adolescents are exposed. Imagine the degree of the nurse's or nutritionist's success in encouraging the adolescent girl to increase her intake of cheese and fish when family or friends tell her that these foods "rot your womb if eaten during pregnancy."

Participation in problem-solving in which her opinions are elicited and respected fosters self-esteem and feelings of worth in the adolescent. Involving both the girl and the boy highlights the reality of the pregnancy for them, portrays childbearing as a cooperative venture, and fosters a positive attitude toward each other, the opposite sex, and people in authority. The adolescents are encouraged to open or to maintain the lines of communication with their parents.

Mothers of unwed pregnant adolescents often feel guilty about the daughter's situation and may use the pregnancy and the baby as a means of controlling the adolescent's behavior. The grandmother-to-be may experience a role conflict when she realizes that her daughter and potential grandchild both need mothering and that her child will also be a mother. Because most young women look to their mothers as a role model, it is vital that the nurse consider the mother in the plan of care.

Career or educational goals may need to be interrupted by the pregnancy. Discussion of these events focuses the adolescent's attention on realistic planning for the future: the realities of parenthood and the drive for self-fulfillment in parenting, social interaction, and career.

In the absence of preparation for parenthood in formal institutions such as school, some responsible professionals have secured community cooperation to develop programs to meet the special needs of adolescent parents while they continue with their formal education. One such program introduces the basics of newborn care during the latter stages of pregnancy (Tankson, 1976). Following delivery, through a day-care program parents earn educational units as they study the growth, development, characteristics, and needs of the infant; the value and techniques of intellectual and social stimulation for the infant; and child care skills. Young parents who participate demonstrate increased self-esteem and confidence, stronger bonds between themselves and their children, and a greater understanding of family relationships. These parents show increased ability to cope with crying, decreased revulsion to changing diapers and cleaning their drooling infants, and a decrease in negative behavior (yelling and screaming) toward the child. Peer support plays a significant role in the progress of these young parents.

Nurses need to examine their attitudes and responses to adolescents. It is important to avoid assuming an authoritarian stance. It is not enough to be knowledgeable and sympathetic and to feel that one is nonjudgmental. The nurse also needs to be able to convey these attributes as well as her interest in and desire to help the pregnant adolescent.

SUMMARY

Pregnancy is an extremely stressful period for the expectant family. Members of the health team can facilitate the resolution of family disequilibrium resulting from this crisis and of associated factors such as body changes, adjustments in family roles and responsibilities, fears related to the unborn child, and fears about labor and delivery. Knowledge about childbirth and childrearing will do much to strengthen the family's ability to cope with fears.

Nurses are often responsible for providing prenatal education to expectant families. Information about the labor and delivery processes is supplied to the childbearing couple. They may be taught communication skills, which will provide them with a means of dealing with their problems. In addition, these skills can be integrated into their parenting method.

The expectant couple can also learn various methods of childbirth preparation that utilize relaxation and breathing techniques to alleviate discomfort.

The pregnant adolescent requires additional attention from the nurse. She is at physical and psychologic risk because of her incomplete development. The expectant adolescent couple must be prepared to assume the role of father and mother before they are independent from their own parents.

If the expectant family is properly prepared for childbirth, this experience can be one of growth and development for all members. The nurse has an important role in ensuring the family of the opportunity to have this positive experience.

SUGGESTED ACTIVITIES

1. List typical family responses to pregnancy and discuss appropriate nursing interventions.
2. Arrange through a prenatal clinic or physician's office to have preschool siblings participate in prenatal care by asking questions and listening to fetal heart sounds. Describe the siblings' prenatal and postpartum reactions.
3. Establish a nursing data base for three expectant families and compare differences requiring individualized nursing intervention.
4. Attend a series of childbirth classes and maintain a diary with cross-references for clinical application of information. Exchange the information with classmates who have attended other kinds of childbirth classes.

REFERENCES

Auerbach, A. 1968. *Parents learn through discussion: principles and practice of parent group education.* New York: John Wiley & Sons, Inc.

Bing, E. 1967. *Six practical lessons for an easier childbirth.* New York: Bantam Books, Inc.

Bradley, R. A. 1974. *Husband-coached childbirth.* 2nd ed. New York: Harper & Row Publishers, Inc.

Childbirth Education Association of the Pikes Peak Region. *Levels of breathing.* Colorado Springs: The Association.

Colman, A. D., and Colman, L. 1972. *Pregnancy: the psychological experience.* New York: Herder & Herder.

Dick-Read, G. 1959. *Childbirth without fear.* 2nd ed. New York: Harper & Row Publishers, Inc.

Duvall, E. 1971. *Family development.* 5th ed. Philadelphia: J. B. Lippincott Co.

Gordon T. 1970. *Parent effectiveness training.* New York: Peter W. Wyden, Publisher.

Hartman, R. 1975. *Exercises for true natural childbirth.* New York: Harper & Row Publishers, Inc.

Heardman, H. 1961. *A way to natural childbirth: a manual for physiotherapists and parents to be.* Edinburgh: E. & S. Rivingsterne.

Karmel, M. 1965. *Thank you, Dr. Lamaze.* New York: Doubleday & Co., Inc.

Poole, C. March–April 1976. Adolescent mothers: can they be helped? *Pediatr. Nurs.* 2:7.

Rubin, R. 1967. Attainment of the maternal role. I. Processes. *Nurs. Res.* 16:272.

Tankson, E. A. May–June 1976. The adolescent parent: one approach to teaching child care and giving support. *J. Obstet. Gynecol. Neonatal Nurs.* 5:9.

Tinterow, M. M. 1972. Techniques of hypnosis. In *Obstetric analgesia and anesthetics*, ed. J. J. Bonica. Philadelphia: F. A. Davis Co.

ADDITIONAL READINGS

Arms, S. 1975. *Immaculate deception.* Boston: Houghton Mifflin Co.

Barnett, C. R., et al. 1970. Neonatal separation: maternal side of interactional deprivation. *Pediatrics.* 45:197.

Bobak, I. M. April 1969. Self-image: a universal concern of women becoming mothers. *CNA Bull.* 9:7.

Bonica, J. J. 1972. *Obstetric analgesia and anesthetics.* Philadelphia: F. A. Davis Co.

Bowlby, J., et al. 1956. The effects of mother-child separation: a follow-up study. *Br. J. Med. Psychol.* 29:211.

Brazelton, T. B.; School, M. L.; and Robey, J. S. 1966. Visual responses in the newborn. *Pediatrics.* 37:284.

Bucove, A. 1964. Postpartum psychoses in the male. *N.Y. Acad. Med.* 40.961.

Cannon, R. March–April 1977. The development of maternal touch during early mother-infant interaction. *J. Obstet. Gynecol. Neonatal Nurs.* 6:28.

Chabon, I. 1966. *Awake and aware.* New York: Dell Publishing Co., Inc.

Chiota, B. J.; Goolkasian, P.; and Ladewig, P. Jan.–Feb. 1976. Effects of separation from spouse on pregnancy, labor, and delivery, and the postpartum period. *J. Obstet. Gynecol. Neonatal Nurs.* 5:21.

Clark, A. 1973. *Leadership technique in expectant parent education.* 2nd ed. New York: Springer Verlag New York, Inc.

Clark, A. L., and Affonso, D. D. 1976. *Childbearing: a nursing perspective.* Philadelphia: F. A. Davis Co.

Clark, A. L., and Affonso, D. D. March–April 1976. Infant behavior and maternal attachment: two sides to the coin. *MCN.* 1:94.

Clausen, J. P., et al. 1977. *Maternity nursing today.* 2nd ed. New York: McGraw-Hill Book Co.

Colman, A. D., and Colman, L. L. Winter 1974. Pregnancy as an altered state of consciousness. *Birth Fam. J.* 1:8.

Edwards, M. Winter 1973–1974. The crises of fourth trimester. *Birth Fam. J.* 1:19.

Ewy, D., and Ewy, R. 1970. *Preparation for childbirth: a Lamaze guide.* Boulder, Colo.: Pruett Publishing Company.

Fein, R. A. Summer 1976. The first weeks of fathering: the importance of choices and supports for new parents. *Birth Fam. J.* 3:53.

Fielding W. L., and Benjamin, L. 1962. *The childbirth challenge: commonsense versus "natural" childbirth.* New York: The Viking Press, Inc., Publishers.

Hawkins, M. 1979. Fitting a prenatal education program into the crowded inner city clinic. *MCN.* 4:226.

Hoprich, P. A. July–Aug. 1977. Assisting the couple through a Lamaze labor and delivery. *MCN.* 2:245.

Hurd, J. M. L. July–Aug. 1975. Assessing maternal attachment: first step toward the prevention of child abuse. *J. Obstet. Gynecol. Neonatal Nurs.* 4:25.

Lamaze, F. 1972. *Painless childbirth.* New York: Pocket Books.

LeMaster, E. E. 1965. Parenthood as crisis. In *Crisis interventions: selected readings*, ed. H. J. Parad. New York: Family Service Association of America.

Pillitteri, A. 1976. *Nursing care of the growing family: a maternal newborn text.* Boston: Little, Brown & Co.

Roberts, J. May–June 1976. Priorities in prenatal education. *J. Obstet. Gynecol. Neonatal Nurs.* 5:17.

Robinson, D. Aug. 1969. Our surprising moral unwed fathers. *Ladies' Home Journal*, p. 49.

Robson, K. S. 1967. The role of eye-to-eye contact in maternal-infant attachment. *J. Child Psychol. Psychiatry* 8:13.

Rubin, R. 1963. Maternal touch. *Nurs. Outlook.* 11:828.

Rubin, R. 1970. Cognitive style in pregnancy. *Am. J. Nurs.* 70:502.

Salk, L. 1970. Critical nature of the postpartum period in the human for establishment of the maternal-infant bond. *Dis. Nerv. Syst.* 31(suppl.):110.

Schroeder, M. A. May–June 1977. Is the immediate postpartum period crucial to the mother-child relationship? *J. Obstet. Gynecol. Neonatal Nurs.* 6:37.

Smako, M. R., and Schoenfeld, L. S. 1976. Hypnotic susceptibility and the Lamaze childbirth experience. *Am. J. Obstet. Gynecol.* 12:631.

Sumner, G. 1979. Giving expectant parents the help they need: the ABC's of prenatal education. *MCN.* 4:220.

Sumner, G., and Fritsch, J. May–June 1977. Postnatal parental concerns: the first six weeks of life (research and studies). *J. Obstet. Gynecol. Neonatal Nurs.* 6:27.

Tanzer, D. 1968. Natural childbirth: pain or peak experience? *Psychology Today.* 2:16.

Vellay, P. 1960. *Childbirth without pain.* New York: E. P. Dutton.

Warrick, L. 1969. Femininity, sexuality, and mothering. *Nurs. Forum.* 8:224.

Wiedenbach, E. 1964. *Clinical nursing; a helping art.* New York: Springer Verlag New York, Inc.

Zalar, M. K. Nov.–Dec. 1975. Human sexuality: a component of total patient care. *Nurs. Dig.* 3:40.

Zalar, M. K. May–June 1976. Sexual counseling for pregnant couples. *MCN.* 1:176.

CHAPTER 13

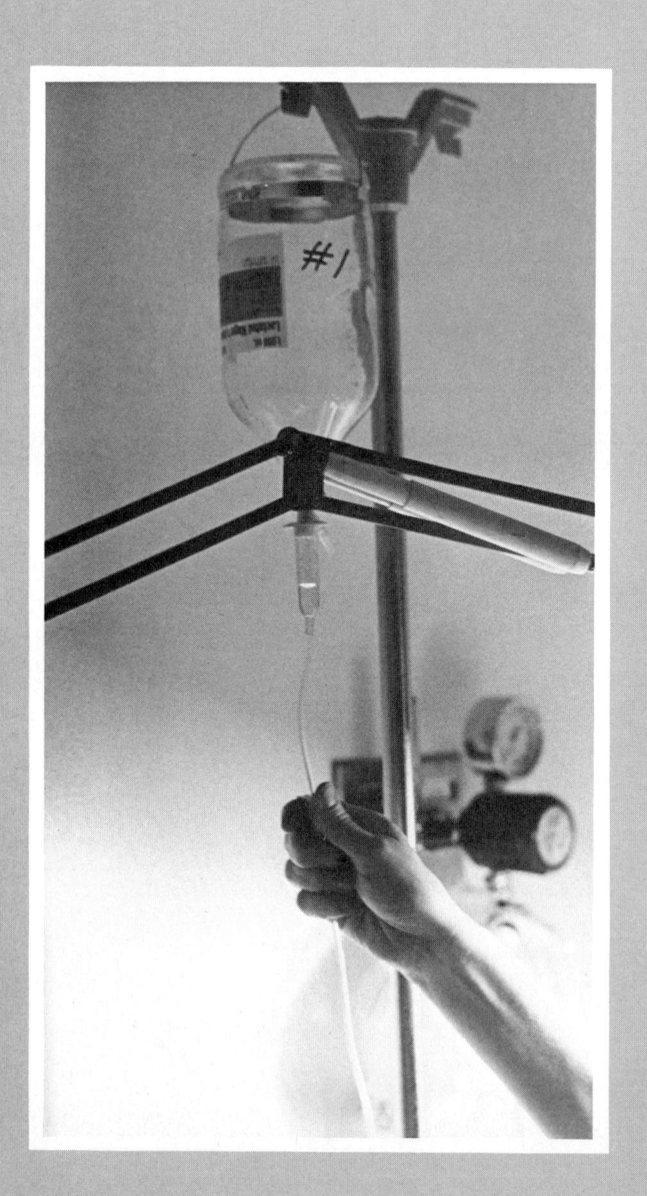

COMPLICATIONS OF PREGNANCY

OBJECTIVES

- Discuss the effects of preexisting medical conditions on pregnancy.
- Differentiate the bleeding problems associated with pregnancy.
- Discuss the development and course of hypertensive disorders associated with pregnancy.
- Discuss some common infections that may be contracted during pregnancy.
- Discuss drug use and abuse during pregnancy.

Within the past few years, scientific and technologic advances in the assessment and diagnosis of maternal well-being and the prognosis of fetal well-being have been furthered as a result of such procedures as amniocentesis for amniotic fluid analysis, amnioscopy, oxytocin challenge test (OCT), ultrasonography, and urinary estriol determinations (see Chapter 14). These advances have succeeded in decreasing perinatal mortality (stillbirths plus neonatal deaths) in this country to its present rate of approximately 15 per 1000 live births. Statistics indicate that perinatal deaths that do occur can be attributed to the category of pregnant patients identified as high risk: those who have predisposing medical disruptions such as cardiopulmonary disease, diabetes mellitus, or thyroid disturbances. The incidence of fetal loss is increased from three to five times in patients with these disorders (Clark and Affonso, 1976).

Pregnancy puts stress on the healthy female biologically, physiologically, and psychologically. In the presence of certain factors, pregnancy may become a life-threatening event. It is therefore imperative that prenatal care be aimed toward specific identification, assessment, and management of the high-risk patient.

In this chapter, the discussion focuses on pregestational medical disorders and specific disorders that are unique to the pregnant condition. The possible effects of these disruptions on the outcome of pregnancy are examined. In addition, infectious processes that may influence maternal and fetal well-being are described.

PREGESTATIONAL MEDICAL DISORDERS

Cardiac Disease

The majority of expectant women with cardiac disease can successfully complete a pregnancy. Statistics demonstrate a progressive decline in maternal mortality with this condition to an incidence in recent years of less than 1%. This significant reduction has evolved as a result of a better understanding of cardiovascular adaptation in pregnancy, more intensive prepregnancy and prenatal assessment and management, and a general improvement in the care of all cardiac patients.

The normal cardiovascular system during pregnancy exhibits several changes. Beginning early in the course of gestation, there is an increase in heart rate, cardiac output, and total blood volume. Cardiac output is increased by 30%–40% and thus affects the increased heart rate. The blood volume begins to increase during the first trimester; the average blood volume increases 30%–50% and shows little change during the last trimester of pregnancy (Burrows and Fettis, 1976).

Rheumatic heart disease lesions account for the greatest number of cases (61%) of cardiac disease in pregnancy. However, with the advent of appropriate prophylactic antibiotic therapy for β-streptococcal infections, the incidence of rheumatic fever is declining. Congenital heart defects account for approximately 31% of cardiac disease in pregnancy. Atherosclerotic, coronary, and thyroid disruptions appear to occur less frequently and together account for the remaining 8% (Messer, 1973).

Classification

To further clarify the severity of cardiac disease in pregnancy, the following classification of functional capacity has been standardized by the Criteria Committee of the New York Heart Association, Inc. (1955):

- Class I. No limitation of physical activity. Ordinary physical activity causes no discomfort; patients do not have anginal pain.
- Class II. Slight limitation of physical activity. Ordinary physical activity causes fatigue, dyspnea, palpitation, or anginal pain.
- Class III. Moderate to marked limitation of physical activity. During less than ordinary physical activity, patients experience excessive fatigue, dyspnea, palpitation, or anginal pain.
- Class IV. Unable to carry on any physical activity without experiencing discomforts. Even at rest, they experience symptoms of cardiac insufficiency or anginal pain.

Patients in classes I and II usually experience a normal pregnancy and have few complications, whereas those in classes III and IV are at risk for more severe complications.

Clinical Manifestations

Clinical signs and symptoms that the pregnant woman with impending cardiac decompensation exhibits include:

1. Coughs (frequent, with or without hemoptysis).
2. Dyspnea (progressive, upon exertion).
3. Edema (progressive, generalized, including extremities, face, eyes).
4. Heart murmurs (heard on auscultation).
5. Palpitations.
6. Rales (auscultated in lung bases).

These progressive symptoms are indicative of congestive heart failure, the heart's signal of its decreased ability to meet the demands of pregnancy. It should be noted that this cycle is *progressive,* because some of these same behaviors are seen to a minor degree in a pregnancy without cardiac involvement.

Careful monitoring of these patients during the prenatal period is essential. If such symptoms appear, prompt medical actions are required to correct the cardiac status. Until cardiac function is improved, no obstetric manipulation should be attempted, because even the slightest stimulus might lead to cardiac failure.

Fetal-Neonatal Implications

Infant mortality increases if maternal cardiac decompensation occurs. Uterine congestion, hypoxia, and elevation of carbon dioxide content of the blood not only compromise the fetus but also frequently give rise to premature labor and delivery (Danforth, 1977). The respiratory and metabolic acidosis suffered in utero as a result of suboptimal oxygenation of the fetus leads to cellular damage and predisposes the traumatized fetus to intrauterine fetal distress once labor begins and oxygen transport and exchange are further reduced. Therefore, optimal fetal outcome can only be achieved through prevention of maternal cardiac decompensation.

The neonate who has suffered hypoxia in utero and during birth is at risk during the neonatal period, particularly if born prematurely. Prognosis for the newborn of the cardiac patient is based on maintenance of normal respiratory and metabolic functioning as determined by observation and laboratory testing. (See Chapter 25 for discussion of the nursing and medical care of the newborn with respiratory compromise.)

Interventions

The primary goal of nursing care is to preserve the cardiac reserve function of the pregnant patient. To do this it is necessary to maintain a balance between cardiac reserve and cardiac work load. Specific goals for nursing management are as follows:

1. Assess the stress of pregnancy on the heart's functional capacity.
   a. Compare the patient's vital signs of pulse and respiration to the normal values expected during pregnancy.
   b. Establish activity level of patient, including rest, and assess any changes in vital signs that may occur.
   c. Identify in order of priority the problems indicating cardiac decompensation.
2. Support the woman's adaptive coping mechanisms to deal with stress.
   a. Allow ample time for the patient to ask questions and encourage her to comment on her pregnancy and its progress.
   b. Answer the patient's questions as fully as possible and in terms that she can understand.
   c. Carefully explain all nursing actions to the woman.
   d. Identify and utilize significant others, such as spouse, mother, or friend, to give physical and psychologic support.
3. Identify the severity of the disease process.
   a. Note cardiac classification of the patient.
   b. Identify problems in order of priority based on nursing diagnosis and patient input.

Nursing management of the pregnant woman with cardiac disease involves varying tasks in the antepartal, intrapartal, and postpartal periods.

Antepartal Period

The following nursing actions are based on the physiologic and psychosocial needs of the pregnant woman with cardiac disease. It is important to note that all these actions are essential for any pregnant cardiac patient. However, the priority of nursing actions varies, depending on the severity of the disease process.

1. *Adequate nutrition.* A diet should be instituted that is high in iron, protein, and essential nutrients to meet the increased demands of pregnancy for increased blood volume and oxygen. However, sodium and calorie intake should be minimized.

2. *Promotion of rest.* Eight to ten hours of sleep is essential, with frequent daily rest periods. The nurse must assist the patient to understand the absolute necessity for this rest.

3. *Protection from infection.* It is vitally important to protect the heart from the additional stress of upper respiratory infections, which could lead to cardiac failure due to overload of the heart's reserve capacity.

4. *Drug therapy.* Besides the iron and vitamin supplements prescribed during pregnancy, the cardiac patient may need additional drug therapy to maintain health. If the woman develops coagulation problems, the anticoagulant heparin may be used because it offers the greatest safety to the fetus. It does not cross the placenta. Digitalis glycosides and common antiarrhythmic drugs may also be used, but they result in known teratogenic or other fetal insult. Penicillin prophylaxis to protect against infection, if not contraindicated by allergy, is encouraged.

5. *Restriction of activity.* Decreased exertion decreases fatigue, thereby promoting adequate ventilation.

6. *Continuous monitoring of pregnancy.* One or two prenatal visits per week for assessment of cardiac status are encouraged.

7. *Psychologic support.* The patient and her family are provided with information concerning her condition and management. This will increase their understanding and decrease anxiety. The nurse can counsel the patient and family regarding their preparation for childbirth and offer them encouragement to boost their morale.

It is the aim of nursing to support the implementation of this care in the home. However, hospitalization may become necessary. The pregnant cardiac patient is most prone to cardiac decompensation between the 28th and 32nd weeks of gestation. It is at that time that the cardiac work load is highest. Careful assessment of the patient's status is necessary to ensure safe culmination of pregnancy.

Intrapartal Period

During labor and delivery, tremendous stress is normally exerted on the unborn fetus. This stress could be fatal to the fetus of a cardiac patient because of the possible decreased oxygen and blood supply to it. It is therefore essential that the intrapartal management of a cardiac patient be aimed at reducing the amount of physical exertion and accompanying fatigue. Nursing actions include the following:

1. *Continuous monitoring.* Routine labor signs should be observed. Monitor FHTs and contractions (see Chapter 16). Assess vital signs frequently, particularly if the pulse rate is 100/min or and respirations are 25/min greater, to determine whether there is progressive tachycardia or hyperventilation.

2. *Assessment of pulmonary function.* Dyspnea, coughing, and rales at the lung bases should be noted.

3. *Proper positioning.* To assure cardiac emptying and proper oxygenation, the semi-Fowler and side-lying positions, with head and shoulders elevated, are recommended.

4. *Supportive therapies.* These include use of prophylactic antibiotics, oxygen by mask if any pulmonary embarrassment such as dyspnea occurs, diuretics to decrease fluid retention, sedatives for rest and reduction of anxiety, analgesics with tranquilizers to potentiate action and reduce pain, and digitalis if signs of cardiac decompensation occur (listed on p. 345).

5. *Assistance during delivery.* Delivery by low forceps is the safest method, using a regional or local anesthetic to maintain controlled vaginal delivery, thereby reducing the stress of pushing and decreasing possible trauma to the infant. The goal of nursing actions is to minimize the duration of the second stage of labor by encouraging and supporting relaxation. Cesarean section should be performed only if fetal or obstetric indications are present and not on the basis of heart disease alone.

6. *Psychologic support.* The nurse should remain with the patient to support and encourage her.

Postpartal Period

This is a most significant time for the cardiac patient. Due to the rapid fluid shift resulting from the physiologic readaptation process, there is an increase in cardiac output and blood volume as the extravascular fluid is returned to the bloodstream for excretion.

After delivery, the intraabdominal pressure is reduced significantly, venous pressure is reduced, the splanchnic vessels engorge, and blood flow to the heart increases. The extravascular fluid moves into the bloodstream. This mobilization of fluid can place a great strain on the heart if excess interstitial fluid is present. This stress on the heart could lead to cardiac decompensation, especially during the first 48 hours postpartum or as late as the sixth postnatal day. Continued nursing care includes the following actions:

1. *Assessment of post-delivery heart status.* The patient remains in the hospital for at least one week to allow for rest and recovery of cardiac function.

2. *Proper positioning.* The semi-Fowler and side-lying positions, with elevation of head and shoulders, assist respiratory and cardiac function.

3. *Planning of activity schedule.* Based on nursing assessment of the patient's cardiac status as indicated by pulse and respirations, the patient begins a gradual and progressive activity program:

   a. Bed rest with nurse performing grooming, hygiene, and nutritional measures. As cardiac status improves, the patient may increase her performance of these activities of daily living.

   b. Progressive ambulation as tolerated. Assess pulse and respirations of patient before and after exercise to evaluate tolerance.

   c. Use of diet, administration of stool softeners, and mild local anesthetic to episiotomy site to facilitate bowel movement and urination without stress or strain.

4. *Psychologic support.* Encourage maternal-infant bonding process.

5. *Education and assistance of mother in infant care.*

6. *Preparation for discharge.* The patient will need education, referrals, and support for her care and that of her infant:

   a. Determine whether there are significant others to assist the mother at home in caring for self and infant.

   b. An activity schedule that is gradual and progressive and appropriate to patient's needs and home environment should be planned with the patient.

   c. Information regarding sexual relations and contraception should be given as appropriate.

Diabetes Mellitus

Another major complication of the maternity cycle is diabetes mellitus, an endocrine disorder of carbohydrate metabolism that results from inadequate production or utilization of insulin. It is characterized by hyperglycemia and glycosuria.

Diabetes mellitus disrupts approximately 1 in 700 pregnancies. Prior to the discovery of insulin in 1921, the maternal mortality reported by Williams was 30% and the fetal mortality was 65% (Hellman and Pritchard, 1971). Since that time the management of the diabetic maternity patient has evolved into an interspecialty team approach, including medical internist, obstetrician, nutritionist, nurse, perinatologist, and pediatrician. This approach has been adopted to decrease maternal and fetal risk of death in a pregnancy complicated by diabetes mellitus.

The overall changes in metabolism during pregnancy are profound in the healthy nondiabetic woman, but her physiologic tolerance for carbohydrate remains normal. This balance in the endocrine system is achieved in the following way. The increased activity of the maternal pancreatic islets results in the increased production of insulin. This is counterbalanced by the placenta's increased production of the hormone human chorionic somatomammotropin (HCS), which diminishes the effectiveness of maternal insulin. HCS is secreted primarily in the third trimester and increases tenfold over the last 20 weeks of gestation. The increase in HCS is paralleled by an increase in insulin production.

Insulin requirements of pregnant women increase because of the insulin antagonism and altered insulin utilization that exists during pregnancy. Just as HCS diminishes the effectiveness of maternal insulin, it has been suggested that human placental lactogen also reduces the physiologic effectiveness of circulating insulin. A rise in the glomerular filtration rate in the kidneys in conjunction with decreased tubular glucose reabsorption results in glycosuria. A decrease in the normal fasting blood sugar occurs in pregnancy, but free fatty acids and ketones are increased. In summary, the delicate system of checks and balances that exists between glucose production and glucose utilization is stressed by the growing fetus, who derives energy from glucose taken solely from maternal stores. This stress is referred to as the *diabetogenic effect* of pregnancy. Thus any preexisting disruption in carbohydrate metabolism is augmented by pregnancy, and any diabetic potential may precipitate *gestational diabetes,* which is defined as diabetes diagnosed during pregnancy but subclinical and unidentifiable in nonpregnant women. Generally, this disorder can be controlled by proper diet during gestation. It should be differentiated from *prediabetes,* which denotes a latent phase of diabetes that may exist prior to the diagnosis of actual diabetes mellitus. It is not a clinical entity and therefore is an inappropriate term in patient management. The classification of diabetes in pregnancy is presented in Table 13–1.

Table 13–1. Classification of Diabetes in Pregnancy*

Class	Description
A	Gestational or chemical diabetes (abnormal glucose tolerance test)
B	Overt diabetes Onset after age 20 Duration less than 10 years No vascular involvement
C	Overt diabetes Onset before age 20 Duration 10 to 20 years No vascular involvement
D	Overt diabetes Onset before age 10 Duration more than 20 years Vascular involvement Benign retinopathy Leg calcification
E	Calcified pelvic vessels (this classification is not generally employed in current practice)
F	Diabetic renal impairment
R	Malignant retinopathy (proliferative)

*From White, P. 1965. Pregnancy and diabetes: medical aspects. *Med. Clin. North Am.* 49:1016.

Influence of Pregnancy on Diabetes

Pregnancy can affect diabetes in the following ways:

1. Diabetic control
    a. Increased insulin requirements, particularly in third trimester, especially labor
    b. Decreased renal threshold
    c. Dietary fluctuations due to nausea, vomiting, and cravings
    d. Increased risk of ketoacidosis, insulin shock, and coma
2. Possible accelerations of vascular disease
    a. Hypertension: increase in blood pressure of greater than 30 mm/Hg systolic and 15 mm/Hg diastolic
    b. Nephropathy: renal impairment
    c. Retinopathy

The primary concern is control of circulating blood glucose levels, which can be affected by severity of the diabetic disease state, emotional condition, and activity level. Awareness of the specific behaviors and stressors is vital to appropriate planning and subsequent implementation of nursing care.

The patient with gestational diabetes has an abnormal glucose tolerance test (GTT) but no clinical symptoms. The indications for performing a GTT in pregnancy include the following: glycosuria (as indicated by more than one urine sample), family history of diabetes, previous large-for-gestational-age (LGA) infant (4000 gm or more at birth), hydramnios, and a history of unexplained stillbirths, neonatal deaths, or congenital anomalies. The GTT involves diet preparation, fasting before glucose ingestion, and three subsequent blood samples taken one hour, two hours, and three hours after ingestion. The norm at three hours should be under 125 mg/100 ml. Diagnosis of gestational diabetes is made when two or more values exceed this norm. The results are most reliable when performed in the second or third trimester.

Influence of Diabetes Mellitus on Pregnancy Outcome

The course of the pregnancy in a diabetic patient is characterized by an increased incidence of maternal, fetal, and neonatal complications. With the team approach to the management of this high-risk pregnancy, the chances for increased maternal and fetal well-being are enhanced. The most important complication is fetal mortality, which occurs at the rate of 10%–20%, or three to six times that for the general population. In contrast, maternal rates are negligible.

Diabetes mellitus can cause the following complications during pregnancy:

1. *Maternal complications:* increased morbidity, acidosis, hydramnios, preeclampsia, dystocia, infection.

2. *Fetal complications:* increased morbidity, congenital anomalies, hyperbilirubinemia, hypocalcemia, hypoglycemia, macrosomatia (LGA), spontaneous abortions, increased fetal mortality (stillbirths—death in utero third trimester).

3. *Neonatal complications:* increased morbidity, hyperbilirubinemia, hypocalcemia, hypoglycemia, hypoxia, respiratory distress syndrome, increased mortality (neonatal deaths due to congenital anomalies and RDS).

Maternal Implications

Hydramnios, or an increase in the volume of amniotic fluid, occurs in almost all diabetic pregnancies. Approximately 25% of diabetic pregnant women will show an increase greater than 1500 ml. The exact mechanism causing the increase is unknown, although osmotic pressure, hypersecretion of amniotic fluid, and diuresis due to fetal hyperglycemia are suspected (Haynes, 1969). Premature rupture of membranes and onset of labor may be a problem, but only occasionally does this pose a threat. Amniocentesis may be utilized to decrease fluid volume; however, this procedure predisposes the diabetic patient to potential infection, possible initiation of premature labor, possible premature separation of the placenta due to manipulation, and hemmorhage due to placental laceration.

If vascular disease is present in the diabetic, the pregnancy is vulnerable to hypertensive disruptions, particularly preeclampsia. Proteinuria and excessive weight gain are also found.

The management of ketoacidosis in the pregnant diabetic deserves special consideration. The risk of fetal death is increased to 50% or more if ketoacidosis is not promptly treated. However, in pregnancy it is vital to differentiate between starvation ketosis and diabetic ketoacidosis. In starvation ketosis, hyperglycemia is not present in the blood sugar. Prompt treatment is with glucose solutions and not insulin (Burrows and Fettis, 1976).

The pregnant diabetic is also at risk for dystocia caused by cephalopelvic disproportion due to macrosomatia (an LGA fetus). Anemia may develop as a result of vascular involvement and of nausea and vomiting caused by hormonal changes. Infections of the urinary tract, particularly monilial vaginitis, commonly develop because of glycosuria. The patient should not be allowed to go past term, because of the increased incidence of intrauterine fetal death. Because of fetal macrosomatia, induction of labor is often not successful; thus cesarean section is frequently performed.

Fetal-Neonatal Implications

It has long been recognized that the incidence of stillbirths increases markedly with gestations carried beyond the 36th week. In some instances, these intrauterine deaths can be attributed to poor diabetic control and acidosis. However, even in well-controlled diabetic patients, fetal jeopardy remains a significant problem. Of the total fetal-neonatal mortality, approximately 50% of the deaths occur during the first five to seven days after delivery. The single most important factor related to these statistics is not the severity of maternal diabetes but the prematurity of the neonate's lungs. Thus the major cause of neonatal deaths is respiratory distress secondary to hyaline membrane disease. Another important cause of neonatal deaths is directly related to lethal congenital anomalies, particularly abnormalities of the heart (ventricular septal defect) and neurologic defects (Burrows and Fettis, 1976). The insulin-dependent diabetic woman has a 10% risk of bearing a child with a congenital anomaly. The risk for a woman who develops gestational diabetes is slightly less but remains higher than that for the general population.

Characteristically, infants of diabetic mothers (classes A, B, and C) are macrosomatic or LGA as a result of the high maternal levels of blood sugar, from which the fetus derives its glucose. These elevated levels provide a relentless stimulus to the fetal islets of Langerhans to produce insulin. The sustained fetal hyperinsulinism and hyperglycemia ultimately lead to excessive growth and deposition of fat. After birth the umbilical cord is severed, and thus the generous maternal blood glucose supply is eliminated. However, continued islet cell hyperactivity leads to excessive insulin levels and depleted blood glucose (hypoglycemia) in two to four hours. See Chapter 24 for discussion of the management of the infant of a diabetic mother.

Interventions

The major goals of nursing care are (a) to maintain a physiologic equilibrium of insulin production and glucose utilization during pregnancy and (b) to deliver an optimally healthy mother and neonate. To achieve these goals, good prenatal care must be of top priority, utilizing the previously discussed team approach. Prenatal nursing care of the diabetic patient is based on the following general principles of care:

1. Thorough clinical assessment of disease process and patient information.
2. Dietary regulation.
3. Urine and blood testing for glucose levels.
4. Determination of insulin requirements.
5. Evaluation of fetoplacental functioning.
6. Assessment of fetal maturity.

In general, the prenatal care of the class A diabetic patient is similar to that of the normal pregnant woman. Assessment of the patient yields information about her ability to cope with the additional stress of a complication to pregnancy and some idea of her ability to follow a recommended regimen of care. Dietary regulation is usually minimal, with a restriction on excessive carbohydrate ingestion. Urine testing is done at each prenatal visit, and results should be validated with blood sugar testing. The two-hour postprandial (after a meal) blood sugar test is most reliable. Fasting blood sugars are often tested prior to a two-hour postprandial test to assess glycemic behaviors, which may be suggestive of hypoglycemia.

A two-hour postprandial blood sugar level of 140 mg/100 ml is indicative of diabetes mellitus, and a level of 110–140 mg/100 ml is suggestive of subclinical diabetes (Danforth, 1977).

Generally, insulin therapy is not indicated for class A diabetics. However, it may occasionally be utilized if fasting blood sugar levels are greater than 120 mg/100 ml and postprandial values are above 180 mg/100 ml. The mode of therapy is usually on a sliding scale as assessed through urine testing, until a daily or twice-daily dosage can be established. Oral hypoglycemics are contraindicated in pregnancy because of the severe damage they can cause in the fetus. The NPH and Lente insulins are commonly used. However, individual patient needs should determine the insulin program utilized.

Patients with overt diabetes, classes B through F, require more frequent and in-depth nursing management. Prenatally they should be seen twice a month up through the second trimester and once a week during the third trimester. Individualization of care is imperative, and this can only be attained through careful assessment of patient knowledge and needs. Utilizing the previously identified nursing care principles, care for this patient includes the following actions:

1. *Strict dietary regulation.* Recommended daily intake includes 30–40 calories/kg, 150–250 gm of carbohydrates, 60–90 gm of protein, and 80–90 gm of fat. The goal is to increase calorie intake, with sufficient insulin therapy to force glucose into the cells.

2. *Urinary and blood sugar determinations.* The nurse should be aware of the correlation between urine glucose results and blood sugar levels. The blood sugar ideally should be maintained at 120–150 mg/100 ml after fasting and 150–180 mg/100 ml

two hours after meals. Fractional urine testing for glucose and acetone levels is done four times a day as needed. In the presence of control, optimum fetal outcome is enhanced, and the risk of ketoacidosis with subsequent fetal demise or retarded fetal growth is minimized.

3. *Establishment of insulin requirements.* Ordinarily, the patient is hospitalized to achieve maximum control of the diabetes and to establish insulin requirements. A team approach is used. Insulins used most frequently are NPH and Lente Iletin. The choice depends on individual patient needs based on urine and blood determinations of blood glucose level. During the second and third trimesters, insulin requirements will always increase because of the insulin-antagonistic hormones (Williams, 1974).

4. *Evaluation of fetoplacental functioning.* Particularly in overt diabetes, assessment of fetal well-being is essential. It is performed throughout the prenatal course, utilizing such clinical and chemical techniques as collection of 24-hour urinary estriols (at about the 32nd week of gestation), monitoring of insulin requirements (failure to require increased insulin dosages after first trimester or sudden drop in requirement should lead to doubt in placental functioning), ultrasound to assess fetal growth, measurement of fundal height, and OCT (attempted at about 34 weeks' gestation to determine the ability of the fetus to withstand stress of contractions).

5. *Assessment of fetal maturity and delivery.* Overtly diabetic patients are usually hospitalized one to two weeks prior to planned delivery to assess diabetic control and fetal maturity. Usually delivery is accomplished between the 36th and 38th weeks of gestation. Fetal maturity is confirmed by obtaining a sample of amniotic fluid by amniocentesis and then determining the lecithin/sphingomyelin (L/S) ratio (see p. 399). Caution must be used in evaluating L/S ratio results since they may be falsely elevated in the diabetic. Pelvic adequacy is ascertained by pelvimetry, and if the cervix is ripe, induction by oxytocin is initiated. Fetal monitoring is continuous, and if labor fails to progress or if fetal distress is noted, a cesarean section is performed immediately. At delivery the pediatric staff is present to assess the neonate for complications.

6. *Support of the expectant couple.* The nurse provides encouragement to the patient and her partner, stresses the concept of the family unit, and provides comfort as well as information to them to decrease anxiety caused by fear and lack of knowledge.

In the postpartal period the maternal insulin requirements fall significantly. The termination of the pregnancy reverses the gestationally induced endocrine changes that demanded additional insulin to be physiologically available for utilization in carbohydrate metabolism. Postpartally the estrogen and progesterone levels fall, thus decreasing the contra-insulin factors that tended to increase blood glucose levels. Therefore, a lowered blood glucose level requires decreased insulin production and availability. The diabetic mother may require no insulin for the first 24 hours. Then a reregulation of insulin needs is necessary, based on blood sugar testing. Diet and exercise levels must also be redetermined. Diabetic control and the establishment of parent-child relationships in light of neonatal needs are the priorities of this period.

In summary, a diabetic pregnancy demands thorough assessment, planning, and follow-through in nursing care. The nursing assessment considers the biologic, psychologic, and sociologic needs of the patient and her family. Planning necessitates a coordinated team approach to assure optimum care and outcome, and follow-through requires the nurse to have knowledge, understanding, and patience to implement and evaluate the required therapies successfully (see the accompanying Nursing Care Plan).

Thyroid Dysfunction

The thyroid gland is affected by the metabolic and hormonal changes that occur in pregnancy. However, thyroid dysfunction is not a common complication of pregnancy. The behaviors that result from pregnancy mimic those of the hyperthyroid state: increased metabolic rate, increased protein-bound iodine values, and increased ^{131}I intake. Evidence has shown that hypothyroid women ovulate irregularly, or, if pregnancy is achieved, their maintenance of the gravid state is difficult. It appears that infertility and high fetal mortality are characteristic of the hypothyroid state. In hyperthyroid women, there is no convincing evidence to support fertility impairment;

(Continued on p. 354)

NURSING CARE PLAN

Diabetes Mellitus in Prenatal and Intrapartal Periods

Patient Data Base

Nursing history

1. Complete assessment: patient and family
2. Identification of patient's predisposition to diabetes
   a. Recurrent preeclampsia-eclampsia
   b. Previous LGA infants ($\geq$4000 gm)
   c. Polyhydramnios
   d. Unexplained fetal death
   e. Obesity
   f. Family history of diabetes

Physical examination

1. Length of gestation
2. Complaints of thirst and hunger
3. Recurrent monilial vaginitis
4. Frequent urination beyond first trimester and prior to third trimester
5. Fundal height greater than expectation for gestation
6. Obesity

Laboratory evaluation

1. Fasting blood sugar (FBS)
2. 2-hour postprandial GTT
3. 3-hour GTT
4. Urine test for glucose
5. 24-hour urinary estriol

Note for diagnosis: 2 hr pp of 140 mg/100 ml is indicative of diabetes mellitus and a level of 110–140 mg/100 ml is suggestive of subclinical diabetes. May be confirmed with GTT.

Nursing Priorities

1. Observe for signs of hypoglycemia, hyperglycemia, preeclampsia.
2. Test urine daily for glucose.
3. Dietary and insulin regulation as needed.
4. Assess patient and family needs for referral.
5. Assess knowledge level of patient relative to disease.
6. During labor, monitor labor and amount and color of amniotic fluid.

Problem	Nursing interventions and actions	Rationale
Hypoglycemia	Observe for signs of hypoglycemia: 1. Palpitations (pulse >100/min). 2. Tachycardia. 3. Hunger. 4. Weakness. 5. Pallor. 6. Sweating. 7. Glycosuria (test urine).	Correction of hypoglycemia and maintenance of controlled state will provide optimal maternal health, thereby providing optimal fetal health.
Dietary regulation	Maintain strict diet: 1. 30–40 calories/kg. 2. 150–250 gm carbohydrate. 3. 60–90 gm fat to provide approximately 35% of fetal stores. 4. Sodium intake may be restricted.	Maintain ideal weight in first trimester and average gain in last two trimesters (no more than 3–3.5 lb/month).
Insulin needs	Assess insulin needs: 1. Check lab results of FBS and 2-hour postprandial.	Sufficient insulin must be present to enable proper carbohydrate metabolism to take place. Pregnancy requires a marked

NURSING CARE PLAN Cont'd

Diabetes Mellitus in Prenatal and Intrapartal Periods

Problem	Nursing interventions and actions	Rationale
	2. Test urine four times daily using Clinitest. Determine amount of insulin based on sliding scale. 3. Administer NPH or Lente insulin as ordered.	increase in circulating insulin to maintain normal blood glucose. Fasting glucose level tends to be lower than nonpregnant value. Effectiveness of insulin may be reduced by presence of human placental lactogen. Insulin requirements fluctuate widely during pregnancy because of factors mentioned in text and because of lowered sugar tolerance, especially in second half of pregnancy, and fluctuate during intrapartal period because of depletion of glycogen stores during labor. Fluctuations during puerperium are a result of involuntary process. In addition, conversion of blood glucose into lactose during lactation may cause marked changes in glucose tolerance and/or hypoglycemia.
Inadequate rest	Instruct patient to rest frequently during day in lateral position.	Lateral position has favorable influence on uteroplacental circulation and diminishes myometrial tone.
Fear and lack of knowledge	Support and encourage patient and husband: 1. Explain procedures. 2. Allow them to ask questions. 3. Assess their level of knowledge of childbirth and utilize this to teach about what is happening. 4. Involve husband as much as possible.	By decreasing fear, the patient will be more effective as a member of the antepartal-intrapartal health team.
	5. Utilize breathing and relaxation techniques to minimize amount of medication needed, especially if gestation is 36 or 37 weeks, to decrease fetal narcosis. For more detailed information, see Nursing Care Plan on labor and delivery, Chapter 17. 6. Administer analgesics as needed in labor.	Fetal narcosis should be avoided.
Compromise of fetoplacental status	Periodic assessments: 1. Level of plasma and/or urine estriol. 2. Creatinine clearance.	Continued slow rise of estriol indicates adequate functioning of maternal system, placental function, and fetal status, because estriol and creatinine require interplay of all three systems.
	3. Regular assessment of fetal size.	Assess fetal growth.
	4. Sonograms.	Evaluate fetal size.
	5. L/S ratio.	2:1 ratio indicates fetal lung maturity sufficient to sustain infant in extrauterine environment. In one-third of insulin-dependent patients, L/S ratio fails to show a terminal rise; others show early excessive rise.
Size of fetus	Assessments: 1. Sonograms.	Increased circulating glucose leads to increased deposition of fatty tissue in fetus.

NURSING CARE PLAN Cont'd
Diabetes Mellitus in Prenatal and Intrapartal Periods

Problem	Nursing interventions and actions	Rationale
	2. Measuring fundal height.	Indicates uterine size, not necessarily size of fetus.
Frequent hospitalization	Orient patient to surroundings and routines: 1. Provide support. 2. Promote rest.	Admit prenatally to assess diabetic status. Admit if there are signs of incipient preeclampsia or infection. Admit for most of third trimester if patient has microvascular disease, so that rest can be maintained and patient can be closely supervised.
Hydramnios	Assess size of uterus. Assess signs of distress from polyhydramnios: 1. Respiratory distress. 2. Stasis of fluid in legs.	Diabetic patients are more prone to polyhydramnios, and it may develop rapidly.
	Slow removal of amniotic fluid by transabdominal amniotomy may be done.	Remove fluid slowly to prevent abruptio placentae and amniotic fluid embolus.
Labor	Admit to unit: 1. Perform routine admission. See Nursing Care Plan on labor and delivery, Chapter 17. 2. Assess size of fetus and capacity of pelvis: sonograms, x-ray pelvimetry. 3. Administer IV fluids to maintain hydration and glucose to avoid depleting glycogen stores. 4. Assess insulin needs. 5. Continuously monitor fetal status. 6. Alleviate induction concerns (see Nursing Care Plan on induction, Chapter 20).	Induction of labor at about 37 weeks, once fetal lung maturity is ascertained, is recommended to ensure safe fetal outcome.

Nursing Care Evaluation

Patient's diabetes will be controlled.

Patient will consume needed calories and nutrients.

Patient will have sufficient insulin to maintain control.

Fetoplacental status will be monitored to avoid complications.

Patient education will be enhanced and patient questions will be answered.

however, there is a slight increase in neonatal mortality rate and a significant increase in the frequency of delivery of small-for-gestational-age infants.

Hyperthyroidism

Diagnosis of hyperthyroidism during pregnancy is difficult because of normal gestational changes. Symptoms that are indicative include (a) a resting pulse rate greater than 100 beats/min, without slowing during Valsalva's maneuver; (b) muscle wasting, particularly of the quadriceps; and (c) separation of the distal nail from its nail bed. Serum thyroxine levels are not accurate determinants because of the influence of pregnancy.

With hyperthyroidism there is an increased incidence of premature delivery, postpartum hemorrhage, and possibly preeclampsia. The major complication for both the hyperthyroid mother and the fetus is that of thyroid storm. This rare but frightening occurrence presents a clinical picture of extremely high fever, tachycardia, severe dehydration, sweating, and possible heart failure. In addition, mental function may be erratic. Prompt medical and nursing intervention include hospitalization and appropriate pharmacologic agents to reduce presenting behaviors and to achieve control. Thyroid storm most commonly occurs in pregnant patients in whom the diagnosis of hyperthyroidism has been missed. It is therefore imperative that a thorough nursing prenatal assessment include careful history-taking and close observation of the patient's physiologic and physical behaviors that may be indicative of increased thyroid function, as well as nervousness, heat sensitivity, fatigue, diarrhea, and insomnia. Hyperthyroidism appears in approximately 2 of every 1000 pregnant women (Haynes, 1969).

Fetal-Neonatal Implications

Hyperthyroidism in newborns is even more uncommon than in the mother. It is seen more often in male neonates, which is contrary to the general trend of hyperthyroid dysfunction. Neonates born to mothers with this complication should have serum thyroxine determinations done at birth and should be observed carefully during the first two weeks of life for signs of hyperthyroidism.

Interventions

Treatment of thyroid dysfunction involves a choice between drug therapy and surgical intervention. These alternatives must be weighed in view of gestational age and thyroid function. A variety of drugs are utilized to control the overactivity of the sympathetic nervous system, to block the uptake of iodine by the thyroid gland, or to inhibit the production of the thyroid hormone. It must be noted that these drugs do cross the placenta and interfere with fetal thyroid function. Overtreatment of the mother with hyperthyroid drugs may result in fetal hypothyroidism and deficient development, especially of the central nervous system. For the patient with mild hyperthyroidism, sedation with phenobarbital is usually effective. If drug therapy is not effective, surgical resection of part or all of the thyroid gland is indicated. In the pregnant patient, the most favorable time would be after the first trimester to decrease the risk of spontaneous abortion.

Hypothyroidism

Hypothyroidism in its extreme form is usually accompanied by amenorrhea or oligomenorrhea, with resultant sterility. However, a less severe deficiency is compatible with pregnancy, although abortion is likely. Generally, diagnosis is made based on the results of laboratory findings of free serum thyroxine concentrations, which are estimated by calculation of the free thyroxine index. Determination of radioactive iodine uptake is contraindicated during pregnancy because the substance is readily taken up by the fetal thyroid.

Additional supportive data include suggestive medical history and physical signs, such as a decreased basal metabolic rate, a firm diffuse goiter (enlarged thyroid gland), fatigability, cold intolerance, myxedema, constipation, dry skin, headache, and delayed deep tendon reflexes.

In pregnancy, relative iodine deficiency may be induced by increased renal iodide clearance and increased hormonogenesis.

Fetal-Neonatal Implications

The infant of a hypothyroid mother has a slightly increased risk of being born with congenital goiter or with true cretinism. There is also an increased risk for development of congenital anomalies (Danforth, 1977).

Interventions

As soon as diagnosis is confirmed, treatment should begin in order to decrease the possibility of fetal mortality. There appears to be a need for replacement thyroid therapy to sustain normal growth and development of the fetus. Replacement doses are prescribed, and the free thyroxine index is used to monitor the adequacy of medication. Iodine administration is desirable as a means of reducing the risk of cretinism in the newborn. Early abortions from multiple causes often exhibit low levels of protein-bound iodine. However, thyroid medication should not be used prophylactically in the hope of reducing fetal death.

MEDICAL DISORDERS ASSOCIATED WITH PREGNANCY

Disruptive conditions that arise during the gestational period are the result of many high-risk factors, such as age, blood type, socioeconomic status, parity, psychologic well-being, and predisposing chronic illnesses (see Chapter 10). The major thrust of prenatal nursing care should be toward screening patients for these complications and toward supportive therapies that will facilitate optimal health for mother and fetus.

Hyperemesis Gravidarum

Hyperemesis gravidarum is pernicious vomiting during pregnancy. In its early stages, it may be difficult to diagnose because initially vomiting does not occur after each feeding. However, true hyperemesis progresses to a point at which the woman not only vomits everything she swallows but retches between meals.

The cause of hyperemesis during pregnancy is still debatable but probably is related to trophoblastic activity and gonadotropin production and is stimulated or exaggerated by psychologic factors. It appears in approximately 1 of every 1000 pregnant women (Jensen et al., 1977).

The pathology of hyperemesis in extreme cases begins with dehydration. This leads to fluid-electrolyte imbalance, particularly acidosis. Starvation causes severe protein and vitamin deficiencies. Characteristic symptoms include jaundice and hemorrhage due to deficiencies of vitamin C and B-complex vitamins and bleeding from mucosal areas due to hypothrombinemia. Fetal or embryonic death may result, and the mother may suffer irreversible metabolic changes or death.

The differential diagnosis may involve infectious diseases such as encephalitis or viral hepatitis, intestinal obstruction, hydatidiform mole, or peptic ulcer.

It is imperative that diagnosis be made so that necessary therapy may be started. In severe cases, hospitalization is required. The objectives of nursing management include control of vomiting, correction of dehydration, restoration of electrolyte balance, and maintenance of adequate nutrition.

Barbiturates usually will control vomiting, but minimal effective doses should be utilized. Parenteral fluid therapy to correct dehydration, electrolytes, and vitamins is also necessary for proper management. As the patient's condition improves, six small dry feedings followed by clear liquids in one hour may be cautiously resumed. Nursing care should be supportive and directed at maintaining a relaxed, quiet environment. Because emotional factors have been found to play a major role in this condition, psychotherapy is recommended. With proper treatment, prognosis is favorable.

Shock

In the antepartal patient, the most common type of shock is caused from hypovolemia, or a reduction of blood volume. When 10%, or approximately 2 units of blood, is lost, objective signs of shock may be noted. As the blood volume decreases, the venous return decreases, and this shortage causes a decrease in cardiac output. The body attempts to compensate by releasing catecholamines, which results in tachycardia and vasoconstriction. The observable signs include a decrease in the blood pressure; increase in the heart rate; cool, clammy skin; air hunger; and restlessness.

The nurse's first responsibility is to assist in identifying patients who may be at risk. Assessment of blood pressure and pulse is important, as these may provide the earliest signs of shock. When shock is suspected, an intravenous infusion should be started. It should be in place with a large bore needle or plastic cannula that will accommodate a blood transfusion if needed. The patient should be lying flat, either in a supine or lateral position. Circulation to the head is better if the patient is lying flat than if she is sitting up. Oxygen may be given by face mask if the shock is worsening or if the patient exhibits air hunger or restlessness.

Treatment of shock involves identification of the cause, supportive therapy to the patient, and blood volume replacement. See Chapter 19 for further discussion and a nursing care plan for hemorrhage and shock.

Bleeding Disorders

During the first and second trimesters of pregnancy, the major cause of bleeding is abortion. This is defined as the termination of a pregnancy prior to the 28th week of gestation or prior to viability of the fetus. Abortions are either *spontaneous,* occurring naturally with no artificial means, or *induced,* occurring as a result of artificial or mechanical interruption (see Chapter 7 for discussion of induced abortion). *Miscarriage* is a lay term applied to abortion. Its usage appears directly related to the negative legal and moral implications that the term *abortion* implies to the general public.

Other complications that can cause bleeding

in the first half of pregnancy are ectopic pregnancy (1 of every 200 pregnancies) and hydatidiform mole (1 of every 2000 pregnancies). In the second half of pregnancy, particularly in the third trimester, bleeding may develop that may be fatal to mother and fetus. Two major causes of bleeding at this time are placenta previa (1 of every 200 pregnancies) and abruptio placentae (1 of every 115 pregnancies) (Jensen et al., 1977).

General Principles of Nursing Intervention

All bleeding during pregnancy should be carefully evaluated. Therefore, antepartal teaching regarding bleeding as a warning sign should be stressed. It is often the nurse's responsibility to make the initial assessment of bleeding. In general, the following nursing measures should be implemented for pregnant patients being treated for bleeding disorders:

1. Constant monitoring of vital signs of blood pressure and pulse is imperative.
2. Observe patient for behaviors indicative of shock, such as pallor, clammy skin, perspiration, dyspnea, or restlessness.
3. Count pads to assess amount of bleeding over a given time period. Any tissue or clots expelled should be saved.
4. Prepare for intravenous therapy.
5. Prepare equipment for examination.
6. Have oxygen therapy available.
7. Collect and organize all data, including antepartal history, onset of bleeding episode, laboratory studies (hemoglobin, hematocrit, and hormonal assays).
8. Assess coping mechanisms of patient in crisis. Give emotional support to enhance her coping abilities by continuous, sustained presence, by clear explanation of procedures, and by communicating her status to her family. Most important, prepare the patient for possible fetal loss. Assess her expressions of anger, denial, silence, guilt, depression, or self-blame.

The nurse's role in the care of the pregnant patient with a bleeding disorder involves assessment of biologic and psychologic factors. With a thorough data base, the nurse can more effectively coordinate the care of such patients and implement the holistic approach of the health team to meet the patient's needs.

Spontaneous Abortion

Many pregnancies are lost in the first trimester as a result of spontaneous abortion. Statistics are inaccurate, because some women may have aborted but were unaware that they were pregnant during the early weeks of gestation (through week 8). The bleeding is seen as a heavy menstrual period.

Approximately 82% of spontaneous abortions occur in the first trimester, with only 18% in the second. The overall figures range from 10% to 30% of all pregnancies (Roth, 1962).

Etiology

When a spontaneous abortion occurs, the woman and her family must search for a cause so that they may plan knowledgeably for future family expansion. However, even with current technology and medical advances, a direct cause cannot always be determined. The genetic findings for a couple may include the following (Danforth, 1977):

1. Chromosomal structure and number are normal in both partners, but abnormal offspring can result sporadically and unpredictably.
2. One member of couple is a carrier of a balanced translocation. Repeated abortion may result.

The most common causes of spontaneous abortion are related to abnormal development of the embryo or fetus. The abnormal development may be due to drugs or genetic makeup, faulty implantation due to abnormalities of the female generative tract, placental abnormalities, chronic maternal diseases, and endocrine imbalances.

Most spontaneous abortions appear to be related to imperfections in sperm or ova or to effects of teratogenic drugs, as discussed later in this chapter. Abnormalities of the woman's generative tract may be a result of organ imperfections, such as an undeveloped uterus, double uterus, or adhesions of the adnexa as a result of pelvic inflammatory disease. Abortion may also result from uterine tremors and retrodisplacement of the fundal portion of the uterus (Clark and Affonso, 1976). Sometimes abortion occurs in midpregnancy as a result of an incompetent cervix. The weakened cervix is unable to remain closed and painlessly dilates, the membranes rupture, and the products of conception are expelled. This is often the cause of second trimester habitual abortion.

Maternal infections, if left untreated, can emit toxins that stimulate abortion. Endocrine imbalances, particularly a reduction in progesterone and estrogen in early pregnancy, can retard the normal growth of the endometrial lining of the uterus. In later pregnancy, a decrease in HCG produced by the placenta can cause loss of pregnancy. Maternal malnutrition has also been implicated in abortion. Other chronic maternal diseases affecting embryonic and fetal growth include essential hypertensive vascular diseases, ABO incompatibility, chronic nephritis, and in the second trimester, syphilis. It is commonly believed that psychic trauma and accidents are the primary causes of abortion, but statistics do not generally support this belief.

Classification

Spontaneous abortions are subdivided into the following categories so that they can be differentiated clinically (see Table 13-2):

Table 13-2. Classification of Spontaneous Abortion (First and Second Trimesters)

Category	Signs and symptoms	Products of conception
Threatened	Vaginal bleeding, cramping, backache	May be partially or totally expelled
Imminent	Vaginal bleeding, cramping, backache, cervical dilatation	Will be partially or totally expelled
Complete	Same as imminent abortion	Totally expelled
Incomplete	Same as imminent abortion	Partially expelled
Missed	Weight loss, decrease in breast size, continued amenorrhea	Remain in utero
Habitual	Loss of three or more successive pregnancies	

1. *Threatened abortion:* The fetus is jeopardized by unexplained bleeding, cramping, and backache. Bleeding may persist for days. The cervix is closed. It may be followed by partial or complete expulsion of pregnancy (Figure 13-1).

2. *Imminent abortion:* Abortion is inevitable. Bleeding and cramping increase. The internal cervical os is dilated and will admit one finger.

3. *Complete abortion:* All the products of conception are expelled.

4. *Incomplete abortion:* Part of the products of conception are retained, most often the placenta. The internal cervical os is dilated and will admit one finger.

5. *Missed abortion:* The fetus dies in utero but is not expelled. It can remain in utero for two or more months with no untoward effects. The cervix is closed.

6. *Habitual abortion:* Abortion occurs consecutively in three or more pregnancies.

Diagnosis

A primary consideration in the differential diagnosis of this condition is to determine whether vaginal bleeding is related to spontaneous abortion or due to other factors. One of the more reliable indices of evaluation is the presence of pelvic cramping and backache. These symptoms are usually absent in bleeding caused by polyps, ruptured cervical blood vessels, or cervical erosion.

Laboratory evaluations do not provide much help in establishing a diagnosis. If there has been significant blood loss, the hemoglobin level will be lowered. Results of pregnancy tests are not particularly helpful, because they may remain positive for as long as two weeks after fetal death.

Interventions

The therapy prescribed for the pregnant patient with bleeding is restriction of activities, bed rest, abstinence from coitus, and perhaps sedation. If bleeding persists and abortion is incomplete, the patient is hospitalized, intravenous therapy or blood transfusions may be utilized to replace fluid, and dilatation and curettage or vacuum curettage is performed to remove the remainder of

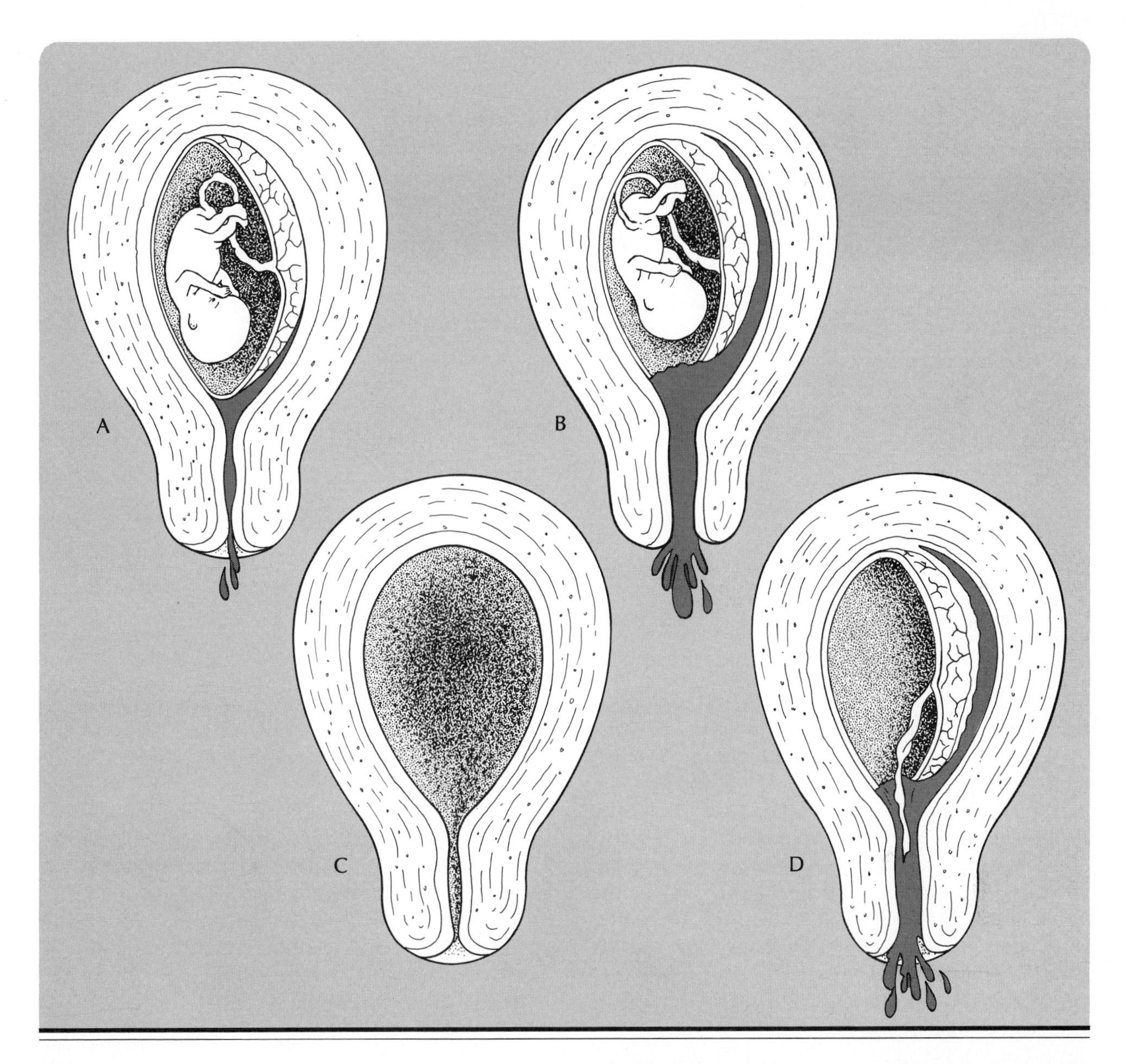

Figure 13–1. Types of spontaneous abortion. **A,** Threatened abortion. **B,** Imminent abortion. **C,** Complete abortion. **D,** Incomplete abortion.

the products of conception. In missed abortions, the products of conception eventually are expelled spontaneously, but if this does not occur, hospitalization for a D and C or induction by intravenous oxytocin is necessary to expel the dead fetus.

The nursing interventions for bleeding disorders listed on p. 357 are implemented for spontaneous abortion with bleeding. Nurses caring for women who have aborted may find that their most significant role is in helping the women and their families to deal with their feelings about this unelected termination of pregnancy and resultant fetal death.

Couples who approached the pregnancy with feelings of joy and a sense of expectancy now feel grief, sadness, and possibly anger. For those who were perhaps less than joyful or even negative about their pregnancy, there may be guilt and blame. The woman may harbor negative feelings about herself, ranging from lowered self-esteem, resulting from a belief that she is lacking or abnormal in some way, to a notion that the abortion may be a punishment for some wrongdoing.

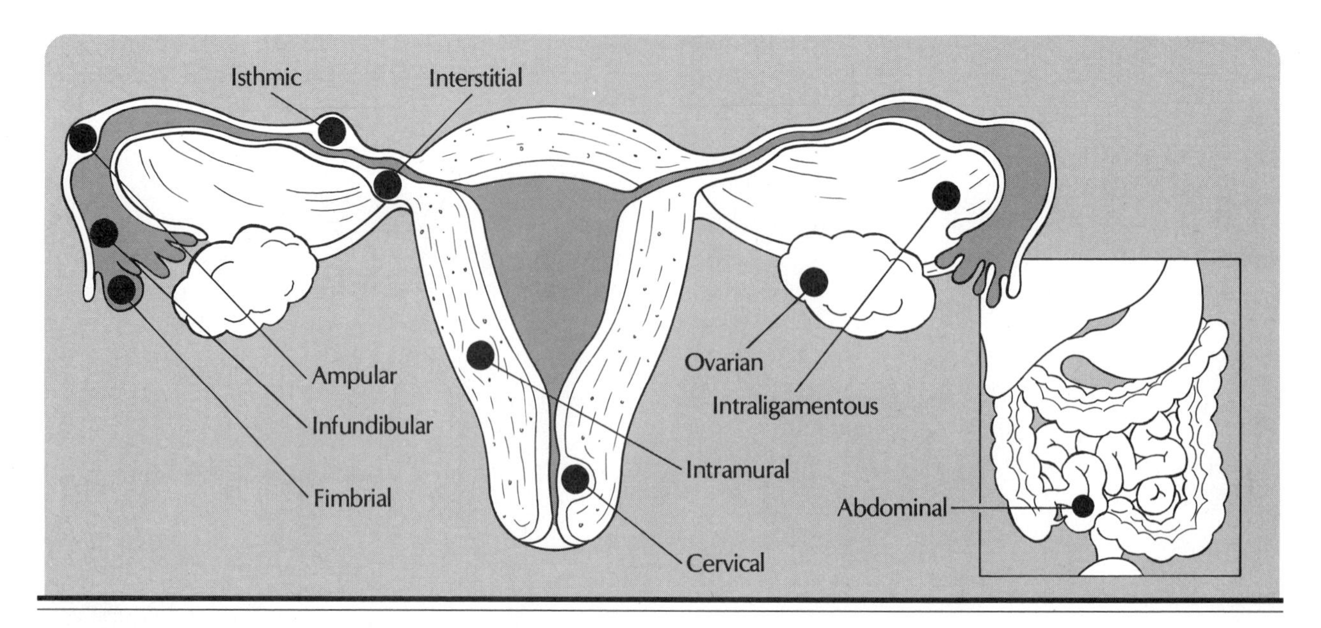

Figure 13–2. Various implantation sites in ectopic pregnancy.

The nurse assesses the responses of the patient and her family to this crisis and evaluates their coping mechanisms and their ability to comfort each other. If the nurse perceives that the patient's reactions are abnormal or pathologic (for example, denial or hostility), the patient should be referred for the proper help.

The nurse can provide invaluable psychologic support to the patient and her family by encouraging them to verbalize their feelings, by allowing them the privacy to grieve, and by sympathetically listening to their concerns about this pregnancy and future ones. The nurse can aid in decreasing any feelings of guilt or blame by supplying the patient and her family with information regarding the causes of spontaneous abortion and possibly referring them to other health care professionals for additional help, such as a genetic counselor if there is a history of habitual abortions.

Ectopic Pregnancy

Ectopic pregnancy is an implantation of the blastocyst in a site other than the endometrial lining of the uterine cavity. It may result from a number of different causes, including tubal damage caused by previous pelvic surgery, hormonal factors that may impede ovum transport and thus mechanically stops the forward motion of the egg in the fallopian tube, tubal atony or spasms, and blighted conceptus. The actual pathogenesis occurs when such conditions are present and the fertilized ovum is prevented or slowed in its progress down the tube.

The most common type is a tubal pregnancy, in which implantation occurs in a fallopian tube. Other less common types of ectopic pregnancy are abdominal and cervical (Figure 13–2).

Incidence of ectopic pregnancy is greater in nonwhite populations (1 in 150 pregnancies) as compared with white populations (1 in 300 pregnancies).

Clinical Manifestations and Diagnosis

Clinical signs and symptoms indicative of ectopic pregnancy include:

1. Lower abdominal pain, which may be sharp or dull, constant or intermittent.
2. Vaginal bleeding.
3. Amenorrhea.
4. Vital signs indicative of shock: a rise in pulse rate or a fall in blood pressure.
5. Urinary frequency.

The clinical picture appears vague in ectopic pregnancy. If these symptoms are present, laboratory tests of hematocrit or hemoglobin value and leukocytes can serve to validate the diagnosis. Pregnancy tests may be negative and therefore of no help in diagnosis. The following procedures are utilized in establishing the diagnosis:

1. A careful assessment of menstrual history, particularly the LMP, should be undertaken.
2. Careful pelvic exam should be performed, with the patient under anesthesia if necessary, to identify any abnormal pelvic masses.
3. Laparoscopy may reveal an extrauterine pregnancy.
4. Culdoscopy may reveal clotted blood, possibly including an aborted conceptus.
5. Laparotomy will give a confirmed diagnosis and allow opportunity for immediate treatment.

It is important to differentiate an ectopic pregnancy from other disorders with similar clinical presenting pictures. Consideration must be given to possible uterine abortion, ruptured corpus luteum cyst, appendicitis, salpingitis, torsion of the ovary, ovarian cysts, and urinary tract infection.

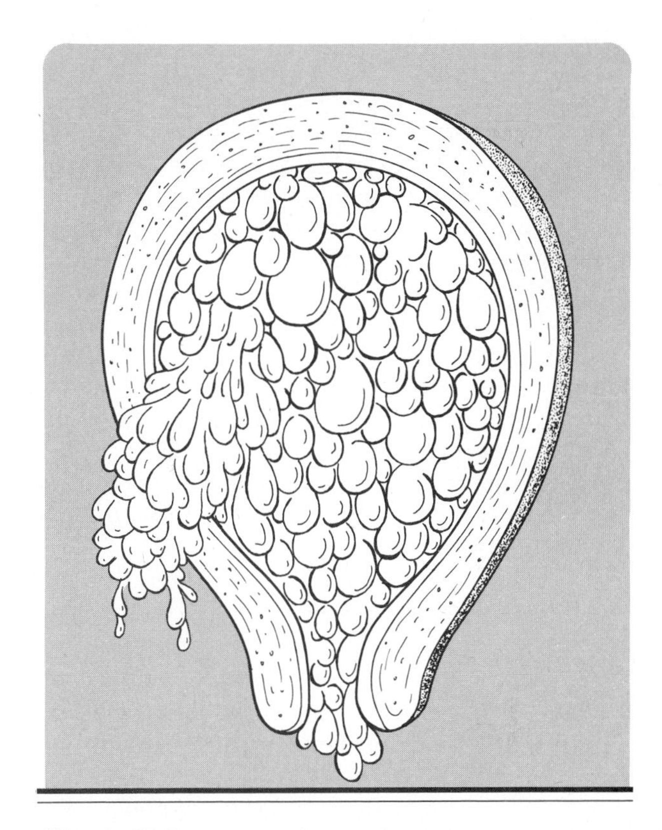

Figure 13–3. Hydatidiform mole.

Interventions

Once the diagnosis has been made, surgical intervention is initiated. Intravenous therapy and blood transfusion are utilized to replace fluid loss. The affected tube and ovary are removed surgically. If massive infection is found, a complete removal of uterus, tubes, and ovaries may be necessary. However, every effort is made to leave a normal tube, ovary, and uterus so that childbearing may be a future possibility. During surgery, the most important risk to be considered is potential hemorrhage. Bleeding must be controlled, and replacement therapy should be on hand. Blood transfusions may be necessary to allay shock.

The patient and her family will need emotional and psychologic support during this difficult time. Their feelings and responses to this crisis will probably be similar to those that occur in cases of spontaneous abortion. As a result, similar nursing actions are required for these patients (see p. 359).

Hydatidiform Mole

Hydatidiform mole (hydatid mole) is a developmental anomaly of the placenta (Figure 13–3). It represents a degeneration of the villi accompanied by a proliferation of the epithelium of the chorion. The degenerating villi become distended with fluid, forming grapelike clusters. Usually no embryo is present. Hydatidiform mole is a rare occurrence but bears discussion because it can present a clinical picture similar to other bleeding complications.

Clinical Manifestations and Diagnosis

Diagnosis is based on a clinical picture of vaginal discharge of grapelike vesicles. Other indicators include uterine fundal height in advance of length of gestation, absence of lightening, either scanty or profuse bleeding, hyperemesis, concomitant uterine infection, and a characteristic brownish vaginal discharge. No fetal heart tone is heard, nor can fetal movement be discerned by abdominal palpation. Clinical results of sonography reveal no fetal skeleton, and the laboratory results of HCG serum levels are high for 100 days or more after the last menstrual period.

Interventions

Therapy consists of complete emptying of uterine contents, careful curettage, prevention of further blood loss, antibiotics to treat infection, and support to the woman who is no longer pregnant. Additional counseling regarding future pregnancies may be necessary in light of the fact that a few of these women develop recurring moles or choriocarcinoma, a rare but highly malignant form of cancer for which survival rates of greater than one year are uncommon.

The patient treated for hydatidiform mole should receive follow-up therapy for one year, including cautions against conception for one year and measurement of HCG at intervals beginning at 60 days postpartum.

Continued high or rising HCG titers are abnormal. Dilatation and curettage are performed, and tissue is examined. If malignant cells are found, chemotherapy for choriocarcinoma is started, using either methotrexate or dactinomycin. If therapy is ineffective, the choriocarcinoma has a tendency to metastasize rapidly.

If, after a year of supervisory therapy, the HCG serum titers are within normal limits, a couple may be assured that subsequent normal pregnancy can be anticipated with low probability of recurrent hydatidiform mole.

Placenta Previa

In placenta previa, the placenta is improperly implanted in the lower uterine segment, perhaps on a portion of the lower segment or over the internal os. As the lower uterine segment contracts and the cervix dilates in the later weeks of pregnancy, the placental villi are torn from the uterine wall, thus exposing the uterine sinuses at the placental site. Bleeding begins, but because its amount depends on the number of sinuses exposed, initially it may be scanty or profuse. The classic symptom is painless vaginal bleeding. See Chapter 19 for an in-depth discussion of placenta previa.

Abruptio Placentae

Abruptio placentae is the premature separation of the placenta from the uterine wall. It occurs prior to delivery and usually during the labor process. See Chapter 19 for an in-depth description of abruptio placentae.

Incompetent Cervix

Cervical incompetence is associated with repeated second trimester abortions. The cervix may become weakened from the birth of a macrosomatic infant, with resultant cervical lacerations, excessive dilatation and curettage, or other obstetric trauma; from congenital structure defect; or from premature initiation of cervical effacement and dilatation.

Diagnosis is established by eliciting a positive history of repeated, relatively painless and bloodless second trimester abortions. Serial pelvic exams reveal progressive effacement and dilatation of the cervix and bulging membranes.

Incompetent cervix is managed surgically with a Shirodkar-Barter operation (cerclage), which reinforces the weakened cervix by adding suture material. A purse-string suture is placed in the cervix between the 14th and 18th week of gestation. The procedure should not be done if any of the following conditions exist: the diagnosis is in doubt, membranes are ruptured, there is vaginal bleeding and cramping, the cervix is dilated beyond 3 cm. Once the suture is in place, a cesarean section may be planned (to prevent repeating the procedure in subsequent pregnancies), or the suture may be released at term and vaginal delivery permitted.

HYPERTENSIVE DISORDERS IN PREGNANCY

Classification

The American College of Obstetricians and Gynecologists has classified the hypertensive states of pregnancy as follows:

> *Gestational edema.* Gestational edema is the occurrence of a general and excessive accumulation of fluid in the tissues of greater than 1^+ pitting edema after 12 hours' rest in bed, or of a weight gain of 5 pounds or more in one week due to the influence of pregnancy.
>
> *Gestational proteinuria.* Gestational proteinuria is the presence of proteinuria during or

under the influence of pregnancy, in the absence of hypertension, edema, renal infection, or known intrinsic renovascular cause.

Gestational hypertension. Gestational hypertension is the development of hypertension during pregnancy or within the first 24 hours postpartum in a previously normotensive woman. . . .

Preeclampsia. Preeclampsia is the development of hypertension with proteinuria, edema, or both due to pregnancy or the influence of a recent pregnancy. It occurs after the 20th week of gestation but may develop before this time in the presence of trophoblastic disease. Preeclampsia is predominantly a disorder of primigravidas.

Eclampsia. Eclampsia is the occurrence of one or more convulsions, not attributable to other cerebral disorders such as epilepsy or cerebral hemorrhage, in a patient with preeclampsia.

Superimposed preeclampsia or eclampsia. Superimposed preeclampsia or eclampsia is the development of preeclampsia or eclampsia in a patient with chronic hypertensive, vascular, or renal disease. When the hypertension antedates the pregnancy, as established by previous blood pressure recordings, a rise in the systolic pressure of 30 mm Hg, a rise in the diastolic pressure of 15 mm Hg, and the development of proteinuria, edema, or both are required during pregnancy to establish the diagnosis.

Chronic hypertensive disease. Chronic hypertensive disease is the presence of persistent hypertension, of whatever cause, before pregnancy or prior to the 20th week of gestation, or persistent hypertension beyond the 42nd day of the postpartum period.*

Preeclampsia and Eclampsia (Toxemia)

Two major disruptions occurring in the third trimester of pregnancy are preeclampsia and eclampsia, also referred to as *toxemia of pregnancy.* They are characterized by the development of hypertension, excessive weight gain caused by fluid retention resulting in edema, and proteinuria. Preeclampsia is seen most often in the last ten weeks of gestation, during labor, or in the first 12 to 48 hours after delivery. Predisposing factors include diabetes mellitus, hypertensive or renal disease, hydatidiform mole, multiple pregnancy, and hydramnios. Teenagers and primigravidas are at risk for the development of this condition, but the incidence of preeclampsia also increases with advancing maternal age. The only cure for preeclampsia is termination of the pregnancy.

Eclampsia is manifested by convulsions and coma. If prompt and intensive antepartal care is given to pregnant women, eclampsia may be prevented.

Preeclampsia may be mild or severe. Women with mild preeclampsia may exhibit an almost asymptomatic pregnancy. They may have little or no peripheral edema evident following bed rest. Their blood pressure may be 140/90 or more, or about 30 mm Hg above their baseline systolic pressure and 15 mm Hg above their baseline diastolic pressure. This is an important consideration, because a young woman who may normally manifest a blood pressure of 90/60 would be hypertensive at 120/80, which is a marked increase above her baseline norm. Therefore, it is an essential part of the nursing assessment to obtain a baseline blood pressure in early pregnancy. Urine testing may show a +1 or +2 albumin in a clean midstream specimen, and a 24-hour urine collection may contain 1 gm of protein.

Severe preeclampsia may develop suddenly. Edema becomes generalized and readily apparent in face, hands, sacral area, lower extremities, and the abdominal wall. It is characterized by an excessive weight gain of more than 0.9 kg (2 lb) over a period of a couple of days to a week. Blood pressure is 160/100 or higher, a dipstick albumin measurement is +3 to +4, and the 24-hour urine protein is greater than 5 gm. Other characteristic symptoms are frontal headaches, blurred vision, nausea, vomiting, irritability, hyperreflexia, cerebral disturbances, oliguria (less than 400 ml of urine in 24 hours), and finally, epigastric pain. The epigastric pain is often the sign of impending convulsion (eclampsia) and is thought to be caused by increased vascular engorgement of the liver.

Preeclampsia occurs in about 7% of all pregnancies. Because of improved antepartal care, preeclampsia has declined considerably and eclampsia rarely occurs.

The cause of preeclampsia-eclampsia is still unknown. Many factors are believed to play a role, including a functioning pregnancy, environ-

*From Danforth, D. N., ed. 1977. *Obstetrics and gynecology.* 3rd ed. Hagerstown, Md.: Harper & Row Publishers, Inc.

mental factors such as climate and socioeconomic status, diet, activity, and health status.

Some of the current theories related to preeclampsia development involve uteroplacental ischemia and nutritional status. Research is being conducted to study causes of the ischemia and specific predisposing factors. Also, investigators are directing their studies to vitamins, minerals, and especially protein and the possible relationship between these nutrients and the preeclampsia-eclampsia syndrome. It is no longer considered valid to restrict weight gain by restricting calories in pregnancy. Salt restrictions have also been lifted, although women with evident pitting edema may not be allowed to increase their salt intake (Danforth, 1977).

Fetal-Neonatal Implications

Perinatal mortality associated with preeclampsia is approximately 10%, and that associated with eclampsia is 30%. When preeclampsia is superimposed on hypertensive vascular disease, the perinatal mortality rate may be as high as 50% (Danforth, 1977).

At the time of delivery, the neonate may be oversedated because of medications administered to the mother. He may also have hypermagnesemia due to treatment of the mother with large doses of magnesium sulfate.

Interventions

The management of the severely preeclamptic patient is aimed at the prevention of convulsions by decreasing the blood pressure, establishing adequate renal function, and continuing the pregnancy until the fetus is mature. The principal cause of fetal death in utero of SGA infants is uteroplacental insufficiency, which causes a decreased blood supply. Therefore, the woman is hospitalized and placed on strict bed rest. Hypotensive drugs and sedatives may be utilized. She is encouraged to lie on her side to increase renal and uterine blood flow, which may encourage diuresis and return her blood pressure to within normal limits. Continuous external fetal monitoring is recommended to assess fetal well-being. Vital signs are recorded regularly, and intake and output are measured daily. Generally, with this strict regimen, the clinical symptoms diminish. During this antepartal crisis, the patient needs continuous nursing support in the form of reassurance that her condition is stabilizing and that the fetus is doing well. She should also have the proposed plan of care explained so that she understands why the procedures are necessary.

Every effort is made to maintain pregnancy until the 36th week of gestation. Urinary estriol determinations and ultrasonography are utilized to monitor the condition of the fetus (see Chapter 14).

The pharmacologic agent most commonly used to lower blood pressure is magnesium sulfate, which is administered intramuscularly in a 50% solution with 1% procaine. Magnesium sulfate acts to depress the myoneural junction, thus decreasing hyperreflexia and resulting in some vasodilatation. It also has a depressing effect on the central nervous system.

Magnesium sulfate is usually given in a dosage of 5–10 gm/10–20 ml of solution and is injected intramuscularly into the gluteal area. Because the solution is irritating, a new needle should be used to administer the medication after it is drawn into the syringe. The needle should be rotated like a wheel as the injection is made, because of the large amount of solution. The dose is divided equally between the two buttocks, and each injection site is massaged well following the injection. Urine output must be maintained so that the medication is excreted properly. Excessive levels of magnesium sulfate can cause respiratory or cardiac depression, but generally this does not occur until the patellar reflex disappears. No more magnesium sulfate is given if respiratory or cardiac depression occurs. Calcium gluconate is an effective metabolic antagonist and should be readily available. If needed, 20 ml of calcium gluconate in a 10% aqueous solution is slowly administered intravenously and repeated every hour until respiratory, cardiac, urinary, and neurologic depression are relieved. In a 24-hour period, no more than eight injections should be administered. Other medications utilized include the antihypertensive hydralazine, morphine, or other sedatives.

In the event of eclampsia, the woman is monitored carefully. Nursing actions include the following:

1. Maintenance of strict bed rest with padded side rails.
2. Institution of intravenous fluid therapy.
3. Maintenance of a central venous pressure line.

4. Insertion of a Foley catheter.
5. Recording hourly intake and output.
6. Frequent monitoring of vital signs and fetal monitoring.
7. Decreased sensory stimulation.

Once convulsions have ceased and the patient has stabilized, termination of pregnancy is indicated. If the cervix is favorable for labor, the membranes are ruptured and oxytocin is given by infusion pump. If the induction fails, if the woman's condition worsens, or if fetal distress is noted, a cesarean section is performed.

Following delivery, the preeclamptic and eclamptic behaviors diminish rapidly. The first sign of recovery in the postpartal period is diuresis, usually occurring approximately 12 hours after delivery. The postpartal hospital stay is extended to about ten days. The edema and proteinuria usually disappear by the fifth postpartal day. This extended stay affords the new mother the opportunity to begin to assume the tasks of mothering. With the continuous support of nursing staff, a progressive activity schedule of self-care, baby care, and relaxation can be planned so as to support the well-being of mother and baby (see the accompanying Nursing Care Plan on preeclampsia-eclampsia).

NURSING CARE PLAN

Preeclampsia-Eclampsia

Patient Data Base

Nursing history

1. Complete assessment: patient and family
2. Identification of patient's predisposition to preeclampsia-eclampsia
   a. Primigravida
   b. Presence of diabetes mellitus
   c. Multiple pregnancy
   d. Polyhydramnios
   e. Hydatidiform mole
   f. Preexisting vascular or renal disease
   g. Adolescent or "elderly" gravida

Physical examination

1. Blood pressure – if possible compare with baseline
2. Observe for edema – note weight gain >1 kg/wk
3. Patient's weight – obtain weekly weight gain if possible
4. Evaluate for hyperreflexia
5. Assess presence of visual disturbances, headache, drowsiness, epigastric pain

Laboratory evaluation

1. Urine for urinary protein: 1 gm protein/24 hr = 1-2+; 5 gm protein/24 hr = 3-4+
2. Hematocrit: Elevation of hematocrit implies hemoconcentration, which occurs as fluid leaves the intravascular space and enters the extravascular space
3. BUN: Not usually elevated except in patients with cardiovascular renal disease
4. Blood uric acid appears to correlate well with the severity of the preeclampsia-eclampsia (Note: Thiazide diuretics can cause significant increases in uric acid levels)

Nursing Priorities

1. Carefully monitor patient's vital signs, urinary output, hyperreflexia.
2. Evaluate fetal status.
3. Provide support to patient and family.
4. Observe for signs of worsening condition:
   a. Increase in BP.
   b. Decrease in hourly urine output ≤30 ml/hr.
   c. Increased drowsiness.
   d. Increased hyperreflexia.
   e. Development of severe headache.
   f. Epigastric pain.
   g. Convulsion.

NURSING CARE PLAN Cont'd

Preeclampsia-Eclampsia

Problem	Nursing interventions and actions	Rationale
Water retention	Weigh patient daily.	Weight gain and evidence of edema are due to sodium and water retention.
	Assess edema (Danforth, 1977): + (1+) Minimal. Slight edema of pedal and pretibial areas. ++ (2+) Marked edema of lower extremities. +++ (3+) Edema of hands, face, lower abdominal wall, and sacrum. ++++ (4+) Anasarca with ascites.	Decreased renal plasma flow and glomerular filtration contribute to retention. The actual mechanisms are not clear.
	Maintain patient on bed rest.	Bed rest produces an increase in the glomerular filtration rate.
	Maintain normal salt intake (4-6 gm/24 hr).	Normal salt intake is now advised, but excessive salt intake may cause the condition to become more severe.
Hypertension	Assess BP every 1-4 hr.	Blood pressure can fluctuate hourly. Blood pressure increases as a result of increased peripheral resistance due to peripheral vasoconstriction and arteriolar spasm. Diastolic pressure is a better indicator of severity of condition.
Proteinuria	Obtain clean voided urine specimen.	Urine contaminated with vaginal discharge or red cells may test positive for protein.
	Test urine for proteinuria, hourly and/or daily.	Helps evaluate severity and progression of preeclampsia. Proteinuria results from swelling of the endothelium of the glomerular capillaries. Escape of protein is enhanced by vasospasm in afferent arterioles.
Decreased urine output	Insert indwelling catheter.	Catheter facilitates hourly urine assessment. Renal plasma flow and glomerular filtration are decreased.
	Determine hourly urine output. Notify physician if urine output ≤30 ml/hr.	Increasing oliguria signifies a worsening condition.
Inadequate protein intake	Provide adequate protein: 1.5 gm/kg/24 hr for incipient and mild preeclampsia. Patients with severe preeclampsia will be NPO ("nothing by mouth").	Plasma proteins affect movement of intravascular and extravascular fluids.
Hyperreflexia	Assess knee, ankle, and biceps reflexes (see Figure 13-4).	Assessing reflexes helps determine level of muscle and nerve irritability.
	Promote bed rest. Allow patient to rest quietly in a darkened, quiet room. Limit visitors.	Rest reduces external stimuli.
	Administer sedation as ordered (phenobarbital orally or IM).	Sedation is frequently ordered.
	Administer magnesium sulfate per physician order: 1. IM dose: 6-10 gm of 50% solution every 4-6 hours. 2. IV dose: 20 ml of 10% solution or as continuous infusion at a rate of 1 gm/hr.	Magnesium sulfate is cerebral depressant. It also reduces neuromuscular irritability and causes vasodilatation and drop in BP. Therapeutic blood level is 6-8 mg/100 ml.

NURSING CARE PLAN Cont'd

Preeclampsia-Eclampsia

Problem	Nursing interventions and actions	Rationale
	Before administering subsequent doses of magnesium sulfate, check reflexes (knee, ankle, biceps).	Knee jerk disappears when magnesium sulfate blood levels are >10 mg/100 ml. Toxic signs and symptoms develop with increased blood levels. Respiratory arrest can be associated with blood levels of 12-15 mg/100 ml.
	Check respirations and measure urine output. Do not give magnesium sulfate if: 1. Reflexes are absent. 2. Respirations are <16/min.	Cardiac arrest can occur if blood levels are 15 mg/100 ml.
	3. <100 ml urine output in past four hours.	Kidneys are only route for excretion of magnesium sulfate.
	Have calcium gluconate available.	Calcium gluconate is antidote for magnesium sulfate.
Convulsions	Provide supportive care during convulsion:	
	1. Place tongue blade or airway in patient's mouth.	Acts to maintain airway and to prevent patient from biting tongue.
	2. Suction nasopharynx as necessary.	Removes mucus and secretions.
	3. Administer oxygen.	Promotes oxygenation.
	4. Note type of seizure and length of time it lasts.	
	After seizure, assess for uterine contractions. Assess fetal status.	Precipitous labor may start during seizures. Continuous fetal monitoring is necessary to identify fetal stress.
	Maintain seizure precautions:	
	1. Quiet, darkened room.	Quiet reduces stimuli.
	2. Have emergency equipment available—O_2, suction, padded tongue blade.	
	3. Pad side rails.	Padding protects patient.
Increased fetal morbidity and mortality	Assess fetal status. Monitor FHTs every 4 hr if patient has mild eclampsia. Patient with severe preeclampsia-eclampsia requires continuous fetal monitoring.	Evaluates fetal status.
Increased risk of abruptio placentae	Assess for signs of abruptio placentae: 1. Vaginal bleeding. 2. Uterine tenderness. 3. Change in fetal activity. 4. Change in fetal heart rate. 5. Sustained abdominal pain.	40%-60% of women with abruptio placentae have preeclampsia. In patients with severe preeclampsia-eclampsia, abruption occurs in 10%-15% of the cases (Danforth, 1977).

Nursing Care Evaluation

Infant delivered.

Blood pressure within normal range.

Absence of protein in urine.

Symptoms of preeclampsia-eclampsia resolved or controlled.

Woman independent in activities of daily living.

Mother able to care for infant.

Mother understands and can verbalize course of condition, diet and medication instructions, infant care, and symptoms to report to physician (Davidson et al., 1977).

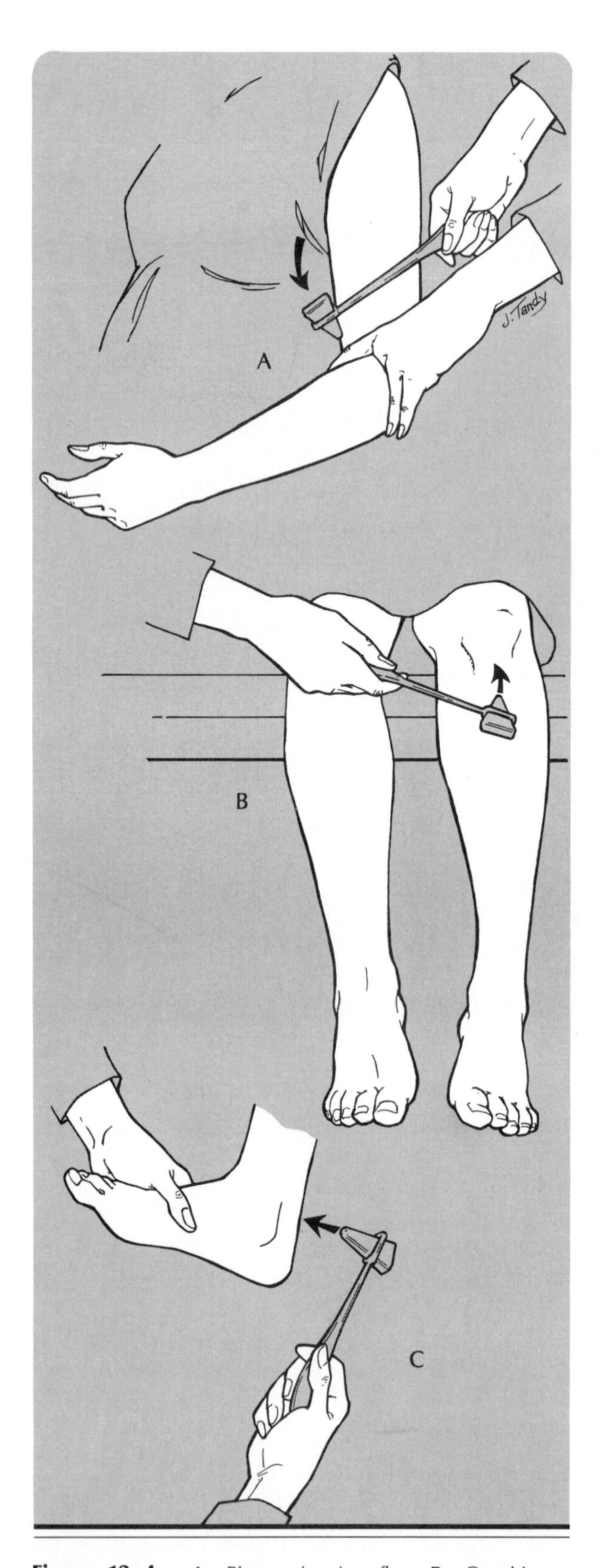

Figure 13–4. **A,** Biceps (arm) reflex. **B,** Quadriceps (knee) reflex. **C,** Achilles (ankle) reflex.

RH SENSITIZATION

As discussed in detail in Chapter 19, Rh sensitization results from an antigenic reaction within the body. Sensitization most commonly occurs when an Rh-negative woman carries an Rh-positive fetus, either to term or terminated by spontaneous or induced abortion. It can also occur if an Rh-negative nonpregnant woman receives an Rh-positive blood transfusion.

The red blood cells from the fetus invade the maternal circulation, thereby stimulating the production of Rh antibodies. Because this usually occurs at delivery, the first baby is not affected. However, in a subsequent pregnancy Rh antibodies cross the placenta and enter the fetal circulation, causing severe hemolysis. The destruction of fetal red blood cells causing anemia in the fetus is proportional to the extent of maternal sensitization.

Fetal-Neonatal Implications

If treatment is not initiated, the anemia resulting from this disorder can cause marked fetal edema, called *hydrops fetalis*. Congestive heart failure may result. This severe hemolytic syndrome is known as *erythroblastosis fetalis*. Hemolytic disease of the newborn is discussed in detail in Chapter 25.

Interventions

As a general part of the prenatal assessment of any pregnant woman, blood is drawn to determine type and Rh factor. In the prenatal history, the father's blood type and Rh factor are elicited. If the mother is Rh-negative, special effort should be made to determine whether sensitization has occurred.

For the Rh-sensitized woman, intensive prenatal care can promote a more positive outcome for the fetus. The severity of sensitization in the mother is assessed by antibody titers measured periodically. The best indicator of fetal well-being is amniotic fluid analysis to determine bilirubin level. Bilirubin is the breakdown product of hemolyzed blood, and the higher its level, the greater the degree of sensitization and the more severe the fetal anemia. Generally, this testing is begun at 26 weeks' gestation and is repeated at intervals until the fetus is ready for delivery. If the amount of bilirubin reaches a level indicating

Procedure 13–1. Intrauterine Transfusion
Intrauterine transfusion is done only between the 23rd and 32nd week of gestation. Amniocentesis is done 24 hours prior to admission, and radiopaque dye is instilled into the amniotic cavity.

Objective	Nursing action	Rationale
Prepare patient	Explain procedure.	
Maintain patient comfort	Administer medications as ordered: 1. Magnesium sulfate 10 mg. 2. Sodium phenobarbital 90 mg. 3. Promethazine 25 mg.	Promotes relaxation and decreases discomfort.
Prepare skin	Cleanse abdomen with 10-min Betadine scrub.	Decreases possibility of infection.
Transport	Transport patient to x-ray unit via stretcher.	Use of stretcher promotes patient comfort and helps maintain cleansed abdomen.
Locate fetal gastrointestinal system	Under sterile technique, physician inserts 17-gauge Touhy needle into fetal peritoneal cavity. Catheter is threaded through needle and needle is removed.	Television fluoroscopy is utilized to visualize peritoneal cavity.
	5–10 ml radiopaque dye is inserted.	Checks placement of catheter in peritoneal cavity.
Perform intrauterine transfusion	Fresh O Rh-negative blood is infused through catheter, and catheter is removed.	Infuse 50 ml in fetus of 24 weeks' gestation. Repeat every 7–10 days until a total of 350 ml is given or fetal maturity is assured.
Monitor vital signs	Assess BP every 10–15 min, pulse and respirations every 2–15 min. Assess FHT every 10–15 min with fetoscope or continuously if using electronic monitoring equipment.	Assists in identification of transfusion reactions or other problems.

serious risk to fetal well-being, the baby is delivered prematurely.

If the prognosis for extrauterine life is poor, intrauterine transfusion using Rh-negative blood cells can be done (see Procedure 13–1). This blood may be obtained from the mother or cross-matched to her blood. The intrauterine transfusion may be repeated every seven to ten days until a total of 350 ml is given or fetal maturity is assured. The procedure for transfusion involves localizing the placenta and passing a needle under fluoroscopic control through the abdominal wall and uterus of the mother and into the amniotic sac. The needle is then localized and the transfusion begun. At delivery, prompt and intensive neonatal care is essential (see Chapter 25). Further extrauterine transfusions may be done utilizing an umbilical vein.

Rh sensitization and the resultant hemolytic disease of the newborn are less common today because of the development of RhoGAM, an immunoglobulin. It is administered to an Rh-negative woman within 72 hours of delivery, abortion, or transfusion. RhoGAM acts to prevent antibody formation. Administration must be repeated after each subsequent delivery, abortion, or transfusion. RhoGAM is not effective for and should not be administered to a previously sensitized woman. Therefore, a woman should have a negative Coombs' test prior to its administration.

INFECTIONS

One of the major factors predisposing to risk in pregnancy is the presence of maternal infection, whether contracted prior to conception or during the gestational period. Frequently abortion is the result of a severe maternal infection. If the pregnancy is carried to term in the presence of infection, the risk of fetal and maternal morbidity and mortality increases. In many instances of fetal risk due to infection, the mother presents few or no signs or symptoms. Therefore, it is essential to maternal and fetal health that diagnosis and treatment be prompt. Therapy must be based on an awareness of possible fetal effects as well as a desire for maternal well-being.

Venereal Diseases

Venereal diseases are a group of infectious disorders contracted through intimate sexual contact, oral or genital, with another person. The most common venereal diseases, syphilis and gonorrhea, are described in this section. Herpes simplex, caused by herpesvirus type 2, can also be acquired by sexual intercourse. This disease is discussed in the section on TORCH (p. 373).

Syphilis

Syphilis is a chronic infection caused by a spirochete, *Treponema pallidum.* Syphilis can be acquired congenitally through transplacental inoculation, resulting from maternal exposure to infected exudate during sexual contact, or from contact with open wounds or infected blood. The incubation period is 10–60 days, and even though no symptoms or lesions are noted during this time, the patient's blood contains spirochetes and is infective.

Syphilis is divided into early and late stages. During the early stage (primary), a chancre appears at the site where the *Treponema pallidum* organism entered the body. Symptoms include slight fever, loss of weight, and malaise. The chancre persists for about four weeks and then disappears. In six weeks to six months, secondary symptoms appear. Skin eruptions called *condylomata,* which resemble wartlike plaques, may appear on the vulva. Other secondary symptoms are acute arthritis, enlargement of the liver and spleen, iritis, and a chronic sore throat with hoarseness. When infected in utero, the newborn will exhibit secondary stage symptoms of syphilis.

The incidence of syphilis declined after discovery of penicillin, but since 1958 the incidence has been increasing. As a result of the increased incidence and the significant morbidity and mortality to the fetus in utero that this disease causes, serologic testing of every pregnant woman is recommended, and required by some state laws, at initial prenatal screening and is repeated in the third trimester. (See the prenatal physical examination in Chapter 10.) If syphilis is detected in the pregnant patient, adequate treatment with penicillin or erythromycin must be instituted immediately. Because the placenta provides a barrier to *Treponema pallidum* until the 18th week of gestation, adequate treatment before the 18th week prevents the development of congenital syphilis.

Fetal-Neonatal Implications

One of the following outcomes can occur in the presence of untreated maternal syphilis: (a) a late abortion at any time after the fourth month of pregnancy, (b) a stillborn infant at term, (c) a congenitally infected infant born prematurely or at term, or (d) an uninfected live infant (Burrows and Fettis, 1976). The clinical manifestations and treatment of the syphilitic newborn are discussed in Chapter 25.

Interventions

If testing of maternal serum is positive, treatment should be started immediately. It has been demonstrated that, in pregnancies treated prior to the 18th week of gestation, the likelihood of fetal infection is diminished. The prescribed treatment for syphilis is antibiotic therapy. Treatment of the mother later in pregnancy also treats the infected fetus because penicillin crosses the placenta.

For women with syphilis of less than one year duration, 2.4 million units of benzathine penicillin G intramuscularly or 4.8 million units of procaine penicillin G are divided into three doses given three days apart. If syphilis is of long (more than one year) duration, these drugs are given but in total dosages of 6 million to 9 million units given intramuscularly in divided doses. Should the woman be allergic to penicillin, erythromycin can be given. Maternal serologic testing may remain positive for eight months, and the newborn may have a positive test for three months.

Gonorrhea

Gonorrhea is an infection caused by the bacteria *Neisseria gonorrhoeae*. The expectant woman can be screened for this infection during her prenatal examination by means of a cervical culture. A chronic infection is usually found in the urethra, Skene's and Bartholin's glands, and the cervix. The infection generally remains localized to those areas until rupture of the membranes, at which time it can spread upward, causing endometritis, salpingitis, oophoritis, and pelvic peritonitis.

In acute gonorrheal infections in a gravid woman, the vulvar area and urethra are acutely inflamed. The discharge from the vagina is greenish yellow, and her vulva may be covered with a grayish exudate or condylomata. The cervix is often swollen and eroded and may secrete a foul-smelling discharge in which the gonococci are present.

Fetal-Neonatal Implications

If untreated, morbidity in the fetus and neonate can result from ascending infectious gonorrhea during prolonged rupture of membranes or as a result of a vaginal delivery through an infected birth canal. The fetus is also at risk for prematurity because an acute gonorrheal infection predisposes to premature labor. For the fetus who is delivered through an infected birth canal, the result is a gonococcal eye infection known as *ophthalmia neonatorum.* Infections of the stomach, external ear canal, oropharynx, and anus can also occur. See Chapter 25 for further discussion on gonorrheal infection of the newborn and its treatment.

Interventions

Therapy consists of antibiotic treatment with aqueous procaine penicillin G given intramuscularly to the infected woman. A total dosage of 4.8 million units is administered, with 2.4 million units injected into each buttock. If the patient is allergic to penicillin, kanamycin or erythromycin may be utilized. Additional treatment using twice the initial dose may be required if the cultures remain positive.

If the woman has a positive culture at the time of labor, a cesarean section should be done to decrease the chances of the fetus contracting the infection in the birth canal.

Vaginal Infections

Monilial (Yeast) Infection

Monilial vaginitis is caused by the fungus *Candida albicans,* which normally is found in the intestinal tract. It can, however, invade the vagina, causing infection. Monilial infection is seen at term in women with poorly controlled diabetes (the organism thrives in a carbohydrate-rich environment) and in those on antibiotic or steroid therapy (these drugs reduce the numbers of Döderlein's bacilli, which are normally present flora). Diagnosis is made on the basis of a speculum exam, which reveals thick, white, tenacious cheeselike patches adhering to the pale, dry, and sometimes bluish vaginal mucosa. Additional symptoms include thick vaginal discharge, itching, dysuria, and dyspareunia.

Fetal-Neonatal Implications

If the infection is not cured prior to delivery, the fetus will contract thrush by direct contact with the organism in the birth canal. The infection can also be contracted from contaminated hands, feeding equipment or breast, and bedding. Therefore, scrupulous cleanliness must be maintained. In most cases, the neonate does not display severe discomfort; however, some newborns have demonstrated difficulty in swallowing. Care of the neonate who has contracted this infection is discussed in Chapter 25.

Interventions

Treatment for monilial vaginitis is the same as for simple vaginitis and involves the following nursing, medical, and self-care actions:

1. Explanation of proper wiping technique (front to back) following elimination.
2. Prescription of drug therapy.
   a. Application of gentian violet (2%) swabs to vaginal mucosa with applicator every two to three days until infection is eliminated (patient should wear perineal pad to safeguard clothing from stains).
   b. Insertion of nystatin (Mycostatin) vaginal tablets (100,000 units twice daily for 14 days) or suppositories (0.5 gm twice daily for 10 days).
3. Abstention of patient from intercourse until infection is cured.
4. Local application of K-Y jelly or gentle bathing of vulva with weak sodium bicarbonate solution to relieve discomfort of pruritus.

Trichomonas Infections

The organism *Trichomonas vaginalis* causes a type of vaginitis. Symptoms include foamy leukorrhea, itching and irritation of the vulva, dyspareunia, and urinary frequency and dysuria. Previously, treatment consisted of metronidazole (Flagyl), which was administered orally three times a day for seven days. However, current research has identified Flagyl as a teratogenic drug that is not recommended for use during pregnancy (Pritchard and MacDonald, 1976).

TORCH

The following group of infections is identified as TORCH: toxoplasmosis *(TO)*, rubella *(R)*, cytomegalovirus *(C)*, and herpesvirus type 2 *(H)*. The effects on the fetus of a mother who is infected with these organisms are severe. The TORCH identification assists health team members to quickly assess the potential risk to each woman in pregnancy.

The importance of understanding what these infections are and identifying risk factors cannot be overemphasized—not only in light of maternal morbidity and mortality but also because of the serious effects on the fetus when the infection crosses the placenta. Exposure of the mother during the first 12 weeks of gestation may cause developmental anomalies. The three major viral infections are caused by rubella, cytomegalovirus, and herpesvirus type 2. Toxoplasmosis is a protozoal infection.

Toxoplasmosis

Toxoplasmosis is caused by the protozoan *Toxoplasma gondii.* It is innocuous in adults, but when contracted in pregnancy, it is transmitted to the fetus in half the cases (Danforth, 1977). The pregnant woman may contract the organism by eating raw or poorly cooked meat or by contact with the feces of infected animals. In the United States the most common carrier is the cat, which transmits the infection by way of its feces. It is therefore strongly recommended that pregnant women avoid cat litter boxes.

The incubation period for the disease is ten days. The mother with toxoplasmosis may be asymptomatic, or she may develop myalgia, malaise, rash, splenomegaly, and posterior cervical lymphadenopathy. Symptoms usually disappear in a few days or weeks. Diagnosis can be made by doing serologic tests, such as the Sabin-Feldman dye test. If diagnosis can be established by physical findings, history, and positive serologic results, the mother may be treated with sulfadiazine and pyrimethamine, which are administered for one month. If toxoplasmosis is diagnosed before the 20th week of gestation, therapeutic abortion should be considered.

The incidence of abortion, stillbirths, and severe congenital anomalies is increased in the affected fetus and neonate. Severe neonatal disorders associated with congenital infection are fever and neurologic abnormalities such as convulsions, coma, hypotonia, microcephaly, or hydrocephalus. Other conditions seen in the infant are chorioretinitis, ecchymosis, hepatosplenomegaly, intracranial calcifications, jaundice, microphthalmia, and pallor (anemia).

Rubella

The effects of rubella are no more severe, nor are there greater complications, in pregnant women than in nonpregnant women of comparable age. But the effects of this infection on the fetus and neonate are great, because rubella causes a chronic infection that begins in the first trimester of pregnancy and may persist for months after birth.

Estimates say that approximately 10%–20% of all pregnant women are susceptible to rubella. The only accurate method of screening is by performing a serology test, the test for hemagglutination inhibition (HAI). The presence of a 1:16 HAI titer or greater is evidence of immunity. A titer less than 1:8 indicates susceptibility, and repeat testing should be done to determine later infection. A fourfold rise in serum HAI titer or a high value initially indicates recent infection and the possibility of damage to the fetus.

Fetal-Neonatal Implications

The period of greatest risk for the teratogenic effects of rubella on the fetus is during the first trimester. If infection occurs between the third and seventh week of pregnancy, damage usually results in death. In the second month, 25% of affected fetuses may have serious defects, and if infection occurs in the third month, 15% of fetuses are affected. If infection occurs early in the second trimester, the resultant fetal effect is most often permanent hearing impairment.

Clinical signs of congenital infection are congenital heart disease, intrauterine growth retardation, and cataracts. Cardiac involvements most often seen are patent ductus arteriosis and narrowing of peripheral pulmonary arteries. Cataracts may be unilateral or bilateral and may be present at birth or develop in the neonatal period. A petechial rash is seen in some infants, and hepatosplenomegaly and hyperbilirubinemia are frequently seen. Other abnormalities may become evident in infancy, such as mental retardation or cerebral palsy. Diagnosis in the neonate can be conclusively made in the presence of these conditions and with an elevated rubella IgM antibody titer at birth.

Frequently, in mothers who had rubella during pregnancy, an infant is born with active viral infection. This is called the *extended rubella syndrome.* It is typified by one or more of the following disorders: cardiac maldevelopment, encephalitis, hepatosplenomegaly, jaundice, ocular abnormalities, pneumonitis, and thrombocytopenia or purpura. A tendency toward the development of leukemia in childhood has been noted. Thus, infected babies often die early in infancy. Others survive longer, and isolation of babies with active viral infection is mandatory; the active rubella has been cultured for as long as one to one and a half years after birth. Treatment involves penicillin by injection or, if sensitivity is suspected, erythromycin or tetracycline may be given.

Interventions

The best therapy for rubella is prevention. All women of childbearing age should be vaccinated, but only when pregnancy is not established or suspected. If a woman who is pregnant becomes infected during the first trimester, therapeutic abortion is an alternative. Nursing support and understanding are vital at this time because such a decision may initiate a crisis for a couple who have planned for this pregnancy. They need objective data to understand the possible effects on their unborn fetus and what the prognosis is for this child.

Cytomegalovirus

Cytomegalovirus (CMV) belongs to the herpesvirus group and causes both congenital and acquired infections referred to as *cytomegalic inclusion disease* (CID). The significance of this virus in pregnancy is related to its ability to be transmitted by asymptomatic mothers across the placenta or by the cervical route.

Accurate diagnosis in the pregnant woman depends on the presence of CMV in the urine, a rise in IgM levels, and identification of the CMV antibodies within the serum IgM fraction. At present, none of the antiviral drugs has been effective in preventing CMV or in treating the congenital disease in the neonate.

For the fetus, this infection can result in extensive intrauterine tissue damage that is incompatible with life, in survival with brain damage, or in survival with no damage at all.

The infected neonate is often SGA and hypoplastic. The principal tissues and organs affected are the blood, brain, and liver. However, virtually all organs are potentially at risk. Hemolysis leads to anemia and hyperbilirubinemia. Thrombocytopenia, with subsequent petechiae and ecchymosis, often occurs. Another commonly seen effect is hepatosplenomegaly. Encephalitis, with signs ranging from lethargy to hypoactivity and convulsions, may occur. Microcephaly may be present at delivery, and chorioretinitis is apparent in 10%–20% of infants displaying symptoms of CMV.

Herpesvirus Type 2

Herpesvirus type 2, which causes the disease herpes simplex, affects the cervix, vagina, and external genitals and can be transmitted through sexual contact. Herpesvirus type 1 is responsible for lip lesions (cold sores) and skin lesions, which are usually found above the umbilicus. The incubation period is two to seven days after exposure. Primary lesions of herpesvirus type 2 (herpes genitalis) consist of multiple vesicles involving the vulva, vagina, and cervix. Couples engaging in oral sex may develop herpesvirus type 2 lesions of the lips and mouth. The lesions easily become infected with other bacteria. Additional symptoms include enlarged regional lymph nodes, fever, and malaise. Diagnosis is made by cytologic examination and evaluation of patient's serum for complement-fixing antibodies (Danforth, 1977).

Herpes simplex can be transmitted to the fetus in retrograde fashion, vaginally to the intrauterine cavity, or it can be contracted during the descent of the fetus down the birth canal. The transplacental infection route is rare.

Fetal-Neonatal Implications

The herpesvirus type 2 is responsible for about 95% of neonatal infections. In the systemic variety of herpesvirus infection, perinatal mortality is approximately 96%. The infection involves the adrenals, blood, brain, liver, and lungs.

In the nonsystemic varieties of herpesvirus infection, neonatal mortality is less severe, about 25%. Involvement occurs in the central nervous system, eyes, and skin. Of those who survive, about half have neurologic or visual abnormalities.

Interventions

Treatment is directed first toward relieving vulvar pain. Bacterial infections may be treated with cream containing sulfonamide. When herpesvirus type 2 is suspected in the pregnant woman, amniocentesis can be performed to determine if there is fetal involvement. The amniotic fluid is tested for the presence of herpesvirus antibodies. If they are present, a cesarean section should not be performed; the presumably infected fetus should be delivered vaginally. If no infection is present on amniotic fluid analysis, a cesarean section is indicated to protect the fetus from possible infection from the birth canal.

DRUG USE AND ABUSE

Indiscriminate drug use during pregnancy, particularly in the first trimester, may adversely affect the normal growth and development of the fetus. Originally it was thought that the placenta acted as a protective barrier to keep the drugs ingested by the mother from reaching the fetal system. This is not true. The degree to which a drug is passed to the fetus depends on the chemical properties of the drug, including molecular weight, and on whether it is administered alone or in combination with other drugs.

Drugs affecting fetal growth are called *teratogens.* They act on the developing organs to retard growth at crucial stages of organogenesis during the first trimester. Other drugs ingested by the expectant woman at other times during the pregnancy may negatively influence the well-being of the fetus as well as produce critical problems in the neonate. Table 13–3 identifies major drugs and their effects on the fetus and neonate.

When pharmacologic agents are prescribed for a pregnant woman, their possible effects on the fetus must be weighed against the need of the patient. She should be cautioned regarding overuse of the drug and should be warned not to take any prescription or nonprescription drugs without first consulting the prenatal health care team. Drugs such as folic acid and vitamins, which are commonly prescribed in pregnancy, can be started after the crucial period of organ development.

Drugs that are commonly misused include alcohol, amphetamines, barbiturates, hallucinogens, and heroin and other narcotics. Abuse of these drugs constitutes a major threat to the successful completion of pregnancy.

Drug Addiction

Maternal Implications

Drug addiction has an adverse effect on the expectant woman. It affects her state of health, nutritional status, susceptibility to infection, and psychosocial condition. A majority of drug-abusing pregnant women are malnourished and receive little or no antepartal care. In addition, the risk of drug toxicity is present. In general, her psychologic and physiologic ability to handle the stress of pregnancy is severely reduced.

Fetal-Neonatal Implications

The fetus of a pregnant addict is at risk in the following ways:

1. The drug may cause chromosomal aberrations or may have a teratogenic effect on the fetus, resulting in congenital anomalies such as limb abnormalities.
2. The drug may induce physiologic and psychologic changes in the pregnant woman, resulting in placental dysfunction or fetal hypoxia or depression.

Table 13–3. Possible Effects of Selected Drugs on Fetus and Neonate*

Maternal drug	Effect on fetus and neonate	Maternal drug	Effect on fetus and neonate
Alcohol	Cardiac anomalies,	Tolbutamide (Orinase)	Teratogenic effect
	growth retardation,	Hematologic agents	
	potential teratogenic	Vitamin K (excessive)	Hyperbilirubinemia
	effect	Coumarin derivatives	Fetal hemorrhage, death
Antibiotics		Sedatives-tranquilizers	
Amphotericin B	Multiple anomalies,	Methadone	Severe withdrawal
(Fungizone)	abortion		symptoms
Tetracycline	Inhibition of bone growth	Narcotics	Withdrawal symptoms,
	in prematures, staining		convulsions, death
	of deciduous teeth	Phenobarbital	
Chemotherapeutic agents		(excessive)	Bleeding
Amethopterin		Phenothiazine	Hyperbilirubinemia
(methotrexate)	Anomalies, retardation	Promethazine	
Aminopterin	Anomalies, retardation	(Phenergan)	Decreased platelet count
Chlorambucil		Stimulants-hallucinogens	
(Leukeran)	Anomalies, retardation	Dextroamphetamine	Congenital heart defects,
Cyclophosphamide			hyperbilirubinemia
(Cytoxan)	Anomalies	LSD	Teratogenic effects,
Mitomycin C			chromosomal damage,
(Mutamycin)	Anomalies, abortion		IUGR
Endocrine agents		Tobacco (nicotine)	IUGR
Androgens	Masculinization	Others	
Estrogens	Feminization, late-onset	Drugs to control	Low level of coagulation
	malignancy in females	epilepsy	factors II, VII, IX, X
Iodine	Congenital	Quinine	Deafness,
	hypothyroidism		thrombocytopenia
Methimazole		Salicylate (excessive)	Bleeding
(Tapazole)	Goiter, mental retardation		
Progestins, oral	Masculinization,		
	advanced bone age		

*Modified from Overbach, A. M. 1974. Drugs used with neonates and during pregnancy. III. Drugs that may cause fetal damage or cross into breast milk. *RN.* 37(12):39.

3. Taking a mixture of drugs may lead to maternal death and thus fetal death.

The effects of drug abuse on the neonate are severe and include withdrawal behaviors, congenital malformations, and prematurity. The withdrawal syndrome is seen shortly after birth in the addicted infant and includes tremors, agitation, sweating, and seizures. With heroin-addicted and methadone-maintained mothers, the level of drug abuse directly correlates with the severity of withdrawal behavior in the infant. Generally, methadone withdrawal is less severe. Barbiturates also cause a withdrawal syndrome in the neonate. The hallucinogens, such as LSD, are frequently taken in combination with other drugs, so it is difficult to determine the causative agents in many of the neonatal anomalies.

Interventions

Antepartal care of the pregnant addict involves medical, socioeconomic, and legal considerations. The use of a team approach allows for the comprehensive management necessary to provide safe labor and delivery for mother and fetus. The essential components of care include the following:

1. Assess the patient's general health status, with specific attention to skin abscesses and infections, as well as evaluation of other body systems.
2. Assess the patient's obstetric condition. Determine whether venereal disease (syphilis or gonorrhea) is present. Estimate the length of gestation and approximate fetal size.
3. Assess drug use as to type and amount through urine testing. Patients are often unaware of actual amounts.
4. The management of heroin addiction includes the use of methadone, the current agent of choice in the treatment or prevention of withdrawal symptoms. Hospitalization is necessary to initiate detoxification. Maintenance and support therapy are given during weekly prenatal visits.

Preparation for labor and delivery should be a part of the prenatal planning. Analgesic use should be avoided if possible, although it is not necessarily contraindicated. Relief of fear, tension, or discomfort may be achieved through nonnarcotic psychologic support and careful explanation of the labor process. Preferred methods of pain relief include the use of psychoprophylaxis and regional or local anesthetics such as pudendal block and local infiltration. These techniques are preferred to decrease further risk of additional fetal respiratory depression. Immediate intensive care should be available for the newborn who will probably be depressed, SGA, and premature. For care of the addicted newborn, see Chapter 24.

Alcoholism

Maternal Implications

Chronic abuse of alcohol can undermine maternal health by causing malnutrition, especially folic acid deficiency, bone marrow suppression, infections, and liver disease. As a result of this alcohol dependency, withdrawal seizures may occur in the intrapartal period as early as 12 to 48 hours after cessation of drinking. Delirium tremens may occur in the postpartal period, and the neonate may suffer a withdrawal syndrome.

Fetal-Neonatal Implications

The offspring of a chronic alcoholic may exhibit intrauterine and extrauterine growth and developmental retardation, which can be evaluated in the infant with the use of such assessment tools as the Gesell evaluation and the Denver Developmental Screening Test. Infants of these mothers are also at risk for anomalies of the heart, head, face, and extremities.

Interventions

It is important that the nursing staff be aware of the manifestations of alcohol abuse so that preparations for expected needs can be made. The care regimen includes sedation to decrease irritability and tremors, seizure precautions, intravenous fluid therapy for hydration, and preparation for an addicted neonate. Although high doses of sedation and analgesics may be necessary for the mother, caution is advised because these can cause fetal depression.

SUMMARY

The diagnosis of high-risk pregnancy can be a shock to an expectant couple. The stress involved may lead to crisis unless appropriate nursing interventions are initiated.

A period of self-questioning follows the shock, during which the couple ask, "Did we make the right decision?" and "Have we done everything we should have to ensure a healthy pregnancy?" The self-doubt and guilt is even more pronounced if the pregnancy is unplanned. In this situation, the couple may think they are being punished for not initially wanting the pregnancy. Nursing care should be planned individually and in depth, depending on each couple's specific needs. The nursing assessment should include delineation of the factors that identify couples as high risk, identification of their level of understanding related to the specific disruption, evaluation of coping mechanisms utilized by the couple, and an awareness of the questions they need answered.

The most crucial aspect of care will be the development of the nurse-patient/family relationship. The trust and rapport that are established will be the supportive structure on which care is based. Specific nursing interventions include teaching and guidance related to necessary treatment and procedures; encouragement of communication among the couple, physician, and nurse; and support of the pregnant patient's self-esteem and body image. In addition, the nurse must support the physiologic function of the maternal-fetal unit as effectively as possible. Through these caring efforts, it is hoped that the high-risk pregnancy will result in a physiologically and psychologically healthy mother and child.

SUGGESTED ACTIVITIES

1. Make arrangements with your instructor to attend a high-risk prenatal clinic. Observe the assessments made, care given, and teaching provided.
2. In a small group, explore your feelings and reactions to a hypothetical situation in which you are three months pregnant with your first child and have just learned that you have recently been exposed to rubella.

REFERENCES

Burrows, G. N., and Fettis, G. F. 1976. *Medical complications during pregnancy.* Philadelphia: W. B. Saunders Co.

Clark, A. L., and Affonso, D. D. 1976. *Childbearing: a nursing perspective.* Philadelphia: F. A. Davis Co.

Criteria Committee of the New York Heart Association, Inc. 1955. *Nomenclature and criteria for diagnosis of diseases of the heart and blood vessels.* 5th ed. New York: The Association.

Davidson, S. V., et al. 1977. *Nursing care evaluation.* St. Louis: The C. V. Mosby Co.

Danforth, D. N., ed. 1977. *Obstetrics and gynecology.* 3rd ed. Hagerstown, Md.: Harper & Row Publishers, Inc.

Haynes, D. 1969. *Medical complications during pregnancy.* New York: McGraw-Hill Book Co.

Hellman, L. M., and Pritchard, J. A. 1971. *Williams obstetrics.* 14th ed. New York: Appleton-Century-Crofts.

Hughes, E. C., ed. 1972. Obstetric-gynecologic terminology. Prepared by the Committee on Terminology of the American College of Obstetricians and Gynecologists. Philadelphia: F. A. Davis Co.

Jensen, M. D., et al. 1977. *Maternity care: the nurse and the family.* St. Louis: The C. V. Mosby Co.

Messer, J. V. 1973. Heart disease in pregnancy. *J. Reprod. Med.* 10:102.

Overbach, A. M. Dec. 1974. Drugs used with neonates and during pregnancy. III. Drugs that may cause fetal damage or cross into breast milk. *RN.* 37(12):39.

Pritchard, J. A., and MacDonald, P. 1976. *Williams obstetrics.* 15th ed. New York: Appleton-Century-Crofts.

Roth, D. 1962. The stale egg concept in spontaneous abortion. *Obstet. Gynecol.* 14:411.

White, P. 1965. Pregnancy and diabetes: medical aspects. *Med. Clin. N. Am.* 49:1016.

Williams, R. H. 1974. *Textbook of endocrinology.* 5th ed. Philadelphia: W. B. Saunders Co.

ADDITIONAL READINGS

Clausen, J. P., et al. 1973. *Maternity nursing today.* New York: McGraw-Hill Book Co.

Feldman, H. A. 1976. Viral infections in pregnancy. Paper presented at the Second Memorial Ignatz Semmelweis Seminar, Cherry Hill, N.J.

Galloway, K. G. 1976. Placental evaluation studies: the procedures, their purposes, and the nursing care involved. *MCN.* 2:300.

Golditch, I., and Boyce, N. E. 1970. Management of abruptio placentae. *JAMA.* 212:288.

Hanson, J. W., et al. 1976. Fetal alcohol syndrome. *JAMA.* 235:1458.

Jasper, M. L. 1976. Pregnancy complicated by diabetes—a case study. *MCN.* 2:307.

Jones, M. B. 1975. Antepartum assessment in high-risk pregnancy. *J. Obstet. Gynecol. Neonatal Nurs.* 4:23.

Kieval, J. 1975. Gestational diabetes: diagnosis and management. *J. Reprod. Med.* 14:70.

Korones, S. B. 1976. *High risk newborn infants: the basis for intensive care nursing.* St. Louis: The C. V. Mosby Co.

Ledger, W. J. 1976. Antibiotic treatment of perinatal infections. Paper presented at the Second Memorial Ignatz Semmelweis Seminar. Cherry Hill, N.J.

Liley, A. W. 1976. The management of the Rh sensitized pregnancy. Paper presented at the Second Memorial Ignatz Semmelweis Seminar. Cherry Hill, N.J.

Luke, B. 1977. Maternal alcoholism and fetal alcohol syndrome. *Am. J. Nurs.* 77:1924.

Marlow, D. R. 1977. *Textbook of pediatric nursing.* 5th ed. Philadelphia: W. B. Saunders Co.

Nolan, G. H. 1974. Exclusive review. In *Ross timesaver: ob world and gynecology,* vol. 3. Columbus, Ohio: Ross Laboratories.

Schuler, K. 1979. When a pregnant woman is diabetic: antepartal care. *Am. J. Nurs.* 79:448.

Tichy, A. M., and Chong, D. March–April 1979. Placental function and its role in toxemia. *MCN.* 4:84.

Tyson, J. E., and Hock, R. A. 1976. Gestational and pregestational diabetes: an approach to therapy. *Am. J. Obstet. Gynecol.* 125:1009.

Walters, T. R. 1976. Changing presentation of maternal-infant blood group incompatability. Paper presented at the Second Memorial Ignatz Semmelweis Seminar. Cherry Hill, N.J.

CHAPTER 14

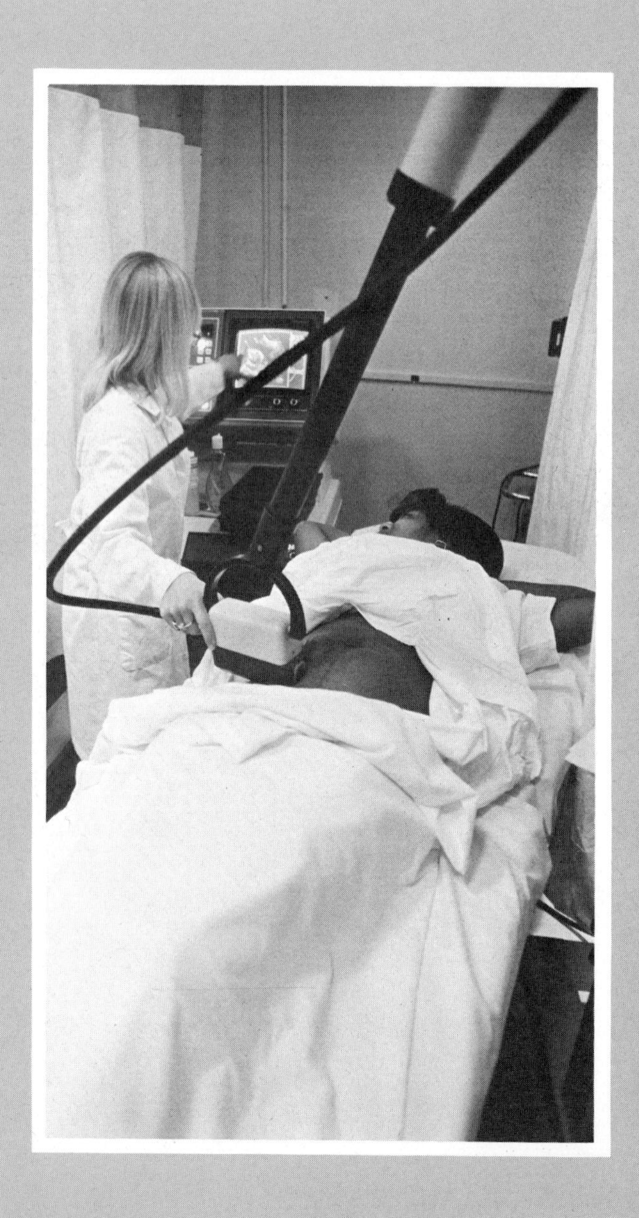

DIAGNOSTIC ASSESSMENT OF FETAL STATUS

AMNIOTIC FLUID ANALYSIS

Clinical Application

Amniocentesis

Types of Amniotic Fluid Tests

AMNIOSCOPY

X-RAY EXAMINATION

IMPLICATIONS OF PRENATAL TESTING FOR DELIVERY

OBJECTIVES

- Discuss noninvasive methods of assessing fetal status.
- Describe the oxytocin challenge test, its use, and interpretation.
- Discuss the method of obtaining estriol determinations and the implications of estriol levels.
- Discuss different aspects of amniotic fluid analysis.

During the past 15 to 20 years, an increasing amount of interest has been focused on the problems of the high-risk pregnant woman, her management, and conditions that might affect her unborn child, because at-risk women and infants have a significantly greater chance of morbidity or mortality before or after delivery. Prematurity, congenital anomalies, mental retardation, cerebral palsy, and other conditions seem to be associated with the presence of certain factors during pregnancy or during delivery. Perinatal morbidity and mortality can be considerably reduced by early skillful diagnosis and appropriate, thorough, and highly intensive antepartal care of the pregnant woman. Thus, health care professionals are beginning to concentrate their efforts on identifying women who are at greater risk for developing problems that may affect their well-being and that of the fetus.

In an attempt to reduce perinatal mortality and morbidity, the field of perinatology has evolved. During the past decade, much knowledge has been acquired concerning the intrauterine environment of the fetus. Physicians, nurses, ultrasonographers, dieticians, social workers, and neonatologists are combining their efforts and expertise to contribute to the growing amount of information about the development of the fetus and the kinds of insult to which the fetus is susceptible.

A variety of tests of placental function and fetal well-being are of value in monitoring the health status of the fetus. These tests include diagnostic ultrasound, measurements of specific hormones and enzymes in maternal plasma and urine, amniocentesis for lung maturity studies, amnioscopy, and fetal stress tests (including the oxytocin challenge test). There is always some risk with each procedure, so fetal morbidity and mortality should be considered before a particular procedure is done. Certainly not all high-risk patients require the same procedures. One must be certain that the advantages outweigh potential risks and added expense. Each of these tests has its limitations in terms of diagnostic accuracy and applicability. No one test should be used to determine fetal status in the management of the high-risk mother, but rather these tests should be used as adjuncts to good clinical judgment by the health care team.

Women who are considered to be at high risk and for whom the physician may order tests of placental function, fetal maturity, or fetal well-being include older primigravidas and patients with chronic hypertension, preeclampsia, diabetes mellitus, pregnancy beyond 42 weeks' gestation, Rh isoimmunization, previous unexplained stillborn or intrapartal loss, sickle cell hemoglobinopathies, suspected IUGR, maternal cyanotic heart disease, or other medical complications. (See Chapter 10 for further discussion of high-risk cases and Chapter 13 for descriptions of various conditions that may threaten the successful termination of pregnancy.)

ULTRASOUND

Valuable information concerning the fetus may be obtained from *pulsed-echo ultrasound.* Intermittent sound waves of extremely high frequency can be transmitted by means of an alternating current to a transducer, which is applied to the maternal abdomen. Ultrasonic sound waves are reflected off tissues of varying densities, and echoes return to the crystal and are changed to electrical signals. These signals are amplified and displayed on an oscilloscope in one of three ways:

1. *A-mode (amplitude mode).* Distance can be measured by deflections of the A-mode. These are shown as spikes on an oscilloscope (Figure 14–1,*A*). The sonographer can measure the exact distance to where the echo is being produced.

2. *B-mode (brightness mode).* Echoes appear as dots, producing a two-dimensional picture that can be photographed or simply visualized on the oscilloscope. This is the method most often used. Gray scale is a refinement of B-mode scanning. Different amplitudes are shown as different levels of brightness. The ability to distinguish internal structures and their various densities or textures is the real advantage of this type of scanning. Instead of just one type of echo, the sonographer can visualize many different levels of density and thereby detect internal structural differences. The picture looks much like that on the screen of a black-and-white television (Figure 14–1,*B*).

3. *M-mode (motion mode or real-time scanning).* By

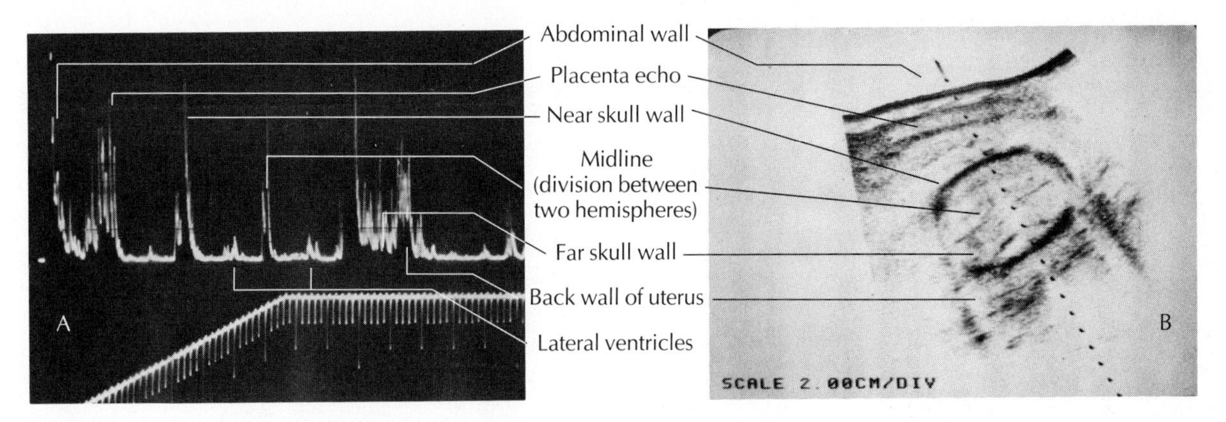

Figure 14–1. Two methods of obtaining information about the fetus. Both scans are of the same fetus and were taken at the same time. The fetus is 24 weeks' gestation. **A,** A-mode. Echo bounces off structures and is recorded as a spike. **B,** B-mode. The abdominal wall, internal structures, and fetal head can be visualized. The lateral ventricles cannot be visualized in the B-mode.

this method, one can demonstrate movements of the fetus, heart valve motion, thumb sucking, fetal hiccups, and fetal breathing. Evaluation of biparietal diameter and location of the placenta or a pocket of amniotic fluid may also be done.

Advantages of diagnostic ultrasound are that it is noninvasive and painless to the patient, the physician can serially study a patient, it is nonradiating to both mother and fetus with no known harmful effects to either, differentiation of soft tissue masses is possible, and immediate information may be gained from its use.

Procedure

Except for the instance of localizing the placenta for amniocentesis, the patient is scanned with a full bladder. This enables the sonographer to assess other structures in relation to the bladder and in particular to determine the relationship of the vagina to the bladder. This is particularly important in the case of vaginal bleeding in which a placenta previa is suspected. The cervical internal os is halfway between the sacral promontory and the base of the bladder. If the lower part of the placenta extends to the internal os, placenta previa is diagnosed. If the lower uterine segment cannot be visualized, the degree of previa cannot be ascertained.

A sonogram requires between 20 and 30 minutes and is uncomfortable to the patient only to the extent that she must lie flat on her back, a position most unphysiologic and uncomfortable for a pregnant woman. Some women, particularly those near term with a large fetus, develop supine hypotension and experience nausea, vertigo, and lightheadedness due to pressure of the gravid uterus on the abdominal aorta and inferior vena cava. This discomfort can be relieved by elevating the feet and turning the body to the lateral recumbent position. Mineral oil is generously spread over the maternal abdomen, and the sonographer slowly scans with a transducer longitudinally and transversely in sections across the abdomen to gain an entire picture of the contents of the uterus. Results are usually immediately available, but unless the physician is at hand, information may be withheld from the patient until the report can be sent to her physician for interpretation.

Clinical Application

B-mode scanning is valuable for monitoring pregnancy in a variety of ways, including the following:

1. Early identification of pregnancy.
2. Identification of multiple fetuses (Figure 14-3).
3. Measurement of the biparietal diameter of the fetal head to date pregnancy or to help identify IUGR (Figure 14-4).
4. Detection of such fetal anomalies as hydrocephaly (Figure 14-5), microcephaly, anencephaly, ascites, myelomeningocele, and polycystic kidneys.
5. Detection of polyhydramnios (Figure 14-6) or oligohydramnios.

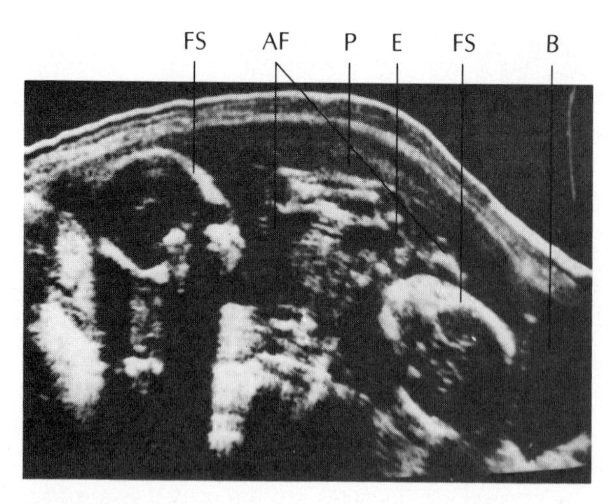

Figure 14–2. Gray scale. Longitudinal scan demonstrating twin gestation, anterior placenta, fetal extremity. Both BPDs are at approximately 25–26 weeks' gestation. (AF = amniotic fluid; FS = fetal skull; E = extremity; B = mother's urinary bladder; P = placenta.) (Courtesy Section of Diagnostic Ultrasound; Department of Diagnostic Radiology, Kansas University Medical Center.)

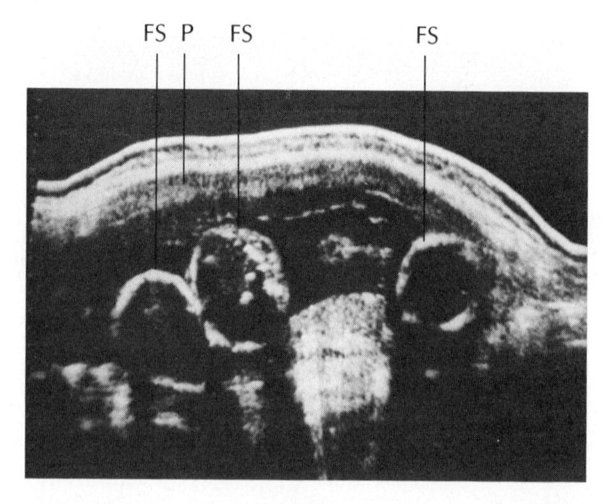

Figure 14–3. Transverse gray-scale scan demonstrating triplets. BPDs of all fetal skulls approximate 27 weeks' gestation. Anterior placenta (P) is shown. (Courtesy Section of Diagnostic Ultrasound, Department of Diagnostic Radiology, Kansas University Medical Center.)

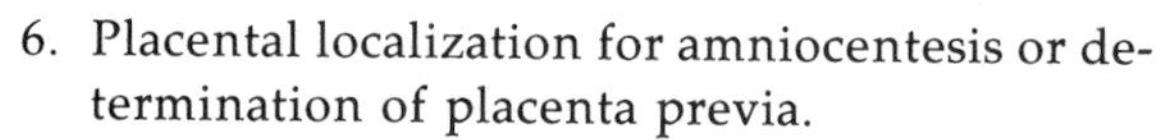

6. Placental localization for amniocentesis or determination of placenta previa.
7. Detection of intrauterine devices.
8. Detection of placental abnormalities.
9. Determination of fetal position and presentation.
10. Detection of fetal death.
11. Observation of fetal heart rate and respiration by real-time scanning.
12. Detection of incomplete or missed abortions and ectopic pregnancies.

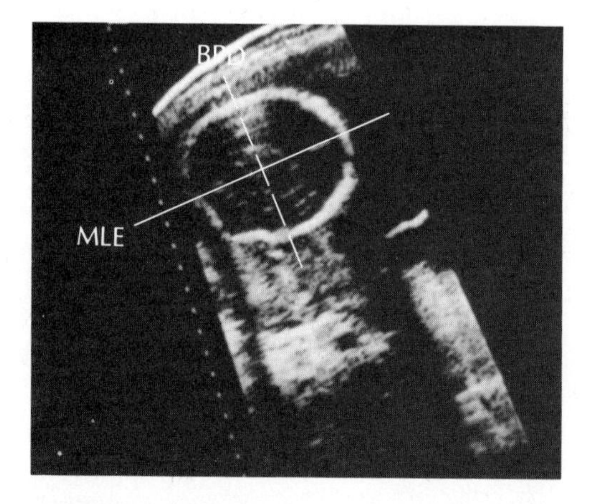

Figure 14–4. Transverse scan of 25–26 weeks' fetal skull. BPD is measured perpendicular to midline echo (MLE). (Courtesy Section of Diagnostic Ultrasound, Department of Diagnostic Radiology, Kansas University Medical Center.)

Early Pregnancy Detection

In managing the high-risk pregnant woman, it is of utmost importance to know the gestational age of the fetus to correlate data from all available tests. Pregnancy may be detected by diagnostic ultrasound as early as the 5th or 6th week following the LMP (Leopold and Asher, 1975; Ragan, 1976). A small collection of ringlike echoes may be seen within the uterus, and this is called the *gestational sac.* By the 8th week, stronger echoes representing the fetus may be seen along with the developing placenta. The placenta may be seen clearly at approximately 11–12 weeks' gestation, the fetal skull at 14 weeks' gestation in 95% of cases (Leopold and Asher, 1975), and the fetal thorax at about 16 weeks' gestation (Ragan, 1976).

The most accurate time for dating a pregnancy by diagnostic ultrasound is between 20 and 30 weeks' gestation. A sonogram obtained during this time can be of great benefit in helping to date a pregnancy if confirmed by a second sonogram a few weeks later.

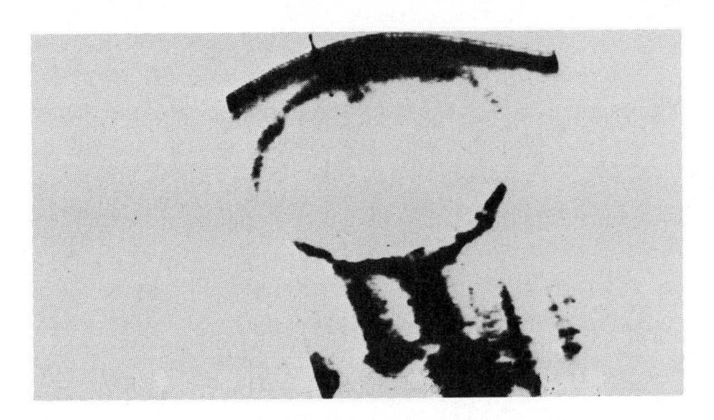

Figure 14–5. Hydrocephalic fetal skull at term. Note the minimal brain tissue in the bottom center. The large clear portion denotes fluid.

Measurement of Biparietal Diameter of Fetal Head

By far the most important application of ultrasound is in the measurement of the biparietal diameter (BPD) of the fetal head. The BPD is the widest diameter of the fetal skull and is perpendicular to the fetal midline echo. This echo is apparently either the falx cerebri or the interhemispheric fissure of the fetus (McQuown, 1977). Measurement of the BPD provides the physician with a useful tool for following fetal development.

Tables correlating the BPD with fetal gestation vary from one institution to the next, undoubtedly because of socioeconomic and geographic factors inherent in the populations for which the tables were derived. Nevertheless, serial determinations on the same fetus using the same tables can be used as a measure of the progress of fetal development. If growth of the fetal head follows a normal curve as gestation advances, one can be assured that the fetus is growing at a normal rate. However, if the curve begins to flatten, the physician must be on the alert for IUGR of the fetus and must then consider this case as high-risk and evaluate the fetus by additional means, such as estriol determinations and oxytocin challenge testing.

Until about the 32nd week, the fetal head grows about 3 mm/week (O'Sullivan, 1976) and thereafter at about 1.8 mm/week (Thompson et al., 1965; McQuown, 1977). One can obtain BPD measurements beginning in the 13th week of gestation. Detection of IUGR and an accurate prediction of fetal age can be most reliably achieved between the 20th and 30th week of gestation, when the most rapid growth in the BPD occurs. After 40 weeks' gestation the BPD shows a growth of less than 1 mm/week; thus sonograms obtained at this point are not of value. Generally, the BPD measurement correlates with gestational age within one to two weeks (see the Appendix for evaluation of biparietal diameters).

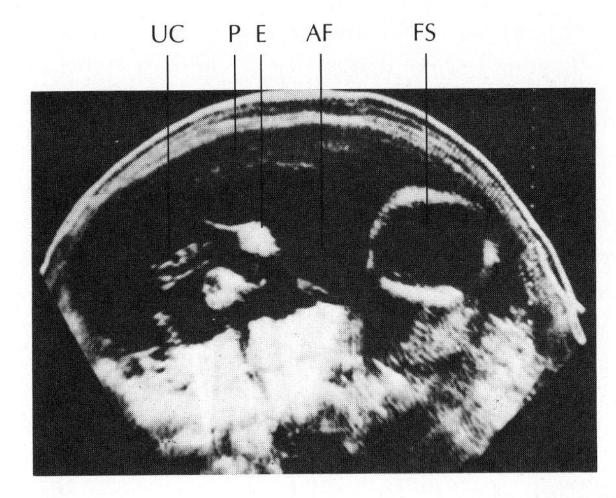

Figure 14–6. Transverse scan demonstrating fetal skull (FS), anterior placenta (P), extremities (E), umbilical cord (UC), and marked polyhydramnios (AF = amniotic fluid). (Courtesy Section of Diagnostic Ultrasound, Department of Diagnostic Radiology, Kansas University Medical Center.)

Detection of Fetal Abnormalities

Only gross abnormalities of the fetus are readily detectable by sonography at present. The two major abnormalities are anencephaly and hydrocephaly. In general, when the BPD is more than 10.8 cm (McQuown, 1977), hydrocephaly should be suspected. Normally there is a 1:1 ratio between the BPD and the measurement of the fetal thorax. If the chest is 5 mm or more smaller than the head size, one should suspect hydrocephaly. Anencephaly may be assumed if the fetal skull cannot be visualized after 14 weeks' gestation. Frequently, polyhydramnios is seen with this condition, and the trunk is able to be well visualized. Occasionally meningomyelocele may be detected, as can hydrops and ascites in the erythroblastotic infant. Polyhydramnios is easily identifiable by the large areas of echo-free spaces.

Localization of Placenta

Ultrasound is valuable in localizing the placenta for amniocentesis and in detecting placenta previa. Placentas appear to be located on the anterior surface of the uterine wall in approximately 40% of the cases (Ragan, 1976), and in some instances the placenta may cover the entire anterior uterine surface. By visualizing its location, the physician can avoid puncturing the placenta during amniocentesis. Ultrasound can also be used to locate a pool of amniotic fluid, thereby showing the physician exactly where and how deep to insert the needle for amniocentesis.

Fetal Growth Determination

As mentioned above, ultrasound provides the physician with a means of monitoring fetal growth. If the BPD of the fetal head is more than two standard deviations less than the mean for that particular gestational age, IUGR is indicated. This type of IUGR may be attributed to malnutrition of the fetus or congenital infection. In a second type of IUGR, the BPD is at first normal for gestational age, but later in the third trimester a decrease or plateau in head growth is noted. This type of curve is seen in patients with vascular disease (Queenan et al., 1976). At some institutions, the fetal thorax can be measured, thereby giving the physician another parameter by which to judge IUGR. Many growth-retarded babies show a difference between head and trunk size. If the head is of normal size and the trunk smaller than would be expected, there may be IUGR.

Fetal Breathing Movements

Fetal breathing movements detected by A-scan and B-mode techniques have been studied over the last decade and are now being suggested as a measure of fetal health. Episodic breathing movements have been reported by Patrick et al. (1978). Manning (1977) reports observing fetal breathing movements as early as the 11th week of gestation. After the 36th week of gestation, the breathing movements are thought to be similar to those of the term neonate.

Three types of patterns of fetal breathing movements have been observed. The first pattern is the most common and is characterized by rapid initial movements, with a gradual decline in number. This pattern is associated with generalized fetal movement before and after the pattern is observed. The second pattern is characterized by rapid breathing movements interspersed with slower movements. Fetal movements occur less frequently. The third pattern is the least frequent in occurrence and consists of isolated fast breathing movements, which occur at the rate of 10–15/min. This pattern is not usually accompanied by fetal movements (Manning, 1977).

Among factors that have been identified as influencing the fetal breathing movements are cigarette smoking, overnight maternal fasting, and uterine activity (Manning, 1977). Platt et al. (1978) report diminished or absent fetal breathing movements in the presence of hypoglycemia, hypoxemia, infection, and fetal distress.

Assessment of the method of collection, assessment of data, and interpretation of results are areas currently being researched. There is an indication that observation and classification of fetal breathing movements may be correlated with fetal distress and with Apgar scores following delivery (Platt et al., 1978). However, further investigation will be necessary to establish clinical significance.

OXYTOCIN CHALLENGE TEST

Kubli et al. (1969) have suggested that placental function may be divided into two components: nutritive, or metabolic, and respiratory. Nutritive deficit may result in IUGR, producing infants who are small for gestational age. IUGR may be suspected when there appears to be a lag in fundal progression of the uterus after approximately 28 weeks' gestation. These fetuses may be followed with serial sonograms, urinary and plasma estriol determinations, and clinical surveillance of fundal progression. The *oxytocin challenge test* (OCT) is a means of evaluating the respiratory function of the placenta and is most helpful in evaluating patients with chronic placental insufficiency and whose estriol values may be abnormally low or difficult to interpret.

The OCT, or contraction stress test (CST), is an external, noninvasive, antenatal means of monitoring the respiratory reserve of the uterine-placental-fetal unit. It enables the health care team to identify the fetus at risk for intrauterine asphyxia by observing the response of the fetal heart rate (FHR) to the stress of uterine contractions (spontaneous or oxytocin-induced) and to intervene if necessary. With an increase in intrauterine pressure during contractions, there is a transient reduction in blood flow to the intervillous space of the placenta and therefore decreased oxygen transport to the fetus. In most instances this reduction is well tolerated by a healthy fetus, but if there is insufficient placental reserve, fetal hypoxia, depression of the myocardium, and late decelerations of the FHR will occur as placental reserve is exceeded. In the intrapartal period, late decelerations of FHR have been associated with fetal metabolic acidosis (low fetal scalp pH), babies with low Apgar scores, and, rarely, fetal intrapartal death (Weingold, 1975). Hon and Quilligan (1967) define *late decelerations* as decreases in the FHR that are uniform and have their onset late in the uterine contraction phase. Late decelerations have their onset at or just following the acme of the contraction and occur repetitively. (See Chapter 16 for further discussion of FHR patterns.)

Procedure

The OCT is performed either on an outpatient basis by qualified perinatal nurses well acquainted with fetal monitoring and the interpretation of various FHR patterns or by a physician in the delivery room or close to it, should adverse reactions to oxytocin stimulation occur. The procedure and reasons for administering the test should be clearly explained to the patient beforehand to alleviate fears and apprehension. Equipment and normal variations in monitoring that occur during the test are also discussed with the patient. It is advisable for the patient to have eaten, so that the fetus remains quiet and bowel sounds do not interfere with the test. The patient should empty her bladder prior to beginning the OCT, because she may be confined to bed for one and a half to two hours.

During the test, the patient assumes a semi-Fowler's position to avoid supine hypotension. For the first 15 minutes the nurse records baseline measurements, including blood pressure, fetal activity, variations of the FHR during fetal movement, and spontaneous contractions. During this time, pertinent medical and obstetric information may be obtained from the patient to aid in her further management. After the area of clearest fetoscopic heart tones is noted, the ultrasonic transducer or phonotransducer is placed over the mother's abdomen so that the FHR may be accurately recorded on the monitoring strip. (See Chapter 16 for further discussion of fetal monitoring.) To record uterine contractions, the tocodynamometer (pressure transducer) is placed over the area of the fundus where there is a good muscle mass (fetal buttocks).

After a 15-minute baseline recording, if no contractions are present or if they are insufficient for interpretation, appropriate intravenous solutions are administered. If the patient is having spontaneous contractions of good quality lasting 40–60 seconds and three occur in a 10-minute period, it is not necessary to administer oxytocin. If there are no contractions, an infusion of 5% dextrose in water or normal saline is begun through a scalp vein needle in the patient's hand. A piggyback infusion of oxytocin in a similar solution is administered by means of a constant infusion pump (not the intravenous drip method) to accurately measure the amount of oxytocin being infused. The infusion is usually started at a rate of 0.5 mU/min, depending on uterine activity already present. Oxytocin infusion is increased at 15–20 minute intervals until the nurse observes three uterine contractions of good quality in 10 minutes. The maximum amount of oxytocin used for an OCT generally does not exceed 20 mU/min. Patients usually experience uterine activity after 5–10 mU/min of oxytocin infusion.

If late decelerations are repetitive, occurring three times regardless of the frequency of the uterine contractions, the oxytocin should be discontinued, as this constitutes a positive test. When criteria for interpreting the test have been met, the oxytocin infusion is discontinued and the patient is monitored until her contractions wane in frequency and amplitude and approach baseline activity. Before dismissing the patient, the monitoring record is reviewed by the physician, the results of the test are explained to the patient, and these results are recorded in her chart.

Indications and Contraindications

The OCT is indicated for those patients at risk for placental insufficiency or fetal compromise because of the following:

1. IUGR.
2. Diabetes mellitus.
3. Heart disease.
4. Chronic hypertension.
5. Preeclampsia-eclampsia.
6. Sickle cell disease.
7. Suspected postmaturity (42 weeks' gestation).
8. History of previous stillborn or intrapartal loss.
9. Rh sensitization with meconium-stained amniotic fluid.
10. Abnormal estriol excretion.
11. Hyperthyroidism.
12. Renal disease.

Contraindications for the OCT are as follows:

1. Third trimester bleeding (placenta previa or marginal abruptio placentae).
2. Previous classical cesarean section.
3. Instances in which the risk of possible premature labor outweighs the advantage of the OCT.
   a. Premature rupture of the membranes.
   b. Incompetent cervix or Shirodkar-Barter operation (cerclage—surgical procedure in which the cervix is encircled with suture to prevent it from dilating before the end of 40 weeks' gestation).
   c. Multiple gestation.

Clinical Application

The survival rate of the prematurely delivered fetus rises from approximately 20% at 28 weeks' gestation to 80% at 34 weeks' (Greenwald, 1970). Therefore, an OCT prior to 28 weeks' gestation has no real clinical value. OCTs are generally begun at approximately 32–34 weeks' gestation and are repeated at weekly intervals until the patient delivers. Should the patient's condition deteriorate, the OCT should be repeated as soon as possible.

A *negative OCT* (Table 14–1) has much prognostic value in that it implies that placental support is adequate. If that is the case, the physician can avoid premature intervention and gain approximately one additional week of intrauterine life for the fetus (Freeman, 1975). A negative test also suggests that the fetus would be likely to tolerate the stress of labor should it ensue within the week (Schifrin et al., 1975).

A woman who exhibits a *positive OCT* (see Table 14–1) may have a fetus whose placental re-

Table 14–1. Interpretation of OCT Results

OCT	Findings
Negative test	Three contractions of good quality in 10 min, lasting 40 or more sec, without late decelerations (Figure 14–7) Contraction of good quality lasting more than 90 sec; hyperstimulation without late deceleration (Figure 14–8) Usually associated with good variability of the FHR and acceleration of FHR with fetal movement
Positive test	Occurrence of repetitive, persistent late decelerations with more than 50% of contractions; frequency of contractions need not be three in 10 min (Figure 14–9) Usually associated with decreased variability and lack of acceleration of the FHR with fetal movement
Hyperstimulation	Contractions closer than every 2 min or lasting more than 90 sec with late decelerations; healthy fetus may show decelerations during a prolonged contraction Repeat in 24 hr
Suspicious test	Nonrepetitive late decelerations occurring with less than 50% of contractions Repeat in 24 hr
Unsatisfactory test	Recording cannot be interpreted or contractions are inadequate, as a result of one or more of following factors: 1. Obesity 2. Excessive maternal or fetal activity 3. Polyhydramnios 4. Fetal hiccups 5. Bowel sounds Repeat in 24 hr (may need to wait one week if unable to obtain contractions)

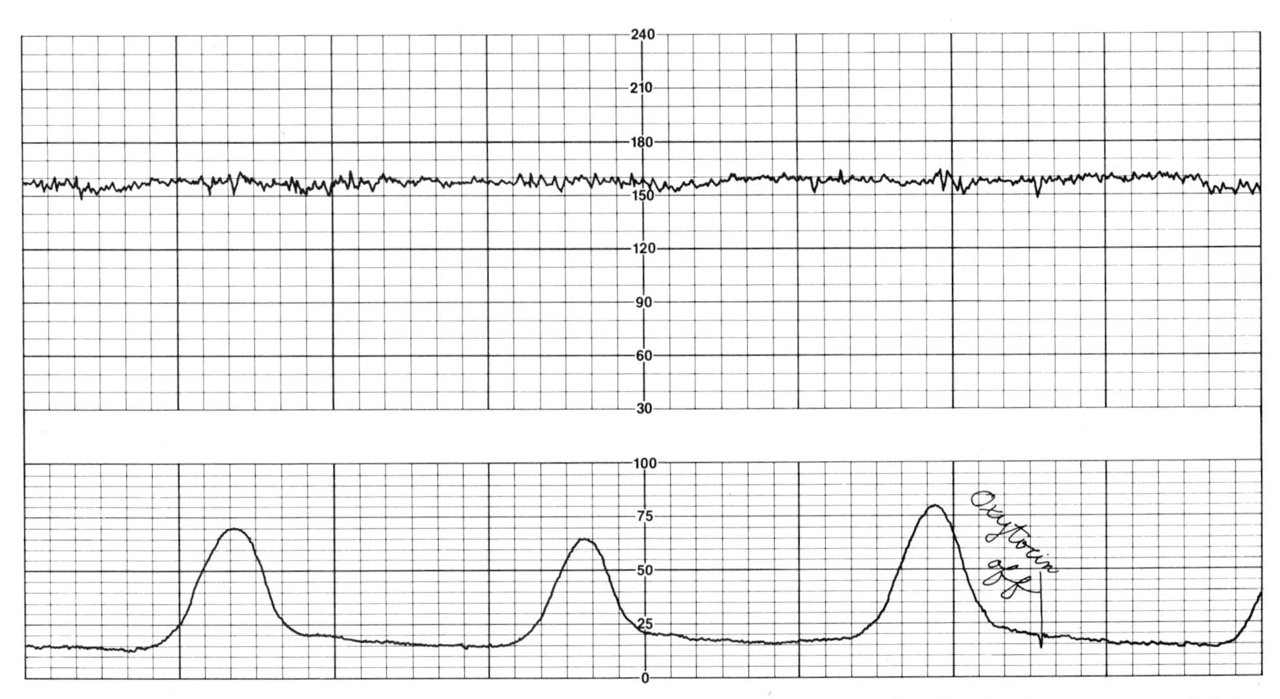

Figure 14–7. Example of a negative OCT using ultrasonic transducer. There are no late decelerations present, and three good contractions within 10 minutes are charted. Variability is minimal due to fetal sleep. (Top of strip = fetal heart rate; bottom of strip = uterine contractions.)

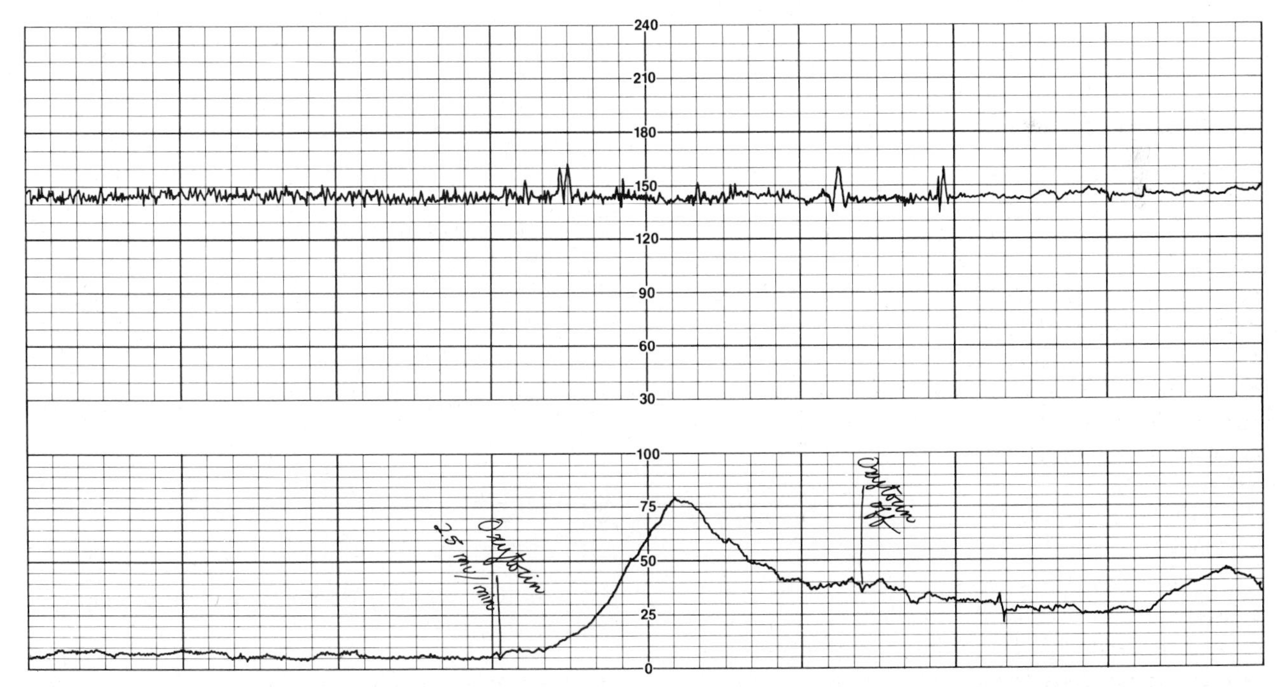

Figure 14–8. Example of hyperstimulation using a phonotransducer. The contraction is of good quality and lasts longer than 90 seconds. There is no deceleration, so this is considered a negative OCT. Note the extreme loss of variability of FHR (which may have been due to the recent ingestion of a narcotic by the patient). (Top of strip = fetal heart rate; bottom of strip = uterine contractions.)

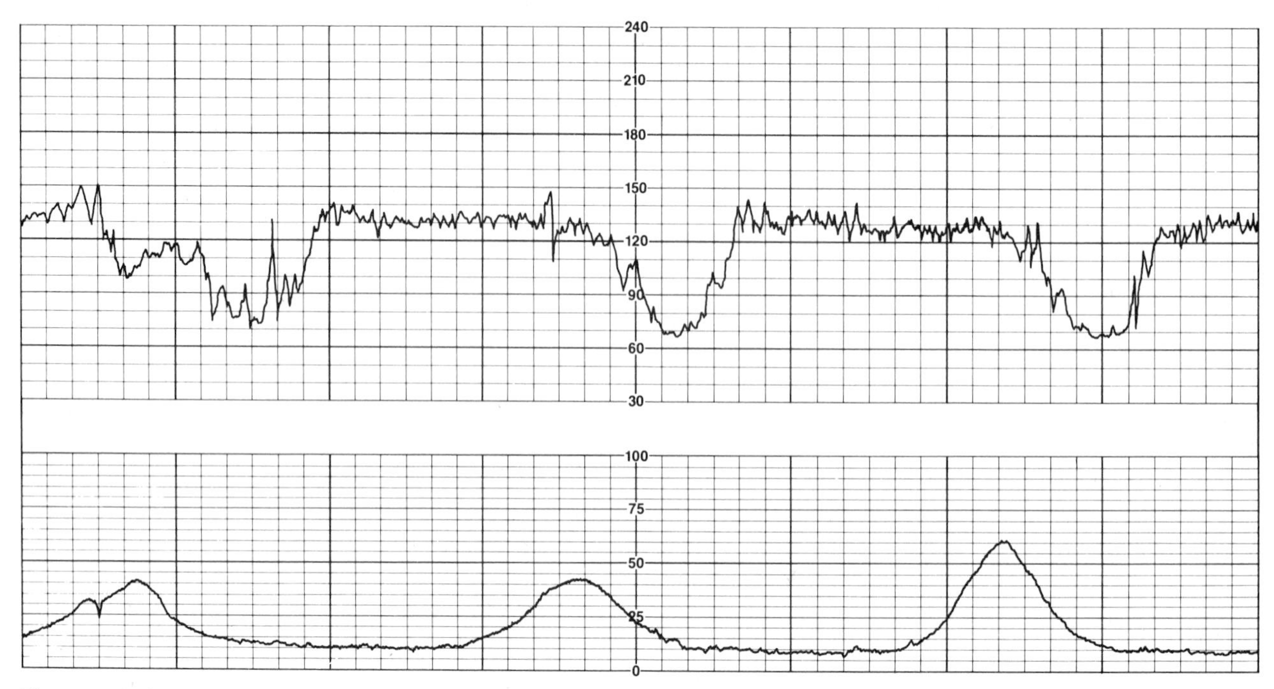

Figure 14–9. Example of a positive OCT. Repetitive late decelerations occur with each contraction. Ultrasonic transducer was used. (Top of strip = fetal heart rate; bottom of strip = uterine contractions.)

serves are compromised. In many instances there is minimal baseline variability of the FHR (a condition that is usually not seen with healthy babies). Most frequently, acceleration of the FHR with fetal movement is absent or diminished, representing inadequate autonomic nervous system control of the fetal heart rate. However, a positive OCT does not appear to be as reliable an indicator of fetal status as a negative one (Freeman, 1975). False positive results may occur due to maternal hypotension during the test, which produces late decelerations. Oxytocin-induced contractions may be more stressful than would normally occur during labor as a result of hyperstimulation, which might not be detected with an external pressure transducer.

Patients with positive test results may be managed differently according to their specific situation. Other parameters of fetal status must be taken into consideration, and on the basis of all available data, the pregnancy may be allowed to continue or labor may be induced. Delivery is usually considered if it has been determined that the fetus's lungs are mature. Whether the patient with a positive OCT should be delivered by cesarean section depends on how rapidly the fetus must be delivered to avoid possible fetal distress, on the adequacy of dilatation, on the softness and effacement of the cervix ("ripeness") at the time, and on the mother's condition.

NONSTRESS TESTING

Much has been written about *nonstress testing* (NST), or *fetal acceleration determinations,* as a predictor of fetal well-being (Trierweiler et al., 1976; Schifrin, 1977). The NST requires less time and fewer qualified personnel than the OCT, can be performed in an outpatient office that is not close to a delivery suite, and can be performed on patients for whom the OCT might be contraindicated.

Procedure

The patient is placed in a semi-Fowler's position and monitored in a similar fashion as for an OCT.

Recordings of the FHR are obtained for approximately 30–40 minutes. Notation is made of fetal activity, acceleration of the FHR with fetal activity, baseline variability of the FHR, and uterine activity.

Classification of FHR Patterns

NST heart rate patterns have been classified as reactive, nonreactive, sinusoidal, combined, and unsatisfactory (Rochard et al., 1976). A reactive pattern exhibits acceleration of the FHR (>15 beats/min) with fetal movement and a good baseline variability (5–15 beats/min). A nonreactive pattern usually shows decreased baseline variability (<5 beats/min) and has minimal (<15 beats/min) or no acceleration of the FHR with fetal movement. Rarely, a sinusoidal pattern may be seen; variability is minimal or absent, and there are uniform periodic oscillations (5–15 beats/min) indicating an undulating heart rate. This pattern may represent an inability of the fetal central nervous system to control its heart rate in certain circumstances, as in Rh-sensitized pregnancies. Combined patterns are those with accelerations of the FHR with some fetal activity and no change in heart rate with remaining activity. On occasion, the test may be unsatisfactory because of uninterpretable registration of the FHR or inadequate fetal activity.

Prognostic Value

Schifrin and Dame (1972) and Lee et al. (1975) have reported that, when acceleration of the FHR accompanies fetal movement and there is good variability, decelerations of the FHR do not occur if there is the added stress of uterine contractions. They claim that this phenomenon can be used as a reliable measure of fetal well-being. Results of studies by Rochard et al. (1976) seem to support the nonstressed form of surveillance as a reliable predictor of fetal well-being. However, others believe that this technique needs further evaluation to prove its absolute predictive value.

ESTRIOL DETERMINATIONS

The amount of estrogen excreted in the urine of a pregnant woman has been used as an indicator of metabolic placental function and a predictor of fetal jeopardy in the management of the high-risk patient. About 90% of the estrogen excreted in urine is in the form of *estriol* (Taylor, 1971; Gobelsmann, 1977), and the presence of this hormone appears to be a reflection of the integrity of the maternal-fetal-placental unit. Estriol levels increase in both urine and blood as pregnancy goes to term, with significant amounts being produced in the third trimester. Estriol excretion during pregnancy may increase as much as a thousandfold over the nonpregnant state, then drops precipitously following delivery or intrauterine fetal death (Gobelsmann, 1977). Estriol determinations are used widely in the obstetric management of women with toxemia, suspected IUGR, chronic hypertension, diabetes, and postmaturity. To maintain optimum estrogen metabolism, there must be a healthy fetus; a normally functioning, intact placenta; and a healthy mother. As the fetus grows and matures, estriol production increases; when growth becomes retarded, production levels off; and when there is fetal distress and the placenta has reached its limit, estriol production decreases.

Estriol Metabolism

Estrogen is produced by the placenta and depends on precursors received from both mother and fetus. There is a constant interplay between mother, fetus, and placenta (Figure 14–10), and all must be healthy and functioning well for estrogen production to be within normal limits.

Estrogen precursors from the mother and placenta (primarily cholesterol and pregnenolone) are transported across the placenta, synthesized by the fetal adrenal glands, and turned into dehydroepiandrosterone sulfate. Hydroxylation occurs in the fetal liver, and the androgens are then converted by the placenta to estriol and other estrogens and are excreted into the mother's circulation. Some of this material is returned to the fetus, and the remainder is conjugated with acids in the maternal liver and excreted by the kidneys.

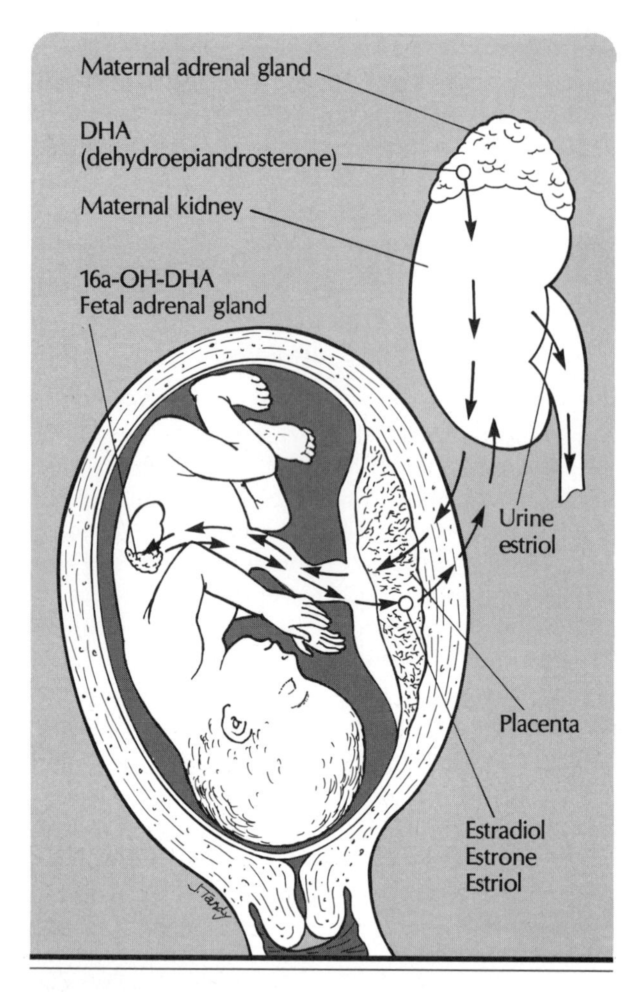

Figure 14–10. Maternal urinary estriol excretion showing interplay of mother, baby, and placenta. (Modified from Duhring, J. L. May 1974. The high risk fetus. *Hosp. Med.*, p. 82.)

Patterns of Excretion

Four patterns of estriol excretion are generally seen, as Figure 14–11 indicates (Green et al., 1969):

- Pattern I: All serial levels fall within the normal range and continue to rise until term.
- Pattern II: Levels are within subnormal range and yet rise so that the critical level of 12 mg is reached at term.
- Pattern III: Values are within the normal range but suddenly fall, either abruptly or gradually. This is an ominous pattern and is seen with fetal death due to a deterioration of the intrauterine environment.
- Pattern IV: Values are never within the normal range. Morbidity and mortality are high with this group. It is questionable whether this pregnancy should continue if fetal lungs are mature.

The range of normal values is broad, and various patterns are seen. A single 24-hour estriol measurement that falls in the normal range does not necessarily indicate fetal well-being, just as a single drop in production does not necessarily indicate fetal jeopardy. Of more significance than any specific value is the general trend in day-to-day or week-to-week values. Estriol production fluctuates daily, so one must be careful not to assume that the fetus is in jeopardy when in fact the fluctuation is normal. Generally, a drop of 50% or more from the previous mean level may signify fetal distress (Tulchinsky, 1975). Decreases of 30% may be due to laboratory variation or normal daily fluctuation. A fall in estriol is usually gradual, except in the case of diabetes, in which the drop may be more dramatic due to abrupt changes in glucose metabolism.

Estriol production reaches a plateau at about 40–41 weeks' gestation and decreases slowly thereafter. Thus, in the case of suspected postmaturity, if estriols are rising, the woman's estimated date for delivery may be incorrect. Urinary excretion of more than 30 mg/24 hr indicates absence of postmaturity, and therefore intervention may be delayed (Gobelsmann, 1977). If values are low but increasing, serial values indicate that the fetus is growing.

Decreasing estriol levels from previously low levels are a poor prognostic sign. Critical levels (lower limits than normal) of estriol excretion are 7 mg/24 hr at 30 weeks' gestation and 12 mg/24 hr at 40 weeks' gestation. A value of 4 mg/24 hr may indicate impending fetal death. Chronically low values may be indicative of IUGR. When low values are obtained, one must consider the following:

1. Laboratory error.
2. Incomplete collection of urine.
3. Incorrect gestational age.
4. Drugs such as ampicillin, heroin, methadone, methenamine mandelate (Mandelamine), neomycin, phenophthalein.
5. Placental steroid sulfatase deficiency.
6. Chronic uteroplacental insufficiency.
7. Anencephaly or hydrocephaly.
8. Maternal pyelonephritis.

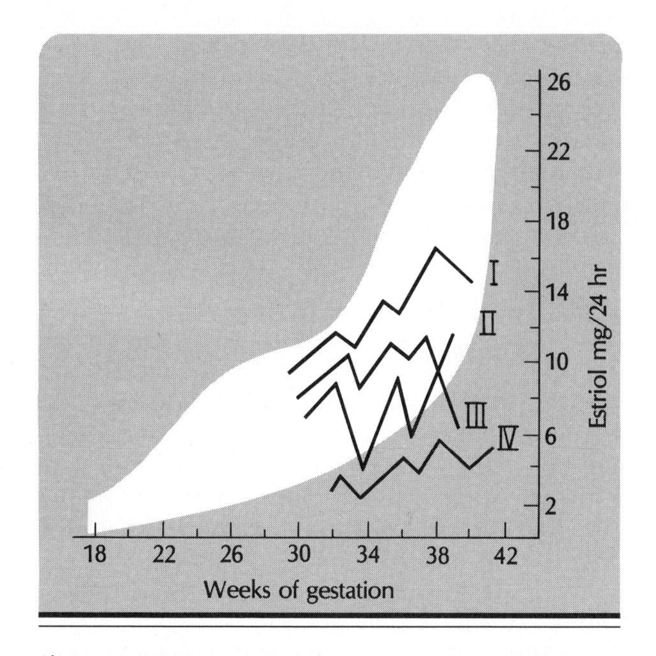

Figure 14–11. Estriol excretion patterns and the range of normal excretion. (From Greene, J. W., et al. 1969. Correlation of estriol excretion patterns of pregnant women with subsequent development of their children. *Am. J. Obstet. Gynecol.* 105:730.)

9. Maternal anemia.
10. Corticosteroids.
11. Fetal congenital adrenal hypoplasia.

Urinary Estriol Determinations

Procedure

Patients must be given a clear explanation by the nurse or physician concerning the urinary collection procedure they must perform for estriol determination. If the test is conducted by a laboratory, one should not depend on the laboratory personnel to explain the procedure. If time is taken with the initial explanation, problems will be kept to a minimum. The patient must understand why all her urine must be saved, why it must be refrigerated, when to bring it to the laboratory, and what the results mean. Specific values need not be her concern.

The patient discards the first urinary specimen of the morning and then collects all urine in a clean container, which is kept refrigerated to prevent formation of bacteria and breakdown of estrogen products. The time that she first empties her bladder the first day is the time she should collect her final specimen the following morning. For example, if the patient first voids at 7 AM on Wednesday, the final specimen to be collected should be at 7 AM on Thursday. The patient must be informed as to the time that she must bring the specimen to the laboratory so that it can be processed the same day to avoid delay in obtaining results. The patient should be told to report any incidence of forgetting to collect a particular voiding, because this will alter test results. It is also advisable to have her begin a second 24-hour urine collection soon after the first to evaluate the results. If the initial estriol level is questionable or low, it will be necessary to confirm this as soon as possible.

Problems in Determining Estriol Levels

Several difficulties may arise in determining estriol levels. If maternal renal function is impaired, as could occur in preeclampsia-eclampsia or chronic hypertensive disease, the test will not be accurate. Creatinine clearance tests should be performed in these cases, and if the levels are decreased, one should suspect impaired renal function.

Certain antibiotics, such as ampicillin, methenamine mandelate, and neomycin, eliminate the normal flora of the maternal intestine and prevent bacterial hydrolysis of estriol conjugates, so that large amounts of estriol are lost in the stools instead of being reabsorbed into the mother's circulation. Thus low estriol values are seen in patients taking such medications.

Estriol production is a function of gestational age. If gestational age is not known or is incorrectly calculated, the values may be confusing or may lead to inaccurate information.

Sulfatase deficiency, an extremely rare sex-linked disorder, may be the reason for exceedingly low estriol levels. Affected infants do well at birth, but the estriol values are minimal. A level of less than 4 mg at term is much cause for concern, probably suggesting sulfatase deficiency, adrenal hypoplasia, anencephaly, or severe illness of the fetus.

In patients with exceedingly high estriol levels, one should suspect the following:

1. More advanced pregnancy than previously determined.

2. Multiple gestation.
3. Macrosomic fetus (if mother is diabetic).

Serial Determinations

In managing the high-risk patient, it is necessary to obtain serial determinations. Estriol determinations are usually instituted at approximately 32–34 weeks' gestation and are collected no more than once or twice a week unless abnormal. Prior to 32 weeks' gestation, delivery is usually not contemplated due to immaturity of the fetus, although the physician may wish to begin to look at estriol excretion as early as 28 weeks in patients with chronic hypertension, preeclampsia, or fetal IUGR.

Estriol determinations may be indicated two to three times each week later in the pregnancy or even daily, as in the case of the diabetic nearing term, because there is a greater risk of missing a significant fall in estriol levels if only twice-weekly determinations are obtained. Estriols tend to fall more slowly in women with chronic hypertension, preeclampsia, and postmaturity. Therefore twice-weekly determinations are usually sufficient.

Some authorities believe that normal levels begin to fall into an abnormal range about 72 hours before the death of the fetus actually occurs. An abrupt fall is an ominous sign of fetal distress, and until proven otherwise by other parameters, it suggests that the condition of the fetus is rapidly deteriorating.

Because of problems in collection, renal disease in the mother, ingestion of medications by the mother, or other factors, estriol determinations should not be used as the sole determining factor in judging the status of the fetal-maternal-placental unit. However, as long as values remain within the normal range for any particular pregnancy, the physician may feel comfortable in allowing the pregnancy to continue (unless there are other indications to suggest that the fetus might be in jeopardy). When values are abnormal or decreased, one must carefully assess the situation to determine whether the fetus is in an unhealthy intrauterine environment and whether intervention is necessary.

Urinary versus Plasma Estriol Determinations

Urinary estriol determinations have been in vogue much longer than plasma determinations. For this reason, many institutions tend to rely more on urinary assays. Both seem to give the same type of information regarding the status of the maternal-fetal-placental unit, although values do vary. One must be aware of normal values within one's own laboratory.

Advantages of plasma over urinary estriol determinations include (a) ease of collection, (b) less difficulty in processing results, (c) less time needed to collect specimens, (d) less time needed to obtain results, (e) probably less expensive, (f) fewer errors in collection, (g) possibility of obtaining two or more plasma samples for analysis in a single day.

Disadvantages of plasma collection are that (a) experience in using them has been limited and techniques are still in the stages of development and refinement, so they are done in only a few centers; (b) erroneously high plasma levels may be obtained with impaired renal clearance; and (c) there is considerable diurnal variation in plasma estriol levels.

Disadvantages of urinary collection include (a) errors in collection of urine (usually incomplete), (b) inconvenience of 24-hour collection, and (c) the amount of time needed to collect urine (24 hours) and to process results (6–8 hours). In addition, low values may be a result of impaired renal function rather than fetal jeopardy.

AMNIOTIC FLUID ANALYSIS

One of the most valuable studies available to the physician in the management of the pregnant woman is the analysis of the amniotic fluid, which is obtained by a technique known as *amniocentesis*. Examination of the fluid can provide information regarding the following:

1. Degree to which Rh-immunization has progressed.
2. Fetal maturity.
3. Presence of meconium, which may indicate fetal distress.

4. Chromosomal analysis (see Chapter 8 for further discussion).
5. Detection of neural tube defects through α-fetoprotein analysis (see Chapter 8 for further discussion).

Clinical Application

Evaluation of Rh-sensitized Pregnancies

The first studies of amniotic fluid were initially done in the early 1950s for the evaluation of bilirubin pigment in the amniotic fluid of Rh-sensitized mothers. By looking at the optical density of the fluid, the analyst could determine the degree to which the fetus was affected.

Bevis in 1956 reported that, by analyzing amniotic fluid of the Rh-sensitized mother, valuable information could be gained concerning the progress of her pregnancy. Liley (1961) produced a graph that is now universally used in determining the severity of hemolytic disease in the fetus (Figure 14–12).

If an Rh-negative woman produces an incompatible Rh-positive fetus, antibodies cross the placenta and cause hemolytic anemia in the fetus. Concentrations of bilirubin and other breakdown products from destroyed red blood cells can be detected in amniotic fluid by spectrophotometry. By plotting their concentration or optical density at 450 nm on a Liley curve, the physician can ascertain the degree to which the fetus is affected and the need for intervention or intrauterine transfusion.

Liley categorized the degree of hemolytic disease into three zones. If the optical density falls in zone I (low zone) at 28–31 weeks' gestation, the fetus either will be unaffected or will have only mild hemolytic disease. Amniocentesis should be repeated in two or three weeks. When the optical density falls in zone II (midzone), amniocentesis is repeated frequently so that the trend can be determined. The age of the fetus and the trend in optical density indicate the necessity for intrauterine transfusion or premature delivery. Optical densities falling in zone III (high zone) indicate that the fetus is severely affected and death is a possibility. The decision concerning delivery or intrauterine transfusion depends on the gestational age of the fetus. After about the 32nd or 33rd gestational week, early delivery and extrauterine treatment are probably preferred to performing intrauterine transfusion.

Evaluation of Fetal Maturity

In managing the patient at risk, the physician is constantly faced with the possibility of having to deliver an infant prior to term and before the onset of labor. There are many indications for early termination of pregnancy, including repeat cesarean section, premature rupture of the membranes, diabetes, hypertensive conditions in the mother, and placental insufficiency. Unfortunately, the most common cause of perinatal mortality is prematurity and complications arising from pulmonary immaturity (Leiker and Hensleigh, 1975); delivery of an infant with immature pulmonary function frequently results in the respiratory distress syndrome (RDS), also known as hyaline membrane disease (see Chapter 25).

Because gestational age, birth weight, and the rate of development of organ systems do not necessarily correspond, before elective delivery of any infant one should determine the lung maturity of the fetus by amniotic fluid analysis. Concentrations of certain substances in the amniotic fluid reflect the pulmonary condition of the fetus (see p. 399). In many cases, delivery of the infant can be delayed until the lungs show maturity.

Identification of Meconium Staining

When the fetus is in utero, any episode of hypoxia may result in an increased fetal peristalsis, relaxation of the anal sphincter, and passage of meconium into the amniotic fluid. The amniotic fluid is normally clear, but the presence of meconium makes the fluid greenish.

Before the amniotic membranes have ruptured, the meconium staining can be observed by amnioscopy. In this procedure, an amnioscope is placed in the vagina and against the fetal presenting part. The amniotic fluid can be visualized through the amniotic membranes.

Meconium staining may also be observed when amniocentesis is done. After the membranes have ruptured, meconium staining may be observed in the drainage from the vagina.

Once meconium staining is identified, more assessments must be made to determine if the fetus is suffering ongoing episodes of hypoxia.

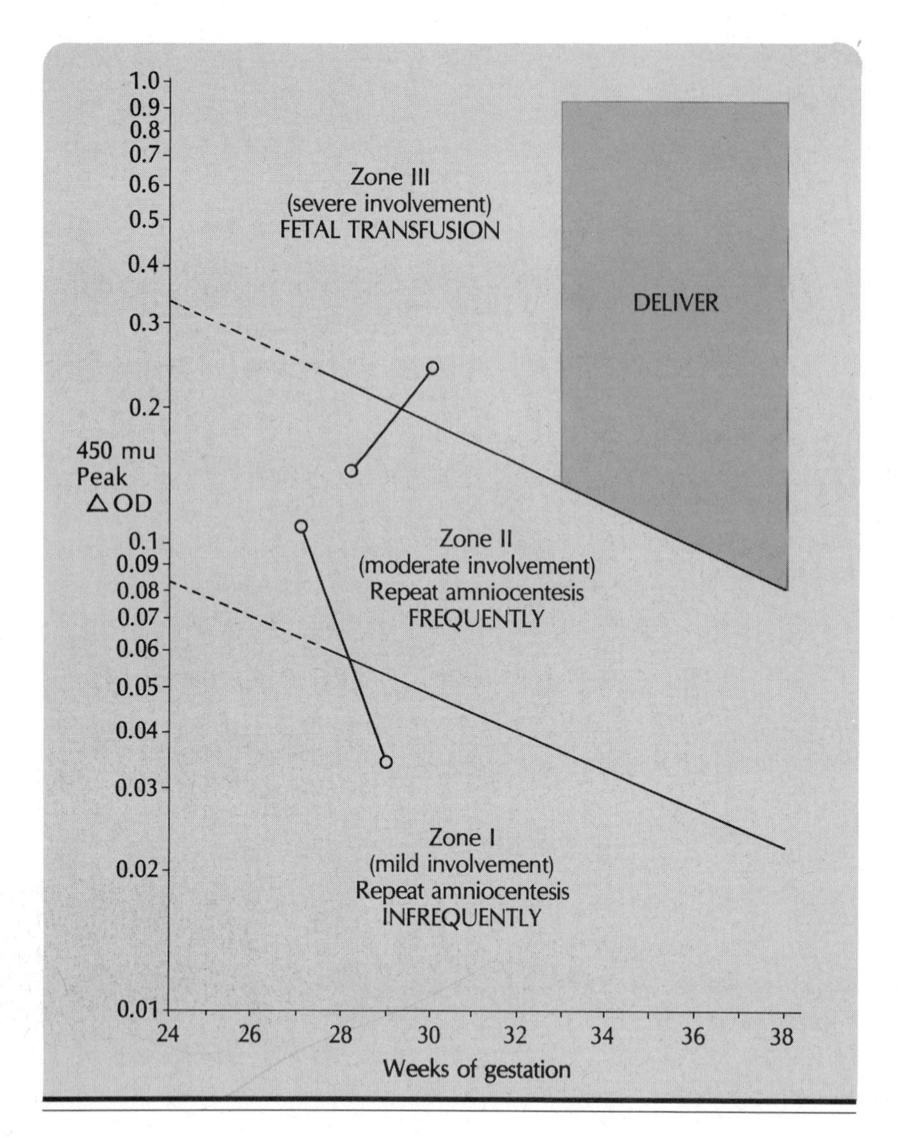

Figure 14–12. The density of amniotic fluid can be useful in determining the severity of erythroblastosis fetalis. There are three zones of optical density, which are correlated with the degree to which the fetus is affected by this condition. In this graph, management of the Rh-sensitized pregnancy is related to the condition of the fetus and gestational age. (Modified from Liley, A. W. 1961. Liquor amnii analysis in the management of the pregnancy complicated by rhesus sensitization. *Am. J. Obstet. Gynecol.* 32:1359.)

Amniocentesis

Amniotic fluid may be obtained by either transabdominal or suprapubic amniocentesis. The procedure is fairly simple, although complications, including trauma, hemorrhage, and infection, do occur rarely (less than 1%). The fetus, umbilical cord, or placenta may be punctured inadvertently, causing injuries ranging from minor scratches of fetal parts to intrauterine hemorrhage, leading to fetal distress and intrauterine death. Fetal pneumothorax and cord hematomas have been reported. Placental perforation could result in hemorrhage from the fetal circulation, which could lead to fetal anemia or to increased sensitization of the Rh-negative mother. Complications are rare, but the mother does need to be informed of them. Generally, an operative permit is signed for this procedure. Intraamniotic infection and induction of premature labor are also hazards.

Amniocentesis may be done on an outpatient basis but should be performed near a delivery suite should acute fetal distress be encountered. The location for needle insertion is determined by sonography, which enables the physician to visualize the placenta and an adequate pocket of fluid, and with the aid of the sonographer, who can instruct the physician concerning the depth with which to insert the needle. All women with anterior placentas should be "tapped" in sonography to avoid puncturing the placenta. The patient should empty her bladder so that the bladder is not en-

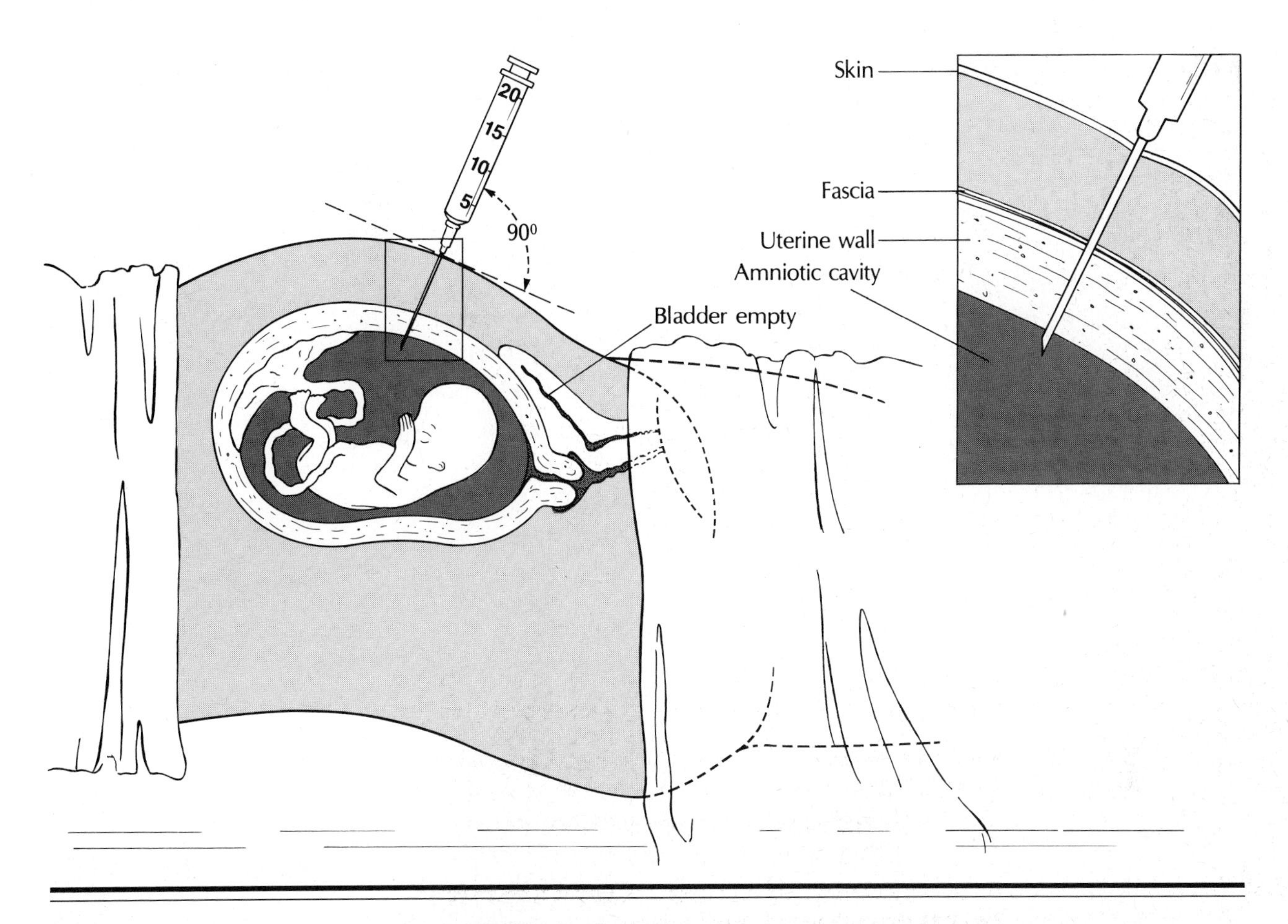

Figure 14–13. Amniocentesis. Patient is usually scanned under ultrasonic direction to determine area of pocket of amniotic fluid. Three levels of resistance are felt as the needle penetrates the skin, fascia, and uterine wall before obtaining amniotic fluid.

tered instead of the uterus. Amniotic fluid and urine may look similar, and if there is a possibility that urine was obtained during a suprapubic tap, the fluid should be checked for pH and protein content with a dipstick. Amniotic fluid has a high protein content (Goldstein, 1977), which is not a normal finding in urine unless the patient has been spilling protein in her urine as a result of preeclampsia or renal disease.

The abdomen is scanned for placental and fetal location, and the amniocentesis, or "tap," is done immediately, before the fetus has the opportunity to move. The needle insertion site is of the utmost importance, because the fetus, placenta, umbilical cord, bladder, and uterine arteries must all be avoided. The importance of locating the placenta cannot be stressed enough, especially in cases of Rh-isoimmunization, in which trauma to the placenta increases fetal-maternal transfusion and worsens the immunization. Except for very late in pregnancy, the fetal head may be displaced upward and the amniocentesis may be done suprapubically. If this is not feasible, it is usually done laterally (Figure 14–13). In the last few weeks of pregnancy, the fetus may occupy what appears to be all the available space in the uterus. There may be a decrease in the amount of available amniotic fluid. With the aid of ultrasound, fluid can usually be located, although in some cases it is impossible.

Procedure

The skin of the maternal abdomen is cleansed with an agent such as thimerosal (Merthiolate), Betadine, or hexachlorophene (pHisoHex). A local anesthetic such as lidocaine (1–2 ml of 1% solution) may be injected just under the skin to anesthetize the area. Many physicians choose not to do this, because it frequently causes more discom-

Procedure 14–1. Amniocentesis

Objective	Nursing action	Rationale
Prepare patient	Explain procedure.	Anxiety of patient will be decreased with information.
Prepare equipment	Collect necessary supplies: 1. 3 ml syringe with 25-gauge needle. 2. Local anesthetic (1% procaine or 1% lidocaine). 3. 4-inch 22-gauge spinal needle. 4. 10 ml syringe. 5. 20 ml syringe. 6. Specimen jar.	
Cleanse abdomen	Scrub abdomen with Betadine (or other cleansing agent).	Incidence of infection is decreased.
Monitor vital signs	Obtain baseline data on maternal BP, pulse, and respirations and on FHR. Monitor every 15 min and immediately after procedure.	Status of patient is assessed.
Collect specimen of amniotic fluid	Physician injects local anesthetic at site of tap (optional). Spinal needle is inserted into amniotic cavity. 15–20 ml of fluid is withdrawn. Place specimen in specimen jar. Send to lab with appropriate request slips. If specimen is bloody, establish whether blood is maternal or fetal in origin. If bleeding is fetal, further evaluation is mandatory. Immediate delivery may be necessary.	
Reassess vital signs	Obtain mother's BP, pulse, and respirations and FHR.	Treatment course can be determined.
Complete patient record	Record type of procedure done, patient and fetal response, and disposition of specimen.	Patient records will be complete and current.
Educate patient	Instruct patient to report any of following side effects: 1. Unusual fetal hyperactivity or lack of movement. 2. Vaginal discharge—clear drainage or bleeding. 3. Uterine contractions or abdominal pain. 4. Fever or chills.	Patient will know how to recognize side effects or conditions that require further treatment.

fort than inserting the spinal needle. A 4-inch 20- or 22-gauge spinal needle is inserted into the uterine cavity with one thrust or slowly, in which case three points of resistance are felt: skin, fascia, and uterine muscle. There is a "give" sensation as the needle enters the amniotic cavity. Generally, fluid immediately flows into the needle, which is attached to a syringe. From 15 to 20 ml of amniotic fluid is withdrawn, placed in test tubes covered with tape (to shield the fluid from light to prevent breakdown of bilirubin and other pigments), and sent to the laboratory for analysis. The needle is withdrawn, and the FHR is measured for approximately 15 minutes. If the patient's vital signs and the FHR are normal, the patient is allowed to leave.

If the amniotic fluid becomes contaminated with blood, the fluid should be centrifuged immediately. The patient is observed closely for 30–40 minutes for alterations in the FHR. The blood should be tested to determine whether it is maternal or fetal by performing an Apt test. Some physicians routinely give Rh-negative mothers RhoGAM after amniocentesis, provided that they are not already sensitized at that time. If the amniotic fluid from these patients is contaminated with blood, the sample should be tested to identify fetal cells. In this situation, a larger dose of immune globulin is required.

Nursing Interventions

The nurse assists the physician during the amniocentesis. Nursing responsibilities are listed in Procedure 14–1. In addition, the nurse supports the patient undergoing amniocentesis. Patients are usually apprehensive about what is about to happen as well as about the information that will be obtained by amniocentesis. The physician generally explains the procedure as it is being performed, but the patient may need additional emotional support. She may become extremely anxious and upset during the procedure. There may be several persons in the room observing, which can be disturbing to the patient. In addition, she may become lightheaded, nauseated, and diaphoretic from lying on her back with a gravid uterus compressing the abdominal vessels. The nurse can provide support to the patient by further clarifying the physician's instructions or explanations, by relieving the woman's physical discomfort when possible, and by responding verbally and physically to the patient's need for reassurance.

Types of Amniotic Fluid Tests

L/S Ratio

The alveoli of the lungs are lined by a substance called *surfactant*, which is composed of phospholipids. Surfactant lowers the surface tension of the alveoli during extrauterine respiratory exhalation. By lowering the alveolar surface tension, surfactant stabilizes the alveoli, and a certain amount of air always remains in the alveoli during expiration. When a newborn with mature pulmonary function takes his first breath, a tremendously high pressure is needed to open the lungs. Upon breathing out, the lungs do not collapse and about half the air in the alveoli is retained. An infant born too early in his development, when synthesis of surfactant is incomplete, is unable to maintain lung stability, resulting in underinflation of the lungs and development of RDS.

Fetal lung maturity can be ascertained by determining the ratio of two components of surfactant—lecithin and sphingomyelin. Early in pregnancy the sphingomyelin concentration in amniotic fluid is more than that of lecithin, resulting in a low *lecithin/sphingomyelin* (L/S) *ratio.* At about 30–32 weeks' gestation, the amounts of the two substances become equal. The concentration of lecithin begins to exceed that of sphingomyelin, rising abruptly at about 35 weeks' gestation (Gluck, 1975). Concurrently, sphingomyelin begins to decrease. Fetal maturity is attained when the L/S ratio is 2:1 or greater; that is, when the amount of lecithin found in the amniotic fluid is at least two times that of sphingomyelin (Figure 14–14).

RDS is associated with pulmonary immaturity; thus RDS does not develop in infants whose L/S ratio is 2:1.

Laboratories vary in their criteria and methods for determining L/S ratios. One must be aware of these differences when interpreting results.

Under certain conditions of stress, premature maturation of the fetal lungs may be seen. The lung seems to react in different ways to acute and chronic stress. Conditions in which one may see accelerated maturation of the lungs include premature rupture of the membranes, acute placental infarction, placental insufficiency, chronic abruptio placentae, renal hypertensive disease due to degenerative forms of diabetes (classes D, E, F, and R), cardiovascular hypertensive disease, and severe chronic preeclampsia-eclampsia of pregnancy. In addition, the smaller of parabiotic twins may manifest lung maturity prematurely. Prolonged rupture of the membranes after 72 hours seems to have an acute effect on lung maturation, causing an abrupt rise in the L/S ratio (signifying lung maturity), independent of previous L/S ratios or gestational age (Richardson et al., 1974).

Delayed maturation is often seen in infants born to mothers with class A, B, and C diabetes, in those born to mothers with nonhypertensive glomerulonephritis or hydrops fetalis, and in the smaller of nonparabiotic twins (Gluck, 1975).

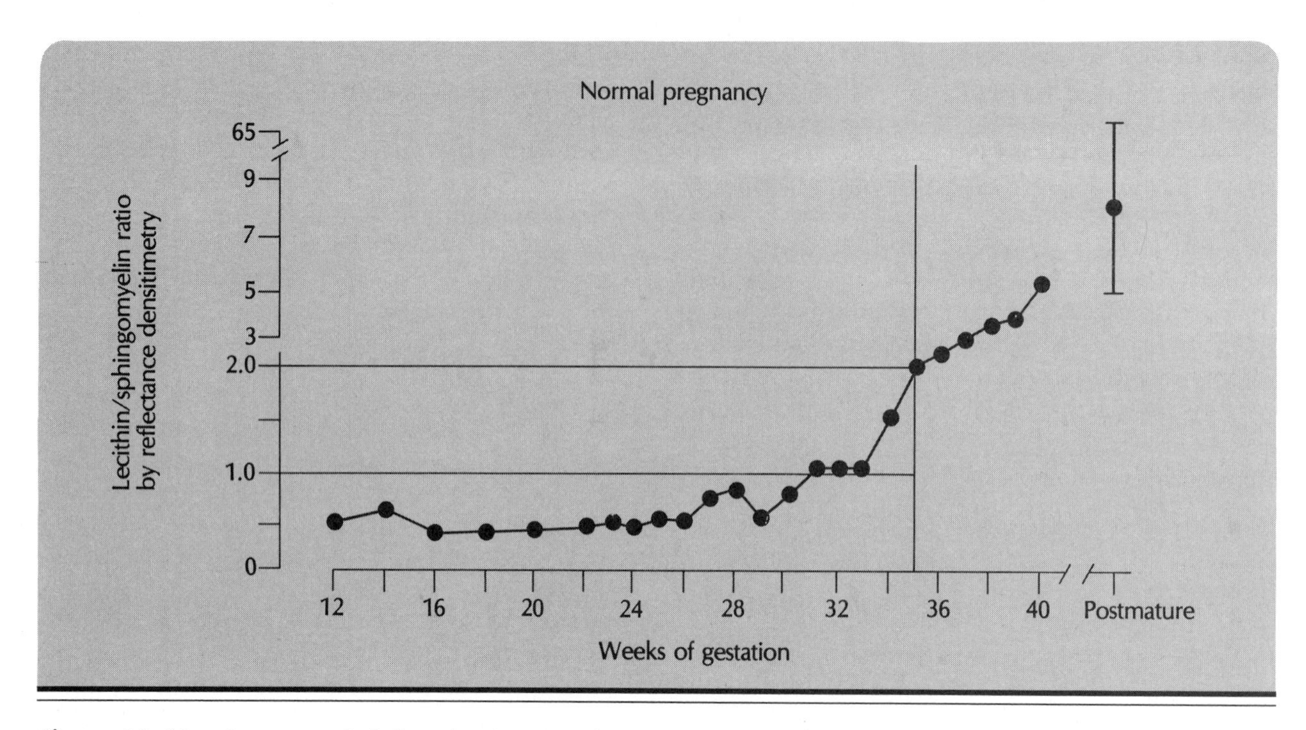

Figure 14–14. Progress of L/S ratio in normal pregnancy. (From Gluck, L., and Kulevich, M. V. 1973. Lecithin/sphingomyelin ratios in amniotic fluid in normal and abnormal pregnancy. *Am. J. Obstet. Gynecol.* 115:541.)

Shake Test (Foam Stability Test)

Introduced by Clements et al. (1972), the shake test is a quick and inexpensive test for prediction of fetal lung maturity. It is based on the ability of surfactant in the amniotic fluid to form bubbles or foam in the presence of ethanol. The test requires 15–30 minutes. Exact amounts of 95% ethanol, isotonic saline, and amniotic fluid are shaken together for 15 seconds. The persistence of a complete ring of bubbles on the surface of the liquid after 15 minutes indicates a positive shake test, indicating lung maturity. There is an extremely high false negative rate but a low false positive rate. Factors that may account for false negativity include dirty glass test tubes and contamination of the reagents or amniotic fluid. The L/S ratio test is normally not done when the shake test is positive, because the shake test indicates fetal lung maturity. If the optical density and creatinine values do not correlate with the shake test finding, the L/S ratio should be obtained regardless of the shake test result.

Optical Density

The measurement of optical density is a reflection of the amount of pigment bilirubin present in the amniotic fluid. Bilirubin may be found in amniotic fluid as early as the 12th week of pregnancy, reaching its highest concentrations between 16–30 weeks' gestation (Leiker and Hensleigh, 1975). As pregnancy continues, the amount of bilirubin progressively decreases, finally disappearing near term.

The amount of bilirubin in amniotic fluid can be determined by a technique described by Liley (1961): evaluation of the optical density (ΔOD) at 450 mu. Although this method cannot be used as an absolute indicator of fetal maturity, many investigators agree that, once the optical density of amniotic fluid falls to zero, fetal maturity is almost assured. Conditions in which increased values are found include anencephaly, intestinal obstruction, and sometimes deteriorating hydrops fetalis. Optical density cannot be used as an indication of fetal maturity in the Rh-sensitized patient.

Creatinine Level

Amniotic creatinine progressively increases as pregnancy advances. This may be due to excretion of fetal urine, reflecting fetal kidney function, or to muscle mass. The use of this value alone to assess maturity is not advisable, because a high creatinine value may be a reflection of muscle mass in a particular fetus and not necessarily indicate kidney maturity. For example, the macrosomic fetus of a diabetic mother may have high creatinine levels due to increased muscle mass, or the small, growth-retarded infant of the hypertensive may demonstrate a low level of creatinine due to decreased muscle mass; in these cases creatinine values can be misleading if used without other data. Nevertheless, when fetal growth (muscle mass) and kidney maturity are at odds, the creatinine is still more indicative of fetal kidney maturity. Creatinine levels of 2 mg/100 ml of amniotic fluid seem to correlate closely with a pregnancy of 37 weeks or more (Pitkin, 1975).

As long as the maternal serum creatinine is not elevated, measurement of creatinine level has a certain degree of reliability when used in conjunction with other maturity studies. An elevated maternal serum creatinine results in increased amniotic fluid levels. The mother's serum creatinine levels should be determined if the creatinine in the amniotic fluid is not what would normally be expected for a particular gestational age.

Cytologic Examination of Fetal Cells

One simple test of maturity, which can be done in the physician's office or at the bedside, is the staining of fetal fat cells in the amniotic fluid with Nile blue sulfate. The fetus sheds cells during its intrauterine life. In the last weeks of pregnancy the sebaceous glands gradually begin to function and cells are sloughed into the amniotic fluid. Sebaceous cells are different from other fetal cells in that they contain lipid globules. The number of these fat cells increases as the fetus matures, and the percentage of these cells present in the amniotic fluid gives an indication of gestational age. When the number of sebaceous cells (which stain orange with Nile blue sulfate) is less than 2%, there is a prematurity rate of about 85%. If more than 20% of the cells in the fluid stain orange, the infant will weigh at least 2500 gm. Andrews (1970) states that, if 10% of the cells stain orange, the gestational age is 36 weeks in about 95% of cases. Others use 20% as the critical level of maturity.

AMNIOSCOPY

Visualization of the amniotic fluid through the membranes with an amnioscope is a technique employed to identify meconium staining of the fluid. As mentioned previously, this staining frequently indicates that there has been an episode of fetal hypoxia, causing relaxation of the rectal sphincter with resultant passage of meconium into the amniotic fluid. In many institutions, evidence of meconium in the amniotic fluid is an indication for delivery. In other centers, additional evidence of fetal distress must be demonstrated before delivery is contemplated.

Problems associated with amnioscopy include the possibility of inadvertently rupturing the membranes during the examination, an insufficiently dilated cervix through which to insert the amnioscope, intrauterine infection, and occasional difficulty in interpreting the color of the amniotic fluid. Amnioscopy may be a difficult procedure to perform if the patient is in active labor, because she may have difficulty maintaining proper position for the examination.

X-RAY EXAMINATION

Because of the increasing popularity and use of diagnostic ultrasound, x-ray examination is not employed as frequently as it was in the past. X-ray examination may be used to measure the diameters of the pelvis (pelvimetry) late in pregnancy or during labor. It can also give information regarding shape and size of the pelvis and the relationship of the baby's presentation, position, and station to the mother's pelvis. An x-ray examination may be performed when clinical pelvimetry is questionable, when abnormal presentation and position is evidenced, when labor is prolonged or arrested, or if abnormal development of the fetus is suspected.

Fetal body length and head diameters are almost impossible to measure, but it is possible to estimate fetal age by the appearance of ossification centers. By the 36th week of pregnancy, the distal femoral epiphysis is present in approximately 80% or more of infants; there is evidence of the proximal tibial epiphysis in 70% to 75% of fetuses at term. The time of appearance of ossification centers seems to be affected by race and sex. The ability to demonstrate these ossification centers by x-ray examination confirms the duration of pregnancy, but their absence does not negate maturity.

Whenever a woman in labor must go to the x-ray department, it is imperative that a nurse accompany her with an emergency delivery pack. The patient is often frightened and worried, because there is obviously something abnormal taking place. The nurse's presence can be reassuring to the patient because the nurse can handle the situation should the patient deliver. Frequently, the patient is left alone by the x-ray technicians or attendants for short periods of time, and the presence of the nurse can be of much comfort to her. The nurse can also be of help in positioning the patient for taking the films. The nurse should at all times be aware of the progress of labor and notify the physician immediately if delivery seems imminent.

IMPLICATIONS OF PRENATAL TESTING FOR DELIVERY

Fainstat (1977) provides guidelines for prenatal testing in relation to timing of delivery for the high-risk mother (Table 14–2). It seems to be the general opinion that when both OCTs and estriol levels indicate fetal jeopardy, whether or not the fetus is mature it should be delivered. If either test indicates jeopardy and if lung maturity has been attained, the physician usually chooses to deliver the infant. If only one of the parameters of fetal health status signifies jeopardy and the fetus is immature, the mother is usually not delivered immediately but rather observed closely and delivered when fetal lung maturity is reached or when further evidence of fetal jeopardy or deterioration of her condition is found.

Table 14–2. Guidelines for Use of Antenatal Tests of Fetal Health As Adjuncts in Timing of Delivery*

Fetal jeopardy				Fetal maturity (L/S; serial sonograms)	Clinical disposition
	OCT		Estriol		
Both	+	and	↓	Mature or immature	Deliver
Either	+	or	↓	Mature	Usually delivered
Either	+	or	↓	Immature	Not delivered; follow closely: daily estriols; repeat OCT and L/S Deliver when L/S mature or estriol ↓ and OCT +

+ signifies positive OCT
↓ signifies low or fallen estriol levels

*From Fainstat, T. Preventing perinatal morbidity and mortality. Reprinted with permission from *Continuing Education for the Family Physician*, vol. 6, May 1977.

NAME ______ HOSP. # ______
ADDRESS ______ PHONE ______
PHYSICIAN ______
GRAVIDA ______ PARA ______ AGE ______
E.D.C ______ L.M.P. ______
DATE ______ WEEKS GEST. ______
INDICATIONS FOR O.C.T. ______

PAST AND PRESENT HISTORY	AMNIOCENTESIS	SONOGRAM	OTHER TESTS
MENSES (regular, irregular) ORAL CONTRACEPTIVES CONCEPTION DATE FHTs HEARD 1ST EXAM PREGNANCY TEST QUICKENING			

O.C.T.						SERUM ESTRIOL	OXYTOCINASE	ESTRIOL (URINE)
DATE	GEST.	ACC. F.M.	METHOD	RESULTS				

REMARKS AND OUTCOME OF PREGNANCY:

Figure 14–15. Sample summary form to be used in monitoring the results of diagnostic procedures performed on the high-risk prenatal patient. (Courtesy N. A. McCluggage, R.N., C.N.M., and M. Imhof, R.N., M.S.)

SUMMARY

It is difficult to assess fetal status in many situations. Each patient must be treated individually in light of her specific circumstances. In addition, there is no one system of care intended for all high-risk patients. Clinical judgment by the attending physician, based on data obtained during the nursing assessment and coupled with appropriate tests of fetal well-being, will ultimately aid in deciding each patient's outcome.

One of the most difficult problems in the management of the high-risk patient is timing of delivery. The physician must weigh the possible disadvantages of delivering a premature infant against the risk to that fetus of remaining in his unhealthy, less than optimal intrauterine environment. For this reason, highly intensive obstetric care and an accurate index of fetal well-being (Figure 14-15) are essential for the management of this patient.

The expert clinical judgment and care rendered by the attending physician and other highly specialized associates is of the greatest significance. The many studies and tests available to the woman at risk are used only as adjuncts to good clinical management, and these tests are of little value if the patient does not understand her condition and assume some of the responsibility for her own management and care. Generally, patients are willing to participate in their care, keep regular appointments, inform their physician about changes in their health status, and cooperate in necessary evaluation procedures. Unfortunately, the group of women in which maternal and infant mortality and morbidity are highest is also the group least motivated or able to cooperate in their health maintenance. These patients are frequently of low socioeconomic status, poorly educated, poorly nourished, and/or teenagers. Much time and effort is required to educate these women to ensure that they receive optimum care and follow-up.

The nurse is in a prime position to offer support and reassurance and to provide valuable input for the care of the high-risk patient. Through the nurse's efforts, the flow of information to and from the patient at risk can be maintained, thus ensuring optimal care for both her and her unborn child. In addition, the establishment of regionalized centers for high-risk pregnant patients, with specialized teams of workers and with electronic and biochemical monitoring of the fetus, will further enhance the potential for a successful childbirth experience.

SUGGESTED ACTIVITIES

1. In a small group discussion, describe how you would provide support to a patient having amniocentesis.
2. Arrange with your instructor to observe an amniocentesis and the various tests performed on the amniotic fluid.
3. With a classmate, role play a situation in which you as the nurse must explain the purpose of an OCT, and the procedure for doing it, to a patient.

REFERENCES

Andrews, B. F. 1970. Amniotic fluid studies to determine maturity. *Pediatr. Clin. N. Am.* 17:49.

Bevis, D. C. A. 1956. Blood pigments in haemolytic disease of the newborn. *J. Obstet. Gynaecol. Br. Emp.* 63:68.

Clements, J. A., et al. 1972. Assessment of the risk of respiratory distress syndrome by a rapid test for surfactant in amniotic fluid. *N. Engl. J. Med.* 286:1077.

Fainstat, T. 1977. Preventing perinatal morbidity and mortality. *Cont. Ed. Family Phys.* 6:67.

Freeman, R. 1975. The use of the oxytocin challenge test for antepartum clinical evaluation of uteroplacental respiratory function. *Am. J. Obstet. Gynecol.* 121:487.

Gluck, L. 1975. Fetal maturity and amniotic fluid surfactant determinations. In *Management of the high-risk pregnancy,* ed. W. N. Spellacy. Baltimore: University Park Press.

Gobelsmann, U. April 1977. The clinical value of estriol determinations. From the proceedings of the Second International Symposium on Perinatal Medicine. Las Vegas, Nev.

Goldstein, A. I. 1977. Amniocentesis: indications, techniques, complications and alpha-fetoprotein. In *Advances in perinatal medicine,* ed. A. Goldstein. New York: Symposia Specialists, Stratton Intercontinental Medical Books Corp.

Green, J. W., et al. 1969. Correlation of estriol excretion patterns of pregnant women with subsequent development of their children. *Am. J. Obstet. Gynecol.* 105:730.

Greenwald, P. 1970. Perinatal death of full-sized and full-term infants. *Am. J. Obstet. Gynecol.* 107:1022.

Hon, E. H., and Quilligan, E. J. 1967. The classification of fetal heart rate. II. A revised working classification. *Conn. Med.* 31:781.

Kubli, R. W., et al. 1969. In *The feto-placental unit,* eds. Pecile and Finzi. Amsterdam: Excerpta Medica Foundation.

Lee, C. Y., et al. 1975. A study of fetal heart rate acceleration patterns. *Obstet. Gynecol.* 45:142.

Leiker, J., and Hensleigh, P. 1975. Amniotic fluid analysis. *J. Kansas Med. Soc.* 76:159.

Leopold, G., and Asher, W. 1975. *Fundamentals of abdominal and pelvic ultrasonography.* Philadelphia: W. B. Saunders Co.

Liley, A. W. 1961. Liquor amnii analysis in the management of the pregnancy complicated by rhesus sensitization. *Am. J. Obstet. Gynecol.* 82:1359.

Manning, F. A. 1977. Fetal breathing movements. *Postgrad. Med.* 61:116.

McQuown, D. 1977. Ultrasound in pregnancy. In *Advances in perinatal medicine,* ed. A. Goldstein. New York: Symposia Specialists, Stratton Intercontinental Medical Books Corp.

O'Sullivan, M. J. 1976. Acute and chronic fetal distress. *J. Reprod. Med.* 17:320.

Patrick, J. E., et al. 1978. Human fetal breathing movements and gross fetal body movements at weeks 34–35 of gestation. *Am. J. Obstet. Gynecol.* 130:693.

Pitkin, R. M. 1975. Fetal maturity: nonlipid amniotic fluid assessment. In *Management of the high-risk pregnancy,* ed. W. N. Spellacy. Baltimore: University Park Press.

Platt, L. D., et al. 1978. Human fetal breathing relationships to fetal condition. *Am. J. Obstet. Gynecol.* 132:514.

Queenan, J., et al. 1976. Diagnostic ultrasound for detection of intrauterine growth retardation. *Am. J. Obstet. Gynecol.* 124:870.

Ragan, W. Sept. 1976. Ultrasound in obstetrics. *Am. Family Physician.* 14(3):130.

Richardson, C. J., et al. 1974. Acceleration of fetal lung maturation following prolonged rupture of the membranes. *Am. J. Obstet. Gynecol.* 118:1115.

Rochard, F., et al. 1976. Nonstressed fetal heart rate monitoring in the antepartum period. *Am. J. Obstet. Gynecol.* 126:699.

Schifrin, B. S. April 1977. Antepartum fetal heart rate monitoring. From the proceedings of the Second International Symposium on Perinatal Medicine. Las Vegas, Nev.

Schifrin, B. S., and Dame, L. 1972. Fetal heart rate patterns: prediction of Apgar score. *JAMA.* 219:1322.

Schifrin, B. S., et al. 1975. Contraction stress test for antepartum fetal evaluation. *Am. J. Obstet. Gynecol.* 45:436.

Taylor, E. S., ed. 1971. *Beck's obstetric practice.* 9th ed. Baltimore: The Williams & Wilkins Co.

Thompson, H. E., et al. 1965. Fetal development as determined by ultrasonic pulse echo technique. *Am. J. Obstet. Gynecol.* 92:44.

Trierweiler, M. W., et al. 1976. Baseline fetal heart rate characteristics as an indicator of fetal status during the antepartum period. *Am. J. Obstet. Gynecol.* 125:623.

Tulchinsky, D. 1975. The value of estrogen assays in obstetric disease. In *Plasma hormone assays in evaluation of fetal well-being,* ed. A. Klopper. Edinburgh: Churchill Livingstone.

Weingold, A. B. 1975. Intrauterine growth retardation: obstetrical aspects. *J. Reprod. Med.* 14:244.

ADDITIONAL READINGS

Aladjem, S., and Brown, A. 1977. *Perinatal intensive care.* St. Louis: The C. V. Mosby Co.

Botella-Liusia, J. 1974. Clinical aspects of placental insufficiency. In *Clinical perinatology,* eds. S. Aladjem and A. K. Brown. St. Louis: The C. V. Mosby Co.

Campbell, S. 1974. Fetal growth. *Clin. Obstet. Gynecol.* 1:41.

Crane, J., et al. 1976. A high risk pregnancy management protocol. *Am. J. Obstet. Gynecol.* 125:229.

Duhring, J. L. 1974. The high risk fetus. *Hosp. Med.* 10:77.

Duhring, J. L., et al. 1976. Amniotic fluid analysis in Rh-sensitized pregnancies. *Am. J. Obstet. Gynecol.* 125:368.

Gluck, L. 1973. Lecithin/sphingomyelin ratios in amniotic fluid in normal and abnormal pregnancy. *Am. J. Obstet. Gynecol.* 115:539.

Gluck, L. 1975. Fetal lung maturity. In *Progress in clinical and biological research, Vol. 2: Preventability of perinatal injury,* eds. K. Adamsons and H. Fox. New York: Alan R. Liss, Inc.

Gluck, L. 1975. *Management of the high-risk pregnancy and intensive care of the neonate.* 3rd ed. St. Louis: The C. V. Mosby Co.

Gluck, L. 1976. Lung maturation and the prevention of hyaline membrane disease. In *Report of the seventieth Ross conference on pediatric research,* ed. T. D. Moore. Columbus, Ohio: Ross Laboratories.

Gluck, L. April 1977. The role of fetal stress in induction of pulmonary maturity. From the proceedings of the Second International Symposium on Perinatal Medicine. Las Vegas, Nev.

Gluck, L., et al. 1971. Diagnosis of the respiratory distress syndrome by amniocentesis. *Am. J. Obstet. Gynecol.* 109:440.

Kantor, G. K. Sept.–Oct. 1978. Addicted mother, addicted baby—a challenge to health care providers. *MCN.* 4:281.

Littlefield, V., and Subert, G. Sept.–Oct. 1978. The group approach to problem-solving for pregnant diabetic women. *MCN.* 4:274.

Lubchenco, L. O., et al. 1963. Intrauterine growth as estimated from liveborn birth weights data at 24 to 42 weeks of gestation. *Pediatrics.* 32:793.

Nelson, G. H. 1969. Amniotic fluid phospholipid patterns in normal and abnormal pregnancies—term. *Am. J. Obstet. Gynecol.* 105:1072.

Pritchard, J. A., and MacDonald, P. C. *Williams obstetrics.* 15th ed. New York: Appleton-Century-Crofts.

Ray, M. et al. 1972. Clinical experience with the oxytocin challenge test. *Am. J. Obstet. Gynecol.* 114:1.

Sabbagha, R. E. 1975. Ultrasound in managing the high-risk pregnancy. In *Management of the high-risk pregnancy,* ed. W. N. Spellacy. Baltimore: University Park Press.

Weingold, A., et al. 1975. Oxytocin challenge test. *Am. J. Obstet. Gynecol.* 123:466.

Wilson, J. R., et al. 1975. *Obstetrics and gynecology.* 5th ed. St. Louis: The C. V. Mosby Co.

UNIT IV

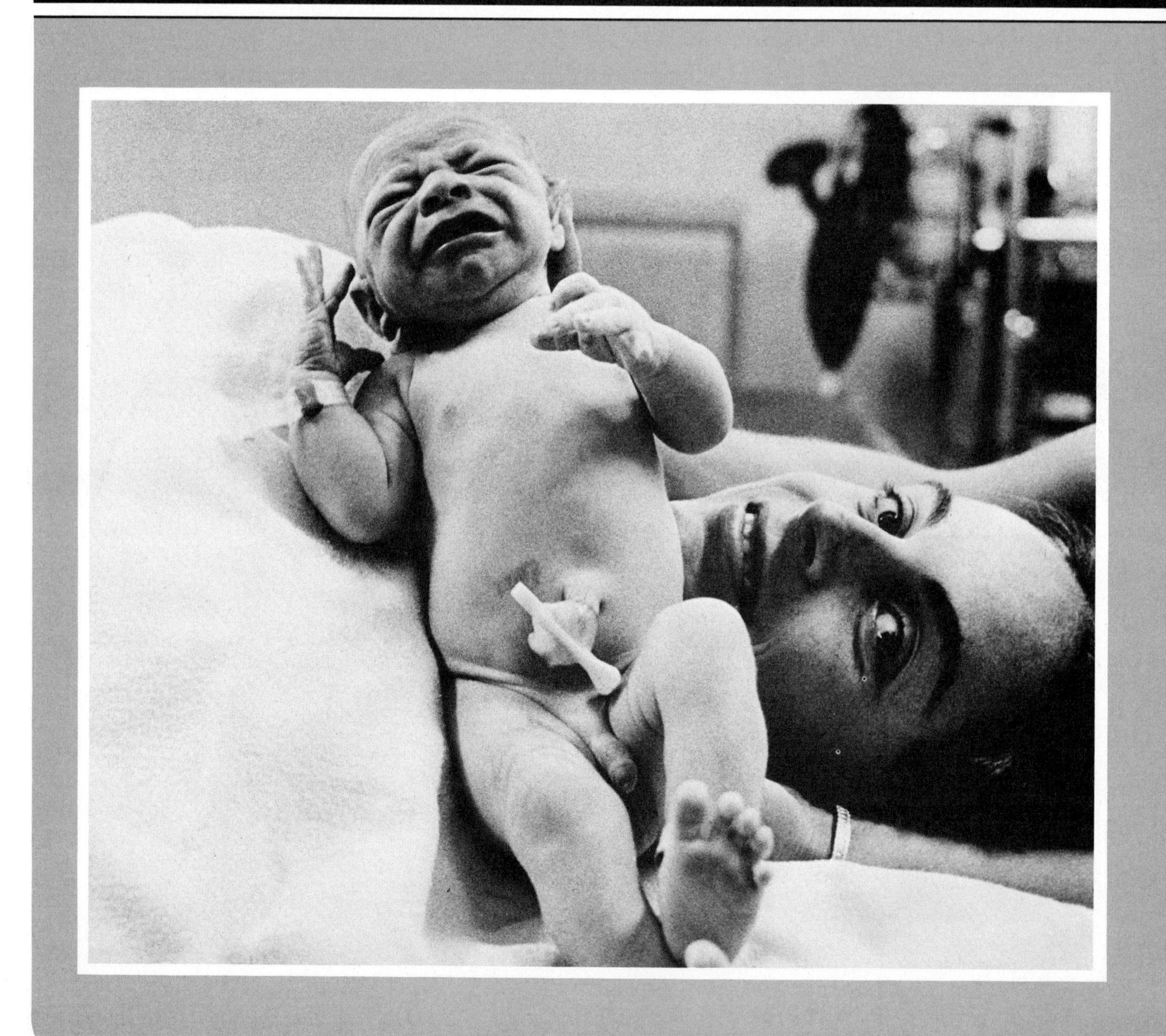

LABOR AND DELIVERY

CHAPTER 15

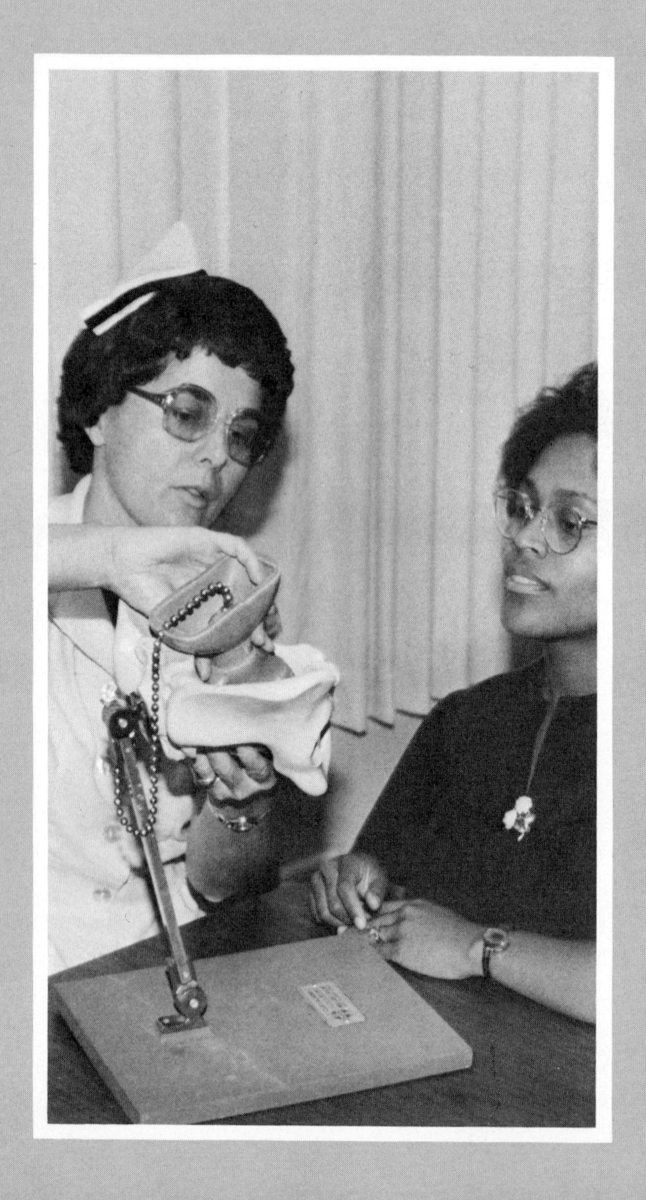

PROCESSES AND STAGES OF LABOR

OBJECTIVES

- Discuss the significance of each type of pelvis to the birth process.
- Discuss the factors that influence labor and the physiology of the mechanisms of labor.
- Differentiate between false and true labor.
- Describe the fetal positional changes that constitute the mechanisms of labor.
- Discuss the probable causes of labor onset and the premonitory signs of labor.
- Describe the physiologic changes occurring in each of the stages of labor.

The process of labor and delivery is the culmination of the entire maternity cycle, and it marks the ultimate crisis to the childbearing woman, the fetus, and the family. The series of events by which the fetus, placenta, amniotic fluid, and fetal membranes (the products of conception) are expelled from the maternal body is appropriately called *labor* because this word implies an expenditure of energy to obtain a goal or product. The terms *childbirth, parturition,* and *confinement* have been used as synonyms for this process.

During the months of gestation, the fetus and the gravid woman prepare to accommodate themselves to each other during the birth process. The fetus progresses through various stages of growth and development, preparing for the independence of extrauterine life. The gravid woman undergoes various physiologic and psychologic adaptations during pregnancy that gradually prepare her for childbirth and the role of mother. For both woman and fetus the onset of labor marks a significant change in their relationship.

CRITICAL FACTORS IN LABOR

Four factors are of critical importance in planning individualized nursing care for the laboring patient: the passage, the passenger, the powers, and the psyche. The "four Ps," as they are commonly known, are defined as follows:

1. Passage
   a. Size of the pelvis (diameters of the pelvic inlet, midpelvis, and outlet)
   b. Type of pelvis (gynecoid, anthropoid, platypelloid, or android)
   c. Ability of the cervix to dilate and efface and ability of the vaginal canal and introitus to distend
2. Passenger
   a. Fetal head (size and presence of molding)
   b. Fetal attitude (flexion or extension of the fetal body and extremities)
   c. Fetal lie
   d. Fetal presentation (the part of the fetal body entering the pelvis in a single or multiple pregnancy)
   e. Fetal position (relationship of the presenting part to the pelvis)
3. Psyche
   a. Physical preparation for childbirth
   b. Racial and sociocultural heritage
   c. Previous childbirth experience
   d. Support from significant others
   e. Emotional integrity
4. Powers
   a. The frequency, duration, and intensity of uterine contractions as the passenger is moved through the passage
   b. The duration of labor

The progress of labor is critically dependent on the complementary relationship of these four factors. Abnormalities in the passage, the passenger, the psyche, or the powers can alter the outcome of labor and jeopardize both the gravid woman and the fetus (Nurses Association of the American College of Obstetricians and Gynecologists, 1974; Jensen et al., 1977). Complications involving the four Ps are discussed in Chapter 19.

The Passage

In both males and females the pelvis provides support for the body weight and for the lower extremities. In the female, however, the pelvis must also adapt to the demands of childbearing (Pritchard and MacDonald, 1976). Because the process of labor essentially involves the accommodation of the fetus to the bony pelvis through which it must descend, the size and shape of the maternal pelvis must be assessed by the health care team.

The obstetric pelvis may be divided into the false pelvis and the true pelvis. The false pelvis helps support the pregnant uterus. The true pelvis, which forms the bony canal through which the baby must pass, is divided into three sections: the inlet, the pelvic cavity (midpelvis), and the outlet. These are described in detail in Chapter 4, as are the pelvic measurements that influence the childbirth outcome. The techniques used to determine these measurements are described in Chapter 16.

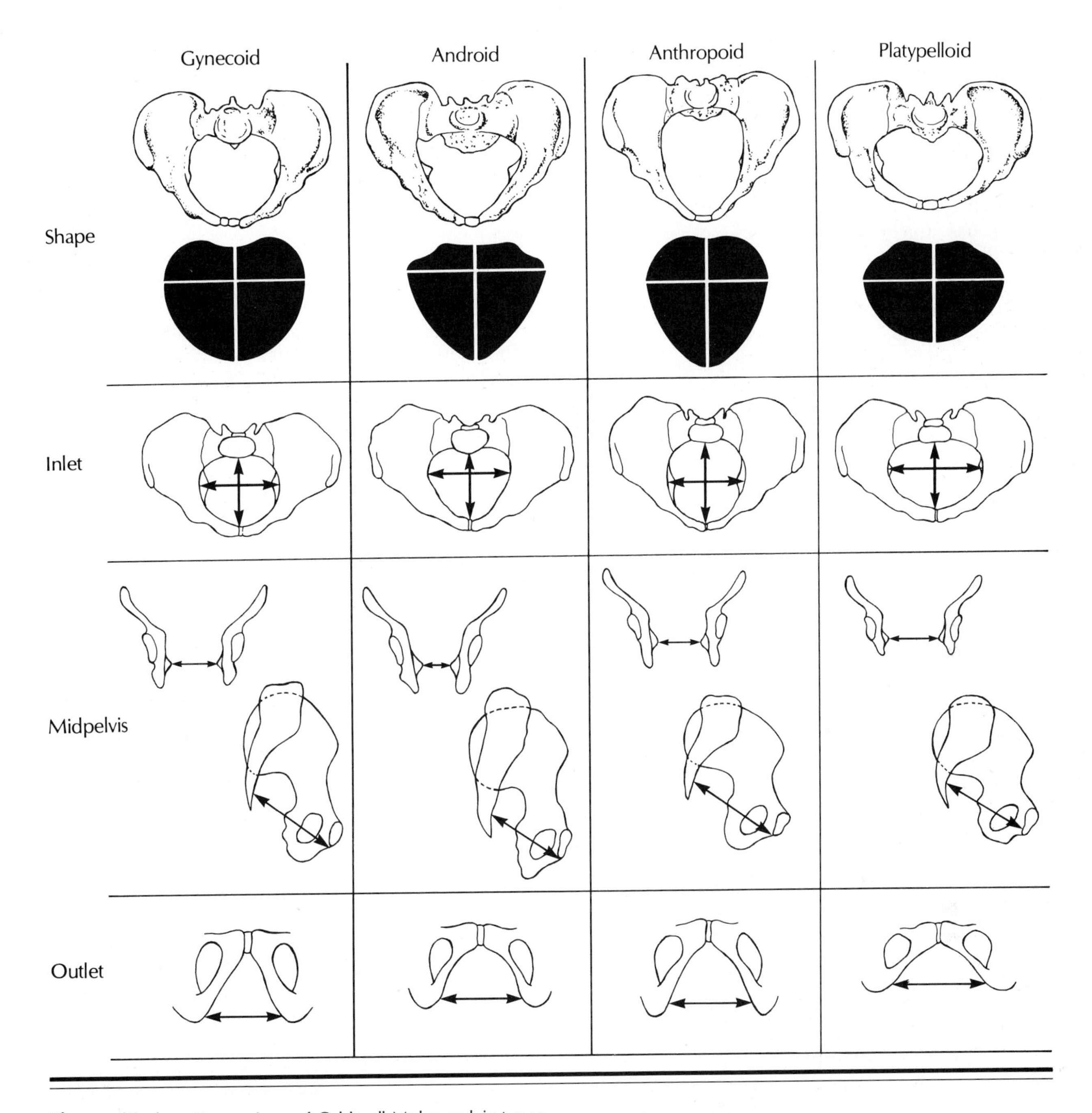

Figure 15–1. Comparison of Caldwell-Moloy pelvic types.

Types of Pelves

Familiarity with the types of pelves contributes to the understanding of the mechanism of labor and of the relationship of passage, passenger, and powers during the intrapartal period. The Caldwell-Moloy classification of the types of pelves is based on pertinent characteristics of both male and female pelves (Caldwell and Moloy, 1933). Consideration is given to the size of the sacrosciatic notch, flaring of the pelvic brim, the shape of the inlet, and the relationship of the greatest anteroposterior diameter to the greatest transverse diameter.

The four classic types of pelves are gynecoid, android, anthropoid, and platypelloid (Figure 15–1). Mixed types of pelvic configurations occur more frequently than pure types.

Gynecoid Pelvis. The normal female pelvis is the gynecoid type (see Figure 15–1). The inlet is rounded, with the anteroposterior diameter a little shorter than the transverse diameter. All the inlet diameters are adequate at least. The posterior segment is broad, deep, and roomy, and the anterior segment is well rounded. The gynecoid midpelvis has nonprominent ischial spines, straight and parallel side walls, and a wide, deep sacral curve. The sacrum is short and slopes backward. All of the midpelvic diameters are at least adequate. The gynecoid pelvic outlet has a wide and round pubic arch; the inferior pubic rami are short and concave. The anteroposterior diameter is long and the transverse diameter adequate. The capacity of the outlet is adequate. The bones are of medium structure and weight.

Approximately 50% of female pelves are classified as gynecoid. The influence of a gynecoid pelvis on labor is favorable. Descent is facilitated and rapid because the fetal head usually engages in the transverse or oblique diameter with adequate flexion and station occurs at midpelvis. The occipital anterior position at delivery is common (Oxorn and Foote, 1975).

Android Pelvis. The normal male type is the android pelvis (see Figure 15–1). The inlet is heart-shaped. The anteroposterior and transverse diameters are adequate for delivery, but the posterior sagittal diameter is too short and the anterior sagittal diameter is long. The posterior segment is shallow because the sacral promontory is indented, resulting in a reduced capacity. The anterior segment is narrow, and the forepelvis is sharply angled. The android midpelvis has prominent ischial spines, convergent side walls, and a long, heavy sacrum inclining forward. All the midpelvic diameters are reduced. The distance from the linea terminalis to the ischial tuberosities is long, yet the overall capacity of the midpelvis is reduced. The android outlet has a narrow, sharp, and deep pubic arch; the inferior pubic rami are straight and long. The anteroposterior diameter is short and the transverse diameter is narrow. The capacity of the outlet is reduced. The bones are of medium to heavy structure and weight.

Approximately 20% of female pelves are classified as android. The influence of an android pelvis on labor is not favorable. Descent into the pelvis is slow. The fetal head usually engages in the transverse or occipital posterior diameter in asynclitism with extreme molding. Arrest of labor is frequent, requiring difficult forceps manipulations (rotation and extraction), and the deep, narrow pubic arch may lead to extensive perineal lacerations. Cesarean section may be required.

Anthropoid Pelvis. The anthropoid pelvis is often described as apelike (see Figure 15–1). The inlet is oval, with a long anteroposterior diameter and an adequate but rather short transverse diameter. Both the posterior and anterior segments are deep; the posterior sagittal diameter is extremely long, as is the anterior sagittal diameter. The anthropoid midpelvis has variable ischial spines, straight side walls, and a narrow and long sacrum that inclines backward. The midpelvic diameters are at least adequate, making its capacity adequate. The anthropoid outlet has a normal or moderately narrow pubic arch; the inferior pubic rami are long and narrow. The outlet capacity is adequate, and the bones are of medium weight and structure.

Approximately 25% of female pelves are classified as anthropoid. The influence of the anthropoid pelvis on labor is favorable. Usually the fetal head engages in the anteroposterior or oblique diameter in the occipital-posterior position. Labor and delivery progress well.

Platypelloid Pelvis. The platypelloid type refers to the flat female pelvis (see Figure 15–1). The inlet is distinctly transverse oval, with a short anteroposterior and extremely short transverse diameter. The posterior sagittal and anterior sagittal diameters are short. Both the anterior and posterior segments are shallow. The platypelloid midpelvis has variable ischial spines, parallel side walls, and a wide sacrum with a deep curve inward. Only the transverse diameter is adequate; thus the midpelvic capacity is reduced. The platypelloid outlet has an extremely wide pubic arch; the inferior pubic rami are straight and short. The transverse diameter is wide but the anteroposterior diameter is short. The outlet capacity is inadequate. The platypelloid bones are similar to the gynecoid type.

Only 5% of female pelves are classified as platypelloid. The influence of the platypelloid pelvis on labor is not favorable. The fetal head usually engages in the transverse diameter with marked asynclitism. If the infant can traverse the inlet, it rotates at or below the spines, and delivery is rapid through the wide arch. But frequently there is delay of progress at the inlet, requiring a cesarean section.

The Passenger

The fetal passenger must accommodate itself to the maternal passage during labor. To pass through the relatively immobile pelvis, the fetus goes through a series of maneuvers to align its body.

Movement of the fetus through the pelvis involves the articulation of the ovoids of the fetus to the ovoids presented by the pelvis. The inlet of the pelvis presents a transverse ovoid, and the midpelvis and outlet present an oval passage that is anteroposterior or perpendicular to the ovoid of the inlet. The fetus brings to the laboring process two oval parts with a movable articulation at the neck. In a cephalic presentation the passenger first presents an anteroposterior ovoid (the head), followed by a second ovoid (the shoulders) in a transverse direction. Herein lies the problem. The fetal head must enter the pelvis in a transverse position and be rotated by the powers of labor to enter the midpelvis in an anteroposterior position. The shoulders of the passenger meanwhile must enter the inlet in a transverse position. As the head is lowered into the outlet, the shoulders are compressed and are rotated into the anteroposterior ovoid of the midpelvis (Oxorn and Foote, 1975).

Fetal Head

The fetal head is composed of bony parts that can hinder or enhance childbirth. Once the head (the least compressible and largest part of the fetus) has been delivered, there is rarely a delay in the birth of the rest of the passenger's body. Occasionally there is difficulty in delivering the fetal shoulders under the pubis symphysis or over the coccyx; this shoulder dystocia (difficult labor) may require increased manipulation by the obstetrician, which may fracture the passenger's clavicle or the mother's coccyx.

The fetal skull is composed of three major divisions: the face, the base of the skull, and the vault of the cranium (roof). The bones of the face and base are well fused and are basically fixed. The base of the cranium is composed of the two temporal bones: the sphenoid and the ethmoid bones. The bones composing the vault are the two frontal bones, the two parietal bones, and the occipital bone (Figure 15-2). These bones are not fused, allowing this portion of the head to adjust in shape as the presenting part of the passenger passes through the narrow portions of the pelvis. This overlapping of the cranial bones under pressure of the powers of labor and the demands of the unyielding pelvis is called *molding* (see Figure 19-5).

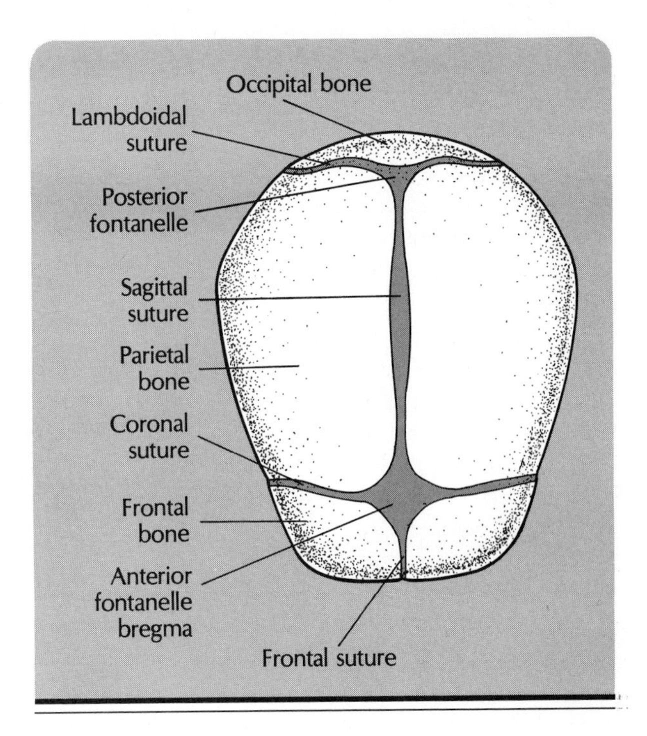

Figure 15-2. Superior view of the fetal skull.

The *sutures* of the fetal skull are membranous spaces between the cranial bones. The intersections of the cranial sutures are called *fontanelles.* Presence of these sutures allows for molding of the passenger's head and assists the examiner in identifying the position of the fetal head on vaginal examination. The important sutures of the cranial vault are as follows (see Figure 15-2):

- *Frontal suture:* Located between the two frontal bones; becomes the anterior continuation of the sagittal suture.
- *Sagittal suture:* Located between the parietal bones; divides the skull into left and right halves; runs anteroposterior, connecting the two fontanelles.

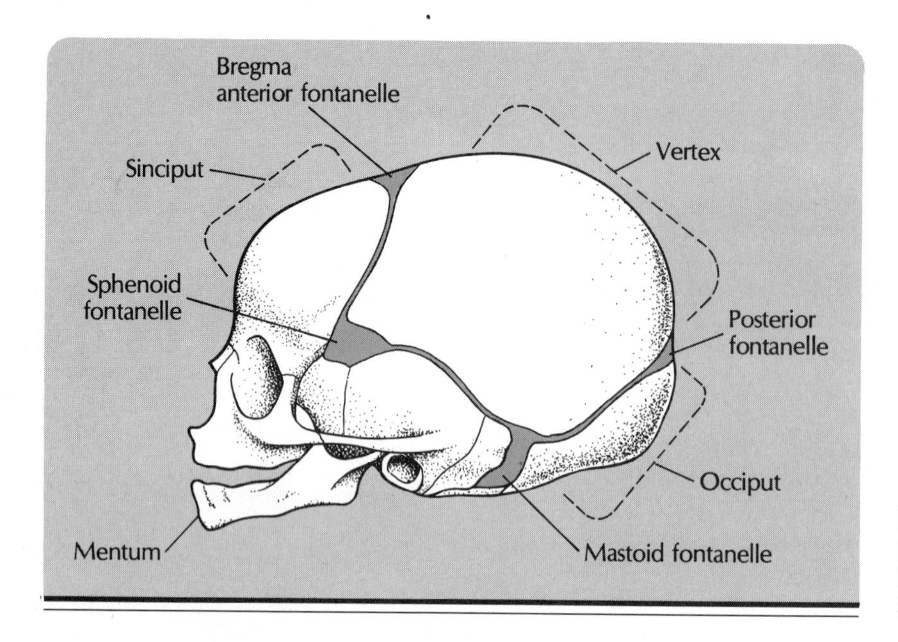

Figure 15-3. Lateral view of the fetal skull. The landmarks that have significance in obstetrics are identified.

- *Coronal sutures:* Located between the parietal and frontal lobes; extend transversely left and right from the anterior fontanelle.
- *Lambdoidal suture:* Located between the two parietal bones and the occipital bone; extends transversely left and right from the posterior fontanelle.

The anterior and posterior fontanelles are clinically useful in identifying the position of the fetal head in the maternal pelvis and in assessing the status of the newborn after birth. The anterior fontanelle is diamond-shaped and measures 2 × 3 cm; it facilitates growth of the brain by remaining unossified for as long as 18 months. The posterior fontanelle is much smaller and closes within 8 to 12 weeks after birth; it is shaped like a small triangle and marks the meeting point of the sagittal suture and the lambdoidal suture (Oxorn and Foote, 1975).

Following are several important landmarks of the fetal skull (Figure 15-3):

- *Sinciput:* The anterior area known as the brow.
- *Bregma:* The large diamond-shaped anterior fontanelle.
- *Vertex:* The area between the anterior and posterior fontanelles.
- *Posterior fontanelle.*
- *Occiput:* The area of the fetal skull occupied by the occipital bone, beneath the posterior fontanelle.
- *Mentum:* The fetal chin.

The diameters of the fetal skull vary considerably within normal limits. Some diameters shorten and others lengthen as the head is molded during labor. Fetal head diameters are measured between the various landmarks on the skull (Figure 15-4). The compound words used to designate the various diameters allow one to decipher which measurement is actually being reported. For example, the biparietal diameter is measured between the parietal bosses, or prominences; similarly, the suboccipitobregmatic diameter notes the distance from the undersurface of the occiput to the center of the bregma, or anterior fontanelle. Fetal skull measurements are given in Figure 15-4.

Much can be learned from these diameters regarding the degree of extension or flexion of the fetal head. Extension of the head results in a larger diameter presenting than if the head is strongly flexed. Alterations in flexion of the fetal head can yield problems during the process of labor. The fetus endeavors to accommodate its most favorable head diameters to the limited measurements of the bony pelvis (Greenhill and Friedman, 1974).

Fetal Attitude

Fetal attitude, or habitus, refers to the relation of the fetal parts to one another. The normal attitude of the fetus, providing there is adequate amniotic

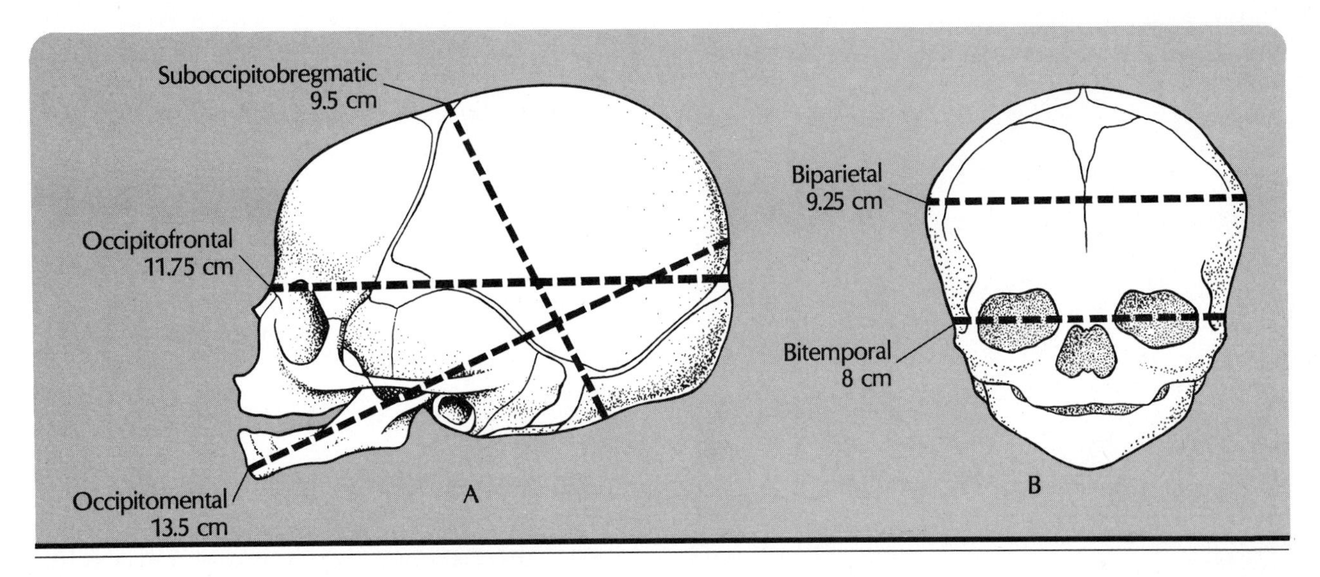

Figure 15-4. **A,** Anteroposterior diameters of the fetal skull. When the vertex of the fetus presents and the fetal head is flexed with the chin on the chest, the smallest anteroposterior diameter (suboccipitobregmatic) enters the birth canal. **B,** Transverse diameters of the fetal skull.

fluid, is one of moderate flexion of the head and extremities on the abdomen and chest. This ovoid attitude has been called the *fetal position.* The back bows outward, the chin rests on the sternum, and the arms and thighs are flexed on the chest and abdomen. The fetus assumes various attitudes during the pregnancy, flexing and extending the arms, legs, and body. A strongly flexed and cramped attitude is maintained if the fetus has insufficient space in which to stretch, such as occurs in oligohydramnios (scant amniotic fluid) (Greenhill and Friedman, 1974; Reeder et al., 1976).

Alterations in fetal attitude cause the fetus to present various diameters of the head to the maternal passage. With increased extension of the passenger's head, a larger diameter of the fetal skull must be accommodated by the pelvis. This alteration from a normal fetal attitude often contributes to a difficult labor. The fetus assumes a military attitude (chin up, shoulders back) when the head is moderately extended. Marked and excessive extension of the fetal head yield brow and face presentations.

Fetal Lie

Fetal lie refers to the relationship of the cephalocaudal axis of the fetus to the cephalocaudal axis of the mother. The passenger may assume either a transverse lie or a longitudinal lie. A *transverse lie* occurs when the long axis of the fetus is perpendicular to the mother's spine. The abdomen appears oval from left to right, with the buttocks of the fetus on one side and the head on the other. A *longitudinal lie* is assumed when the cephalocaudal axis of the fetus is parallel to the mother's spine. Depending on the fetal part entering the pelvis first, a longitudinal lie may either be a cephalic (head) or breech (buttocks) presentation.

Fetal Presentation

Fetal presentation is determined by the body part of the passenger that enters the pelvic passageway first. This portion of the fetus is referred to as the *presenting part.* Depending on the attitude of the fetal extremities to its body and the fetal lie, the presentation is either cephalic, breech, or shoulder.

Cephalic Presentations

The fetal head presents itself to the passage in approximately 95% of term deliveries (Danforth, 1977). The cephalic presentations are classified according to the degree of flexion or extension of the fetal head. Thus the fetal attitude becomes critical in determining the type of cephalic presentation in each case.

There are four types of cephalic presentation. *Vertex presentation,* in which the head is completely flexed on the chest, is the most common

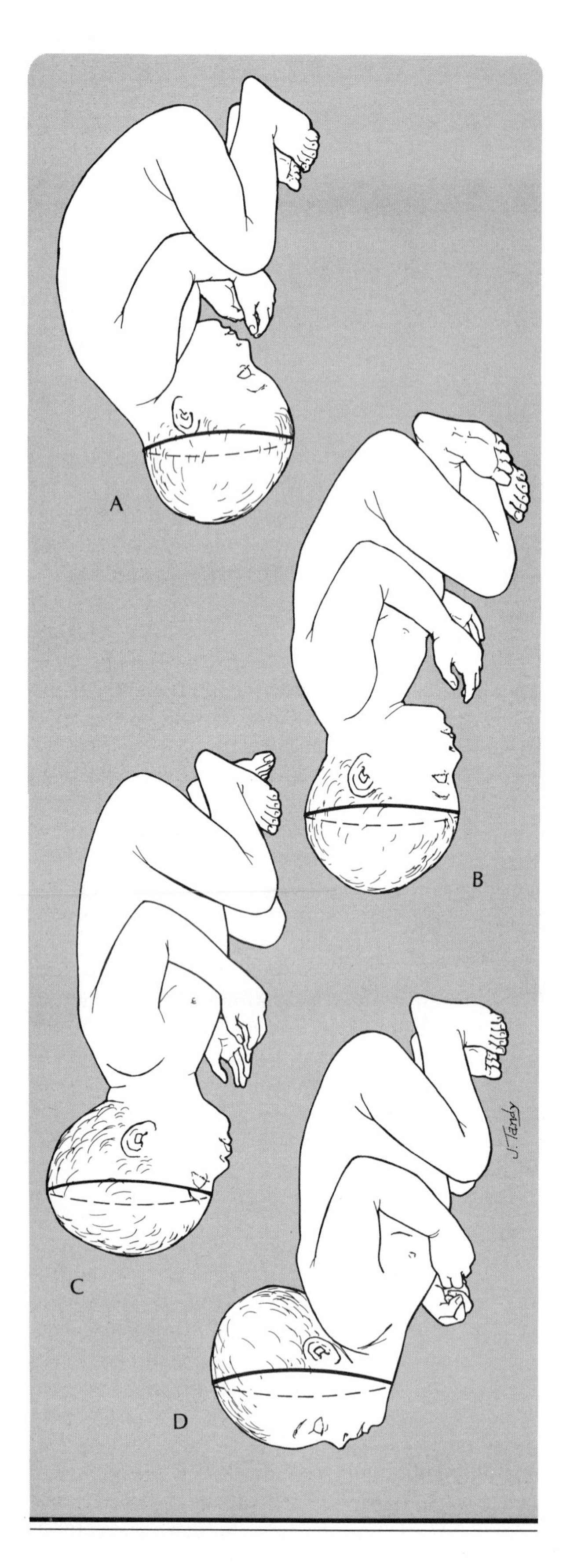

cephalic presentation; the smallest diameter of the passenger's head enters the passage in this presentation (Figure 15–5,*A*). Moderate flexion of the fetal head yields a *sinciput presentation* (Figure 15–5,*B*). A *brow presentation* is assumed when the fetal head is partially extended (Figure 15–5,*C*). The most extreme cephalic presentation is the *face presentation* (Figure 15–5,*D*), in which the head is hyperextended and the mentum (chin) is the presenting part. The mentum is the landmark on the fetal head used to note the relationship of the fetal head to the maternal pelvis.

Breech Presentations

Breech or pelvic presentations occur in 3% of term births. These presentations are classified according to the attitude of the passenger's hips and knees (see Figure 15–9 and Figure 19–11). A *complete breech* occurs when the knees and hips are both flexed, placing the thighs on the abdomen and the calves on the posterior aspect of the thighs. On vaginal examination both buttocks and feet can be palpated. Flexion of the hips and extension of the knees changes a complete breech to a *frank breech*. This presentation causes the fetal legs to extend onto the abdomen and chest, presenting the buttocks alone to the pelvis. The buttocks and genitals are palpable on vaginal examination when the passenger assumes a frank breech presentation. A *footling breech* presentation occurs when there is extension both at the knees and at the hips. A *single footling breech* presentation occurs if only one foot is presenting; a *double footling breech* occurs if both feet enter the pelvis first. In all variations of the breech presentation the sacrum is the landmark to be noted. See Chapter 19 for further discussion on the implications of the breech presentations for labor and delivery.

Figure 15–5. Cephalic presentations. **A,** Vertex presentation. Complete flexion of the head allows the suboccipitobregmatic diameter to present to the pelvis. **B,** Sinciput presentation. There is moderate flexion of the fetal head (military attitude). The occipitofrontal diameter, which is one of the larger anteroposterior diameters, must enter the pelvis. **C,** Brow presentation. The fetal head is partially extended (deflexion). The occipitonasal diameter is a relatively large anteroposterior diameter. **D,** Face presentation. The fetal head is completely extended. The occipitomental diameter is the largest diameter, and engagement is prevented.

Shoulder Presentation

A shoulder presentation, usually referred to as a *transverse lie,* is assumed by the fetus when its cephalocaudal axis lies perpendicular to the maternal spine. The fetus appears to lie crosswise in the uterus. Most frequently the shoulder is the presenting part in a transverse lie. In this case the acromion process of the scapula is the landmark to be noted. However, an arm, the fetal back, abdomen, or side may present in a transverse lie. This presentation may be caused by placenta previa (implantation of the placenta over the cervical os), small pelvic measurements, or excessive relaxation of the abdominal walls in women who have borne many children (grandmultiparas). Unless the fetus rotates during labor to a longitudinal lie, the delivery must be accomplished by cesarean section. See Chapter 19 for further discussion on the transverse lie and its effects on the labor and delivery processes.

Consequences of Malpresentations

Presentation other than the cephalic may affect the laboring woman, the fetus, and the powers of labor. The efficiency of labor may be greatly reduced by the presentation of a body part less symmetrical and less forceful than the round, bony head. The presenting part usually takes longer to descend into the pelvis, the cervix may dilate slowly and incompletely, uterine contractions tend to be irregular and less strong in the presence of the malpresentation, and a greater degree of fetal rotation is necessary for delivery. The fetus is also subjected to greater risk of trauma as a result of necessary obstetric intervention, such as forceps rotation or midforceps delivery. Disproportion between the maternal pelvis and the fetus is greater in presentations other than a vertex presentation. This disproportion, coupled with a greater incidence of premature rupture of the membranes in the presence of malpresentations, causes an increase in the need for an operative delivery with a malpresentation.

The mother may experience a prolonged labor with accompanying maternal exhaustion when there is an altered fetal presentation. A malpresentation necessitates greater contractile efforts by the uterus, and the mother must push harder to deliver the passenger. The maternal soft tissues and perineum must undergo more stretching, and the incidence of lacerations of the uterus, cervix, or vagina increases.

The fetus may experience grave consequences with a face, breech, or shoulder presentation. Fitting less perfectly into the passage, the fetus may have a more difficult descent through the pelvis. A prolonged labor increases the risk of fetal anoxia, asphyxia, or intrauterine death. Fetal compromise occurs more with malpresentations, since there is an increased incidence of prolapsed cord in the absence of a symmetrical head to cover the cervical os (Oxorn and Foote, 1975).

See Chapter 19 for further discussion about malpresentations and their management.

Functional Relationships of Presenting Part and Passage

Engagement of the presenting part takes place when the largest diameter of the presenting part passes through the pelvic inlet (Figure 15-6). The biparietal diameter is the largest dimension of the fetal skull to pass through the pelvis in a cephalic presentation. The intertrochanteric diameter is the largest to pass through the inlet in a breech presentation. Once the criteria for engagement have been met, the bony prominences of the presenting part are usually descending into the midpelvis (near the level of the ischial spines).

A vaginal examination determines whether engagement has occurred. In primigravidas, engagement usually occurs two weeks before term. Multiparas, however, may experience engagement several weeks before the onset of labor or during the process of labor. If engagement has occurred, the adequacy of the pelvic inlet has been validated. Engagement does not suggest that the midpelvis and outlet are also adequate.

The presenting part is said to be *floating* when it is freely movable above the inlet. When the presenting part begins to descend into the inlet, before engagement has truly occurred, it is said to be *dipping* into the pelvis.

Station refers to the relationship between the ischial spines in the passage and the presenting part of the passenger. In a normal pelvis, the ischial spines mark the narrowest diameter of the pelvis that the fetus must encounter. These spines are not sharp protrusions that harm the fetus but rather are blunted prominences at the midpelvis. The ischial spines as a landmark have been designated as zero station (Figure 15-7). If the presenting part is higher than the ischial spines, a negative number is assigned, noting centimeters above zero station. Station −5 is at the inlet, and station

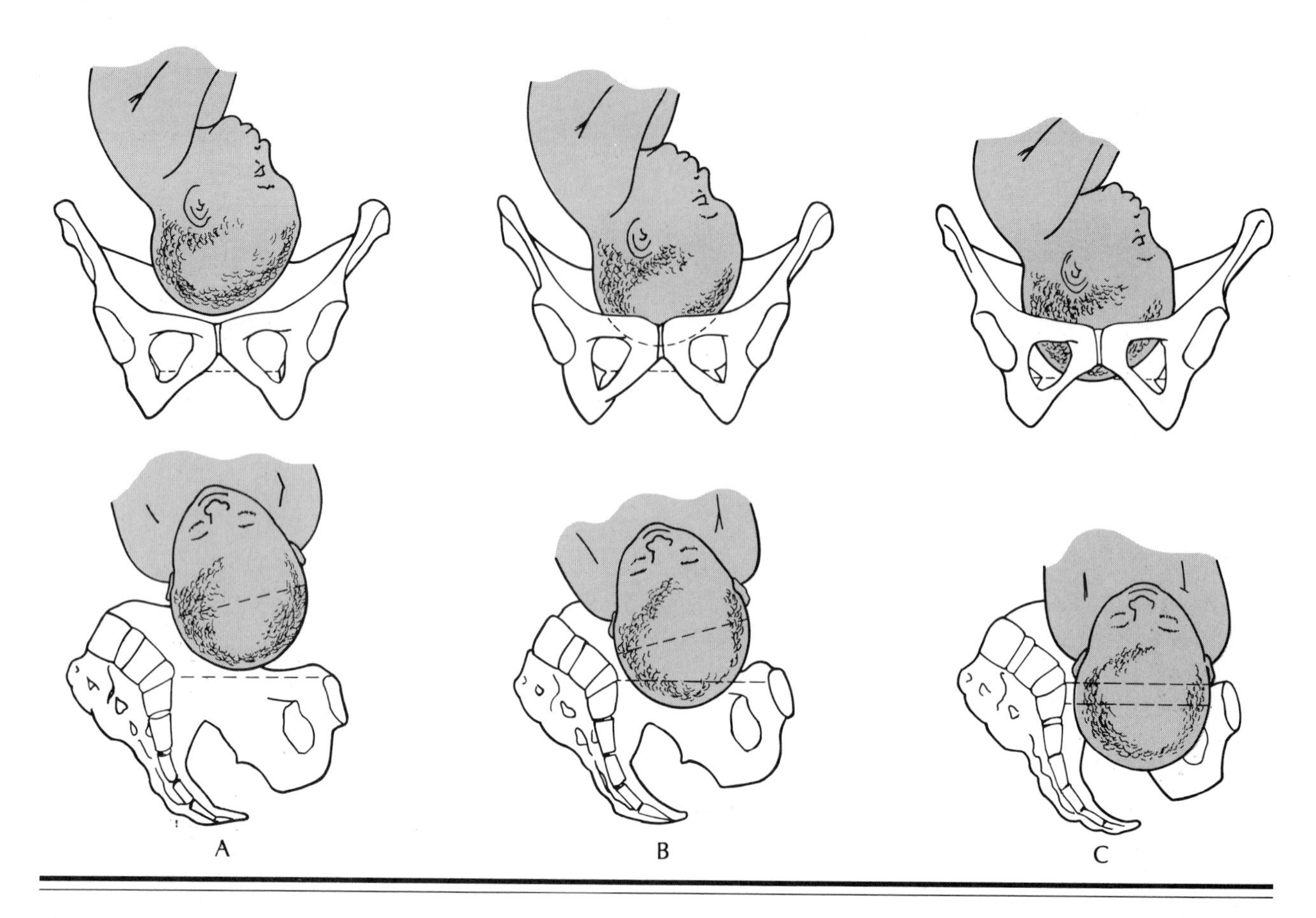

Figure 15–6. Process of engagement. **A,** Floating. **B,** Dipping. **C,** Engaged.

+4 is at the outlet; the presenting part is at the outlet and can be visualized upon viewing the mother's perineum, and delivery is imminent. During the process of labor, the presenting part should move progressively from the negative stations to the midpelvis at zero station and into the positive stations. If the presenting part does not descend in the presence of strong contractions, the maternal pelvis and the presenting diameters of the passenger may not be in proportion.

When both pelvic and fetal planes are parallel, the relationship is said to be *synclitic* (Figure 15–8,*A*). Thus in a cephalic presentation, engagement occurs in synclitism when the biparietal diameter of the fetal head is parallel to the sacrum and the symphysis pubis. Engagement in synclitism takes place when the uterus is perpendicular to the inlet, not retroflexed or anteflexed. Synclitic engagement also indicates that the pelvis is roomy.

Asynclitism indicates that the uterus is not perpendicular to the inlet and that the fetal head is not parallel to the planes of the pelvis (Figure 15–8,*B*, Figure 15–8,*C*). This usually occurs with small pelvic diameters or with weak abdominal musculature that allows the uterus to tilt anteriorly or posteriorly. When there is a large fetal head or small pelvic diameters, asynclitism facilitates engagement by allowing a smaller diameter of the fetal head to enter the pelvis. Persistent asynclitism may cause difficulties, however, preventing normal rotation of the head in the pelvis (Oxorn and Foote, 1975).

Fetal Position

Fetal position refers to the relationship of the landmark on the presenting fetal part to the front, sides, or back of the maternal pelvis. The landmark on the fetal presenting part is related to four imaginary quadrants of the pelvis: left anterior, right anterior, left posterior, and right posterior. These quadrants assist in designating whether the presenting part is directed toward the front, back, left, or right of the passage. The landmark chosen

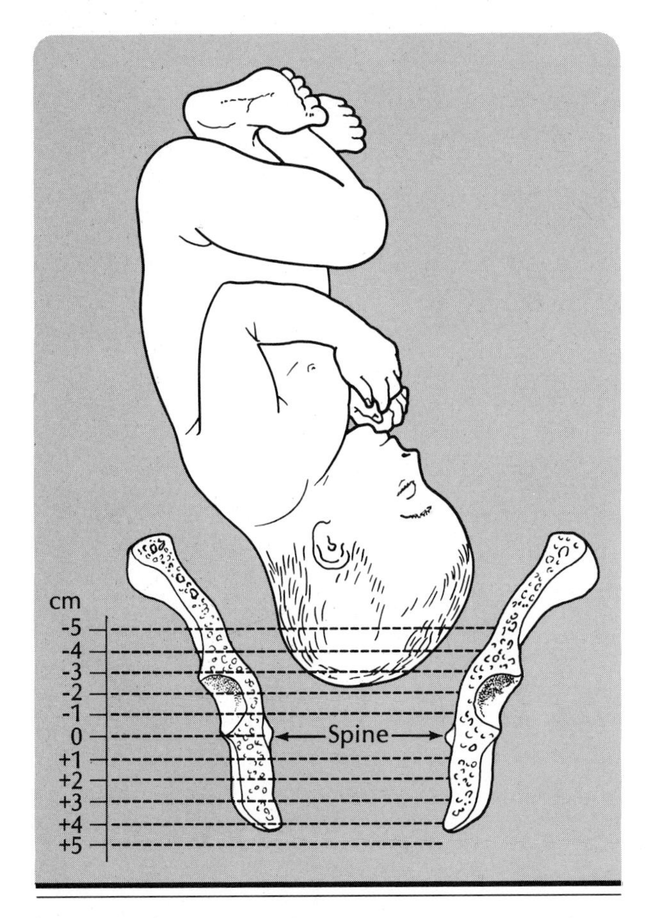

Figure 15–7. Measuring station of the fetal head while it is descending.

for cephalic presentations is the occiput in vertex presentations and the mentum in face presentations. Breech presentations use the sacrum as the designated landmark, and the acromion process on the scapula is noted in shoulder presentations. If the landmark is directed toward the center of the side of the pelvis, it is designated as a *transverse position,* rather than anterior or posterior.

Three notations are used to describe the fetal position:

1. Right (R) or left (L) side of the maternal pelvis.
2. The landmark of the fetal presenting part: occiput (O), mentum (M), sacrum (S), or acromion process (A).

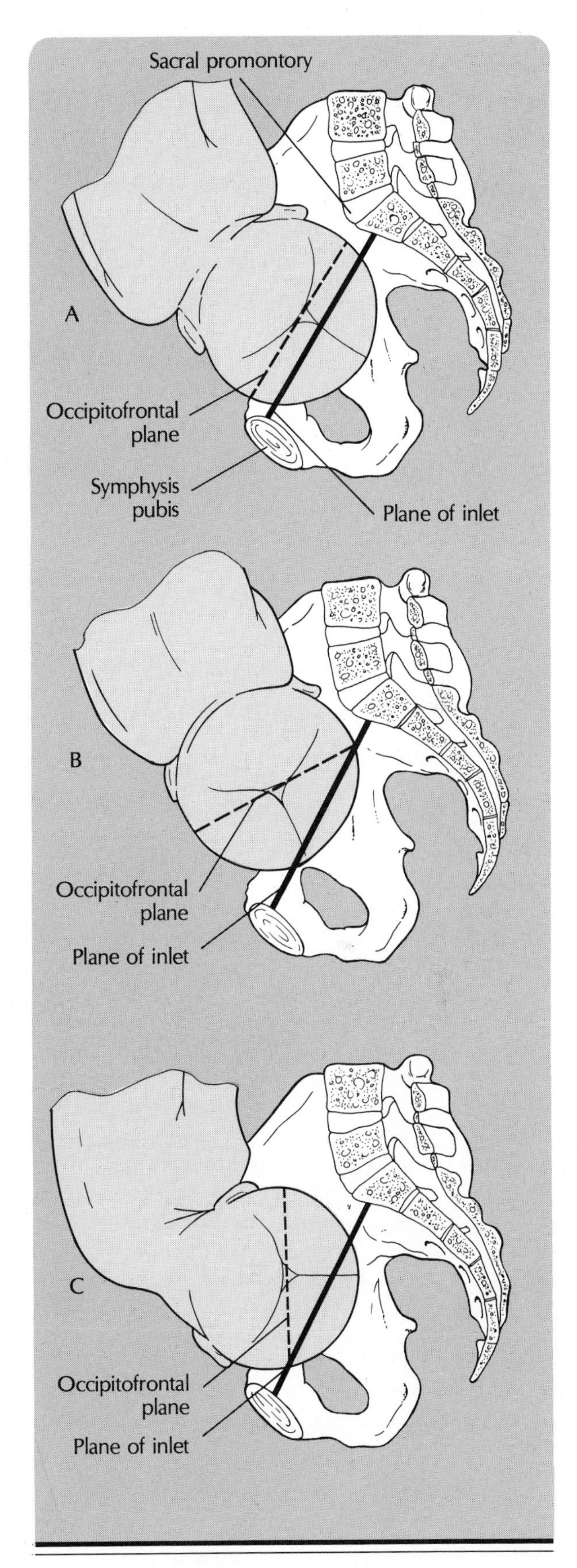

Figure 15–8. **A,** Synclitism. Fetal occipitofrontal plane and pelvic superior strait are in concordance. **B,** Asynclitism with uterus and fetus tilted posteriorly. **C,** Asynclitism with uterus and fetus tilted anteriorly.

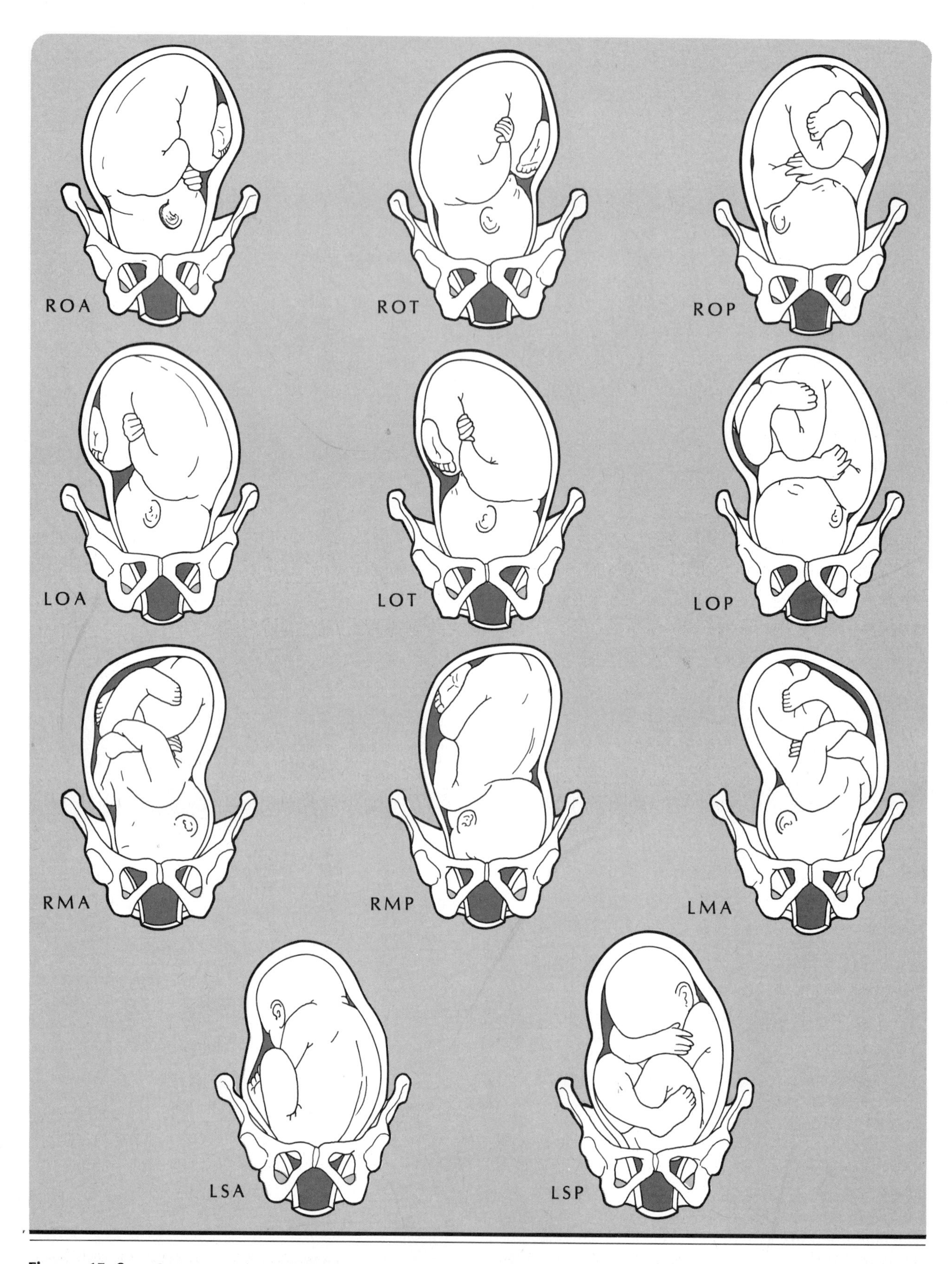

Figure 15-9. Categories of presentation. (Courtesy Ross Laboratories, Columbus, Ohio.)

3. Anterior (A), posterior (P), or transverse (T), depending on whether the landmark is in the front, back, or side of the pelvis.

Abbreviations are formed from these notations to assist the health care team in communicating the fetal position. Hence, when the fetal occiput is directed toward the back and to the left of the passage, the abbreviation used is LOP (left-occiput-posterior). The term *dorsal* (D) is used when denoting the fetal position in a transverse lie; it refers to the fetal back. Thus the abbreviation RADA indicates that the acromion process of the scapula is directed toward the mother's right and the passenger's back is anterior.

Following is a list of the positions for various fetal presentations, some of which are illustrated in Figure 15–9:

Positions in vertex presentation:

ROA	Right-occiput-anterior
ROT	Right-occiput-transverse
ROP	Right-occiput-posterior
LOA	Left-occiput-anterior
LOT	Left-occiput-transverse
LOP	Left-occiput-posterior

Positions in face presentation:

RMA	Right-mentum-anterior
RMT	Right-mentum-transverse
RMP	Right-mentum-posterior
LMA	Left-mentum-anterior
LMT	Left-mentum-transverse
LMP	Left-mentum-posterior

Positions in breech presentation:

RSA	Right-sacrum-anterior
RST	Right-sacrum-transverse
RSP	Right-sacrum-posterior
LSA	Left-sacrum-anterior
LST	Left-sacrum-transverse
LSP	Left-sacrum-posterior

Positions in shoulder presentation:

RADA	Right-acromion-dorsal-anterior
RADP	Right-acromion-dorsal-posterior
LADA	Left-acromion-dorsal-anterior
LADP	Left-acromion-dorsal-posterior

The fetal position influences labor and delivery. For example, posterior position causes a larger diameter of the fetal head to enter the pelvis than an anterior position. With a posterior position, pressure on the sacral nerves is increased, causing the laboring woman backache and pelvic pressure and perhaps encouraging her to bear down or push earlier than normal. (See Chapter 19 for an in-depth discussion of malpositions and their management.)

Fetal position is determined by a combination of methods, utilizing various senses and technology. Assessment of the maternal abdomen for fetal position may be done by inspection, palpation, auscultation of FHTs, vaginal examination, and x-ray examination. (See Chapter 16 for further discussion of assessment of fetal position.)

The Psyche

Colman and Colman (1971) describe labor as a journey into the unknown that is uncertain, irrevocable, and uncontrollable. Primigravidas face a totally new experience, and multiparas cannot be certain what each new labor will bring.

Various factors influence a woman's reaction to the physical and emotional crisis of labor. A major factor is what the experience means to the individual involved. When viewed as a positive experience, the couple usually seeks childbirth education and participates in such a group. The labor and delivery process may be viewed as a termination of one phase but the beginning of another. Viewing the childbirth experience as a positive one is also influenced by whether the culture looks on childbirth as a worthwhile experience and whether children are valued as a part of society.

The mother's expectations of her own self and her performance are another important factor. Her expectations are more likely to be realistic if she has attended childbirth education classes or has had other children.

A woman's response to labor and the discomfort she experiences is in particular affected by her physical preparedness for labor, racial influences and cultural expectations, psychologic experiences from her past, and the coping mechanisms and support systems that she brings to the labor experience.

Physical Preparedness for Labor

Because labor is a physical event, muscle toning and controlled breathing exercises during labor are taught in prepared childbirth classes (Chapter 12). Women who use these physical techniques along with other components of preparedness need less medication during labor and report less pain in labor than do unprepared mothers.

Erkkola and Rauramo (1976) have reported a correlation between physical fitness of the mother and levels of maternal and newborn pH at the time of delivery. Acidic pHs are postulated to be due to lactic acid metabolites, which cross the placenta rapidly. Physiologically, in any muscular work, the more physically fit the subject the less the increase in acidic products (Cogan, 1975; Zax, 1975).

Muscle relaxation is also taught to women to prepare them for labor. According to Dick-Read's theory (1972), fear = tension = pain, and one way to reduce tension is through education for childbirth and conscious relaxation.

Past Psychologic Experiences and Coping Mechanisms

If a mother has had an unpleasant or traumatic labor experience, she may anticipate another such experience. Stories shared by friends and relatives of their unpleasant experiences also color a mother's expectations. Mothers who bring to the labor experience knowledge of the birth process, techniques to use during contractions, a person to coach them through the experience, and a positive outlook toward childbirth tend to have a better and more satisfying experience, physically and mentally.

The Powers

Primary and secondary powers work complementarily to deliver the fetus, the fetal membranes, and the placenta from the uterus into the external environment. The primary power is uterine muscular contractions, which effect the changes of the first stage of labor—complete effacement and dilatation of the cervix. The second power is abdominal musculature contractions, which add to the primary power after full dilatation has occurred.

Uterine Response

Contractions are divided into an increment, acme (peak), and decrement. They are described according to the duration of each contraction, which begins at the beginning of the increment and ends with the completion of decrement. In beginning labor, contractions last about 30 seconds and, as labor continues, increase to 60–90 seconds. Their duration remains relatively stable at 60 seconds until delivery.

The frequency of contractions is the amount of time from the beginning of one contraction to the beginning of the next contraction. The frequency diminishes as birth becomes more imminent. Initially the interval between contractions may be 20–30 minutes. Primigravidas are often told to contact their physician or to come to the hospital when their contractions are 8–12 minutes apart. During the height of the expulsive stage, contractions are usually 2–3 minutes apart. All contractions should have a resting phase between them. This resting phase allows uterine muscles to rest and restores a compromised uteroplacental circulation, which is important to fetal oxygenation and adequate circulation in the uterine blood vessels.

The intensity of each contraction is measured by the rise in the intrauterine pressure above the normal resting tone of the uterus, which is between 0 and 15 mm Hg. During labor, intensity is estimated, because true intensity can only be measured with an intrauterine electronic monitor. On palpation, the intensity is estimated to be mild if one can indent the uterus slightly and the contraction lasts about 45–55 seconds; it is considered strong if the uterus cannot be indented and the contraction lasts 65–75 seconds (Figure 15–10). The contractions demonstrate fundal dominance in that the contraction is initiated at the top and radiates down over the body of the uterus. Although the contraction initiates in the fundus, the pregnant woman may perceive the contraction as suprapubic pressure, back discomfort, or pressure in other areas. Contractions that begin elsewhere may indicate pathology. As labor progresses, a rhythmic pattern is seen. Contractions increase in force (intensity) and last longer (duration).

Musculature Changes in the Pelvic Floor

The levator ani muscle and fascia of the pelvic floor draw the rectum and vagina upward and forward with each contraction, along the curve of the pelvic floor. As the fetal head descends to the pelvic floor, the pressure of the presenting part causes the perineal structure that was once 5 cm in thickness to change to a structure of less than a centimeter, and a normal physiologic anesthesia is produced as a result of the decreased blood supply to the area. The anus everts, exposing the interior rectal wall as the head descends forward (Pritchard and MacDonald, 1976).

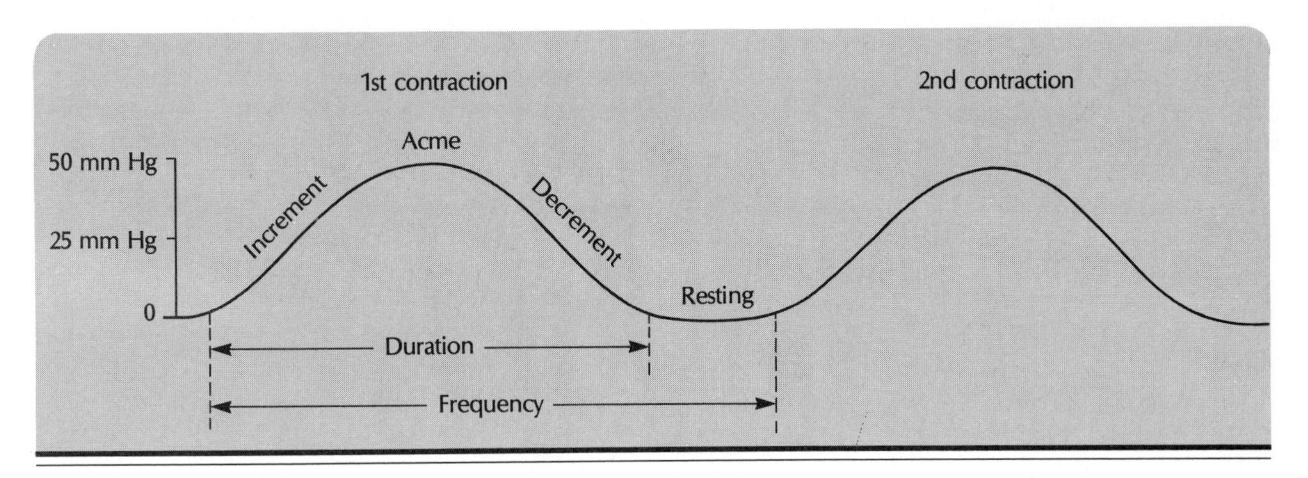

Figure 15-10. Characteristics of uterine contractions.

PHYSIOLOGY OF LABOR

Biochemical Interaction

The contraction wave of the uterus is controlled by pacemakers, the normally dominant one being at the uterine end of the right fallopian tube. The impulses are conducted quickly in a wavelike manner to the uterine myometrium cell membrane, which is activated and continues to propagate the stimuli (Assali, 1968). Because of the quickness of the propagation of the stimuli, the myometrium appears to contract as a unit. The concentration of the contractile proteins, actin and myosin, is greatest at the fundus, diminishing gradually toward the cervix. Thus the strongest myometrial activity occurs at the fundus.

Myometrial contraction efficiency depends on four basic systems: (a) the contractile substance, (b) a source of energy, (c) a stimulus, and (d) a conduction system (Figure 15-11). The contractile substance is composed of the proteins actin and myosin. The conduction system is under hormonal control. Under the influence of progesterone, calcium is bound to the cell membrane, rendering it impermeable to sodium and potassium exchange and cellular depolarization. The cell, in the presence of progesterone, is under the domination of the β-inhibitory effects of epinephrine and norepinephrine. With the α-excitatory effect of epinephrine and norepinephrine, estrogen activates acetylcholine at the neuromuscular junction. Acetylcholine is reported to generate myometrial activity through propagation of the stimuli, to assist in rhythmic control of contractions, to regulate uterine perfusion with blood, and to liberate calcium from the cell membrane. When the membrane becomes more permeable, a sudden influx of sodium occurs, which rapidly depolarizes the cell (Bonica, 1967).

Myometrial Activity

For reasons not clearly understood, stretching of the cervix increases myometrial activity. This is known as the *Ferguson reflex.* Pressures exerted by the contracting uterus vary from 20 to 60 mm Hg with an average of 40 mm Hg.

In true labor the uterus divides into two portions. This division is known as the *physiologic retraction ring.* The upper portion, which is the contractile segment, becomes progressively thicker as labor advances. The lower portion, which includes the lower uterine segment and cervix, is passive. As labor continues, the lower uterine segment expands and thins out.

With each contraction the musculature of the upper uterine segment shortens and exerts a longitudinal traction on the cervix, causing effacement. *Effacement* is the taking up of the internal os and the cervical canal into the uterine side walls.

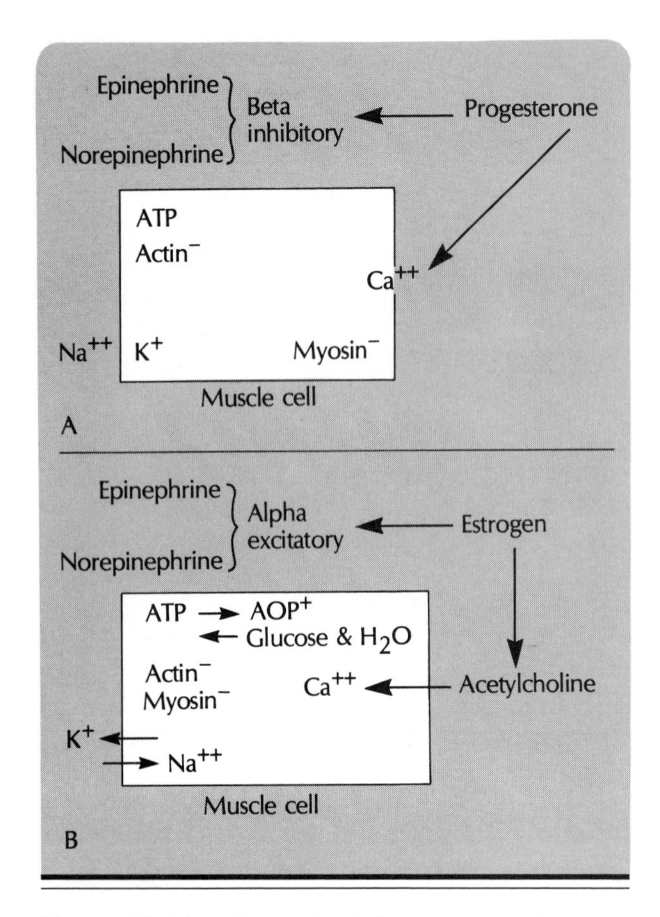

Figure 15-11. Biochemical influences on uterine myometrial cells during contractions. **A,** Resting cell. **B,** Contracting cell.

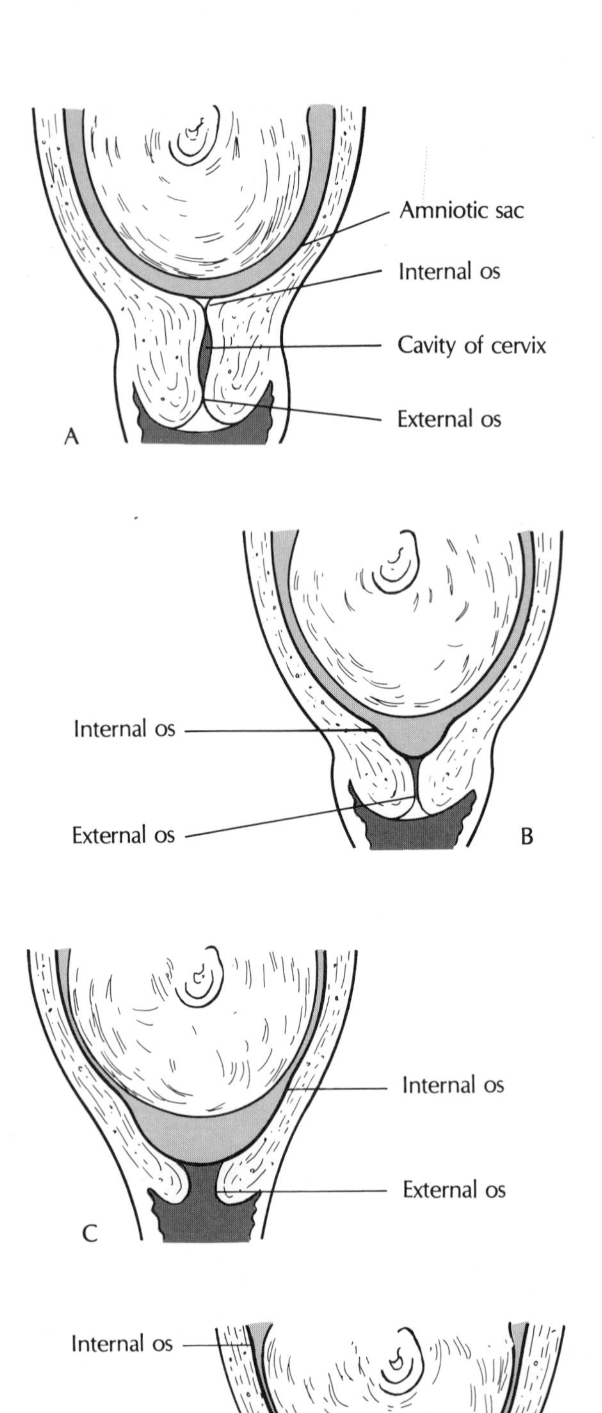

Figure 15-12. Effacement of the cervix in the primigravida. **A,** At the beginning of labor there is no cervical effacement or dilatation. **B,** Beginning cervical effacement. **C,** Cervix is about one-half effaced and slightly dilated. **D,** Complete effacement and dilatation.

The cervix changes progressively from a long, thick structure to a structure that is tissue-paper thin (Figure 15-12). In primigravidas, effacement usually precedes dilatation. This musculature remains shorter and thicker and does not return to its original length. This phenomenon is known as *brachystasis.* The space in the uterine cavity decreases as a result of brachystasis.

The uterus elongates with each contraction, decreasing the horizontal diameter. This elongation causes a straightening of the fetal body, pressing the upper pole against the fundus and thrusting the presenting part down toward the lower uterine segment and the cervix. The pressure exerted by the fetus is called the *fetal axis pressure.* As the uterus elongates, the longitudinal muscle fibers are pulled upward over the presenting part. This action, plus the hydrostatic pressure of the fetal membranes, causes cervical dilatation. The cervical os and cervical canal widen from less than a centimeter to approximately 10 cm, allowing delivery of the fetus. When the cervix is completely dilated and retracted up into the lower uterine segment, it can no longer be palpated.

The round ligament contracts with the uterus, pulling the fundus forward, thus aligning the fetus with the bony pelvis. In preparation for labor, the cohesiveness of collagen fibers of the cervix decreases. This decrease in cohesiveness is due to a decrease in the hydroxyproline content of the cervix, but the mechanism of action is poorly understood (Pritchard and MacDonald, 1976).

Intraabdominal Pressure

After the cervix is completely dilated, the abdominal musculature of the mother contracts with forced respiratory efforts. The glottis is closed with these efforts. The pushing that the mother does in reponse to this pressure aids in expulsion of the infant and the placenta after delivery. If the cervix is not completely dilated, bearing down can cause cervical edema, which retards dilatation, and can cause maternal exhaustion as a result of straining. Tearing and bruising will also result from bearing down upon an incompletely dilated cervix.

MATERNAL SYSTEMIC RESPONSE TO LABOR

Cardiovascular System

Contractions cause an increase in the blood pressure, pulse pressure, and mean venous pressure. These changes are less severe with the mother in the lateral Sims position. In the second stage during bearing-down efforts, the cardiac output may increase up to 40% above prelabor values. Arterial and central venous pressures also rise significantly. During delivery there is another change in cardiac volume as a result of the normal blood loss of about 500 ml (Burrow and Ferris, 1975).

Fluid and Electrolyte Balance

Diaphoresis and hyperventilation occur during labor, which alters electrolyte and fluid balance from insensible loss. The muscle activity increases the body temperature, which increases sweating and evaporation from the skin. The increase in the respiratory rate as the mother responds to the work of labor increases the evaporative water volume, because each breath of air must be warmed to the body temperature and humidified (Dukes and Bowen, 1976). With the increased evaporative water volume, adequate hydration via parenteral fluids during labor becomes increasingly important.

Gastrointestinal System

During labor, gastrointestinal motility and absorption decrease, resulting in the need to restrict oral intake. It is not uncommon for a mother to vomit stomach contents that had been ingested 12 hours previously.

Respiratory System

Oxygen consumption in labor increases to equal that of moderate to strenuous exercise.

Hemopoietic System

There is an elevation of leukocytes to as much as 25,000 to 35,000 which equals the elevation that occurs during strenuous exercise.

Renal System

It is not uncommon to have a trace of proteinuria during labor as a result of muscle breakdown from exercise. This proteinuria should not be greater than 2+, which is suggestive of pathology. Bladder atony may also occur, with distention and the inability to void. Bladder atony is caused by compression of the urethra by the uterus and infant and by overall decreased tone from the progesterone influence during pregnancy. During labor, the nurse should encourage the mother to void at regular intervals, should observe for bladder distention, and should catheterize as needed.

Discomfort of Labor

According to Bonica (1960), discomfort in labor can be caused by a number of sources. Throughout labor the contracting uterus can cause pain, from stretching of ligaments and muscle cell anoxia (Greenhill and Friedman, 1974). In the first stage of labor, the dilating cervix is the primary source of pain. These pain impulses travel from the cervix by way of (a) the uterine plexus, (b) the pelvic plexus, (c) the hypogastric plexus, (d) the superior hypogastric plexus, (e) the lumbar and thoracic chain, and (f) the white rami communicantes associated with the 11th and 12th thoracic nerves. Women describe these sensations as cramping, coliclike pressure sensations. Pressure on nerves radiating from the lumbar and sacral plexus results in pain in the lumbosacral area of the back.

After complete dilatation, when the fetal head descends into the vaginal canal, ischemia of the muscle cells of the vaginal canal and perineal floor produces discomfort by way of the pudendal nerves. These nerves enter the spinal cord by way of the posterior roots of the S2-3-4. Women describe the sensations as burning, stinging, or tearing. Contraction of the uterus continues to contribute to the discomfort (Bonica, 1960; Greenhill and Friedman, 1974). Pain during childbirth and its management are discussed in depth in Chapter 18.

FETAL RESPONSE TO LABOR

In the presence of a normal fetus the mechanical and hemodynamic changes enforced by normal labor have no adverse fetal effect (Aladjem and Brown, 1974).

Biomechanical Changes

High pressures are exerted on the fetal head during contractions and to an even greater extent after rupture of the membranes. During the second stage, the pressures may rise as high as 200 mm Hg (Aladjem and Brown, 1974).

Cardiac Changes

It has been demonstrated by researchers that fetal heart rate decelerations can occur with intracranial pressures of 40 to 55 mm Hg. The currently accepted explanation for this is hypoxic depression of the central nervous system, which is under vagal control. The absence of these head compression decelerations in some mothers is explained by the existence of a threshold that is more gradually reached in the presence of intact membranes and lack of maternal resistance. These changes are innocuous in the normal fetus (Aladjem and Brown, 1974).

Hemodynamic Changes

The adequate exchange of nutrients and gases to and from the fetal capillaries and the intervillous space depends on a number of factors, one of which is the fetal blood pressure. Fetal blood pressure serves as a protective mechanism for the normal fetus for the stresses of the anoxic period, which are enforced by the contracting uterus during labor. The fetal and placental reserve is enough to see the fetus through these anoxic periods without adversity (Aladjem and Brown, 1974).

Positional Changes

So that the fetus can make the transition from intrauterine life to extrauterine life, the fetal head and body must accommodate to the passage by certain positional changes, often called *cardinal movement* or *mechanics of labor.* These changes are described in the order in which they occur (Figure 15–13).

Descent

Descent is thought to occur because of four forces: (a) pressure of the amniotic fluid, (b) direct pressure of the fundus on the breech, (c) contraction of the abdominal muscles, and (d) extension and straightening of the fetal body. The head enters the inlet in the occiput transverse or oblique position, because the pelvic inlet is widest from side to side.

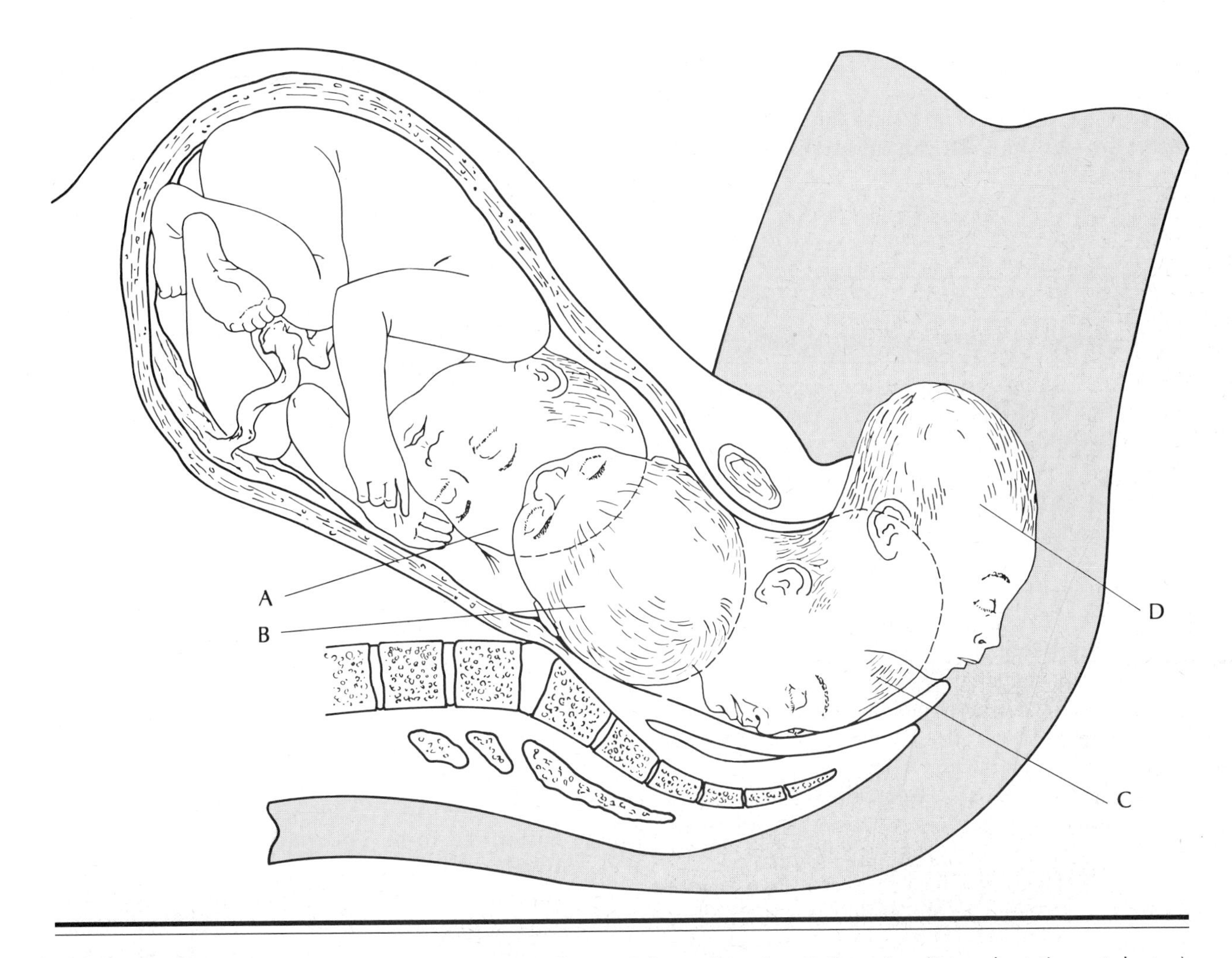

Figure 15–13. Mechanism of labor. **A,** Descent. **B,** Flexion. **C,** Internal rotation. **D,** Extension. (External rotation not shown.)

Flexion

Flexion occurs as the fetal head descends and meets resistance from the soft tissues of the pelvis, the musculature of the pelvic floor, and the cervix.

Internal Rotation

The fetal head must rotate to fit the diameter of the pelvic cavity, which is widest in the anteroposterior diameter. The sagittal suture aligns in the anteroposterior pelvic diameter, which is the plane of least resistance.

Extension

The resistance of the pelvic floor and the mechanical movement of the vulvar opening anteriorly and forward assists with extension of the fetal head as it passes under the symphysis pubis. With this positional change, the head emerges from the introitus.

Restitution and External Rotation

The shoulders of the infant enter the pelvis obliquely and remain oblique when the head rotates to the anteroposterior diameter through internal rotation. Because of this rotation the neck becomes twisted. Once the head delivers and is free of pelvic resistance, the neck untwists and aligns with the shoulders. It returns to the original position that it had held in utero. For the shoulders to deliver they must align in the anteroposterior diameter of the pelvic outlet. Therefore, the head externally rotates to maintain its normal position with the shoulders.

Expulsion

After the external rotation and through expulsive efforts of the mother, the anterior shoulder appears under the symphysis pubis. With lateral flexion the posterior shoulder delivers over the perineum. The body quickly follows (Oxorn and Foote, 1975).

ONSET OF LABOR

Possible Causes of Labor Onset

For some reason, usually at the appropriate time for the uterus and the baby, the process of labor begins. Although medical researchers have been conducting numerous studies to determine the exact cause, it still remains a mystery. Some of the more widely accepted theories are as follows:

1. *Oxytocin stimulation theory.* Oxytocin can be administered in minute quantities to a mother at term to initiate labor because the myometrium is increasingly sensitive to oxytocin prior to and during labor. Therefore, it is theorized that endogenous oxytocin from the mother's pituitary gland is responsible for labor's onset. Supportive evidence for oxytocin being the sole initiator of labor is scarce (Pritchard and MacDonald, 1976).

2. *Progesterone withdrawal theory.* Progesterone has been reported to inhibit uterine activity by rendering the cell membrane stable from depolarization, and it is essential in maintaining pregnancy. As placental production of progesterone decreases, uterine contractions are able to proceed. However, clinicians have been unable to stop premature labor effectively with the use of progesterone, and there is no documented evidence that blood and tissue levels of progesterone are altered prior to labor. Progesterone may have an indirect effect on the onset of labor and may be coupled with other factors (Pritchard and MacDonald, 1976).

3. *Estrogen stimulation theory.* Estrogen causes hypertrophy of the myometrium and an increase in concentrations of actin and myosin (contractile proteins) and adenosine triphosphate (ATP), which is the energy source for contractions. This hormone has been shown to abet the depolarization of the muscle cell membrane. Estrogen probably also plays an important role in labor in combination with other factors (Greenhill and Friedman, 1974).

4. *Fetal cortisol theory.* In the past ten years, Liggins (1973) has found that the removal of the fetal lamb's pituitary gland and adrenal cortex delays the onset of labor (Pritchard and MacDonald, 1976). Thus he has postulated that the fetus may play an important role in the initiation of labor. He also has reported premature labor in sheep that were infused with cortisol or ACTH. This phenomenon has not been confirmed in humans.

5. *Fetal membrane phospholipid–arachidonic acid–prostaglandin theory.* According to this theory, estrogen promotes storage of esterified arachidonic acid in the fetal membranes. Withdrawal of progesterone activates phospholipase A_2, which is an enzymatic liberator. Phospholipase A_2 hydrolyzes phospholipids to liberate arachidonic acid in a nonesterified form. The arachidonic acid acts on prostaglandins E_2 or F_{2a} or both in the decidual membranes. Prostaglandin stimulates the smooth muscle to contract, especially in the myometrium. Prostaglandin is present in increased quantities in the blood and amniotic fluid just prior to and during labor. The exact relationship of prostaglandins to the initiation of labor has yet to be established (Pritchard and MacDonald, 1976).

6. *Distention theory.* This theory proposes that there is pressure from an overdistended uterus on nerve endings, stimulating contractions and increasing irritability of the uterus. This theory seems to have some basis when one looks at premature labor in multiple pregnancies and at cases of polyhydramnios.

Premonitory Signs

Most primigravidas and many multiparas experience warning signs that labor is about to begin.

Lightening

The majority of primigravidas experience the phenomenon of *lightening* before the onset of labor.

This feeling occurs because the fetus begins to settle into the pelvic inlet. With its descent, the uterus moves downward, and the fundus no longer presses on the diaphragm. The mother can breathe easier. However, as the fetus descends, increased pressure on the bladder by the fetal head results in increased urinary frequency. Leg pain may be noted because of pressure on the sciatic nerve. In theory, primigravidas experience lightening because of the bracing action of abdominal muscles of good tone. Engagement then results, and the vaginal secretions become more profuse. In one study, the mean interval between engagement and delivery in primigravidas was found to be 1.39 weeks (Weekes and Flynn, 1975).

Braxton Hicks Contractions

Prior to the onset of labor, the irregular, intermittent contractions that have been occurring throughout the pregnancy may become uncomfortable. The pain seems to be in the abdomen and groin but may feel like the "drawing" sensations experienced by some with dysmenorrhea. These prelabor sensations, called *false labor,* assist in the ripening process of the cervix. In this process the cervix softens, effaces, and moves anteriorly. With effacement the mucous plug (accumulated cervical secretions that have closed off the opening of the uterine cavity) is often lost, resulting in a bloody show from the exposed cervical capillaries. Some dilatation also occurs (Greenhill and Friedman, 1974).

Sudden Burst of Energy

Some women report a sudden surge of energy before labor. They may do their spring housecleaning or rearrange all the furniture (referred to as the "nesting instinct"). The nurse in prenatal teaching should warn prospective mothers not to overexert themselves at this time so that they will not be excessively tired at labor's onset. This energy may result from a decrease in progesterone production by the placenta.

Other Signs

Additional premonitory signs may be loss of weight resulting from fluid loss and electrolyte shifts produced by changes in estrogen and progesterone levels, increased backache and sacroiliac pressure from the influence of relaxin hormone on the pelvic joints, and increased vaginal secretions resulting from vaginal mucous membrane congestion. Some mothers report loose bowel movements or diarrhea just prior to the onset of labor.

Differences Between True and False Labor

The contractions of true labor produce progressive dilatation, effacement, and descent. They occur regularly and increase in frequency, intensity, and duration. The discomfort of true labor is in the back and abdomen and is not relieved by ambulation (in fact, it may intensify).

The contractions of false labor do not produce progressive dilatation, effacement, and descent. Classically they occur irregularly and do not increase in frequency, intensity, or duration. However, in the clinical setting, it is sometimes difficult to distinguish false labor from true labor until the woman has been assessed for a period of hours. The discomfort of false labor is most often experienced in the lower abdomen and groin and may be relieved by ambulation. Sedation alleviates this discomfort.

It is helpful for the mother to know the characteristics of true labor contractions as well as the premonitory signs of ensuing labor. However, sometimes the only way to accurately differentiate between true and false labor is by assessment of dilatation. The mother must feel free to come in for accurate assessment of labor and must not feel foolish if it is false labor. The nurse must reassure the woman that false labor is common and that it often cannot be distinguished from true labor except by vaginal examination.

STAGES OF LABOR AND DELIVERY

There are three stages of labor. The first stage begins with the beginning of true labor and ends when the cervix is completely dilated at 10 cm. The second stage begins at that time and ends with the birth of the infant. The third stage begins with the expulsion of the infant and ends with the delivery of the placenta.

Some clinicians identify a fourth stage of labor. During this stage, which lasts one to four hours after delivery of the placenta, the uterus effectively contracts to control bleeding at the placental site (Pritchard and MacDonald, 1976).

The management of the laboring patient is discussed in Chapter 17.

First Stage

For management purposes the first stage of labor is divided into the latent phase and the active phase. The *latent phase* begins with the onset of regular contractions and, when plotted on the Friedman graph (Chapter 16, p. 457), is represented by a flat slope that curves upward slightly. The latent phase is considered the effacing phase. It averages 8.6 hours in primigravidas and 5.3 hours in multiparas and should not exceed 20 hours in primigravidas and 14 hours in multiparas. Uterine contractions may be mild, lasting for 10–30 seconds and following a regular pattern every 15–20 minutes. In this phase the cervix is effacing and some dilatation is occurring. Abdominal cramps, backache, rupture of membranes, and perhaps bloody show accompany this phase.

The *active phase*, called the *dilatation phase*, may be divided into the acceleration phase, the maximum slope of dilatation, and the deceleration phase. The acceleration phase is slower than the maximum slope of dilatation but does not last long. Contractions are stronger and longer (30–45 seconds), more frequent (every 3–5 minutes), and may be accompanied by pain. The mother may become restless, have labored respirations, and have a tendency to hyperventilate.

The acceleration phase heralds the onset of the maximum slope of dilatation, which normally averages 3 cm/hr but not less than 1.2 cm/hr in primigravidas and 5.7 cm/hr but not less than 1.5 cm/hr in multiparas.

The culmination of the maximum slope of dilatation is the deceleration phase, in which the cervix retracts around the fetal head. The deceleration phase is also referred to as the *transitional phase of labor* (8–10 cm cervical dilatation). Uterine contractions last 45–60 seconds and occur every 1–2 minutes. They may be accompanied by amnesia between contractions; leg cramps; nausea and possible vomiting; hiccups and unexpected belches; perspiration on the forehead and upper lip; profuse, dark, heavy show; irritable abdomen; and a pulling or stretching sensation deep in the pelvis. The mother may demonstrate emotional irritability or panic. Her attention and response to external environmental stimuli become progressively limited as labor progresses, necessitating repetition and simplicity of instructions and explanations given by health personnel. The deceleration phase averages 2 hours in primigravidas but should not be longer than 3½ hours for both primiparas and multigravidas.

At the beginning of labor the membranes bulge through the cervix in the shape of a cone. As labor progresses and dilatation occurs, the membranes assume the shape of a large watch crystal. They may rupture before labor or any time during labor. If the chorion ruptures and the amnion remains intact, the infant may deliver with the amnion covering its head. The child is then born with a *caul*. Rupture of membranes (ROM) generally occurs at the height of an intense contraction with a gush of the fluid out the introitus. If this occurs in transition, then descent of the fetal head will follow (Greenhill and Friedman, 1974).

Second Stage

The second stage of labor, called the *pelvic phase* or *expulsive stage*, begins with complete dilatation of the cervix and ends with the delivery of the baby. Contractions last 50–90 seconds and may be only 1–2 minutes apart. Intraabdominal pressure is exerted from contraction of the maternal abdominal musculature, and the mother has the urge to push because of the pressure of the fetal head on the sacral and obturator nerves. As the fetal head descends, the perineum begins to bulge, flatten, and move anteriorly. There is an increase in bloody show. The labia begin to part with each contraction. Between contractions the head appears to recede. As the head descends further, crowning occurs, signifying that delivery is imminent (Figure 15–14) (Greenhill and Friedman, 1974).

Spontaneous Delivery (Vertex Presentation)

As the head distends the vulva with each contraction, the perineum becomes extremely thin and the anus stretches and protrudes. With assistance from the physician or nurse-midwife, the head is delivered slowly under the symphysis pubis, with

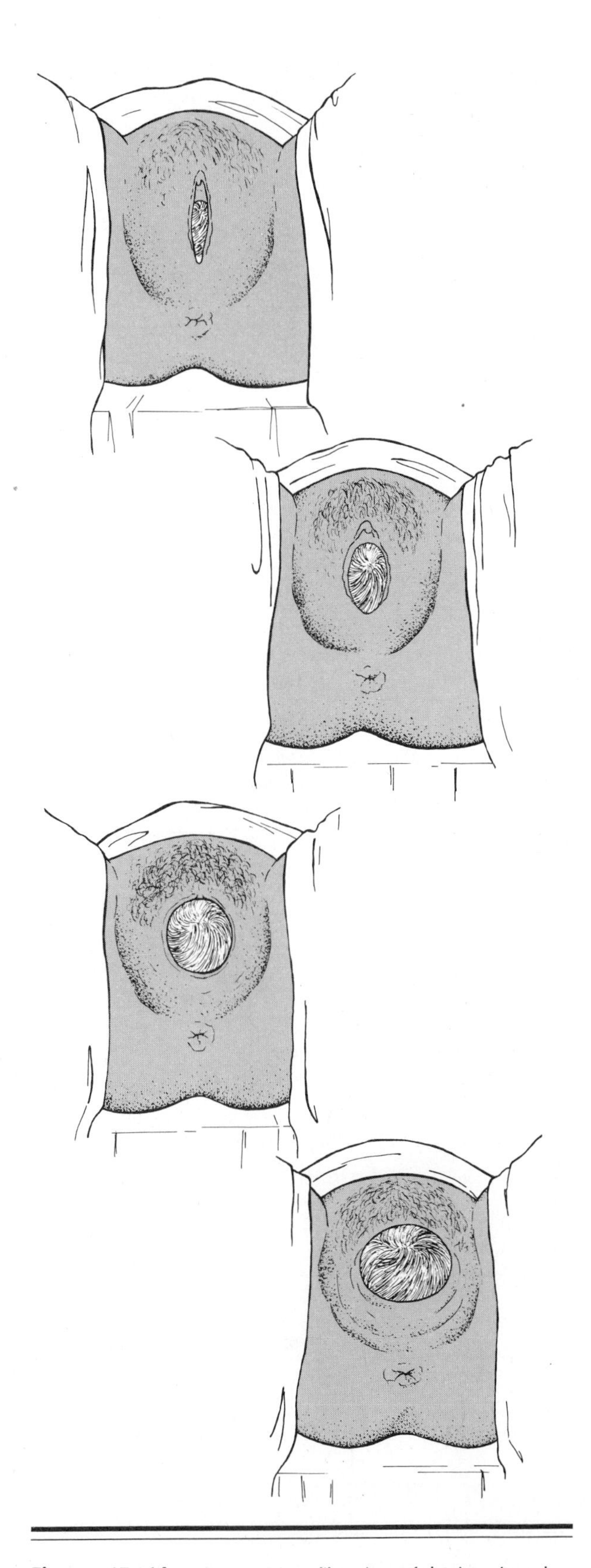

Figure 15–14. Progressive dilatation of the introitus during the second stage of labor.

the face sliding over the perineum. (See Chapter 17 for medical and nursing interventions to facilitate the delivery process.) After delivery of the head, restitution and external rotation of the infant occurs. When the shoulders appear at the symphysis pubis, gentle traction applied to the infant's head aids in their delivery. The body then follows.

Delivery of infants in presentations other than the vertex is discussed in Chapter 19.

Third Stage

Placental Separation

After the infant is delivered, the uterus firmly contracts, diminishing its capacity and the surface area of placental attachment. The decidua spongiosa begins to separate because of this decrease in surface area. As this separation occurs, bleeding results in the formation of a hematoma between the placental tissue and the remaining decidua. This hematoma accelerates the separation process. The membranes are the last to separate. They are peeled off the uterine wall as the placenta extrudes into the vagina.

Signs of placental separation usually appear around 5 minutes after delivery of the infant. These signs are (a) a globular-shaped uterus, (b) a rise of the fundus in the abdomen, (c) a sudden gush or trickle of blood, and (d) further protrusion of the umbilical cord out the introitus.

Placental Delivery

When the signs of placental separation appear, the mother may bear down to aid in placental expulsion. If this fails and the clinician has ascertained that the fundus is firm, gentle traction may be applied to the cord while pressure is exerted on the fundus. The weight of the placenta as it is guided into the placental pan aids in the removal of the membranes from the uterine wall. Even though a placenta is not considered retained until after 30 minutes have elapsed from completion of the second stage of labor, Pritchard and MacDonald (1976) recommend manual removal if the placenta has not separated in 5 minutes after the birth, in order to reduce the blood loss of the

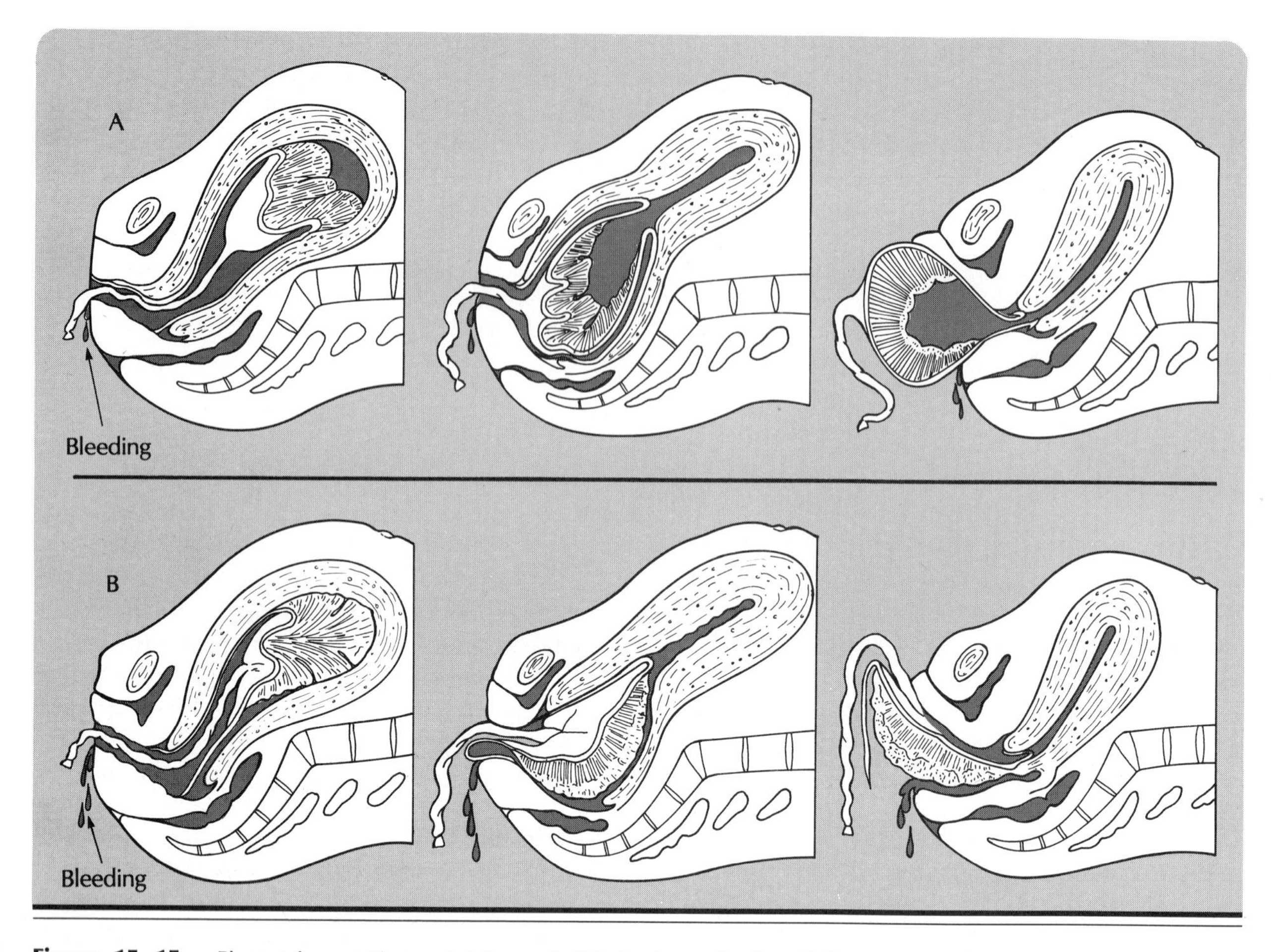

Figure 15–15. Placental separation and delivery. **A,** Schultze's mechanism. **B,** Duncan's mechanism.

third stage. The danger of this method is the introduction of pathogens into the uterine cavity.

If the placenta separates from the inside to the outer margins, it is delivered with the fetal or shiny side presenting (Figure 15–15). This is known as *Schultze's mechanism* of placental delivery, or more commonly *shiny Schultze's.* If the placenta separates from the outer margins inward, it will roll up and present sideways with the maternal surface delivering first. This is known as *Duncan's method* of placental delivery, and is commonly called *dirty Duncan* because the placental surface is rough appearing.

Nursing and medical interventions during the third stage of labor are discussed in detail in Chapter 17.

Fourth Stage

The period of time from 1 to 4 hours after delivery, in which physiologic readjustment of the mother's body begins, is designated as the fourth stage of labor. During this stage the mother's systemic responses stablize and the uterus contracts. Management of this stage is discussed in Chapter 17.

EXTRAUTERINE ADAPTATIONS OF THE NEONATE

There is elastic recoil of the infant's chest as it emerges from the birth canal, and air is drawn in to replace the fluid that was squeezed out during the latter part of labor. After the first inspiration, the newborn expires against a partially closed glottis, which creates a positive intrathoracic pressure of up to 40 cm H_2O. With the initiation of respiration and lung expansion, pulmonary vascular resistance falls. This decrease is thought to be a direct effect of oxygen and carbon dioxide on the blood vessels. There is a gradual transition from fetal to adult circulation. The ductus arteriosus constricts in response to an increase in the arterial oxygen tension.

The immediate care of the newborn is discussed in Chapters 17 and 23.

SUMMARY

The wonderful phenomenon of labor—the process of birth—is a period of transition for the pregnant woman, because it is the climax of her waiting. A competent maternity nurse understands the factors that influence the actual mechanical process of labor and the various emotional changes that take place.

SUGGESTED ACTIVITIES

1. Your neighbor is expecting her first child and asks you what causes labor to begin. Explain the theories of labor to her.
2. Review a case study of a labor and delivery patient, identifying the factors that influenced her progress in labor and the approximate length of time in each stage of labor.
3. Design a crash course for a primipara in your care who knows nothing about labor. Consider the factors that influence her learning.

REFERENCES

Aladjem, S., and Brown, A. K. 1974. *Clinical perinatology.* St. Louis: The C. V. Mosby Co.

Assali, N. S. 1968. *Biology of gestation.* Vol. 1. New York: Academic Press, Inc.

Bonica, J. J. 1960. *Mechanisms and pathways of pain in labor.* Chicago: Abbott Laboratories.

Bonica, J. J. 1967. *Principles and practices of obstetric analgesia and anesthesia.* Philadelphia: F. A. Davis Co.

Burrow, G. N., and Ferris, T. F. 1975. *Medical complications during pregnancy.* Philadelphia: W. B. Saunders Co.

Caldwell, W. E., and Moloy, H. C. 1933. Anatomical variations in the female pelvis and their effect on labor with a suggested classification. *Am. J. Obstet. Gynecol.* 26:479.

Cogan, R. 1975. Comfort during prepared childbirth as a function of parity reported by four classes of participant observers. *J. Psychosom. Res.* 19:33.

Colman, A. D., and Colman, L. L. 1971. *Pregnancy: the psychological experience.* New York: Herder & Herder.

Danforth, D., ed. 1977. *Textbook of obstetrics and gynecology.* 3rd ed. New York: Harper & Row Publishers, Inc.

Dick-Read, G. 1972. *Childbirth without fear.* 4th ed. New York: Harper & Row Publishers, Inc.

Dukes, J. H., and Bowen, J. C. 1976. Fluid and electrolytes: basic concepts and recent developments. *Contemp. OB/Gyn.* 8:173.

Erkkola, R., and Rauramo, L. 1976. Correlation of maternal physical fitness during pregnancy with maternal and fetal pH and lactic acid at delivery. *Acta Obstet. Gynecol. Scand.* 55:441.

Greenhill, J. P., and Friedman, E. A. 1974. *Biological principles and modern practice of obstetrics.* Philadelphia: W. B. Saunders Co.

Jensen, M., et al. 1977. *Maternity care: the nurse and the family.* St. Louis: The C. V. Mosby Co.

Liggins, G. C. 1973. Fetal influences on myometrial contractility. *Clin. Obstet. Gynecol.* 16:148.

Nurses Association of the American College of Obstetricians and Gynecologists (NAACOG). April 24, 1974. The four Ps. Postgraduate course. Las Vegas, Nev.

Oxorn, H., and Foote, W. 1975. *Human labor and birth.* New York: Appleton-Century-Crofts.

Pritchard, J., and MacDonald, P. C. 1976. *Williams obstetrics.* 15th ed. New York: Appleton-Century-Crofts.

Reeder, S., et al. 1976. *Maternity nursing.* Philadelphia: J. B. Lippincott Co.

Weekes, A. R., and Flynn, M. J. 1975. Engagement of fetal head in primigravidae and its relationship to duration of gestation and onset of labor. *Br. J. Obstet. Gynecol.* 82:7.

Zax, M., et al. 1975. Childbirth education, maternal attitudes and delivery. *Am. J. Obstet. Gynecol.* 123:185.

ADDITIONAL READINGS

Clark, A. L., and Affonso, D. D. 1976. *Childbearing: a nursing perspective.* Philadelphia: F. A. Davis Co.

Duigan, N. M., et al. 1975. Characteristics of normal labour in different racial groups. *Br. J. Obstet. Gynecol.* 82:593.

Friedman, E. A. 1967. *Labor: clinical evaluation and management.* New York: Appleton-Century-Crofts.

Friedman, E. A. July 1970. An objective method of evaluating labor. *Hosp. Pract.* 5:82.

Kennell, J. 1974. Evidence for a sensitive period in the human mother. In *Maternal attachment and mothering disorders: a round table,* ed. M. Klaus et al. Sausalito, Calif.: Johnson & Johnson Baby Products Company.

Korones, S. 1976. *High risk newborn infant: the basis for intensive nursing care.* 2nd ed. St. Louis: The C. V. Mosby Co.

Roberts, J. E. Jan. 1973. Suctioning the newborn. *Am. J. Nurs.* 73:63.

Ross Laboratories. 1976. Clinical education aids no. 13 and no. 18. Columbus, Ohio.

Willson, J. R., et al. 1975. *Obstetrics and gynecology.* St. Louis: The C. V. Mosby Co.

CHAPTER 16

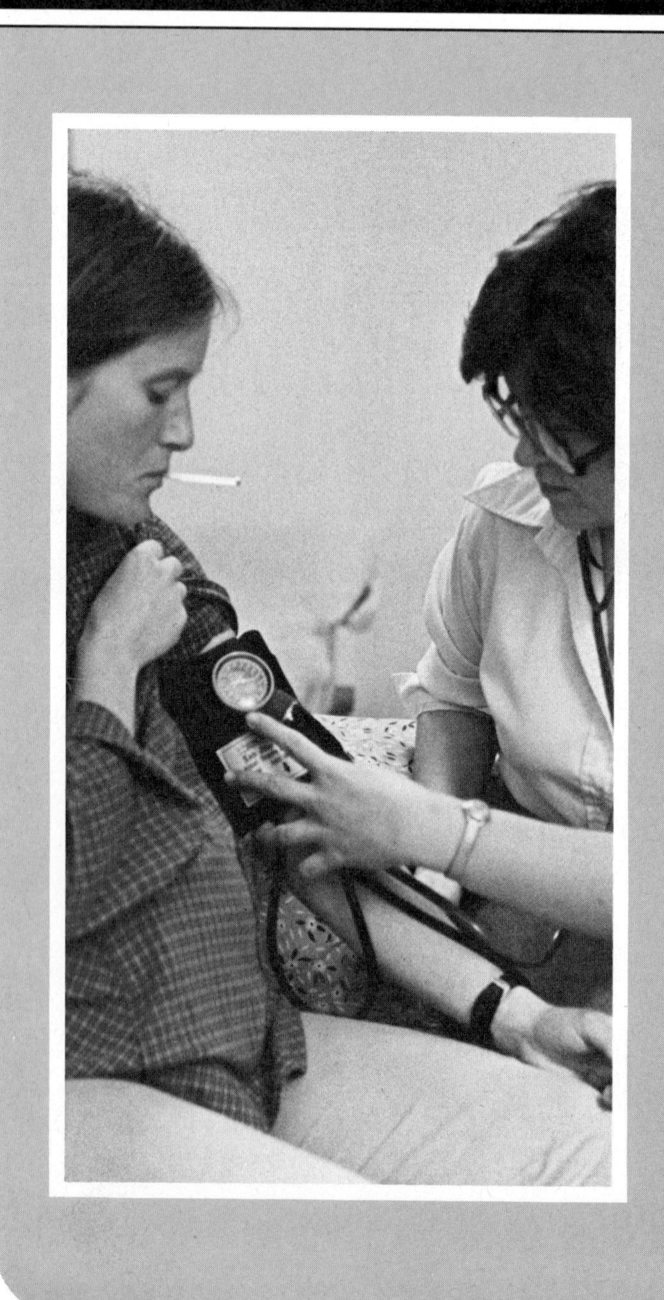

INTRAPARTAL NURSING ASSESSMENT

MATERNAL ASSESSMENT

History

Intrapartal High-Risk Screening

Intrapartal Physical Assessment

Intrapartal Psychologic Assessment

Methods of Evaluating Labor Progress

FETAL ASSESSMENT

Determination of Fetal Position

Evaluation of Fetal Status During Labor

OBJECTIVES

- Identify the methods used to evaluate the progress of labor.
- Explain the parts of, functions of, and indications for use of the internal and external electronic monitors.
- Discuss the procedures used to ascertain fetal presentation and position and the information obtained by each method.
- Describe the three periodic fetal heart rate patterns and differentiate them from baseline fetal heart rate.
- Discuss the indications for fetal scalp blood sampling and related blood values.

The physiologic changes that occur during the process of labor call for many adaptations of the mother and fetus. Assessment becomes more crucial because the changes are rapid and involve two patients, mother and child, both of whom require frequent reevaluation and intervention.

Most labors are uncomplicated for the mother and fetus. However, the potential for risk is great because of the rapidity of the changes. Thus the nurse must be aware of factors that can change a normal labor to a high-risk one.

The number and efficacy of intrapartal assessment techniques have increased over the years. In the past, nurses assessed the mother and fetus in labor by palpation and auscultation. These methods gave the nurse only intermittent information about the mother and fetus. Uterine contractions were estimated to be mild, moderate, or strong, and judgments varied according to the palpating hand.

FHTs were auscultated between contractions and usually for only 15 seconds. The 15-second rate was multiplied by 4 for the rate per minute. The nurse who was wise enough to auscultate right after the end of a contraction could hear what is termed *late decelerations.* However, many nurses would listen through the deceleration period and record the best rate. Nurses could also ascertain tachycardia and bradycardia by auscultation.

Assessment of abnormal labor through FHTs is best accomplished by continuous monitoring. With the advent of electronic monitors, this is now possible. Electronic and other techniques to assess maternal and fetal status during labor are discussed in this chapter.

MATERNAL ASSESSMENT

History

A patient history may be obtained in an abbreviated format when the patient is admitted to the labor and delivery area. Figure 16–1 is a sample hospital admission form. The information at the top of the form needs to be obtained for each patient. The rest of the form is used to record data that are pertinent to the labor process.

Intrapartal High-Risk Screening

Hobel (1976) determined that high-risk mothers deliver high-risk newborns. He developed an assessment form for the intrapartal period in which risk factors are identified and totaled (Figure 16–2). On this record, a mother with a score greater than 10 has a good chance of delivering a sick newborn. The nurses and physicians use this record, beginning with a careful history obtained by the nurse. The medical and nursing assessment is ongoing throughout the intrapartal period. It is important that this assessment form be sent to the nursery and postpartal unit for continuity of care.

Patients in the high-risk category include mothers who are younger than 16 or older than 35 years of age, who are over gravida 4, who are classified as overweight or underweight, or who smoke. Women who have an Rh-negative blood type, who received blood transfusions at one time, or who had a pregnancy loss should also be considered high risk. Also at risk are those mothers with less than a high school education, who are in the poverty-level income group, who are unmarried, who have an unplanned pregnancy, and who have had little or no antepartal care. Other risk factors are given in Table 16–1.

Any combination or multiple occurrence of these risk factors increases the dangers for the mother and fetus. Any mother with a medical or pregnancy-induced disease should be monitored throughout labor. Whenever a risk factor occurs during labor, even if the mother has had an uneventful antepartal period, she becomes high risk and should be monitored electronically.

Intrapartal Physical Assessment

A physical examination is included as part of the admission procedure and as part of the ongoing care of the patient. The assessment becomes the basis for initiating nursing interventions.

The intrapartal physical assessment is not as complete and thorough as the initial prenatal physical examination (Chapter 10), but it does involve assessment of some body systems and of the actual labor process. The accompanying Intrapartal Physical Assessment Guide provides a framework for the maternity nurse's examination of the laboring woman.

Admission Date	Time	Admitting nurse		
Patient name	Age	E.D.C.	L.M.P.	Length of gestation by dates
Attenting physician	Pediatrician			
Gravida	Para	Abortions	Neonatal deaths	
Blood type-RH	Serology	Date of serology testing	Prepregnant weight	Present weight
Onset of labor: ☐ Spontaneous ☐ Induced Date Time	Membranes ruptured: ☐ Spontaneous ☐ Artificial Date Time			
Bleeding:	Nursing: ☐ yes ☐ no			
Allergies: Medications	Foods or substances			
History of previous illness: (e.g., TB, heart disease, diabetes, convulsive disorder)				
Problems in prenatal course: (e.g., elevated blood pressure, bleeding problems)				
Patient requests: (e.g., no anesthesia, father in delivery room, rooming-in)				
Prenatal education classes Yes ____ No ____ Type				
Admission urinalysis	Prep	Enema		

		Maternal			
Date	Hour	Temp	Pulse	BP	Type Exam

		Fetus			
Date	Hour	Fetal Heart	Type Exam	Presenting Part	Membranes

		Labor Progress					
Date	Hour	Dilatation	Effacement	Position	Contractions (quality, duration)	Medications	Nurse Notes

Figure 16–1. Sample hospital admission form.

PATIENT WEIGHT	AGE	TERM	PREMI	Ab	LIVE	PRENATAL CARE ☐ NO ☐ YES	CLINIC OR PHYSICIAN	CODE

ADMISSION DATE __/__/__ TIME ____	LMP	CONDENSED PRENATAL PROBLEM LIST / PROB. NO. / PROB. NO.
MEMBRANES RUPTURED __/__/__ TIME ____	EDC	
ONSET LABOR __/__/__ 1 TIME ____		

	+ −	Risk Value	Prob. No.	PRENATAL HOSPITALIZATION ☐ No ☐ Yes PRENATAL SCORE ► / PATIENT TRANSFERRED FROM ANOTHER HOSPITAL ☐ NO ☐ YES - specify:
EARLY PROBLEMS		10	101	PREMATURE LABOR <37 ► Lung Maturity: ☐ Immature ☐ Interm. ☐ Mature Treatment: ☐ Alcohol ☐ B-Mimetic ☐ Other:
		10	102	HYDRAMNIOS—A clinical estimate of excessive amniotic fluid.
		10	103	MULTIPLE PREGNANCY
		10	104	ABN PRESENTATION ☐ Breech ☐ Face ☐ Brow ☐ Compound ☐ Transverse Lie ☐ Other
		10	105	MODERATE SEVERE PRE-ECLAMPSIA—B.P. ≥160/110 or Proteinuria >2+ after 26 wks. Gest. Age
		5	106	MILD PRE-ECLAMPSIA #1 required for the Diagnosis ☐ 1 BP ≥140/90 or +30 mm in systolic or 15 mm in diastolic ☐ 2 Proteinuria 1+ or 2+ ☐ 3—Persistent edema of Hands or Face
		5	107	INDUCTION ☐ Medical ☐ Elective ☐ Amniotomy ☐ Oxytocin
		5	108	PREMATURE RUPTURE OF MEMBRANES—Rupture 12 hours or more prior to labor onset.
		5	109*	C-SECTION ☐ Primary ☐ Repeat
		10	110	HEAVY MECONIUM—Dark stained Amniotic Fluid—usually dark green and tenacious
		5	111	LIGHT MECONIUM—Light stained Amniotic Fluid—yellow or greenish
		5	112	PROLONGED LATENT PHASE—Over 13 hours Multipara, over 20 hours Nullipara
INTERIM PROBLEMS		5	113	PRIMARY DYSFUNCTIONAL LABOR—W/O Oxytocin after 4 cm dilatation ☐ 1—Nullipara—at least 1 cm per hour ☐ 2—Multipara—1.5 cm per hour
		1	114	SECONDARY ARREST OF DILATATION—Failure to progress after 5 cm Cervical Dilatation
		5	115	PITOCIN AUGMENTATION OF LABOR—Use of Oxytocin to improve uterine contractions
		10	116	CORD PROLAPSE
		10	117*	UTERINE BLEEDING ☐ Abruption ☐ Previa ☐ Marginal Separation
		10	118	FETAL TACHYCARDIA >160 beats per minute lasting more than 30 minutes.
		10	119	AMNIONITIS ☐ Mat. Temp. ≥100.4° ☐ Bacteria in Amniotic Fluid
		10	120	FETAL BRADYCARDIA—<120 Beats/min. or abnormal heart rate patterns (HRP) persisting over 30 min ☐ Mild ☐ Mod ☐ Sev. cord comp. or ☐ Mild ☐ Mod ☐ Sev. late decel. HRP
		10	121	DECREASE BASE LINE VARIABILITY DUE TO ☐ Medication ☐ Acidosis ☐ Unknown
COMPLETE DILATION DATE __/__/__ 2 TIME ____		5	122	EXCESSIVE MEDICATION ☐ Demerol, greater than 150 mg ☐ Phenobarbitol, greater than 60 mg ☐ Magnesium Sulfate, greater than 25 grams ☐ Other
LATE PROBLEMS		10	123	SEIZURE ☐ Eclampsia ☐ Previous Seizure Disorder ☐ Unknown
		10	124*	BREECH DELIVERY (VAGINAL) METHOD: ☐ Spontaneous ☐ Assisted ☐ Breech Ext. TYPE: ☐ Single Footling ☐ Double Footling ☐ Frank
		10	125	SHOULDER DYSTOCIA
		5	126*	☐ OPERATIVE FORCEPS ☐ VACUUM EXTRACTION ☐ FAILED VACUUM
		1	127*	OUTLET FORCEPS ☐ Simpson ☐ Tucker McLane ☐ Luikart ☐ Other
		5	128	LATE PASSAGE OF MECONIUM—Any stained fluid after previously clear fluid
		10	129	COMPLICATIONS OF ANESTHESIA ☐ Convulsion ☐ Fetal Bradycardia ☐ Hypotension ☐ Other:
		5	130	SECOND STAGE >2.5 HOURS
		5	131	PRECIPITOUS LABOR <3 HOURS TOTAL
DELIVERY DATE __/__/__ 3 TIME ____		5	132	LABOR >20 HOURS TOTAL
			133	MOTHER-INFANT BONDING ☐ Excellent ☐ Good ☐ Poor
PLACENTA DATE __/__/__ 4 TIME ____			134	DELIVERED ☐ Home ☐ In Transit ☐ Elsewhere in Hospital
			135	STILLBIRTH ☐ Antepartum ☐ Intrapartum

	HOURS	MIN	
STAGE I 1 (−2)	__	__	**FINAL SCORE**
STAGE II 2 (−3)	__	__	SIGNATURES 1-
STAGE III 3 (−4)	__	__	2-
TOTAL LABOR TIME			3-

4 B R INTRAPARTUM PROBLEM LIST

Figure 16–2. Intrapartal problem list. (From Hobel, C. 1976. Problem-oriented risk assessment during labor. *Contemp. OB/Gyn.* 8:120.)

Table 16–1. Guidelines for Intrapartum Monitoring*

Factors	Risk value	Factors	Risk value
Prenatal historical factors		Intrauterine growth retardation	10
Age >35 or <16	5	Vaginal spotting	10
Diabetes	10	Abnormal fetal-placental tests	10
Chronic hypertension	10	Multiple pregnancy	10
Cardiac disease	10	*Early intrapartum problems*	
Rh sensitization	5	Induction of labor	5
Sickle cell disease or trait	5	Premature labor	10
Previous cesarean section	5	Premature rupture of membranes	5
Prenatal developing factors		Meconium-stained fluid	10
Anemia	5	Abnormal fetal heart tones by auscultation	10
Preeclampsia	10	Prolonged latent phase of labor	5
Postterm >42 weeks	10		
Polyhydramnios	10		

*From Hobel, C. 1976. Problem-oriented risk assessment during labor. *Contemp. OB/Gyn.* 8:121.

INTRAPARTAL PHYSICAL ASSESSMENT GUIDE: FIRST STAGE OF LABOR

Assess	Normal findings	Deviations and possible causes*	Nursing interventions†
Vital signs			
Blood pressure	90–140/60–90	High blood pressure (essential hypertension, preeclampsia, renal disease, apprehension or anxiety)	Evaluate history of preexisting disorders and check for presence of other signs of preeclampsia.
Pulse	60–90 beats/min	Increased pulse rate (excitement or anxiety, cardiac disorders)	Evaluate cause. Report to physician.
Respirations	16–24/min (or pulse rate divided by 4)	Marked tachypnea (respiratory disease)	Report to physician. (Note: Do not assess respirations during a uterine contraction.)
Temperature	36.2–37.6C (98–99.6F)	Elevated temperature (infection, dehydration)	Assess for other signs of infection or dehydration.
Weight	15–30 lb greater than prepregnant weight	Weight gain > 30 pounds (fluid retention, obesity, large infant)	
Breasts	Slightly firm	Mass in any area of breasts (cysts, neoplasms)	Withhold hormones that prevent lactation from women who have breast masses or a history of problems.

*Possible causes of deviations are placed in parentheses.
†Nursing interventions are primarily for identified deviations.

INTRAPARTAL PHYSICAL ASSESSMENT GUIDE Cont'd

Assess	Normal findings	Deviations and possible causes*	Nursing interventions[†]
Lungs	Normal breath sounds (see irregular breath sounds Procedure 10-1)	Rales, rhonchi, friction rub (infection)	Refer to physician.
Heart	Normal heart sounds (see Procedure 10-3); grade II/VI systolic ejection murmur is normally found in pregnant woman due to extra blood volume passing through heart valves	Murmurs	Refer to physician.
Fundus	At 40 weeks' gestation, located just below xyphoid process	Uterine size not compatible with gestational age (SGA, polyhydramnios, multiple pregnancy)	Reevaluate history regarding pregnancy dating. Refer to physician for assessment of gestational age.
Edema	Slight amount of dependent edema	Pitting edema of face, legs, abdomen (preeclampsia)	Refer to physician. Check patella, deep tendon reflexes, and feet for clonus.
Hydration	Normal skin turgor (see Prenatal Initial Physical Assessment Guide, Chapter 10)	Poor skin turgor (dehydration)	Assess skin turgor. Refer to physician for deviations.
Perineum	Tissues smooth, pink color (see Prenatal Initial Physical Assessment Guide, Chapter 10)	Varicose veins of vulva	Exercise care while doing a perineal prep. Note on patient record need for follow-up in postpartal period. Reassess after delivery.
	Presence of small amount of bloody show	Profuse, purulent drainage	Suspect gonorrhea. Report to physician. Initiate care to newborn's eyes. Notify newborn nursing staff and pediatrician. (Note: Gaping of vagina and/or anus and bulging of perineum are suggestive signs of second stage of labor.)
Pelvic adequacy			
Inlet	Diagonal conjugate, 12.5 cm Obstetric conjugate, 11 cm True conjugate, 11.5 cm	Inadequate measurements	Determine fetal presentation, lie, and position. Inform physician if cephalopelvic disproportion is suspected.

*Possible causes of deviations are placed in parentheses.
[†]Nursing interventions are primarily for identified deviations.

Table 16–2. Correlation of Cervical Dilatation and Uterine Activity During Phases of First Stage

	Latent phase	Active phase	Transition
Dilatation	0–3 cm	4–7 cm	7–10 cm
Contractions			
Frequency	Every 15–30 min	Every 3–5 min	Every 1½–3 min
Duration	10–30 sec	30–45 sec	45–60 sec
Intensity	Mild	Moderate	Strong

INTRAPARTAL PHYSICAL ASSESSMENT GUIDE Cont'd

Assess	Normal findings	Deviations and possible causes*	Nursing interventions†
Cavity	Midplane, 12.45 cm Anteroposterior, 11.5–12 cm Posterior sagittal, 4.5–5 cm Transverse, 10.5 cm		
Outlet	Bituberous width, 8 cm Mobile coccyx height <6 cm	Contractures, immobile coccyx	
Symphysis pubis	Mobile coccyx height, 6 cm Inclination: 85°–90°		
Labor status			
Uterine contractions	Regular pattern (Table 16–2 shows normal characteristics during first stage)	Failure to establish a regular pattern Hypertonicity Hypotonicity	Evaluate whether patient is in true labor. Evaluate patient status and contractile pattern.
Cervical dilatation	Progressive cervical dilatation from size of fingertip to 10 cm (Figure 16–3 and Table 16–2)	Rigidity of cervix (frequent cervical infections, scar tissue, failure of presenting part to descend)	Evaluate contractions, fetal engagement, and position. (Note: Sterile vaginal examination is done to assess dilatation and effacement of cervix, fetal station, position, and presentation, and condition of membranes.)

*Possible causes of deviations are placed in parentheses.
†Nursing interventions are primarily for identified deviations.

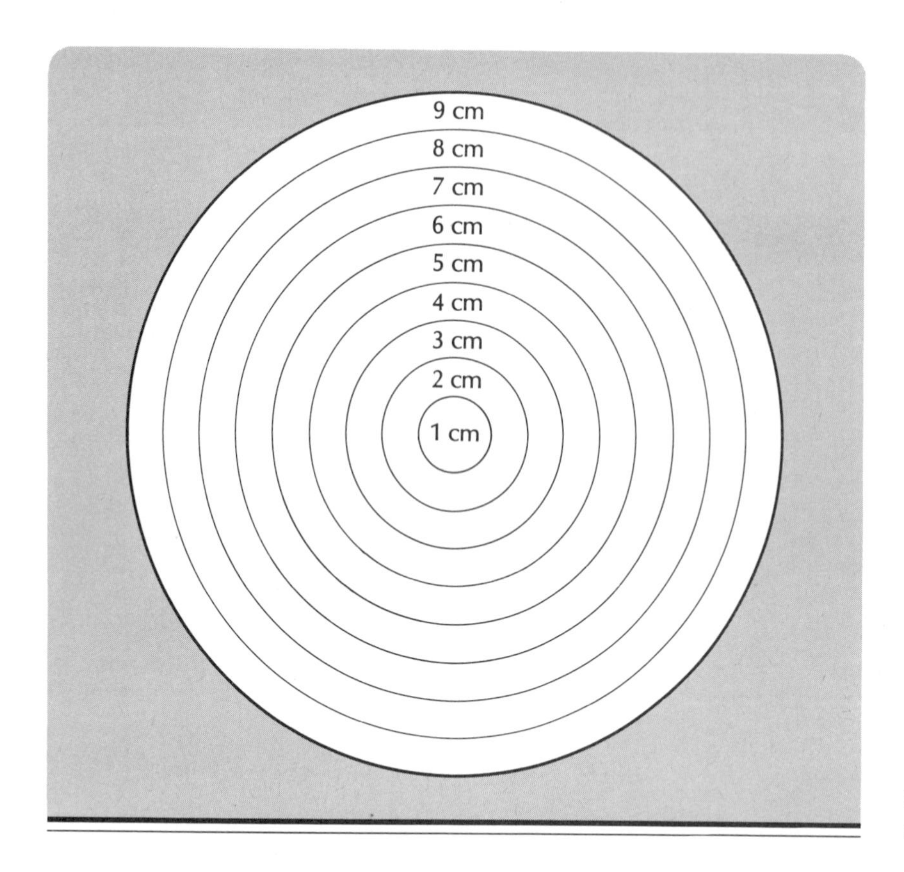

Figure 16–3. Cervical dilatation measurement tool.

INTRAPARTAL PHYSICAL ASSESSMENT GUIDE Cont'd

Assess	Normal findings	Deviations and possible causes*	Nursing interventions†
Cervical effacement	Progressive thinning of cervix (see Figure 15–12 and Figure 16–4)	Failure to efface (rigidity of cervix, failure of presenting part to engage) Cervical edema (pushing effort by woman before cervix is fully dilated and effaced, trapped cervix)	Evaluate contractions, fetal engagement, and position.
Fetal descent	Progressive descent of fetal presenting part from station −5 to +4 (see Figures 16–4 and 16–11)	Failure of descent (abnormal fetal position or presentation, a macrosomic fetus, inadequate pelvic measurement)	Evaluate fetal position, presentation, and size. Evaluate maternal pelvic measurements.
Membranes	May rupture before or during labor	Rupture of membranes increases before engagement of presenting part or with abnormal fetal position	Assess for ruptured membranes using Nitrazine test tape before doing vaginal exam. Instruct patients with ruptured membranes to remain on bed rest.

*Possible causes of deviations are placed in parentheses.
†Nursing interventions are primarily for identified deviations.

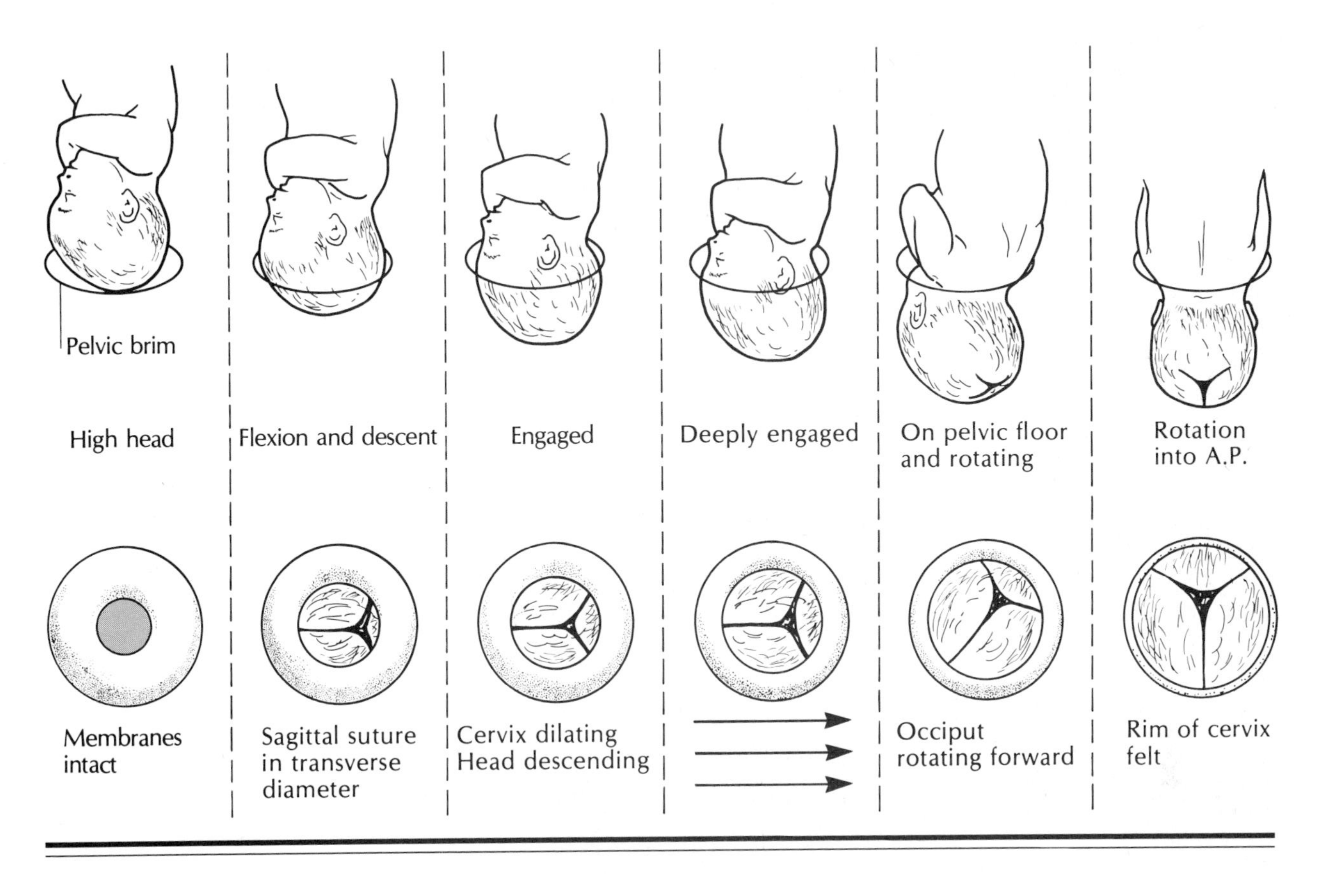

Figure 16–4. *Top,* the fetal head progressing through the pelvis. *Bottom,* The changes that the nurse will detect on palpation of the cervix. (From Myles, M. F. 1975. *Textbook for midwives.* Edinburgh: Churchill Livingstone, p. 246.)

INTRAPARTAL PHYSICAL ASSESSMENT GUIDE Cont'd

Assess	Normal findings	Deviations and possible causes*	Nursing interventions†
	Findings on Nitrazine test tape: Probably intact membranes yellow pH 5.0 olive pH 5.5 olive green pH 6.0 Probably ruptured membranes blue-green pH 6.5 blue-gray pH 7.0 deep blue pH 7.5	False positive results may be obtained if large amount of bloody show is present or if previous vaginal examination has been done using lubricant	
	Amniotic fluid clear, no odor	Greenish amniotic fluid (fetal distress)	Assess FHR and report to physician.
		Strong odor (amnionitis)	Take patient's temperature and report to physician.

*Possible causes of deviations are placed in parentheses.
†Nursing interventions are primarily for identified deviations.

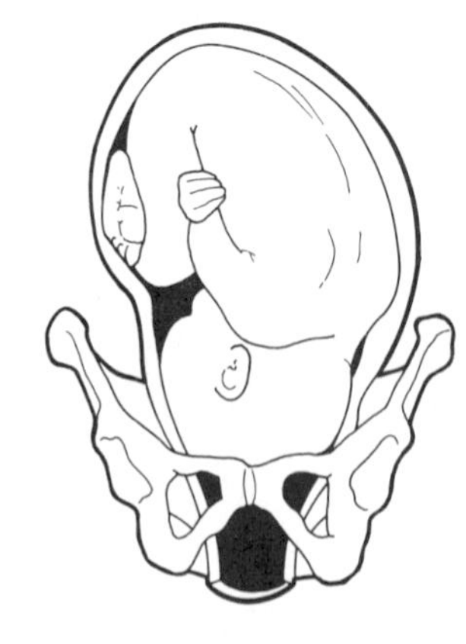

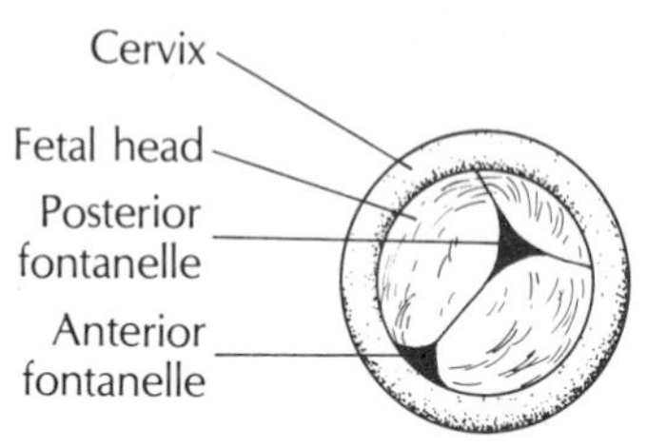

Figure 16-5. Palpation of presenting part in LOA position. Posterior fontanelle is in upper right.

INTRAPARTAL PHYSICAL ASSESSMENT GUIDE Cont'd

Assess	Normal findings	Deviations and possible causes*	Nursing interventions[†]
			Assess fluid at regular intervals for presence of meconium staining.
Fetal status			
FHR	120-160 beats/min	< 120 or > 160 beats/min (fetal distress); abnormal patterns on fetal monitor: decreased variability, late decelerations, variable decelerations (p. 473)	Initiate interventions based on particular FHR pattern (p. 473).
Presentation	Cephalic, 97% Breech, 3%	Face or brow presentation	Report to physician. After presentation is confirmed as face or brow, patient may be prepared for cesarean section.
Assessment methods 1. Visualization of abdomen (p. 458) 2. Leopold's maneuvers (p. 460) 3. Vaginal examination (Procedure 17-1)		Transverse lie	Report to physician. Prepare patient for cesarean section.
Position	LOA most common (Figure 16-5)	Persistent occipital-posterior position; transverse arrest	Carefully monitor maternal and fetal status.
Activity	Fetal movement	Hyperactivity (may precede fetal hypoxia)	Carefully evaluate FHR.
		Complete lack of movement	Carefully evaluate FHR.

*Possible causes of deviations are placed in parentheses.
[†]Nursing interventions are primarily for identified deviations.

INTRAPARTAL PHYSICAL ASSESSMENT GUIDE Cont'd

Assess	Normal findings	Deviations and possible causes*	Nursing interventions†
Laboratory evaluation			
Hematologic tests			
Hemoglobin	12-16 gm/100 ml	< 12 gm (anemia, hemorrhage)	Evaluate woman for problems due to decreased oxygen-carrying capacity caused by lowered hemoglobin.
CBC			
Hematocrit	38%-47%	Presence of infection or blood dyscrasias	Evaluate for deviations.
RBC	4.2-5.4 million/μl		
WBC	4,500-11,000/μl		
WBC differential			
Neutrophils	56%		
Bands	3%		
Eosinophils	2.7%		
Basophils	0.3%		
Lymphocytes	34%		
Monocytes	4%		
Serologic testing			
STS or VDRL test	Nonreactive	Positive reactive (see Chapter 10, Initial Prenatal Physical Assessment Guide)	For reactive test, notify newborn nursery and pediatrician.
Urinalysis			
Glucose	Negative	Glycosuria (low renal threshold for glucose, diabetes mellitus)	Assess blood glucose. Test urine for ketones. Ketonuria and glycosuria require further assessment of blood sugars.‡
Ketones	Negative	Ketonuria (starvation ketosis)	
Proteins	Negative	Proteinuria (urine specimen contaminated with vaginal secretions, fever, kidney disease); proteinuria of 2+ or greater found in uncontaminated urine may be a sign of ensuing preeclampsia	Instruct patient in collection technique. Chance of contamination from vaginal discharge is common.
Red blood cells	Negative	Blood in urine (calculi, cystitis, glomerulonephritis, neoplasm)	Assess collection technique.
White blood cells	Negative	Presence of white blood cells (infection in genitourinary tract)	Assess for signs of urinary tract infection.
Casts	None	Presence of casts (nephrotic syndrome)	

*Possible causes of deviations are placed in parentheses.
†Nursing interventions are primarily for identified deviations.
‡Glycosuria should not be discounted. The presence of glycosuria necessitates follow-up.

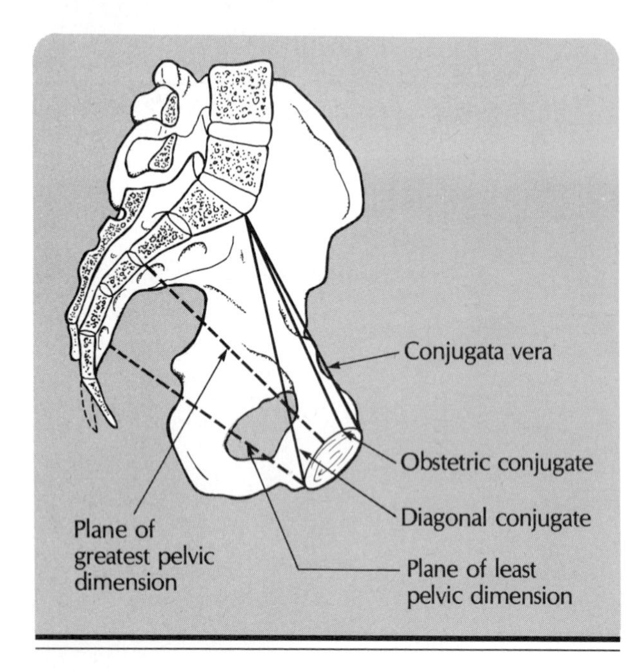

Figure 16-6. Anteroposterior diameters of the pelvic inlet and their relationship to the pelvic planes.

Assessment of Pelvic Adequacy

The pelvis may be assessed by x-ray pelvimetry at the discretion of the obstetrician but should always be assessed vaginally. Nurses prepared in an expanded role may perform the vaginal assessment and interpret pelvimetry findings.

1. *Pelvic Inlet.* The important anteroposterior diameters of the inlet for childbearing are the diagonal conjugate, the obstetric conjugate, and the true conjugate, or conjugata vera (Figure 16-6). Others are the transverse (13.5 cm) and the oblique diameters (12.5 cm).

The anteroposterior diameter of the pelvic inlet may be assessed by attempting to reach from the lower border of the symphysis pubis to the sacral promontory with the middle finger. The clinician should determine the length of the finger before attempting this. The diagonal conjugate can then be measured by marking the place where the proximal part of the hand makes contact with the pubis (Figure 16-7). Then the distance is measured (about 12.5 cm). The obstetric conjugate can be estimated by subtracting 1.5 from the length of the diagonal conjugate. At about 11 cm in length, it is the smallest and thus the most important anteroposterior diameter through which the fetus must pass. It is measured by x-ray examination from the sacral promontory to the upper inner point on the symphysis that extends farthest back into the pelvis. The true conjugate extends from the upper border of the symphysis pubis to the sacral promontory. It can be determined by subtracting 1.0 cm from the diagonal conjugate.

2. *Pelvic cavity (midpelvis).* Important measurements include the plane of greatest dimension, or midplane (12.75 cm), and the planes of least dimension (anteroposterior diameter, 11.5–12 cm; posterior sagittal diameter, 4.5–5 cm; and transverse diameter, 10.5 cm). These latter diameters can be measured digitally.

Location of the sacrospinous ligament, a firm ridge of tissue, makes location of the ischial spines easier. When this ligament is located, the examiner should run the fingers along it bilaterally toward the anterior portion of the pelvis. The spines may range from a small firm bump like the knuckle of a finger (termed *not encroaching*) to a very prominent bone. The space between the ischial spines (transverse diameter) is estimated according to the prominence of the spines. The sacrosciatic notch should admit two fingers. A wide notch means that the sacrum curves back posteriorly, giving the anteroposterior diameter of the midpelvis a greater length. A narrow notch indicates a decreased diameter. The width of the sacrosciatic notch is more accurately evaluated through x-ray examination but can be estimated through vaginal examination.

The length of the sacrospinous ligament is measured by tracing the ligament from its origin on the ischial spines to its insertion on the sacrum. It is usually 4 cm or two to three finger breadths long.

The capacity of the cavity can be assessed by sweeping the fingers down the side walls bilaterally to evaluate the shape of the pelvic side walls—whether convergent, divergent, or straight. The curvature, inclination, and hollowness of the sacrum help indicate the capacity of the posterior pelvis. It is estimated digitally by palpating the sacrococcygeal junction and by inching up toward the promontory. The examiner then estimates the hollowness of the sacrum, which is normally hollow.

If the lumbar curve changes, it can increase or decrease the pelvic inclination and influence the progress of labor, because the fetus has to adapt

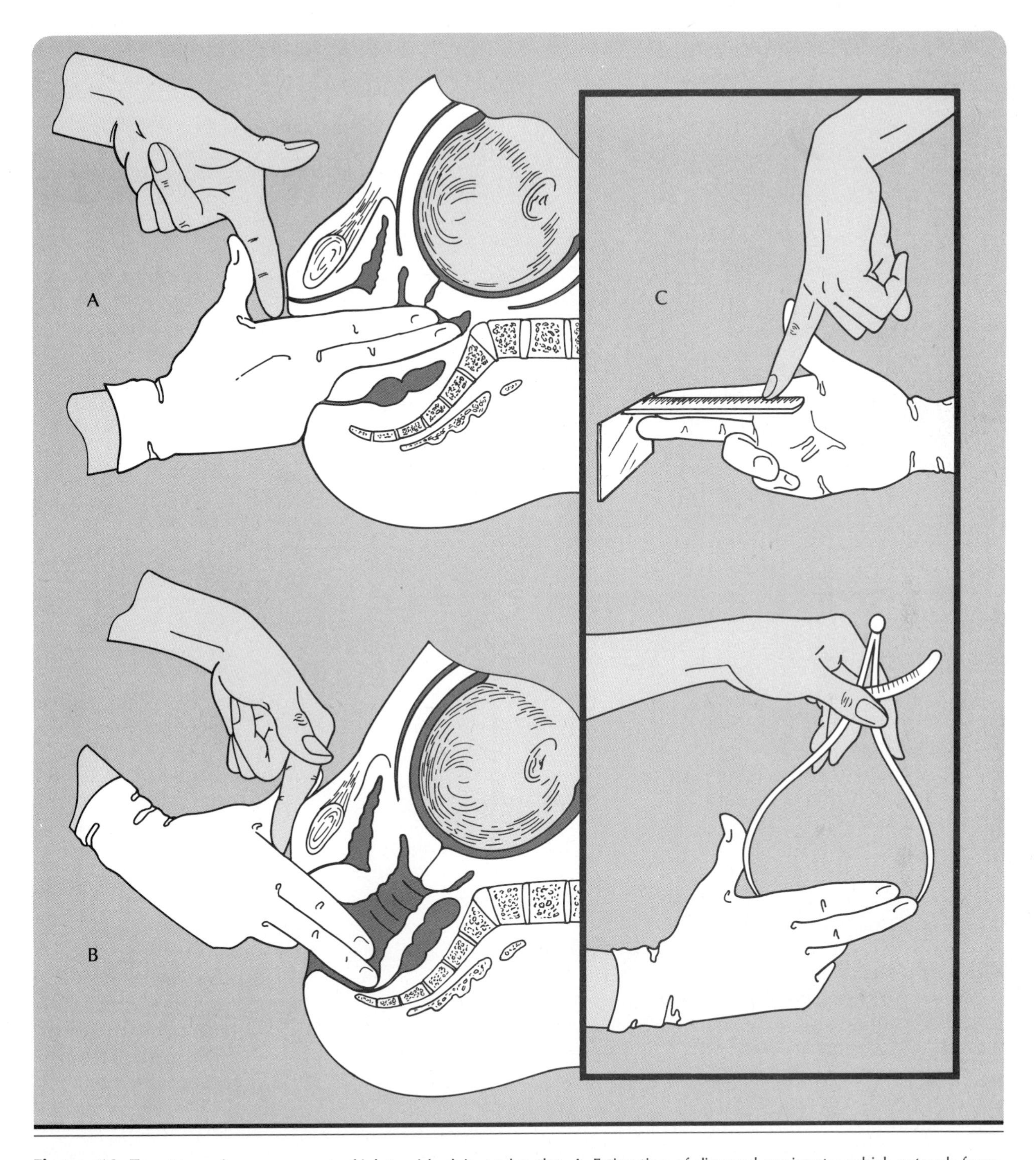

Figure 16–7. Manual measurement of inlet, midpelvis, and outlet. **A,** Estimation of diagonal conjugate, which extends from lower border of symphysis pubis to sacral promontory. **B,** Estimation of anteroposterior diameter of the outlet, which extends from the lower border of the symphysis pubis to the tip of the sacrum. **C,** Methods that may be used to check manual estimation of anteroposterior measurements.

itself to a curved path as well as to the different diameters of the true pelvis.

3. *Pelvic Outlet.* The anatomic anteroposterior diameter of the outlet, which is normally 9.5 cm, may be measured digitally (Figure 16–8). The mobility of the coccyx is determined by grasping the coccyx between the thumb externally and the

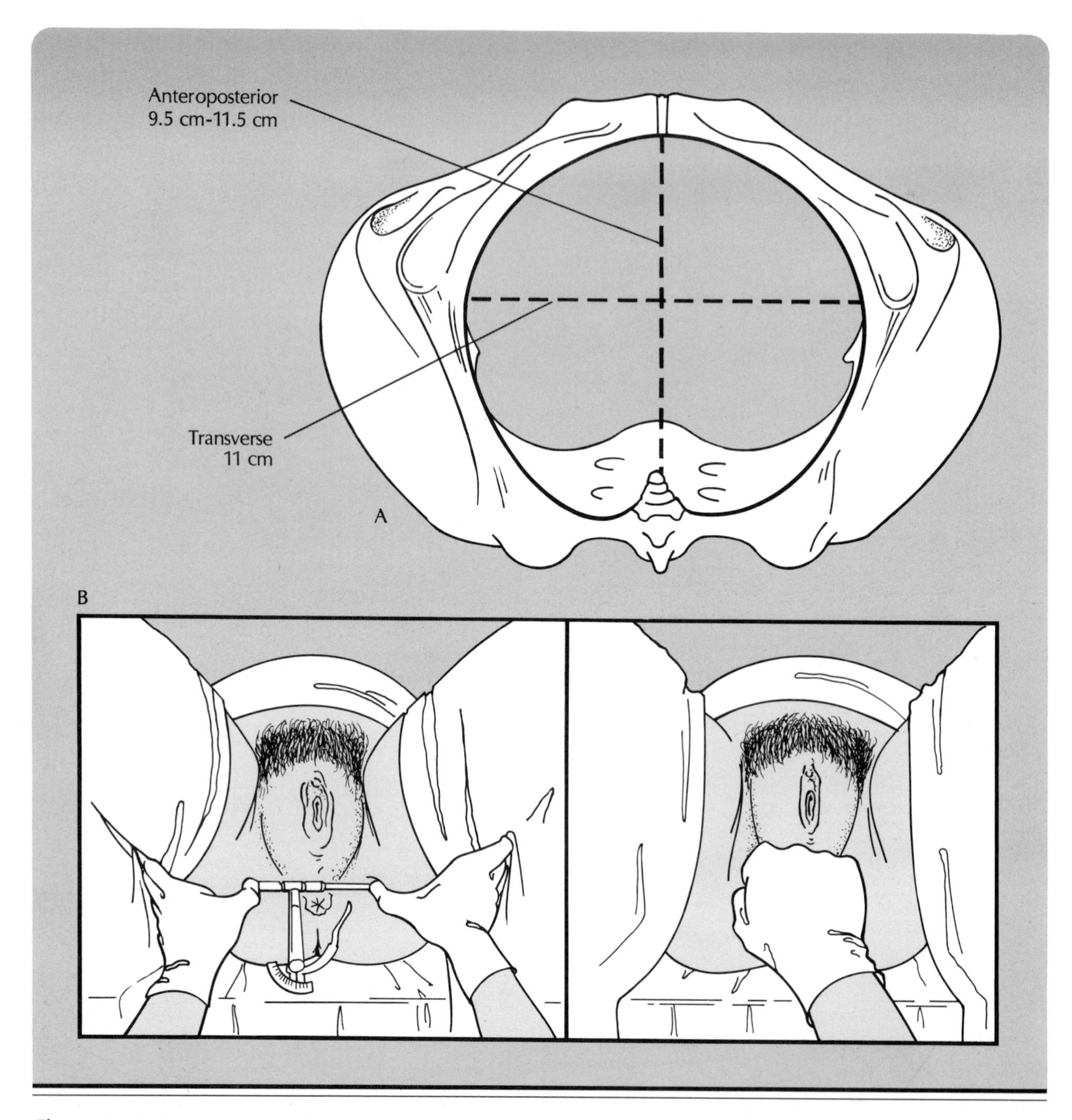

Figure 16–8. **A,** Diameters of the pelvic outlet. **B,** Measurement of the transverse diameter of the outlet. *Left,* use of Thom's pelvimeter; *right,* use of closed fist.

forefinger, which is inserted in the rectum. An immobile coccyx can decrease the diameter of the outlet. The obstetric anteroposterior diameter of the outlet is normally 11.5 cm.

The transverse diameter of the outlet is measured by placing the fist between the ischial tuberosities. Another method of measurement is to use the Thom's pelvimeter. The transverse diameter normally meaures 8 cm.

The suprapubic angle is estimated by palpating the bony structure externally. It should be 85°–90°. The suprapubic angle is estimated by placing two fingers side by side at the border of the symphysis (Figure 16–9). It is probably reduced if the examiner cannot separate his or her fingers.

The length and shape of the pubic rami affect the transverse diameter of the outlet. The pubic ramus is expected to be short and concave inward, as opposed to straight and long.

The height and inclination of the symphysis pubis are measured and the contour of the pubic arch is estimated. Excessively long or angulated bone structure shortens the diameter of the obstetric conjugate. Height can be determined by placing the index finger of the gloved hand up to the superior border of the symphysis. The examiner should measure the length of the first phalanx of the index finger (normally about 2.5 cm). Inclination may be determined by externally placing one finger on the top of the symphysis while the internal finger palpates the internal margin. An imaginary line is drawn between the fingers and the angle is estimated.

A posterior inclination with the lower border of the pubis slanting inward decreases the anteroposterior diameter. The anteroposterior sagittal diameter is the most significant diameter of the outlet, as it is the shortest diameter through which the baby must pass as he is delivered. Estimating the contour of the pubic arch provides information on the width of the angle at which these bones come together. The pubic arch has obstetric importance; if it is narrow the baby's head may be pushed backward toward the coccyx, making extension of the head difficult. This condition is called *outlet dystocia,* and forceps (outlet) delivery is required. (See Chapter 20 for further discussion.) Fetal head injury or deep perineal laceration may occur.

In questionable situations some pelvic measurements should be determined by means other than digital methods, for example, by ultrasound or x-ray pelvimetry. X-ray pelvimetry reveals the shape and type of pelvis, the true internal measurements, the fetopelvic relationship, and the estimated fetal size (Oxorn and Foote, 1975).

X-ray evaluation is recommended in the following cases:

a. During most dysfunctional labors, particularly if the physician is considering using oxytocin.

b. In patients with abnormal clinical measurements if there is a question as to pelvic adequacy after vaginal examination has been performed during early labor.

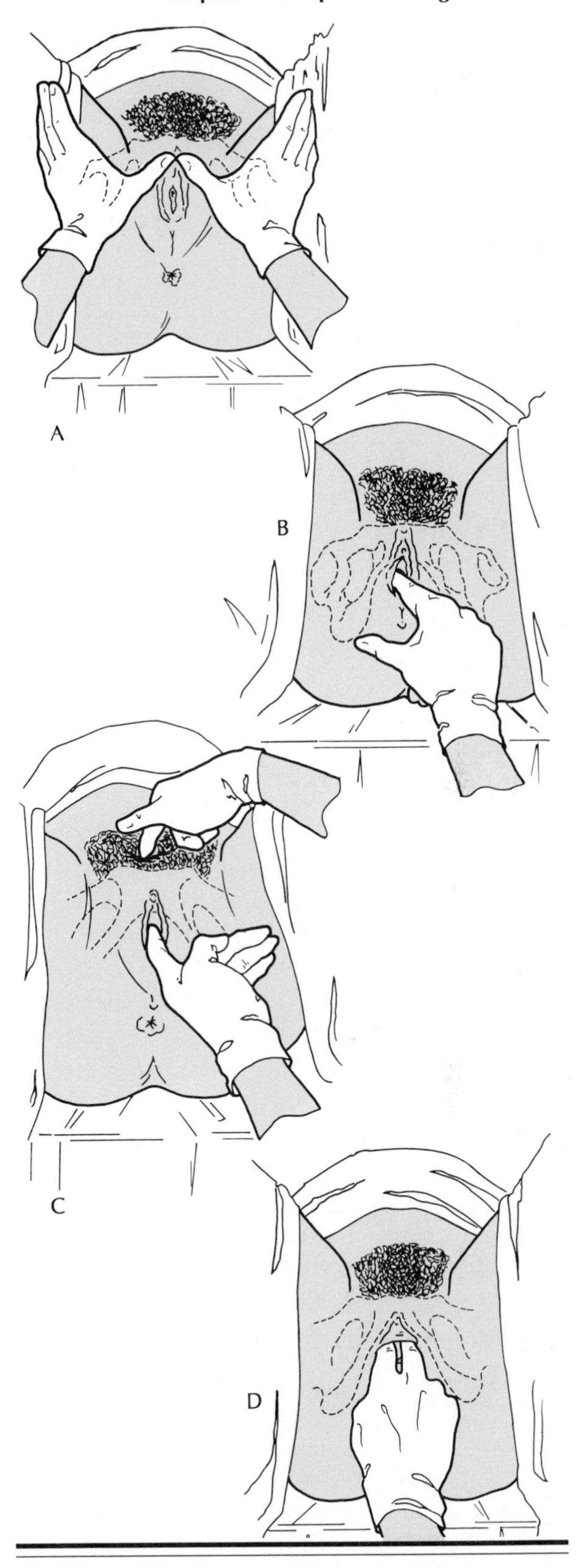

Figure 16–9. Evaluation of outlet. **A,** Estimation of subpubic angle. **B,** Estimation of length of pubic ramus. **C,** Estimation of depth and inclination of pubis. **D,** Estimation of contour of suprapubic angle.

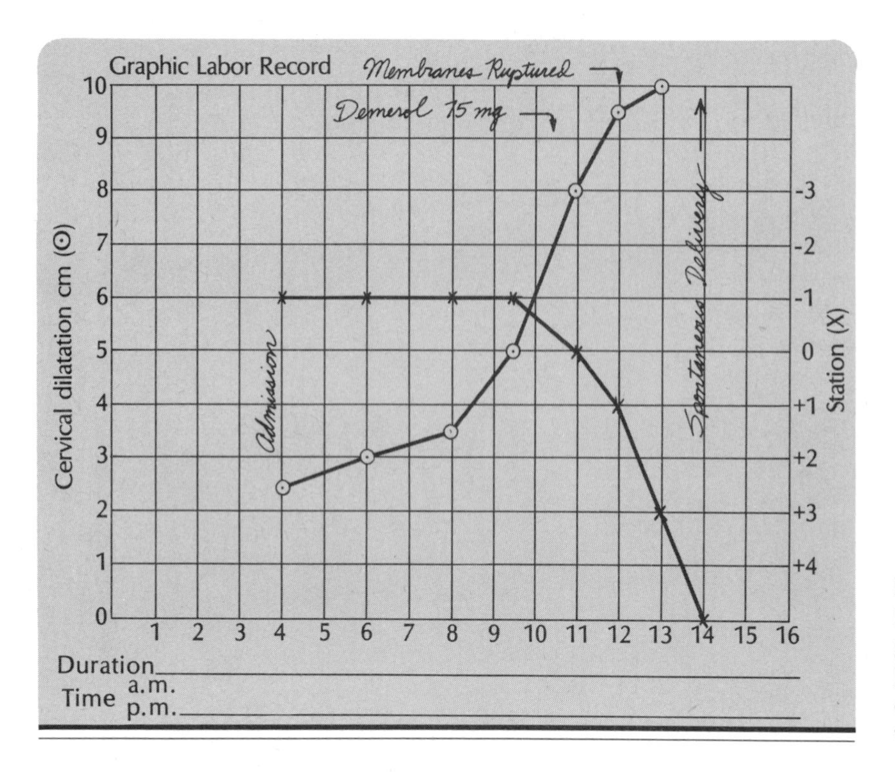

Figure 16–10. Example of charting labor progress on a Friedman graph. (Modified from Friedman, E. July 1970. An objective method of evaluating labor. *Hospital Practice,* vol. 5, no. 7, p. 87.)

c. During a trial labor for contracted pelvis before a decision to administer oxytocin or to perform cesarean section is made.
d. In breech positions during labor at term or whenever an abnormal fetal position is suspected.
e. In patients who have had disease or injury involving the bony pelvis or hips.
f. In patients who have had difficult labors or large infants previously.
g. Whenever there is suggestive evidence of disproportion, such as a floating head during early labor in a primigravida.*

Intrapartal Psychologic Assessment

Assessment of the laboring woman's psychologic status is an important part of the total assessment. The woman brings to labor previous ideas, knowledge, and fears. Assessment of her psychologic status enables the nurse to meet her informational and support needs. The nurse can support the mother and her partner, or in the absence of a partner, the nurse may become the significant other. See the accompanying Intrapartal Psychologic Assessment Guide.

Methods of Evaluating Labor Progress

Friedman Graph

Evaluation of the intensity, frequency, and duration of contractions does not present the entire birthing picture. Nurses can document labor progress objectively by using the Friedman graph, which evaluates uterine activity, cervical dilatation, and fetal descent.

To use this method, one needs special graph paper and skill in determining cervical dilatation and fetal descent. The numbers at the bottom of the graph in Figure 16–10 are hours of labor from 1 to 16. Vertically, at the left, cervical dilatation is measured from 0 to 10 cm. The vertical line on the right indicates fetal station in centimeters, from −5 to +5 (Friedman, 1970). When one plots cervical dilatation and descent on the basic graph, a characteristic pattern emerges: an S curve repre-

*From Willson, J. R., and Carrington, E. 1979. *Obstetrics and gynecology.* 6th ed. St. Louis: The C. V. Mosby Co., p. 468.

INTRAPARTAL PSYCHOLOGIC ASSESSMENT GUIDE: FIRST AND SECOND STAGES OF LABOR

Assess	Normal findings	Deviations and possible causes*	Nursing interventions[†]
Patient education	Prenatal education course	Lack of education	Give patient information regarding process, procedures, and breathing techniques.
Patient support	Presence of a significant person who will be available for encouragement and support	Lack of support	Provide support and encouragement.
Response to labor	Latent phase: relaxed, excited, anxious for labor to be well established Active phase: becomes more intense, begins to tire Transitional phase: feels tired, may feel unable to cope, needs frequent coaching to maintain breathing patterns	Inability to cope with contractions (fear, anxiety, lack of education)	Provide support and encouragement. Establish trusting relationship.

*Possible causes of deviations are placed in parentheses.
[†]Nursing interventions are primarily for identified deviations.

sents dilatation and an inverse S curve represents descent.

When the laboring woman enters the hospital, she is asked at what time regular contractions began. A sterile vaginal examination determines cervical dilatation and the station of the presenting part of the fetus. This information is plotted on the graph. To determine the appropriate point to begin plotting data, the nurse must know how many hours the patient has been having regular contractions. In the example shown in Figure 16–10, on admission the cervix was dilated 2–3 cm after four hours of labor, and the station was −1. Later examinations are noted on the graph. When the patient was in the 11th hour of labor, the graph indicates that cervical dilatation was 8 cm and the station was zero. At 14 hours of labor, the graph indicates spontaneous delivery.

Active descent should be 1 cm/hr for primiparas and 2 cm/hr for multiparas. Active descent normally begins after active cervical dilatation has been in progress for some time.

Three phases of cervical dilatation take place in the first stage of labor: (a) the latent phase, (b) the active phase, and (c) the deceleration phase. During the latent phase, also called the *preparatory phase* or *division* by Friedman (1970), effacement and coordination of contractions occur. The latent phase usually lasts about 20 hours for primiparas and about 14 hours for multiparas. In the active phase of labor, also referred to as the *dilatational phase* or *division,* active cervical dilatation occurs. In the active phase, primiparas progress at a rate of 1.2 cm/hr and multiparas progress at a rate of 1.5 cm/hr. During the deceleration phase, referred to as the *pelvic division,* active descent occurs and terminates with delivery. Normal values for this phase are 3 hours for primiparas and 1 hour for multiparas.

When utilizing the Friedman graph, the following method may be used to calculate the progress in centimeters of cervical dilatation per hour (or maximum slope of active dilatation). Divide the difference between two consecutive observations by the intervening time interval to obtain the value for the slope in centimeters per hour. For example, in the case illustrated in Figure 16–10, at 9½ hours of labor there is 5 cm cervical dilatation. At 11 hours of labor there is 8 cm cervical dilatation. The difference between these two observations is 3 cm. Divide the difference by the intervening time interval, which is 1½ hours: 3 cm ÷ 1½ = 2 cm/hr.

Differences in labor progress for primiparas and multiparas are illustrated in Figure 16–11. (Note: The correct term for a woman pregnant for the first time is nullipara; however, in the clinical situation the term primipara is in common usage.)

During these phases or functional divisions of dilatation, certain dysfunctions may occur. The latent phase may be prolonged. Two disorders are possible in the dilatational phase: (a) protraction of dilatation and (b) protraction of descent. In the pelvic division there are three disorders: (a) prolonged deceleration, (b) secondary arrest of dilatation, and (c) arrest of descent. An additional abnormal pattern occurs when dilatation is greater than 5 cm/hr in primiparas and 10 cm/hr in multiparas; this is known as a *precipitate labor.* Nursing and medical interventions for these dysfunctional labor patterns are discussed in Chapter 19.

Friedman (1970) has demonstrated that certain factors can affect the course of labor. Analgesic agents given in the latent phase can prolong that phase of labor. However, if the analgesic is given in the active phase of labor when dilatation is progressing normally, it will have a minimal effect on labor progress. Oxytocin induction or stimulation tends to shorten all phases of labor after administration. A manifestation that occurs in patients of increased parity is a decrease in the lengths of the latent and deceleration phases of the first stage of labor and the second stage. The fetus in occipital-posterior position may cause the deceleration phase to be prolonged.

Electronic Monitoring

All patients classified as high risk (see p. 440) should be electronically monitored during labor. In addition, women who receive any form of oxytocin stimulation or induction should be continuously monitored.

Tocodynamometer

An indirect method for monitoring uterine activity is by use of the tocodynamometer, which contains a flexible disk that responds to pressure. This disk is strapped to the mother's abdomen directly over the fundus, which is the area of greatest contractility, and it records the external tension exerted by contractions (Figure 16–12). The pressure is amplified and recorded on graph paper. The advantages to this method are that (a) it may be used prior to rupture of membranes antepartally and intrapartally and (b) it provides a continuous recording of the duration and frequency of contractions. The major disadvantage is that this method does not record the magnitude or intensity of a contraction. Another disadvantage to this method is that sometimes the strap bothers the mother, because it requires frequent readjustment as the mother changes position.

Pressure Transducer

Uterine activity may be monitored directly with the use of an intrauterine catheter. The catheter is threaded into the plastic catheter guide and then flushed with about 5 ml of sterile water to check for patency and to remove air. A sterile vaginal examination is done to locate the presenting part of the fetus, and then the catheter is inserted alongside the examining hand about 2 cm beyond the examining fingers. While the guide is held in place, the catheter is advanced until the black mark is even with the introitus. If resistance or bleeding is encountered, the catheter should be withdrawn and reinserted. After the catheter is placed properly, the guide is carefully removed and the catheter is taped to the mother's thigh. The catheter is attached to a three-way stopcock, which is attached to a strain gauge on the side of the fetal monitor that has been adjusted to the height of the mother's xiphoid process.

When the contracting uterus exerts pressure on the water-filled catheter, the pressure transducer receives the message. The pressure is then amplified and recorded on graph paper. (See p. 467 for care of monitoring equipment.) The pressure transducer is used conservatively because of increased chance of uterine infection and perforation of the uterus.

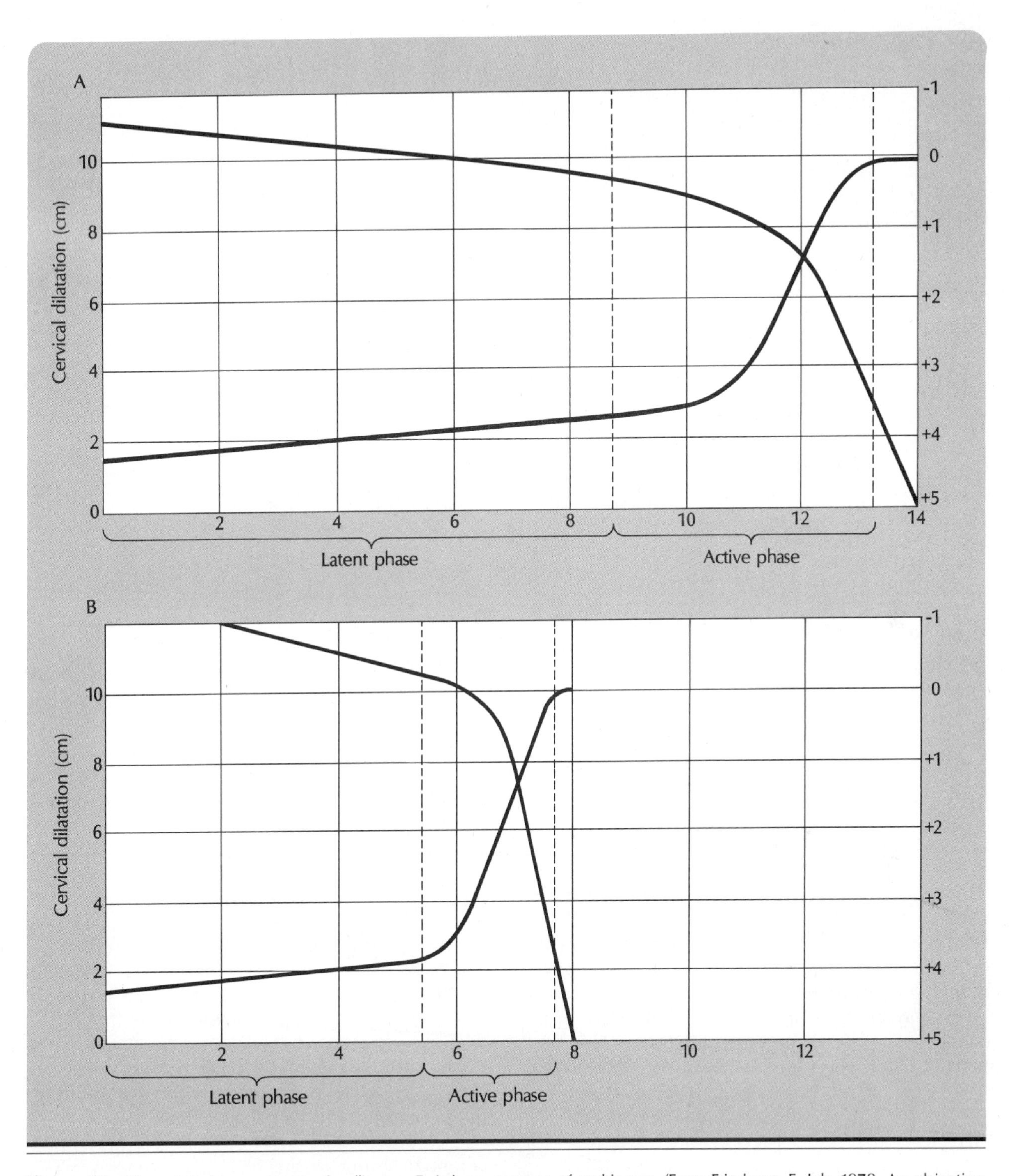

Figure 16–11. **A,** Labor progress of nulliparas. **B,** Labor progress of multiparas. (From Friedman, E. July 1970. An objective method of evaluating labor. *Hospital Practice,* vol. 5, no. 7, pp. 83 and 82.)

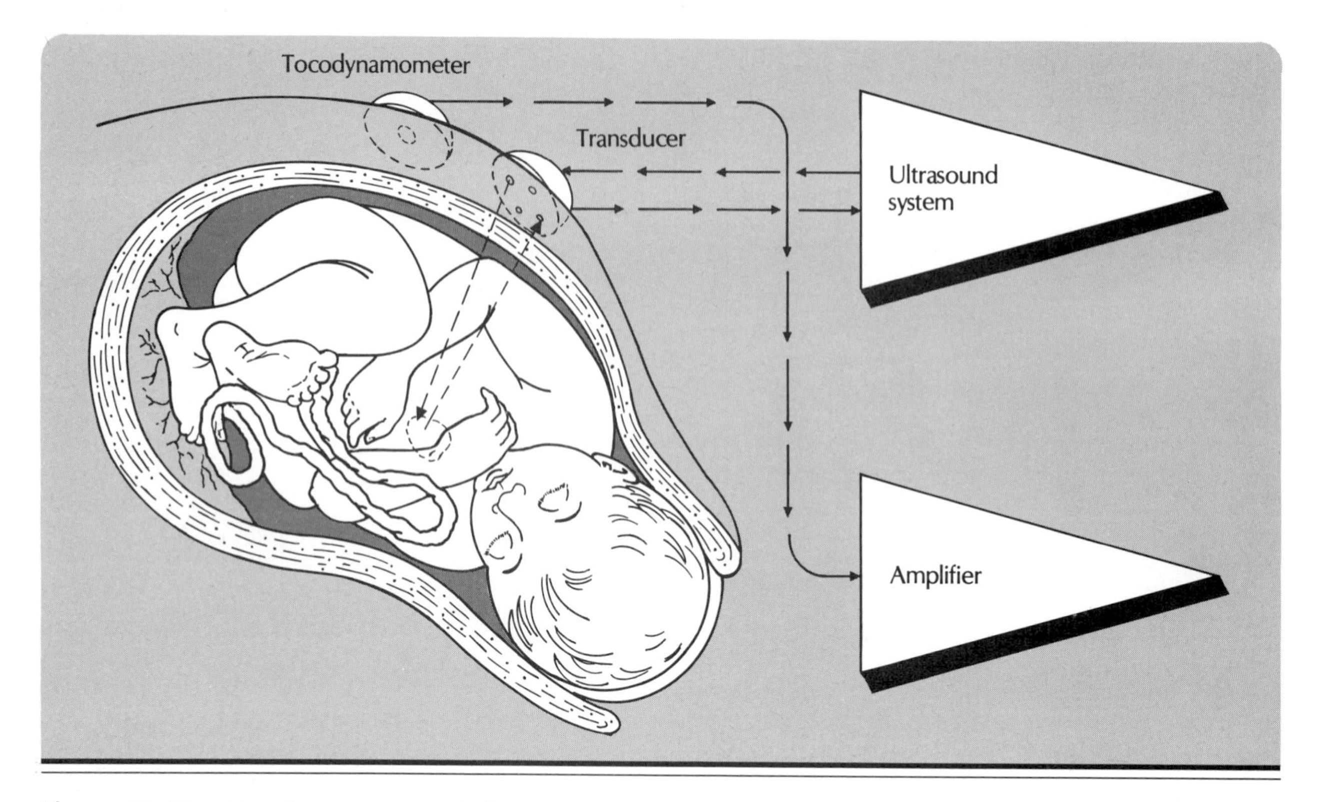

Figure 16–12. Tocodynamometer and ultrasonic technique to monitor maternal and fetal status during labor. (From Hon, E. 1972. *An introduction to fetal heart monitoring.* Los Angeles: University of California School of Medicine, p. 65.)

FETAL ASSESSMENT

Determination of Fetal Position

Fetal position is determined by a combination of factors, using various senses and technology. Assessment of the maternal abdomen for fetal position may be done by inspection, palpation, auscultation of fetal heart tones, determination of presenting part by vaginal examination (discussed in Chapter 17), and utilization of radiographs.

Inspection

The nurse should observe the pregnant abdomen for size and shape. Attention should be given to the lie of the fetus by assessing whether the shape of the uterus projects up and down (longitudinal lie) or left and right, which indicates a transverse lie (Figure 16–13).

Palpation

Use of Leopold's maneuvers provides a systematic evaluation of the maternal abdomen. Frequent practice with these maneuvers increases the proficiency of the examiner in determining fetal position by palpation. Difficulty may be encountered in performing these techniques on an obese patient or on a patient who has excessive amniotic fluid (polyhydramnios).

Leopold's maneuvers should be performed before listening to the fetal heart tones (FHTs). Auscultation of the FHTs is facilitated by locating the fetal back, because the sound of the heart tones is carried with more intensity through the fetal back and the uterine wall; it becomes diffused as it passes through the amniotic fluid.

Care should be taken to ensure the mother's comfort during Leopold's maneuvers. The patient

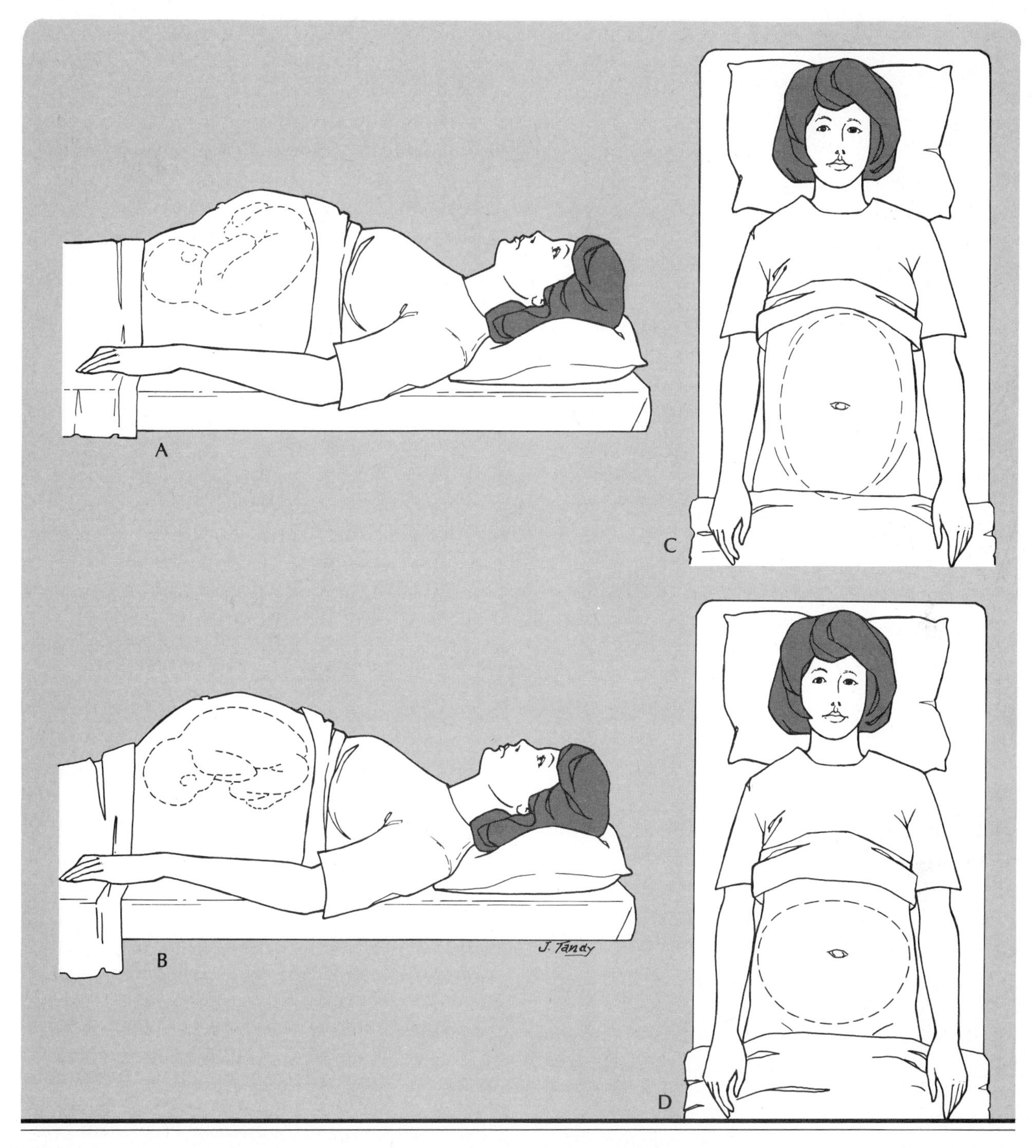

Figure 16–13. Variations in appearance in maternal abdomen with different fetal positions and presentations. **A,** Occiput posterior position. **B,** Occiput anterior position. **C,** Cephalic or breech presentation. **D,** Transverse lie.

should have recently emptied her bladder and should lie on her back with her abdomen uncovered. To aid in relaxation of the abdominal wall, the shoulders should be raised slightly on a pillow and the knees drawn up a little. The procedure should be completed between contractions. The examiner's hands should be warm.

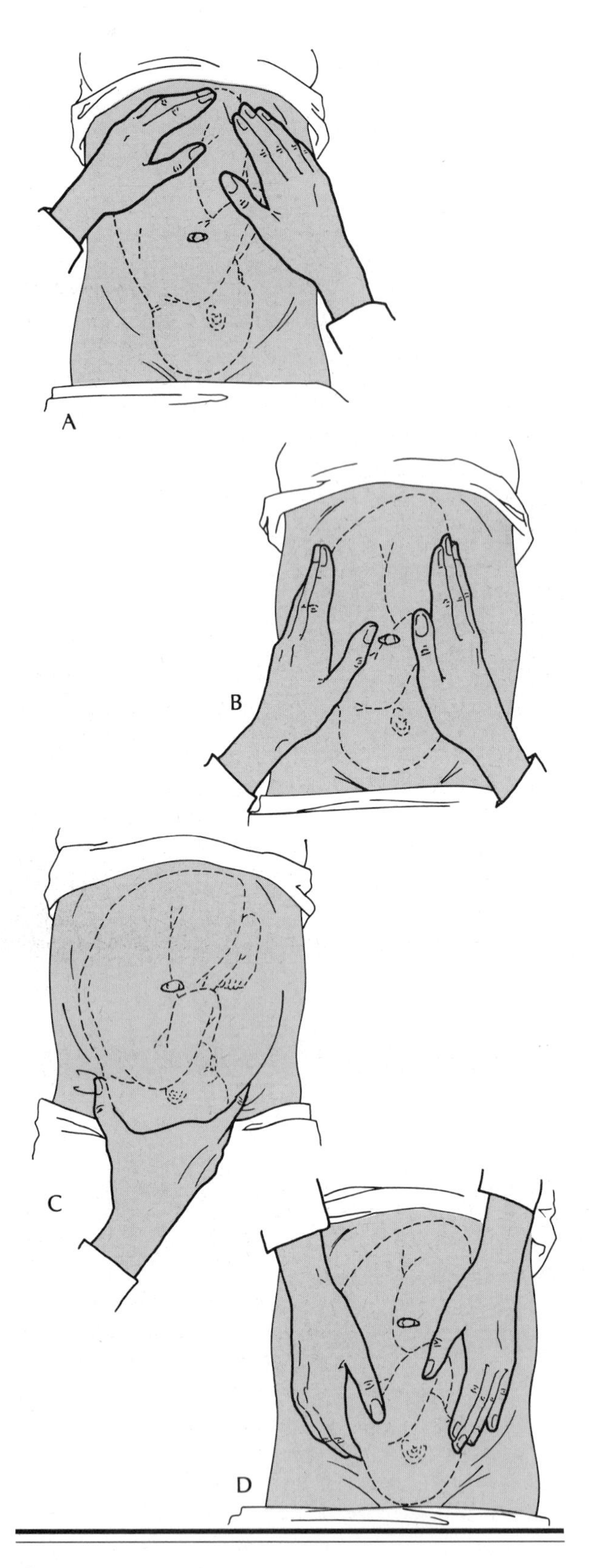

Figure 16–14. Leopold's maneuvers to determine fetal position. **A,** First maneuver. **B,** Second maneuver. **C,** Third maneuver. **D,** Fourth maneuver.

Consideration should be given to several questions while inspecting and palpating the maternal abdomen:

- Is the fetal lie longitudinal or transverse?
- What is in the fundus? Am I feeling buttocks or head?
- Where is the fetal back?
- Where are the small parts or extremities?
- What is in the inlet? Does it confirm what I found in the fundus?
- Is the presenting part engaged or floating?
- Is there fetal movement?
- How large is the fetus?
- Is there one fetus or more than one?
- Is fundal height proportionate to the estimated gestational age?

1. *First maneuver.* Facing the patient, palpate the upper abdomen with both hands (Figure 16–14,*A*). What is the shape, size, consistency, and mobility of the form that is found? The fetal head is firm, hard, and round and moves independently of the trunk. The breech feels softer and symmetrical and has small bony prominences; it moves with the trunk.

2. *Second maneuver.* After ascertaining whether the head or the buttocks occupies the fundus, the nurse tries to determine the location of the fetal back and notes whether it is on the right or left side of the mother. Still facing the mother, the nurse palpates the abdomen with deep but gentle pressure, using her palms (Figure 16–14,*B*). The right hand should be steady while the left hand explores the right side of the uterus. The maneuver should be repeated, probing with the right hand and steadying the uterus with the left hand. The fetal back should feel firm and smooth and should connect what was found in the fundus with a mass in the inlet. Once the back is located, the nurse validates the finding by palpating the extremities (small knobs and protrusions) on the opposite uterine wall.

3. *Third maneuver.* Next the nurse should determine what fetal part is lying over the inlet by gently grasping the lower portion of the abdomen just above the symphysis pubis with the thumb and fingers of the right hand (Figure 16–14,*C*). This maneuver yields the opposite information

from what was found in the fundus and validates the presenting part. If the head is presenting and is not engaged, it may be gently pushed back and forth.

4. *Fourth maneuver.* For this portion of the examination, the nurse faces the patient's feet and attempts to locate the cephalic prominence or brow. Location of this landmark assists in assessing the descent of the presenting part into the pelvis. The fingers of both hands are moved gently down the sides of the uterus toward the pubis (Figure 16–14,*D*). The cephalic prominence (brow) is located on the side where there is greatest resistance to the descent of the fingers toward the pubis. It is located on the opposite side from the fetal back if the head is well flexed. However, when the fetal head is extended, the occiput is the first cephalic prominence felt, and it is located on the same side as the back. Therefore, when completing the fourth maneuver, if the first cephalic prominence palpated is on the same side as the back, the head is not flexed. If the first prominence found is opposite the back, the head is well flexed and a normal labor can be anticipated (Oxorn and Foote, 1975).

Auscultation of FHTs

Location of FHTs assists in confirming the diagnosis of fetal position. However, locating the area of maximum intensity of the FHTs is not totally reliable because a loop of the umbilical cord may be near the uterine wall. In cephalic presentations, FHTs are loudest midway between the umbilicus and the symphysis pubis. Thus, if an emergency situation exists and there is no time to complete Leopold's maneuvers, one should attempt to find the FHTs in the midline between the pubis and umbilicus.

The FHTs are heard best in the lower quadrants of the abdomen in cephalic presentations. When the head is in a posterior position, the FHTs are heard most easily toward the maternal flank; in an occipital-anterior position, the heart tones are auscultated best toward the midline and left or right lower quadrant (Figure 16–15). The location of the FHTs tends to descend and move toward the midline as the presenting part descends and rotates in the pelvis. In a breech presentation, FHTs are best heard in the upper quadrants or at the level of the umbilicus (Oxorn and Foote, 1975).

Vaginal and X-ray Examinations

Vaginal and x-ray examinations assist in determining fetal position. During the vaginal examination, the presenting part may be palpated if the cervix is dilated, and information about the position of the fetus and the degree of flexion of its head (in cephalic presentations) can be obtained.

X-ray examination is not usually advised to determine normal fetal presentations because of the potential risks to the fetus. For obese women or women in whom abdominal palpation is difficult, x-ray evaluation assists in identifying possible problem situations because x-ray film gives accurate information concerning position, presentation, flexion, and degree of descent of the fetal part.

Evaluation of Fetal Status during Labor

Electronic Monitoring

Fetal monitoring should be instituted in cases classified as high risk. In addition, oxytocin administration is an indication for electronic monitoring.

There are two methods of electronic evaluation of the fetus: the indirect and the direct.

Indirect Methods

The indirect methods for monitoring the fetus include phonocardiography, ultrasound, and indirect fetal electrocardiography.

1. *Phonocardiography.* This method is one of the earlier attempts to continuously monitor the fetus. A microphone is secured to the maternal abdomen with a belt, and the first and second heart sounds are recorded. The advantages of this method are that (a) the membranes do not have to be ruptured, (b) the cervix does not have to be dilated, and (c) the fetal part does not have to be in the pelvis. In addition, phonocardiography may be used antepartally and intrapartally. It is easy to apply, and there are no known fetal hazards. The major disadvantage of this method is the microphone's ability to record artifacts. The mother should be instructed to remain totally quiet, because any movement may be recorded as a heart sound. Therefore, this method is not suit-

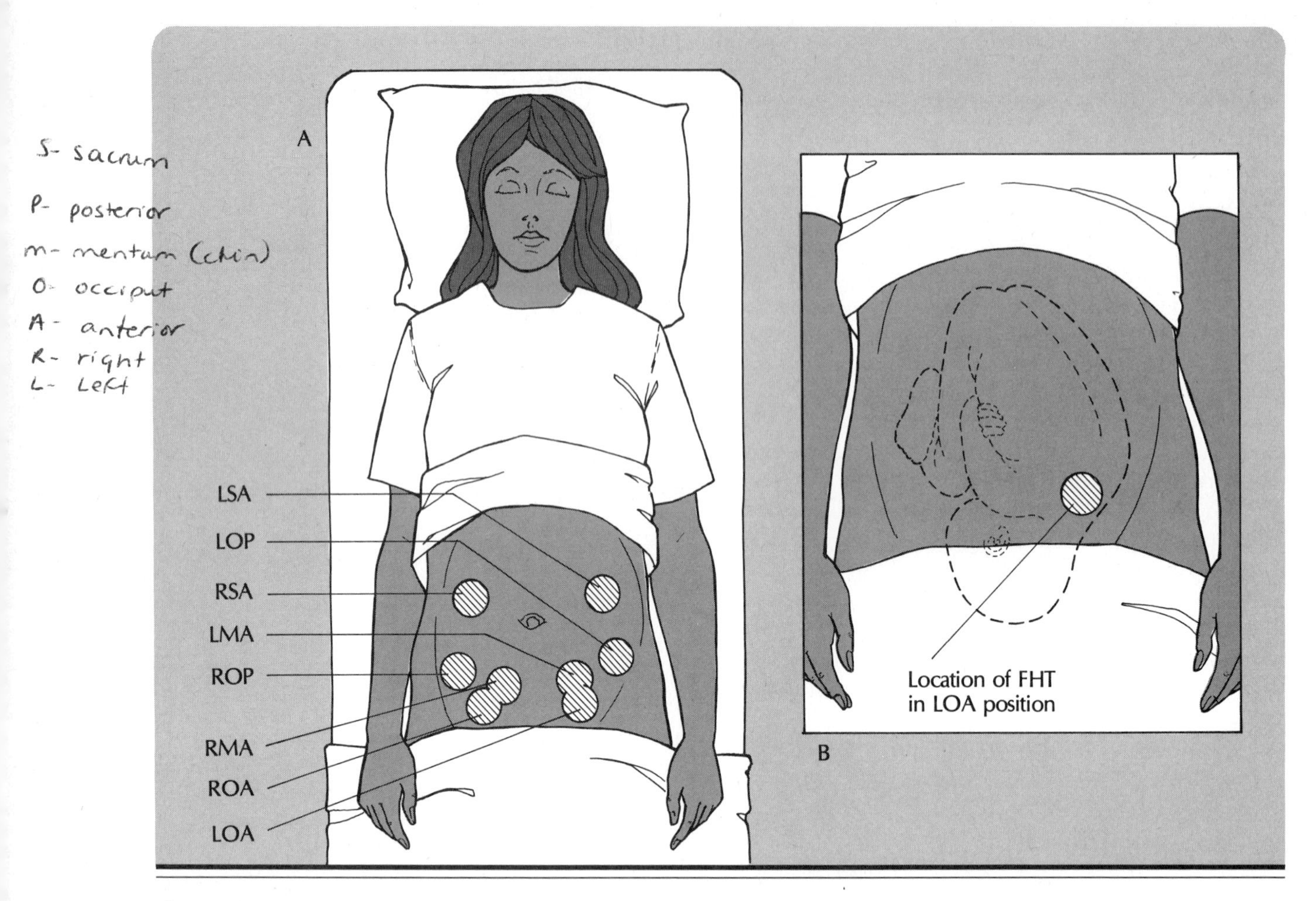

Figure 16–15. **A,** Location of FHTs in relation to various fetal positions. **B,** Location of FHTs in LOA position.

able for active labor. As an indirect method, it is being replaced by ultrasound (Hon, 1976).

2. *Ultrasound.* An ultrasonic transducer is strapped to the mother's abdomen at the site of the loudest auscultated heart tone. A conducting gel is applied to the transducer, which improves the tone pickup. A continuous ultrasonic beam is then emitted from transmitting crystals. This beam bounces off the blood moving in the fetal cardiovascular system and is reflected back to receiving crystals. The cardiotachometer uses the time intervals between the audible signals that are received to measure the fetal heart rate. The rate is then graphically recorded. Advantages of this system are that (a) a continuous fetal heart rate recording can be obtained in conjunction with uterine activity, demonstrating periodic changes, (b) the membranes do not have to be ruptured, (c) cervical dilatation and fetal descent do not have to be present, (d) it is easy to apply, and (e) there are no known detrimental maternal-fetal effects. Disadvantages of this method are that (a) accurate baseline variability cannot be obtained because of the monitor counting noise averages; (b) mothers in active labor move often and the Doppler beam is narrow; therefore, readjustment of the Doppler mechanism is mandatory; (c) there may be difficulty in getting a signal if the mother is obese; and (d) the signal is lost as the conducting gel dries out.

3. *Fetal electrocardiography.* This method records electrical fetal impulses by way of electrodes

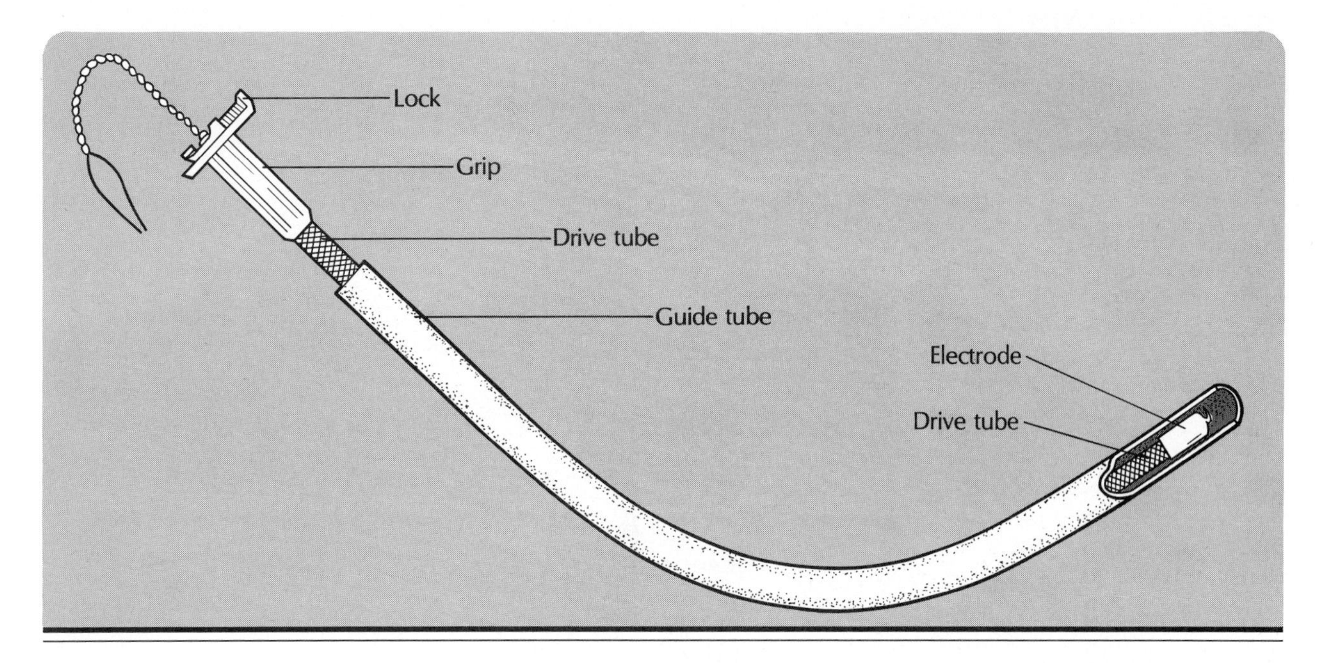

Figure 16–16. Internal fetal electrode.

placed on the maternal abdomen. Unfortunately, it also records maternal electrocardiography (ECG) impulses, so the fetal impulses must be interpreted between the larger maternal signals. The advantages to this method are the same as with the other indirect techniques, but the disadvantages are many. Patient movement is recorded, and it obiterates the fetal ECG signal. The fetal signal may occur at the same time as the maternal signal, which makes the fetal signal impossible to read. It is also difficult to pick up a maternal abdominal ECG signal in obese mothers. This method has been used successfully at the University of Mississippi Hospital for stress testing but cannot be used with mothers in active labor (Hon, 1976).

Direct Methods

Currently, the direct method of monitoring the fetus is by an internal spiral electrode (Figure 16-16). When the fetus is accessible—membranes ruptured, cervix dilated at least 2-3 cm, and presenting part at the cervix—a small electrode may be applied to the fetal epidermis using sterile technique. The electrode is in a guide tube that is inserted into the cervix and placed against the fetal scalp. It is best to apply the electrode to the parietal portion of the fetal scalp, because then one avoids inserting the electrode into the fontanelle. The electrode is unlocked from the guide tube, advanced, and rotated until it is attached to the fetal scalp. The guide tube is then removed, and the end wires are connected to a leg plate attached to the mother's leg. The electrode is then connected to the proper connection on the monitor. The fetal ECG signals are amplified and recorded on a cardiotachometer and on an oscilloscope.

Prior to insertion of the guide tube, the maternal vulva should be cleansed according to the institutional procedure, and sterile technique should be maintained throughout the insertion. Characteristics of the presenting part may be identified while doing a vaginal examination. Locate the suture lines and anterior fontanelle (diamond-shaped) and posterior fontanelle (triangle-shaped). Care must be taken not to insert the electrode into a suture, a fontanelle, or the infant's face.

The scalp electrode provides a continuous recording of the fetal heart rate and shows periodic changes associated with contractions. The direct method also provides true baseline variability. Disadvantages of this method are that ruptured fetal membranes and dilatation are necessary and that a presenting part must be in the pelvis. Also,

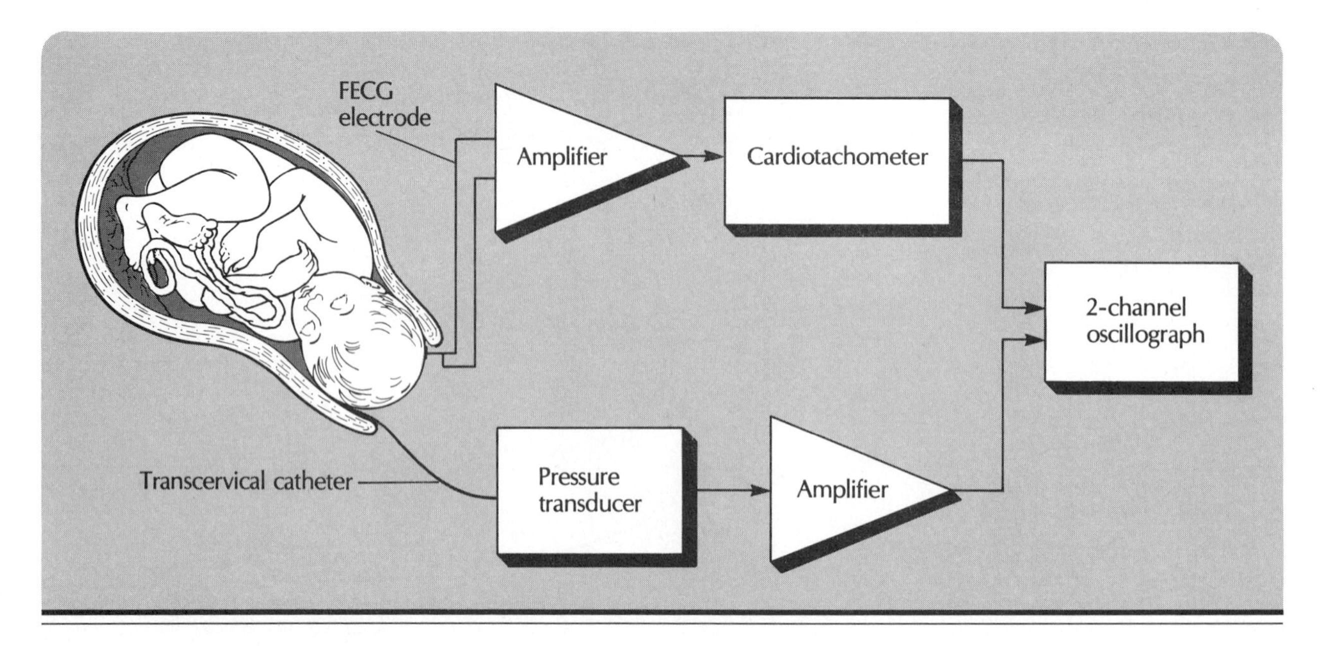

Figure 16–17. Direct monitoring of the fetus by scalp electrode. The pressure of the uterine contractions is being measured by transcervical catheter. (From Hon, E. 1976. *An introduction to fetal heart monitoring.* 2nd ed. Los Angeles: University of Southern California School of Medicine, p. 72.)

in the presence of fetal death, the monitor may record the maternal heart rate as it is transmitted through the fetus. There may be a risk of infection in the fetal scalp at the electrode attachment site (Figure 16–17).

Limitations and Pitfalls of Electronic Monitoring

The nurse must beware of the temptation to focus on the electronic monitor and thereby forget the laboring couple. Labor coaches also have been caught up in the dramatics of the lights and beeps of this equipment.

The nurse can use the monitor as a valuable assistant. With the internal monitor, the mother does not have to be disturbed for palpation of contractions or repositioned for auscultation of fetal heart rate. The labor coach can use the monitor in determining when to begin controlled breathing exercises.

Use of electronic monitoring may be disturbing to the laboring couple. It is frustrating and frightening for the laboring couple to experience the noises emitted from the external monitor when the mother and fetus change positions. Attachment to the monitor limits the mother's mobility. In addition, the external monitor must be continually adjusted, which further disturbs the mother. The nurse must provide the couple with information about the value and idiosyncrasies of the electronic equipment being used.

Electronic monitors do have limitations, as illustrated in Figures 16–18 to 16–20. Figure 16–18 demonstrates a "dirty" tracing, according to Freeman (1974b). The physician has to decide whether this pattern indicates rapid beat changes in the FHR, as with premature ventricular contractions or electrical interference. Sometimes one can see premature ventricular contractions on the oscilloscope; but if the arrhythmia is atrial in origin, it is not possible to detect this without a fetal ECG strip. In the case illustrated in the figure, an ECG was obtained and the tracings were determined to be due to interference.

In Figure 16–19 the fetal heart rate baseline was determined to be around 120 beats/min. At delivery the fetus was dead, and complete placental abruption was found. The heart rate recorded was the maternal heart rate being transmitted through the dead fetus (Paul and Petrie, 1973).

Figure 16–20 illustrates the limitations of the external monitor using the Doppler device. Whenever the rate in this tracing dropped below 90 beats/min, the monitor automatically doubled the rate. Halving also can occur with the external monitor with rates in excess of 180. When the

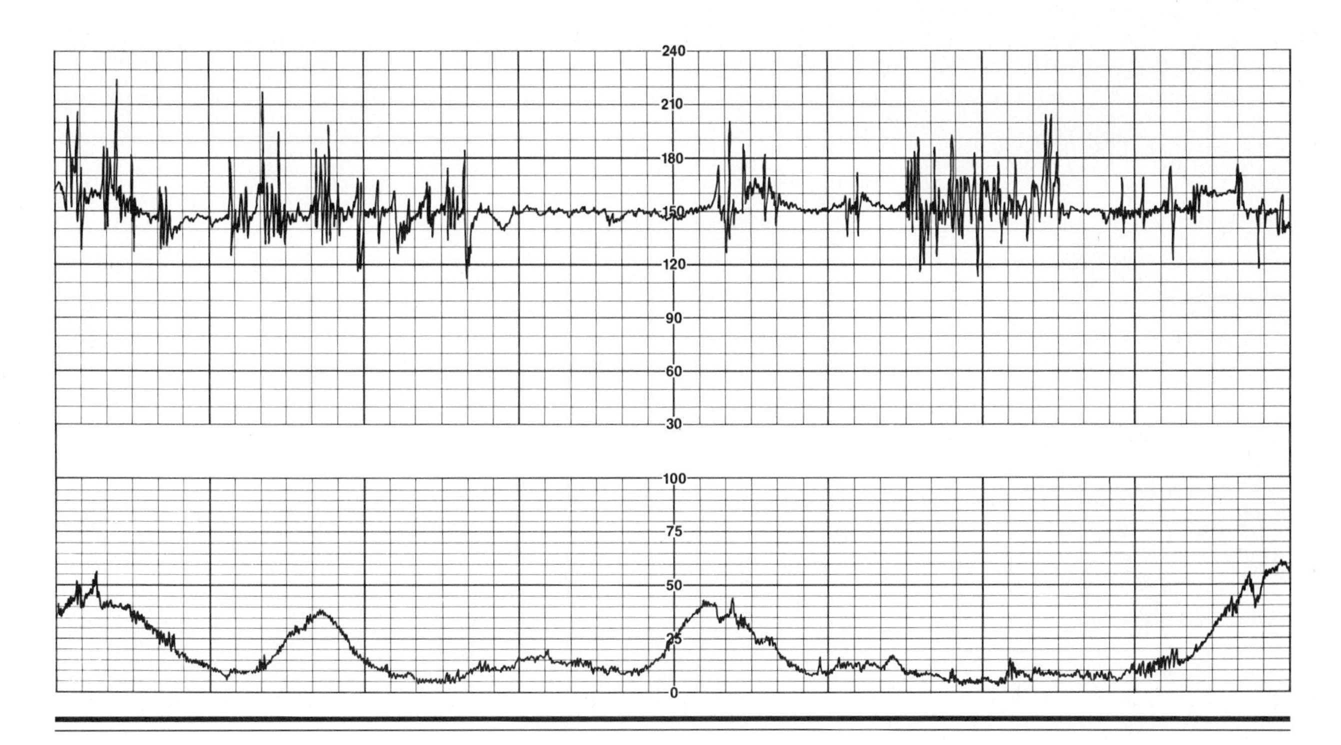

Figure 16–18. Noisy direct monitoring. (From Barden, T. F. 1976. *Selected pattern interpretations.* Slide No. 4. Wallingford, Conn.: Corometrics Medical Systems, Inc.)

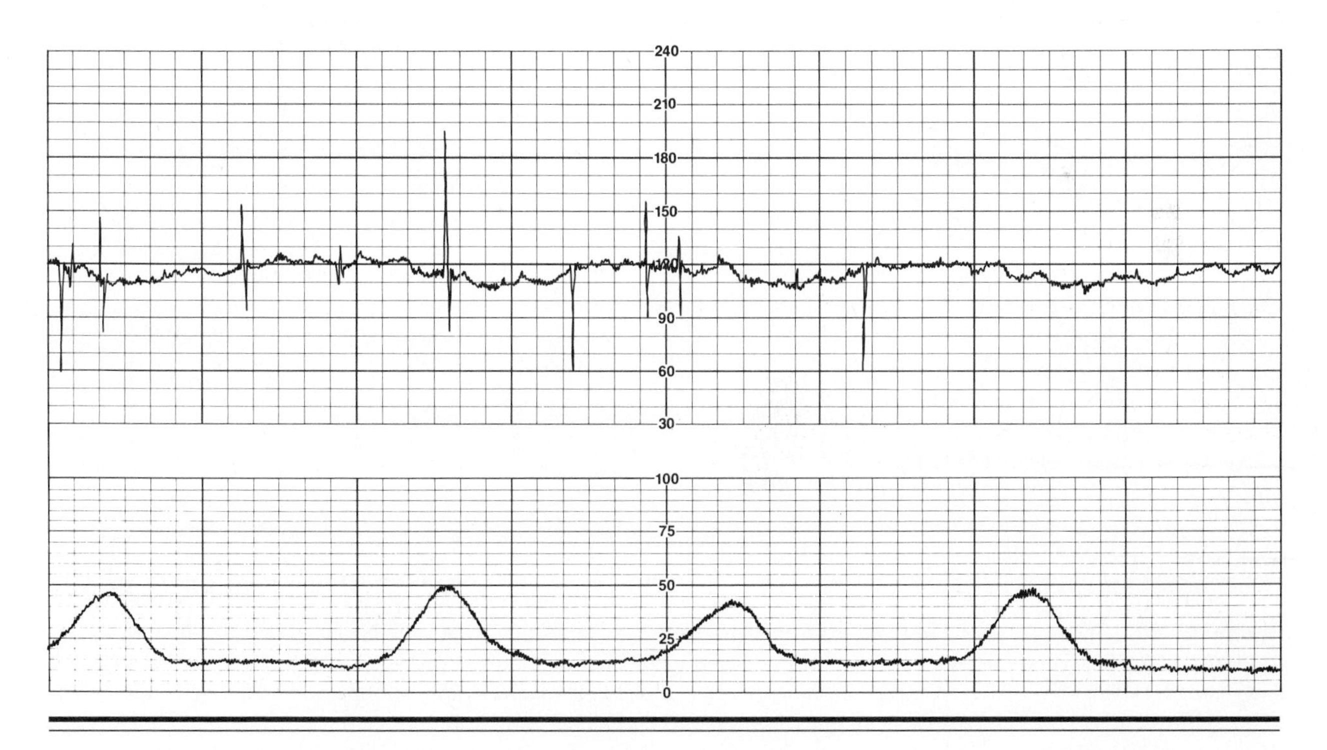

Figure 16–19. Erroneous fetal heart rate tracing. Fetal heart rate was actually the maternal heart rate. (Modified from Paul, R. H., and Petrie, R. H. 1973. *Fetal intensive care: Current concepts—monitoring records with self instruction.* Los Angeles: University of Southern California School of Medicine, Postgraduate Division, p. 65.)

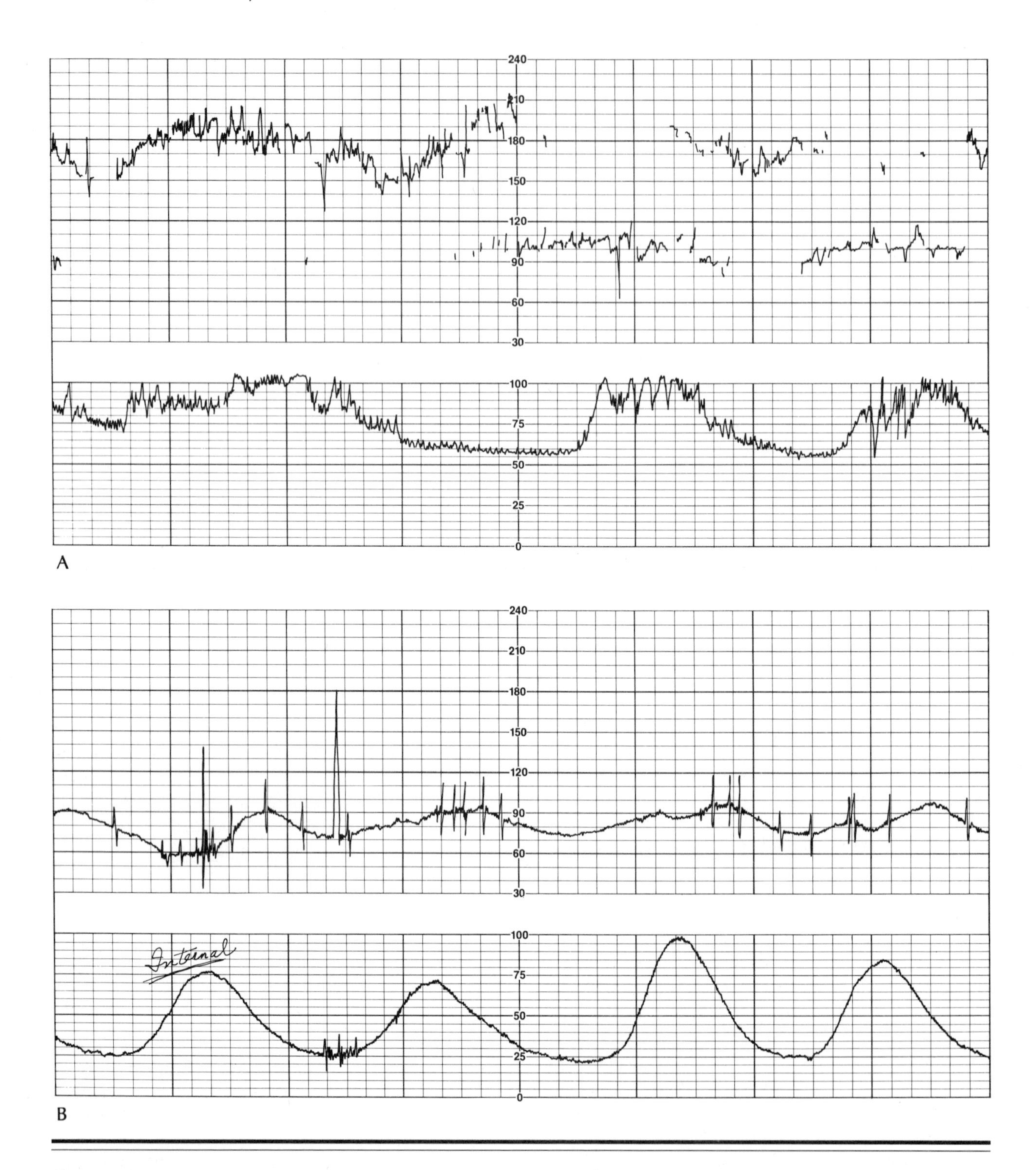

Figure 16–20. Incorrect tracing resulting from doubling. Fetal heart rate tracing in **A** was obtained using an indirect method (external monitor). Fetal heart rate tracing in **B** was obtained with direct method (internal device). (Modified from Paul, R. H., and Petrie, R. H. 1973. *Fetal intensive care: Current concepts—monitoring records with self instruction.* Los Angeles: University of Southern California School of Medicine, Postgraduate Division, p. 21).

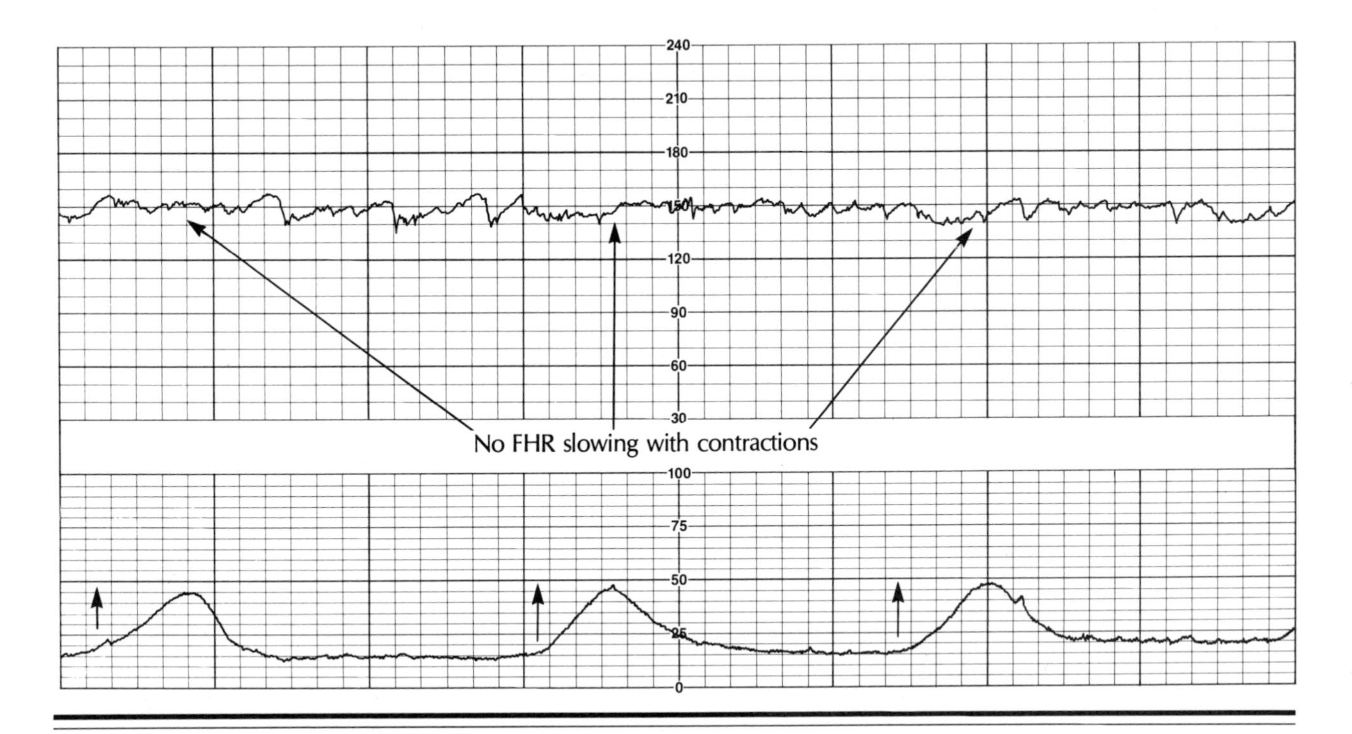

Figure 16–21. Normal fetal heart rate pattern.

internal monitor was applied to the fetus in which the tracings were being doubled, a rate of 90 beats/min was discovered (Barden and Freeman, 1977.)

Care of Equipment

There are several varieties of internal-external electronic monitor combinations. Before a model is used, the physician and nurse must become thoroughly familiar with its operations manual to prevent damage to expensive equipment as a result of misuse. The cleaning and disinfecting of the equipment are clearly explained by the manufacturers of the monitors. The procedure for loading the monitoring paper (Z paper) is also outlined in the operations manual. The paper on the fetal monitor should run at 3 cm/min, as this is the rate that most medical and nursing managers have learned to use and provides better data for interpretation. It is a good policy for a nurse to be assigned daily to check the equipment for electrical hazards, cleanliness, and working order.

Fetal Heart Rate Patterns

The baseline fetal heart rate is recorded between contractions for a ten-minute segment. The normal baseline rate is between 120 and 160 beats/min (Figure 16–21) and is influenced by autonomic control and various factors that affect it directly, such as maternal drugs. The more mature the fetus, the slower the heart rate—a phenomenon related to the maturity of the fetal autonomics (Martin and Gingerich, 1976).

Baseline Changes

Baseline fetal heart rate changes are defined in terms of ten-minute time periods. These changes are tachycardia, bradycardia, and baseline variability (beat-to-beat variability).

Tachycardia. Fetal tachycardia is a rate of more than 160 beats/min for a ten-minute period. Moderate tachycardia is between 160 and 179 beats/min, and severe tachycardia is 180 beats/min or above. Although tachycardia can occur for no apparent reason (Martin and Gingerich, 1976), possible causes of fetal tachycardia include the following:

1. Prematurity, which results in an immature fetal autonomic nervous system.
2. Maternal fever, which results in an increase in sympathetic nervous system stimulation

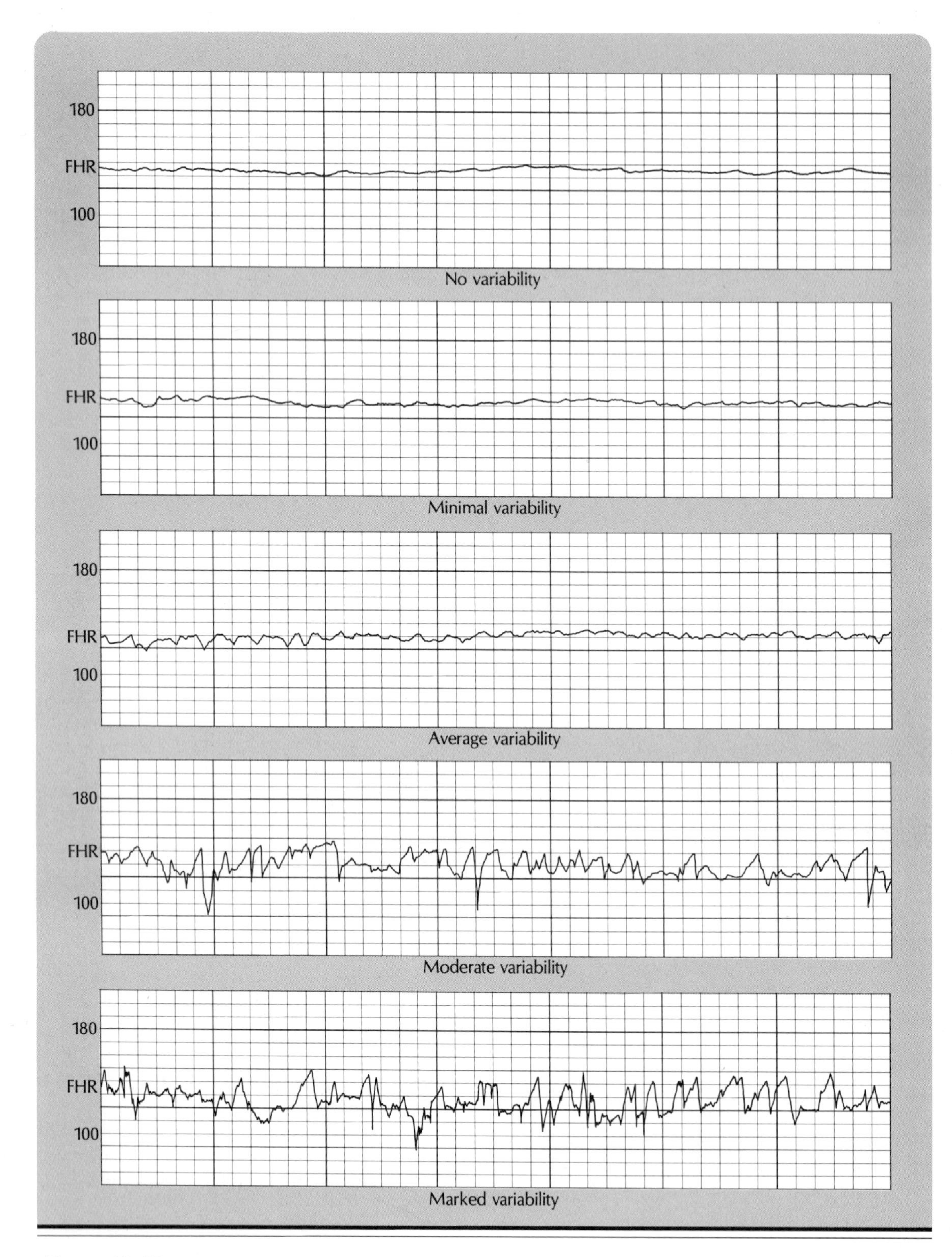

Figure 16–22. Types of variability. No variability = 0–2 beats/min; minimal variability = 3–5 beats/min; average variability = 6–10 beats/min; moderate variability = 11–25 beats/min; marked variability = more than 25 beats/min. (From Hon, E. 1976. *An introduction to fetal heart rate monitoring.* 2nd ed. Los Angeles: University of Southern California School of Medicine, p. 41.)

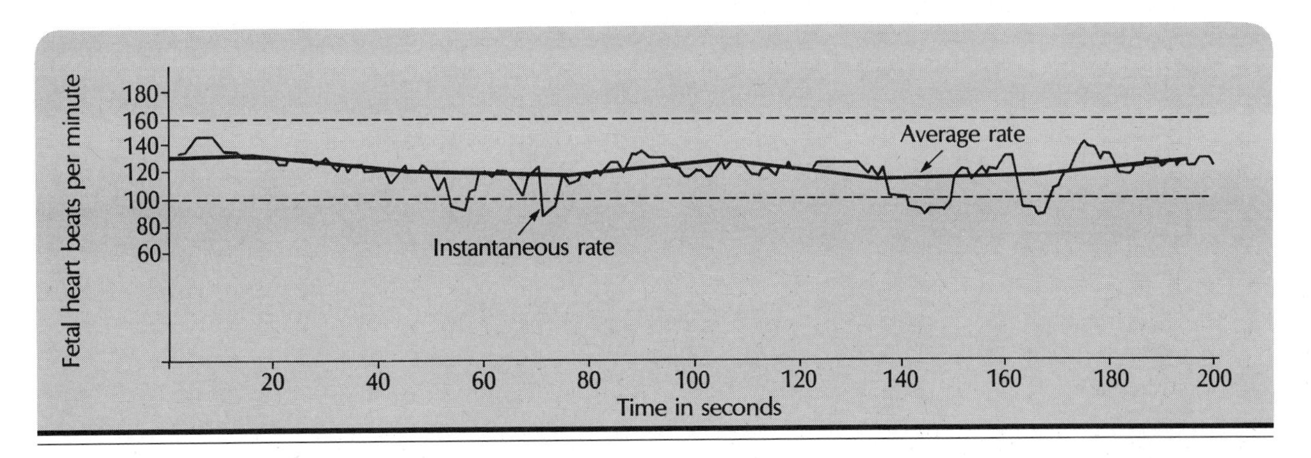

Figure 16–23. Comparison of instantaneous and average fetal heart rates. (From Hon, E. 1976. *An introduction to fetal heart rate monitoring,* 2nd ed. Los Angeles: University of Southern California School of Medicine, p. 9.)

and an increase in the maternal metabolic rate, thus increasing the oxygen demand.

3. Mild or chronic fetal hypoxia, which results in an effort by the fetus to compensate for the oxygen deficit with increased sympathetic nervous system stimulation.
4. Fetal infection, which results in a fetal stress reaction to pathogens.
5. Frequent repetitive fetal movements.
6. Maternal anxiety, which causes maternal epinephrine to cross the placenta.
7. Arrhythmias (these are uncommon).
8. Maternal drugs, which inhibit the transmission of the vagal response to the SA node.

Bradycardia. Fetal bradycardia is a rate of less than 120 beats/min for a ten-minute period. Moderate bradycardia is 90 to 120 beats/min and is benign. Marked bradycardia is 70 to 89 beats/min and is associated with fetal acidosis. Severe bradycardia is a rate of less than 70 beats/min and is associated with a rapidly occurring fetal acidosis. Whenever a bradycardia is preceded by a deceleration, one should be aware that the fetal reserve is diminishing.

Causes of fetal bradycardia are as follows (Martin and Gingerich, 1976):

1. Hypoxia.
2. Persistent increases in vagal tone, which may be due to a sudden hypoxemia with a reflex fetal response.
3. Arrhythmias as seen with congenital heart block.
4. Hypothermia due to maternal hypothermia, reflecting a slowed cardiac metabolism.
5. Drugs such as β-adrenergic (sympathetic) blocking agents (these include anesthetic agents used as paracervical and epidural blocks).

Baseline Variability. Generally, a healthy fetus has an irregular baseline, which is caused by the action of the sympathetic and parasympathetic nervous systems. *Variability* refers to the interval between beats (Figure 16–22). Average variability is a good indication that the fetus will be well, even with abnormal patterns. Increased variability does not seem to indicate a serious condition; however, experience with this situation is somewhat limited. Decreased variability must be assessed in relation to change, duration, and the presence of other ominous patterns. A variability of less than 5 beats/min is considered ominous; loss of variability occurs prior to fetal death. Decreased or absent variability is an important warning sign of fetal jeopardy.

It should be remembered that true variability can only be evaluated by direct monitoring; the external monitor exhibits only an average (Figure 16–23).

A reduction in variability is demonstrated with the following:

1. Maternal hypnotics, analgesics, parasympathetic blockers, and magnesium sulfate.
2. Fetal rest (decreased variability should not last longer than 15 minutes).

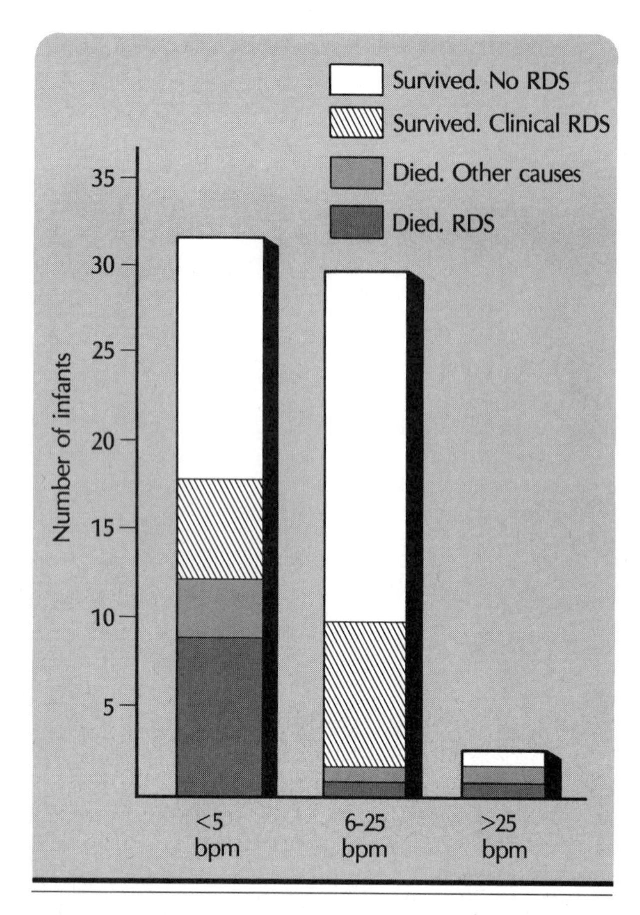

Figure 16–24. Correlation between different degrees of baseline fetal heart rate variability and the incidence of respiratory distress syndrome and death from this cause. (From Hon, E., Zanini, B., and Cabal, L. A. 1975. *An introduction to neonatal heart rate monitoring,* p. 11. © 1975 by E. H. Hon.)

3. An immature fetus (prior to 32 weeks' gestation).
4. Fetal hypoxia and acidosis.
5. Fetal malformation.

Stimuli such as maternal activity, abdominal palpation, and myometrial contractions increase the variability. Sometimes a complete loss of variability occurs with complete heart block. If tachycardia or bradycardia occurs with the loss of variability, the outcome is usually poor (Boehn, 1977).

Recent research has shown that the amount of variability in the fetal heart rate correlates with the incidence of respiratory distress syndrome (RDS) in the neonate and is predictive of those who will die of this condition. As shown in Figure 16–24, as the beat-to-beat variability decreases, the number of infants who develop RDS and die increases. The increase is substantial with variability of less than 5 beats/min.

Based on current research with the fetal ECG (abdominal or internal electrodes), the following observations can be made:

1. If average FHR variability is present, the probability of delivering a nondepressed infant is high.
2. One cannot compare externally monitored variability with internal monitoring data.
3. If the baseline is smooth, the probability of delivering a depressed infant is high.
4. One must consider the modifying effects of maturity, drugs, and sleep.
5. The fetal nervous system is more sensitive to hypoxia than the myocardium is.
6. The time-course change of the variability must be considered.
7. Minimal variability in a premature fetus indicates a nine-times greater chance of developing RDS.

Variability is becoming more important as an area of assessment for fetal distress and prediction of fetal outcome.

Changes Relative to Contractions

Two types of changes occur relative to contractions: accelerations and decelerations. An acceleration is a periodic increase in the baseline. There are two types of accelerations: *Type I acceleration* is associated with a variable deceleration, coming either before or after it. The significance of this pattern is unknown. *Type II acceleration* is not related to a deceleration pattern. It may occur with the contraction, which is probably the fetal response to the contracting uterine musculature, or between contractions, which is associated with fetal movement. These heart rate responses are not pathologic. If, however, the acceleration occurs late in the contraction cycle and the baseline variability is smooth, a late deceleration may follow it. This pattern is a sign of fetal acidosis (Martin and Gingerich, 1976).

A deceleration is a periodic decrease in the baseline fetal heart rate. There are three types of decelerations (Table 16–3). *Type I decleration* is also called an *early* or *head compression deceleration. Type*

II deceleration may be called a *late deceleration. Type III deceleration* is referred to as the *variable deceleration.*

Type I deceleration is a smooth-curve wave form that inversely mirrors the contraction (Figure 16–25). It begins with the beginning of the contraction and ends within 15 seconds after the contraction ends. The nadir (lowest point) comes at the contraction's peak. Generally, these patterns are benign and are seen late in labor when the head is on the perineum. According to Sherline (1976), two events can render this pattern ominous. If the pattern occurs early in labor, head compression may be a result of bony pelvis dystocia and cephalopelvic disproportion. Occasionally the pattern is actually a late deceleration. With a severely compromised fetus, the beginning of the contraction initiates the deceleration. A decrease in the baseline variability should be noted if the latter is the cause.

Type II or late deceleration is a smooth uniform curve that inversely mirrors the contraction but is late in its onset (see Figure 16–25). The nadir occurs after the peak of the contraction, usually about the time the contraction is over. A late deceleration of any magnitude is ominous. It is

Table 16–3. Fetal Responses Related to Decelerations in Fetal Heart Rate

	Type I (early deceleration)	Type II (late deceleration)	Type III (variable deceleration)
Physiologic response	Pressure on fetal head ↓ Change in blood flow ↓ Vagal stimulation ↓ Changes in nervous mechanism altering heart condition ↓ Decrease in heart rate	Cause (e.g., hypertonic contractions) ↓ Hypoxia → acidosis ↓ Hypercarbia ↓ Changes in nervous control of heart ↓ Decreased heart rate	Transitory pressure on cord ↓ Change in blood flow ↓ Signal to vagus ↓ Signal to cardiac nervous system ↓ Sudden drop in FHR OR Profound pressure on cord ↓ Hypoxic changes ↓ Myocardial changes ↓ Cardiac arrest
FHR pattern			
Shape	Waveform consistently uniform	Waveform uniform; shape reflects contractions	Waveform variable, generally sharp drops and returns
Onset	Just prior to or early in contraction	Late in contraction	Immediate with fetal insult; not related to contraction
Lowest level	Consistently at or before midpoint of contraction	Consistently after the midpoint of the contraction	Variable around midpoint
Range	Usually within normal range of 120–160 beats/min	Usually within normal range with a high baseline (120–130 beats/min); when severe may drop to 60 beats/min	Usually within normal range but can drop low
Ensemble	Can be single or repetitive	Occasional, consistent, gradually increase	Variable—single or repetitive

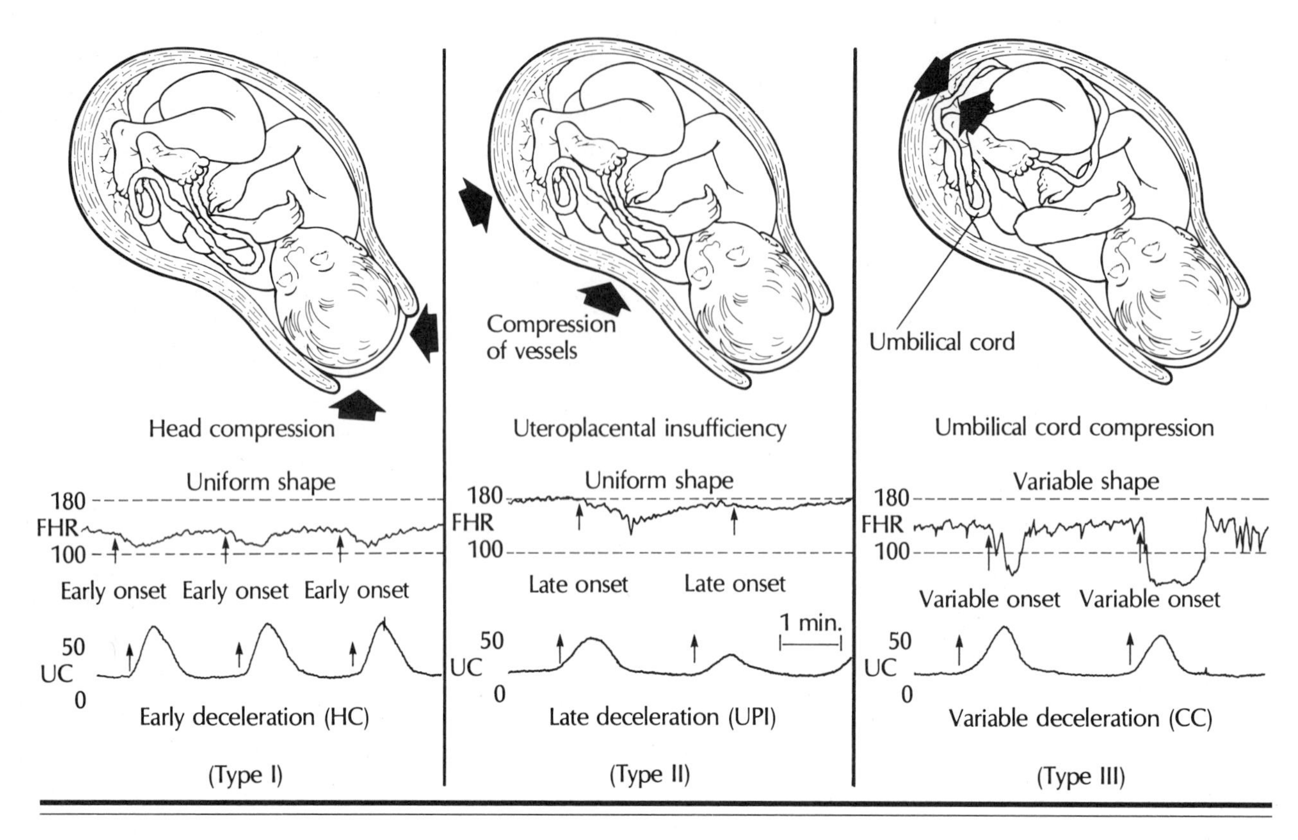

Figure 16–25. Types of decelerations (From Hon, E. 1976. *An introduction to fetal heart rate monitoring.* 2nd ed. Los Angeles: University of Southern California School of Medicine, p. 29.)

due to fetal hypoxia associated with a decrease in uteroplacental blood flow. Usually a well-oxygenated fetus is not pathologically affected by labor. However, a fetus with a compromised pO_2 becomes further compromised with labor. This fact provides the basis of the oxytocin challenge test, which is discussed in Chapter 14. If late decelerations are allowed to continue, fetal bradycardia, reduced baseline variability, and eventual fetal death will result.

Variable or type III deceleration is a nonuniform, periodic change that may or may not occur with contractions. The deceleration falls abruptly in a jagged line and returns to baseline either abruptly or slowly (see Figure 16–25). This is the most common deceleration pattern, and according to research conducted by Tejani (1977), it occurs in 52% of fetuses with abnormally positioned cords. Variable decelerations may be classified as severe, in which the FHR falls below 70 for longer than 60 seconds, or moderate, in which the rate falls below 70 for 30–60 seconds or falls between 70 and 80 beats for more than 60 seconds. These patterns may be ominous. A pattern with a slow return to baseline is also ominous. A mild variable deceleration is a fall to any level for less than 30 seconds or a fall to 80 beats/min of any duration. Unless the fetus is already compromised, a mild variable deceleration is benign. If allowed to continue, moderate and severe variable decelerations can result in progressive fetal acidosis, loss of baseline variability, and fetal death. It is not uncommon to see severe variable decelerations just prior to delivery. The duration is brief, and the fetus can usually tolerate it.

Mixed Patterns

A combination of patterns is probably the most confusing of all the monitoring tracings. Mixed and unusual patterns should be considered pathologic, especially if associated with a loss of baseline variability. It can be helpful for the medical manager to check the fetal scalp pH, as it provides additional data in assessing the significance of various FHR patterns.

Reassuring and Nonreassuring Patterns

A systematic way to approach fetal monitoring tracings is to assess whether they are reassuring or nonreassuring patterns. With reassuring patterns, it has been found that five-minute Apgar scores are 9 to 10. In nonreassuring patterns there is a low Apgar infant score in 20% of infants, but almost all low-Apgar infants exhibit nonreassuring monitoring patterns.

Reassuring patterns are those with (a) no periodic change, (b) accelerations, (c) early decelerations, and (d) mild variable decelerations (Table 16–4).

Nonreassuring patterns are (a) late decelerations, (b) severe variable decelerations with rising baselines, decreasing baselines, rates that remain below 70 beats/min for over 30 seconds, and variable decelerations with a slow return to baseline, and (c) decelerations that last more than 60 seconds (Table 16–5). It should not be forgotten that any loss of baseline variability makes the pattern

Table 16–4. Management of Reassuring Patterns*

Pattern	Treatment	Intervention
No periodic change	None	None
Acceleration	None	None
Early deceleration	None	None
Mild variable deceleration	Attempt correction with maternal position change	None

*From Freeman, R. K. 1974a. Management of acute fetal distress. In *A clinical approach to fetal monitoring.* San Leandro, Calif.: Berkeley BioEngineering, Inc.

Table 16–5. Management of Nonreassuring Patterns*

Pattern	Treatment	Intervention
Late deceleration of any magnitude	1. Turn on side	
	2. Administer 100% O_2	If corrected → None
	3. Discontinue oxytocin	If not corrected → Expeditious delivery
		or
	4. Correct maternal hypotension	If fetal pH >7.25 → Repeat every 10–15 min
		If fetal pH <7.25 → Expeditious delivery
Severe variable deceleration		
1. FHR <70 beats/min, longer than 30 sec	Maternal position change	If corrected → None
		If not corrected → Administer O_2; expeditious delivery
2. Rising baseline FHR		
3. Decreasing variability		
4. Slow return to baseline		
Prolonged decelerations	Correct identifiable cause	If FHR returns → None
		If no identifiable cause → Expeditious delivery after recovery

*From Freeman, R. K. 1974a. Management of acute fetal distress. In *A clinical approach to fetal monitoring.* San Leandro, Calif.: Berkeley BioEngineering, Inc.

†Decreased variability or rising baseline FHR makes late deceleration more ominous.

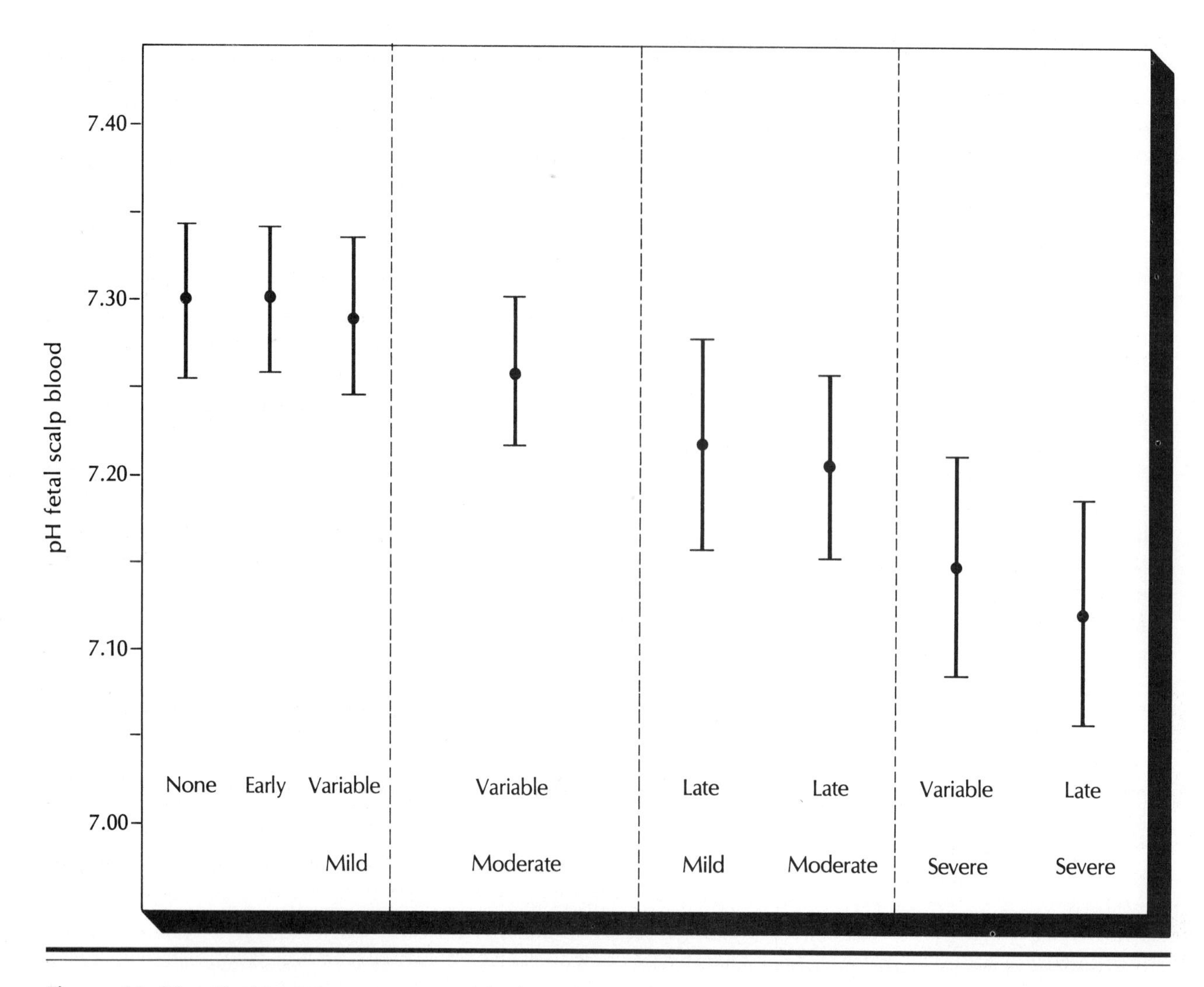

Figure 16–26. Fetal heart rate patterns and fetal acid-base status. (From Hon, E., Zanini, B., and Cabal, L. A. 1975. *An introduction to neonatal heart rate monitoring,* p. 6. © 1975 by E. H. Hon.)

a nonreassuring pattern. Mixed patterns are also classified as nonreassuring (Freeman, 1974a).

Fetal Blood Sampling

Fetal blood sampling is a valuable method to aid in identifying fetal hypoxemia and acidosis. When oxygen exchange is compromised, the fetus develops hypoxia and changes from aerobic to anaerobic metabolism. The anaerobic metabolism results in the production of lactic acid, which causes acidosis and therefore a drop in pH.

The normal range of pH in a fetus is 7.30 to 7.35 (Tucker, 1978). A pH value between 7.20 and 7.25 is considered borderline, and the sample may be repeated in 15 minutes. A pH value below 7.20 requires immediate delivery of the fetus by low forceps or cesarean section (Tucker, 1978).

Indications for fetal blood sampling include (a) late decelerations with decreasing variability, (b) a smooth baseline with minimal variability, (c) fetal bradycardia or tachycardia, and (d) persistent moderate or severe variable decelerations (Figure 16–26).

Collecting fetal scalp blood is a sterile procedure with certain prerequisites: ruptured membranes, cervical dilatation adequate for visualization of fetal scalp, and engagement of the presenting part. (The buttocks can be used in a breech presentation.) The vulvar area should be cleansed, and sterile drapes should be applied. A conical vaginal endoscope is then inserted in the vagina and through the cervix to facilitate scalp visualization. The endoscope should rest on the fetal scalp but not over a fontanelle or suture line.

Working through the scope, one should clean the site to remove vernix, blood, amniotic fluid, and other material. Silicone is then applied to the scalp to enhance visualization and to provide a surface for the formation of a blood globule. The fetal scalp is punctured with a 2 × 2 mm microscalpel in a plastic guard. Blood from the fetal scalp flows more freely if the scalp is punctured at the beginning of a uterine contraction. With the aid of gravity, the blood is collected in a heparinized glass capillary tube.

After sufficient blood is obtained, one should apply pressure to the site with a sponge on a holder. Pressure is maintained through the next two contractions, and the site is observed during a third contraction. The acid-base determinations are then done immediately.

SUMMARY

Effective, thorough assessment of the mother and fetus during the intrapartal period requires an understanding of normal physiologic values and risk factors, the effective utilization of monitoring equipment, and the development of specific assessment skills.

SUGGESTED ACTIVITIES

1. In a prenatal setting and with assistance, carry out Leopold's maneuvers, auscultation of fetal heart tones, and an intrapartal assessment for high-risk factors.
2. In the classroom laboratory, using actual labor patient fetal monitor tracings, identify the various types and significant aspects of uterine contraction patterns and fetal heart patterns.
3. Plot a patient's progress on a Friedman graph.
4. Role-play preparation of the patient and family for external or internal monitoring.

REFERENCES

Barden, T. P., and Freeman, R. K. 1977. *Interpreting labor tracings.* New York: Academic Press, Inc.

Boehn, R. H. 1977. FHR variability, key to fetal well-being. *Contemp. OB/Gyn.* 9:52.

Freeman, R. K. 1974a. Management of acute fetal distress. In *A clinical approach to fetal monitoring.* San Leandro, Calif.: Berkeley BioEngineering, Inc.

Freeman, R. K. 1974b. Monitoring records from selected clinical cases. In *A clinical approach to fetal monitoring.* San Leandro, Calif.: Berkeley BioEngineering, Inc.

Friedman, E. A. 1970. An objective method of evaluating labor. *Hosp. Pract.* 5:82.

Hobel, C. J. 1976. Problem-oriented risk assessment during labor. *Contemp. OB/Gyn.* 8:120.

Hon, E. H. 1976. *An introduction to fetal heart rate monitoring.* 2nd ed. Newport Beach, Calif.: Corometrics Medical Systems, Inc.

Martin, C. B., and Gingerich, B. 1976. Factors affecting the fetal heart rate: genesis of FHR patterns. *J. Obstet. Gynecol. Nurs.* 5(supp.):305.

Oxorn, H., and Foote, W. 1975. *Human labor and birth.* New York: Appleton-Century-Crofts.

Paul, R. H., and Petrie, R. H. 1973. *Fetal intensive care: current concepts.* Los Angeles: University of Southern California School of Medicine.

Sherline, D. M. 1976. Lecture (videotape) at the University of Mississippi Medical Center. Jackson, Miss.

Tejani, N. A. 1977. The association of umbilical cord complications and variable decelerations with acid-base findings. *Obstet. Gynecol.* 49:159.

Tucker, S. M. 1978. *Fetal monitoring and fetal assessment during high-risk pregnancy.* St. Louis: The C. V. Mosby Co.

Willson, J. R., and Carrington, E. 1979. *Obstetrics and gynecology.* 6th ed. St. Louis: The C. V. Mosby Co.

ADDITIONAL READINGS

Babaknia, A., and Niebyl, J. 1976. The effects of magnesium sulfate on fetal heart rate baseline variability. *Obstet. Gynecol.* 51 (supp.): 25.

Clark, A. L., and Affonso, D. D. 1976. *Childbearing: a nursing perspective.* Philadelphia: F. A. Davis Co.

Danforth, D., ed. 1977. *Textbook of obstetrics and gynecology.* 3rd ed. New York: Harper & Row Publishers, Inc.

Erkkola, R., and Rauramo, L. 1976. Correlation of maternal physical fitness during pregnancy with maternal and fetal pH and lactic acid at delivery. *Acta Obstet. Gynecol. Scand.* 55:441.

Friedman, E. A. 1967. *Labor: clinical evaluation and management.* New York: Appleton-Century-Crofts.

Greenhill, J. P., and Friedman, E. A. 1974. *Biological principles and modern practice of obstetrics.* Philadelphia: W. B. Saunders Co.

Jensen, M. D., et al. 1977. *Maternity care: the nurse and the family.* St. Louis: The C. V. Mosby Co.

Myles, M. F. 1975. *Textbook for midwives.* Edinburgh: Churchill Livingstone.

Parer, J. T. 1976. Physiological recognition of fetal heart rate. *J. Obstet. Gynecol. and Neonatal Nurs.* 5(supp.):265.

Pritchard, J. A., and MacDonald, P. C. 1976. *Williams obstetrics.* 15th ed. New York: Appleton-Century-Crofts.

Weeks, A. R. L., and Flynn, J. J. 1975. Engagement of fetal head in primigravidae and its relationship to duration of gestation and onset of labor. *Br. J. Obstet. Gynecol.* 82:7.

CHAPTER 17

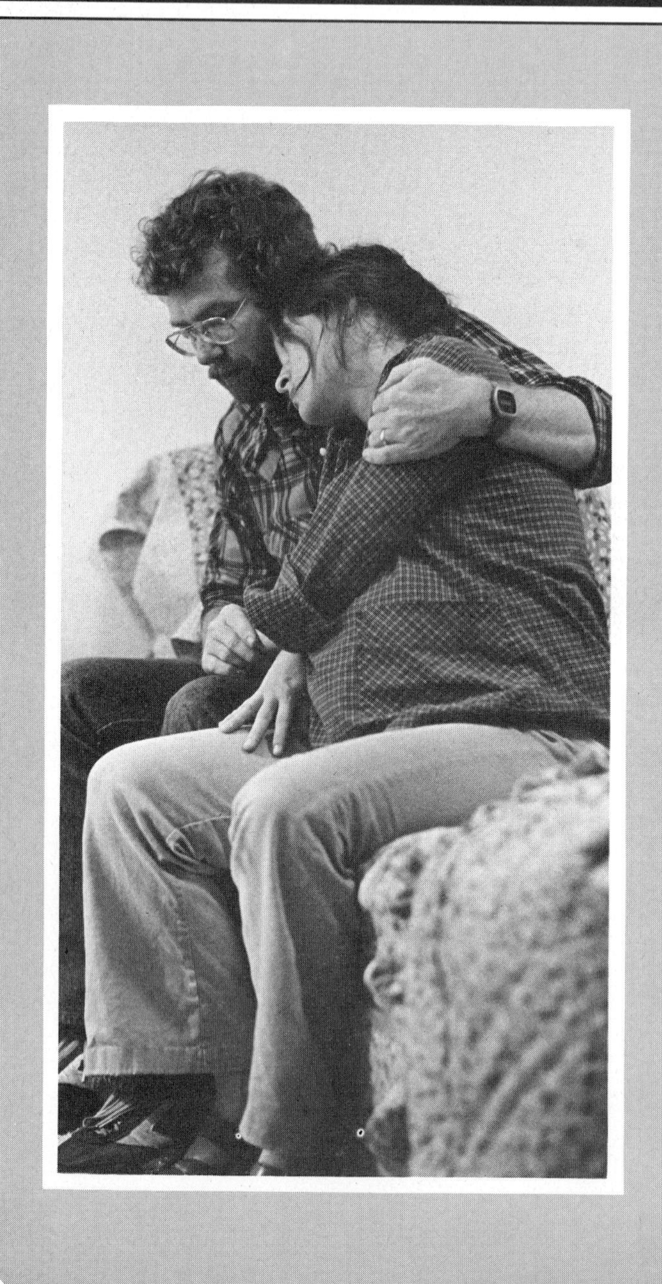

THE PARENTS IN CHILDBIRTH: NEEDS AND CARE

OBJECTIVES

- Identify the key questions to ask when admitting a labor patient.
- Discuss the psychologic and physiologic alterations seen in the patient during each of the stages of labor and delivery.
- Identify the appropriate nursing interventions during each stage of labor and delivery.
- Discuss the immediate care to the mother after delivery.
- Describe the individual assessment components of the Apgar scoring system.
- Identify the immediate needs of the neonate.

It is time for a child to be born. The waiting is over; labor has begun. The dreams and wishes of the past months fade as the expectant parents face the reality of the tasks of childbearing and childrearing that are ahead.

The couple is about to undergo one of the most meaningful and stressful events in their life together. The adequacy of their preparation for childbirth will receive its trial. The coping mechanisms and communication and support systems that they have established as a couple will be put to the test. In particular, the childbearing woman may feel that her psychologic and physical limits are about to be challenged.

The care rendered to all couples during labor and delivery can affect their feelings about this childbirth as well as future births. The nurse who can apply the concepts of the nursing process to her practice enhances the chances for each couple to have a positive childbearing experience.

The quality of nursing care received by the laboring couple depends on the accuracy of the nurse's assessment, diagnosis, and plan of care; her skill in implementing that plan; and whether the outcomes of her interventions are desirable, expected, and positive. If the interventions are not successful, the nurse must evaluate her application of the nursing process and question whether the assessment and diagnosis were accurate, whether the objectives of the plan of care are realistic for that couple, and whether the interventions are appropriate for the identified problems.

Providing nursing care to the childbearing couple is challenging and rewarding. The nurse is participating in one of the most emotional experiences in life. Childbirth is usually joyous; sometimes it is a time of grief and sadness. In the event of complications, labor and delivery can be an extremely tense and stressful time for both the parents and the health care team. The needs of the childbearing couple in the event of crisis during or after labor and delivery are discussed in later chapters. In this chapter, however, the needs of the couple during normal labor and delivery are described.

NURSING MANAGEMENT OF ADMISSION

The patient is instructed during her prenatal visits to come to the hospital if one or both of the following occur:

1. Rupture of amniotic membranes.
2. Uterine contractions (primiparas, 8–12 minutes apart; multiparas, 10–15 minutes apart).

Early admission means less discomfort for the laboring woman when traveling to the hospital and more time to prepare for the delivery. Sometimes the labor is advanced and delivery is imminent, but usually the patient is in early labor at admission.

The manner in which the patient and her partner are greeted by the maternity nurse influences the course of the woman's hospital stay. It should be remembered that the sudden environmental change and sometimes impersonal technical aspects of the admission procedures can produce additional sources of stress. If she is greeted in a brusque, harried manner, she will be less likely to look to the nurse for support. A calm, pleasant manner is preferred when greeting the new admission. This calm manner indicates to the patient that she is an important person and may instill in the couple a sense of confidence in the staff's ability to provide quality care during this critical time.

After the initial greeting, the patient is taken into the labor room. Some couples prefer to remain together during the admission process, and others prefer to have the partner wait outside the labor room. As the nurse helps the patient undress and get into a hospital gown, the nurse can begin conversing with the patient to establish the nursing data base (see the Nursing Care Plan for labor and delivery). The experienced labor and delivery nurse can obtain essential information regarding the patient and her pregnancy within a few minutes after admission (see Figure 16–1), initiate any immediate interventions needed, and establish individualized priorities.

A major challenge for nurses is the formulation of realistic objectives for laboring mothers. Each woman has different coping mechanisms and support systems. The unmarried 14-year-old primigravida who has had no prenatal care and comes to the hospital alone does not bring the same coping mechanisms to the labor room as does the couple with a planned pregnancy who have attended prepared childbirth classes. The nurse may be the 14-year-old girl's support system, whereas the nurse may be needed only minimally by the couple.

After the patient is assisted into bed, she is prepared for a sterile vaginal examination (Procedure 17–1). The patient should be informed about the procedure and the purpose of it. She is instructed to lie on her back, pull up her knees, put her heels together, and let her knees fall out to the side. Privacy is maintained by draping the patient with a sheet or bath blanket during this procedure. If the patient states that the membranes are ruptured, the Nitrazine tape test is administered before applying lubricant to the sterile glove, because the lubricant may change the reaction of the test tape (see p. 447 for pH values). The vaginal examination provides information about cervical effacement and dilatation, the status of membranes, the presenting part, station, the position of the presenting part, the umbilical cord, and the bloody show. If the patient is in advanced labor, preparations for delivery need to be made quickly. If the patient is in early labor, the preparation can be accomplished at a more relaxed pace.

The nurse obtains the mother's blood pressure, oral temperature, pulse, and respirations, and she auscultates the FHTs. (Detailed information on FHR is presented in Chapter 16.)

Procedure 17–1. Intrapartal Vaginal Examination

Objective	Nursing action	Rationale
Prepare patient	Explain procedure, indications for carrying out procedure, and what information is being obtained.	Explanation of procedure decreases anxiety and increases relaxation of patient during procedure.
	Position patient in lithotomy position with thighs flexed and abducted. Instruct patient to put heels of feet together.	Prevents contamination of area during examination and provides for visualization of external labor progress signs.
	Drape so she is covered but so perineal area is exposed.	Provides as much privacy as possible.
	Encourage her to relax her muscles and legs during procedure.	
Assemble and prepare equipment	Have following equipment easily accessible: • Sterile disposable gloves. • Lubricant. • Nitrazine tape test prior to first examination.	Examination is facilitated and can be done quickly.
Use aseptic technique during examination	Put on both gloves. Using thumb and forefinger of left hand, spread labia widely, insert well-lubricated second and index fingers of right hand into vagina until they touch the cervix, without touching surrounding vulvar structures.	Avoid contaminating hand by contact with anus. Positioning of hand with wrist straight and elbow tilted downward allows fingertips to point toward umbilicus and find cervix.
Determine status of fetal membranes	Palpate for movable bulging sac through the cervix. Observe for expression of amniotic fluid during exam. Perform Nitrazine paper test first.	If bag of waters is intact, it will feel like a bulge. If the membranes have ruptured, amniotic fluid may be expressed while performing the vaginal examination. Nitrazine paper test (unless a lubricant has been used) registers a change in pH if amniotic fluid is present. Determination of membrane integrity is important, as membranes can act as dilating wedge during labor and safeguard against ascending infection to fetus in utero.

Procedure 17–1. Cont'd

Objective	Nursing action	Rationale
Determine status of labor progress during and after contractions	Carry out vaginal examination during and between contractions.	Examination between contractions reveals degree of cervical dilatation and effacement when presenting part is not under pressure of contractions. During a contraction, examination reveals information about the maximum amount of thinning, dilatation, and descent possible under influence of contractions.
Identify degree of: 1. Cervical dilatation	Palpate for opening or what appears as a depression in the cervix with a surrounding circular ridge of tissue. Estimate diameter of cervical opening in centimeters (0–10 cm) (Figure 17–1).	Estimation of the diameter of the depression identifies degree of dilatation. One finger is approximately 1.5–2 cm cervical dilatation.
2. Cervical effacement	Palpate the thickness of the surrounding circular ridge of tissue. Estimate degree of thinning in percentages.	Degree of thinning determines the amount of lower uterine segment that has been taken up into the fundal area.
Determine presentation and position of presenting part	As cervix opens, palpate for presenting part and identify its relationship to the maternal pelvis (Figure 17–2): • In vertex presentation, palpate for sutures and fontanelles and relate the occiput to one of the four quadrants of the maternal pelvis. • In face presentation, palpate facial features. • In breech presentation, palpate buttocks and sacrum.	Presenting part is easier to palpate through a dilated cervix, and differentiation of landmarks is easier. Molding can make identification of landmarks more difficult.
Determine station and whether engagement has occurred	Locate lowest portion of presenting part, then palpate the side walls of the pelvis for the ischial spines. Estimate in centimeters the relationship of the lowest portion of presenting part to the ischial spines (see Figure 15–7).	Identification of station provides information as to degree of descent and some information about adequacy of maternal pelvis. Engagement occurs when the presenting part is at or below the level of the ischial spines.

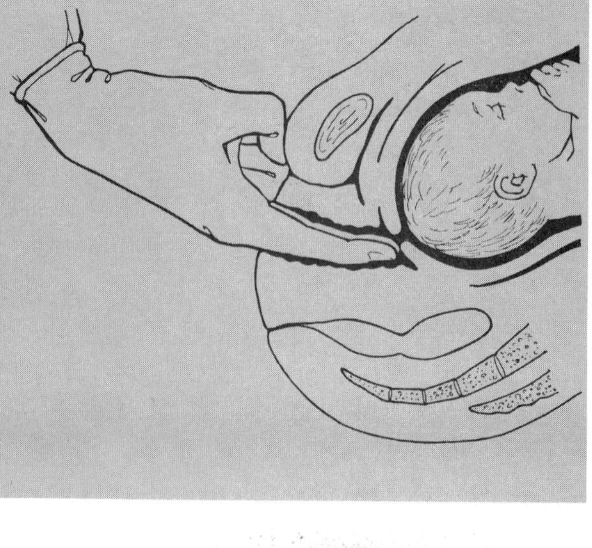

Figure 17–1. Vaginal palpation of cervical dilatation, effacement, amniotic membranes, and presenting part.

Procedure 17–1. Cont'd

Objective	Nursing action	Rationale
Inform patient about progress in labor	Discuss with patient findings of the vaginal examination and correlate them to her progress in labor.	Assists the patient in identifying progress and reinforces need for frequency of procedure. Information is reassuring and supportive for patient and family.
Identify possible complications	Observe for: 1. Signs of bleeding. 2. Prolapse of cord into vaginal canal.	Any bleeding, no matter how slight, may make vaginal examination contraindicated.

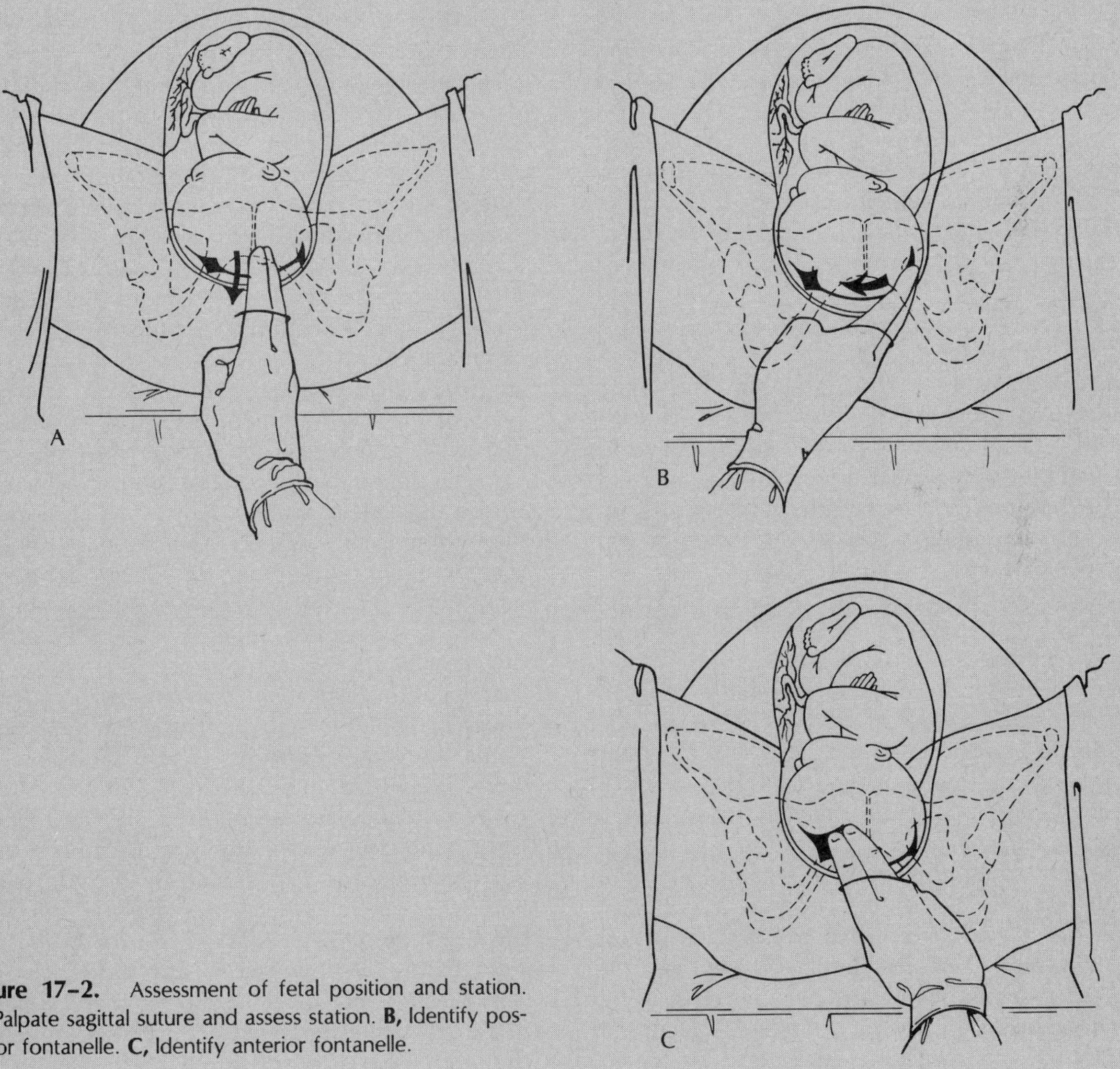

Figure 17–2. Assessment of fetal position and station. **A,** Palpate sagittal suture and assess station. **B,** Identify posterior fontanelle. **C,** Identify anterior fontanelle.

Ascertainment of fetal position by vaginal examination and abdominal palpation (Leopold's maneuvers) is an aid in locating the FHTs (see Chapter 16). If the fetal position is questionable, the nurse begins auscultation with the fetoscope at the midline of the abdomen below the umbilicus and moves the fetoscope in an ever-widening circle until the FHTs are located. As soon as the FHTs are located, the nurse palpates the mother's pulse. The mother's pulse rate should range from 70 to 100 beats/min and the FHR from 120 to 160 beats/min. By determining both rates, the nurse can be assured that she is listening to the FHTs and not to the uterine souffle. The FHR is counted for one full minute. While the nurse listens, she notes the presence of any unusual fetal activity.

In addition to the physical labor admission procedures, laboratory tests are carried out. Hemoglobin and hematocrit values may be obtained to help determine the oxygen-carrying capacity of the circulatory system and the ability of the mother to withstand blood loss at delivery. Elevation of the hematocrit may indicate hemoconcentration of blood, which occurs with edema or dehydration, while a low hemoglobin, in the absence of other evidence of bleeding, suggests anemia.

The blood of the woman is typed and crossmatched if she is in a high-risk category or if she is to receive oxytocin stimulation or induction. In some hospitals, blood is drawn on all laboring mothers for blood typing, and a clot may be held in the laboratory in case it is needed.

A serology test for syphilis is obtained if one has not been done in the last three months or if antepartal serology was positive.

During the admission process, the nurse assesses the uterine contractions. Contraction status is evaluated by placing the fingertips of one hand on the fundus of the uterus and waiting for the pressure of the contraction to begin. The uterus may be tender, so it is important to palpate gently. The frequency, intensity, and duration of uterine contractions and patient response are determined.

After this information is obtained, a clean-voided midstream urine specimen is collected. The patient with intact membranes may walk to the bathroom. If the membranes are ruptured, the patient remains in bed and the specimen is obtained in a clean bedpan to decrease the chance of prolapsed cord. The urine may be tested for the presence of protein, ketones, and glucose by using a dipstick before it is sent to the laboratory. This procedure is especially important if edema or elevated blood pressure is noted on admission. Proteinuria may be a sign of ensuing preeclampsia if it is 2+ or greater and not contaminated with blood or amniotic fluid. Ketonuria is a good index of starvation ketosis. Glycosuria is found frequently in pregnant women because of the increased glomerular filtration rate in the proximal tubules and the inability of these tubules to increase reabsorption of glucose. Glycosuria should not be discounted, however. Researchers have demonstrated that 20% of pregnant women with glycosuria and with a strong family history of diabetes are class A, or latent, diabetics (Burrow and Ferris, 1975). Presence of glycosuria necessitates follow-up.

While the patient is obtaining the urine specimen, the equipment for shaving the pubic area (referred to as the *prep*) and for the enema, if ordered, may be prepared. Many physicians leave standing orders for prep measures and enema administration. Prep orders vary from physician to physician, but most believe that some form of skin preparation facilitates their work in the delivery room, makes perineal repair easier, and facilitates cleansing of the perineum in the postpartal period. When a *complete prep* is performed, all pubic, perineal, and rectal hair is shaved. During a *miniprep*, perineal hair is shaved from the level of the clitoris down, including around the rectum. If *no prep* is ordered, no hair is shaved.

The nurse performing a prep washes her hands and then positions the patient in the same manner as for a vaginal examination. A towel is placed under the patient's buttocks. Lighting is adjusted so that the area may be well seen. The patient is questioned about the presence of any moles or warts while the nurse is applying the soap solution with a gauze square or sponge provided in the prep set. The (right-handed) nurse holds the skin taut with the left hand, using a towel from the prep set to protect her fingers, and shaves in short strokes, holding the razor in the right hand. She works downward to the vagina. Soap solution and hair should not be allowed to enter the vagina. When the perineum has been prepared, the patient is asked to turn to her left side and to assume the lateral Sims position. Again using the towel to protect the hand, the nurse pulls the upper buttock upward to expose the rectal area. After sudsing, the area around the rectum is shaved. The nurse must take care to prevent contaminants from the rectal area from entering the vaginal area.

While the patient is lying on her left side, the enema may be administered, unless the patient's obstetric history or findings during vaginal examination contraindicate it, such as vaginal bleeding or rapid labor progress and imminent delivery. The purposes of an enema are to evacuate the lower bowel so that labor will not be impeded, to stimulate uterine contractions, to avoid patient embarrassment if bowel contents are expelled during pushing efforts, and to prevent contamination of the sterile field during delivery. The nurse explains this procedure to the patient as it is being performed. If the membranes are intact and labor is not far advanced, the patient may expel the enema in the bathroom; otherwise she is positioned on the bedpan in bed.

Before leaving the labor room, the nurse must be sure that the patient knows how to operate the call system so that she can obtain help if she needs it. After the enema is expelled, the nurse monitors the FHTs again to assess any changes. If the partner has been out of the labor room, the couple are reunited as soon as possible.

In many hospitals, the admission process also includes signing a delivery permit, fingerprinting the mother on the infant records, and fastening an identification bracelet to the patient's arm.

Depending on how rapidly labor is progress-

Table 17–1. Normal Progress, Psychologic Characteristics, and Nursing Support During First Stage of Labor

Phase	Cervical dilatation	Uterine contractions	Patient response	Support measures
Latent phase	0–4 cm	Every 15–20 min 10–30 sec duration Mild intensity	Usually happy, talkative, and eager to be in labor	Get acquainted with patient (and partner, if present) and ascertain her preparation and needs. Instruct her in breathing techniques if she has not had prenatal classes.
			Exhibits need for independence by taking care of own bodily needs and seeking information	Allow patient to participate in care. Provide information needed.
Active phase	4–8 cm	Every 3–5 min 30–45 sec duration Moderate intensity	Exhibits increased fatigue and may begin to feel restless and anxious as contractions become stronger	Encourage patient to maintain breathing patterns. Provide quiet environment to reduce external stimuli. Inform couple of patient's progress.
			Becomes more dependent as she is less able to meet her needs	Anticipate needs. Allow patient to assist in her care as she desires or is able to.
Transition	8–10 cm	Every 1½–2 min 45–60 sec duration Strong intensity	Tires and may exhibit increased restlessness and irritability; may feel she cannot keep up with labor process and is out of control	Encourage patient to rest between contractions. If patient sleeps between contractions, wake her at increment of contraction so she can begin breathing pattern. This measure decreases her feeling that she is out of control. Praise couple's efforts and inform them of progress.

ing, the nurse notifies the clinician before or after she has completed the admission procedures. As many data as possible are reported, particularly data concerning cervical dilatation and effacement, station, presenting part, status of the membranes, contraction pattern, FHR, any vital signs that are not in the normal range, and the patient's reaction to labor.

The laboring couple can give cues about the support they want from the attending nurse. Many prospective parents have attended childbirth education classes and need minimal support to maintain breathing patterns. Many feel comfortable in asking for items that they need, such as extra pillows. Specific support measures the nurse should take are presented in Table 17-1.

Admission of Patient Who Had Planned Home Birth

Occasionally a couple who had decided to deliver at home without assistance must come to the hospital. The nurse must be cognizant of several important considerations.

First, the couple may be feeling defensive about having to undergo hospital-assisted birth and may be hostile toward the staff. A nonjudgmental attitude on the nurse's part is a necessity. This nonjudgmental attitude must also be carried over into the postpartal period.

Second, the couple have probably come to the hospital because they suspect a complication. The nurse should reinforce the couple's good judgment in seeking additional help and refrain from any comment about the couple's original intention.

Finally, many physicians are opposed to home births and may lack the understanding to deal with the couple in a sympathetic manner. In this instance, the nurse needs to be the buffer between the couple and the physician. If necessary, the physician should be informed that the delivery room is not the appropriate place to discuss the relative merits of home births. A woman who is about to give birth should not be submitted to a lecture about her decisions.

NURSING MANAGEMENT OF LABOR

The nurse continually assesses and supports maternal and fetal status throughout labor. The Nursing Care Plan for labor and delivery is based on the following factors:

1. Physiologic maintenance patterns.
2. Labor progress (changes associated with parturition, such as dilatation and effacement, contractile patterns, bloody show, rupture of membranes).
3. Fetal status patterns (physical responses of fetus to labor and fetal well-being).
4. Activity state of patient.
5. Discomforts of labor—patterns of sleep or rest (relaxation and amnesia-sleep).
6. Sustenance (oral or parenteral intake and toleration of fluids).
7. Elimination (all forms of output).
8. Giving and receiving care (care the couple can perform for themselves or measures with which they need assistance).
9. Psychologic maintenance patterns (progressive changes manifested during labor).

Many of the physical and psychologic changes that occur during labor and delivery are normal and predictable, and the outcome depends on the mother's internal system and the external support measures available to and used by the laboring couple. For example, the psychologic changes include manifestations of happiness, fear, anxiety, hostility, frustration, and success. As changes are exhibited, they should be identified and evaluated in terms of their normalcy, because occasionally deviations occur. Table 17-2 summarizes the immediate nursing action for physical problems that may occur. More specific intervention is detailed in Chapter 19.

NURSING CARE PLAN

Labor and Delivery

Patient Data Base

History (see Figure 16-1)

Mother's and father's names

Age of mother

Obstetric history: gravida, para, abortions, fetal deaths, birth weight of previous children, complications during previous labors and deliveries

EDC, calculated gestational age, and LMP (first day of last menstrual period)

Maternal and family medical history: health status of living children, medications taken during pregnancy, recent infections

Prenatal care: type and amount, any significant antepartal problems

Prenatal education: type of childbirth preparation

Pediatrician

Chosen method of infant feeding

Status of labor: when contractions began, when they became regular, quality of contractions; how patient seems to be coping with contractions at this time

Status of membranes: intact, ruptured, time ruptured, fluid characteristics, amount of fluid

Last time woman ate

Physical examination
(see Intrapartal Physical Assessment Guide, Chapter 16)

General appearance of mother and partner (calm appearance or anxious)

Height and weight

Vital signs

Heart and lungs

Breasts

Presence of edema

Abdomen and fundus (size and contour)

Hydration

Perineum

Uterine contractions

Nitrazine test

Vaginal examination: cervical dilatation and effacement, presentation and position of fetus, membranes

Fetal status (FHR)

Laboratory evaluation

Hemoglobin

Hematocrit

CBC

Maternal blood type

Serologic tests

Urinalysis

Nursing Priorities

1. Assess physical and psychologic status of mother.
2. Assess uterine contractile patterns.
3. Assess status of fetus (FHR, position, presence of meconium, hyperactivity).
4. Assess labor progress.
5. Prepare mother for delivery.
6. Support laboring mother and coach (or partner) as needed.

Nursing Interventions

The interventions given here are based on common needs of laboring couples per stage of labor. Couples prepared in the psychoprophylactic method of childbirth are taught to begin the first concentrated breathing exercise when needed and to change to the next one only when the first one is not serving its purpose. Consequently, some couples may be able to use one or two breathing exercises throughout the entire labor experience. Although certain exercises are suggested with different labor phases, the couple need not use this particular breathing exercise if the need is not there. Similarly, nursing actions performed in one phase or stage of labor may need to be performed in other phases or throughout labor. The intervention depends on the problems identified with continued assessment.

NURSING CARE PLAN Cont'd

Labor and Delivery

Problem	Nursing interventions and actions	Rationale
First stage LATENT PHASE *Admission*	Greet couple warmly; orient couple to environment and admission procedures.	Conveys acceptance, reduces anxiety, and establishes rapport.
	Obtain history (see Figure 16-1).	Provides data base.
	Assess maternal vital signs and FHR.	Provides baseline values.
	Notify physician or nurse-midwife of admission.	
	Perform Intrapartal Physical Assessment (see Chapter 16).	
	Administer enema as ordered.	Enema empties lower bowel, which stimulates uterine contractions, prevents contamination of sterile field during delivery, and facilitates descent of presenting part.
	Perform perineal prep as ordered.	Shaving of skin in pubic and perineal areas facilitates perineal repair and cleansing of perineum in postpartal period.
	Obtain urine specimen.	*Proteinuria of 2+ or more found in urine that is not contaminated with blood or amniotic fluid may be sign of ensuing preeclampsia.
	Check FHR after mother expels enema.	A change in fetal station may cause fetal distress if cord has progressed before presenting part.
Physiologic maintenance	Assess vital signs: 1. Temperature every 4 hr unless >37.5C (99.6F), in which case check every 2 hr. 2. Check BP, pulse, and respirations every hour; if BP >140/90, pulse >100, and/or respiration >22/min, notify physician.	Maternal vital signs provide information on state of dehydration, development of infection or maternal fetal complications. BP >140/90 requires more frequent reassessment and additional assessments of signs and symptoms of preeclampsia.
Labor progress 1. Dilatation a. Cervix 1-4 cm dilated b. Effacement occurring	Begin charting on Friedman graph (see Figure 16-10). Assess dilatation and effacement by vaginal examination.	Confirms normal or detects abnormal labor progression.
2. Contractions a. Becoming regular b. Frequency: every 15-20 min c. Duration: 10-30 sec d. Intensity: mild to moderate	Assess contractions by palpation and/or electronic methods.	
3. Bloody show and mucous plug	Ascertain presence of bloody show and passage of mucous plug.	As labor begins, mucous plug is shed. Beginning dilatation of cervix causes rupture of small capillaries in cervix, which results in blood-tinged mucus.
Fetal status	Check FHR every 30 min as long as it remains between 120-160/min. If FHR is outside these parameters, continuous monitoring is recommended. At some time during early labor, attach external monitor for at least 15 min to assess fetal status. Monitor may be removed and reapplied later or allowed to remain throughout labor, depending on findings.	Evaluates fetal well-being, and provides information concerning fetal response to labor.

NURSING CARE PLAN Cont'd

Labor and Delivery

Problem	Nursing interventions and actions	Rationale
	Palpate abdomen (Leopold's maneuvers, p. 460).	Determines fetal position.
	Perform vaginal examination to assess degree of engagement of presenting part.	Presenting part may be engaged in the primigravida and entering the inlet in the multipara.
Activity	Allow woman to ambulate if desired unless any of following are present:	Provides diversion.
	1. Ruptured membranes.	Prolapse of cord is possible.
	2. Malpresentation and/or malposition of fetus.	
	3. Vaginal bleeding.	
	4. Advanced labor.	Patient may deliver suddenly.
	5. Administration of analgesic agent.	Patient may feel dizzy or drowsy.
Discomfort (back or lower abdomen)	Assist in diversional activities—e.g., conducted tour of facilities—if her membranes are intact and she can ambulate.	Woman's attention is diverted away from her discomfort and contractions. Tour familiarizes couple with the territory.
	Assess couple's coping mechanisms for labor and answer their questions.	Provides information; reduces fear of unknown. Provides labor coping mechanism.
	Anticipatory guidance may be needed for unprepared couple.	
	Suggest to couple that they begin the following measures if needed:	Provides focus for attention and other busy work for the brain.
	Effleurage.	Stimulation eases abdominal discomfort.
	Pelvic rocking or the OB back rub.	Eases back discomfort.
Sleep/rest	Encourage woman to relax.	Reduces tension, conserves energy, and decreases discomfort.
Sustenance	If clinician permits, woman may have clear liquids or ice chips.	Provides energy and maintains hydration.
	Do not give woman solid foods.	Gastrointestinal absorption is decreased during labor. Patient may vomit and aspirate gastric contents while under medication or anesthesia.
Elimination	Encourage patient to void every 2 hr or as needed.	A full bladder can cause discomfort, impede descent of the fetus, and cause dysfunctional labor.
	Check for bladder distention.	Patient may not have urge to void due to decreased tone of bladder from the hormones of pregnancy, pressure from the presenting part, and analgesia.
	If catherization is necessary, use small flexible catheter (no. 14 French) and lubricate well so it slides in easily. Insert catheter between contractions, because during contraction fetal head presses down and makes insertion difficult and painful.	Bladder trauma may predispose to postpartal urinary retention and cystitis.
	Record intake and output.	Evaluates hydration status.
Care giving and receiving	Couple can usually manage during this phase of labor. Nurse should periodically see if she can be of assistance.	

NURSING CARE PLAN Cont'd
Labor and Delivery

Problem	Nursing interventions and actions	Rationale
Psychologic maintenance	Listen and convey acceptance of behavior and attitudes. Give correct information and support. Inform couple of any procedures. Answer any questions.	Couple usually is happy and relieved that this day has finally arrived. They may have some fear of the unknown and may anticipate problems.
ACTIVE PHASE *Physiologic maintenance*	Assess vital signs: 1. Temperature every 4 hr unless >37.5C (99.6F), in which case check every 2 hr. 2. BP, pulse, and respirations every hour.	Evaluates maternal status.
Labor progress 1. Dilatation	Chart data on Friedman graph.	Provides objective means of assessing progress and detecting abnormal patterns.
a. Cervix 4-8 cm (active dilatation) b. Effacement complete (100%)	Perform vaginal examination to assess dilatation and effacement. Encourage shallow chest breathing during examination.	Promotes relaxation.
2. Contractions a. Regular b. Frequency: every 3-5 min c. Duration: 30-45 sec d. Intensity: moderate	Assess contractions every 15 min.	
3. Increase in bloody show and vaginal discharge	Change bed pads frequently.	Promotes hygiene and comfort. Keeps contaminants from reaching the vagina.
Fetal status	Check FHR every 15 min by fetal monitor or by auscultation (immediately after contractions).	Evaluates effect of active labor on fetus.
Activity	Institute bed rest if patient has been ambulatory up to this point. Assist coach in helping the mother into comfortable position (lateral position is recommended). Observe for signs of vena caval syndrome, such as drop in BP; elevation of pulse; air hunger; pallor; moist, clammy skin; marked change in baseline FHR.	Quality of contractions is better due to increased placental perfusion and increased O_2 transport to fetus. When patient is on her back, uterus lies on vena cava and obstructs venous return from extremities. Reduction of blood volume results in signs and symptoms of shock.
Discomfort 1. Feelings of pain increasing	Coach may suggest that patient switch to another level of breathing. Offer pharmacologic support. If analgesic is administered: 1. Instruct patient to remain in bed. 2. Keep side rails up. 3. Check maternal vital signs, FHTs, and fetal activity.	Promotes safety. Medication may make patient dizzy and/or drowsy. Patient and/or fetus may respond poorly to medication.
2. Backache	Administer or encourage coach to administer back rub (see Chapter 12).	Relieves discomfort.
Sleep/rest	Provide environment conducive to relaxation (e.g., dim lights, decreased noise and activity in and out of room, soft music). Assist coach in identifying factors interrupting relaxation.	Relaxation enhances labor experience, conserves energy, and lessens pain.

NURSING CARE PLAN Cont'd

Labor and Delivery

Problem	Nursing interventions and actions	Rationale
	Offer to relieve labor coach.	Coach needs rest and sustenance.
Sustenance	Provide ice chips. Assess following parameters of hydration status: 1. Measure pulse and temperature for elevation. 2. Check skin for dryness. 3. Check patient's lips for cracking and apply petroleum jelly or similar agent.	Determines presence of dehydration and development of hypoglycemia. Labor depletes the glycogen stores and thereby increases the chance of hypoglycemia.
	Intravenous electrolyte solution may be given at this time. Monitor rate.	Provides energy and prevents dehydration or corrects a dehydrated state.
Elimination (bladder)	Continue to encourage mother to void every 2 hr. Check for bladder distention.	Prevents distention, discomfort, and trauma to bladder.
Care giving and receiving 1. Dry mouth	Provide ice chips, mouth wash, glycerine swabs.	Promotes comfort.
2. Cracked lips	Apply petroleum jelly to lips.	Promotes comfort.
3. Vaginal discharges	Change linen and bed pads frequently. Provide perineal care.	Promotes hygiene and comfort and relieves discomforts from secretions.
4. Diaphoresis	Sponge body and face.	Relieves discomfort.
Psychologic maintenance	Assure couple that efforts of labor are effective.	Couple becomes more serious and purposeful and less talkative. Patient is less receptive to instructions other than those given by her partner.
	Provide information about labor progress.	Decreases anxiety, because woman may begin to have fears or doubts about coping.
	Avoid using words like *slow* when talking about progress.	Connotations of the word *slow* can be discouraging.
	Praise accomplishments of patient and labor coach.	Promotes confidence of laboring couple.
TRANSITION (DECELERATION PHASE)	Continue graphic analysis of labor and physiologic parameters. Assess vital signs.	Provides objective data about labor patterns.
Labor progress 1. Dilatation pattern a. Cervix 8-10 cm	Continue graphic analysis. Assess by vaginal examination.	
b. Effacement complete (100%)	Multipara may be taken to delivery room at 8 cm cervical dilatation. Primipara may stay in labor room until dilatation is complete, fetus has descended, and there is perineal bulging. Remain with couple.	Tissues and muscles of birth canal in multipara are more relaxed, and birth process is more rapid. Deceleration phase in multiparas lasts about 30 min.
2. Contractions a. Regular b. Frequency: every 1-2 min c. Duration: 50-60 sec d. Intensity: strong	Assess each contraction.	This is most active phase of first stage.
3. Heavy bloody show	Change bed pad and administer perineal care.	Decreases chances of infection and provides comfort.
4. Rupture of membranes	Monitor FHR immediately after membranes rupture (spontaneously or due to amniotomy).	Determines presence of prolapsed cord, which can occur with rupture of membranes if pelvic inlet is not occluded.

NURSING CARE PLAN Cont'd
Labor and Delivery

Problem	Nursing interventions and actions	Rationale
	Inspect amniotic fluid for color, odor, amount, and consistency.	To detect presence of meconium staining and infection.
	Report and record observations.	
	Perform vaginal examination, assessing dilatation, fetal position, and station.	Rupture of membranes is usually sign of advanced progress.
	Palpate for cord.	Confirms absence of cord prolapse.
	Dry perineum and change bed pad.	Promotes comfort and good hygiene.
Fetal status	Monitor fetal heart rate every 15 min or more frequently, especially in event of bradycardia or tachycardia.	This is most active phase for fetus. Uterus is contracting frequently, increasing anoxic periods for fetus.
Discomfort		
1. Generalized discomfort	Coach should try variation of pant-blow exercise.	Highly complex breathing pattern involves more mental concentration, thus decreasing pain reception at cerebral level.
2. May have severe abdominal back pain or irritable abdomen	Apply firm pressure to lower abdomen and/or lower back.	Alleviates some discomfort by producing counterpressure.
	Apply heat to abdomen or back by using k-pad or hot water bottle.	Warmth soothes muscle discomfort.
	Palpate contractions lightly.	
	Avoid pressure.	
	Assist patient to change position.	
3. Trembling		May be due to very rapid labor.
Sleep/rest	Assist coach in watching for tension and keeping mother relaxed.	
	Encourage coach to awaken mother at beginning of contraction to begin her breathing exercises.	Woman dozes between contractions and wakens at peak of contraction. Breathing exercises provide focus of concentration, reducing perception of pain.
Sustenance	Continue to observe for hypoglycemia.	Deceleration phase of labor requires much energy.
	Increase rate of parenteral fluids if signs of dehydration occur. Due to great activity of this labor phase, patient will probably not tolerate any quantity of oral intake.	Fluid is lost by means of diaphoresis.
	Offer sips or chips at frequent intervals.	Breathing patterns tend to dry out the mouth.
Elimination	Check for bladder distention.	
Nausea and vomiting	Apply cold cloth to woman's throat.	Helps alleviate nausea.
	Elevate head of bed.	
Care giving and receiving		
1. Diaphoresis (especially on upper lip and forehead)	Wash face.	Promotes comfort.
2. Hiccups, holding breath, urge to push	Check to see if complete dilatation has occurred; if it has not, urge mother to blow.	Pushing on cervix that is not completely dilated results in cervical edema and increases danger of cervical lacerations and fetal head trauma. Blowing exercise inhibits breath holding and pushing efforts.
3. Leg tremors	Assure couple that this is normal and explain cause.	Fetal head is pressing on nerves and blocks vessels to extremities.

NURSING CARE PLAN Cont'd

Labor and Delivery

Problem	Nursing interventions and actions	Rationale
4. Muscle cramps in lower extremities	Place blankets over legs and feet.	Circulation is diverted to uterus and upper body. Because of decreased circulation, extremities become cold.
	Extend mother's leg and dorsiflex foot.	Counteracts spasm, promoting relaxation.
Hyperventilation	Encourage slow breathing, breathing with her if necessary. Mother may breathe into paper bag.	Hyperventilation increases loss of carbon dioxide and leads to respiratory alkalosis. Woman may complain of tingling and numbness of lips, face, hands, and feet or may develop carpopedal spasms.
Psychologic maintenance	Praise and encourage the laboring couple. Help them through one contraction at a time.	Reinforces couple's ability to cope.
	Convey an accepting, caring attitude. Coach (or nurse) should call mother by name, speak with firm, short commands, breathe with her, and maintain eye contact.	Woman may become angry at nurse and labor coach. Loss of control can occur.
Second Stage (Expulsion Phase)		
Physiologic maintenance	Assess vital signs.	
Labor progress	Perform vaginal examination to assure complete dilatation (10 cm and 100% effaced).	
	Primipara is taken to delivery room when perineal bulging is noted. After patient is in delivery room, check BP every 5-15 min and FHT after each contraction. When mother is taken to delivery room, provide scrub suit, boots, hat, and mask for partner if he is going into delivery room with her. Assess physiologic parameters of expulsion phase. Assist mother to a comfortable position for pushing.	Abdominal musculature contracts to assist with expulsion. Mother feels strong urge to push (similar to urge to defecate). Anal eversion occurs, as does perineal bulging and flattening. Introitus gradually opens wider with each contraction.
	Elevate head of bed or delivery table 30° to 60° degrees or place pillows under head and torso. Woman's legs should be spread slightly and knees slightly flexed.	Faciliates expulsion. When mother's shoulders are raised, use of abdominal muscles is facilitated.
	If woman's feet are to be placed in stirrups, lift both legs simultaneously to reduce muscle strain. Feet should be supported with stirrups in low position with no pressure on popliteal area or calf of leg.	Pressure on popliteal area or calf of leg may lead to thromboplebitis.
	Adjust handles so that mother may pull back on them while pushing and so there is slight flexion of arm. At beginning of the contraction, mother should be instructed to take two short breaths, holding third breath while leaning forward and thinking the letter "J" as she steadily bears down. Encourage woman to exhale and inhale and repeat bearing-down effort until contraction ends.	Pushing adds the forces of intraabdominal pressure to the existing intrauterine pressure which moves the baby through the birth canal.

NURSING CARE PLAN Cont'd

Labor and Delivery

Problem	Nursing interventions and actions	Rationale
	Encourage use of blowing exercise when pushing is undesirable.	
Fetal status	Observe perineum for appearance of fetal vertex.	Primigravida is transported to delivery room when vertex is visible at introitus without spreading labias.
	Monitor FHTs.	Pressure is being exerted on fetal head with each expulsive effort.
	Electronic monitoring device may be moved to delivery room with patient to assess fetal response to efforts of delivery. If electronic monitoring device is not in use, auscultate FHR after each contraction.	
Discomfort 1. May be decreasing 2. Stretching, burning sensations as infant moves into vagina and compresses perineal nerves	Praise pushing efforts. Inform couple when head becomes visible. (Some delivery rooms have mirrors for couple to see infant emerge.)	Communicates success of couple's hard work. Shows that mother can work with forces of labor.
Sleep/rest	Encourage mother to rest between contractions.	Efforts of labor and delivery are exhausting.
Psychologic maintenance	Praise and support couple.	Mother feels relief that she can push. Couple often feels satisfaction after each pushing effort.
Third Stage		
Immediate postdelivery	Note and record following: 1. Time of delivery of infant and position. 2. Type of episiotomy and kind of suture used to repair incision.	Maintains correct delivery records.
	3. Analgesic or anesthetic agents used.	Some anesthetics and blocking agents increase uterine relaxation, which may lead to hemorrhage.
	4. Complications (excessive bleeding, uterine inertia, neonatal complications).	Complications may increase risk of hemorrhage or infection.
Delivery of placenta	Record delivery time and mechanism of placenta.	Duncan delivery of placenta increases chance of incomplete separation, which in turn increases chance of hemorrhage due to retained placental fragments.
	Administer and record oxytocic drugs.	Increases uterine contractility.
	Administer Deladumone or Ditate if woman is not breast-feeding.	Suppresses letdown of breast milk.
	Inspect intactness of placenta and check for irregularities of cord insertion.	Duncan delivery of placenta increases chances of retention of placental tissue.
	Check maternal blood pressure and pulse.	Assesses physiologic status.
	Obtain cord blood.	If mother is Rh negative, send cord blood for direct Coombs' test. If mother is Rh positive, cord blood may be sent to laboratory to determine blood type and Rh.
	Clinician does manual and visual examination of vagina to determine presence of lacerations.	Prevents hemorrhage from undetected lacerations.
Fourth Stage First Hour	Assess vital signs:	Evaluates physiologic parameters for homeostatic adjustment.

NURSING CARE PLAN Cont'd
Labor and Delivery

Problem	Nursing interventions and actions	Rationale
Physiologic maintenance	1. Temperature every hour. If it is not elevated, check every 4 hours. 2. Check BP, pulse, and respirations every 15 min.	Detects complications such as hemorrhage, hypovolemia, infection, and others.
Assessment		
1. Fundus	Check firmness and position of fundus every 15 min for the first hour—should be firm at midline at level of umbilicus or two finger-breadths below.	Fundus must stay contracted to close off vessels at placental implantation site and to prevent hemorrhage.
2. Perineum	Inspect perineum for redness, swelling, bruising, discharge, gapping, every 15 min for the first hour.	Identifies excessive trauma that may hinder healing.
3. Lochia	Check lochia for amount, color, presence of clots every 15 min for the first hour.	Presence of clots may indicate retained placental fragments or uterine relaxation. Saturation of more than one or two perineal pads in the first hour is considered excessive.
4. Bladder	Palpate bladder for distention. Encourage patient to void.	Distended bladder can cause uterine atony and postpartal bleeding.
Chilling	Cover mother with warmed blankets.	Sudden release of intra-abdominal pressure after emptying of uterus, reaction to fatigue, and exhaustion associated with stress of labor may cause chilling.
SECOND TO FOURTH HOUR AFTER DELIVERY		
Physiologic and physical maintenance	Perform previous assessment every 30 min as long as findings are within normal parameters.	
	Give bed bath and prepare mother to transfer to postpartal unit. Utilize time to assess learning needs with regard to self-care: massaging fundus, changing pads, perineal care after elimination.	Promotes hygiene.
Psychologic maintenance	Evaluate emotional status. Provide quiet rest periods.	

Nursing Care Evaluation

Mother has had safe labor and delivery with no undue trauma or problems.

Infant is delivered without undue trauma.

Mother is transferred to postpartal unit when the following criteria are met:

1. Vital signs are stable.
2. Uterus is firm, in the midline, and at the umbilicus.
3. Blood flow is moderate.
4. Bladder is not distended.

Mother understands self-care measures:

1. Massaging fundus and assessing its firmness.
2. Changing pads.
3. Care after elimination.

Table 17–2. Deviations from Normal Labor Process Requiring Immediate Intervention

Problem	Immediate action
Patient admitted with vaginal bleeding or history of painless vaginal bleeding	1. Do not perform vaginal examination. 2. Assess FHTs. 3. Evaluate amount of blood loss. 4. Evaluate labor pattern. 5. Notify physician immediately.
Presence of greenish amniotic fluid	1. Continuously monitor FHR. 2. Evaluate dilatation status of cervix and determine whether umbilical cord is prolapsed. 3. Maintain patient on complete bed rest. 4. Notify physician immediately.
Absence of FHT and fetal movement	1. Notify physician. 2. Provide emotional support to laboring couple (patient has an idea that "something is wrong").
Prolapse of umbilical cord	1. Relieve pressure on cord manually. 2. Continuously monitor FHTs; watch for changes in FHR pattern. 3. Notify physician.
Patient admitted in advanced labor; delivery imminent	1. Proceed directly to delivery room. 2. Obtain necessary information: a. Physician's name. b. Bleeding problems. c. Obstetric problems. d. FHR and maternal vital signs, if possible. e. Length of labor and last time she ate. 3. Direct ancillary personnel to telephone physician. *Do not leave patient alone.* 4. Provide support to couple.

MANAGEMENT OF SPONTANEOUS DELIVERY

Delivery Room

The instrument table, which is set up in advance, generally includes a linen pack containing a buttocks drape, two leg drapes, one abdominal drape, and several towels. Many delivery rooms are now using disposable linen packs. The delivery instruments can be sterilized in a large basin and are added to the table at the time it is set up. Equipment required in preparation for delivery varies somewhat from hospital to hospital but should include the following items or their equivalent:

1 large basin with cotton balls kept in a ring stand (sterile water is added at the time of delivery)

1 placenta basin

1 iodine cup

1 pair suture scissors

1 pair episiotomy scissors

3 sponge forceps

3 Kelly clamps

3 hemostats

3 towel clips

3 Allis clamps

00 or 000 chromic sutures (may be added at delivery if needed)

1 needle holder

1 right-angle retractor
1 uterine dressing forceps
1 thumb forceps with teeth
1 thumb forceps without teeth
2 ear bulb syringes wrapped in gauze
1 cord clamp
3 cord blood tubes
1 5-yard vaginal pack
4 × 4 sponges

The solution to be used for the perineal scrub is placed in a warm place so it will be warmed before using on the patient. Two gowns with towels, two pairs of gloves or more, and a sterile baby blanket should be added to the table when it is set up. Some delivery setups include a French catheter in a small basin. This may be wrapped separately and added if needed.

An instrument table is set up under sterile precautions, and it may be covered with sterile side sheets, labeled with the time and date, and initialed by the person who set it up. The table may be left for up to eight hours.

Most delivery rooms are equipped with a radiant-heated infant care unit, which is equipped with oxygen, suction, and an intermittent positive pressure breathing (IPPB) system that can be used with a mask or connected directly to an endotracheal tube. Before each delivery, this unit should be checked to make sure it is working and that a sterile area is available in which to place the infant. Two sterile towels are opened and placed in the unit for drying the infant. If not left on continuously, the radiant heater is turned on at this time so that there will be a warm environment for the newborn infant.

It is suggested that the following equipment be available for infant care: a soft rubber ear bulb syringe for suctioning of the nose and mouth (this may be brought with the baby from the delivery table); a DeLee mucus suction trap; suction catheters (sizes 10, 12, and 14 French and sizes 8, 10, 12, and 14 disposable plastic catheters with finger control); a laryngoscope with a working light; Miller size 0 premature and size 1 blade; and 2.5–4 mm or size 10, 12, and 14 endotracheal tubes with stylets for those physicians who use them. A bag resuscitator should also be available if the heated unit does not have one (Roberts, 1973; Korones, 1976).

Nursing Interventions

The nurse has responsibilities to four people in the delivery room: the mother, her partner/coach, the infant, and the clinician (physician or nurse-midwife).

The delivery is conducted under strict sterile precautions. Therefore, all those who enter the delivery room wear scrub apparel, caps, and masks and wash their hands. The mask is changed when it becomes damp because it does not provide an effective bacterial barrier when wet. The nurse assists the labor coach in donning the appropriate apparel for accompanying the mother to the delivery room.

Nursing duties include assisting with the transport of the mother to the delivery room and helping her onto the delivery table. Before she is placed in stirrups, the nurse ascertains the type of anesthesia, if any, that may be used. Women receiving spinal anesthesia are not placed in stirrups until after the procedure is complete and permission is given by the anesthesiologist, because the level of the block is affected by the mother's position.

Preparing the Woman and the Coach for Delivery

When placing the woman in stirrups, the nurse should lift both legs simultaneously to avoid strain on abdominal and perineal muscles. Wrappers covering the delivery table may be used to pad the stirrups. The stirrups should be adjusted to fit the length of the mother's lower extremities (Figure 17–3). The feet are supported in the stirrup holders, and the height and angle of the stirrups are adjusted so there is no pressure on the popliteal or calf area of the mother's legs, which might cause discomfort and possible postpartal vascular problems. The expulsive efforts of the mother will be aided if the back of the delivery table is elevated about 30 to 60 degrees and the handles on the delivery table are adjusted so she may pull back on them.

The mother's vulvar and perineal area is prepared in the following manner: A sterile prep tray containing two small basins with at least six large cotton balls in each cup should be set up. One cup contains a surgical scrub solution in sterile water, and the other cup contains sterile water. After thoroughly washing her hands, the nurse dons sterile gloves and cleans the vulva and perineum with the scrub solution (Figure 17–4), then rinses

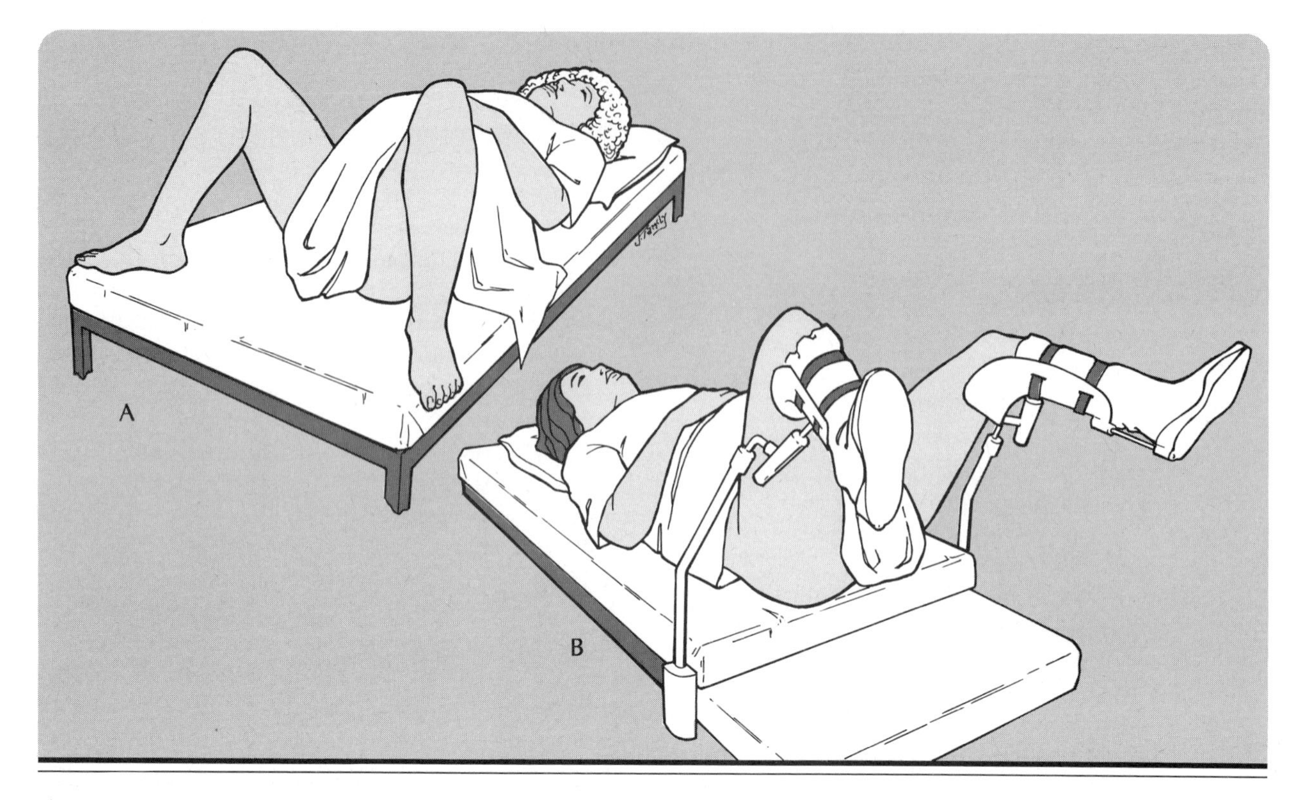

Figure 17–3. Positioning of women on the delivery table. **A,** Dorsal recumbent position. **B,** Lithotomy position.

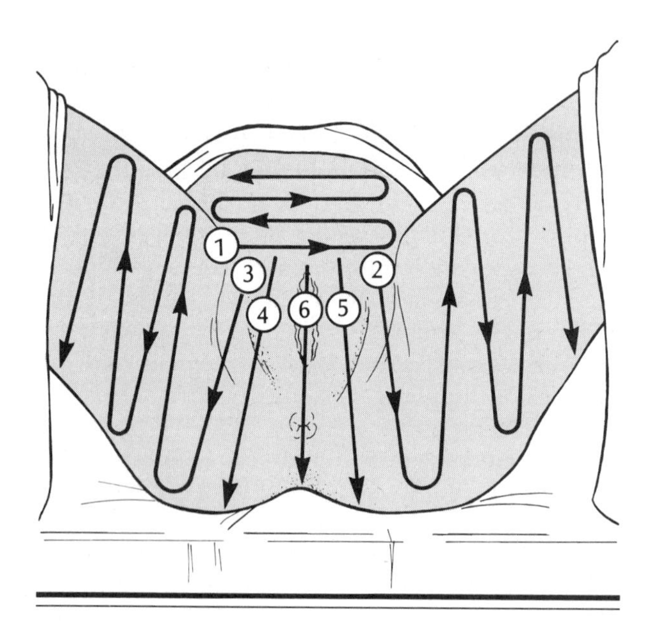

Figure 17–4. Cleansing the perineum prior to delivery. The nurse follows the numbered diagram, using a new cotton ball for each area.

with sterile water. Beginning with the mons, the area is scrubbed up to the lower abdomen. The second ball is used to scrub the inner groin and thigh of one leg, and the third cotton ball is used to scrub the other leg, moving outward to avoid carrying material from surrounding areas to the vaginal outlet. The last three cotton balls are used to scrub the labia and vestibule with one downward sweep each. The used cotton balls are then discarded.

The labor coach is provided a stool to sit on if desired. Both the mother and the coach are informed of procedures and progress and are supported throughout the delivery. Some delivery rooms come equipped with a mirror on the overhead light so that the couple may watch the delivery.

The mother's blood pressure and the fetal heart rate are monitored between contractions, and contractions are palpated until delivery to assess status. In spontaneous deliveries, the mother is encouraged to push until the fetal chin clears the perineum. The nurse instructs her to use the "blow-blow-blow" pattern of breathing until expulsion is complete. This procedure prevents a too-rapid delivery, which may traumatize or tear the maternal tissues. The head is often delivered between contractions, when control is easiest. Sometimes a gentle push from the mother is required for expulsion of the shoulders. Easy, gradual traction effects complete delivery of the infant.

Assisting the Clinician

The end third of the delivery table is retractable but should remain unretracted until the clinician is present so that a ready surface is available in the event that the infant arrives suddenly and unassisted. The nurse observes the perineum until the clinician is ready and keeps the clinician informed as to the advancement of the delivery.

The clinician scrubs and dons a gown, which the nurse is responsible for tying. The nurse ensures that enough gown and towel packs are available for all assistants who are scrubbing. After the clinician puts on sterile gloves, he or she is then ready to proceed with draping the patient. One sterile drape is placed under the mother's buttocks, one over each leg, and one over the abdomen. The mother should be cautioned not to touch the drapes so a sterile field can be maintained. The clinician takes care not to touch the skin of the perineum or anal area with the sterile gloves.

The nurse needs to anticipate the clinician's needs during the entire delivery and to listen closely for requests for such items as extra sponges or sutures. A stool for the clinician to sit on is provided if desired. The overhead light is adjusted so that the maternal perineal area and introitus are well lighted.

Clinician Interventions

When the fetal head has distended the perineum about 5 cm, the clinician may perform certain hand maneuvers to prevent undue trauma to the fetal head and maternal soft tissues. With a towel draped over one hand, the clinician applies pressure on the chin of the fetus through the maternal perineum. The other hand exerts gentle pressure on the occiput. This is the modified Ritgen maneuver (Figure 17-5). This maneuver permits the head to be delivered slowly under the symphysis pubis, with the face sliding successfully over the perineum. If the infant is too large and tearing of the perineum is possible, an episiotomy may be performed (see Chapter 20). After the infant's head is delivered, the clinician palpates the infant's neck for the presence of a cord, which can be slipped over the infant's head if it is loose. If the cord is tight, it is double-clamped and cut.

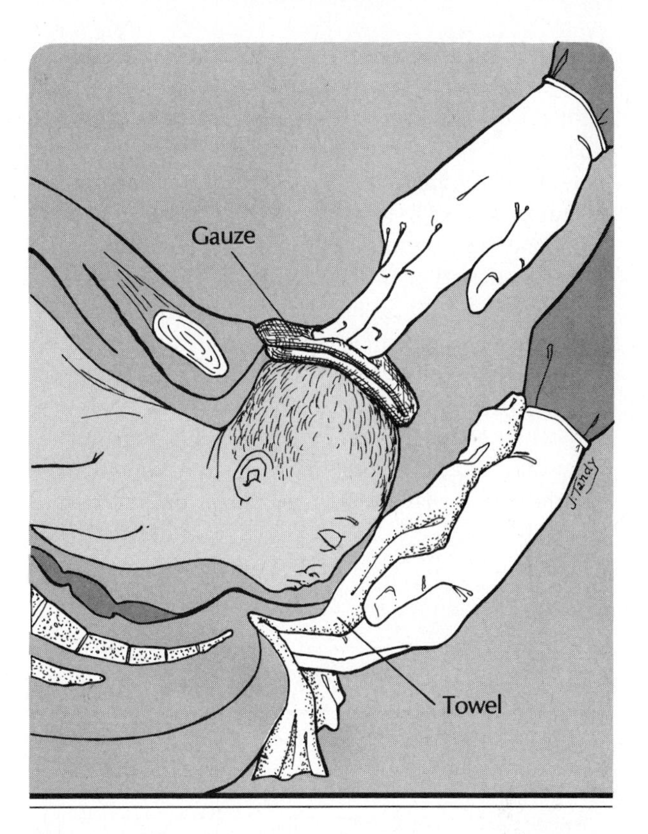

Figure 17–5. Delivery by modified Ritgen maneuver.

Restitution and external rotation occur after the head is delivered. The only assistance needed during this time is support of the maternal perineum. While awaiting completion of external rotation, the clinician suctions the infant's nose and mouth to remove mucus. When the infant's shoulder appears at the symphysis pubis, the clinician may use both hands to grasp the infant's head gently and push downward for delivery of the anterior shoulder. Gentle upward traction facilitates delivery of the posterior shoulder.

Delivery of the infant's body may be controlled by grasping the posterior shoulder with one hand, palm turned toward the perineum. The left hand may be used for this if the infant is LOA. The right hand then follows along the infant's back, and the feet are grasped as they are delivered. The infant's head is kept down and to the side as the infant's feet, legs, and body are tucked under the clinician's left arm in a football hold. The clinician's right hand is then free for further care of the infant, and the infant is securely held. The nose and mouth are suctioned with a bulb syringe, and respiratory passages are cleared.

There is considerable controversy about when to clamp and cut the cord. If the infant is held at or below the introitus, as much as 100 ml of blood may be shifted from the placenta to the fetus. If the infant is held 50 to 60 cm above the introitus, a negligible amount of blood is transferred to the infant, even after three minutes. The extra amount of blood added to the infant's circulation may reduce the frequency of iron-deficiency anemia, which can occur later in infancy—or the circulatory overload may produce polycythemia and favor hyperbilirubinemia. Pritchard and MacDonald (1976) advocate clamping the cord after clearing the infant's airway, which takes about 30 seconds. The infant is not elevated above the introitus.

The cord is clamped with two Kelly clamps and cut between them. The clamp on the placental side is placed on the mother's abdomen. A plastic cord clamp or umbilical tape may be applied on the infant's cord about 2 cm from the infant's abdomen, and then the Kelly clamp on the infant's side may be removed.

Figures 17-6 to 17-13 on pp. 502-503 depict the labor and delivery experience of one family.

MANAGEMENT OF THE THIRD AND FOURTH STAGES OF LABOR

Third Stage

Immediately after the delivery, the clinician palpates the uterus for placental separation. As discussed in Chapter 16, the following signs suggest placental separation:

1. The uterus rises upward in the abdomen because the placenta settles downward into the lower uterine segment.
2. As the placenta proceeds downward, the umbilical cord lengthens.
3. A sudden trickle or spurt of blood appears.
4. The uterus changes from a discoid to a globular shape.

While waiting for these signs, the nurse palpates the uterus to check for ballooning of the uterus caused by uterine relaxation and subsequent bleeding into the uterine cavity.

After the placenta has separated, the mother may be asked to bear down to facilitate delivery of the placenta. As discussed on p. 501, oxytocics are frequently given at the time of the delivery of the placenta. Methylergonovine maleate (Methergine) 0.2 mg may be given intravenously along with oxytocin (Pitocin), 10 units intramuscularly. The nurse assesses and records maternal blood pressure before and after administration of oxytocics. The medications used vary with different clinicians. It is the nurse's responsibility to clearly understand and carry out the orders of the clinician and to record all medications on the delivery room record.

After the delivery of the placenta, the clinician inspects the placental membranes to make sure they are intact and that all cotyledons are present. This inspection is especially important with Duncan placentas. If there is a defect or a part missing from the placenta, a digital uterine examination is done. The vagina and cervix are inspected for lacerations, and any necessary repairs are made. The episiotomy may be repaired now if it has not been done previously. The fundus of the uterus is palpated; normal position is at the midline and below the umbilicus. If the fundus is displaced, it may be because of a full bladder or a collection of blood in the uterus. The uterus may be emptied of blood by grasping it anteriorly and posteriorly and squeezing.

The time of delivery of the placenta and the mechanism (Schultze or Duncan) is noted on the delivery record.

The uterine fundus is palpated at frequent intervals to ensure that it remains firmly contracted. The maternal blood pressure is monitored at 5-15 minute intervals to detect any untoward elevation, which may occur because of oxytocic drugs, or any decrease, which may be associated with excessive blood loss.

The patient may be transferred to the recovery room after any active bleeding has subsided, the uterus is firm and well retracted, and maternal blood pressure and pulse are within normal limits.

Use of Oxytocics

Clinicians advocate the use of oxytocic drugs to promote homeostasis through the stimulation of myometrial contractility after delivery. Oxytocin (Pitocin, Syntocinon) is a synthetic product of the posterior pituitary oxytocin hormone. Each ampule of oxytocin contains 10 USP units/ml. The halflife of the compound is three minutes when given intravenously. Oxytocin should not be given by intravenous push in a large bolus because of the danger of maternal hypotension. It may be given intravenously or intramuscularly. Oxytocin may be added to 1000 ml fluid and given intravenously over a period of hours.

The clinician may request that oxytocin (10 units) be given intramuscularly at the time of delivery of the anterior shoulder of the infant; some believe that this facilitates delivery of the placenta. At other times, oxytocin may be administered intramuscularly as the placenta delivers.

Oxytocin also has an antidiuretic effect. If given rapidly in an electrolyte-free solution, water intoxication could occur. Pritchard and MacDonald (1976) advocate the use of a solution that contains electrolytes coupled with an increase of the hormone's concentration rather than merely increasing the intravenous flow rate.

Controlling Postpartal Hemorrhage

Ergonovine (Ergotrate) and methylergonovine (Methergine) are alkaloids derived from lysergic acid from the rye plant fungus. They may be given parenterally or orally and are used to control postpartal hemorrhage. Tetanic contractions are produced, with little tendency toward uterine relaxation. Transient but severe hypertension is a dangerous side effect with these drugs. For this reason they should not be given to mothers with hypertensive problems or to mothers who have received conduction anesthesia (Pritchard and MacDonald, 1976).

Fourth Stage

As soon as the placenta is delivered and the episiotomy or any vaginal lacerations are repaired, the delivery drapes may be removed. The nurse washes the perineum with gauze squares and sterile solution and dries the area with a sterile towel before placing the maternity pads. The legs of the mother are removed from the stirrups at the same time to decrease muscle strain. The mother is transferred to a recovery room bed, and the nurse helps her don a clean gown. The mother may feel cold and begin shivering. She can be covered with a warmed bath blanket, which may be covered by a second blanket. If the mother has not had a chance to hold her infant, she may do so before she is removed from the delivery room. The nurse ensures that the mother and father and newborn are provided with time to begin the attachment process. (See Chapter 28 for further discussion of attachment.)

The mother is transferred to the recovery room, remaining there for a minimum of two hours, and in some institutions she remains until she has voided for the first time. The recovery period requires close observation. The mother's oral temperature is taken once unless it is elevated. Her blood pressure, pulse, respirations, consistency and position of fundus, and amount and character of vaginal flow are checked every 15 minutes for the first hour. Deviations from the normal ranges require more frequent checking. Blood pressure should return to the prelabor level, and pulse rate should be slightly lower than it was in labor. The return of the blood pressure is due to an increased volume of blood returning to the maternal circulation from the uteroplacental shunt. Baroceptors cause a vagal response, which slows the pulse. A rise in the blood pressure may be a response to oxytocic drugs or may be caused by toxemia. Blood loss may be reflected by a lowered blood pressure and a rising pulse rate.

The fundus should be firm at the umbilicus or lower and in the midline. It should be palpated (Figure 17-14) but not massaged unless atonic. If it becomes boggy or appears to rise in the abdomen, the fundus should be massaged until firm; then with one hand supporting the uterus at the symphysis, the nurse should attempt to express retained clots. Overmassaging of the fundus causes an increased tendency toward uterine relaxation due to muscle exhaustion.

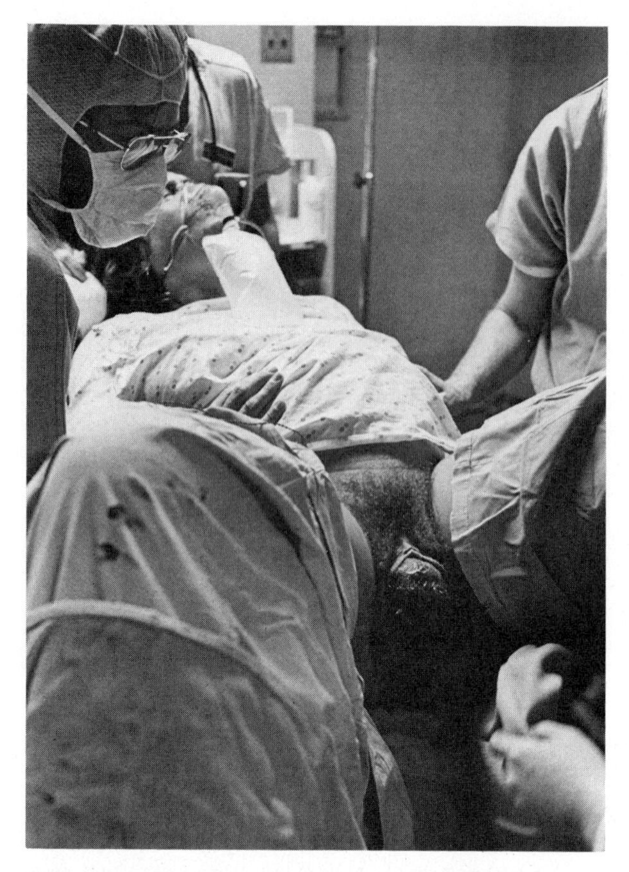

Figure 17–6. The fetal head is crowning. The father is by the mother's side. She is wearing an oxygen mask to facilitate her breathing.

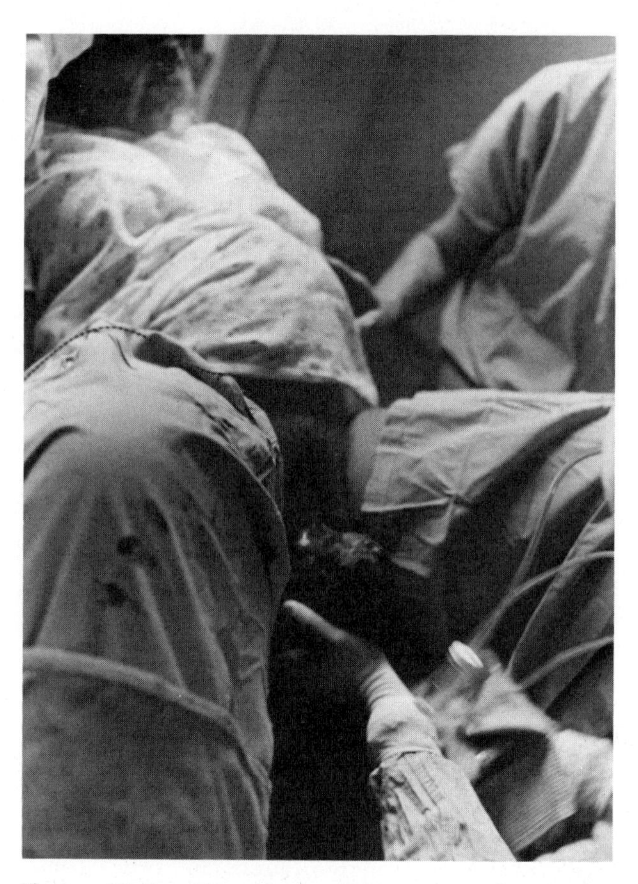

Figure 17–7. Note that the clinician is controlling the delivery of the head by supporting the perineum.

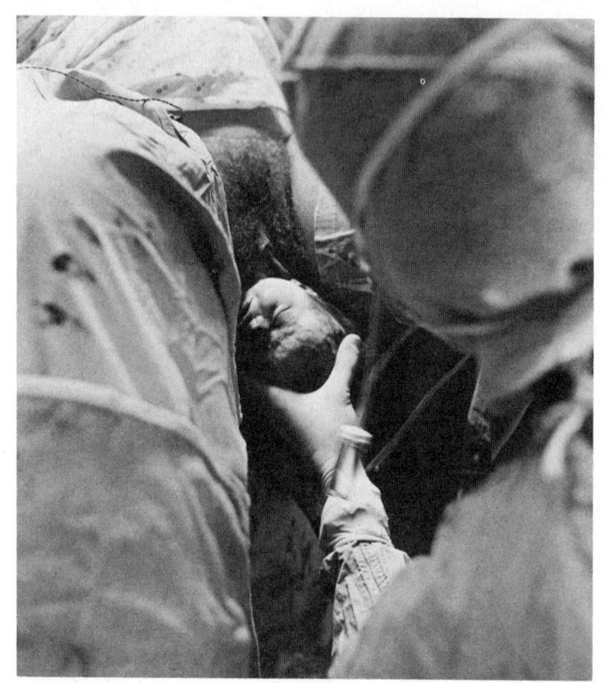

Figure 17–8. The head is delivered.

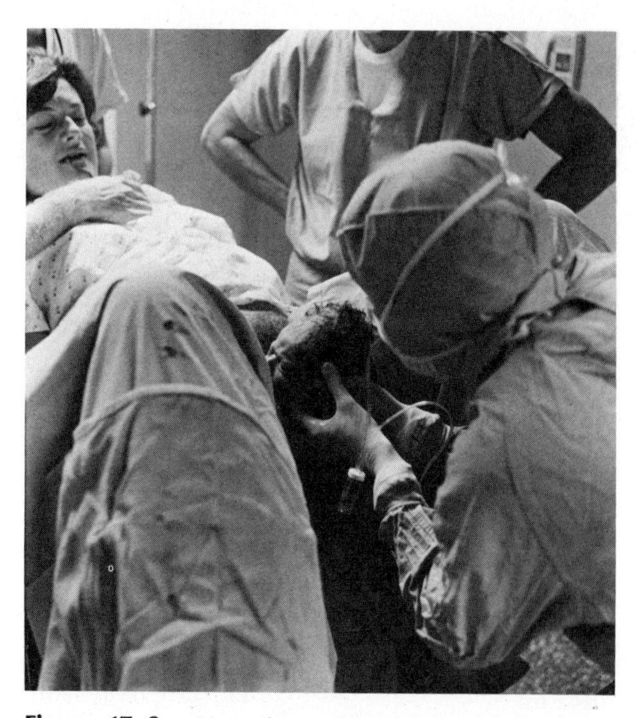

Figure 17–9. Note the molding of the infant's head. Restitution and external rotation has occurred.

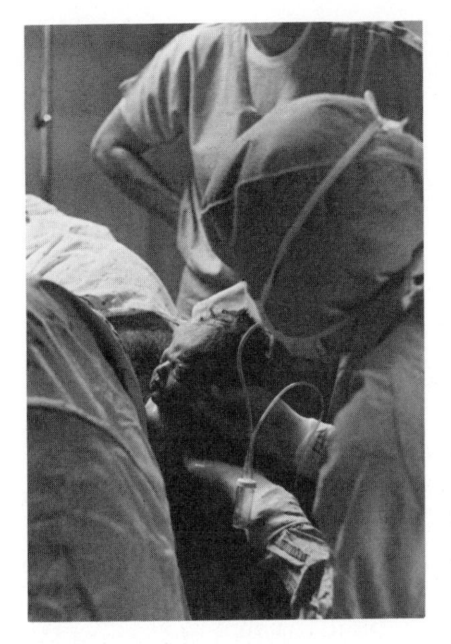

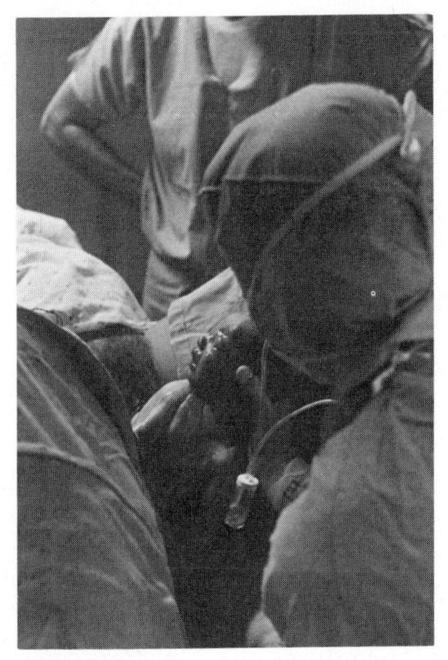

Figure 17–10. Delivery of the baby's shoulders.

Figure 17–11. Delivery of the baby's body.

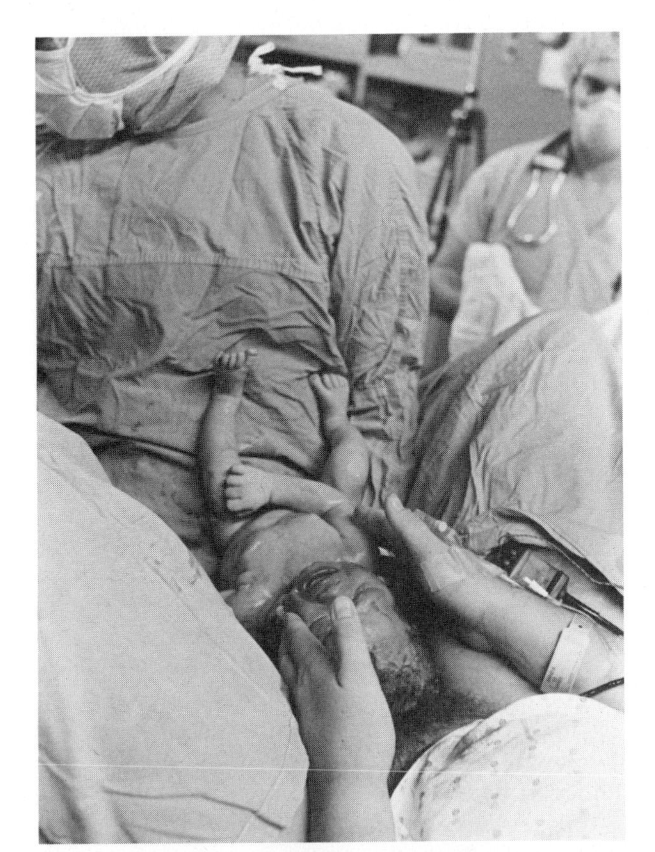

Figure 17–12. The infant rests between his mother's legs. Note that she is able to touch her baby immediately. The infant is held with his head lowered to facilitate drainage and to prevent aspiration of blood, amniotic fluid, and mucus.

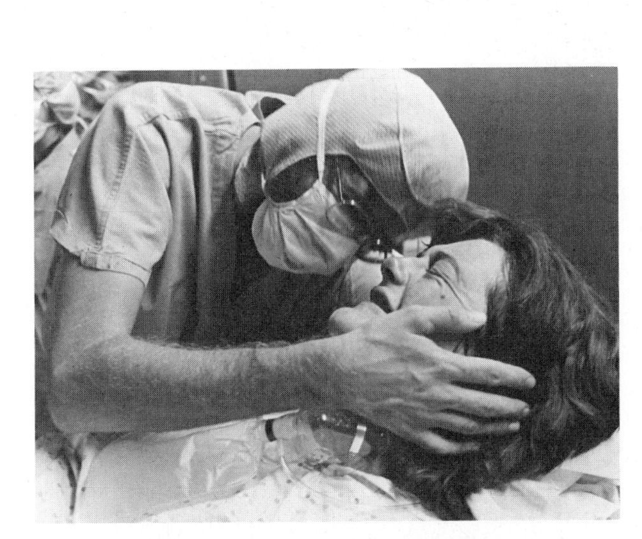

Figure 17–13. The new father and mother.

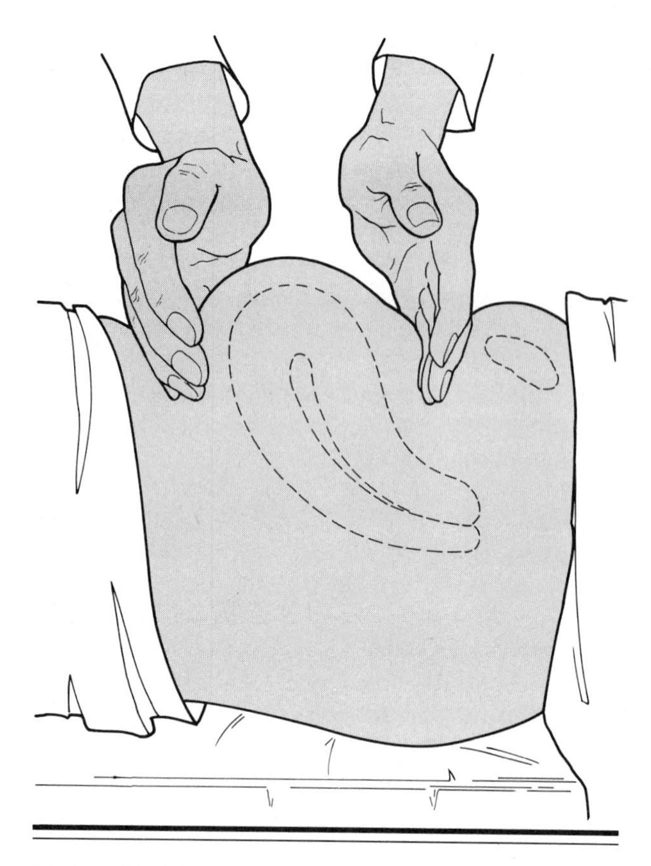

Figure 17–14. Suggested method of palpating the fundus of the uterus during the fourth stage. The left hand is placed just above the symphysis pubis, and gentle downward pressure is exerted. The right hand is cupped around the uterine fundus.

The nurse inspects the bloody vaginal discharge for amount and charts it as minimal, moderate, or heavy and with or without clots. This discharge, or *lochia rubra,* should be bright red. A soaked perineal pad contains approximately 100 ml of blood. If the perineal pad becomes soaked in a 15-minute period or if blood pools under the buttocks, continuous observation is necessary. Laceration of the vagina, cervix, or an unligated vessel in the episiotomy may be indicated by a continuous trickle of blood even though the fundus remains firm.

If the fundus rises and displaces to the right, the nurse palpates the bladder to determine whether it is distended. All measures should be taken to enable the mother to void. If she is unable to void, catheterization is necessary. Postpartal women have decreased sensations to void as a result of the decreased tone of the bladder, enforced by the hormones of pregnancy, and as a result of the trauma imposed on the bladder and urethra during childbirth. The bladder fills rapidly as the body attempts to rid itself of the extra fluid volume returned from the uteroplacental circulation and of intravenous fluid that may have been received during labor and delivery. If the mother is unable to void, a warm towel placed across the lower abdomen or warm water poured over the perineum may help the urinary sphincter to relax and may thus facilitate voiding. A distended bladder can cause uterine atony and postpartal bleeding.

The perineum is inspected for edema and hematoma formation. With episiotomies, an ice pack often reduces swelling and alleviates discomfort.

The following conditions should be reported to the clinician: hypotension, tachycardia, uterine atony, excessive bleeding, or a temperature over 100F or 38C. The nurse should be aware that the blood pressure may not fall rapidly in the presence of dangerous bleeding in postpartal mothers because of the extra systemic volume. A normal blood pressure with the mother in the Fowler position is a good confirmation of a normotensive mother.

Frequently mothers have tremors in the immediate postpartal period. It has been proposed that this shivering response is caused by a difference in internal and external body temperatures (higher temperature inside the body than on the outside). Another theory proposes that the maternal organism is reacting to the fetal cells that have entered the maternal circulation at the placental site. A heated bath blanket placed next to the mother tends to alleviate the problem.

The couple may be tired, hungry, and thirsty. Some hospitals serve the couple a meal. The tired mother will probably drift off into a welcomed sleep. The father should also be encouraged to rest, because his role as one of the mother's major support systems is tiring physically and mentally.

After two hours, if the mother's vital signs are stable with no bleeding, if her bladder is not distended, if her fundus is firm, and if her sensorium is fully reactive from any anesthetic agent that she may have received during delivery, she is usually transferred from the delivery unit to the postpartal floor.

IMMEDIATE CARE OF THE NEWBORN

Preparing to Receive the Newborn

As soon as the infant is delivered, the nurse notes on the delivery room record the time and sex and reports to the couple. If the mother is awake, she can be supported in a position to see the infant. The clinician clears the newborn's airway and then clamps and cuts the cord. At this time the nurse approaches the instrument table and picks up a baby blanket by one corner, taking care not to contaminate the instrument table. The blanket is unfolded and draped over the nurse's arms and chest, again taking care not to contaminate the inner surface of the blanket. The clinician places the newborn on the blanket that covers the nurse's outstretched arms. The bulb syringe and any equipment that may be needed if the umbilical cord needs further attention are also handed to the nurse. As soon as the newborn is received, the nurse folds him toward her chest to maintain a secure hold and holds one leg through the blanket. The infant is then placed in the radiant-heated unit and dried immediately. After drying, he is placed on a clean, dry blanket and allowed to be exposed to the radiant heat. Radiant heat warms the outer surface of objects; thus if the newborn is wrapped in blankets, the outer surface of the blanket is warmed instead of the infant's skin.

The newborn is placed in modified Trendelenburg position to facilitate drainage of mucus from the nasopharynx and trachea by gravity.

Apgar Scoring System

The Apgar scoring system (Table 17–3) was designed in 1952 by Dr. Virginia Apgar, an anesthesiologist. The purpose of this system is to evaluate the physical condition of the infant at birth and the immediate need for resuscitation. The newborn is rated one minute after birth and again at five minutes and receives a total score ranging from 0 to 10 based on the following criteria:

1. The *heart rate* is auscultated or palpated at the junction of the umbilical cord and skin. This is the most important assessment. A newborn heart rate of less than 100 beats/min indicates the need for immediate resuscitation.

2. The *respiratory effort* is the second most important Apgar assessment. Complete absence of respirations is termed *apnea.* A vigorous cry is indicative of good respirations.

3. The *muscle tone* is determined by evaluating the degree of flexion and resistance to straightening of the extremities. A normal infant demonstrates flexion of the elbows and the hips, with the knees positioned up toward the abdomen.

4. The *reflex irritability* is evaluated by flicking the soles of the feet. A cry merits a full score of 2. A grimace is 1 point, and no response is 0.

5. The *color* is inspected for cyanosis and pallor. Generally, infants have blue extremities, and the rest of the body is pink, which merits a score of 1. This condition is termed *acrocyanosis* and is present in 85% of normal newborns at one minute after birth. A completely pink infant scores a 2 and a totally cyanotic, pale infant is scored 0.

A score of 7–10 indicates an infant in good condition who requires only nasopharyngeal suctioning (Figure (17–15).

Table 17–3. The Apgar Scoring System*

	Score		
Sign	**0**	**1**	**2**
Heart rate	Absent	Slow—below 100	Above 100
Respiratory effort	Absent	Slow—irregular	Good crying
Muscle tone	Flaccid	Some flexion of extremities	Active motion
Reflex irritability	None	Grimace	Vigorous cry
Color	Pale blue	Body pink, blue extremities	Completely pink

*From Apgar, V. Aug. 1966. The newborn (Apgar) scoring system, reflections and advice. *Pediatr. Clin. N. Am.* 13:645.

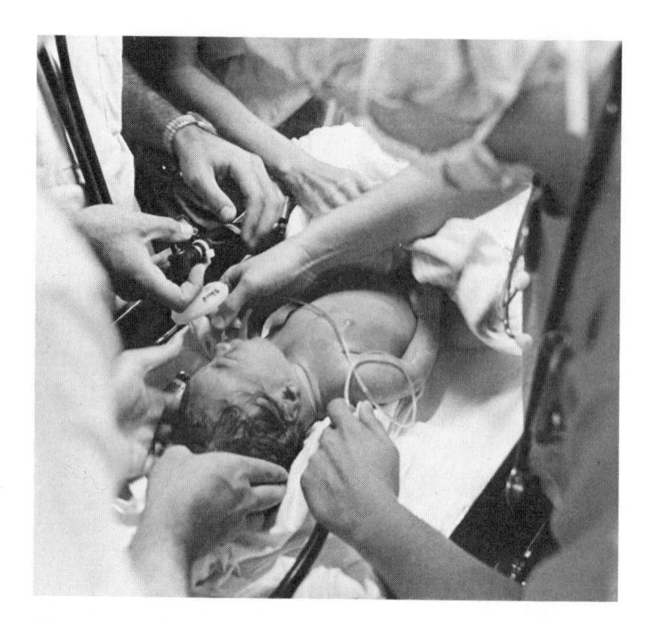

Figure 17–15. Nasopharyngeal suctioning.

A score of 3–6 indicates a moderately depressed infant. Such infants may have a normal heart rate but are cyanotic or pale, dyspneic, and limp. Respirations are irregular and shallow and there is some reflex irritability. The larynx should be examined with a laryngoscope, and endotracheal suctioning should be performed to remove blood, meconium, vernix, and mucus. An airway should then be inserted and the infant bagged with 100% oxygen. If there is no response after one minute or if the heart rate falls below 100 beats/min, the infant is intubated.

An Apgar score of 0–2 indicates a severely depressed infant. Such infants are blue and limp with no reflex irritability and have a heart rate less than 100 beats/min. Immediate intubation and suctioning is required. The nurse attaches oxygen to the endotracheal tube and breathes for the neonate at a rate of 50 times/min. Positive pressures should be maintained at 25 to 40 mm Hg. Greater pressures may produce a pneumothorax. With continued absence of the heart rate after three or four insufflations, external cardiac massage is begun at the rate of 120 beats/min. The sternum is depressed with the index and middle fingers about 1 inch three to four times, alternating with a breath of oxygen (Korones, 1976; Pritchard and MacDonald, 1976). (See Chapter 24 for more detailed information on newborn resuscitation.)

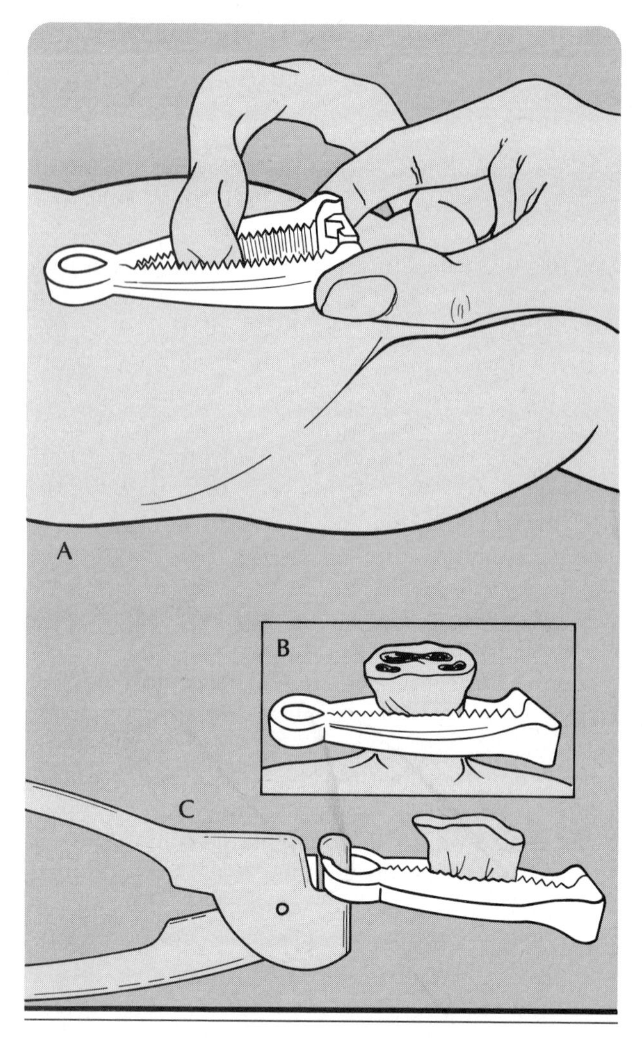

Figure 17–16. Hollister cord clamp. **A,** Clamp is positioned ½ to 1 inch from the abdomen and then secured. **B,** Cut cord. **C,** Plastic device for removing clamp after cord has dried.

Care of the Umbilical Cord

If the clinician has not placed a cord clamp (Hollister or Hesseltine, Figures 17–16 and 17–17) on the newborn's umbilical cord, it becomes the responsibility of the nurse to do so. Before applying the cord clamp, the nurse should examine the cut end for the presence of two arteries and one vein. The umbilical vein is the largest vessel, and the arteries are seen as smaller vessels. The number of vessels must be recorded on the delivery room and newborn records. The cord is clamped approximately ½–1 inch from the abdomen to allow room between the abdomen and clamp as the cord dries. The clamp must not catch any abdomi-

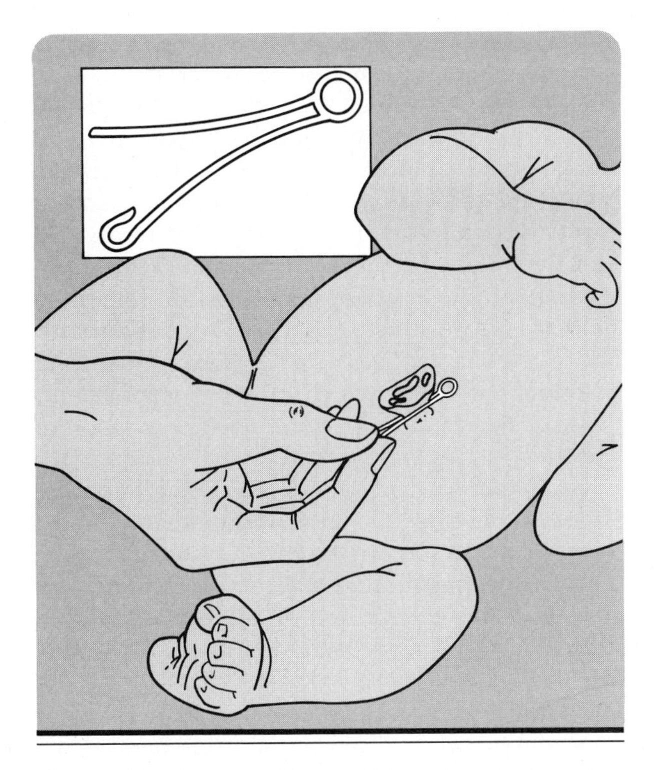

Figure 17-17. Hesseltine cord clamp is applied in a similar manner. When the cord has dried, the clamp may be removed manually.

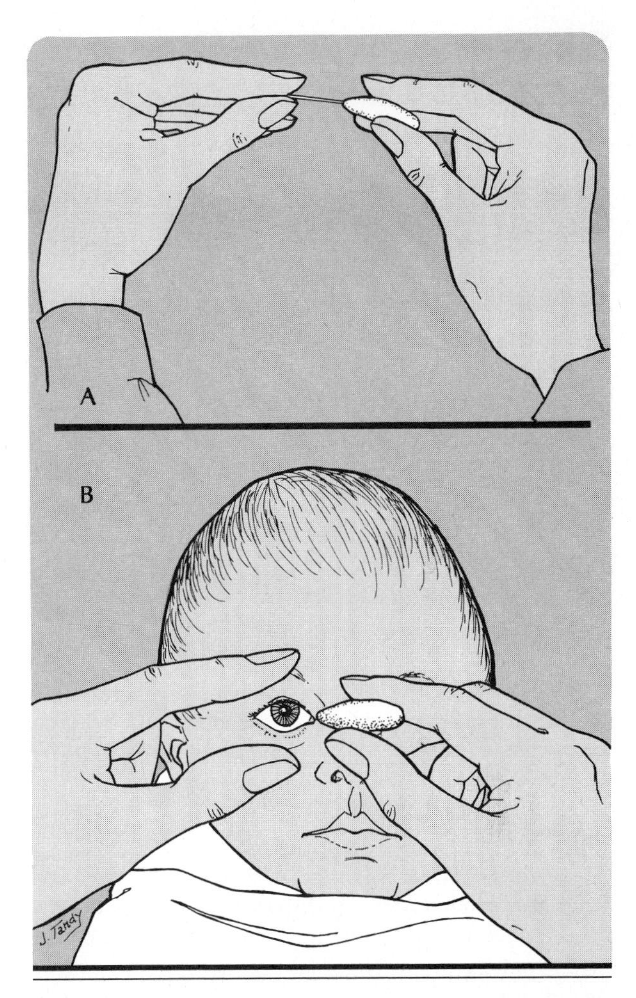

Figure 17-18. Silver nitrate instillation. **A,** Wax container is punctured with a needle. **B,** One or two drops of 1% silver nitrate solution are instilled in the lower conjunctival sac.

nal skin as this will cause necrosis of the tissue. The clamps are removed in the newborn nursery approximately 24 hours after the cord has dried.

Care of the Eyes

The newborn's eyes may become infected during the birth process if gonococci are present in the birth canal. Proper eye care can prevent infection. Therefore, it is a legal requirement for all newborns to have eye treatment. A 1% solution of silver nitrate or ophthalmic antibiotic ointment such as Ilotycin (erythromycin) are currently in use (Figure 17-18). To instill 1% silver nitrate, the nurse punctures the wax container of 1% silver nitrate with a sterile needle, pulls down the infant's lower eyelid, and administers one or two drops in the lower conjunctival sac. The eye is closed to spread the medication. The other eye is treated in the same manner. Controversy exists as to the value of flushing the eye with sterile water following the instillation of the silver nitrate.

The instillation of the ophthalmic ointment is accomplished by pulling down the lower lid and instilling the ointment along the lower lid, starting at the inner canthus. This procedure is repeated on the second eye. In some hospitals, it is the practice to instill the ophthalmic ointment just prior to removing the newborn to the nursery or after admission to the newborn nursery so that there can be maximal eye contact as the mother and father hold the newborn in the delivery room.

Physical Assessment of the Newborn by the Delivery Room Nurse

An abbreviated systematic physical assessment is performed by the nurse in the delivery room to detect any abnormalities (Figure 17-19). First, the size of the infant and the contour and size of the

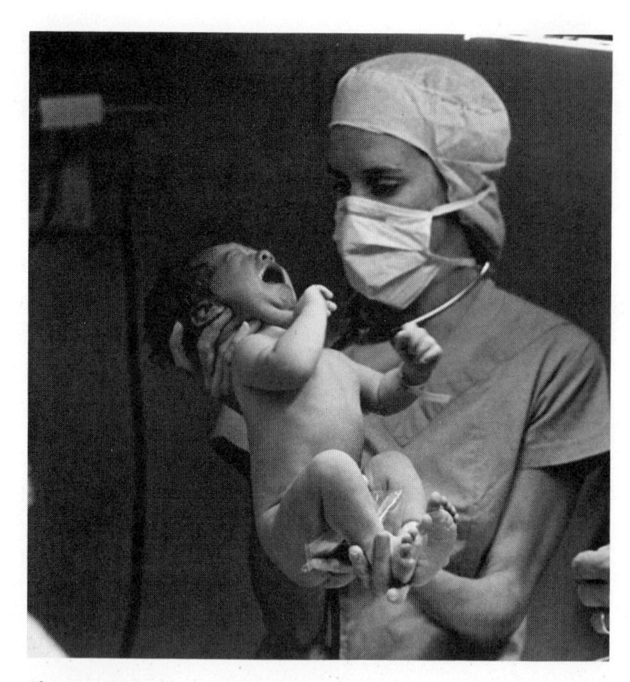

Figure 17–19. The delivery room nurse assesses the newborn. Notice the urine bag on the infant. (In most institutions, a urine collection is not done in the delivery room.)

head in relationship to the rest of the body are noted. The infant's posture and movements indicate tone and neurologic functioning. A flaccid or flexed upper extremity could mean a brachial plexus palsy.

The skin is inspected for discoloration, presence of vernix caseosa and lanugo, and evidence of trauma and desquamation. Vernix caseosa is a white, cheesy substance found normally on newborns. It is absorbed within 24 hours after delivery. Vernix is present in abundance on preterm infants and not at all on postterm infants. A large quantity of fine hair (lanugo) is often seen on preterm infants, especially on their shoulders, foreheads, back, and cheeks. Desquamation of the skin is seen in postterm infants.

Facial symmetry should be inspected. A one-sided cry may mean facial paralysis. A wide-eyed stare by an agitated infant is a sign of intrauterine hypoxia.

The chest is inspected for retraction, grunting, or stridor, and the respiratory rate is counted before the infant is disturbed. A normal rate is 30–40 respirations/min.

The fontanelles and cranial sutures are palpated, and the fontanelles are measured if they appear excessively large. The widest point of the anterior fontanelle should be no greater than 5 cm. The posterior fontanelle should be no greater than 1 cm. Any molding or caput succedaneum is noted. The hair is felt for texture. The eyes are gently opened and inspected for the presence and clarity of pupils. The nose is inspected for flaring, and the nares are checked for patency by introducing a catheter in each nostril. The mouth is palpated for intactness of the soft and hard palate, and the gums are inspected for the presence of membranous teeth, which must be removed because of the danger of aspiration. The location of the ears is checked by laying the finger at the edge of the eye and drawing an imaginary line back to the ears. The pinna should be located above the line. Ears set below the line are associated with congenital mental retardation and kidney problems. The pinna of the ears should be folded forward. They will stay folded or slowly return back in preterm infants.

The infant's neck is palpated bilaterally for size and presence of webbing. The clavicles are then palpated for intactness. Sometimes fractures occur in difficult deliveries. The breast tissue is measured for thickness, and any discharge is noted. Breast tissue that is 7 mm thick is seen in infants over 39 weeks' gestation. About 4 mm is found in infants who are of 37–38 weeks' gestation and 2 mm in infants of less than 36 weeks' gestation. Any supernumerary nipples are noted.

The heart is auscultated for murmurs. About 90% of newborn murmurs are transient. The lungs are auscultated bilaterally for breath sounds. Absence of breath sounds on one side could mean a pneumothorax. Rales may be heard immediately after birth because of the presence of a small amount of fluid in the lungs, which will be absorbed. Ronchi indicate aspiration of oral secretions.

The infant's abdomen is inspected for shape, size, contour, and abnormal pulsations. A pulsation around the epigastrium could indicate an enlarged heart. Distention could be a sign of congenital malformation. Localized flank enlargement is seen with enlarged kidneys. The edge of the liver is normally palpable below the right costal margin, and the tip of the spleen may also be palpated. The lower pole of each kidney may be felt abdominally 1 or 2 cm above the umbilicus. Anything below this level is enlargement. Distention of the bladder that occurs with obstructions may be palpated in the suprapubic region.

The genitals are inspected for sex verification, and any ambiguity is noted. Full rugation on the male scrotum indicates 39 weeks' gestation or more. Intermediate rugation is seen from 37 to 38 weeks. The scrotum is palpated for descended testes. Preterm infants may have testes located in the inguinal canal. In female infants, the clitoris is inspected for enlargement. Sometimes an enlarged clitoris may resemble a penis. The labia minora of preterm infants are more prominent than the labia majora.

The anus is inspected for patency. If the infant passes meconium or voids while in the delivery room, this is recorded on the delivery record and reported to the newborn nursery staff, because they are concerned about the first voiding and defecation, which indicate normal system functioning.

The upper and lower extremities are inspected for the correct number of digits. Long fingernails are seen in the postterm infant. To check for "hip click," which occurs with congenitally dislocated hips, the nurse flexes the legs at the knees and rotates them laterally. The soles of the feet are examined for creases. On infants who are 39 weeks of gestational age or more, the creases cover the entire foot. Creases on the anterior two-thirds of the feet are seen in infants who are 37–38 weeks' gestation. In infants less than 36 weeks, a single anterior transverse crease is found (Korones, 1976; Pritchard and MacDonald, 1976).

This brief examination reveals any gross abnormalities and permits a quick determination of gestational age. Most of this examination is accomplished by visual assessment. Further neurologic assessment and an in-depth physical examination are performed in the newborn nursery (see Chapter 22).

After physiologic homeostatic patterns are established, the newborn is weighed and measured in the newborn nursery.

Newborn Identification Procedures

To assure that the parents are given the correct newborn, the mother and baby are tagged with identical bands or bracelets before the newborn is separated from the mother. One bracelet is applied to the mother's wrist, and two bracelets are applied to the newborn—one on each wrist, one on a wrist and one on an ankle, or one on each ankle. The bands must be applied snugly to prevent loss.

Most hospitals footprint the baby and fingerprint the mother for further identification purposes. When preparing to footprint the newborn, the nurse wipes the soles of both the infant's feet to remove any vernix caseosa, which interferes with the placement of ink on the foot creases.

See the accompanying Nursing Care Plan on the immediate care of the newborn.

NURSING CARE PLAN

Immediate Care of Newborn

Patient Data Base

History

Maternal prenatal history

Fetal status in utero (FHR, presence of meconium, hyperactivity)

Progress of labor and status of membranes

Type of delivery (spontaneous, forceps, etc.)

Physical examination

Estimation of infant's status utilizing the Apgar scoring system at 1 and 5 min (score of 7–10: respirations present, cry strong, heart rate over 100, reflexes present, muscle tone good, and color dusky to pink)

Examination of cord for number of vessels, any hemorrhagic areas, and length

Complete short physical examination (see Neonatal Physical Assessment Guide, Chapter 22 for complete exam)

1. Sex of infant determined
2. No observable congenital anomalies

Nursing Priorities

1. Establish a clear airway and adequate respiratory and cardiac effort.

NURSING CARE PLAN Cont'd

Immediate Care of Newborn

2. Stabilize temperature.
3. Prevent infection.
4. Identify newborn.
5. Facilitate parent-newborn bonding.

Problem	Nursing interventions and actions	Rationale
Apgar assessment	Record time of delivery of infant and position.	Apgar score indicates need for possible resuscitative efforts.
	Determine and record Apgar score for infant at 1 and 5 min after birth.	
	Gently suction nose and mouth with bulb syringe. If respirations are depressed, suction with a Defee catheter.	Vagus nerve runs behind throat. Vigorous suctioning can cause vagal stimulation, which leads to bradycardia.
	Place infant in modified Trendelenburg position (lateral position).	Assists in gravity drainage of mucus.
	Administer O_2 by marks at 4-7 liters/min if marked pallor or cyanosis is present.	Supports respirations.
	Provide tactile stimulation. Institute appropriate resuscitative efforts as needed (Chapter 24).	
Temperature maintenance	Dry newborn thoroughly and place infant uncovered under radiant heat.	Radiant heat works most efficiently on a dry surface. Newborn remains naked so that radiant heat warms his skin surface.
Infection control	Administer 1% silver nitrate solution in drops or place antibiotic ointment in newborn's eyes.	Prevents ophthalmia neonatorum.
	Place clamp on umbilical cord using aseptic technique.	Clamping cord also prevents bleeding. Aseptic technique reduces chance of infection.
Identification	Apply two bracelets to infant (both wrists, both ankles, or one of each). Note: Newborn loses 5%-10% of birth weight, so bracelets must be snug.	
Congenital abnormalities	Assess for presence of malformations. Observe and record number of vessels in cord.	One artery in the umbilical cord is associated with genitourinary abnormalities.
Bonding	Allow mother and father to hold the newborn as soon as possible.	Facilitates formation of relationship between parents and child.

Nursing Care Evaluation

Infant is delivered without undue trauma.

Adequate respiratory effort is established.

Neutral thermoregulation is provided.

Measures to prevent infection are instituted.

Identification of the newborn is accomplished.

Attachment process is facilitated.

Any congenital abnormalities are noted.

FACILITATION OF ATTACHMENT

Dramatic evidence indicates that a sensitive period for attachment of mother and infant exists in the first few hours and even minutes after birth (Kennell, 1974). Separation during this critical period not only delays attachment but also affects maternal and child behavior over a much longer

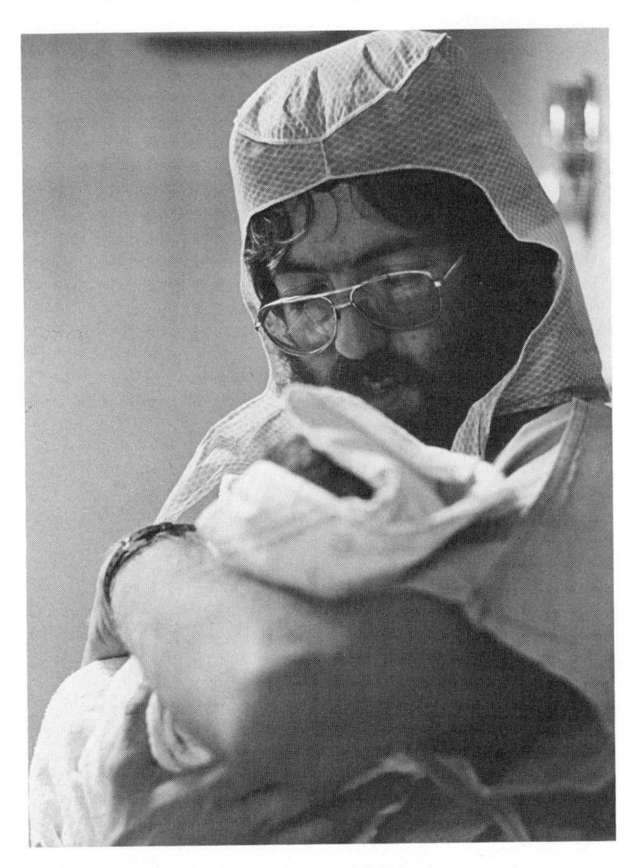

Figure 17–20. The father holds his son.

period. At one month and one year after childbirth, mothers who were merely shown their infants after delivery and had them only briefly for 15- to 20-minute feeding periods demonstrated less eye contact and less soothing behavior during physical examination than did mothers who were allowed to hold their infants for one hour beginning one or two hours after delivery and for five hours on each of three succeeding days. The mothers with this extended contact asked twice as many questions about their children and used fewer commands at two years (Kennell, 1974). The results of this and other research indicate that as soon as feasible the newborn needs to be united with his parents.

The infant can be placed in direct skin contact with the mother soon after delivery and covered with a warm blanket so that no heat loss occurs. Breast-feeding may begin on the delivery table and is encouraged because of the natural release of oxytocin stimulated by sucking. Oxytocin causes uterine contractions, which prevent post-delivery hemorrhage. Even if the infant does not actively nurse, he can lick, taste, and smell the mother's skin, which stimulates the release of milk (referred to as the *letdown reflex*). This physical contact also serves to acquaint the infant and his mother. The father may also hold his child and is given time to get acquainted with the infant (Figure 17–20). The nurse praises the couple for their accomplishment, helps them to become comfortable with the infant, and listens to their expressions of elation or disappointment.

SUMMARY

Labor and delivery can be a time of anxious or eager anticipation. The nurse must remember that the care she renders to the patient and family at this time has an impact not only on the patient's feelings about and reactions to this labor and delivery but also on future childbearing plans and expectations.

The nurse must be adept at intrapartal assessment; must be cognizant of the physiologic changes that are occurring and the wide range of emotional reactions to labor and delivery; and must incorporate these into her plan of care for meeting the needs of the childbearing couple.

The first hour after delivery is critical for both mother and infant from both a physiologic and psychologic viewpoint, and it demands continued knowledgeable and caring nursing management.

SUGGESTED ACTIVITIES

1. A neighbor calls to tell you she is having contractions every five minutes and that she has bloody mucus mixed with green fluid. How would you advise her?
2. While observing a delivery, assign your own Apgar score to the infant, identifying the factors that influenced your score.
3. During observation of a labor and delivery, identify the factors that promote or hinder the parent-infant attachment process. What could the nurse do to promote healthy bonding attitudes throughout the labor and delivery process?

REFERENCES

Apgar, V. Aug. 1966. The newborn (Apgar) scoring system: reflections and advice. *Pediatr. Clin. N. Am.* 13:645.

Burrow, G. N., and Ferris, T. 1975. *Medical complications during pregnancy.* Philadelphia: W. B. Saunders Co.

Kennell, J. 1974. Evidence for a sensitive period in the human mother. In *Maternal attachment and mothering disorders: a round table,* ed. M. Klaus et al. Sausalito, Calif.: Johnson & Johnson Baby Products.

Korones, S. 1976. *High risk newborn infants: the basis for intensive nursing care.* 2nd ed. St. Louis: The C. V. Mosby Co.

Pritchard, J., and MacDonald, P. C. 1976. *Williams obstetrics.* 15th ed. New York: Appleton-Century-Crofts.

Roberts, J. E. 1973. Suctioning the newborn. *Nursing* 73:63.

ADDITIONAL READINGS

Aladjem, S., and Brown, A. K. 1974. *Clinical perinatology.* St. Louis: The C. V. Mosby Co.

Assali, N. S. 1968. *Biology of gestation.* Vol. 1. New York: Academic Press, Inc.

Bonica, J. J. 1960. *Mechanisms and pathways of pain in labor.* Chicago: Abbott Laboratories.

Bonica, J. J. 1967. *Principles and practice of obstetric analgesia and anesthesia.* Philadelphia: F. A. Davis Co.

Brown, M. S. Oct. 1976. A cross-cultural look at pregnancy, labor, and delivery. *J. Obstet. Gynecol. Neonatal Nurs.* 5:35.

Clark, A. L. 1975. Labor and birth expectations and outcomes. *Nurs. Forum.* 14:77.

Cogan, R. 1975. Comfort during prepared childbirth as a function of parity reported by four classes of participant observers. *J. Psychosom. Res.* 19:33.

Colman, A. D., and Colman, L. L. 1971. *Pregnancy: the psychological experience.* New York: Herder & Herder.

Dick-Read, G. 1972. *Childbirth without fear.* 4th ed. New York: Harper & Row Publishers, Inc.

Duignan, N. M., et al. 1975. Characteristics of normal labour in different racial groups. *Br. J. Obstet. Gynecol.* 82(8):593.

Erkkola, R., and Rauramo, L. 1976. Correlation of maternal physical fitness during pregnancy with maternal and fetal pH and lactic acid at delivery. *Acta Obstet. Gynecol. Scand.* 55:441.

Friedman, E. A. 1967. *Labor: clinical evaluation and management.* New York: Appleton-Century-Crofts.

Friedman, E. A. July 1970. An objective method of evaluating labor. *Hosp. Pract.* 5:82.

Greenhill, J. P., and Friedman, E. A. 1974. *Biological principles and modern practice of obstetrics.* Philadelphia: W. B. Saunders Co.

Henneborn, W. J., and Cogan, R. 1975. The effect of husband participation on reported pain and probability of medication during labor and birth. *J. Psychosom. Res.* 19:39.

Huprich, P. July–Aug. 1977. Assisting the couple through a Lamaze labor and delivery. *MCN.* 2:245.

Landry, K. E., and Kilpatrick, D. M. May–June 1977. Why shave a mother before she gives birth? *MCN.* 2:189.

Leonard, L. Feb. 1977. The father's side: a different perspective on childbirth. *Can. Nurse.* 73:16.

McCaffery, M. 1972. *Nursing management of the patient with pain.* Philadelphia: J. B. Lippincott Co.

Myles, M. F. 1975. *Textbook for midwives.* Edinburgh: Churchill Livingstone.

Newton, N., and Newton, M. 1972. Childbirth in cross-cultural perspective. In *Modern perspectives in psycho-obstetrics,* ed. J. G. Howells. New York: Brunner/Mazel.

Oxorn, H., and Foote, W. R. 1975. *Human labor and birth.* New York: Appleton-Century-Crofts.

Weekes, A. R. L., and Flynn, M. J. 1975. Engagement of the fetal head in primigravidae and its relationship to duration of gestation and onset of labour. *Br. J. Obstet. Gynecol.* 82:7.

Willson, J. R., et al. 1975. *Obstetrics and gynecology.* 5th ed. St. Louis: The C. V. Mosby Co.

Zax, M., et al. 1975. Childbirth education, maternal attitudes and delivery. *Am. J. Obstet. Gynecol.* 123:185.

CHAPTER 18

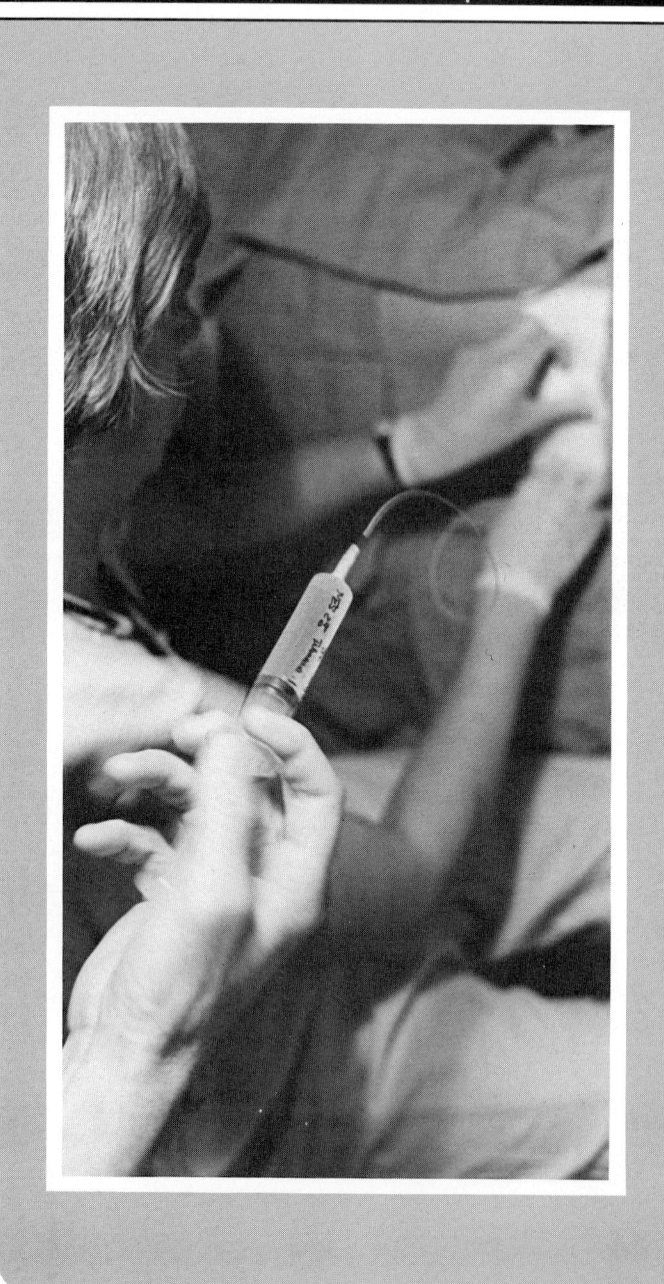

PAIN RELIEF AND OBSTETRIC ANESTHESIA

THEORIES OF PAIN

PAIN DURING LABOR

Factors Influencing Perception of Pain

Methods of Pain Relief During Labor

Nursing Management of Pain Relief

OBSTETRIC ANESTHESIA

General Anesthesia

Regional Analgesia and Anesthesia

OBJECTIVES

- Define pain.
- Compare the specificity theory, the pattern theory, and the gate control theory of pain.
- Discuss the factors influencing an individual's perception of pain.
- Describe the use of systemic drugs to promote pain relief during labor.
- Relate psychologic preparation for childbirth to the relief of pain during labor.
- Identify appropriate nursing interventions that may be used to promote the relief of pain during labor.
- Briefly describe the major inhalation anesthetics used to provide general anesthesia.
- List the major complications of general anesthesia.
- Identify the advantages and disadvantages of the major types of regional analgesia and anesthesia.
- Discuss the complications of regional anesthesia that may occur.

The management of pain during parturition is an important aspect in the health care of the childbearing woman. The discomfort associated with labor and delivery has been a subject of concern throughout history. A woman's attitude toward childbirth and pain reflects her culture. During the early Greek, Roman, and Egyptian civilizations, the art of assisting women in childbirth was highly developed. Unfortunately, the practices from these cultures were displaced during the Dark Ages by ignorance and superstition.

It was not until the nineteenth century that health care for mothers and babies began to improve. One significant clinical advance was the introduction of anesthetic agents into obstetrics. Ether and chloroform were first used for labor and delivery in Great Britain by Sir James Simpson of the University of Glasgow. An outraged clergy claimed that the pain of childbirth was decreed by God as punishment for the fall from grace in the Garden of Eden. They cited the Bible (Genesis 3:16) as proof that women must suffer: "Unto the woman He said, I will greatly multiply thy sorrow and thy conception; in sorrow thou shalt bring forth children . . ." In his defense of the practice, Simpson also used the Bible (Genesis 2:21) to propose that God used anesthesia for the creation of Eve: "And the Lord God caused a deep sleep to fall upon Adam . . ."

The use of chloroform by Queen Victoria for the birth of her seventh child was the event that finally stopped the controversy and sanctioned the use of anesthetic agents for childbearing. Since that time, many agents and techniques have been introduced. The goal of pain relief in childbirth is alleviation of discomfort in the mother while ensuring the safety of both mother and fetus. To date, no method or agent has been discovered that can meet these criteria. The search for a safe, effective method of pain relief during labor and delivery thus continues in the twentieth century.

THEORIES OF PAIN

Pain is a universal experience but is extremely complex. The word is derived from the Latin word *poena,* the Greek word *poine,* and the old French *peine,* which all mean "a penalty" or "punishment." The ancients thought of pain as something inflicted by the gods on anyone who incurred their displeasure. There is an echo of this attitude in the modern lament about pain: "What have I done that I must suffer this way?" It has been difficult to depart from our cultural view of pain as a penalty.

Many disciplines have attempted to define pain, but each has approached it from a different point of view. The sociologist sees pain or the threat of pain as a powerful instrument of learning and social preservation. A biologist views it as a sensing signal that warns the individual when a harmful stimulus threatens injury. An existentialist philospher regards pain as a phenomenon that unites an individual with the rest of humanity in its existential suffering. To the psychologist, pain is the brain's translation of a signal into a sensory experience.

As early as 1943, Livingston proposed that pain is a subjective, individualized experience modified by one's degree of attention, by one's emotional state, and by one's past experience. Psychologic evidence supports the view of pain as a perceptual experience in which the quality and intensity are affected by past history, the meaning of the experience, and the state of mind of the person experiencing pain. Melzack (1973) believes that all these factors play a part in determining the pattern of the nerve impulses going to the brain and of transmission within the brain. Pain becomes a function of the total individual. This approach is consistent with the nursing profession's view of the patient as a holistic being.

Many theories of pain have evolved during the past century. The traditional theory of pain is known as the *specificity theory.* It proposes that a specific pain system carries messages from pain receptors in the body to a pain center in the brain. However, too many clinical facts do not fit this model of a rigid, closed system. The amount and quality of pain experienced by an individual is modified by psychologic and environmental variables.

The simplest form of response to stimuli is a protective mechanism, the withdrawal reflex that occurs in the sensorimotor arc. For example, when the hand is placed on a hot object, pain fibers

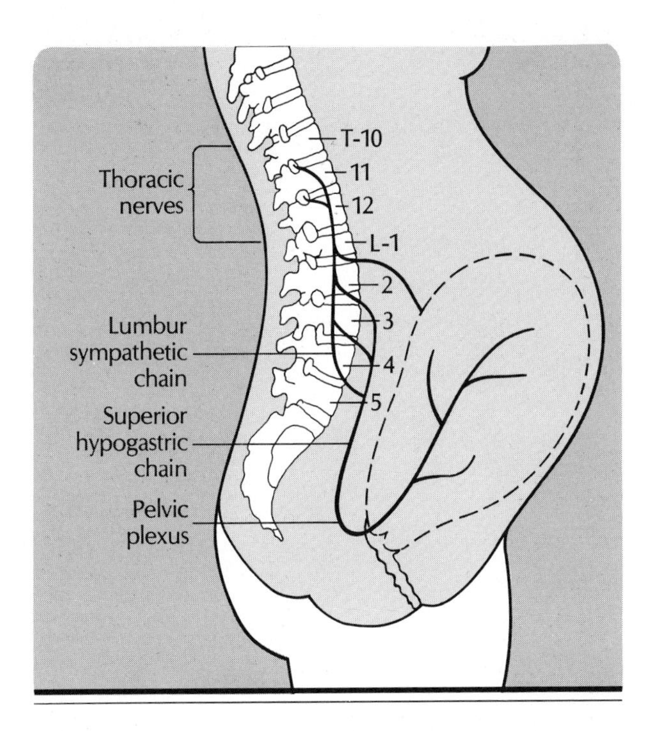

Figure 18–1. Pain pathway from uterus to spinal cord. Nerve impulses travel through the uterine plexus, pelvic plexus, inferior hypogastric plexus, middle and superior hypogastric plexus, and the lumbar sympathetic chain and enter the spinal cord through the 12th, 11th, and 10th thoracic nerves. (Modified from Bonica, J. J. 1972. *Principles and practice of obstetric analgesia and anesthesia.* Philadelphia: F. A. Davis Co., p. 492.)

transmit impulses to the dorsal root of the spinal cord. Each impulse synapses to the ventral root and returns to the local muscles as a motor impulse causing a jerking movement away from the hot object. This reaction occurs before the sensory information is processed by the brain; the hand is lifted before pain is perceived. Even this simple mechanism does not occur in isolation. The individual is thrown off balance by the reflex action, and immediately the entire body moves to restore equilibrium. This is the type of reflex action that occurs during an intramuscular injection—the patient flinches as the skin is penetrated.

The *pattern theory* attempts to incorporate the psychologic aspects of pain left out by the specificity theory. The pattern theory proposes that particular patterns of nerve impulses are produced by the summation of sensory input at the dorsal horn cells. Pain results when the total output of these cells exceeds a critical level as a result of excessive stimulation of receptors or of pathologic conditions that enhance the summation of impulses. The patterns of impulses travel over multiple pathways and go to widespread regions of the brain.

When the mechanisms suggested by the specificity and pattern theories are examined, valuable complementary concepts come to light. The *gate-control theory* proposed by Melzack (1973) has attempted to integrate all aspects of pain into a comprehensive theory. According to this view, pain results from activity in several interacting specialized neural systems.

The gate-control theory proposes that a mechanism in the dorsal horn of the spinal column, probably the substantia gelatinosa, serves as a gate that increases or decreases the flow of nerve impulses from the periphery to the central nervous system. The pain pathway along a single sensory tract is illustrated in Figure 18–1. The gate mechanism is influenced by the size of the transmitting fibers and by the nerve impulses that descend from the brain. Psychologic processes such as past experiences, attention, and emotion may influence pain perception and response by activating the gate mechanism. The gates may be opened or closed by central activities, such as anxiety or excitement, or through selective, localized activity (Melzack, 1973). The gate-control theory has two important implications for obstetrics: Pain may be controlled by tactile stimulation, and pain can be modified by "maximizing central control factors by means of special training in childbirth education, using suggestion, distraction and behavioral conditioning" (Clark and Affonso, 1976).

PAIN DURING LABOR

The pain associated with the first stage of labor is unique in that it accompanies a normal physiologic process. Even though perception of the pain of childbirth is greatly determined by cultural patterning, there is a physiologic basis for discomfort during labor. Pain during the first stage of

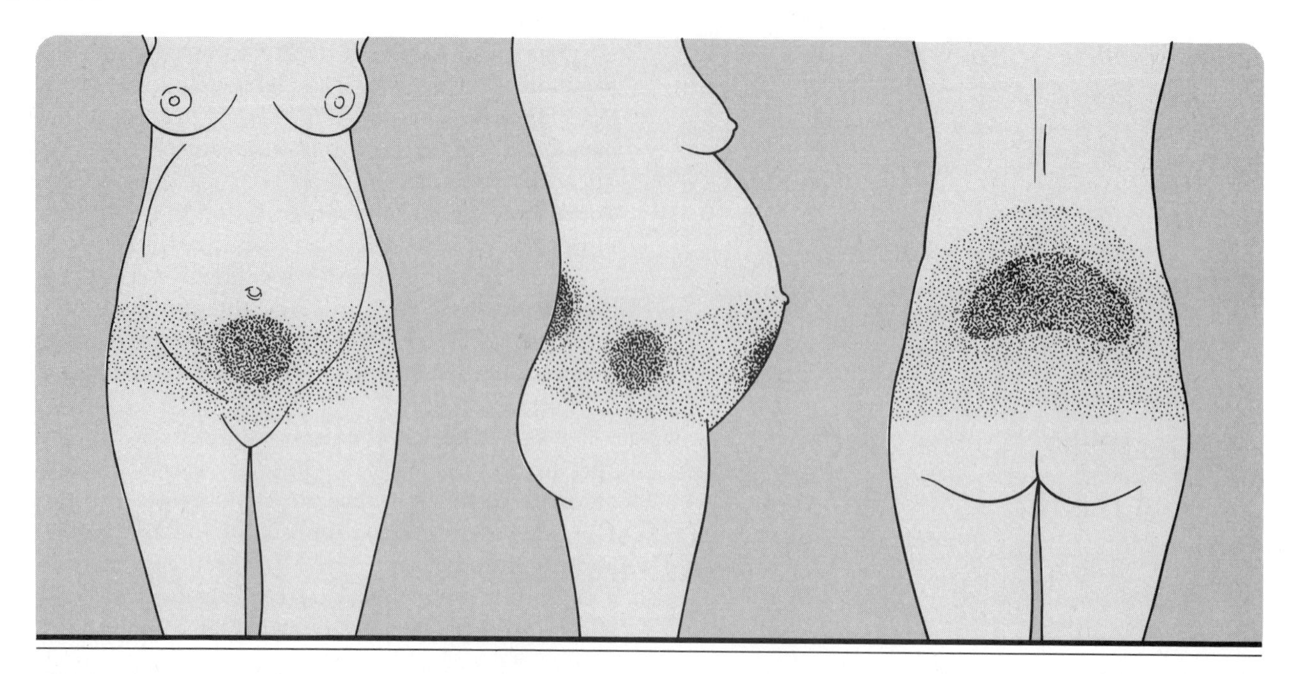

Figure 18–2. Area of reference of labor pain during the first stage. Density of stippling indicates intensity of pain. (From Bonica, J. J. 1972. *Principles and practice of obstetric analgesia and anesthesia.* Philadelphia: F. A. Davis Co., p. 108.)

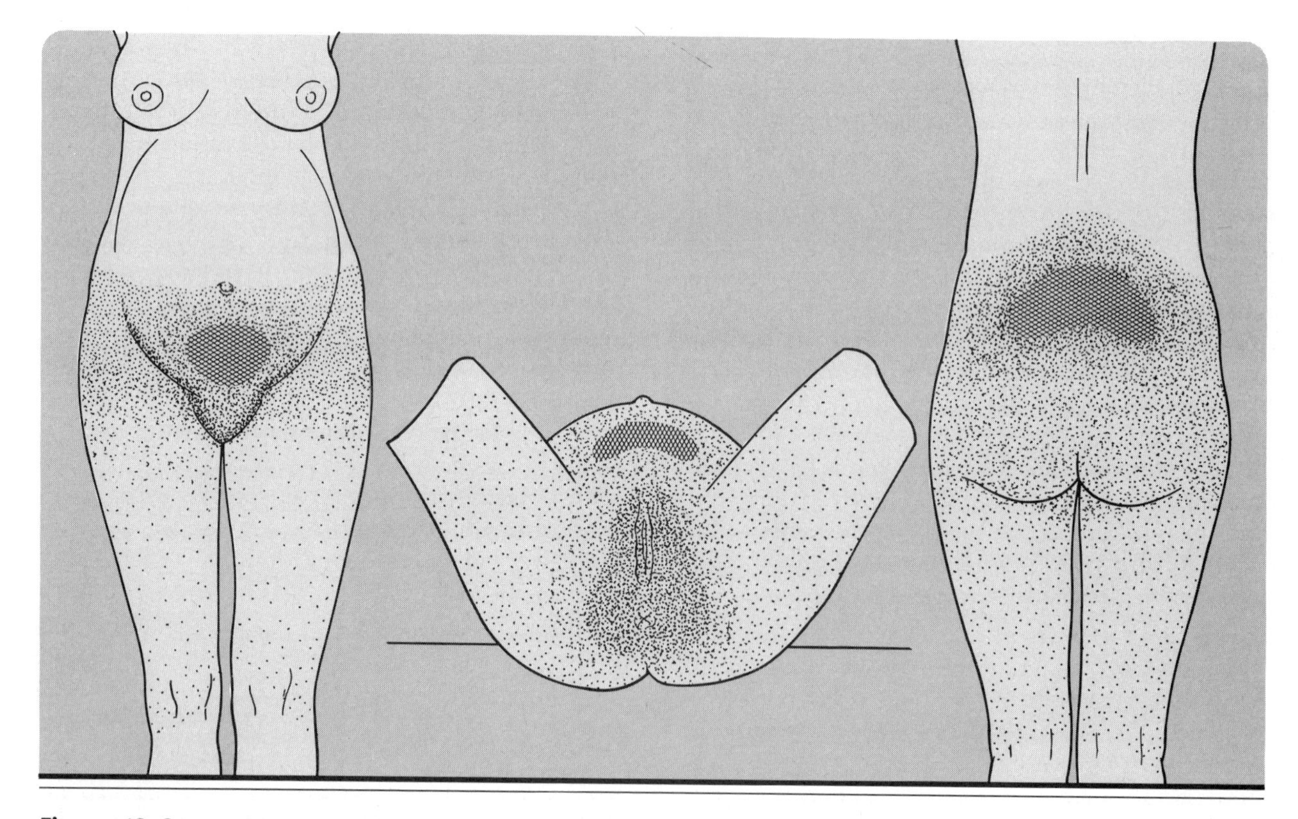

Figure 18–3. Distribution of labor pain during the later phase of the first stage and early phase of the second stage. Cross-hatched areas indicate location of the most intense pain; dense stippling, moderate pain; and light stippling, mild pain. Note that the uterine contractions, which at this stage are very strong, produce intense pain. (From Bonica, J. J. 1972. *Principles and practice of obstetric analgesia and anesthesia.* Philadelphia: F. A. Davis Co., p. 109.)

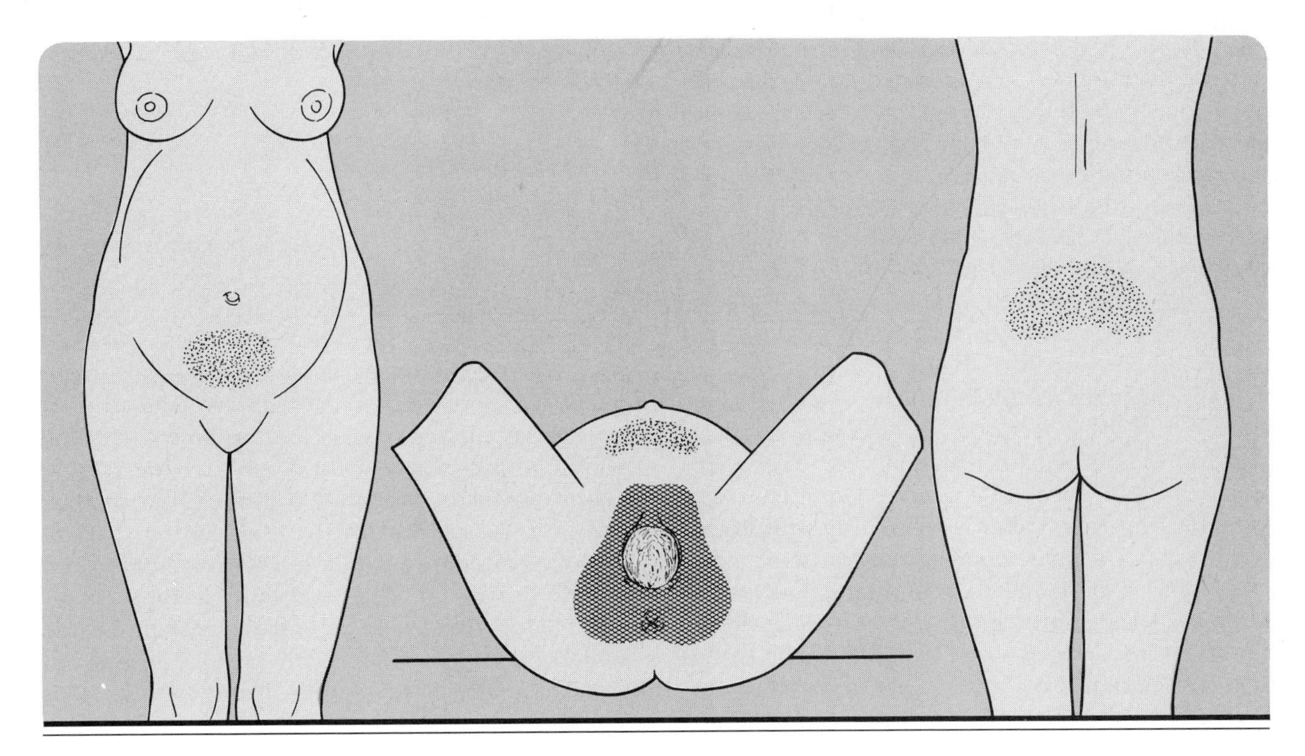

Figure 18–4. Distribution of labor pain during the later phase of the second stage and actual delivery. The perineal component is the primary cause of discomfort. Uterine contractions contribute much less. (From Bonica, J. J. 1972. *Principles and practice of obstetric analgesia and anesthesia.* Philadelphia: F. A. Davis Co., p. 109.)

labor arises from (a) hypoxia of the uterine muscle cells during contraction, (b) stretching of the lower uterine segment, (c) dilatation of the cervix, and (d) pressure on adjacent structures. The primary source of pain is stretching of the cervix. Nerve impulses travel through the uterine plexus, inferior hypogastric (pelvic) plexus, middle hypogastric plexus, superior hypogastric plexus, and the lumbar and lower thoracic chain and enter the spinal cord through the posterior roots of the 10th, 11th, and 12th thoracic nerves. As with other visceral pain, pain from the uterus is referred to the dermatomes supplied by the 10th, 11th, and 12th thoracic nerves. The areas of referred pain include the lower abdominal wall and the areas over the lower lumbar region and the upper sacrum (Figure 18–2).

During the second stage of labor, discomfort is due to (a) hypoxia of the contracting uterine muscle cells, (b) distention of the vagina and perineum, and (c) pressure on adjacent structures. The nerve impulses from the vagina and perineum are transmitted by way of the pudendal nerve plexus and enter the spinal cord through the posterior roots of the 2nd, 3rd, and 4th sacral nerves (Figure 18–3).

Pain during the third stage of labor results from uterine contractions and cervical dilatation as the placenta is expelled (Figure 18–4). The mechanism for the transmission of nerve impulses is the same as for the first stage of labor. This stage of labor is short, and the primary need for anesthesia after this phase of the labor process is for episiotomy repair.

Factors Influencing Perception of Pain

Because pain is a total psychosomatic experience, many factors affect the individual's perception of pain impulses. All human societies have developed patterns of behavior for the maternal role during childbirth. Some psychologic and environmental influences particularly appropriate to labor are discussed here.

Cultural Background

Individuals tend to respond to painful stimuli in the way that is acceptable in their culture. It is important to realize the many varieties of response to pain to assess a patient's need for assistance. The absence of crying and moaning does not necessarily mean that pain is absent, nor does the presence of crying and moaning necessarily mean that pain relief is desired at that moment. Some cultures believe it is natural to communicate the pain experience, no matter how mild. Members of other cultures stoically accept pain out of fear or because it is expected of them. Women of the Chagga tribe in Africa believe the baby will die if they scream during labor, despite the fact that ritual clitoridectomy scars interfere with delivery and increase pain (Raum, 1940).

The attitudes about childbirth of a particular culture may be a factor in the reaction to pain. The San Blas Indians of Panama view childbirth as a shameful event that must be hidden from men and children. Labor is frequently prolonged and so painful that women lose consciousness (Newton, 1964). At the other extreme, the Navajo Indians of the southwestern United States view childbirth as an open social event. All who come to give support are invited to stay and eat (Lockett, 1939). The sensations of labor are not thought of as painful by Navajo women. In fact, the language has two words for labor, one meaning painful labor and the other meaning labor (McCammon, 1951). Acculturation has no doubt modified these attitudes since the original studies were done.

It is interesting to note that in our own culture, there has been a surge of interest in psychoprophylactic preparation and partner participation in childbirth following a liberalized attitude toward sexuality and childbearing.

Fatigue and Sleep Deprivation

Exhaustion may be so great that attention wanders from the physical stimuli of childbirth, or it may have the opposite effect, lowering the powers of resistance and self-control to produce an exaggerated response. Fatigue from sleep deprivation affects an individual's response to pain in several ways. The fatigued person has less energy and a decreased ability to use such usual strategies as distraction or imagination as coping mechanisms in dealing with pain. The fatigued patient may choose a less demanding alternative, such as analgesia (McCaffery, 1972). This is a particularly important factor in laboring patients, because prolonged prodromal labor may interfere with sleep. A woman may begin the active phase of labor in an exhausted state and have difficulty coping with the discomfort of frequent intense contractions.

Personal Significance of Pain

The significance of pain is closely related to the woman's self-concept as well as to cultural expectations. She may view labor as a fearful event, one she has dreaded throughout pregnancy, or she may view it as the happiest event of her life. Pain may be interpreted by some women as punishment for perceived sins, such as engaging in premarital intercourse or feeling ambivalent toward the pregnancy. Others who have had psychoprophylactic preparation for childbirth may consider the pain a test of their ability to cope with a challenging event. If such women do not handle the pain of labor according to their expectations, they tend to experience a sense of failure, which threatens not only their self-concept but also their ability to mother. Consequently, it is vital that childbirth instructors and nurses stress to each woman that the reaction to childbirth is varied and individual. A woman should feel no sense of failure if she requires analgesia to assist her in coping. The primary goal of psychoprophylactic preparation is not totally unmedicated childbirth but a childbirth experience that is satisfying to both father and mother.

Previous Experience

One's previous experience with pain affects one's ability to manage current and future pain. Particularly painful experiences can condition one to expect the same degree of pain in a similar situation. All persons, with very few exceptions, have experienced pain. It appears likely that those who have had more experience with pain are more sensitive to painful stimuli.

Anxiety

Anxiety related to pain must be approached on two levels, that associated with anticipation of pain and that associated with the presence of pain. Studies suggest that a moderate degree of anxiety about impending pain is necessary for the person to handle the pain experience (Janis, 1958). Anxiety during the pain experience should be reduced as much as possible by nursing intervention. Anxiety during labor produces tension, which increases the intensity of the pain.

Anxieties unrelated to the pain can intensify the pain experience. For many young women, the admission to labor and delivery is their first hospitalization. Routine procedures, rules and regulations, equipment, and the general environment are unfamiliar and anxiety-provoking. For many women the spontaneous onset of labor has an element of surprise. Even though the event is expected and even anticipated, few women are totally prepared for the actual onset of labor and hospitalization. Last-minute details must be completed. Arrangements for the care of other children have usually been made but now must actually be carried out. Having to leave young children for a few days is accompanied by varying degrees of anxiety for any mother.

Separation from loved ones is another major source of anxiety. Unfortunately, some institutions throughout the United States do not allow husbands and significant others to be with patients during labor and delivery. One study of postoperative pain revealed that married persons seem to experience less pain than unmarried persons, possibly because of the emotional support given by the spouse (Bruegel, 1971). The implications of this study are not related solely to the married state, because many stable relationships are formed outside the bond of marriage, but to the probability that the presence of the partner decreases anxiety. When anxiety is decreased by the support of a significant person, pain perception is decreased.

Attention and Distraction

Both attention and distraction have an influence on the perception of pain. When pain sensation is the focus of attention, the perceived intensity is greater. Preoccupation with an activity lessens pain perception. The classic example is the football player who is unaware of an injury until the game is over. Only then does he experience painful sensations from the injury.

A sensory stimulus can serve as a distractor because the person's attention is focused on the stimulus rather than the pain, for example, providing a patient with a back rub. Cutaneous sensations are carried by large-diameter afferent fibers, which can inhibit the pain sensation carried by small-diameter fibers. This is a component of the gate-control theory of pain. Cutaneous stimulation to relieve pain may also be explained by the theory of extinction or perceptual dominance. It is possible that sensory input may extinguish pain or raise its threshold.

Methods of Pain Relief During Labor

The reduction or relief of pain during labor is achieved by several different methods, including (a) systemic drugs, (b) regional nerve blocks, and (c) psychoprophylactic methods. This classification provides a convenient framework for exploring various alternatives for pain relief.

No method is mutually exclusive. The agents used for regional nerve blocks may enter general circulation and cause unwanted side effects. Systemic drugs such as meperidine (Demerol) or diazepam (Valium) may assist the tense psychoprophylactically prepared woman to regain control and to progress to a satisfying childbirth experience. Regional nerve blocks with analgesic doses of anesthetic agents administered during the course of labor are not incompatible with the goals of prepared childbirth.

In this section, systemic drugs and narcotic antagonists are discussed, as is the psychologic preparation for childbirth. Also considered are nursing responsibilities in the area of pain relief during labor. A discussion of obstetric anesthesia appears later in the chapter.

Systemic Drugs

The goal of pharmacologic pain relief during labor is to provide maximal analgesia with minimal risk for the mother and fetus. Three factors must be considered in the use of analgesic agents: (a) the effects on the mother, (b) the effects on the contractions of labor, and (c) the effects on the fetus.

Maternal drug action is of primary importance because the well-being of the fetus depends on adequate functioning of the maternal cardiopulmonary system. Any alteration of function that disturbs the mother's homeostatic mechanism affects the fetal environment. Maintaining the respiratory rate and blood pressure within normal range is thus of prime importance. The use of electronic fetal monitoring has provided a means of accurately assessing the effects of pharmacologic agents on uterine contractions. The Friedman labor curve provides a basis for determining the effects of drugs on the overall course of labor. (See Chapter 16 for discussion of the Friedman graph and electronic monitoring.)

All systemic drugs used for pain relief during labor cross the placental barrier by simple diffusion, with some agents crossing more readily than others. Drug action in the body depends on the rate at which the substance is metabolized by liver enzymes and excreted by the kidneys. The fetal liver enzymes and renal systems are inadequate to metabolize analgesic agents, so that high doses remain active in fetal circulation for a prolonged period of time. The fetal brain receives a greater amount of the cardiac output than the neonatal brain (Yaffee and Catz, 1971). The percentage of blood volume flowing to the brain is increased even further during intrauterine stress, so that the hypoxic fetus receives an even larger amount of a depressant drug. The blood-brain barrier is more permeable at the time of birth, a factor that also increases the amount of drug carried to the central nervous system. Depressed infants may have a decrease in sucking effort, visual attentiveness, and overall activity for as long as four days after birth (Moore, 1972).

Sedatives. Sedatives formerly played an important role in the pharmacologic management of labor. However, barbiturates have the disadvantage of producing restlessness in the presence of moderate to severe pain, and they readily cross the placental barrier, causing respiratory depression in the newborn.

The principal use of barbiturates in current obstetric practice is in false labor or in the early stages of prodromal labor. An oral dose of 100 mg of secobarbital (Seconal) or pentobarbital (Nembutal) promotes relaxation and allows the patient to sleep a few hours. If the patient is in false labor, the contractions usually stop. Women in prodromal labor enter the active phase of labor in a more relaxed and rested state.

Amnesics. Scopolamine is mentioned for historic purposes and to demonstrate the change in the management of labor that has occurred in recent years. This alkaloid of belladonna produces amnesia. It was administered many years ago in conjunction with morphine to produce "twilight sleep" during labor. In the presence of inadequate analgesia, scopolamine caused delirium, hallucinations, and uncontrolled behavior. Close observation was necessary to protect the patient from injury. Even though the patient screamed and thrashed about during strong contractions, she had little or no recollection of the experience after delivery. Depressed infants frequently resulted from this combination of scopolamine and morphine. Fortunately, scopolamine is no longer used in most areas of North America because women want to participate in their deliveries and to be fully aware of the event.

Ataractics. Ataractic drugs do not relieve pain but are reported to decrease apprehension and anxiety, to relieve nausea, and to potentiate the effects of narcotics. Agents frequently used in labor include promethazine (Phenergan), promazine (Sparine), hydroxyzine (Vistaril), and diazepam (Valium). There is still a great deal of controversy about the use of these drugs during labor. Many of the favorable reports are not from controlled studies. Evidence suggests that tranquilizers do not significantly affect the contractions of active labor.

The effects on the fetus are being questioned. Benson (1974) states that the drugs affect the attention span of the infant after delivery because these agents are poorly metabolized in the fetal and neonatal system. Many times, untoward fetal effects go unrecognized. Hypothermia and hypotonia in the newborn following intrapartal administration of diazepam (Valium) have recently been noted (Pritchard and MacDonald, 1976).

Ataractics may be given alone to reduce tension, or they may be combined with narcotics to potentiate the analgesic effect. The dosage of the narcotic is decreased by half. These agents may be given intramuscularly or intravenously. The peak action occurs within minutes when given intravenously and within 30–60 minutes when given intramuscularly.

Analgesics. Although many agents have been used to produce analgesia, the most common drug used in the United States is the synthetic narcotic meperidine (Demerol). In general, a narcotic is not administered until the patient is in active labor. It has been suggested that analgesic agents not be given until the cervix of a primipara is 5–6 cm dilated and that of a multipara is 3–4 cm dilated. More important than precise figures is an assessment of the characteristics of the contractions and the progress of labor.

Narcotics cross the placental barrier and depress the fetus. There is some disagreement as to the safe time for administration. In one study, peak depression of the infant occurred during the second or third hour after intramuscular injection of meperidine, with little or no effect when the infant was delivered during the first hour or after the fourth hour (Snider and Moya, 1964). Demerol may be given intramuscularly or intravenously in doses of 25–100 mg. The intravenous dose is 25–50 mg, with the onset of analgesia within 3–5 minutes and a duration of 1½–2 hours. It has been suggested that the intravenous injection be given during a contraction, when blood flow to the uterus and the fetus is decreased.

Narcotic Antagonists. Narcotic antagonists are available to counteract the respiratory depressant effects of opiate-type narcotics. Levallarphan (Lorfan), nalorphine (Nalline), and naloxone (Narcan) are effective only against respiratory depression caused by narcotic analgesics. When these drugs are administered intravenously in an appropriate dose, the marked depression of respiration from excessive doses of narcotics is dramatically reversed. Nalorphine (2.5–5 mg), levallarphan (0.1 mg), or naloxone (0.4 mg) may be administered intravenously to the mother five to ten minutes before delivery to prevent respiratory depression of the newborn. If time does not permit this method, nalorphine (0.05 mg/kg body weight), levallarphan (0.1 mg/kg body weight), or naloxone (0.01 mg/kg body weight) may be diluted and given directly to the neonate through the umbilical vein immediately after delivery.

The anatagonists act by competing with narcotics in the respiratory center receptors and by displacing the narcotic molecules form the receptor sites. If the receptors are not occupied by narcotics, nalorphine and levallarphan produce respiratory depression by occupying these sites. For this reason, these agents increase the depression caused by barbiturates, tranquilizers, and other sedative drugs. Naloxone exhibits little pharmacologic activity in the absence of narcotics, so it is less likely to potentiate nonnarcotic respiratory depression. Bauer (1971) advocates treating the depression by assisted ventilation and oxygen rather than by narcotic antagonists.

Psychologic Preparation for Childbirth

A positive attitude toward pregnancy and motherhood is probably the most significant preparation for a satisfying labor and delivery experience. Even though the pain of labor reaches great intensity at transition, the gradual increase in intensity throughout the first stage and the intermittent nature of the pain allow the prepared mother time to utilize and renew her coping mechanisms.

It is more positive to refer to the uterine contractions of labor as contractions rather than as pains. The use of the term *pain* suggests that the entire labor is expected to be painful. McCaffery (1972) states that "most mothers are not so suggestible that they would actually feel unbearable pain during contractions simply because the nurse used the term *pains* rather than *contractions.* But the use of the term *pains* may generate needless anxiety about the sensations of labor." Thus anxiety could be increased in the unprepared patient, and doubt in her ability to cope could be created within the mind of the prepared patient.

There are currently many methods of formal preparation for childbirth. Variations can be found between methods and even within a specific method. It is almost impossible to be completely knowledgeable about all the techniques. Generally, one or two types of preparation predominate in a given geographic area, so a practitioner can become familiar with the programs in her area.

Regardless of variations, each method usually includes a support person, positioning during labor, relaxation techniques, distraction or concentration techniques, breathing patterns, and specific physical activities. The need for analgesia and anesthesia is minimized and may be eliminated completely. (Sources for obtaining information about the various methods are included in the Additional Readings.) Despite the differing philosophies and techniques, the goal of all the methods is to assist the childbearing couple to have a safe, rewarding childbirth experience. See Chapter 12 for descriptions of various prepared childbirth methods.

Nursing Management of Pain Relief

One of the most important factors in determining a patient's emotional reaction to labor and delivery is the manner in which she is received by hospital personnel on admission to the unit. A woman approaches childbirth with a mixture of apprehension, excitement, reluctance, and relief. The event for which she has been preparing, both physically and emotionally, for the past nine months has begun—the transition to motherhood. Her life-style will never be the same again. It is sometimes difficult for the nurse, who may be admitting the seventh patient toward the end of a busy shift, to share the enthusiasm and excitement of the expectant couple.

A labor and delivery nurse is in the unique position of assisting during one of the most profound experiences of human existence. She has the privilege of sharing in each couple's personal miracle.

It is interesting to note that no other society has delegated the care of the laboring mother to total strangers. The rapidity with which family-centered childbirth is sweeping the country and the trend toward home delivery are results of inadequate emotional support from professional personnel during hospital delivery. There are too many people in the maternal-newborn health care system who do not possess the personal characteristics or commitment necessary to provide the emotional support a childbearing woman needs. A warm and supportive nurse helps set the stage for a satisfying childbirth experience.

Assessment

The first step in planning care for the patient is assessment of factors that may contribute to discomfort in labor. Identification and validation of these factors provide a basis for nursing intervention that can decrease the degree of discomfort the patient experiences. Assessment of the pain experience has been categorized into eight possible types of behavioral response (McCaffery, 1972):

1. Physiologic manifestations.
2. Body movement.
3. Facial expression.
4. Verbal statements.
5. Vocal behavior.
6. Physical contact.
7. Response to environment.
8. Patterns of handling pain.

Many of these behaviors overlap in the total response to pain. The most frequent physiologic manifestations are increases in pulse, respiration, and blood pressure; dilated pupils; and an increase in muscle tension. In labor these reactions are transitory because of the intermittent nature of the pain. The increase in muscle tension is the most significant in labor because it may impede the progress of labor. Patients are frequently seen voluntarily tightening skeletal muscles during a contraction and remaining motionless. Facial grimacing is also a common observation. Verbal statements relating to pain are generally reliable because requests for intervention usually mean that the woman has reached her tolerance level. Vocalization may take many forms during the first stage of labor. A grunting sound typically accompanies the bearing-down effort during the second stage of labor.

Some patients desire body contact during a contraction and may reach out to grasp the supporting person. As the intensity of the contractions increases with the progress of labor, the woman is decreasingly aware of the environment and may have difficulty hearing verbal instructions. The pattern of coping with the contractions of labor varies from the use of highly structured breathing techniques to loud vocalizations. Irritability and refusal of touch are common responses to the discomfort of the second stage of labor. The tense and frightened patient is more likely to lose control during any stage of labor.

Intervention

A decrease in the intensity of discomfort is one of the goals of nursing intervention during labor. The total elimination of pain can only be accomplished with selected regional anesthetic techniques. Nursing measures used to decrease pain include (a) increasing general comfort, (b) decreasing anxiety, (c) providing information, (d) utilizing specific supportive techniques, and (e) administering pharmacologic agents as ordered by the physician. These measures are not mutually exclusive but are interrelated in the total management of care during labor.

General Comfort

General comfort measures are of utmost importance throughout labor. The patient should be assisted to any position that she finds the most comfortable. A side-lying position is generally the most advantageous for the laboring woman. Care should be taken that all body parts are supported, with the joints slightly flexed. If the patient is more comfortable on her back, the head of the bed should be elevated to relieve the pressure of the uterus on the vena cava. Back rubs and frequent change of position contribute to comfort and relaxation.

Fresh, smooth, dry bed linen promotes patient comfort. Diaphoresis and the constant leaking of amniotic fluid contribute to discomfort. Changing the bed linen and gown of the patient who has intravenous fluids in place and is attached to the fetal monitor can be rather overwhelming to the beginning nurse and may be considered too much trouble by the experienced labor and delivery nurse, but the degree of effort required is far outweighed by the benefit to the patient. The need to change the bottom sheet following rupture of the membranes can be decreased by changing incontinent pads (chux) at frequent intervals. The perineal area should be kept as clean and dry as possible to prevent infection as well as to promote comfort.

Particular attention should be focused on the bladder. It should be kept as empty as possible. Even though the patient is voiding, it is not unusual for urine to be retained because of the pressure of the fetal presenting part. A full bladder can be detected by palpation and percussion directly over the symphysis pubis. Some of the regional procedures for analgesia during labor contribute to the inability to void, and catheterization may be necessary. A full bladder adds to the discomfort during a contraction and may prolong labor by interfering with the descent of the fetus.

The patient may experience dryness of the oral mucous membranes, as she is usually allowed no food or liquids by mouth. Even though the patient may have intravenous fluids, the mouth still becomes dry. A lemon glycerine swab, ice chips, or a wet 4 × 4 sponge helps relieve the discomfort. Some prepared childbirth programs advise the patient to bring lollipops to help combat the dryness that occurs with some of the breathing patterns. By relieving some of these minor discomforts the patient is better able to use her coping mechanisms for dealing with pain.

Handling Anxiety

The anxiety experienced by women entering labor is related to a combination of factors inherent to the process. According to McCaffery (1972), anxiety is necessary during the anticipation of pain. She states that "during the anticipation of pain, pain relief is enhanced if the patient experiences a moderate amount of anxiety and this anxiety is channeled into methods of coping with pain." Note that she says moderate and not a high degree of anxiety and that the anxiety should be related only to the pain experience.

This concept can be correlated with the theory that a moderate degree of anxiety improves student performance on an examination whereas a high degree of anxiety decreases test performance. An excessive degree of anxiety interferes with one's ability to cope. Anxieties relating to other aspects of labor also inhibit coping mechanisms. One way to decrease anxiety that is not related to pain is to eliminate the unknown quality of labor by patient teaching and by establishing a good rapport with the couple to preserve their personal integrity. In addition to being a good listener, it is important for the labor and delivery nurse to demonstrate genuine concern for the patient. Remaining with the woman as much as possible conveys a caring attitude and decreases the fear of abandonment. Praise for correct breathing, relaxation efforts, and pushing efforts not only provides positive reinforcement for repetition of the behavior but also decreases anxiety about the ability to cope with the process of labor.

Patient Teaching

Providing information about the nature of the discomfort that will occur during labor is important. Stressing the intermittent nature and maximum duration of the contractions can be most helpful. It is much easier to cope with pain when a period of complete relief is assured. Describing the type of discomfort and specific sensations that will occur as labor progresses helps the woman recognize these sensations as normal and expected when she does experience them.

Rectal pressure during the second stage may be interpreted as the need for a bowel movement. The instinctive response is to tighten muscles rather than bear down. A sensation of splitting apart also occurs in the latter part of the second stage, which tends to retard bearing-down efforts. If the woman expects these sensations and has been counseled that bearing down contributes to progress at this stage, she is more likely to listen to instructions and to make her best effort to control her responses. Descriptions of sensations should not be given unless the woman is also given instructions as to what she can do when the sensations occur. Some patients experience the urge to push during transition when the cervix is not fully dilated and effaced. This sensation can be controlled by panting, and instructions should be given prior to the time that panting is required.

A thorough explanation of procedures and equipment being used also decreases anxiety, thereby decreasing pain. Most women are prepared for the perineal shave and enema, but few are prepared for the artificial rupturing of the membranes unless they have experienced it before. Assurance that it is no more uncomfortable than a vaginal examination decreases anxiety. Attachment to a fetal monitor can produce fear, because equipment of this type is associated with critically ill patients. Many labor and delivery units routinely monitor all women in labor. The beeps, clicks, and other strange noises should be explained, and a simplified explanation of the monitor strip should be given. The nurse can emphasize that the use of the monitor provides a more accurate way to assess the well-being of the fetus during the course of labor.

Specific Supportive Techniques

Tense muscles increase resistance to the descent of the fetus and contribute to maternal fatigue. This fatigue increases pain perception and decreases the ability to cope with the pain experience. Comfort measures, techniques for decreasing anxiety, and patient teaching have been identified as factors that contribute to relaxation. Other factors are adequate rest and sleep. The woman must be encouraged to use the period between contractions for rest and relaxation. A prolonged prodromal phase of labor may have prevented the woman from sleeping. An aura of excitement is usually present, with the onset of labor making it difficult to sleep, even though the contractions are mild and infrequent. The administration of a mild, short-acting sedative may enable the woman to sleep between contractions. During the active phase of labor, an analgesic to decrease pain perception during contractions also promotes relaxation and sleep between contractions. An exhausted mother may be less enthusiastic about the delivery process and about holding her newborn.

Distraction is a specific method of coping with discomfort. During early labor, conversation or such activities as light reading, bridge, or Scrabble serve as distractors. One technique that is effective with moderate pain is to have the patient concentrate on a pleasant experience she has had in the past. This requires a good imagination, but some women can close their eyes and recreate the pleasant experience. Another type of distraction is touch. Some women have the desire to touch another person during a painful experience, whereas others regard touching as an invasion of privacy or a threat to their independence. When an assessment does not reveal this information about a patient, the nurse can make herself available to the patient who desires this support. One way to do this is by placing one's hand on the side rail of the bed within the patient's reach. The person who needs touch will reach out for contact, and the nurse can pick up and follow through with this behavioral cue. Touch may be used to communicate to the patient that dependency is allowed in stressful situations.

A specific type of cutaneous stimulation used prior to the transitional phase of labor is known as *abdominal effleurage.* Pain impulses are carried by small-diameter nerve fibers, and cutaneous sensations are carried by large-diameter nerve fibers. The theory is that the transmission of pain impulses is inhibited by the competing input from the large fibers. The light abdominal stroking used in the Lamaze method is effective for mild to moderate pain but is not effective for intense pain. Deep pressure over the sacrum is more effective for relieving back pain.

Administration of Analgesic Agents

The optimal time for administering analgesia is determined after making a complete assessment of many factors. In general, an analgesic agent is administered to primiparas when the cervix has dilated to 5–6 cm, and to multiparas when the cervix has reached 3–4 cm dilatation. This is only a generalization, however; the character of the labor must be taken into account. Analgesia given too early may prolong labor, and analgesia given too late is of no value to the patient and may harm the fetus. In many institutions the nurse makes the decision as to when the analgesic ordered by the physician is given. This decision is based on a complete assessment of the patient as well as the progress of labor.

Currently a minimal amount of an analgesic agent is given in labor. Oral analgesics are not used because of poor absorption and decreased gastric-emptying time. The intramuscular and intravenous routes are most frequently utilized. When the prescribed route is intramuscular, a needle of sufficient length to penetrate the muscle is a necessity. One study revealed that blood levels of a drug were more than doubled when injected intramuscularly by physicians rather than by nurses. The physicians in the study used larger and longer needles, so that the agent entered the muscle rather than the subcutaneous fat (Dundee et al., 1974). When an agent is given intravenously, it should be administered no faster than 1 ml/min. Whatever the route of administration, the power of suggestion on the part of the nurse greatly increases the effectiveness of the agent.

Even though minimal amounts of medication may make some of the steps unnecessary, the general principles for administering analgesic drugs are as follows:

1. The patient should be in an individual labor room.
2. The environment should be free from sensory stimuli, such as bright lights, noise, and irrelevant conversation, to allow the patient to focus on the drug action.
3. An explanation of the effects of the medication should be given, including how long the effects will last and how the drug will make the patient feel.
4. The patient should be encouraged to empty her bladder prior to administration of the drug.
5. The baseline FHR should be recorded prior to administration.
6. Dentures, glasses, contact lenses, and jewelry should be removed from the patient.
7. The physician's written order should be checked and the medication prepared.
8. The medication should be signed out on the narcotic or control sheet.
9. The patient should be asked again if she is allergic to any medication.
10. The patient's arm band should be checked for identification.
11. The drug should be administered by the route ordered, using correct technique.
12. The side rails should be pulled up for patient safety, and the reasons should be explained to the patient.
13. The medication, dosage, time, route, and site of administration should be charted on the nurse's notes and on the monitor strip.
14. The FHR should be monitored to assess the effects of the medication on the fetus.
15. The effectiveness of the analgesic agent should be evaluated.
16. The patient should not be left alone. If it is necessary for the nurse to leave, the patient should be given a short explanation and assurances that the nurse will return.

There is no completely safe and satisfactory method of pain relief. When analgesia is used judiciously, however, it can be beneficial to the mother and do little harm to the fetus. The woman who is free from fear and who has confidence in the medical and nursing personnel usually has a relatively comfortable first stage of labor and requires a minimum of medication. A positive attitude on the part of the professional nurse and the expectant parents is an essential part of pain relief.

OBSTETRIC ANESTHESIA

The goal of obstetric anesthesia is to provide maximal pain relief with minimal side effects to the fetomaternal unit. Anesthetic techniques and drugs should be selected to meet the needs of the mother and her infant. Prior to the anesthetic procedure, intravenous fluids should be initiated so that access to the intravascular system is immediately available in case of emergency. Women who have had fluids withheld throughout the course of labor need an infusion for hydration and energy.

General Anesthesia

When used, general anesthesia is usually administered at the time of delivery, although some agents serve as analgesic agents during labor. The method used to produce general anesthesia may be intravenous injection or inhalation.

No method or agent is without maternal and fetal hazards. All agents for general anesthesia cross the placental barrier and depress the nervous system of the fetus in varying degrees. Anesthetic deaths are the fifth leading cause of maternal mortality in the United States, and half of the deaths are attributable to aspiration during general anesthesia (Moya, 1975). Despite the maternal and fetal hazards, general anesthesia is still popular in much of North America.

General anesthesia is indicated for a woman with certain obstetric complications. When hemorrhage or the threat of hemorrhage is present, general anesthesia may be the method of choice, because regional anesthesia with resulting sympathetic blockage and peripheral vasodilatation compounds the problem of hypovolemia. Any obstetric condition requiring uterine relaxation, such as delivery of the head in a breech presentation, internal version with a second twin, and tetanic contractions, is an indication for general anesthesia. Bonica (1972) states, "The potent inhalation anesthetics are the best uterine relaxants currently available because they act more rapidly and are better controlled than any other drugs." It is the procedure of choice in emergency cesarean section for fetal distress. General anesthesia is also used for patients with central nervous system disease and allergies to local anesthetic agents and for those who are emotionally unsuited for regional procedures.

Many drugs have been used as obstetric anesthetic agents since chloroform was first used. Ether and nitrous oxide were first introduced in the mid-eighteenth century for the relief of pain. Inhalation anesthetics depress the central nervous system in varying degrees, which correlate to the concentration of the agent in arterial blood entering cerebral circulation. By balancing the amount of a drug entering arterial circulation by way of the lung against the amount returning chemically intact to the lung by way of venous circulation, the anesthesiologist can control the concentration in the brain and keep the patient at the level of anesthesia desired. Inhalation anesthetics are considered to be safer than intravenously administered drugs because the circulating concentrations can be more quickly and better controlled. Once injected, intravenous agents cannot be retrieved and must be metabolized by the body for excretion.

The reticular activating system, which relays sensory impulses to the cerebral cortex, is the first structure to be affected. Very small anesthetic doses decrease sensory perception. The characteristic pattern of symptoms reflecting central nervous system depression is the basis for the various stages and planes of anesthesia (Table 18-1). Plane 1 of Stage III is usually adequate for both vaginal and abdominal delivery. Planes 2 and 3 may be used for short periods of time when greater perineal and uterine relaxation are necessary. Plane 4 is never required in obstetric anesthesia.

Nurses who care for anesthetized patients in the delivery and recovery rooms must be able to assess the patient's level of anesthesia to provide appropriate intervention. Patients in Stage I anesthesia respond to verbal orders even though sensorium is altered. It is important that only one person give commands. Otherwise, confusion results and the patient cannot respond appropriately.

It must also be remembered that the patient in Stage II anesthesia is actually unconscious and unable to control behavior. The higher cortical centers are depressed by the anesthetic agent, releasing the lower motor and emotional centers from control. The patient is not responsible for her actions at this level.

Inhalation Anesthetics

Nitrous Oxide

Nitrous oxide is the oldest analgesic and anesthetic gaseous agent. It provides rapid and pleasant induction; it is nonirritating, nonexplosive, and inexpensive; and it provides less disturbance in physiologic functioning than any other agent (Bonica, 1972). At a concentration of 40%, it produces excellent analgesia yet permits the patient to cooperate. Little or no fetal depression occurs with this concentration. When used alone, there is no effect on the maternal respiratory center.

Nitrous oxide is generally used in combination with other agents for anesthesia. Although it is an excellent analgesic, nitrous oxide provides poor muscular relaxation. The main use of nitrous oxide is as an analgesic agent during the second stage of labor, as an induction agent or supplement to more potent inhalation anesthetics, and as a part of balanced anesthesia.

Methoxyflurane (Penthrane)

Of the more recent halogenated anesthetics, methoxyflurane is the most potent and the most widely used in obstetrics. Analgesic doses may be

Table 18–1. Stages of Anesthesia

Stage	Respiration	Eye	Muscle tone
Stage I			
Plane 1	Regular	Normal pupils, voluntary control of eye movement	No loss
Plane 2	Regular	Normal pupils, voluntary eye movement	No loss
Plane 3	Regular	Normal pupils, voluntary eye movement, lid reflex lost	No loss
Stage II	Irregular	Dilated pupils	Increased, tense, struggling
Stage III			
Plane 1	Normal, deep, regular	Pupils constricted, lid reflex lost	Loss of tone in small muscles
Plane 2	Normal, deep, regular	Pupils in mid-dilation, cessation of eyeball movement, corneal reflex lost	Decreased muscle tone, visceral and pharyngeal reflexes lost
Plane 3	Shallow, progressive intercostal paralysis	Pupils moderately dilated, light reflex lost	All muscles relaxed except diaphragm
Plane 4	Abdominal breathing, progressive diaphragmatic paralysis	Pupils completely dilated	All muscle tone lost
Stage IV	None	Widely dilated	No muscle tone

self-administered with an inhaler to provide pain relief during transition and the second stage of labor without significantly affecting the course of labor. Masks designed for self-administration should *never* be held over the patient's face by nursing personnel, because the agent is not to be administered continuously.

Anesthetic doses provide smooth induction and emergence with minimal irritation of the tracheobronchial tree, although fetal depression occurs with high concentrations for a prolonged period of time. The addition of nitrous oxide and oxygen decreases the amount of methoxyflurane needed for effective anesthesia. When required for emergency conditions, a higher concentration can produce good uterine relaxation. One of its disadvantages, although enhancing its wide margin of safety, is the slow induction time. The emergence from anesthesia is also slow, and the patient must be carefully supervised in the recovery room by nursing personnel.

Trichloroethylene (Trilene)

Trichloroethylene is a self-administered anesthetic agent that is effective and has no notable toxic effects for the mother or fetus, provided it is used intermittently. However, some specific disadvantages render it an anesthetic agent to use only when no alternative exists. If general anesthesia follows administration of trichloroethylene, agents employing a soda lime absorption cannister are contraindicated—a neurotoxic substance (dichloroacetylene) may be formed, and cranial nerve palsy may develop.

Cyclopropane

Cyclopropane is generally the agent of choice in the presence of hemorrhage or shock because of the speed of induction and the tendency to increased vascular tone. Fetal depression does occur, however, so duration of anesthesia before delivery should not exceed 12 minutes.

Halothane (Fluothane)

The agent halothane produces good uterine relaxation and is therefore useful for intrauterine manipulations. Postpartal hemorrhage frequently occurs because of the sustained uterine relaxation.

Intravenous Anesthetics

Thiopental Sodium (Pentothal)

Thiopental sodium is an ultrashort-acting barbiturate that produces narcosis within 30 seconds after intravenous administration. Induction and emergence are smooth and pleasant, with little incidence of nausea and vomiting. The patient goes from the first stage of anesthesia to the first plane of the third stage so rapidly that the clinical signs of the levels in between are difficult to detect. Barbiturates are nonirritating to the respiratory tract and are nonexplosive. They differ from the inhalation anesthetics in two major ways: (a) little or no analgesia occurs, and (b) the method of administration is less controllable.

Thiopental sodium is extremely irritating to tissues, and sloughing may result if infiltration occurs with high concentrations of the agent. Because of this effect, the integrity of the intravenous line must be checked prior to administration. The rapidity of action makes it valuable in convulsive states, particularly those that occur as side effects of local anesthetics. Maternal peak plasma concentration after injection may fall as much as 90% in one minute, so injection at the onset of a contraction prevents the fetus from receiving the transient high concentration of the agent.

Thiopental sodium is rarely used alone, because the dosage required for anesthesia produces profound central nervous system depression. It is most frequently used for induction and as an adjunct to other more potent anesthetics. Significant neonatal depression does not occur with administration of single doses of less than 250 mg (Danforth, 1977).

Balanced Anesthesia

A current trend in the management of delivery is to use balanced anesthesia. Balanced anesthesia is induced with nitrous oxide or thiopental sodium (Pentothal), which provides good induction but little muscle relaxation, and another agent is added to produce relaxation. The patient benefits from the most useful characteristics of each agent without the problems associated with the higher concentration necessary if either agent is used individually.

Complications of General Anesthesia

The primary dangers of general anesthesia are as follows:

1. *Fetal depression.* Most general anesthetic agents reach the fetus in about two minutes. The depression in the fetus is directly proportional to the depth and duration of the anesthesia. The long-term significance of fetal depression in a normal delivery has not been determined. The poor fetal metabolism of general anesthetic agents is similar to that of analgesic agents administered during labor. General anesthesia is not advocated in cases in which the infant is considered to be at high risk, particularly the premature infant.

2. *Uterine relaxation.* The majority of agents cause some degree of uterine relaxation, thereby increasing the incidence of cesarean section and forceps delivery as well as postpartal uterine atony.

3. *Vomiting and aspiration.* These can occur with both regional and general anesthetics, but they occur most frequently during emergence from general anesthesia and are always a danger in obstetrics. Pregnancy results in decreased gastric motility, and the onset of labor halts the process almost entirely. Food eaten many hours earlier may still be in the stomach undigested. Even when food and fluids have been withheld, fasting gastric juice is highly acidic and can produce a fatal chemical pneumonitis if aspirated. The nurse should ascertain when the patient last ate and record this information. All delivery suites should have emergency equipment available to deal with complications such as aspiration.

Signs of aspiration include respiratory obstruction and laryngoscope visualization of solid particles of food in the tracheobronchial tree. Aspiration of liquid gastric contents may be undetected until the patient complains of chest pain and has respiratory embarrassment, cyanosis, fever, and tachycardia in the postanesthetic stage, referred to as *Mendelson's syndrome.*

Interventions

The immediate medical treatment of acute respiratory obstruction includes the following measures:

1. Place the delivery table in a 30-degree head down position, with the patient on her right side.
2. Quickly suction pharynx and larynx or remove food with gauze-wrapped finger.
3. Perform laryngoscopy and endotracheal intubation. If the jaws cannot be forced open, succinylcholine may be given intravenously to facilitate removal of emesis and intubation. Cricoid pressure may be applied by the delivery room nurse.
4. Give 100% oxygen for pulmonary ventilation.
5. Perform bronchoscopy.
6. Tracheobronchial lavage is advocated by some, but this procedure remains controversial.

Follow-up care includes these measures:

1. *Broncholytic agents:* Aminophylline, 500 mg, slowly injected intravenously to produce bronchodilatation.
2. *Adrenocorticosteroids:* Cortisone, 100 mg, to decrease inflammatory response.
3. *Antibiotics:* Broad-spectrum agent to decrease secondary infection.
4. *Oxygen:* IPPB.

The use of a respirator and tracheostomy should not be delayed until the patient is moribund. Should cardiac failure occur, it must be treated promptly and thoroughly (Bonica, 1972).

Regional Analgesia and Anesthesia

Regional analgesia and anesthesia are achieved by injecting local anesthetic agents into an area that will bring the agent into direct contact with nervous tissue. Local agents stabilize the cell membrane, preventing initiation and transmission of nerve impulses. The methods most commonly utilized in obstetrics include local infiltration, paracervical block, pudendal block, peridural block (lumbar epidural and caudal), and subarachnoid block. The nerve blocks may be accomplished by a single injection or continuously by means of an indwelling plastic catheter. Regional techniques have gained widespread popularity in recent years and are particularly compatible with the goals of psychoprophylactic preparation for childbirth.

Although there are advantages and disadvantages specific to each technique, in general the advantages of regional procedures are as follows:

1. Relief from discomfort is complete in the area blocked.
2. Depression of maternal vital signs rarely occurs.
3. Aspiration of gastric contents is virtually eliminated if the parturient has not received adjunct sedation.
4. Administration at the optimal time does not significantly alter the course of labor.
5. The mother remains alert and able to participate in the childbirth process.

The disadvantages include:

1. A high degree of skill is required for proper administration of most procedures.
2. Failures such as no effect or unilateral or incomplete anesthesia can occur even with experienced operators.
3. Side effects do occur with some techniques.
4. Systemic toxic reactions are more common than with agents used for general anesthesia.

Essential prerequisites for the administration of regional analgesia and anesthesia are knowledge of the anatomy and physiology of pertinent structures, of techniques for administration, of the pharmacology of local anesthetics, and of potential complications. With the exception of nurse anesthetists and nurse-midwives, who may perform procedures for which they have been trained, nurses may *not* legally administer anesthetic agents. This admonition includes the reinjection of agents through indwelling catheters. However, it is important for the nurse to have an adequate knowledge of all aspects of regional anesthesia to provide patient support and to give appropriate reinforcement of the administrator's explanation to the patient. The nurse who has a thorough understanding of the techniques and agents can also provide more efficient assistance to the administrator. Patient safety is increased when the nurse recognizes complications and immediately initiates appropriate intervention.

The relief of pain associated with the first

stage of labor can be accomplished by blocking the sensory nerves supplying the uterus with the techniques of paracervical, lumbar sympathetic, and peridural blocks. The relief of pain associated with the second stage and delivery can be alleviated with pudendal, peridural, and subarachnoid blocks (Figure 18–5).

Regional Anesthetic Agents

The local agents most commonly used for obstetric analgesia and anesthesia are procaine (Novocaine), dibucaine (Nupercaine), lidocaine (Xylocaine), tetracaine (Pontocaine), mepivacaine (Carbocaine), chloroprocaine (Nesacaine), and bupivacaine (Marcaine).

This group of anesthetic drugs blocks the conduction of nerve impulses from the periphery to the central nervous system. Although the mechanism of their action is not fully understood, it is thought that the agents do not allow sodium ions to enter the cell, thereby preventing depolarization. The neuronal membrane is stabilized in its resting state so that nerve impulses from the source of pain are not transmitted. Motor and sympathetic fibers of mixed spinal nerves may be blocked in the attempt to achieve loss of sensation. The types of peripheral nerve fibers are differentially sensitive to the agents. The smaller the fiber, the more sensitive it is to local anesthetics. It is possible to block the small C and A-Δ fibers, which conduct the sensations of pain, temperature, pressure and touch, without affecting the large, heavily myelinated A-α, A-β, and A-γ fibers, which continue to maintain muscle tone, position sense, and motor function (Bonica, 1972).

Absorption of local anesthetics depends primarily on the vascularity of the area of injection. The agents also contribute to increased blood flow by causing vasomotor paralysis. Higher concentration of drugs causes greater vasodilatation. Good maternal physical condition or a high metabolic rate aids absorption. Malnutrition, dehydra-

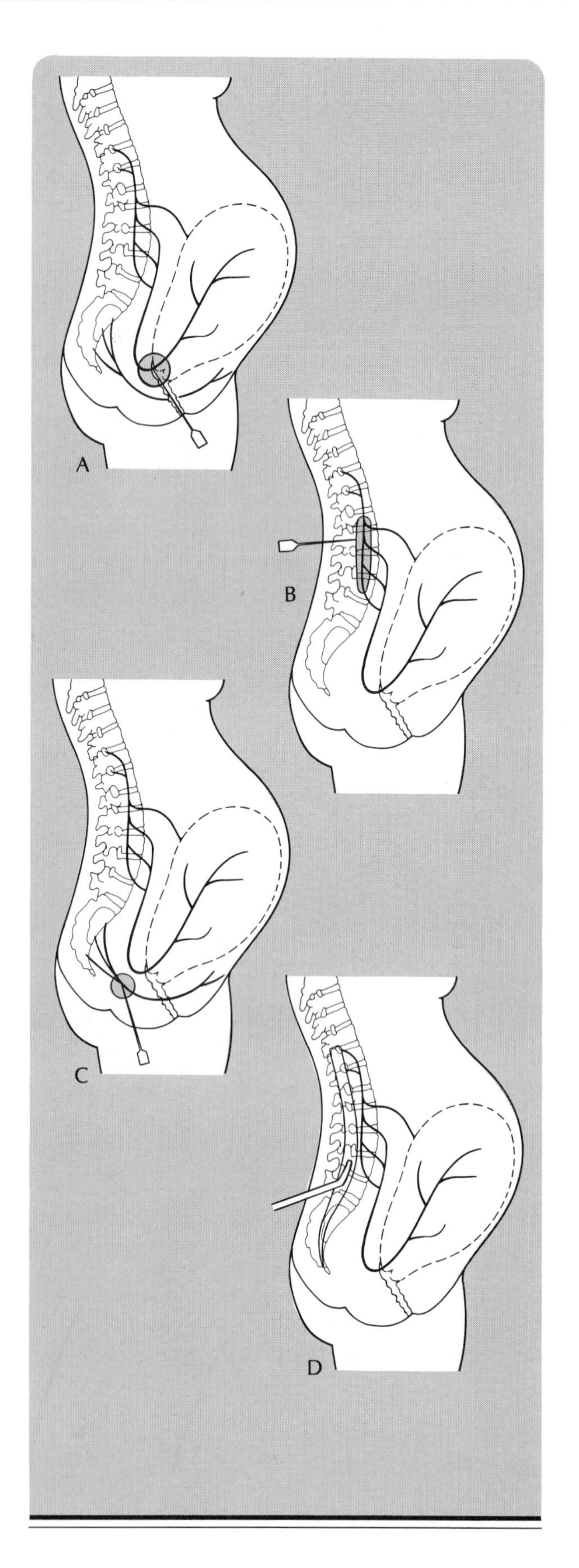

Figure 18–5. Schematic diagram showing pain pathways and sites of interruption. **A,** Paracervical block: relief of uterine pain only. **B,** Lumbar sympathetic block: relief of uterine pain only. **C,** Pudendal block: relief of perineal pain. **D,** Lumbar epidural block: dark area demonstrates peridural space and nerves affected, and white tube represents continuous plastic catheter. (From Bonica, J. J. 1972. *Principles and practice of obstetric analgesia and anesthesia.* Philadelphia: F. A. Davis Co., pp. 492, 512, 521, and 614.)

tion, electrolyte imbalance, and cardiovascular and pulmonary problems lower the threshold for toxic effects. The pH of tissues affects the rate of absorption, which has implications for fetal complications. The addition of vasoconstrictors such as epinephrine delays absorption and prolongs the anesthetic effect. Recent studies have demonstrated that epinephrine decreases uteroplacental blood flow, making it an undesirable additive in many situations. The breakdown of local anesthetics in the body is accomplished by the liver and plasma esterase, with the resulting substance being eliminated by the kidneys.

The weakest concentration and the smallest amount necessary to produce the desired results is advocated.

Adverse Maternal Reactions

Reactions to local anesthetic agents range from mild symptoms to cardiovascular collapse. The signs and symptoms of toxic reactions to local anesthetic agents are summarized in the box below. Mild reactions include palpitations, vertigo, tinnitus, apprehension, confusion, headache, and a metallic taste in the mouth. Moderate reactions include more severe degrees of mild symptoms plus nausea and vomiting, hypotension, and muscle twitching, which may progress to convulsions and loss of consciousness. The severe reactions are sudden loss of consciousness, coma, severe hypotension, bradycardia, respiratory depression, and cardiac arrest. Local toxic effects on tissues may also result with high concentrations of the agents. Anesthetic agents should not be used unless an intravenous line is in place.

Systemic toxic reactions most commonly occur with an excessive dose through too great a concentration or too large a volume. Accidental intravenous injection that suddenly increases the amount of the drug in maternal circulation results in depression of vasomotor, respiratory, and other medullary centers of the brain. It also depresses the heart and peripheral vascular bed. A massive intravascular dose can result in sudden circulatory collapse within 1 minute. Reactions to subcu-

SUMMARY OF SIGNS AND SYMPTOMS OF SYSTEMIC TOXIC REACTIONS FROM LOCAL ANESTHETIC DRUGS*

Central nervous system effects

A. Stimulation of
   1. Cerebral cortex → excitement, disorientation, incoherent speech, convulsions
   2. Medulla
      a. Cardiovascular center → increased blood pressure and pulse
      b. Respiratory center → increased respiratory rate and/or variations in rhythm
      c. Vomiting center → nausea and/or vomiting

B. Depression of
   1. Cerebral cortex → unconsciousness
   2. Medulla
      a. Vasomotor → fall in blood pressure and rapid or absent pulse (syncope)
      b. Respiratory → variations in respiration and/or apnea

Peripheral effects

A. Cardiovascular (syncope)
   1. Heart → bradycardia, i.e. depression from direct action of local anesthetic agent on myocardium
   2. Blood vessels → vasodilatation from direct action of local anesthetic agent on blood vessels

Allergic responses

A. Skin → urticaria, etc.
B. Respiration → depression ("clinical anaphylactic shock")
C. Circulation → depression ("clinical anaphylactic shock")

Miscellaneous reactions

A. Psychogenic
B. To other drugs, e.g. vasoconstrictors

*From Danforth, D., ed. 1977. *Textbook of obstetrics and gynecology.* 3rd ed. New York: Harper & Row Publishers, Inc., p. 608; modified from Moore, D. C. 1967. *Regional block.* 4th ed. Springfield, Ill.: Charles C Thomas, Publisher.

taneous and extradural injection occur between 5 and 40 minutes. The short-acting agents can produce toxic reactions in 10–15 minutes (procaine), and the long-acting agents (mepivacaine), in 20–40 minutes. It is imperative that the patient be under close supervision by knowledgeable personnel throughout the time that the agent is being used.

If epinephrine has been added to the anesthetic agent to prolong the anesthesia, it is necessary to differentiate between reaction to the anesthetic agent and to the epinephrine. Reaction to epinephrine is characterized by pallor, perspiration, a greater increase in blood pressure and pulse than occurs with reactions to anesthetic agents, and dyspnea.

Psychogenic reactions can occur, with symptoms similar to systemic toxic reactions. This phenomenon may occur as the procedure is begun and prior to the injection of the anesthetic agent. Regardless of the cause, the symptoms must be treated.

Allergic reactions to anesthetic agents may also occur. The manifestations of the antigen-antibody reaction include urticaria, laryngeal edema, joint pain, swelling of the tongue, and bronchospasm. An antihistamine such as diphenhydramine (Benadryl) should be administered intravenously to treat allergic reaction (Bonica, 1972).

Interventions

Treatment of systemic toxicity. In the treatment of mild toxicity, the administration of oxygen and intravenous injection of a short-acting barbiturate is advocated. Preparation must be made to treat convulsions or cardiovascular collapse. Specific interventions in the treatment of systemic toxicity are listed in the box on p. 535.

Treatment of convulsions. The best treatment for convulsions is administration of oxygen, administration of 40–60 mg of succinylcholine, and intubation (Bonica, 1972). This method is quick, and succinylcholine can be given intramuscularly if necessary. It does not depress myocardial and medullary centers, nor does it depress the fetus. This treatment has an advantage over treatment with short-acting barbiturates such as thiopental or pentobarbital, which depress myocardial and medullary centers as well as the fetus. Overdosage is also more frequent with the short-acting barbiturates.

Treatment of sudden cardiovascular collapse. In sudden collapse, assisted ventilation with 100% oxygen through an endotracheal tube is indicated. The rate of intravenous fluids may be increased to support circulation. Vasopressors with inotropic action may be given, and in extreme cases, epinephrine and closed cardiac massage may be indicated.

Paracervical Block

The paracervical block is useful during the first stage of labor. It anesthetizes the inferior hypogastric plexus and ganglia to provide relief of pain from cervical dilatation but does not anesthetize the lower vagina or perineum. Indwelling catheters may be used for repeated injections. The patient should be in active labor and the cervix dilated 4–5 cm prior to injection. Uterine contractility may be inhibited for a short period of time. It has been postulated that this method may facilitate cervical dilatation by inhibiting muscular contraction of the lower uterine segment (Jensen et al., 1977). The addition of epinephrine to the anesthetic agent is not recommended for this method because of its inhibitory effect on the myometrium. The agents advocated for this procedure are procaine and Pontocaine (tetracaine), because they are better metabolized by the placenta with less transfer to the fetus.

The disadvantages of the paracervical block include the following: The vascularity of the area increases the possibility of rapid absorption, with resulting systemic toxic reaction. Hematomas may occur as a result of uterine vessel damage. Fetal bradycardia frequently follows paracervical block, with a reported incidence of 25%–85% (Pritchard and MacDonald, 1976). It is recommended that an injection be no deeper than 3 mm and that two injections be made on each side in order to reduce the possibility of injecting a large volume into venous circulation or the fetal scalp (Jagerhorn, 1975).

Fetal bradycardia is relatively common and is increased in premature infants, in the fetuses of primiparas, and in births where large doses of anesthetic agents are administered. The amide group of agents—bupivacaine, mepivacaine, and lidocaine—have the potential to produce direct fetal myocardial depression. The ECG of the fetus with bradycardia, in the absence of maternal hypotension or increase in uterine activity, resembles that of a conduction defect due to vagal stim-

SUMMARY OF ACTIVE TREATMENT OF SYSTEMIC TOXIC REACTIONS FROM HIGH BLOOD LEVEL OF LOCAL ANESTHETIC AGENT

Although the following measures apply specifically to toxic reaction from high blood levels of local anesthetic agent, they are general principles of resuscitation and are applicable to any reaction that may progress to shock (Moore, 1967):

1. Be sure airway is clear. If patient becomes unconscious, establish clear airway with oropharyngeal airway or, preferably, cuffed endotracheal tube.

2. Clear vomitus from pharynx, larynx, and trachea. If cuffed endotracheal tube is in trachea and cuff is inflated when vomiting occurs, no emergency exists. Vomitus may be cleared from mouth and pharynx when time permits—cuffed endotracheal tube prevents vomitus from entering tracheobronchial tree. If endotracheal tube is not in place when the patient vomits, a true emergency may exist; vomitus must be cleared from mouth.

3. Administer oxygen. Oxygen administration should be performed with bag and mask apparatus and inadequate respirations should be supplemented.

4. Start intravenous fluids. This is an essential part of the initial treatment of the reaction and should be done when the first signs of reaction occur, because it assures the physician a means of intravenous administration of drugs even if reaction progresses to cardiovascular collapse.

5. Stop convulsions.

a. Administer oxygen. Oxygen alone may stop convulsion.

b. If oxygen alone does not stop convulsion, use intravenous injections of succinylcholine, 2 ml (40 mg), and oxygenate parturient. If convulsions recur after succinylcholine is dissipated (0–8 min), repeat dose. Then if convulsions recur, give d-tubocurarine, 3–5 ml (9–15 mg).

c. If muscle relaxants are not available or anesthetist is not familiar with their actions and uses, give small amounts of short-acting barbiturate, thiopental, 50 mg at 0.5- to 1-min intervals. In obstetrics a single dose of succinylcholine and oxygenation is preferred. A barbiturate should not be used unless convulsions are persistent, because it merely adds to the depression of both mother and fetus.

6. Raise blood pressure. When peripheral vascular collapse starts, immediate steps must be taken to raise blood pressure to approximately the preoperative level; use vasoconstrictor drugs.

7. Institute manual systole. If cardiac arrest or fibrillation occurs, closed manual systole (cardiac massage) must be rapidly instituted.

---

ulation instead of direct depression (Ettiger and McCant, 1976). Greiss et al. (1976) propose that the fetal bradycardia is caused by reduced placental blood flow associated with anesthetic drug action.

Paracervical block should be used only in normal labor with an uncompromised fetus.

Technique. The proper method for administering a paracervical block is illustrated in Figure 18–6:

1. The patient is placed in the dorsal recumbent position with knees flexed.
2. A 12.7–15.24 cm, 22-gauge needle is placed in a guide such as the Iowa trumpet, Kobak device, or Kohl's instrument, which allows the needle to extend 1–1½ cm beyond the tip.
3. The guide is placed in the lateral fornix of the vagina, and the needle is inserted through the vaginal mucosa.
4. Aspiration is done to make sure the needle is not in a blood vessel.

5. Between 5 and 10 ml of the anesthetic solution is injected.
6. The procedure is repeated on the opposite side.
7. If a continuous block is done, the plastic catheters are taped to the abdomen.

This technique provides adequate anesthesia until the patient reaches delivery, when another technique, such as pudendal block, becomes necessary.

Lumbar Sympathetic Block

Lumbar sympathetic block is used to relieve the discomfort of the first stage of labor. Like the paracervical block, it is administered during the active stage of labor when the patient is 4–6 cm dilated and having good-quality contractions. In this technique a long needle is used to inject an anesthetic agent into the lumbar portions of the sympathetic ganglionic cords that extend from the first to the fifth lumbar vertebras (see Figure 18–7). The chains lie alongside the anterior portion of the vertebras. The bilateral nerve block is simple to administer, is relatively safe, and provides good pain relief. Despite its advantages, the technique has not been popular in the United States. It is now being reintroduced into the practice of obstetric anesthesia in some parts of the country.

As with all types of conduction anesthesia, mild maternal hypotension occurs in 15%–20% of patients having a lumbar sympathetic block (Bonica, 1972). Uterine hypertonus may occur for a short period of time. An early study demonstrated conversion of abnormal uterine contractions (midsection dominance) in 75% of cases when a sympathetic block was used (Hunter, 1963). The fetus is not affected unless maternal complications develop.

Technique. Figure 18–7 shows how a lumbar sympathetic block is administered:

1. The patient is placed in a sitting position with her spine flexed.
2. The skin is prepared and left and right wheals are made at the level of the spinous process of the second lumbar vertebras.
3. A 10 cm, 22-gauge needle with a long sharp bevel is inserted through the wheal and maneuvered through the vertebral processes into the sympathetic ganglion and chain.
4. When the needle is in the proper place, the axis is at a 15° angle with the sagittal plane.
5. Aspiration is done to ensure that the needle is not within the subarachnoid space or a blood vessel.
6. Approximately 10 ml of solution is injected into the area, which is sufficient to block the chain that innervates the uterus.
7. Continuous sympathetic block may be done with specially designed needles and plastic catheters.

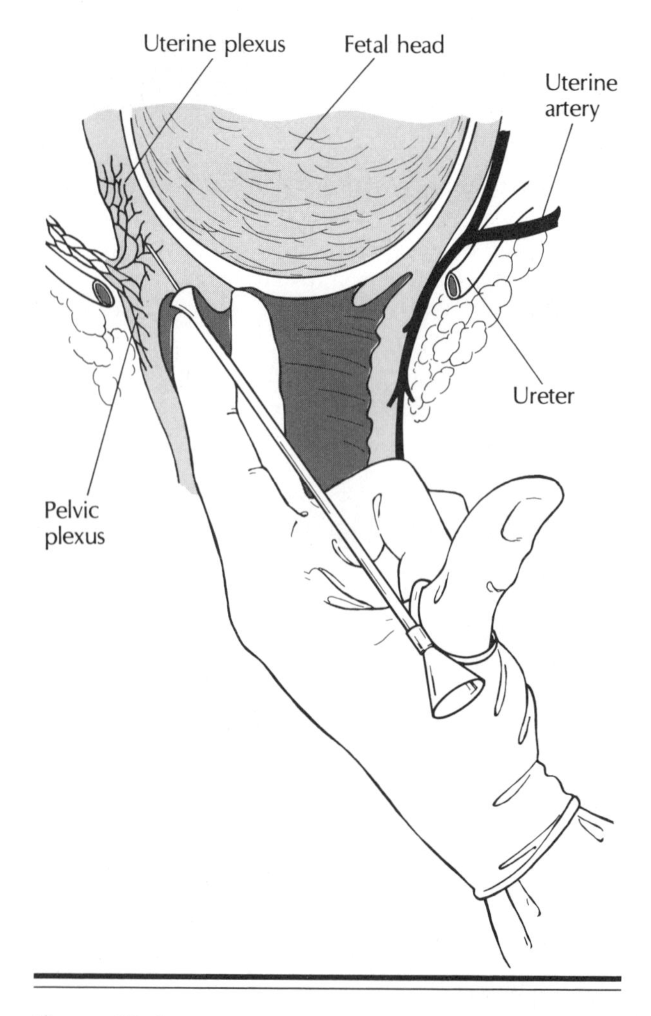

Figure 18–6. Technique for paracervical block from needle in place at appropriate distance beyond guide. (From Bonica, J. J. 1972. *Principles and practice of obstetric analgesia and anesthesia.* Philadelphia: F. A. Davis Co., p. 515.)

An injection of 1% mepivacaine or 1% lidocaine lasts approximately 1–1½ hours. The addi-

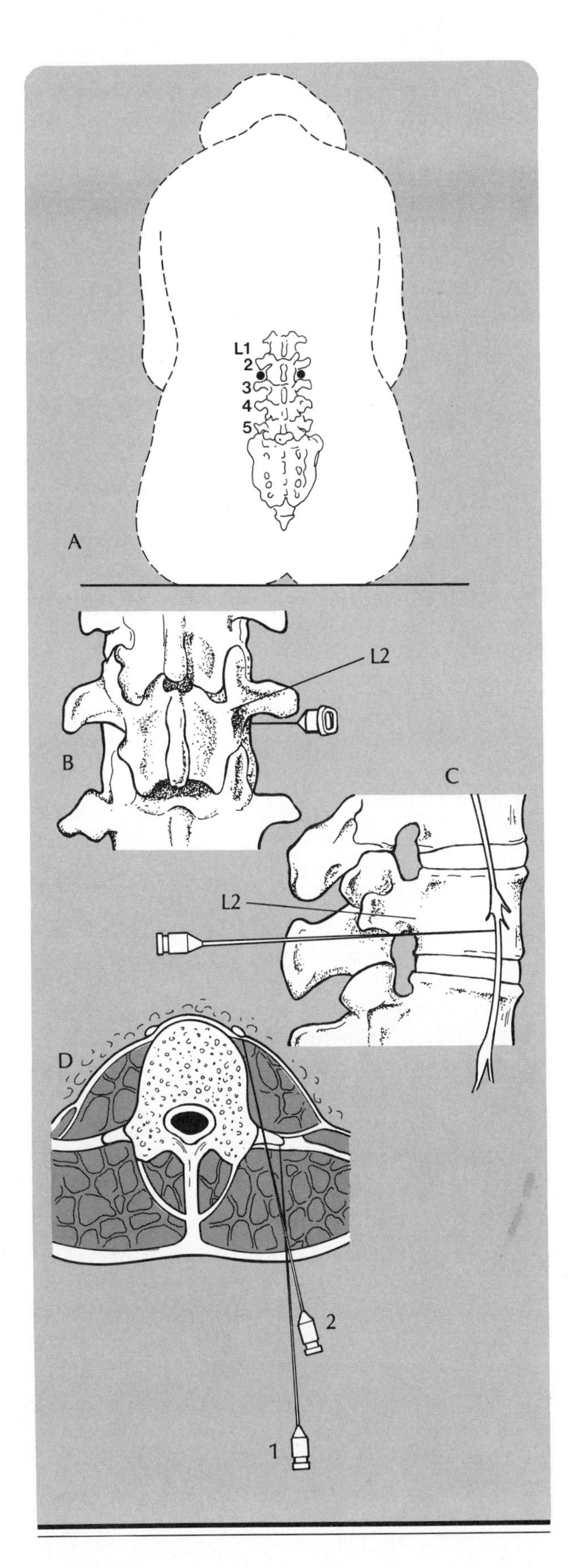

tion of 0.15% tetracaine to the solution increases the duration so that continuous administration is not necessary.

Peridural Block

Peridural anesthesia can provide pain relief throughout the entire course of labor. The peridural space (or the epidural space) is a potential space between the dura mater and the ligamentum flavum that extends from the base of the skull to the end of the sacral canal (Figure 18–8). It contains areolar tissue, fat, lymphatics, and the internal vertebral venous plexus. Access to the space may be through the lumbar or caudal area. The technique is most frequently used as a continuous block to provide analgesia and anesthesia from active labor through episiotomy repair. This method, particularly continuous lumbar epidural block, has become the obstetric anesthesia of choice in many areas of the United States (Figure 18–9).

Peridural anesthesia is advocated for premature labor and in the presence of maternal heart disease, hypertension, diabetes, and pulmonary disease (Greenhill and Friedman, 1974).

Disadvantages of peridural block are varied. Considerable skill is required for peridural techniques, and the incidence of success correlates highly with the skill and experience of the administrator. Pain relief is slower than with other methods, and a higher volume of anesthetic agent is required than for spinal anesthesia. Lumbar epidural has a slight advantage over the caudal method in that anesthesia is more rapid and a smaller volume is necessary. There are also fewer bony abnormalities in the lumbar vertebras than in the sacrum. The administrator must guard against accidental perforation of the dura mater, particularly with the lumbar epidural method, and against the injection of an epidural dose into the spinal canal, with resultant high spinal anesthesia.

Perineal relaxation is another disadvantage; it interferes with internal rotation. There is an in-

Figure 18–7. Techniques for lumbar sympathetic block. **A,** Patient in sitting position with spine reflex. **B,** Enlarged posterior view of vertebral column. **C,** Side view showing relation of needle to bones. **D,** Cross section showing two of the steps in insertion. (From Bonica, J. J. 1972. *Principles and practice of obstetric analgesia and anesthesia.* Philadelphia: F. A. Davis Co., p. 524.)

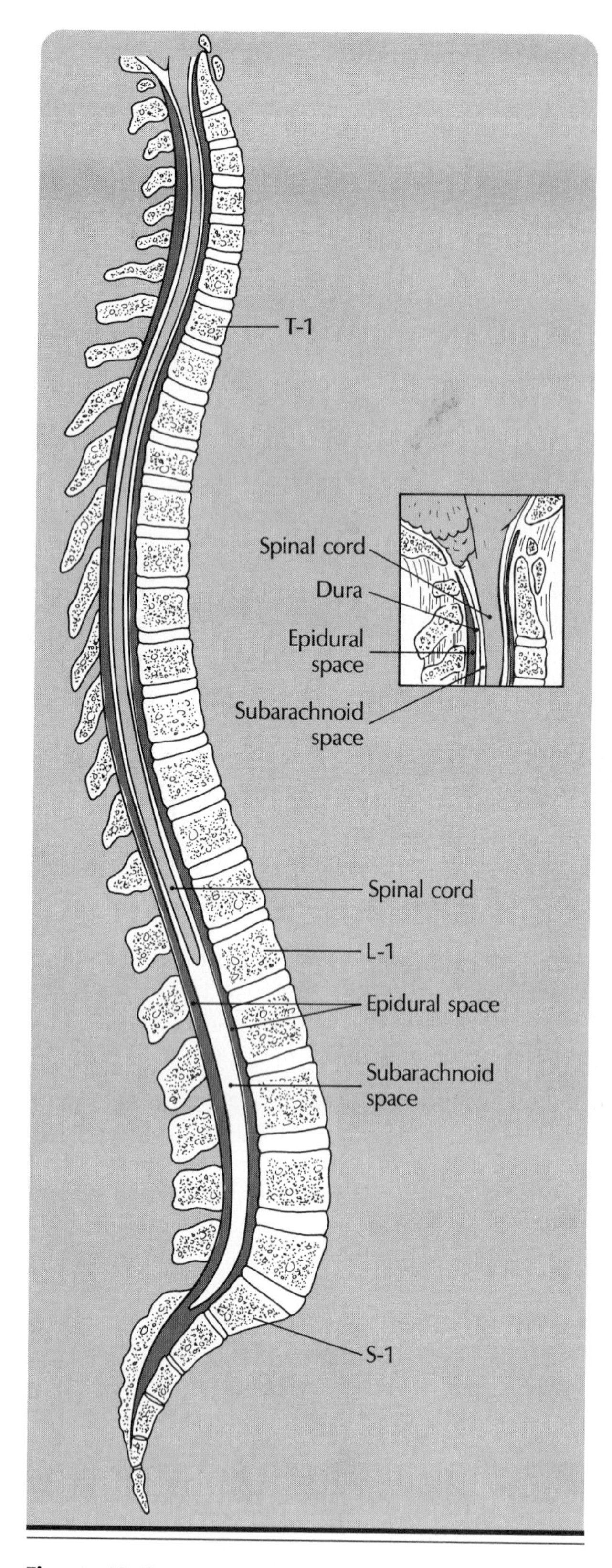

Figure 18–8. Epidural space.

crease in persistent occipital-posterior and occipital-transverse positions. The patient may also find it difficult to bear down effectively. As a result, there is an increase in operative deliveries. Schifrin (1972) has reported that fetal heart rate patterns resembling uteroplacental insufficiency occur in about 25% of the cases who have peridural anesthesia during labor. These FHR patterns are related to maternal hypotension. The incidence of late deceleration increases to 72% when maternal hypotension is present (Greenhill and Friedman, 1974). This conditon is readily corrected by administering oxygen, turning the patient on her left side, and increasing the flow rate of intravenous fluids.

Peridural anesthesia is contraindicated when hemorrhage is present or likely to occur, if there is local infection at the site of injection (such as a pilonidal cyst), and in the presence of central nervous system disease or any condition in which a convulsive seizure or hypotension might have serious effects (cardiac or pulmonary disease). It is also contraindicated when the patient is emotionally unsuited for the procedure.

Technique for Lumbar Epidural Block. The following steps must be taken in administering this type of peridural block:

1. The patient is placed on her left side, shoulders parallel, with her legs slightly flexed. The spinal column is not kept convex, as it is for a spinal, because that position reduces the peridural space to a greater degree and stretches the dura mater, making it more susceptible to puncture. (The epidural space is decreased during pregnancy because of venous engorgement. It is also smaller in obese and short individuals.)
2. The skin is prepared with an antiseptic agent.
3. A skin wheal is made to anesthetize the supraspinous and interspinous ligaments.
4. A short beveled 18-gauge needle is passed to the ligamentum flavum of the second, third, or fourth lumbar interspace (Figure 18–9). The ligamentum flavum is identified by its resistance to injection of saline or air. A rebound effect takes place.
5. Resistance disappears as the peridural space is entered.
6. Aspiration rules out penetration of a blood vessel.

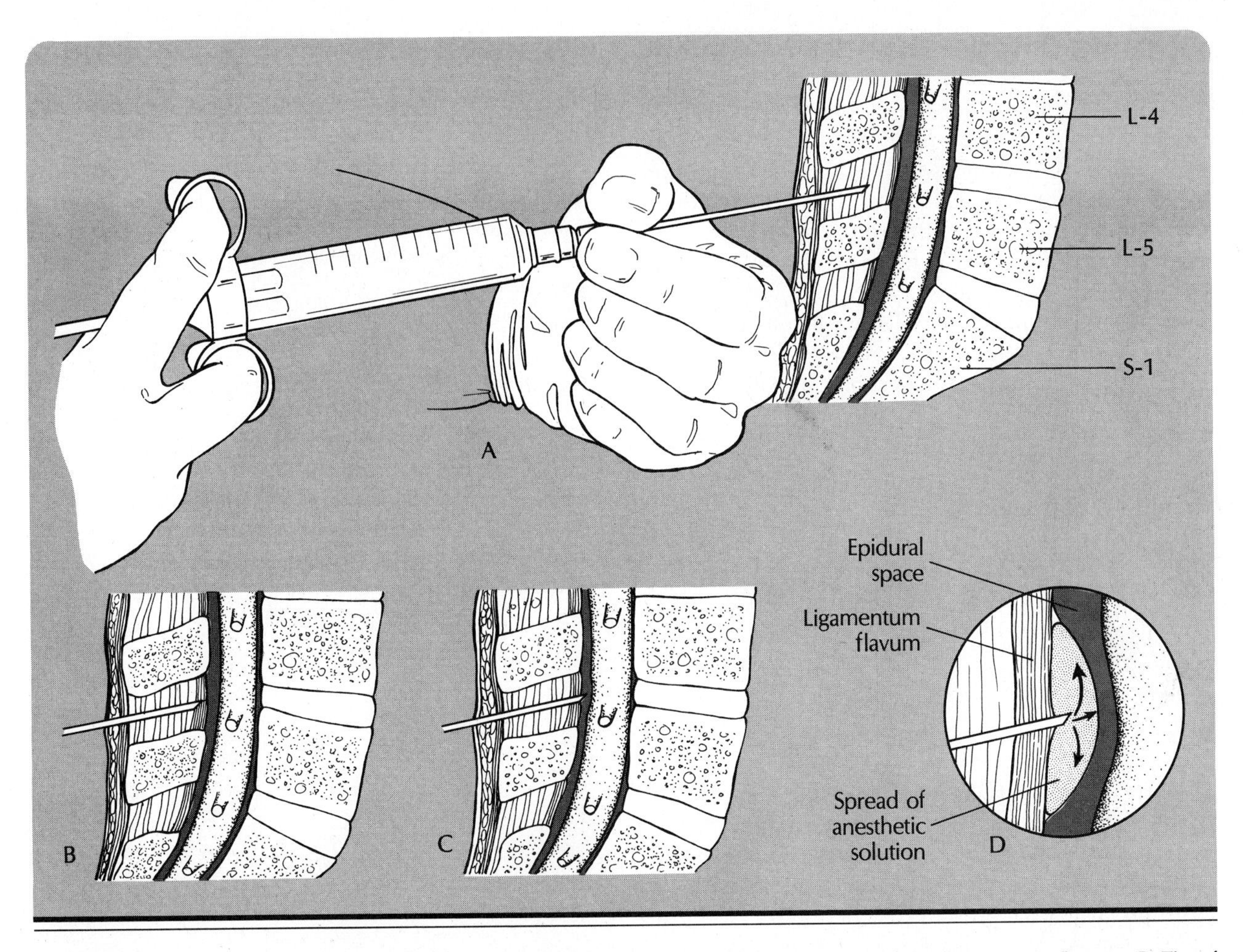

Figure 18–9. Techniques of epidural block. **A,** Proper position of insertion. **B,** Needle in the ligamentum flavum. **C,** Tip of needle in epidural space. **D,** Force of injection pushing dura away from tip of needle. (From Bonica, J. J. 1972. *Principles and practice of obstetric analgesia and anesthesia.* Philadelphia: F. A. Davis Co., p. 631.)

7. A test dose of 2–3 ml of anesthetic agent is injected.
8. A test period of at least five minutes is allowed. During this time, vital signs and levels of anesthesia are checked.
9. After checking again to make sure the dura has not been perforated, a single dose of 10–12 ml is injected to provide anesthesia for delivery.

Technique for Continuous Lumbar Epidural Block. The procedure is the same as for a lumbar epidural block through step 5, after which the following steps are taken:

6. A plastic catheter is threaded 3–5 cm beyond the tip of the needle. Hyperesthetic response in the leg, hip, or back is sometimes elicited if the soft catheter touches a nerve in the peridural space. The needle is removed. (The plastic catheter is *never* pulled back through the needle. Risk of shearing plastic catheters must be kept in mind.)
7. The catheter is taped in place.
8. A test dose of 2–3 ml of anesthetic agent is injected.
9. An analgesic dose of 5–6 ml is given for relief of uterine pain during the first stage of labor. Additional injections are made through the catheter as necessary.
10. An anesthetic dose of 10–12 ml is given just prior to delivery, with the patient sitting in an upright position.

Although any agent may be used for the epidural block, bupivacaine is preferred because each injection produces analgesia for 2½–3 hours

(Akamatsu and Bonica, 1974). A low concentration of the agent of choice is used to provide analgesia during labor, which avoids interference with internal rotation due to paralysis of the perineal muscles. Reinforcing doses should be administered before the anesthetic level has fallen considerably—otherwise tolerance to the agent and a reduction in the effectiveness of the block can occur. High concentrations are given for the "sitting dose" just prior to delivery to ensure good perineal relaxation.

After each dose of anesthetic agent, the patient must be observed constantly. Her blood pressure, pulse, and respiration should be recorded every one or two minutes. The patient should also be engaged in conversation to permit recognition of cerebral dysfunction associated with systemic toxic reaction or hypotension. For maximum safety, the fetal heart should also be monitored continuously. An example of a Nursing Care Plan for a patient receiving regional anesthesia is provided here.

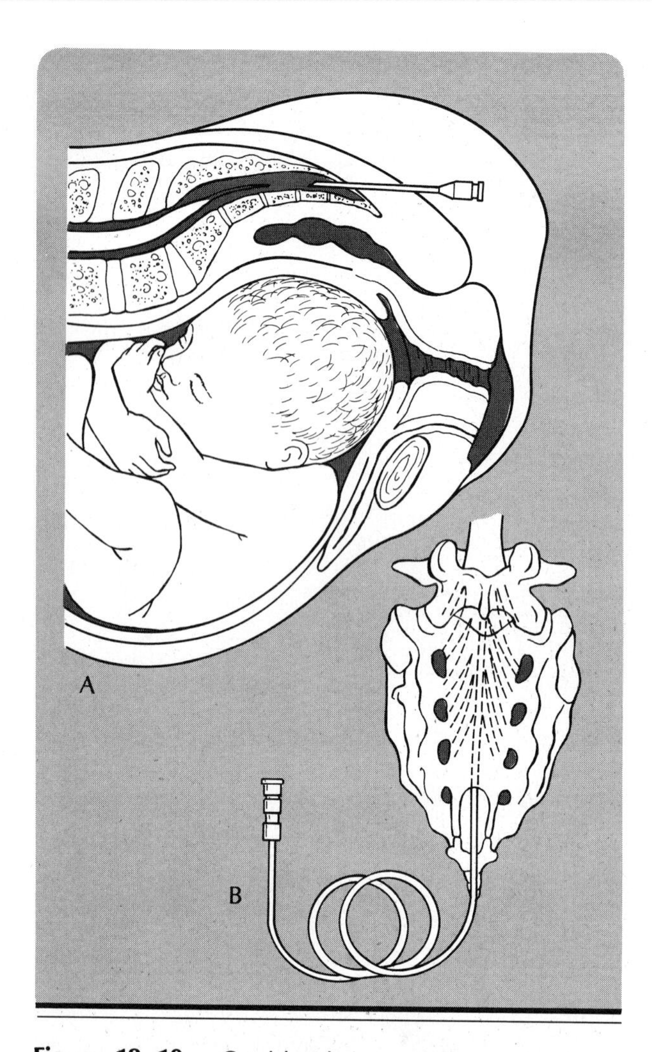

Figure 18–10. Caudal technique. **A,** Placement of needle in caudal canal. **B,** Plastic catheter in caudal canal. (From Regional Anesthesia in Obstetrics, Clinical Education Aid No. 17, Ross Laboratories, Columbus, Ohio.)

Technique for Caudal Block. The caudal approach to the peridural space was formerly a popular procedure, particularly when a catheter was used for administration of additional doses of anesthetic agent. At the lower end of the sacrum on the posterior surface of the fourth sacral vertebra is a U-shaped foramen covered by a thick layer of fibrous tissue that leads into the caudal portion of the peridural space.

The technique is as follows:

1. Although the knee-chest position makes the bony landmarks more prominent, it is most uncomfortable for the patient. A lateral Sims position is better tolerated.
2. The skin is prepared with a suitable antibacterial agent.
3. A skin wheal is raised over the sacral hiatus and into the fascia.
4. An 18-gauge thin-walled stylet for a plastic catheter needle is passed through the skin at a 70° or 80° angle into the sacral hiatus until the sacrum is reached (Figure 18–10).
5. The needle hub is depressed toward the skin at a 35° or 40° angle and advanced into the sacral canal 2–3 cm.
6. Aspiration for blood or spinal fluid is done. If spinal fluid is obtained, the procedure should be discontinued at once. If blood is obtained, the needle is advanced a short distance.
7. While palpating over the sacrum to detect crepitation from a needle that is improperly placed, 3 ml of air is rapidly injected. If major resistance to injection occurs, subperiosteal placement is indicated.
8. A test dose of 3 ml is given, and vital signs are monitored for at least five minutes. The level of hypoesthesia is also checked.
9. The agent is injected slowly into the caudal space for a single dose. A dose of 8–10 ml provides a low block affecting dermatomes S-1–S-5; 20–30 ml sensitizes spinal nerves from T-10–S-5.

NURSING CARE PLAN

Regional Anesthesia

Patient Data Base

History

1. Maternal information
   a. Allergies to drugs (specifically anesthetic agents)
   b. Psychologic status
      (1) What type anesthesia does the patient want and what kind will she accept?
      (2) Does the patient understand the procedure?
      (3) What does she expect it to accomplish?
      (4) Is the patient able to cope with the labor process and can she follow directions?
   c. Prenatal preparation and education
   d. Presence of other disease states, i.e., cardiovascular, pulmonary, and central nervous system disorders, and metabolic diseases
   e. Time at which patient last ate
2. Fetal assessment
   a. Gestational age
   b. Status
   c. Stability of FHR

Physical examination

1. Determine whether site to be used for injection is free from infection
2. Determine whether hemorrhage is present or imminent
3. Evaluate blood pressure for evidence of hypotension
4. Note evidence of URI (upper respiratory infection), which is a contraindication for general anesthesia

Laboratory evaluation

1. No specific tests required for mother
2. Fetal scalp samples may be obtained in presence of fetal distress

Nursing Priorities

1. Maintain a safe environment for maternal-fetal unit.
2. Continuously monitor maternal status to recognize and to treat potential problems.
3. Monitor fetal status.
4. Promote thorough understanding of procedure through education of both parents.

Problem	Nursing interventions and actions	Rationale
Patient's fear and anxiety	Thoroughly explain procedure, its effects, and its value to patient and significant other. Provide an opportunity for questions and discussion. Utilize charts and other teaching aides as necessary. Evaluate emotional significance of regional anesthesia to the patient and intervene appropriately.	Regional anesthesia is frequently poorly understood and frightening for patients. Thorough explanation during procedure ensures patient cooperation.
Adequate preparation for procedure	Have legal permits signed. Have patient empty bladder.	Regional anesthesia interferes with patient's urge to void.
	Begin intravenous fluids.	Intravenous fluids maintain adequate hydration and provide systemic access in the event of untoward reactions or severe hypotension.

NURSING CARE PLAN Cont'd

Regional Anesthesia

Problem	Nursing interventions and actions	Rationale
		Patients receiving subarachnoid or peridural block are to be overhydrated for 5 min prior to the procedure. Increased intravenous fluid intake decreases the possibility of maternal hypotension.
	Position patient correctly for procedure (see text for proper positioning for individual procedures).	
	Assess maternal status: 1. Obtain baseline vital signs before any anesthetic agent is given.	Baseline reading allows more complete evaluation of maternal status.
	2. Monitor blood pressure every 5 min for 30 min following administration of anesthetic agent.	Hypotension is a frequent complication of regional anesthesia.
	3. Monitor pulse and respiration.	Pulse may slow following spinal anesthesia due to decreased venous return, decreased venous pressure, and decreased right heart pressure. Respiratory paralysis is a potential complication of regional anesthesia.
	Assess fetal status: 1. Utilize fetal monitoring to establish a baseline reading of FHR and FHTs. 2. Monitor FHR continuously.	Maternal hypotension may interfere with fetal oxygenation and is evidenced by fetal bradycardia.
	Observe, record, and report complications of anesthesia, including hypotension, fetal distress, respiratory paralysis, changes in uterine contractility, decrease in voluntary muscle effort, trauma to extremities, nausea and vomiting, loss of bladder tone, and spinal headache.	
Hypotension	Observe, record, and report symptoms of hypotension, including systolic pressure <100 mg or a 25% fall in systolic pressure, apprehension, restlessness, dizziness, tinnitus, headache.	
	Institute treatment measures: 1. Place patient with head flat and foot of bed elevated.	Gravity increases venous filling of the heart and the pulmonary blood volume. The result is an increase in stroke volume and cardiac output with a rise in blood pressure.
	2. Increase IV fluid rate.	Blood volume increases and circulation improves.
	3. Administer O_2 by face mask.	Oxygen content of circulating blood increases.
	4. Administer vasopressors as ordered.	Vasoconstriction occurs. Vasopressors are not used in pregnant women unless absolutely necessary because they may further compromise the fetus.

NURSING CARE PLAN Cont'd

Regional Anesthesia

Problem	Nursing interventions and actions	Rationale
	Specific interventions for treatment of hypotension following peridural anesthesia: 1. Raise knee gatch on bed. 2. Manually displace uterus laterally to left. 3. Administer O_2 by face mask at 4-7 liters/min. 4. Increase rate of IV fluids. 5. Keep patient supine for 5-10 min following administration of block to allow drug to diffuse bilaterally. After 5-10 minutes, position patient on side.	 Increases venous return (vena cava is usually to the right). Face mask is method of choice, because woman in labor breathes through her mouth.
	Specific interventions for hypotension following spinal anesthesia: 1. Administer O_2 by face mask at 4-7 liters/min. 2. Manually displace uterus to left. 3. Increase rate of IV fluids. 4. Place legs in stirrups.	BP drops following spinal anesthesia, probably because of paralysis of the sympathetic vasoconstrictor fibers to blood vessels. Increases venous return.
Fetal distress	Observe, record, and report fetal bradycardia (FHR <120/min) and loss of beat-to-beat variability.	Maternal hypotension causes decreased blood circulation to fetus and results in fetal hypoxia.
	Institute treatment measures for maternal hypotension.	
	(Note: Paracervical blocks commonly cause a drop in FHTs for a short period of time.)	Amide group of anesthetic agents (bupivacaine, mepivacaine, and lidocaine) have potential to produce direct fetal myocardial depression. Bradycardia may be caused by reduced placental blood flow.
Respiratory paralysis and spinal blockade	Monitor respirations. If respiratory function is compromised, patient exhibits restlessness, dizziness, drowsiness, dyspnea, and an inability to speak; lapse into unconsciousness, hypotension, and apnea quickly follows. Immediate treatment includes following: 1. Support of ventilation. 2. Increase in IV fluid rate. 3. Preparation for cardiac resuscitation.	Respiratory paralysis may occur with total spinal blockade and results from too concentrated a dose (e.g., injected during a contraction) or too large a dose.
Change in uterine contractility	Monitor uterine contractions manually or electronically. If uterine contractions cease, oxytocic agent may be administered.	Anesthetic agents generally decrease uterine contractility (although increased contractility occasionally occurs). This decrease frequently prolongs labor for the patient.
Decrease in voluntary muscle effort	Monitor contractions. Coordinate patient's pushing effort with pressure of uterine contraction. Delivery by forceps may be necessary.	Loss of muscle control results in loss of ability to push. Patient does not have sensation of having contractions. Pushing without contractions decreases effectiveness and tires the mother.
Trauma to extremities	Support extremity during movement.	Regional block anesthesia produces vasomotor paralysis.

NURSING CARE PLAN Cont'd

Regional Anesthesia

Problem	Nursing interventions and actions	Rationale
	Position legs securely so they cannot fall off stirrups or delivery table.	
	Move legs slowly.	Sudden movement in patient with vasomotor paralysis may precipitate hypotensive episode.
Nausea and vomiting	Protect patient from aspiration of vomitus.	Nausea and vomiting may accompany hypotension and are related to hypoxia and excessive rise in BP following administration of vasopressor.
	Move patient slowly and gently.	Nausea and vomiting are often related to sudden changes in position.
Loss of bladder tone	Evaluate bladder distention.	Regional anesthesia reduces feeling and control of sphincter muscles.
	Insert Foley catheter if distention is present.	Full bladder during second stage of labor increases chance of bladder trauma.
Spinal headache	1. Preventive measures include: a. Use of small (25–26) gauge needle.	Spinal headache is related to the leakage of spinal fluid. A small needle permits less fluid loss.
	b. Maintenance of recumbent position for 6–12 hr following delivery.	Headache, which commonly occurs when the patient is upright, is related to decreased intracranial pressure.
	c. Adequate hydration—IV fluids during labor and delivery, oral fluids following delivery.	Aids in fluid replacement.
	2. Administer analgesics as ordered.	
	3. Use of "blood patch" for severe and incapacitating headache.	

Nursing Care Evaluation

Mother has not suffered injury.

Mother's BP, pulse, and respiration are within her normal limits.

Fetus has not been compromised. FHTs remained fairly stable.

Mother understands type of regional block administered and possible side effects.

For continuous caudal block the procedure is the same, but once the needle is placed correctly, a plastic catheter is threaded through the needle and advanced 15 cm into the caudal space (see Figure 18–10). Initially 15–30 ml is given, with reinforcement doses every 45–90 minutes.

The patient should be watched carefully for at least 20 minutes. Side effects that occur with lumbar epidural can also occur with caudal block. Accidents unique to this procedure include perforation of the rectum and of the fetal scalp.

Subarachnoid Block

In subarachnoid block, a local anesthetic agent is injected directly into the spinal fluid in the spinal canal to provide anesthesia for vaginal delivery and cesarean section. For vaginal delivery, blockade to the T-10 dermatome is usually effective, whereas cesarean section requires anesthesia to the T-8 dermatome (Figure 18–11). The term *saddle block* has been used to describe the subarachnoid block procedure used for vaginal delivery,

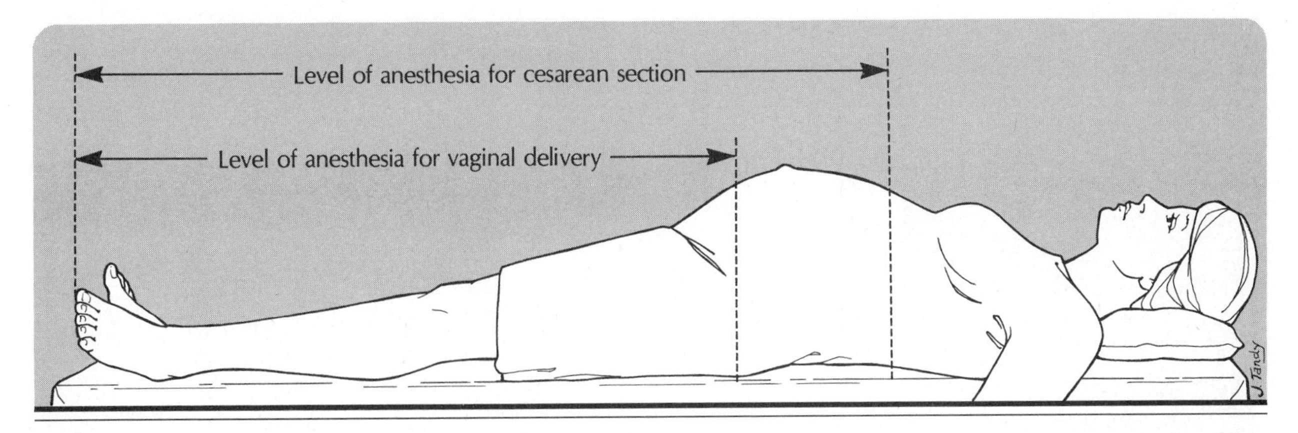

Figure 18–11. Levels of anesthesia for vaginal and cesarean section. (From Regional Anesthesia in Obstetrics, Clinical Education Aid No. 17, Ross Laboratories, Columbus, Ohio.)

but the term is incorrectly used in most cases because the area of the anesthesia is greater than the area anesthetized with a true saddle block (Pritchard and MacDonald, 1976). However, "saddle block" is a more acceptable term to the general public than "low spinal block."

The subarachnoid space is the fluid-filled area between the dura and the spinal cord. During pregnancy, the space decreases because of the distention of the epidural veins. Thus a specific dose of anesthetic produces a much higher level of anesthesia in the pregnant woman than in the nonpregnant woman. The procedure is usually done when the fetal head is on the perineum. Bearing down during the second stage of labor increases the anesthetic level higher than desired, so the injection must not be made while the patient is having a contraction.

When a low spinal is properly administered, there is a low failure rate. The disadvantages include an extremely high incidence of maternal hypotension with resultant fetal hypoxia, maternal postspinal headaches, and maintenance of uterine tone, which makes intrauterine manipulation very difficult. Spinal anesthesia is contraindicated for patients with severe hypovolemia, regardless of the cause; central nervous system disease; infection over the site of puncture; and severe hypotension or hypertension. It is also contraindicated for patients who do not wish to have spinal procedures.

Technique. The following steps are followed in administering a subarachnoid block:

1. The patient is placed in a sitting position with feet supported on a stool.
2. Intravenous infusion should be checked for patency.
3. The patient places her arms between her knees, bows her head, and arches her back to widen the intervertebral space.
4. Careful skin preparation is done, maintaining sterility.
5. A skin wheal is made over L-3 or L-4.
6. The double-needle technique is advocated (Figure 18–12). A 20- or 21-gauge needle, with stylet used as an introducer, is passed through the wheal into the interspinous ligament, ligamentum flavum, and epidural space.
7. A 25- or 26-gauge needle is inserted into the larger needle and advanced through the dura into the subarachnoid space.
8. Upon removal of the stylet, a drop of fluid can be seen in the hub of the needle if the spinal canal has been entered.
9. The appropriate amount of anesthetic agent is injected slowly, and both needles are removed.
10. With hyperbaric solutions, the patient remains sitting up for 45 seconds.
11. The patient is placed on her back with a pillow under her head. Position changes can alter the dermatome level if done within three to five minutes. After ten minutes, a position change will not affect the level of anesthesia.
12. Blood pressure, pulse, and respiration must be monitored every five minutes.

If the patient is unable to move because of motor paralysis, great care must be observed in

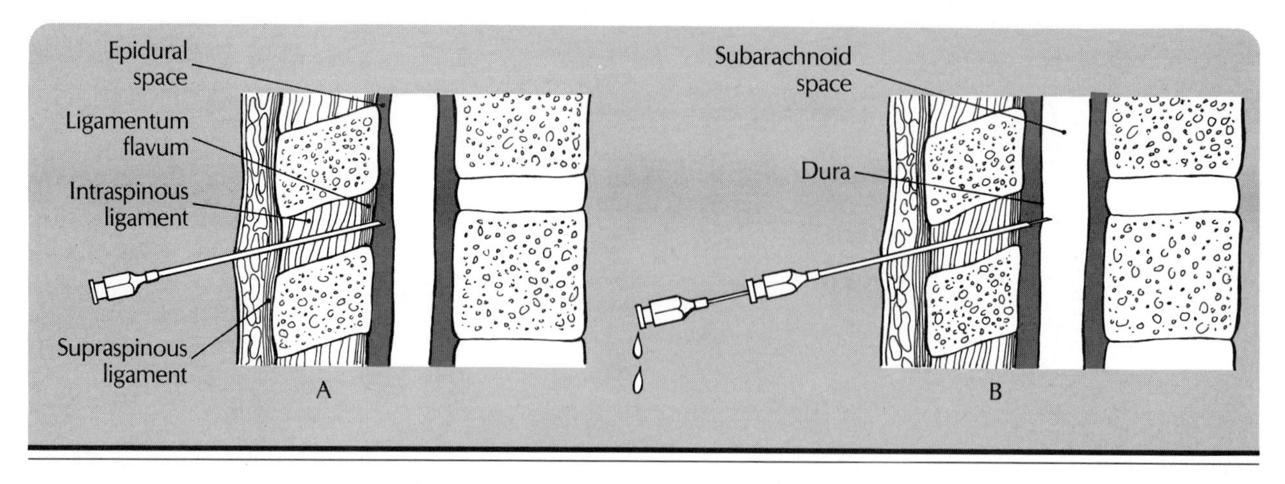

Figure 18–12. Double needle technique for spinal injection. **A,** Large needle in epidural space. **B,** 25–26 gauge needle in larger needle entering the spinal canal. (From Bonica, J. J. 1972. *Principles and practice of obstetric analgesia and anesthesia.* Philadelphia: F. A. Davis Co., p. 563.)

the lifting technique to avoid injury to the patient's muscles and ligaments. Sudden movement in any patient with vasomotor paralysis may precipitate a hypotensive episode.

Pudendal Block

The pudendal block technique provides perineal anesthesia for the latter part of the first stage, the second stage of labor, delivery, and episiotomy repair. An anesthetic agent is injected below the pudendal plexus, which arises from the anterior division of the second and third sacral nerves and the entire fourth sacral nerve. The pudendal nerve crosses the sacrosciatic notch and passes the tip of the ischial spine, where it divides into the perineal, dorsal, and inferior hemorrhoidal nerves. The perineal nerve, which is the largest branch of the pudendal plexus, supplies the skin of the vulvar area, the perineal muscles, and the urethral sphincter. The dorsal nerve supplies the clitoris, and the inferior hemorrhoidal nerve supplies the skin and muscles of the perianal region as well as the internal anal sphincter. Pudendal block provides relief of pain from perineal distention but does not relieve pain of uterine contractions.

Pudendal block is a relatively simple procedure but requires a thorough knowledge of pelvic anatomy to block the pudendal nerve adequately. A moderate dose of anesthetic agent (10 ml per side) has minimal effect on the mother and the course of labor. The urge to bear down during the second stage of labor may be eliminated, but the patient is able to do so with appropriate coaching. There is little effect on the uncompromised fetus unless overly rapid or intravascular injection occurs. The block may be done by a transvaginal or transperineal approach. Transvaginal injection is simpler, safer, and more direct, making it the procedure of choice.

Technique. A pudendal block is administered as follows:

1. The patient is placed in a lithotomy or dorsal recumbent position with the knees flexed.
2. A 12.7–15.24 cm, 22-gauge needle with guide is used to protect the vaginal wall and control needle depth.
3. The instrument is guided into the vagina until the ischial spine is reached (Figure 18–13).
4. The needle is advanced through the vaginal wall and, by the technique of individual operator preference, into the space where the pudendal nerve passes.
5. Following aspiration to make sure that the needle is not in a blood vessel, 3–5 ml of solution is injected.
6. The needle is advanced 1 cm more, aspiration is repeated, and another 3–5 ml of the agent is injected.
7. Injection of the agent into the pudendal nerve on the opposite side follows the same procedure.

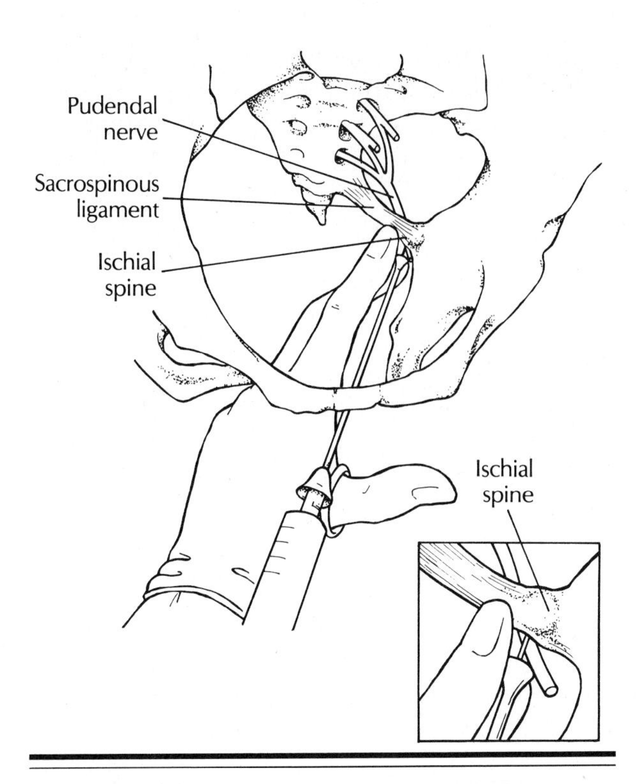

Figure 18–13. Technique for pudendal block. Inset shows needle extending beyond guide. (Modified from Bonica, J. J. 1972. *Principles and practice of obstetric analgesia and anesthesia.* Philadelphia: F. A. Davis Co., p. 495.)

Chloroprocaine, which has a low toxicity, may be used if prompt but brief anesthesia is needed. Lidocaine has prompt effect and intermediate action, whereas dibucaine has a prolonged effect. The possible complications specific to pudendal block include broad ligament hematoma, perforation of the rectum, and trauma to the sciatic nerve. Pudendal block is frequently used in conjunction with paracervical block, or it may be the sole anesthetic technique used. It is compatible with the goals of psychoprophylactic preparation for childbirth. The transvaginal technique must be done before the fetal head has advanced too far in the birth canal.

Local Anesthesia

Local anesthesia is accomplished by injection of an anesthetic agent into the intracutaneous, subcutaneous, and intramuscular areas of the perineum. It is generally used at the time of delivery for episiotomy repair and is especially useful for patients delivering by psychoprophylactic methods of childbirth. The procedure is technically simple and is practically free from complications.

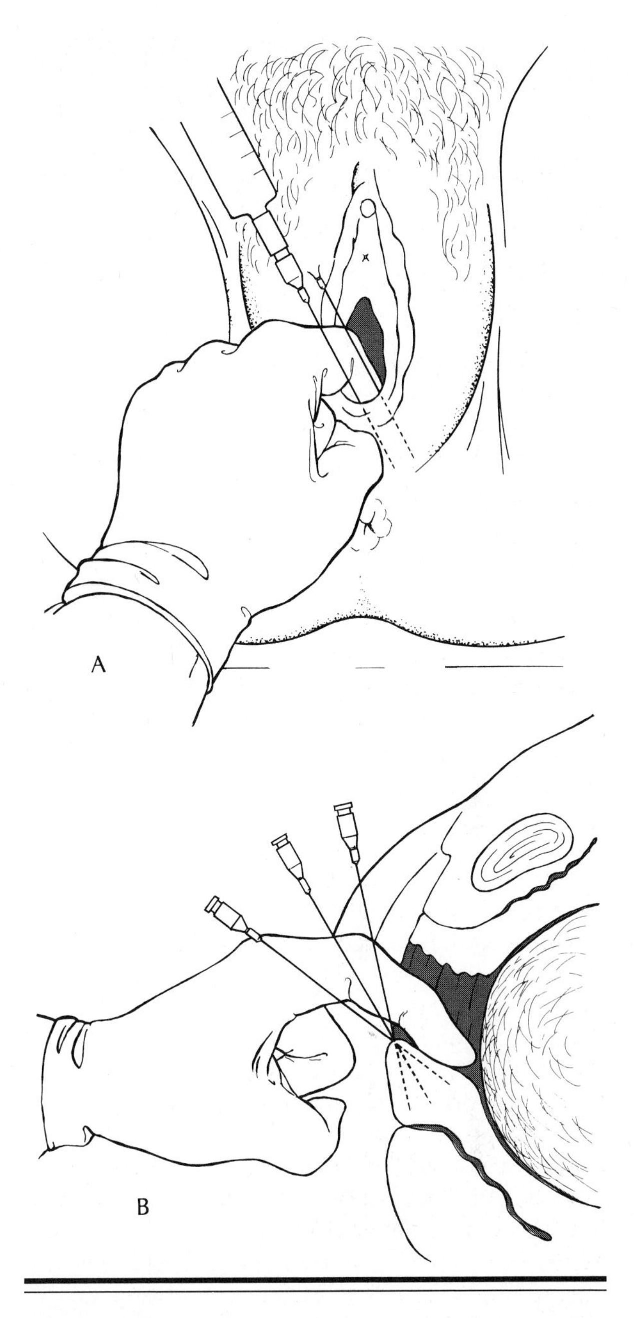

Figure 18–14. Local anesthesia. **A,** Technique of local infiltration for episiotomy and repair. **B,** Technique of local infiltration showing fan pattern for the fascial planes. (From Bonica, J. J. 1972. *Principles and practice of obstetric analgesia and anesthesia.* Philadelphia: F. A. Davis Co., p. 505.)

A disadvantage is that large amounts of solution must be used. Although any local anesthetic may be used, chloroprocaine, lidocaine, and mepivacaine are the agents of choice in local infiltration because of their capacity for diffusion.

The technique consists of injecting the agent with a long, sharp, beveled 22-gauge needle into the various fascial planes of the perineum (Figure 18–14). The procedure is deceptively simple; however, overdose may occur because the anesthetist does not wait for the anesthetic to take effect before injecting more solution. An excessive volume or concentration contributes to systemic toxic reactions and local toxic effects (Greenhill and Friedman, 1974).

Complications of Regional Anesthesia

Hypotension

Anesthetic agents interrupt the preganglionic segments, causing vasodilatation and a decrease in peripheral resistance. There is actual dilatation of peripheral veins and venules, with pooling of blood. This condition, combined with loss of muscular "milking" action on the veins (because of paralysis of skeletal muscles in the lower extremities), leads to a decrease in venous pressure. The decreased peripheral resistance and venous return lead to a decrease in cardiac output, and the blood pressure falls.

The aim of treatment is to reestablish normal tissue perfusion, which can be accomplished by increasing cardiac output, raising tissue perfusion pressure and flow, and increasing blood oxygen content.

Meningitis and Arachnoiditis

These complications have become very rare with strict aseptic technique. Chemical irritation has been virtually eliminated with the use of single-dose disposable equipment.

Postspinal Headache

Although much less serious than other complications, headache is an unpleasant aftermath of spinal anesthesia. Leakage of spinal fluid at the site of dural puncture is thought to be the cause. Several techniques have been suggested to decrease the possibility of headache. The use of a 25- or 26-gauge needle and avoidance of multiple perforations of the dura reduce the incidence. Hyperhydration and keeping the patient flat in bed for 6–12 hours after delivery have been recommended as preventive measures, but there is no evidence that these procedures are effective (Pritchard and MacDonald, 1976). Not all postpartal headaches in patients who had spinal anesthesia are a result of the procedure.

The postspinal headache usually begins on the second postpartal day and lasts one to three days. It may be of varying degrees of severity. The pain occurs or becomes worse when the patient sits or stands and decreases or ceases when the patient lies down or flexes and extends her head (Bonica, 1972).

Treatment consists primarily of bed rest and analgesics for the mild or moderate forms. Severe and incapacitating headache has been treated recently by a "blood patch" over the site of dural puncture. About 10 ml of blood is drawn from the patient and immediately injected into the epidural space over the site of the perforation; the clot applies pressure and seals off the leak. In many cases, this procedure has dramatically relieved symptoms. Injection of saline in larger volumes has also been claimed to provide relief.

SUMMARY

The complications that may occur during obstetric anesthesia are serious. Anyone who performs these procedures should be proficient in preventing, detecting, and managing all possible complications. Nursing personnel in labor and delivery suites must have a thorough understanding of anesthetic techniques, because nurses provide continual and direct care to patients and because the early detection of an incipient complication contributes to the success of medical management.

Psychoprophylactic preparation for childbirth has increased the use of regional procedures for delivery and episiotomy repair. There is every indication that this trend is increasing in popularity. The regional techniques are not without maternal and fetal hazards, however.

According to Bonica (1972), "High quality analgesic and anesthetic management requires observation of the five cardinal C's: Communication, Coordination, Cooperation, Courtesy, and (sometimes) Compromise by every member of the obstetric team." It is obvious that certain safeguards are required for the maximum protection of the mother and fetus. These include (a) continuing education in obstetric analgesia and anesthesia for physicians and nurses; (b) better communication and cooperation among obstetricians, anesthesia personnel, nurses, and pediatricians; (c) establishment of department protocol for the administration of regional procedures, with input from all members of the obstetric team; and (d) the procurement of all equipment necessary to provide safe and effective obstetric anesthesia.

SUGGESTED ACTIVITIES

1. In a small group, compare your feelings and perceptions about the nature of pain. Share with one another approaches you personally find helpful in alleviating pain.
2. Arrange with your instructor to observe the administration of general anesthesia to obstetric patients. Note the reactions of the patient, and attempt to identify the stages through which your patient passes.
3. Formulate drug cards containing pertinent information about analgesics you may administer to a patient in labor.

REFERENCES

Akamatsu, T. J., and Bonica, J. J. June 1974. Spinal and extradural analgesia-anesthesia for parturition. *Clin. Obstet. Gynecol.* 17:2.

Bauer, R. O. 1971. Obstetrical analgesia and anesthesia and resuscitation of neonates. *Int. Anesthesiol. Clin.* 9:77.

Benson, R. C. 1974. *Handbook of obstetrics and gynecology.* 5th ed. Los Altos, Calif.: Lange Medical Publications.

Bonica, J. J. 1972. *Principles and practice of obstetric analgesia and anesthesia.* Philadelphia: F. A. Davis Co.

Bruegel, M. A. 1971. Relationships of post-operative anxiety to perceptions of postoperative pain. *Nurs. Res.* 20:26.

Clark, A. L., and Affonso, D.D. 1976. *Childbearing: a nursing perspective.* Philadelphia: F. A. Davis Co.

Danforth, D. 1977. *Textbook of obstetrics and gynecology.* 3rd ed. New York: Harper & Row Publishers, Inc.

Dundee, J. W., et al. Dec. 1974. Plasma-diazepam levels following intramuscular injections by nurses and doctors. *Lancet.* 2:1461.

Ettiger, B., and McCant, D. Sept.-Oct. 1976. Effects of drugs on the fetal heart rate during labor. *J. Obstet. Gynecol. Nurs.* 5:3.

Greenhill, J. P., and Friedman, E. A. 1974. *Biological principles and modern practice of obstetrics.* Philadelphia: W. B. Saunders Co.

Greiss, F. C., et al. 1976. Effects of local anesthetic agents on the uterine vasculatures and myometrium. *Am. J. Obstet. Gynecol.* 124:8.

Hunter, C. A. 1963. Uterine motility studies during labor: observations on bilateral sympathetic nerve block in the normal and abnormal first stage of labor. *Am. J. Obstet. Gynecol.* 85:681.

Jagerhorn, M. 1975. Paracervical block in obstetrics: an improved injection method. *Acta Obstet. Gynecol. Scand.* 52:13.

Janis, I. L. 1958. *Psychological stress.* New York: John Wiley & Sons, Inc.

Jensen, M. J., et al. 1977. *Maternity care: the nurse and the family.* St. Louis: The C. V. Mosby Co.

Livingston, W. K. 1943. *Pain mechanisms.* New York: The Macmillan Co.

Lockett, C. 1939. Midwives and childbirth among the Navajo. *Plateau* (Northern Arizona Society of Science and Art). 12:15.

McCaffery, M. 1972. *Nursing management of the patient with pain.* Philadelphia: J. B. Lippincott Co.

McCammon, C. S. 1951. Study of 475 pregnancies in American Indian women. *Am. J. Obstet. Gynecol.* 61:1159.

Melzack, R. 1973. *The puzzle of pain.* New York: Basic Books, Inc.

Moore, D. C. 1967. *Regional block.* 4th ed. Springfield, Ill.: Charles C Thomas, Publisher.

Moore, M. L. 1972. *The newborn and the nurse.* Philadelphia: W. B. Saunders Co.

Moya, F. Dec. 1974; Jan. 1975; Feb. 1975. Obstetric analgesia and anesthesia. Parts I, II, III. *Anesthesiol. Rev.*

Newton, N. June 1964. Some aspects of primitive childbirth. *J.A.M.A.* 188:10.

Pritchard, J. A., and MacDonald, P. C. 1976. *Williams obstetrics.* 15th ed. New York: Appleton-Century-Crofts.

Raum, O. F. 1940. *Chagga childhood.* London: Oxford University Press.

Schifrin, B. S. April 1972. Fetal heart rate patterns following epidural anaesthesia and oxytocin infusion during labour. *J. Obstet. Gynaecol. Br. Commonw.* 79:332.

Snider, S. M., and Moya, F. Aug. 1964. Effects of meperidine on the newborn infant. *Am. J. Obstet. Gynecol.* 36:1011.

Yaffee, S. J., and Catz, C. S. Sept. 1971. Pharmacology of the perinatal period. *Clin. Obstet. Gynecol.* 14:725.

ADDITIONAL READINGS

Bean, C. A. 1974. *Methods of childbirth.* New York: Dolphin Books.

Bonica, J. J. 1974. Acupuncture anesthesia in the Peoples' Republic of China: implications for modern medicine. *JAMA.* 229:1317.

Bradley, R. A. 1974. *Husband-coached childbirth.* New York: Harper & Row Publishers, Inc.

Brown, W. U., et al. July 1976. Acidosis, local anesthetics and the newborn. *Am. J. Obstet. Gynecol.* 48:1.

deJong, R. H., and Wagner, I. H. 1963. Physiological mechanism of peripheral nerve block by local anesthesia. *Anesthesiology.* 24:684.

DeLyser, F. 1973. *A professional's guide to prepared childbirth.* Washington, D.C.: American Society for Prophylaxis in Obstetrics.

Dick-Read, G. 1972. *Childbirth without fear.* New York: Harper & Row Publishers, Inc.

Fisher, D., and Paton, J. 1974. The effect of maternal anesthetic and analgesic drugs on the fetus and newborn. *Clin. Obstet. Gynecol.* 17:275.

Floyd, C. C. May 1977. Drugs for childbirth: your guide to their risks and benefits. *RN.* 5:41.

Grad, R. K., and Woodside, J. Feb. 1977. Obstetrical analgesics and anesthesia: methods of relief for the patient in labor. *Am. J. Nurs.* 2:242.

Karmel, M. 1959. *Thank you, Doctor Lamaze.* Philadelphia: J. B. Lippincott Co.

Kitzinger, S. 1973. *Experience of childbirth.* Baltimore: Penguin Books.

Kroger, W. S. 1965. *Childbirth with hypnosis.* North Hollywood, Calif.: Wilshire Book Co.

Lamaze, F. 1972. *Painless childbirth: the Lamaze method.* New York: Pocket Books.

McDonald, J., et al. 1974. Epidural analgesia for obstetrics: a maternal, fetal and neonatal study. *Am. J. Obstet. Gynecol.* 120:1055.

Niswander, K. R. 1976. *Obstetrics: essentials of clinical practice.* Boston: Little, Brown & Co.

Oxorn, H., and Foote, W. R. 1975. *Human labor and birth.* 3rd ed. New York: Appleton-Century-Crofts.

Pilliteri, A. 1976. *Nursing care of the growing family: a maternal-newborn text.* Boston: Little, Brown & Co.

Reeder, S. R., et al. 1976. *Maternity nursing.* 13th ed. Philadelphia: J. B. Lippincott Co.

Roberts, F. B. 1977. *Perinatal nursing: care of newborns and their families.* New York: McGraw-Hill Book Co.

Ruder, S., et al. 1976. The nurses' contribution to pain relief during labor. In *Maternity nursing,* ed. M. McCaffery. 13th ed. Philadelphia: J. B. Lippincott Co.

Wallis, L., et al. 1974. An evaluation of acupuncture analgesia in obstetrics. *Anesthesiology.* 41:596.

Wright, E. 1966. *The new childbirth.* New York: Hart Publishing Co., Inc.

CHAPTER 19

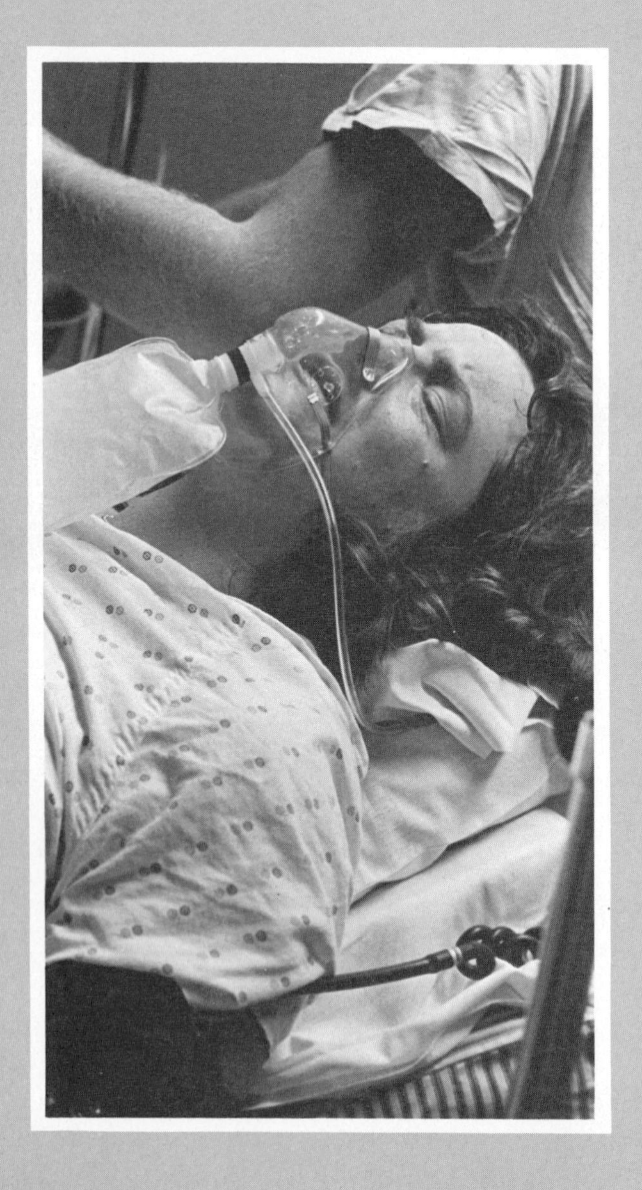

COMPLICATIONS OF LABOR AND DELIVERY

OBJECTIVES

- Describe the psychologic factors that may contribute to complications during labor and delivery.
- Define the term *dystocia*.
- Compare hyperactive labor patterns with hypoactive labor patterns.
- Briefly describe the appearance of a tracing of the maternal contractions in a patient with hypotonic uterine motility.
- Discuss the general nursing interventions indicated for a laboring patient who is hemorrhaging.
- List factors that may contribute to the onset of premature labor.
- Identify the warning signs and symptoms of impending uterine rupture.
- Delineate factors that may contribute to inversion of the uterus.
- Relate deviations that may occur in a "normal labor" to types of malposition of the fetus.
- List the types of malpresentation that result in dystocia associated with the passenger.
- Describe two accepted methods of vaginally delivering a fetus in breech presentation.
- Briefly describe nursing care for mother and infant in the event of fetal macrosomia.
- Relate the occurrence of multiple gestation to commonly occurring maternal-fetal-neonatal complications.
- Discuss the nursing care that is indicated in the event of fetal distress.
- Compare abruptio placentae and placenta previa.
- Define the terms used to identify developmental problems of the placenta.
- Identify, in order of priority, appropriate nursing actions in caring for the mother and fetus in the event of prolapse of the umbilical cord.
- List factors that contribute to the diagnosis of hydramnios during a pregnancy.
- Discuss the effects of a complicated childbirth on the involved family.

The successful completion of the 40-week gestational period requires the harmonious functioning of four components: the passenger, passage, powers, and psyche. (These components are described in depth in Chapter 15.) Briefly, the passenger includes all the products of conception: the fetus, placenta, cord, membranes, and amniotic fluid. The passage comprises the vagina, introitus, and bony pelvis, and the powers are the myometrial forces of the contracting uterus. The psyche is the intellectual and emotional processes of the mother as influenced by heredity and environment and includes her feelings about pregnancy and motherhood.

Disruptions of the passenger, passage, and psyche may be reflected in the functioning of the powers. If there is any cessation or slowing of dilatation, effacement, and descent, the other three components should be carefully assessed.

COMPLICATIONS INVOLVING THE PSYCHE

Stress, anxiety, and fear have a profound effect on the mother. Dick-Read (1972) proposed that "fear equals tension equals pain" in labor. He sought to relieve the pain by reduction of the fear and tension through controlled breathing exercises and education (Chapter 12). Others have reported that labor is lengthened in the scared, tense mother (Erickson, 1976). The physiologic subsystem may in fact become disrupted in the presence of fear and anxiety.

Erickson (1976) reported that the following complications can result in the mother's fear for herself and for her baby and in fear of dependency:

1. Uterine inertia.
2. Prolonged first stage of labor.
3. Prolonged second stage of labor.
4. Rotation of the infant's head.
5. Indicated low forceps.
6. Apgar scores of less than 5.
7. Apgar scores of 5 to 7.

It was noted in this study that many of these factors are interrelated.

Stress produces neural and endocrine responses. The liver releases glucose to satisfy the body's increased energy needs. The bronchial tree dilates for increased oxygen intake, and the anterior pituitary is stimulated, which results in an increase in production of glucocorticoids and mineralocorticoids by the adrenal cortex. These hormones promote the retention of sodium and the excretion of potassium and also stimulate the posterior pituitary to release antidiuretic hormone for the conservation of water. The loss of potassium is postulated to assist in the reduction of myometrial activity. The reduction of glucose stores from stress and anxiety can drain the stores needed for the contracting uterus (Assali, 1972).

The sympathetic nervous system stimulates the adrenal medulla, resulting in the secretion of epinephrine, which increases the heart rate, cardiac output, and blood pressure. The sympathetic nervous system also stimulates the adrenals to release norepinephrine, which increases peripheral vasoconstriction and the blood flow to the vital organs. This physiologic reaction can adversely affect the contracting uterus. The uterus responds to α excitatory and β inhibitory effects of epinephrine. Through baroceptor stimulation, epinephrine inhibits myometrial activity (β receptors). Norepinephrine stimulates the α excitatory receptors. The uterine musculature is then stimulated (Reid et al., 1972).

The anxiety, fear, and laboring pain experienced by the parturient may produce a vicious cycle, resulting in increased fear and anxiety because of continued central pain perception. This leads to enhanced catecholamine release, which in turn increases physical distress and results in myometrial dysfunction. Ineffectual labor and myometrial dysfunction may occur, especially when epinephrine is the predominant substance released (Assali, 1972).

Interventions. Antepartal classes provide education about the developmental and psychologic changes that can be expected during childbirth. Couples learn coping mechanisms in the form of physical and emotional comfort measures, controlled breathing exercises, and relaxation techniques.

Unprepared couples can be taught many of these activities at the time of admission to the delivery room, especially if active labor has not begun. Information about the labor process, medical procedures, the environment, simple breathing exercises, and relaxation techniques can be given, thereby relieving some apprehension and fear. Even a mother in active labor who has had no prior preparation can achieve a good deal of relaxation from physical comfort measures, touch, constant attendance, and possibly pharmacologic support.

If the laboring woman is suffering from complications such as those previously listed, the nurse should try to determine whether fear and stress are causative factors. Support measures can then be instituted to alleviate the psychologic distress, which will be helpful in relieving the physical distress.

COMPLICATIONS INVOLVING THE POWERS

Bonica (1967) describes four basic contractile systems:

1. The energy source adenosine triphosphate (ATP).
2. The ionic exchange of electrolytes: sodium (the major extracellular electrolyte), potassium (the major intracellular electrolyte), and calcium, which is bound to the cell membrane and renders the cell stable and resting.
3. The contractile proteins: negatively charged actin and myosin.
4. The endocrine sources: epinephrine, norepinephrine, acetylcholine, oxytocin, and prostaglandins.

These four systems must interact for effective labor to occur. Any disruption in the interaction of these four systems may result in ineffective, dysfunctional labor.

Dysfunctional labor is referred to as *dystocia.* Dystocia causes a delay in the delivery of the infant and is due to problems with the mechanisms of parturition. Dystocia can have a profound effect on the mother as well as the fetus. Prolonged labor of over 24 hours' duration is associated with an increase in maternal and infant mortality, usually resulting from infection.

Fetal problems caused by dystocia include (a) fetal hypoxia; (b) bone fractures, especially of the skull, shoulders, and clavicles; (c) internal hemorrhage; and (d) neurologic damage from compression. Friedman et al. (1977) conducted a study on the effects of dysfunctional labor on the fetus and infant. They demonstrated a significant increase in perinatal mortality. At eight months of age, there was a greater incidence of motor developmental abnormalities in infants born to mothers who experienced dysfunctional labor. This finding was not verified when the children were one year of age.

General Principles of Nursing Intervention

The nurse can identify patients who have the potential for labor dysfunction by assessing the adequacy of their contractile system and by determining the source of any imbalance or disruption. Nursing interventions are directed toward restoring or maintaining the proper functioning and interactions of the physiologic components of labor as follows:

1. *Fluid-electrolyte imbalance and inadequate glucose level.* Exhaustion associated with prolonged labor can decrease the energy source, resulting in inadequate glucose replacement or diabetic hypoglycemia. Electrolyte imbalances may be caused by vomiting or profuse perspiration, both of which are common occurrences during labor. Intravenous fluids containing electrolytes and glucose are often recommended, because oral fluids are poorly tolerated in labor. The nurse can screen the maternal urine for ketones. Women with dehydration and ketosis exhibit an increase in pulse rate and temperature, a fruity odor of the breath, and a rise in the hematocrit. The diabetic mother may need increased amounts of insulin for the utilization of the glucose.

2. *Imbalance in the contractile proteins.* This situation can occur in a number of medical disorders,

such as anemia, pregnancy-induced hypertension (preeclampsia), and kidney disease. In preeclampsia and kidney disease, proteins are lost because of damage to the renal tubules from the disease processes. The nurse can effectively help to lessen these potential problems through early prenatal counseling. Interventions may include dietary counseling, encouragement of adequate prenatal care, and early detection of problems. In addition, the nurse can encourage the mother to rest in a lateral position to increase uterine and kidney perfusion.

3. *Endocrine imbalance.* Epinephrine-norepinephrine imbalances may result from anxiety, stress, fear, or pain. Nursing interventions are aimed at relieving discomfort and at meeting the patient's psychologic needs. Teaching appropriate breathing and relaxation techniques, administering analgesic or anesthetic agents, positioning the patient, and communicating clearly and sympathetically are helpful nursing measures that can reduce the patient's fears and discomfort.

In general, nursing actions are aimed toward resolving the physiologic imbalances that can affect the powers. However, the nurse must be able to identify the complications that result from these imbalances. In the following pages, specific conditions involving the powers are examined in terms of their effects on the mother and child, and specific nursing and medical interventions are described.

Dysfunctional Labor Patterns

The two major types of dysfunctional labor patterns are hyperactive and hypoactive labor. In hyperactive labor patterns, contractions are too strong, resulting in progression that is too rapid. In hypoactive labor patterns, contractions are ineffective in dilating the cervix and propelling the infant.

Hyperactive Labor Patterns

There are two types of hyperactive labor patterns (Figure 19–1). In the first type, uterine contractility increases in intensity and frequency. Myometrial contractions exert pressures of 50–70 mm Hg, and the frequency of contractions is greater than five in a ten-minute period (Assali, 1972). The second type is a myometrial tachysystole with only increased frequency. Both these labor patterns may result in a precipitous delivery.

Possible causes of hyperactive labor and delivery are (a) multiparity, (b) large pelvis, (c) lax, unresistant maternal soft tissues, and (d) a small baby in a favorable position. One or more of these factors, plus strong contractions, result in a rapid transit of the infant through the birth canal (Pritchard and MacDonald, 1976). In addition, hyperactive labor may be caused by oxytocin overdose, which can occur during induction of labor (Chapter 20). In this case, dysfunctional labor is caused by medical error.

Maternal Implications. If the cervix is effaced and the maternal soft tissues are not resistant to stretching, maternal complications may be few. However, if the cervix is not ripe (soft) and the maternal soft tissues are resistant, lacerations of the cervix, vagina, perineum, and periuretheral area may occur, because the tissues do not stretch adequately. There is also a possibility of uterine rupture. When resistance is present, amniotic fluid embolism may occur (p. 594). The mother is also at risk for postpartal hemorrhage due to expanded uterine fibers (Pritchard and MacDonald, 1976).

Fetal-neonatal Implications. Decreased periods of uterine relaxation result in fetal hypoxia and hypercarbia. Clinically, an acidotic fetus demonstrates decreased beat-to-beat variability and eventually bradycardia. Vagal stimulation is elicited through hypoxic brain tissues, which causes the bradycardia. The same vagal stimulation causes an increase in intestinal motility, resulting in release of meconium in utero (Paul and Petrie, 1973).

Any resistance of the maternal soft tissues to the fetal head, as can occur in precipitous labor, may cause cerebral trauma to the infant. If the birth is unattended and unassisted, the newborn infant may suffer from lack of care in the first few minutes of life. Suffocation and aspiration are possible complications (Paul and Petrie, 1973).

Interventions. During the intrapartal nursing assessment, the labor patient who is at risk for hyperactive labor can be identified. The presence of any of the following factors may indicate potential problems:

1. Previous history of rapid labor.

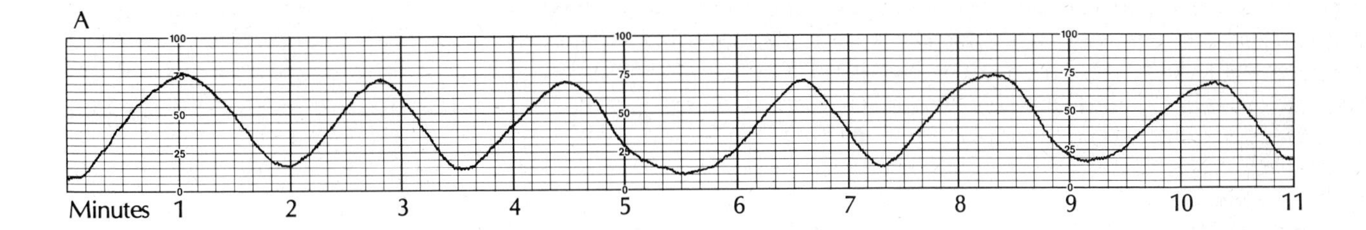

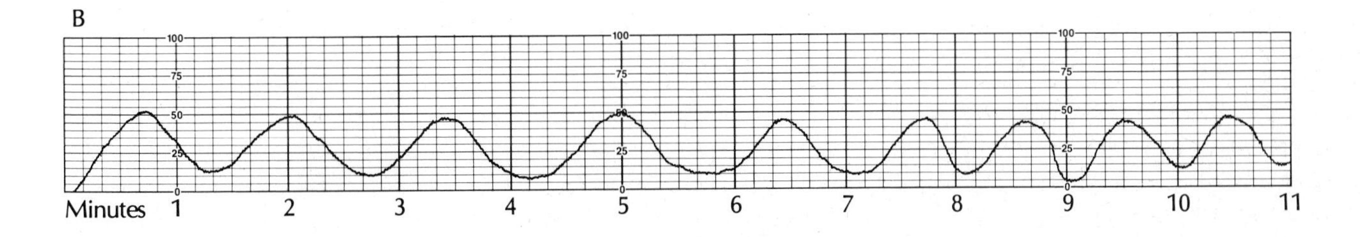

Figure 19–1. **A,** Hyperactive labor. **B,** Myometrial tachysystole.

2. Abnormal findings on the Friedman graph.
3. Uterine contractile patterns in which there is no uterine relaxation between contractions.
4. Pain that seems out of proportion to the contractions.

If the patient has a history of precipitous delivery, she should be closely monitored, and an emergency delivery pack should be close at hand. The physician should be informed of any unusual findings on the Friedman graph. Comfort and rest may be promoted by assisting the patient to a comfortable position, providing a quiet environment, and administering sedative as needed.

Drugs that suppress labor also suppress fetal bodily functions. General anesthetics and other drugs such as magnesium sulfate have been used in cases of hyperactive labor. The benefits and effectiveness of these agents are questionable.

If the mother is receiving oxytocin, it should be discontinued immediately and the mother turned on her left side to improve uterine perfusion. Oxygen may be started to increase the available oxygen in the maternal circulating blood; this increases the amount available for exchange at the placental site.

The ensuing delivery may be slowed by having the mother pant or blow with contractions. This method can be taught to the unprepared mother before active labor begins. It is also helpful for the nurse to breathe with the mother during this time. If delivery is imminent, the nurse can proceed with the emergency delivery procedure (Chapter 21).

In case of oxytocin overdosage during induction of labor, nursing intervention includes constant attendance, electronic monitoring of contractions, palpation of the intensity of contractions if the external monitor is used, and strict control of the infusion rate with an infusion pump.

The nurse should never attempt to stop a delivery by holding the mother's legs together. This may cause trauma to the infant's head.

For nursing interventions in the event of fetal distress, see the Nursing Care Plan on p. 582.

Hypoactive Labor Patterns

Hypoactive labor is prolonged, protracted, or arrested (Figure 19–2) and is manifested in the following ways (Greenhill and Friedman, 1974):

1. *Prolonged latent phase.* Active cervical dilatation has not begun more than 20 hours after the

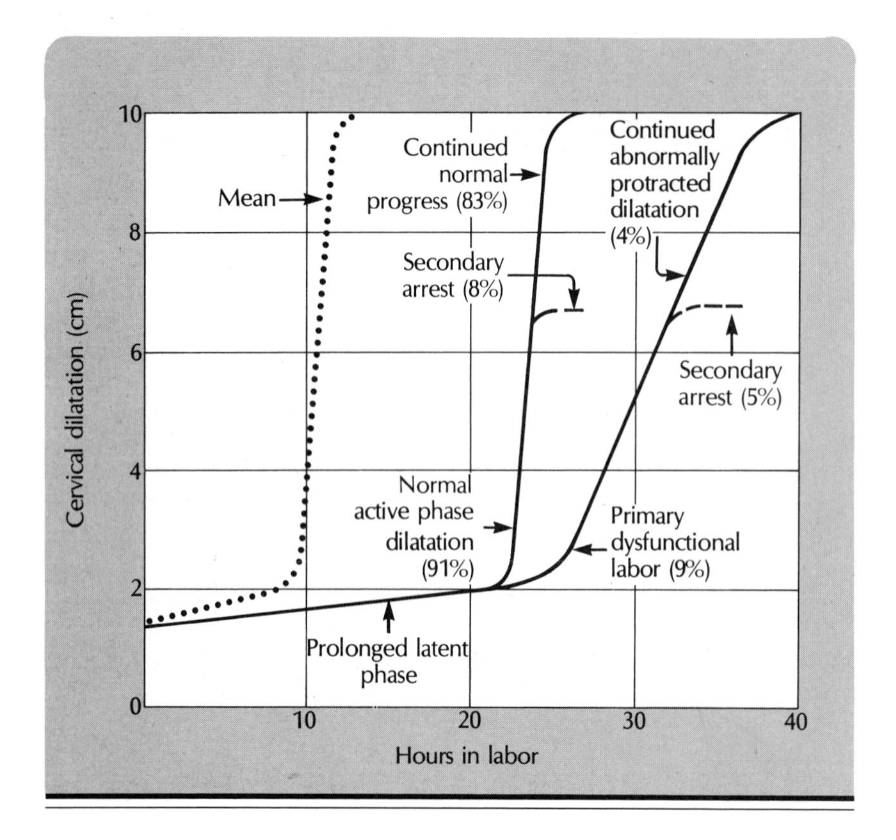

Figure 19–2. Friedman curve. Prolongation of latent phase. (From Friedman, E. July 1970. An objective method of evaluating labor. *Hospital Practice,* vol. 5, no. 7, p. 84. Reproduced with permission.)

onset of labor in primiparas and 14 hours in multiparas.

2. *Prolonged active phase dilatation.* The rate of cervical dilatation is abnormally slow, below the following critical limits: 1.2 cm/hr in primiparas and 1.5 cm/hr in multiparas.

3. *Prolonged deceleration phase.* Progressive cervical dilatation ceases during the active phase of labor before full dilatation is reached. This diagnosis is made if dilatation activity has ceased for a minimum of two hours.

4. *Arrest of descent.* Progressive linear descent of the fetus ceases, most often in the second stage of labor. Usually one hour of inactivity is sufficient to make the diagnosis.

5. *Protracted descent.* The rate of fetal descent is slow: less than 1 cm/hr in primiparas and 2 cm/hr in multiparas in the active phase of labor.

There are three hypoactive labor patterns, classified according to the characteristics of contractions. They are hypertonic uterine motility, incoordinated uterine motility, and hypotonic uterine motility.

Hypertonic and Incoordinated Uterine Motility

In hypertonic uterine motility the resting tone of the myometrium increases more than 15 mm Hg and may increase as much as 50–85 mm Hg. The frequency of contraction is usually increased, whereas the intensity may be decreased (Figure 19–3). The number of fibers in the myometrium that are not contracting and free to receive new impulses from the pacemakers is diminished, which results in an increased resting tone due to premature interruption of the refractory period.

There are two degrees of incoordinated uterine motility (Figure 19–4). First-degree incoordinated uterine motility occurs when two different pacemakers in the uterus are sending stimuli. In

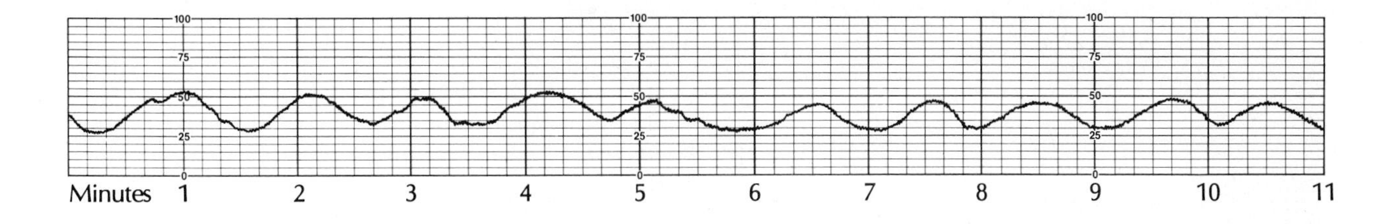

Figure 19–3. Hypertonic uterine motility.

second-degree incoordinated uterine motility, the numerous foci in the uterus that receive stimuli are operating independently (Assali, 1972).

Maternal Implications. Hypertonic and incoordinated labor patterns are extremely painful because of uterine muscle cell anoxia. There is an increase in uterine muscle tone but little cervical dilatation and effacement. Because hypertonic labor often occurs in the latent phase of labor, when dilatation may be no more than 2–3 cm, the mother may be accused of overreacting to her labor.

The mother may be aware of the lack of progress and become anxious and discouraged. Women who have prepared for their labor and delivery may feel frustrated as their coping mechanisms are severely tested.

Fetal-neonatal Implications. Fetal distress occurs early, because contractions interfere with the uteroplacental exchange. If this distress goes unidentified, the fetus may be lost. In any situation in which there is prolonged pressure on the fetal head, cephalhematoma, caput succedaneum, or excessive molding may occur (Figure 19–5). Cephalhematoma is caused by pressure of the fetal head against the bony prominences of the pelvis during labor. It results from the rupture of capillaries under the periosteum. It may be apparent at birth or develop in the next two days. Caput succedaneum is a swelling of the soft tissues of the presenting portion of the scalp area, which is encircled by the cervix during labor. It is apparent at birth.

Interventions. Management of hypertonic labor may include bed rest and sedation to promote relaxation. Oxytocin may be administered to a patient suffering from incoordinated labor to initiate or stimulate a more effective contractile pattern.

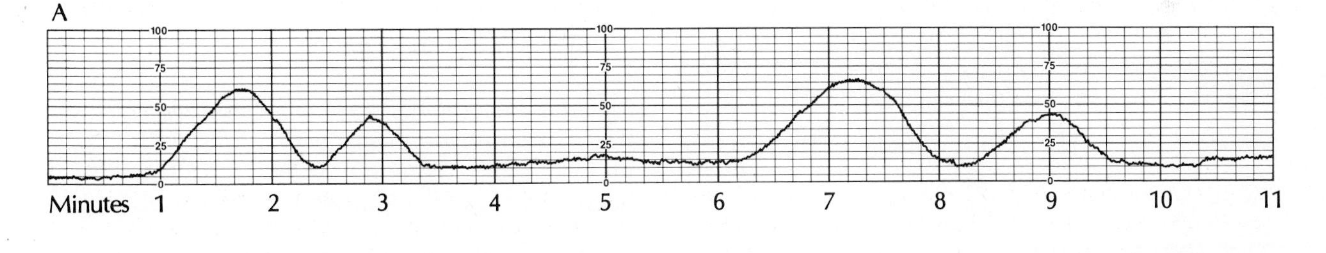

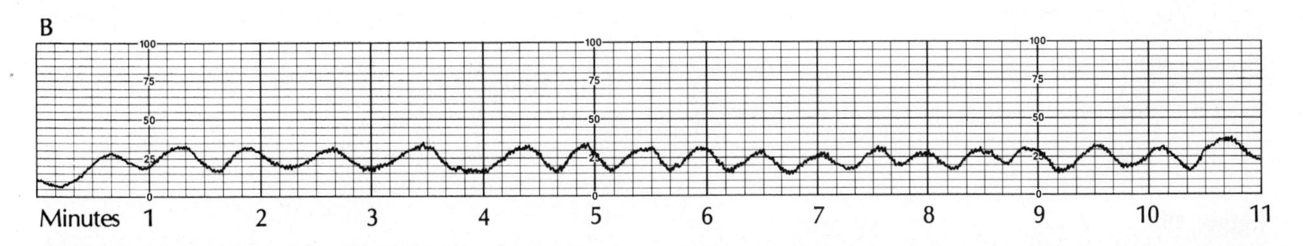

Figure 19–4. Incoordinated uterine motility. **A,** First degree. **B,** Second degree.

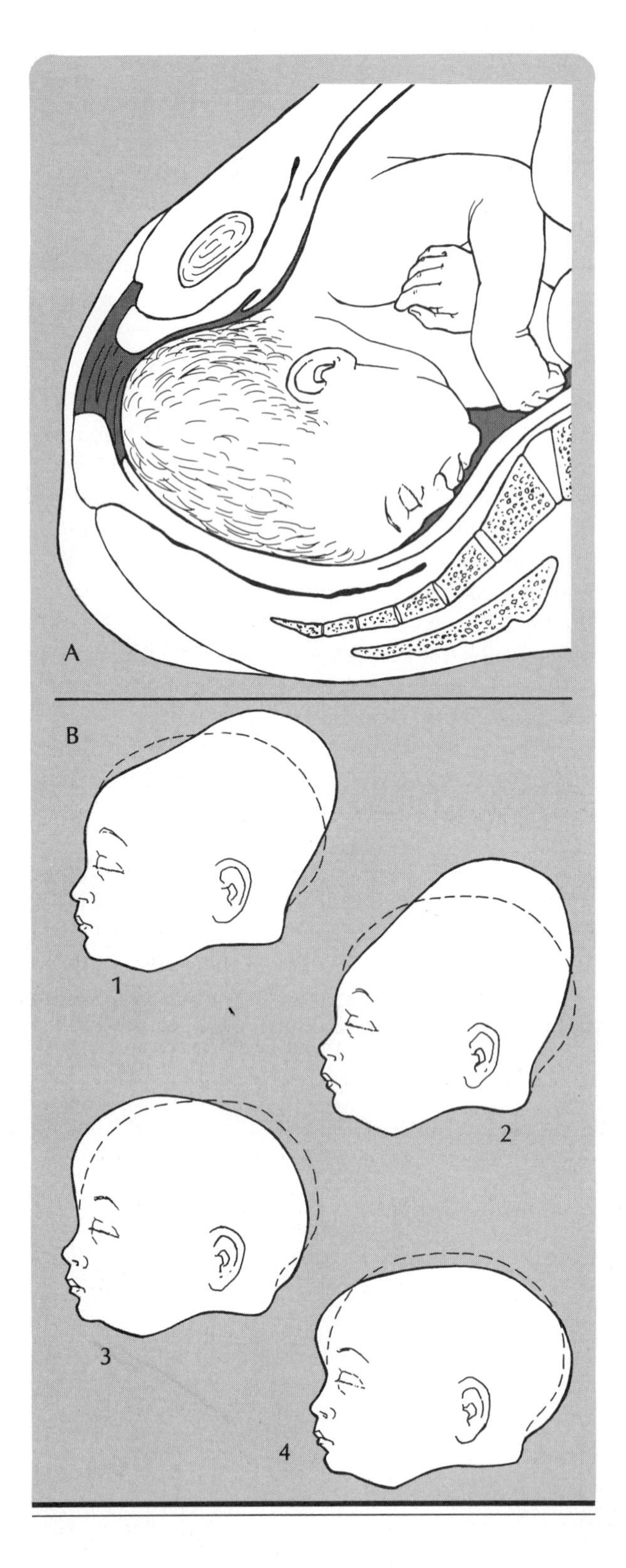

Figure 19–5. Effects of labor on fetal head. **A,** Caput succedaneum formation. **B,** Molding of fetal head in cephalic presentations: *1,* occiput anterior; *2,* occiput posterior; *3,* brow; *4,* face.

Nursing measures include identification and reporting of a dysfunctional labor pattern, provision of information to the laboring family, provision of an environment conducive to relaxation if sedation is ordered, and any supportive technique that the nurse can devise. The nurse may wish to try a change of position for the mother, mouth care, effleurage, back rub, and change of linens. In addition, the labor coach may need assistance in helping the mother to cope.

It is imperative that maternal exhaustion be prevented through adequate hydration. Urine ketones should be monitored hourly. The couple should be kept informed of labor progress.

Nursing measures in the event of fetal-neonatal distress are given in the Nursing Care Plan on p. 582.

Hypotonic Uterine Motility

In this pattern the myometrial resting tone is below 8 mm Hg. There are fewer than two to three contractions in a ten-minute period (Figure 19–6). This type of labor may occur when uterine fibers are overstretched from twins, large singletons, polyhydramnios, and grandmultiparity. Hypotonic uterine motility also occurs when sedation such as meperidine (Demerol) is given in the latent phase of labor or in the presence of various degrees of cephalopelvic disproportion. It may also occur with bladder and bowel distention. Clinically, hypotonic uterine motility may occur in the latent or active phase but is most often seen in the active phase. It is painless and responds to oxytocin if conditions permit its use (Assali, 1972).

Maternal Implications. If labor is prolonged, intrauterine infection can result, along with maternal exhaustion. Any mother with a dysfunctional labor pattern is a candidate for postpartal hemorrhage, but the mother with hypotonic labor is especially at risk. The uterus is demonstrating a weakened muscle power from the onset of labor.

Fetal-neonatal Implications. Fetal distress usually occurs late in hypotonic labor and most often is due to ascending maternal pathogens (Paul and Petrie, 1973). Fetal tachycardia is observed on the electronic monitor or auscultated by the nurse.

The infant delivered of a mother with prolonged labor should be observed closely for signs of sepsis in the nursery.

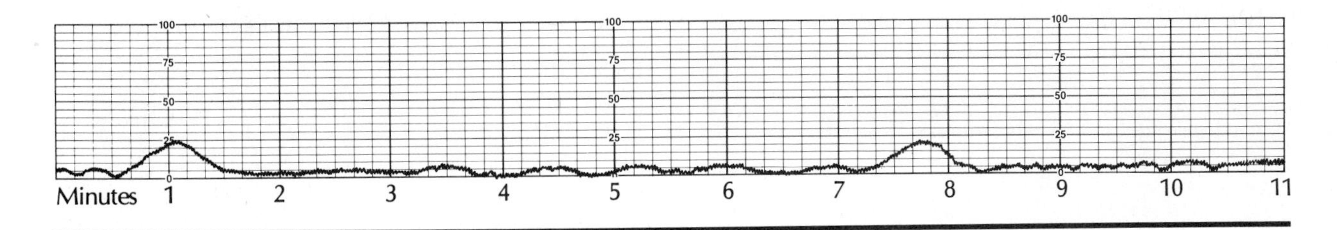

Figure 19-6. Hypotonic uterine motility.

Interventions. Oxytocins are frequently given intravenously in a controlled intravenous infusion to improve the quality of uterine contractions. The IV is also useful because adequate hydration should be maintained to prevent maternal exhaustion. In addition, the mother's vital signs should be monitored closely after delivery and her uterus should be palpated for atony at frequent intervals. Nursing actions for fetal distress are given on p. 582.

Hemorrhage

Dystocia predisposes to maternal hemorrhage. Because the uterine musculature is overtired or overstretched or its contractile ability is dysfunctional, the uterus may not clamp off the blood vessels at the placental separation site, resulting in postpartal hemorrhage.

Hemorrhage shock is due to hypovolemia resulting from a reduction of blood volume. Venous return to the heart and cardiac output are lowered. The immediate compensatory response is the reflex activation of adrenergic receptors and the release of increased amounts of catecholamines, which cause tachycardia and vasoconstriction. There is an attempt to maintain circulating blood volume as the fluids from the extravascular spaces pass into the intravascular space (Danforth, 1977).

The signs and symptoms of the various degrees of hemorrhage are given in Table 19-1. The various sources of hemorrhage are given in Table 19-2.

Maternal Implications. Mild hemorrhage generally results in few, if any, maternal complications. A slight decrease in the hemoglobin and hematocrit levels may be apparent, and the mother may complain of fatigue.

Table 19-1. Degree of Hemorrhage*

Severity	Signs and symptoms	Reduction in blood volume
Mild hemorrhage	Minimal tachycardia Slight decrease in BP Mild evidence of vasoconstriction, with cool hands and feet	15%-25% (750-1250 ml)
Moderate hemorrhage	Tachycardia (100-120 beats/min) Decrease in pulse pressure Systolic BP 90-100 mm Hg Restlessness, increased sweating, pallor, oliguria	25%-35% (1250-1750 ml)
Severe hemorrhage	Tachycardia >120 beats/min Systolic BP decreased to 60 mm Hg and frequently unobtainable by cuff Mental stupor, extreme pallor, cold extremities, anuria	Up to 50% (2500 ml)

*Modified from Danforth, D., ed. 1977. *Obstetrics and gynecology.* Hagerstown, Md.: Harper & Row Publishers, Inc., p. 685.

Table 19–2. Causes and Sources of Hemorrhage

Causes and sources	Signs and symptoms
Antepartal period	
Abortion	Vaginal bleeding Intermittent uterine contractions Rupture of membranes
Placenta previa	Painless vaginal bleeding after seventh month
Abruptio placentae	
Partial	Vaginal bleeding; no increase in uterine pain
Severe	No vaginal bleeding Extreme tenderness of abdominal area Rigid, boardlike abdomen Increase in size of abdomen
Intrapartal period	
Placenta previa	Bright red vaginal bleeding
Abruptio placentae	Same signs and symptoms as listed above
Uterine atony in stage III	Bright red vaginal bleeding, ineffectual contractility
Postpartal period	
Uterine atony	Boggy uterus Dark vaginal bleeding Presence of clots
Retained placental fragments	Boggy uterus Dark vaginal bleeding Presence of clots
Lacerations of cervix or vagina	Firm uterus Bright red blood

Moderate to severe hemorrhage results in hemorrhagic shock, which may ultimately prove fatal to the mother if not reversed.

Fetal Implications. Maternal hemorrhage diminishes the amount of oxygenated blood available to the fetus. Changes in the fetal heart rate and meconium-stained amniotic fluid may appear. If the fetal hypoxia progresses unchecked, it may ultimately result in irreversible brain damage or fetal demise.

Interventions. See the accompanying Nursing Care Plan on hemorrhage.

Premature Labor

Labor that occurs after the 28th week but before the 37th week of pregnancy is referred to as *premature labor.* The causes may be fetal, maternal, or placental factors. Premature rupture of the membranes occurs in 20%–30% of the cases of premature labor. In the other 70%–80% of cases, no known cause has been identified (Danforth, 1977). Maternal factors include cardiovascular or renal disease, diabetes, preeclampsia-eclampsia, abdominal surgery, a blow to the abdomen, uterine anomalies, cervical incompetence, and maternal infection. Fetal factors include multiple pregnancy, hydramnios, and fetal infection.

Maternal Implications. In certain situations, such as preeclampsia-eclampsia, severe renal disease, or cardiovascular disease, continuation of the pregnancy would place the mother in jeopardy, and so no effort is made to prevent labor.

Maternal abdominal surgery is only performed when absolutely necessary and requires the awareness of the possibility that uterine manipulation or displacement may contribute to the early onset of labor.

The major implications for the mother relate to psychologic stress factors related to the welfare of her unborn child.

Fetal-neonatal Implications. Mortality rates increase for infants born before the 37th week of gestation. Although the preterm infant is faced with many maturational deficiencies (fat storage, heat regulation, immaturity of organ systems), the most critical factor is the lack of development of the respiratory system—to the extent that life cannot be supported. In some instances, such as severe maternal diabetes or serious isoimmunization, continuation of the pregnancy may be more life-threatening to the fetus than the hazards of prematurity are. See Chapter 24 for in-depth consideration of the premature infant.

Interventions. Immediate diagnosis is necessary so that premature labor can be stopped before it has advanced to a stage where intervention will be ineffective. Labor is not interrupted if one or more of the following conditions are present:

1. Active labor with cervical dilatation of 4 cm or more.

NURSING CARE PLAN
Hemorrhage

Patient Data Base

History

Identify factors predisposing to hemorrhage:

1. Presence of preeclampsia-eclampsia
2. Overdistention of the uterus
   a. Multiple pregnancy
   b. Polyhydramnios
3. Grandmultiparity
4. Advanced age
5. Uterine contractile problems
   a. Hypotonicity
   b. Hypertonicity
6. Painless vaginal bleeding after seventh month
7. Presence of hypertension
8. Presence of diabetes
9. History of previous hemorrhage or bleeding problems, blood coagulation defects
10. Retained placental fragments
11. Lacerations

Determine religious preference to establish whether patient will permit a blood transfusion

Physical examination

Severe abdominal pain

Revealed or concealed bleeding

Shock symptoms (decreased blood pressure, increased pulse, pallor)

Lack of uterine relaxation or uterine atony

Degree of hemorrhage (see Table 19-1)

Laboratory evaluation

Hemoglobin and hematocrit

Type and cross-match

Fibrinogen levels

Nursing Priorities

1. If IV is not present, start one in large vein with large bore plastic cannula.
2. Evaluate blood loss (if possible, measure or weigh blood-soaked pads to facilitate adequate replacement).
3. Monitor vital signs.
4. Measure urine output.
5. Administer oxygen as necessary.
6. Evaluate fetal status.
7. Maintain fetal life-support mechanisms.

Problem	Nursing interventions and actions	Rationale
Blood loss	Observe, record, and report blood loss.	Hypovolemia causes decreased venous return to the heart and subsequent decrease in cardiac output. Decreased cardiac output initiates sympathoadrenal response, which leads to increased peripheral resistance and tachycardia in an effort to maintain adequate tissue perfusion. Decreased blood flow to kidney causes stimulation of juxtaglomerular apparatus to release hormones. This leads to retention of sodium ions and water (mechanism to increase blood volume) and increased reabsorption of water by distal tubules, which increases intravascular volume. Cells do not receive sufficient O_2 or nutrients because of vasoconstriction of venules and arterioles (caused by increased catecholamines).

NURSING CARE PLAN Cont'd

Hemorrhage

Problem	Nursing interventions and actions	Rationale
	Assess patient experiencing decrease in blood volume using following parameters:	Release of catecholamines and cortisol during shock also stimulates release of fatty acids for energy production. As fatty acids are metabolized, there is increase in ketones. Ketones are normally oxidized in the liver, but the hypoperfused liver cannot do this adequately, resulting in increase in metabolic acidosis.
	1. Monitor rate and quality of respirations continuously.	Initially respiratory rate increases as a result of sympathoadrenal stimulation, resulting in increased metabolic rate. Pain and anxiety may cause hyperventilation.
	2. Measure pulse rate.	Increased pulse rate is an effect of increased epinephrine.
	3. Assess pulse quality by direct palpation. Determine pulse deficit by comparing apical-radial rates.	Reflects circulatory status. Thready pulse indicates vasoconstriction and reflects decreased cardiac output. Peripheral pulses may be absent if vasoconstriction is intense. Bounding pulse may indicate overload.
	4. Compare present BP with patient's normal BP; note pulse pressure.	Hypotension indicates loss of large amount of circulatory fluid or lack of compensation in circulatory system. As cardiac output decreases, there is usually a fall in pulse pressure. Peripheral vasoconstriction may make accurate readings difficult.
	5. Monitor urine output (decrease to less than 30 ml/hr is sign of shock): a. Insert Foley catheter. b. Measure output hourly.	Vasoconstrictor effect of norepinephrine decreases blood flow to kidneys, which decreases glomerular filtration rate and the output of urine.
	c. Measure specific gravity to determine concentration of urine.	Inability to concentrate urine may indicate renal damage from vasoconstriction and decreased blood perfusion.
	6. Assess skin for presence of following: a. Pallor and cyanosis: *Pallor* in brown-skinned persons appears yellowish-brown. Black-skinned individuals appear ashen gray. Generally pallor may be observed in mucous membranes, lips, and nail beds.	Skin reflects amount of vasoconstriction. Pallor is determined by intensity of vasoconstriction.
	a. *Cyanosis* is assessed by inspecting lips, nail beds, conjunctiva, palms, and soles of feet at regular intervals. Evaluate capillary refilling by pressing on nail bed and observing return of color. Compare by testing your own nail bed.	Cyanosis occurs when the amount of reduced hemoglobin in the blood is $\leqq$ 5 gm/100 ml blood.
	b. Coldness.	Produced by slow blood flow.
	c. Clamminess.	Caused by sympathetic stimulation of sweat glands.
	Assess state of consciousness frequently.	Diminished cerebral blood flow causes restlessness and anxiety. As shock progresses, state of consciousness decreases.

NURSING CARE PLAN Cont'd

Hemorrhage

Problem	Nursing interventions and actions	Rationale
	Measure central venous pressure (CVP): Insert catheter into superior vena cava. Intravenous fluid should run freely through catheter before measuring, and baseline zero mark should be marked on patient's chest. Normal CVP is 5-10 cm H_2O.	Provides estimation of volume of blood returning to heart and ability of both chambers in right heart to propel blood. Low CVP indicates a decrease in the circulating volume of blood (hypovolemia).
	Assess amount of blood loss: 1. Count pads. 2. Weigh pads and chux (1 gm = 1 ml blood approximately). 3. Record how much flow there is in specific amount of time (e.g., 50 ml bright red blood on pad in 20 min).	In obstetric patients, blood is replaced according to estimates of actual blood loss, rather than using parameters of increased and decreased BP.
Reduction of hemoglobin	Position patient in supine position.	Position keeps more blood volume available to vital centers.
	Avoid Trendelenburg position.	Trendelenburg position shifts heavy uterus against diaphragm and may compromise respiratory function.
	Administer whole blood.	Corrects reduced oxygen-carrying capacity.
	Administer O_2 by face mask at 4-7 liters/min.	Woman in labor is mouth breather. Using face mask assures better oxygen delivery.
Hypovolemia	Relieve decreased blood pressure by administration of whole blood.	Hypotension results from decreased blood volume.
	While waiting for whole blood to be available, infuse isotonic fluids, plasma, plasma expanders, or serum albumin.	Degree of hypovolemia may be assessed by CVP, hemoglobin, and hematocrit.
Fluctuations in blood perfusion to vital organs	Monitor urine output hourly: 1. 50 ml/hr or more indicates safe renal perfusion. 2. Less than 25 ml/hr indicates inadequate renal perfusion (tubular ischemia and necrosis can result). Monitor adequacy of fluid volume by evaluating CVP.	Provides excellent measure of organ perfusion.
Presence of hemorrhage	Observe for signs and symptoms of hemorrhage (see Tables 19-1 and 19-2).	Bleeding often stops as shock develops but resumes as circulation is restored.
	If partial abruptio placentae is diagnosed: 1. Evaluate blood loss. 2. Assess uterine contractile pattern and tenderness. 3. Monitor maternal vital signs. 4. Assess fetal status. 5. Assess cervical dilatation and effacement. 6. Rule out placenta previa. 7. Perform amniotomy and begin oxytocin infusion if labor does not start immediately or is ineffective.	
	If severe abruptio placentae is diagnosed: 1. Perform same assessments as for partial abruptio placentae.	

NURSING CARE PLAN Cont'd

Hemorrhage

Problem	Nursing interventions and actions	Rationale
	2. Measure CVP. 3. Replace blood loss. 4. Effect immediate delivery. 5. Observe for signs and symptoms of disseminated intravascular coagulation (DIC).	
	If uterine atony is diagnosed intrapartally, assess contractility of uterus and amount of vaginal bleeding. Postpartally, massage uterus until firm and administer ergonovine intramuscularly or orally.	Muscle fibers that have been overstretched or overused do not contract well. Contraction of muscle fibers over open placental site is essential. Slight relaxation of uterus muscle fibers leads to continuous oozing of blood.
	If placental fragments have been retained, assess uterine contractility and vaginal flow.	Interferes with contractility of uterus.
	Massage uterus and scrape out uterine contents.	Couvelaire uterus does not contract well because of presence of blood around muscle fibers.
	If cervical or vaginal lacerations are found, they are repaired by the clinician.	
Fetal distress	Assess and monitor fetal heart rate (range 120-160 beats/min).	Hemorrhage from mother disrupts blood flow pattern to fetus, possibly compromising fetal status.
	Observe for meconium in amniotic fluid.	Hypoxia causes increased motility of intestines and relaxation of abdominal muscles, with release of meconium into amniotic fluid.
	Obtain fetal blood sample (pH <7.2 indicates severe jeopardy).	
Fear	Instruct patient about procedures.	Fear and anxiety affect release of catecholamines.
	Remain calm.	Increases patient's confidence.
Depletion of fibrinogen	Evaluate blood levels. At term, normal fibrinogen level is 375-700 mg/100 ml. Critical level required to clot blood is 100 mg/100 ml. Observe for signs and symptoms of DIC.	Fibrinogen and fibrin are lost because of their accumulation in a retroplacental clot. Further fibrinogen loss and additional coagulation failure may result from intravascular clotting and fibrinolysis.
	Determine whether fetal demise is cause of fibrinogen depletion. Conduct coagulation studies and measure fibrinogen levels. Induce labor if patient is at risk.	Dead fetus releases thromboplastin, which interferes with the clotting mechanism and lowers fibrinogen level.

Nursing Care Evaluation

Blood loss is corrected.

Vital signs remain within normal range.

Fetal heart tones are present and within normal range.

2. Presence of severe preeclampsia-eclampsia, which creates risk for the mother if the pregnancy continues.
3. Fetal complications (isoimmunization, gross anomalies).
4. Ruptured membranes, which increase the risk of uterine infection.

In the recent past, alcohol was given to arrest premature labor. Current information regarding the development of fetal alcohol syndrome and its relationship to elevated maternal blood alcohol levels has contributed to the discontinued use of this treatment regimen.

The drugs currently in use to arrest premature labor are ritodrine, isoxsuprine (Vasodilan), and terbutaline sulfate (Brethine). Ritodrine (a β-mimetic agent) is given intravenously at a dosage of 100 μg/min and the rate is increased by 50 μg every 10 minutes until labor ceases or until a level of 350 μg/min is attained (Spellacy et al., 1978). After labor ceases, ritodrine is given by intramuscular or oral route. Maternal effects include an elevation of maternal blood glucose and plasma insulin. Hyperglycemia may occur in women with abnormal carbohydrate metabolism, because of their inability to release more insulin, so the drug must be used with caution (Spellacy et al., 1978). Other maternal effects may include a slight lowering of serum iron resulting from the action of β-mimetics to activate hematopoiesis and also a decrease in serum potassium following treatment. This hypokalemia may "result from a displacement of the extracellular potassium into the intracellular space. This may be caused by beta-adrenergic induced release of insulin or/and pituitary vasopressin, which are both known to transport potassium ions into the cells" (Kauppila et al., 1978).

Isoxsuprine (Vasodilan), a β-mimetic compound, is given intravenously with a loading dose of 0.2–1.0 mg/min for about 24 hours. After premature labor is arrested, isoxsuprine may be given orally. Side effects include hypotension and maternal and fetal tachycardia (Csapo and Herczeg, 1977). Brazy and Pupkin (1979) report fetal effects of isoxsuprine as increased incidence of hypotension, hypoglycemia, hypocalcemia, ileus, and death.

Terbutaline sulfate (Brethine), a selective B_2-receptor stimulator, may be given intravenously to arrest premature labor. Treatment is initiated at 10 μg/min and may be increased by 5 μg/min to a maximum of 25 μg/min. When contractions cease, the effective infusion rate should be continued for one hour and then decreased by 5 μg/min until the lowest effective maintenance dose is reached. The infusion is continued for eight hours. Subsequent treatment of 0.25 mg is given subcutaneously every six hours for three days, plus 5 mg orally three times a day. Maternal side effects include tachycardia (with little effect on the blood pressure), nervousness, tremor, and headache. Some researchers have indicated an additional side effect of pulmonary edema (Stubblefield, 1978). A mild fetal tachycardia may result. Neonatal hypoglycemia has also been noted (Epstein et al., 1979).

Supportive treatment of the mother in premature labor consists of bed rest, monitoring vital signs, and continuous monitoring of fetal heart rate and uterine contractions. Vaginal examinations are kept to a minimum.

Currently, an additional treatment may be recommended. Administration of glucocorticoids has an effect on the maturation of premature lung membranes, and if given more than 24 hours prior to delivery, the incidence of respiratory distress syndrome may be reduced by 50% (Thornfeldt et al., 1978). Dexamethasone (Decadron) and/or betamethasone (Celestone) may be administered intramuscularly to the mother and delivery is delayed at least 24 hours if possible. Specific fetal side effects are not known; however, the long-term effects of steroid treatment on the fetus still require investigation (Thornfeldt et al., 1978).

When labor cannot be arrested, the decision as to type of delivery is made. Cesarean section is considered if fetal presentation is breech or transverse lie. If vaginal delivery is the method of choice, it is recommended that the amount of analgesics administered be kept to a minimum. Artificial rupture of membranes is usually deferred until the cervix is dilated at least 6 cm in order to reduce the possibility of cord prolapse. During the delivery, the fetal head is protected by the use of forceps and an episiotomy to reduce pressure. Qualified personnel who can assist the premature infant in his respiratory effort should be in attendance.

Emotional support of the mother is imperative during labor and delivery. The mother should be kept informed about labor progress and treatment so that her full cooperation can be elicited.

Vena Caval Syndrome (Supine Hypotensive Syndrome)

When the pregnant woman assumes a supine position, the weight of the gravid uterus may cause partial occlusion of the vena cava (Figure 19–7). This occlusion results in shocklike symptoms as venous return to the heart is impaired, which produces hypotension, tachyardia, sweating, nausea and vomiting, and air hunger.

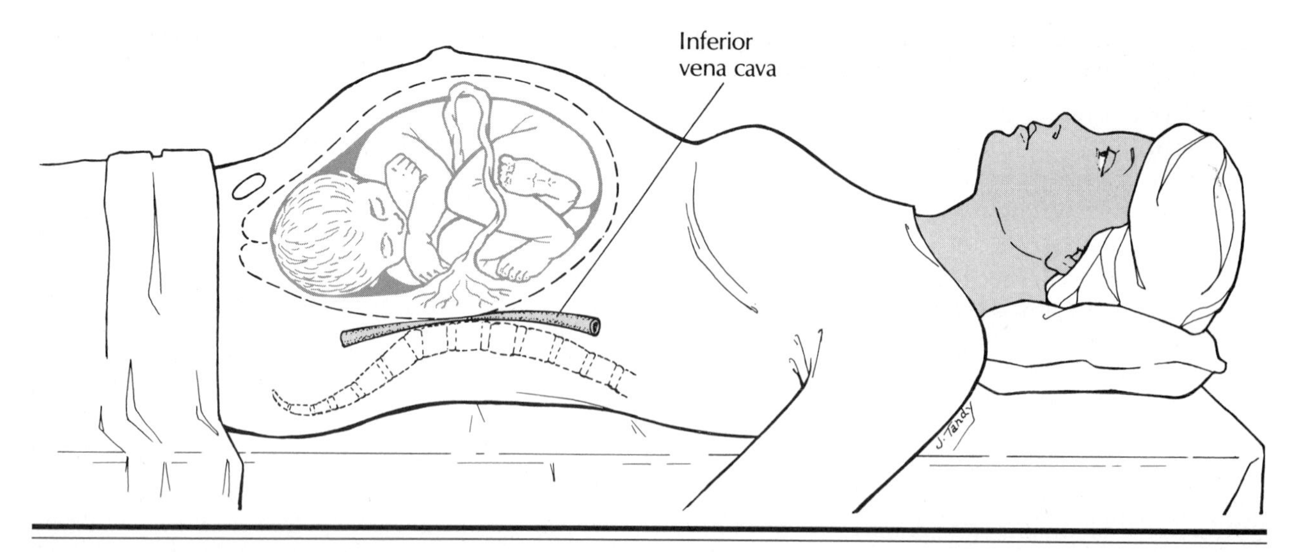

Figure 19–7. Vena caval syndrome. Gravid uterus compresses vena cava when the patient is in a supine position. The blood flow returning to the heart is reduced, and maternal hypotension may result.

Interventions. Recovery is immediate when the patient is positioned on her side. The left side is favored because more pressure is removed from the vena cava, which is located slightly to the right of the midline. If recovery is not immediate, oxygen may be started by tight face mask, and intravenous fluids may be started. Occasionally a change in position to the other side is beneficial. The fetal heart rate should be closely monitored to assess fetal status.

Ruptured Uterus

A ruptured uterus is the tearing of previously intact uterine musculature or an old uterine scar after the period of fetal viability, as opposed to uterine perforation. The rupture may be through the three muscular layers of the uterus, which is termed a *complete rupture,* or through the endometrium and myometrium, which is called an *incomplete rupture.* The rupture can be caused by (a) a weakened cesarean section scar, usually from a classic incision (Chapter 20); (b) obstetric trauma, such as may occur with any undue manipulation of the infant at the time of delivery; (c) mismanagement of oxytocin induction or stimulation during labor; or (d) obstructed labor.

Signs and symptoms of a complete rupture include excruciating pain and cessation of contractions. Vaginal hemorrhage may appear, but bleeding is usually not profuse. The mother exhibits signs of shock, and the uterus can be palpated as a separate mass. An incomplete rupture may not be evident until after the birth of the baby, when shock is profoundly out of proportion to the evident blood loss at the time of delivery.

The nurse should remember the warning signs of impending uterine rupture. The following may mean that the lower uterine segment is becoming acutely thin:

1. Restlessness and anxiety from severe pain and strong uterine contractions may occur.
2. No indication of labor progress is found by vaginal examination.
3. The lower uterine segment balloons out, simulating the appearance of a full bladder, and a pathologic retraction ring may be evident. This ring occurs when there is an abnormal division between the upper and lower uterine segments and is manifested by an indentation across the lower abdominal wall with acute tenderness above the symphysis.
4. On vaginal examination the cervix is found to stretch tautly around the presenting part, and a caput succedaneum may bulge out the cervix into the vagina.

Maternal Implications. If a ruptured uterus remains untreated, irreversible shock and death may occur. Occasionally when the rupture goes undetected for a period of time, peritonitis results.

Fetal Implications. In acute uterine rupture, the fetus extrudes into the abdominal cavity. The fetus, as it faces asphyxia, may become excessively active and exhibit bradycardia, which progresses to absence of heartbeat as it succumbs. All of this may take place within a few minutes.

Interventions. The nurse may be the one to identify the warning signs of impending rupture or postpartal hemorrhage if rupture has occurred. In acute rupture, the nurse quickly mobilizes the staff for an emergency laparotomy. When the physiologic needs of the mother and fetus are met, the nurse can focus on the emotional needs of the family. The family must have a clear understanding of the procedure and its implications for future childbearing. In addition, if fetal death has occurred, the parents should be given an opportunity to grieve and should be permitted to see their infant if they desire.

In the presence of a threatened rupture, cesarean section should be performed. If the rupture has already occurred, the abdomen is opened and the uterus removed. Some physicians will repair a smooth tear if the bleeding is controllable. Greenhill and Friedman (1974) recommend sterilization if a hysterectomy is not done, because there is a danger of repeated rupture with subsequent pregnancies. Low incomplete ruptures or extension of cervical tears may be repaired through the vagina. Women who have ruptured uteruses are advised to have elective cesarean sections with future pregnancies.

Inversion of Uterus

Uterine inversion occurs when the uterus turns inside out. This rare occurrence can be caused by a lax uterine wall coupled with undue tension on an umbilical cord when the placenta has not separated. Forceful pressure on the fundus with a dilated cervix and sudden emptying of the uterine contents may be contributing factors. Maternal bleeding with shock is rapid and profound. The fundus is absent from the abdominal cavity on palpation.

Interventions. The uterus must be replaced manually by grasping the vaginal mass, spreading the cervical ring with the fingers and thumb, and steadily forcing the fundus upward. The patient is under deep anesthesia (Greenhill and Friedman, 1974).

Nursing interventions should be directed at management of shock. Volume replacement should be a priority. The nurse ascertains whether a vein is patent for intravenous infusion and initiates the collection of a blood sample for type and cross-matching. Careful monitoring of the intake and output is vital. An indwelling catheter is usually inserted into the bladder after the uterus is replaced. Kidney function is a good indicator of adequate tissue perfusion and tissue damage from anoxia. Blood pressure and pulse rate should be monitored every five minutes by the nurse until the anesthesiologist arrives and is ready to assume this duty.

COMPLICATIONS INVOLVING THE PASSENGER

Complications involving the passenger include any abnormality of the fetus, placenta, umbilical cord, or amniotic fluid.

Fetal Problems

The progress of labor and delivery can be affected by the position and presentation of the fetus, fetal developmental abnormalities, and the presence of more than one fetus in the uterus.

Malpositions

Occiput-Posterior Position

Persistent occiput-posterior position of the fetus is probably one of the most common complications encountered in obstetrics. Although this position may be normal in some races because of a genetically small transverse diameter of the midpelvis, it is considered a malposition because of the maternal and fetal difficulties that may result. It should be remembered that the fetus generally tries to accommodate to the passage it has to travel through. For a fetus in an occiput-posterior position to rotate to an occiput-anterior position, it must rotate 135 degrees, and most fetuses accomplish this. But some do not, and in those cases labor progress may cease or the fetus may be delivered in a posterior position.

Signs and symptoms of a persistent occiput-posterior position are a dysfunctional labor pattern, a prolonged active phase, secondary arrest of dilatation or arrest of descent, and the complaint of intense back pain by the laboring mother. This back pain is caused by the fetal occiput compressing the sacral nerves. Further assessment may reveal a depression in the maternal abdomen above the symphysis (see Figure 16–13). FHTs will be heard far laterally on the abdomen, and on vaginal examination one will find the wide diamond-shaped anterior fontanelle in the anterior portion of the pelvis. This fontanelle may be difficult to feel because of molding of the fetal head.

Interventions. According to Pritchard and MacDonald (1976), vaginal delivery is possible as follows:

1. Await spontaneous delivery.
2. Forceps delivery with the occiput directly posterior.
3. Forceps rotation of the occiput to the anterior position and delivery.
4. Manual rotation to the anterior position followed by forceps delivery.*

If the pelvis is roomy and the perineum is relaxed, as found in grandmultiparity, the fetus may have no particular problem delivering spontaneously in the occiput-posterior position. If, however, the perineum is rigid, the second stage of labor may be prolonged. A prolonged second stage is one that lasts over an hour in multiparas and two hours or more in primiparas. One of the complications of the fetus delivering in the occiput-posterior position is the possibility of a third- or fourth-degree perineal laceration or extension of a midline episiotomy.

In the event of a prolonged second stage with arrest of descent due to occiput-posterior position, a midforceps or manual rotation may be done if no cephalopelvic disproportion is present. In cases of cephalopelvic disproportion, cesarean section is the treatment of choice.

In the past, a primary nursing intervention in cases of a persistent occiput-posterior fetal position has been the repositioning of the woman. The mother is turned from side to side; the force of gravity supposedly affects rotation. Whether the side position affects rotation is unknown; there is no documentation supporting this management. Turning the mother on her side does allow the labor coach the opportunity to administer counterpressure over the sacral area, which helps relieve the intense back pain experienced by the patient. The modified knee-chest position tends to decrease some of the pressure on the sacral nerves, thereby decreasing discomfort. In addition, the side position increases uterine perfusion, which results in better labor and fetal oxygenation. The knee-chest position provides a downward slant to the vaginal canal, directing the fetal head down on descent.

Transverse Arrest

In mothers with hypoactive labor or a diminished anteroposterior pelvic diameter (as seen with the platypelloid pelvis and diminished transverse diameter in the android pelvis), an incomplete rotation may occur, resulting in a transverse arrest. This may also result in arrest of descent and a prolonged second stage of labor. If the mother's labor is effective, spontaneous rotation may occur if she is allowed to continue to labor. If labor is poor and no cephalopelvic disproportion is present, the delivery may be accomplished by midforceps, manual rotation, or vacuum extractor. Occasionally the head is visible at the introitus even though the biparietal diameters have not entered the inlet. This situation is seen in cases of severe molding and caput formation. Cesarean section is the management of choice if the station is above +2 (Pritchard and MacDonald, 1976).

Maternal Implications. Manipulation during delivery can cause maternal soft tissue damage. If the physician elects to deliver the patient when the fetus is in the occiput-posterior position, a mediolateral episiotomy may be performed. Any prolonged pressure by the fetal head in one posi-

---

*From Pritchard, J. A., and MacDonald, P. C. 1976. *Williams obstetrics.* 15th ed. New York: Appleton-Century-Crofts.

tion may cause the mother later gynecologic problems, such as fistulas resulting from tissue anoxia. Postpartal hemorrhage may result from undetected lacerations or atony if the labor was hypoactive.

Fetal-neonatal Implications. Unless a protraction or arrest disorder is present or an operative delivery is performed, fetal mortality is not increased with an occiput-posterior or transverse position, because most fetuses do rotate spontaneously. Perinatal and neonatal mortality also are not significantly increased when the second stage is longer than three hours in the absence of cephalopelvic disproportion (Cohen, 1977). Cerebral damage may be caused in cases of undetected cephalopelvic disproportion. The fetus should be observed in utero closely by the nurse, and at the time of delivery a pediatrician should be present if a midforceps delivery is anticipated.

Interventions. The nurse continues her efforts to support and comfort the laboring woman. Continuous monitoring of contractions (character and frequency), amount of maternal discomfort, maternal vital signs, and fetal response to labor are important nursing interventions. The nurse notifies the physician in case of distress or dysfunctional labor.

The parents are prepared by the nurse for the extreme molding of the infant's head. The nurse remains alert for signs of postpartal hemorrhage.

Malpresentations

Three vertex attitudes of the fetus are classified as abnormal presentations: the sinciput, brow, and face. The fetal body straightens out in these presentations from the classic fetal position to an S-shaped position. The sinciput presentation is probably the least problematic for the mother and fetus. In most cases, as soon as the head reaches the pelvic floor, flexion occurs and a vaginal delivery results.

In addition to the vertex malpresentation, the breech, shoulder (transverse lie), and compound presentations can cause significant difficulty during labor. These and the vertex presentations are discussed here.

Brow Presentation

The brow presentation occurs more often in the multipara than the primigravida and is thought to be due to lax abdominal and pelvic musculature. The largest diameter of the fetal head, the occipitomental, presents in this type of presentation. The primigravida who has a brow presentation commonly has a small infant. Upon descent into the inlet, the brow presentation frequently converts to an occiput position. Some brow presentations convert to face presentations. Leopold's maneuvers reveal a cephalic prominence on the same side as the fetal back. A brow presentation can be detected on vaginal examination by palpation of the diamond-shaped anterior fontanelle on one side and the orbital ridges and root of the nose on the other side.

Maternal Implications. Delivery should be accomplished by cesarean section in the presence of cephalopelvic disproportion or failure of the brow to convert to an occiput or face presentation.

Fetal-neonatal Implications. Fetal mortality is increased due to injuries received during delivery and/or infection because of prolonged labor. The fetus should be observed closely during labor for signs of hypoxia as evidenced by type II decelerations and bradycardia. Trauma during the birth process can include tentorial tears, cerebral and neck compression, and damage to the trachea and larynx.

Interventions. As long as dilatation and descent is occurring, active interference is not necessary. In the presence of labor problems but no cephalopelvic disproportion, a manual conversion may be attempted. Midforceps delivery in the presence of complete dilatation and fetal station at +2 is advocated by some medical experts. In the presence of failed conversions, cephalopelvic disproportion, or secondary arrest of labor, cesarean section is the management of choice.

Nursing management of abnormal cephalic presentations includes close observation of the mother for labor aberrations and of the fetus for signs of distress. The nurse may need to explain the position to the laboring couple or to interpret what the physician has told them. The nurse should stay close at hand to reassure the couple, inform them of any changes, and assist them with labor-coping mechanisms.

At the time of delivery, adequate resuscitation equipment and pediatric assistance should be available.

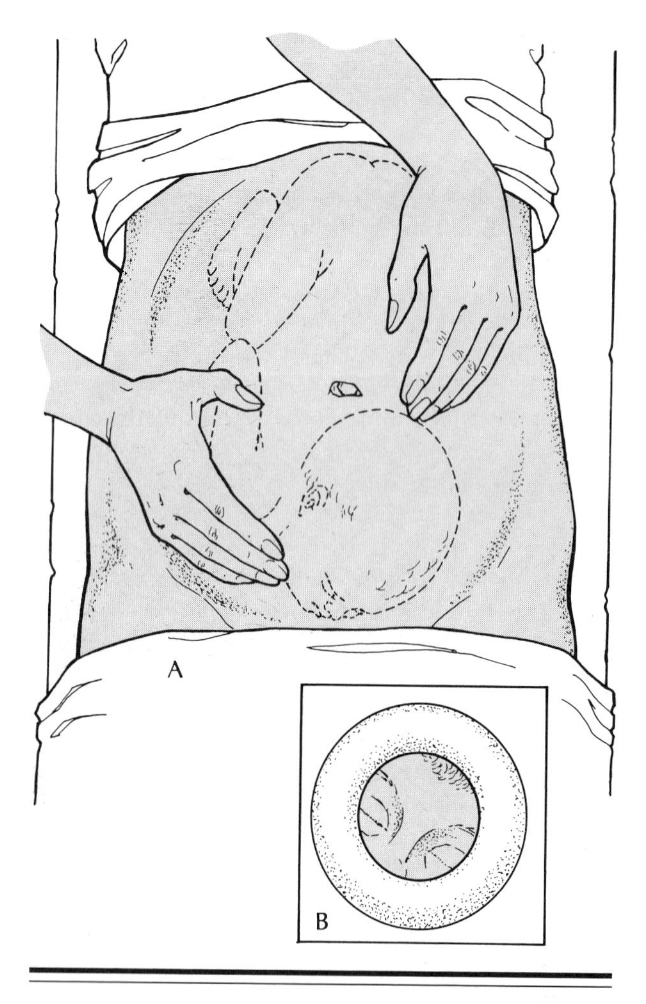

Figure 19–8. Face presentation. **A,** Palpation of the maternal abdomen with the fetus in RMP. **B,** Vaginal examination may permit palpation of facial features of the fetus.

In face and brow presentations, the appearance of the infant may be affected. The couple may need help in beginning the attachment process because of the infant's facial appearance. After the infant is inspected for gross abnormalities, the pediatrician and nurse can assure the couple that the facial edema is only temporary and will subside in three or four days.

Face Presentation

Face presentation of the fetus occurs most frequently in multiparas and in the presence of prematurity and anencephaly. When performing Leopold's maneuvers, one finds that the back of the fetus is difficult to outline, and a deep furrow can be palpated between the hard occiput and the fetal back (Figure 19–8). FHTs may be heard on the side where the fetal feet are palpated. It may be difficult to determine by vaginal examination whether a breech or face is presenting, especially if facial edema is already present. During the vaginal examination, palpation of the saddle of the nose and the gums should be attempted. When assessing engagement, one must remember that the face has to be deep within the pelvis before the biparietal diameters have entered the inlet.

Maternal Implications. The risks of cephalopelvic disproportion and prolonged labor are increased with this presentation. With any prolonged labor, there is an increased chance of infection.

Fetal-neonatal Implications. The fetus may develop caput succedaneum of the face during labor, and after delivery the edema gives the newborn a grotesque appearance. As with the brow presentation, the neck and internal structures may swell due to the trauma received during descent. Petechiae and ecchymoses are often seen in the superficial layers of the facial skin because of the birth trauma.

Interventions. If no cephalopelvic disproportion is present, if the chin (mentum) is anterior, and if there is an effective labor pattern, the mother may deliver vaginally (Figure 19–9). Mentum posteriors can become wedged on the anterior surface of the sacrum (Figure 19–10). In this case as well as in the presence of cephalopelvic disproportion, cesarean section is the management of choice for the delivery.

Nursing interventions are the same as for brow presentation.

Breech Presentations

The exact cause of breech presentation (Figure 19–11) is unknown. This malpresentation occurs in 3%–4% of all pregnancies and is associated with prematurity, placenta previa, hydramnios, multiple pregnancies, grandmultiparity, fetal hydrocephaly, and fetal anencephaly. It has been postulated that in cases of prematurity the fetus is small

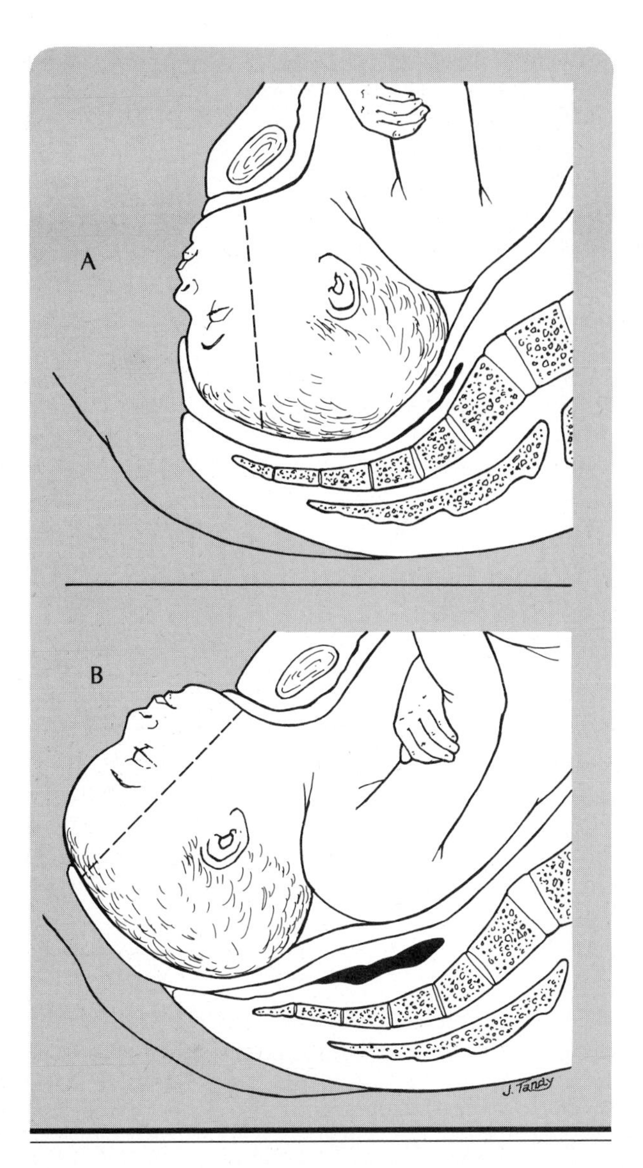

Figure 19–9. Mechanism of birth in mentoanterior position. **A,** The submentobregmatic diameter at the outlet. **B,** The fetal head is born by movement of flexion.

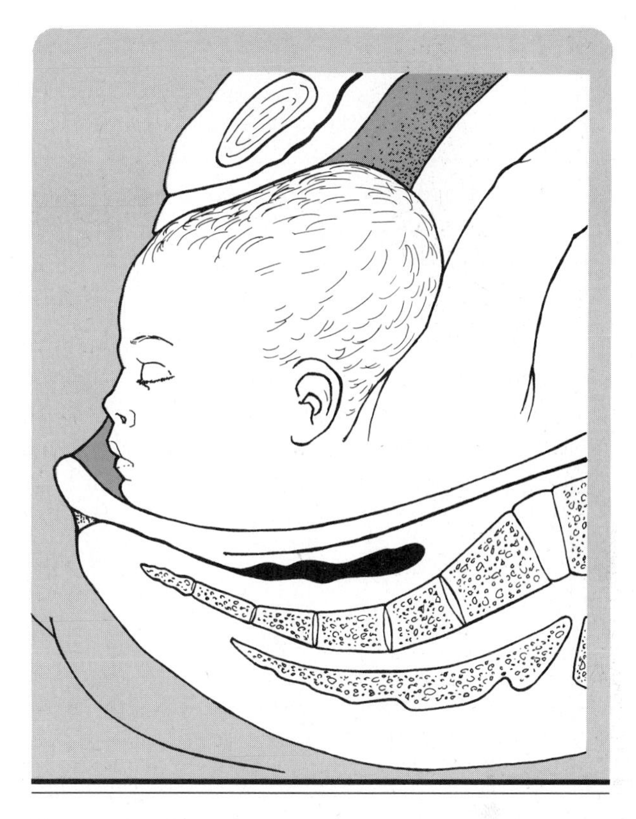

Figure 19–10. Mechanism of birth in mentoposterior position. Fetal head is unable to extend further. The face becomes impacted.

in relation to the overall size of the uterine cavity and has much room to move around. Consequently it may more easily assume any presentation. An incomplete breech, or footling, presentation prolongs labor because an effective dilating wedge is lacking (see Figure 19–11). The most critical problem with a breech presentation is that the largest part of the infant delivers last. In the presence of cephalopelvic disproportion, the pelvis is not really tried until it is virtually too late to salvage the fetus.

Frequently it is the nurse who first recognizes a breech presentation. On palpation the hard vertex is felt in the fundus and ballottement of the head can be done independently of the fetal body. The wider sacrum is palpated in the lower part of the abdomen. If the sacrum has not descended, on ballottement the entire fetal body will move. Furthermore, FHTs are usually auscultated above the umbilicus. Passage of meconium from compression of the infant's intestinal tract on descent is common.

There is a danger of prolapsed umbilical cord, especially in incomplete breeches, because space is available between the cervix and presenting part through which the cord can slip. If the infant is small and the membranes rupture, there is even greater danger. This is one reason why any woman admitted to the labor and delivery suite with a history of ruptured membranes should not be ambulated until a full assessment, including vaginal examination, is performed.

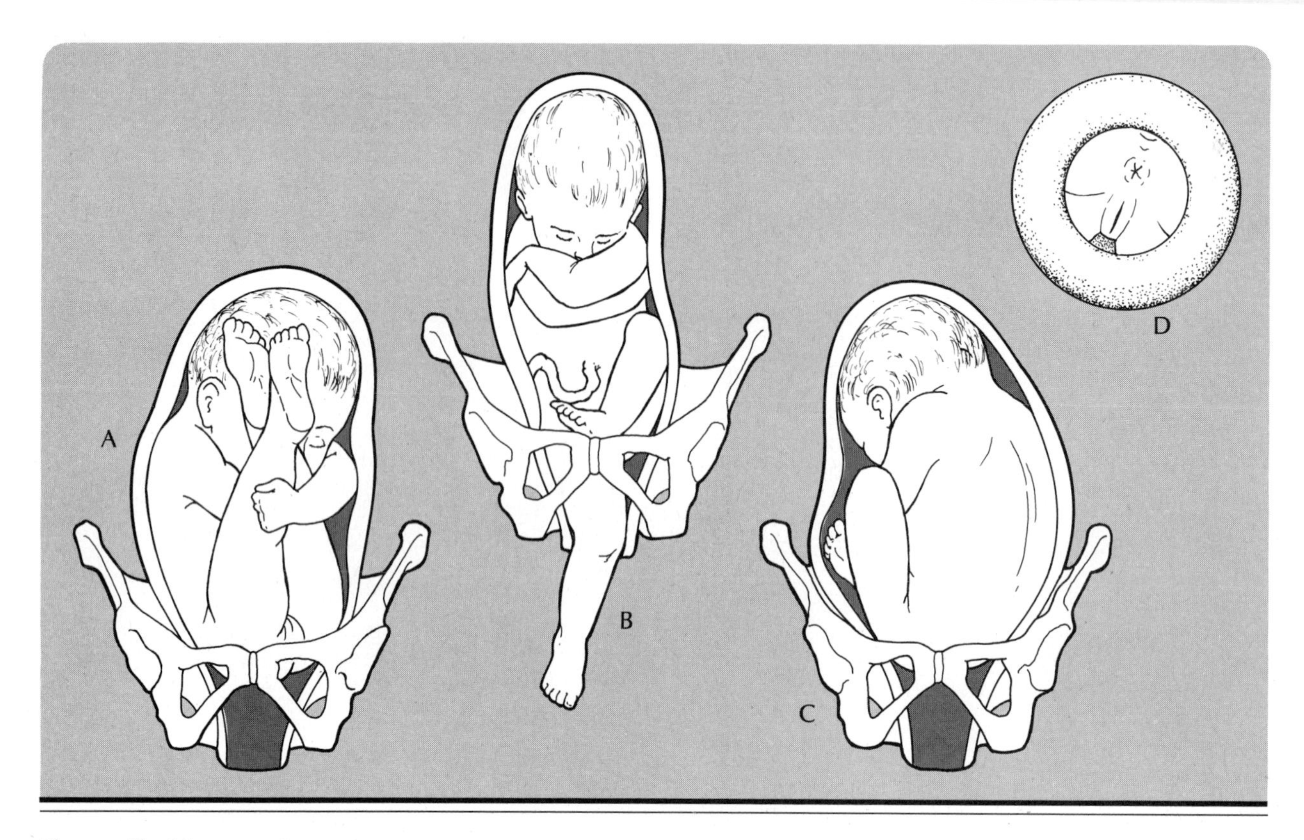

Figure 19–11. Breech presentation. **A,** Frank breech. **B,** Incomplete (footling) breech. **C,** Complete breech in LSA position. **D,** On vaginal examination, the nurse may feel the anal sphincter, which grips her finger. The tissue of the fetal buttocks feels soft.

Maternal Implications. Frequently a breech presentation necessitates delivery by cesarean section. The mother should have a clear understanding of the rationale for electing to deliver her child by this method.

In the event of vaginal delivery there is less maternal risk. The mother should, however, be carefully examined for lacerations or tears.

Fetal-neonatal Implications. The incidence of perinatal mortality increases in breech presentations. Hyperextension of the fetal head can occur at the time of delivery if delivery is vaginal and can result in cervical cord injuries (Kochenour, 1977). Other fetal and neonatal dangers include the following (Korones, 1976):

1. Increased possibility of intracranial hemorrhage from a traumatic delivery of the head.
2. Spinal cord injuries caused by stretching and manipulation of the infant's body.
3. Hemorrhage into the fetal abdominal viscera, particularly the kidneys, liver, and spleen.
4. Brachial plexus palsy.
5. Fracture of the upper extremities.

According to Kochenour:

> Unsuspected cephalopelvic disproportion remains one of the leading causes of perinatal morbidity and mortality. The perinatal morbidity is increased when the pelvis is not radiographically adequate. Several investigators have shown that the infant morbidity with a breech presentation is greater in the multiparous than in the primigravid patient. A factor may be that the primigravid patient may be evaluated more carefully whereas the multiparous patient is assumed to have an "adequate pelvis." Breech presentations do not prolong labor. It has been shown that when oxytocin is used to stimulate a dysfunctional labor associated with a breech presentation that the perinatal morbidity and mortality rate increases.*

*From Kochenour, N. 1977. The management of breech presentations. *PCC News.* 3(5):32.

Interventions. Cesarean section is being performed more in cases of breech presentation because of the increasing documentation of perinatal mortality and morbidity. Kochenour (1977) lists the following criteria for vaginal delivery:

> (1) The fetus should be presenting as a frank breech with an estimated fetal weight of less than 3500 grams, (2) the patient should have an adequate pelvis shown by x-ray pelvimetry, (3) a flat plate of the abdomen must exclude a hyperextended fetal head, (4) labor must progress normally and oxytocin should not be used for an arrested labor, (5) the second stage of labor should be less than one hour in duration, and (6) the patient should not be an elderly primigravida.*

There are two methods of delivering a breech fetus vaginally: partial breech extraction (assisted breech) and total breech extraction.

In the presence of strong uterine contractions, many breech deliveries may be accomplished spontaneously. As the force of the contractions and the mother's bearing-down efforts push the breech against the vulva, a generous episiotomy is made to give adequate room. As the baby is delivered, the physician supports the body and applies gentle downward traction. Flexion of the head is to be maintained. The shoulders emerge with continued pushing effort. The body is held slightly upward, and the head is delivered with the face directed back at the perineum.

In a number of breech presentations, more assistance is required to facilitate delivery. If there is any delay of proper flexion or descent of the head, it may be necessary to use forceps on the aftercoming head. The forceps commonly used are Piper forceps. As assistant (physician or nurse) holds the infant's body, which has been wrapped in a towel to provide handling ease. The physician's hands are then free to apply the Piper forceps and extract the head.

The nurse should include Piper forceps as a part of the delivery table setup. During the delivery process, the nurse may have to assist in the support of the infant's body if the obstetrician elects to use forceps. The circulating nurse should monitor the fetal heart rate closely during the delivery.

*From Kochenour, N. 1977. The management of breech presentations. *PCC News.* 3(5):32.

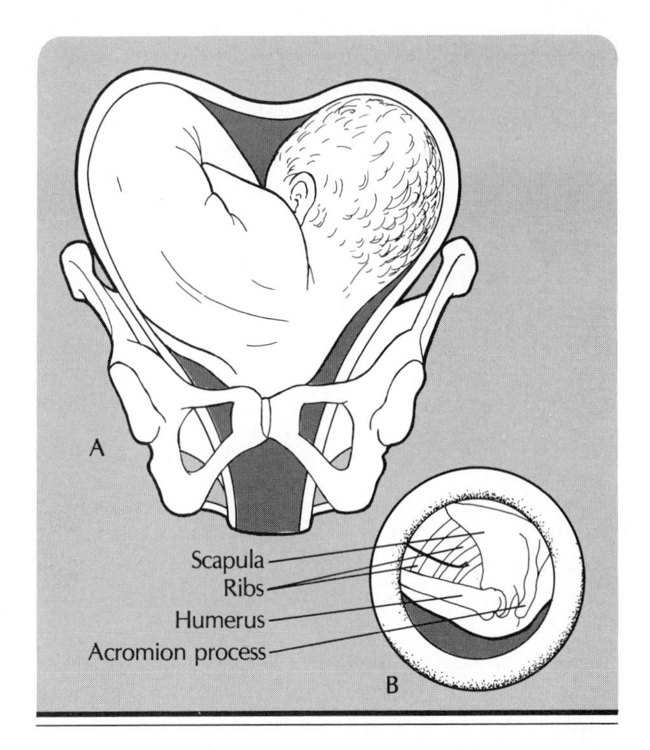

Figure 19–12. **A,** Shoulder presentation. **B,** On vaginal examination, the nurse may feel the acromiom process as the fetal presenting part.

Pediatric assistance should be available at the time of delivery. If meconium has been passed in utero, the pediatrician may want to examine the infant's vocal cords to check for meconium aspiration.

Transverse Lie (Shoulder Presentation)

A transverse lie occurs in approximately one in every 300 to 400 deliveries (Greenhill and Friedman, 1974). The infant's long axis lies across the mother's abdomen, and on inspection the contour of the maternal abdomen appears widest from side to side (Figure 19–12).

On palpation no fetal part is felt in the fundal portion of the uterus or above the symphysis. The head may be palpated on one side and the breech on the other. FHTs are usually auscultated just below the midline of the umbilicus. On vaginal examination, if a presenting part is palpated, it is the ridged thorax or possibly an arm that is compressed against the chest.

Maternal conditions associated with a transverse lie are grandmultiparity with lax uterine musculature; obstructions such as bony dystocia, placenta previa, neoplasms, and fetal anomalies; polyhydramnios; and prematurity. It is not uncommon in multiple gestations for one or more of the fetuses to be in a transverse lie. The nurse must be aware that careless vaginal examinations in the presence of unengagement may convert a dipping fetal head or breech presentation into a transverse lie. Also, premature amniotomy may assist a fetus that has not firmly entered the inlet into assuming this presentation.

Maternal Implications. Labor can be dysfunctional in the presence of a transverse lie. Uterine rupture can occur. As in any case of prolonged labor, the mother is more prone to infection.

Fetal-neonatal Implications. One danger of transverse lie is a prolapsed umbilical cord because there is nothing in the pelvic inlet to serve as a blocking agent. Prolapse of a fetal arm may also occur. If the mother is allowed to labor in the presence of a transverse lie, the fetus may succumb from asphyxia and trauma.

Interventions. The nurse can identify a transverse lie by inspection and palpation of the abdomen, by auscultation of FHTs in the midline of the abdomen (not conclusive), and by vaginal examination. The primary nursing actions are to assist in interpretation of the fetal presentation, to provide information and support to the couple, and to quickly prepare the mother for an operative delivery.

With a live fetus at term, cesarean section is the treatment of choice. External version may be attempted if the following criteria are met:

1. There is no indication for rapid termination of labor.
2. The fetus is highly movable.
3. Contractions are not strong and frequent.
4. There is no cephalopelvic disproportion.
5. The membranes are intact.

When the required criteria are met, attempts at external version are appropriate prior to the onset of labor or in early labor. If the patient is in active, well-established labor, the chance of success is minimal. If the clinician succeeds in manipulating the fetal head into the maternal pelvis, it should be held in place for several contractions in an attempt to fix it in place. In order to eliminate the possible use of undue force, anesthesia is not used (Pritchard and MacDonald, 1976).

Compound Presentation

A compound presentation is one in which there are two presenting parts. It can occur when the pelvic inlet is not totally occluded by the primary presenting part. If the prolapsed part is a hand, the delivery generally is not difficult. Sometimes the hand slips back and occasionally it is delivered alongside the head (Greenhill and Friedman, 1974).

A compound presentation becomes a medical emergency when one of the presenting parts is the umbilical cord (see the discussion on prolapse of the umbilical cord on p. 591).

Developmental Abnormalities

Macrosomia

Fetal macrosomia occurs when an infant weighs more than 4000 gm at birth. This condition is more common among offspring of large parents and diabetic mothers and in cases of grandmultiparity and postmaturity.

Maternal Implications. The pelvis that is adequate for an average-sized fetus may be disproportionately small for an oversized fetus. Distention of the uterus causes overstretching of the myometrial fibers, which may lead to dysfunctional labor and an increased incidence of postpartal hemorrhage. If the oversized fetus acts as an obstruction, there is an increased chance of uterine rupture during labor.

Fetal-neonatal Implications. Fetal prognosis is guarded. If a macrosomic fetus is unsuspected and labor is allowed to continue in the presence of disproportion, the fetus can receive cerebral trauma from intermittent forceful contact with the maternal bony pelvis. During difficult operative procedures performed at the time of vaginal delivery, the fetus may become asphyxiated or receive neurologic damage from pressure exerted on its head (Greenhill and Friedman, 1974).

Shoulder dystocia can occur if the shoulders become wedged between the sacrum and the pubic bone. During manual attempts to facilitate delivery, there is a danger of overstretching the fetal neck. If the cord has also been brought down into the bony pelvis, and there is a delay in the delivery, asphyxia from cord compression can occur.

Interventions. The maternal pelvis should be evaluated carefully if a large infant is suspected. An estimation of fetal size can be made by palpating the crown-rump length of the fetus in utero, but the greatest errors in estimation occur on both ends of the spectrum—the macrosomic and the very small infants. Fundal height can give some clue. Ultrasound or x-ray pelvimetry may give further information about fetal size. Whenever the uterus appears excessively large, hydramnios, an oversized infant, or multiple pregnancies must be considered as possible causes.

If shoulder dystocia occurs and delivery cannot be completed by various manual maneuvers, the physician may find it necessary to fracture the clavicles to save the infant's life.

The nurse should monitor these labors closely for dysfunction, utilizing the Friedman graph. The fetal monitor is applied for continuous fetal evaluation. Early type I head compression dips could mean disproportion at the bony inlet. Any sign of labor dysfunction or fetal distress should be reported to the obstetrician.

The nurse inspects these infants after delivery for skull fractures, cephalhematoma, and Erb's palsy and informs the nursery of any problems. If the nursery staff is aware of a difficult delivery, the newborn will be observed more closely for cerebral and neurologic damage.

Postpartally, the nurse checks the uterus for potential atony and the maternal vital signs for deviations suggestive of shock.

Hydrocephaly

In hydrocephaly 500–1500 ml of cerebrospinal fluid accumulates in the ventricles of the fetal brain. When this occurs before delivery, severe cephalopelvic disproportion results, because of the enlarged cranium of the fetus.

Abdominal palpation reveals the presence of a hard mass just above the symphysis; this is the unengaged head. If the presentation is breech, it is difficult on external palpation to discern between the breech and an enlarged head. A fetogram or sonogram is indicated in the presence of breech presentations to evaluate the cranium. Vaginal examination with a vertex presentation reveals wide suture lines and a globular cranium.

Maternal Implications. Obstruction of labor can occur, and if the uterus is allowed to continue contracting without medical interference, uterine rupture can result.

Fetal-neonatal Implications. Outlook for the fetus is poor. Frequently, other congenital malformations accompany this condition, such as spina bifida and myelomeningocele. The infant is severely brain damaged and often succumbs during delivery or afterward in the nursery because of his malformations and the presence of an infection.

Interventions. Vaginal delivery cannot be accomplished without intervention. The treatment of choice is withdrawal of the cerebrospinal fluid, thus collapsing the fetal skull. If the fetus is in a cephalic presentation, this is accomplished by introduction of a 17-gauge needle into the ventricle after the cervix is 3 cm dilated. With a breech presentation, this may be accomplished on the aftercoming head after it has entered the inlet. If cesarean section is performed, a transabdominal method of drainage is advocated to prevent excessive extension of the incision (Pritchard and MacDonald, 1976).

The nurse assists the physician with the procedures involved in the accomplishment of this delivery. The nurse also helps the couple to cope with this crisis and to deal with their grief.

Other Fetal Malformations

Enlargement of various fetal parts could result in dystocia. These fetal problems include enlargement of fetal organs, such as a liver or distended bladder, and incomplete twinning, in which a partially developed twin is attached to the fetus. It is not uncommon for malpresentations and malpositions to accompany this type of gestation. Hydramnios (see p. 594) often accompanies the pregnancy that has a neurologically damaged fetus with defective swallowing.

Interventions. Cesarean section is recommended to avoid a difficult vaginal delivery if a developmental problem is diagnosed early. Connected fetuses are often joined by movable tissue that can be manipulated without dismembering a fetus.

Nursing tasks fall in the realm of physical and emotional support of the laboring couple. Physical support includes physiologic maintenance of the mother's body functions during labor and assistance with comfort measures. Emotional support includes assisting the couple with the grief process if there is a fetal loss. If the couple wishes to see the infant, the body should be made as attractive as possible. Cleaning the body of offensive odors and substances that cause disfigurement can be helpful. The infant can be wrapped in a colorful blanket and presented to the couple with gentle, loving care, which can make the acceptance easier.

Multiple Pregnancies

When two fetuses develop from the fertilization of one ovum, the twins are categorized as *monozygotic*. The twins are further classified as diamniotic, dichorionic, or monochorionic, depending on the period in which the division of the ovum occurs (Figure 19–13). If the division occurs before the outer cell mass is formed (within the first 72 hours after fertilization), the twins are dichorionic and diamniotic. Each fetus has its own placenta or the two placentas are fused. If, however, the division occurs after 72 hours and the chorionic cells have distinguished themselves, the twins are monochorionic and diamniotic. One placenta serves both fetuses, and they share a chorion. Monozygotic twins are identical and thus the same sex.

Dizygotic twins result from the fertilization of two separate ova. They are diamniotic, dichorionic, and fraternal. They may or may not be the same sex and are not identical. If the twins are of the same sex, the placenta is sent to pathology for examination to determine whether they are monozygotic or dizygotic twins.

According to Pritchard and MacDonald (1976) the incidence of monozygotic twins is independent of race, heredity, age, parity, and fertility therapy. However, the incidence of dizygotic twinning is highly influenced by these factors.

Identification of Multiple Gestations. When obtaining a maternal history, it is important to identify a family history of twinning. Equally important is a history of medication taken to enhance fertility. These facts should be noted on the antepartal record.

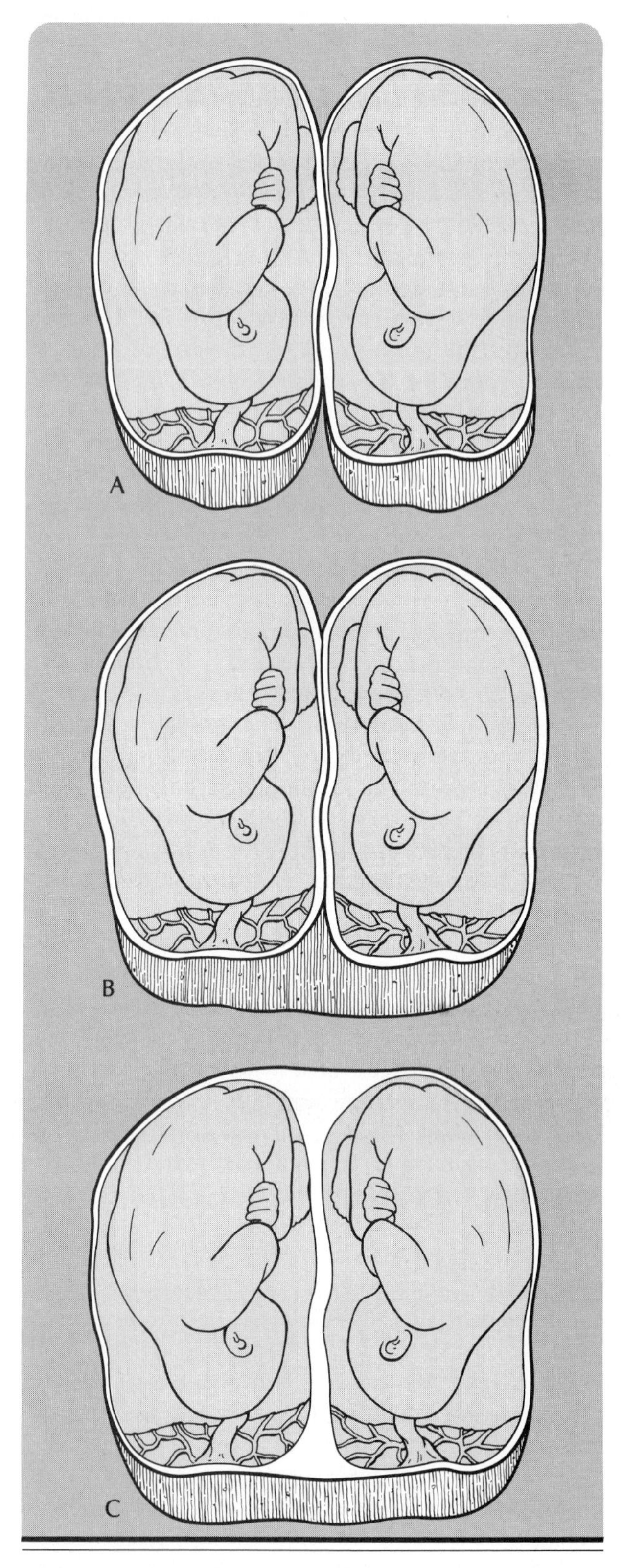

Figure 19–13. Twin pregnancies: placental and membrane development. **A,** Two placentas, two amnions, two chorions. **B,** Single placenta, two amnions, and two chorions. **C,** One placenta, one chorion, and two amnions.

At each antepartal clinic visit, the nurse should measure the fundal height. With any growth, fetal movement, or heart tone auscultation out of proportion to gestational age by dates, twins should be suspected. During palpation, many small parts on all sides of the abdomen may be felt. If twins are suspected, the nurse should attempt to auscultate two separate heartbeats in different quadrants of the maternal abdomen. Use of the Doppler device may be helpful. Conclusive evidence of twins is found on sonography or x-ray examination.

Maternal Implications. The increased incidence of pregnancy-induced hypertension (preeclampsia) associated with multiple gestations is thought to result from an oversized uterus and increased amounts of placental hormones. Abortions are more common in multiple gestations, possibly because of genetic defects or poor placentation or implantation. Maternal anemia is more common, because the maternal system is nurturing more than one fetus. Third trimester bleeding from placenta previa occurs more frequently, as does hydramnios. Hydramnios may be due to increased renal perfusion from cross-vessel anastomosis of monozygotic twins. Placenta previa may be due to a decreased area of choice for implantation.

Complications during labor include (a) uterine dysfunction due to an overstretched myometrium, (b) abnormal fetal presentations, and (c) premature labor. With rupture of membranes and hydramnios, abruptio placentae can occur (Pritchard and MacDonald, 1976). There is also a danger of placental abruption after the delivery of the first twin because of a decrease in the surface area of the uterus to which the placenta is still attached.

The mother with twins may experience more physical discomfort during her pregnancy, such as shortness of breath, dyspnea on exertion, backaches, and pedal edema, because of the oversized uterus.

Occasionally multiple pregnancies are not diagnosed until the time of delivery; this occurs most often in cases of prematurity. If the family has physically, psychologically, and financially prepared for one baby, problems can arise when they are suddenly confronted with more than one child. In addition, infants of multiple pregnancies frequently require intensive care, and this may cause financial and emotional stress.

Fetal-neonatal Implications. Fetal problems in the presence of multiple gestations are numerous. These infants are usually delivered prematurely. In addition, in the presence of monochorionic placentas with artery-to-artery anastomosis, fetoplacental circulation is compromised. One twin is overperfused and is born with polycythemia and hypervolemia and may have hypertension with an enlarged heart. This twin's amniotic sac exhibits hydramnios because of the increased renal perfusion and excessive voiding. The other twin has hypovolemia and exhibits IUGR. In the newborn period the infant with increased perfusion has an increased chance of hyperbilirubinemia as his system tries to rid itself of the extra red blood cells. The other twin is anemic, with all the problems that small-for-gestational-age infants exhibit.

The cytoplasmic mass of all organs is diminished in multiple gestations, and the growth rate is decreased. Therefore, twins may suffer from intellectual and motor impairment.

The high rate of prematurity is associated with an increased incidence of respiratory distress syndrome (RDS). The incidence of fetal anomalies is also greater with twin gestations (Pritchard and MacDonald, 1976).

Interventions. Antepartally, the mother may need counseling about diet and daily activities. The nurse can help her plan meals to meet her increased needs. An increase of 300 calories or more over the recommended daily dietary allowance established by the Food and Nutrition Board of the National Research Council is advised for uncomplicated pregnancy (see Table 11-2). The daily intake of protein should be increased as much as 1.5 gm/kg of body weight. Daily iron supplements of 60–80 mg and an additional 1 mg of folic acid are recommended.

Maternal hypertension is treated with bed rest in the lateral position to increase uterine and kidney perfusion. The nurse can help the mother schedule frequent periods of rest during the day. Family members or friends may be willing to care for this mother's other children periodically to allow her time to get rest. Back discomfort can be alleviated by pelvic rocking, good posture, and good body mechanics.

Occasionally in multiple pregnancies mothers exhibit nausea and vomiting past the first trimester. A diet consisting of dry, nongreasy foods may be helpful. Antiemetics may be necessary to provide relief. The mother is more prone to have a

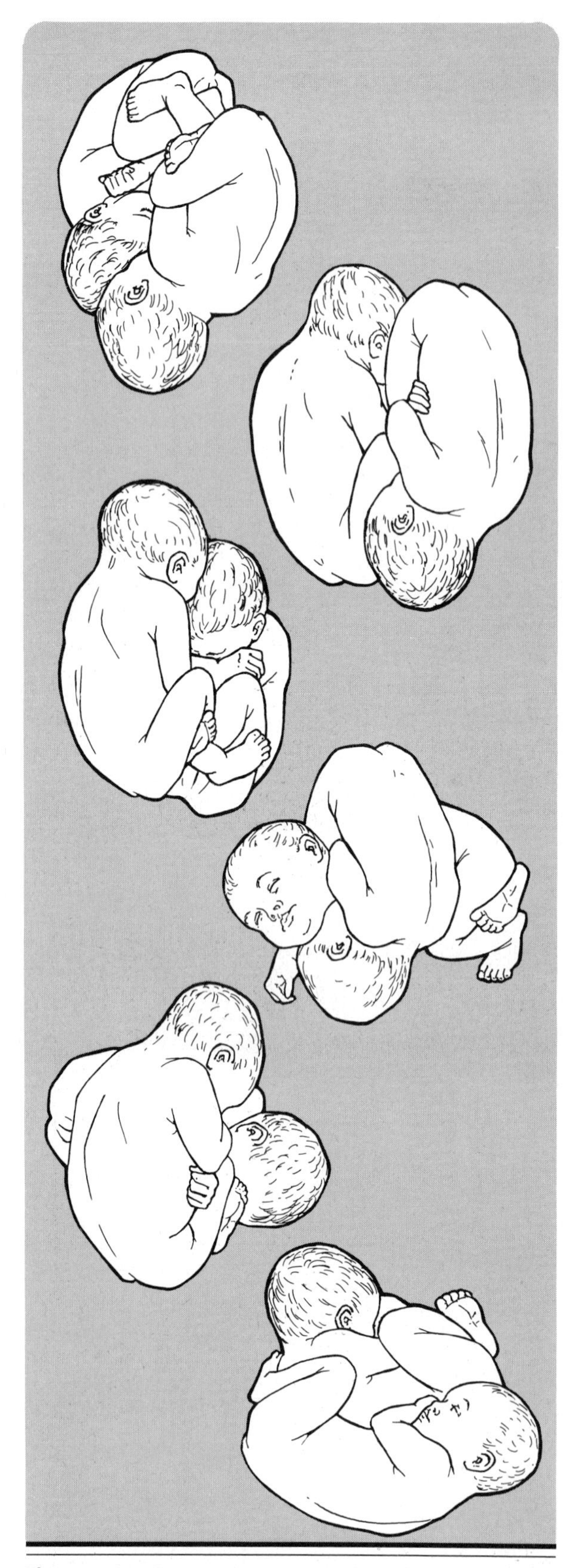

Figure 19–14. Types of twin presentations.

feeling of fullness after eating, and this may be alleviated by eating small but frequent meals.

In the event of fluid and electrolyte imbalance due to hypertension or hyperemesis, hospitalization may be necessary so that appropriate therapy may be instituted.

During labor, it is important to monitor both fetuses. An external electronic monitor can be applied to both fetuses, or if conditions permit, the internal monitor can be applied to the presenting twin and the external monitor can be applied to the other infant. The heart rate may be auscultated on different quadrants of the maternal abdomen, but continuous monitoring is more beneficial. Signs of distress should be reported immediately. The mother's labor should be plotted on the Friedman graph, and any sign of dysfunction should be reported to the physician.

With twins, any combination of presentations and positions can occur (Figure 19–14). A fetogram assists in determining these presentations and positions.

Vaginal delivery is facilitated when the largest fetus is in vertex presentation and is the first to be born. However, in the event that the first fetus is in a breech position, the following can occur:

1. If the fetus is large, the head can be a problem to the bony pelvis.
2. If the fetus is small, its body can descend into the birth canal before complete dilatation has occurred.
3. There is the danger of a prolapsed cord.

If these problems are overcome, the delivery can proceed as any other breech delivery.

The presentation, position, and lie of the second twin must be assessed quickly after the delivery of the first twin. If the breech or vertex is fixed in the pelvic inlet, the membranes may be ruptured and the mother allowed to labor under close supervision. The fetal heart rate of the second twin should be assessed closely. Occasionally diluted oxytocin is given if myometrial activity has not resumed within a ten-minute period.

Delivery in the presence of dysfunctional labor due to overstretched uterine fibers can be managed with cesarean section or infusion of diluted oxytocin. Obstetricians do not agree on the benefits and dangers of the two methods. Nor do physicians agree on the most beneficial type of analgesia and anesthesia to employ for the labor and delivery. In the presence of an unstable maternal circulatory system, as found with pregnancy-induced hypertension, regional anesthetic agents such as epidurals or caudals can cause hypovolemic shock due to the blocking of the sympathetic nervous system. Large and continuous doses of narcotics can cause neonatal respiratory depression, especially if these infants are premature, as twins frequently are. Paracervical blocks have been known to cause transient fetal bradycardia. Pritchard and MacDonald (1976) advocate the use of the pudendal block at the time of delivery. Uterine relaxation can be obtained with halothane if internal podalic version is required.

Cesarean section is advocated in the presence of fetal distress, previous cesarean sections, cephalopelvic disproportion, placenta previa, and sometimes severe pregnancy-induced hypertension. If the second twin is larger than the first and disproportion exists, a cesarean section should be performed (Pritchard and MacDonald, 1976).

The nurse has to prepare to receive two infants instead of one. This means a duplication of everything, including the resuscitation equipment, heated Krieselman units, and infant identification papers and bracelets. Two staff members need to be available for infant resuscitation.

If twins are discovered at the time of delivery, the nurse must move quickly to prepare for the second infant. The pediatric team may need to be notified at this time. While one nurse is monitoring the second twin in utero, the other nurse is caring for the already delivered infant and preparing for the second infant. Special precautions should be observed to ensure correct identification of the infants. The first born is usually tagged Baby A and the second, Baby B.

The matter of suppression of premature labor is under debate. If the labor has been established, little can be done other than to proceed with the deliveries. The labor pattern and fetuses should be continuously monitored, whole blood prepared in case it is needed, and a functioning intravenous route established. Two scrubbed obstetricians, a pediatrician, and an anesthesiologist should be present at the time of premature delivery.

After multiple deliveries, mothers are closely monitored for postpartal hemorrhage. In addition, the nurse assesses these women and their families to determine their need for referral to social welfare agencies or public health clinics for follow-up care. The family may be unprepared financially and psychologically for the arrival of twins and thus at risk for further difficulties.

Three or More Fetuses

When three or more fetuses are present, maternal and fetal problems are potentiated. The more fetuses conceived, the smaller they tend to be at the time of delivery. Generally, delivery of more than two fetuses is accomplished by cesarean section.

Superfecundation and Superfetation

Superfecundation is defined as the fertilization of two ova within a short period of time but not with the same act of intercourse. It occurs commonly in lower animals. *Superfetation* involves the fertilization of ova from two different ovulatory cycles. Superfecundation has been demonstrated in humans, but the occurrence of superfetation is doubtful.

Conjoined Twins

Conjoined or Siamese twins occur when the division of the embryonic disk is incomplete. Labor dystocia is common. Vaginal delivery can be accomplished if the joining is pliable. When essential organs are shared, separation after delivery is usually not successful.

Fetal Distress

The most commonly observed initial signs of fetal distress include meconium-stained amniotic fluid (in a vertex presentation) and decelerations in fetal heart rate. Fetal scalp blood samples demonstrating a pH of 7.20 or less provide a more sophisticated indication of fetal problems and are generally obtained when questions about fetal status arise.

A variety of factors may contribute to fetal distress. The most common are related to cord compression, placental abnormalities, and preexisting maternal disease.

Maternal Implications. Indications of fetal distress greatly increase the psychologic stress a laboring mother must face. The professional staff may become so involved in assessing fetal status and initiating corrective measures that they fail to provide explanation and emotional support to the mother and her partner. It is imperative to provide full explanations of the problem and interventions to the parents. In many instances, if delivery is not imminent the mother must undergo cesarean section. This operation may be a source of fear for the parents and of frustration, too, if they were committed to a shared, prepared delivery experience.

Fetal-neonatal Implications. Prolonged fetal hypoxia may lead to mental retardation or cerebral palsy and ultimately to fetal demise.

Interventions. When evidence of possible fetal distress develops, initial interventions include changing the maternal position and administering oxygen by mask at 6–7 liters/min. If fetal monitoring has not been used prior to this time, it is usually instituted. Fetal scalp blood samples are also taken. The patient is evaluated as to probable cause, and further actions are based on a complete assessment of maternal-fetal status. The accompanying Nursing Care Plan on fetal distress provides a framework for dealing with fetal distress caused by various conditions.

NURSING CARE PLAN

Fetal Distress

Patient Data Base

History

Assess mother for presence of predisposing factors:

1. Preexisting maternal diseases
2. Maternal hypotension, bleeding
3. Placental abnormalities

Physical examination

Asphyxia is suggested when one or more of the following are present:

1. Fetal heart rate decelerations
2. Presence of meconium in amniotic fluid
3. Fetal scalp blood pH determination ≤ 7.20

Laboratory evaluation

Maternal hemoglobin and hematocrit

Urinalysis

Nursing Priorities

1. Evaluate maternal and fetal status for variations requiring immediate intervention.
2. Identify and correct interferences with transplacental gas exchange.
3. Identify and report fetal heart rate decelerations and lack of baseline variability.
4. In presence of fetal asphyxia, prepare mother for immediate delivery (either vaginally or by cesarean section).

Problem	Nursing interventions and actions	Rationale
Fetal asphyxia	Observe and record the signs of fetal axphyxia:	Fetal asphyxia implies hypoxia (reduction in Po_2), hypercapnia (elevation of Pco_2), and acidosis (lowering of blood pH). Anaerobic glycolysis (breakdown of glycogen) takes place in the presence of hypoxia, and the end product of this process is lactic acid, resulting in metabolic acidosis.

NURSING CARE PLAN Cont'd

Fetal Distress

Problem	Nursing interventions and actions	Rationale
	1. Presence of meconium in amniotic fluid.	Fetal hypoxic episode leads to increased intestinal peristalsis and anal sphincter relaxation.
	2. Decelerations in fetal heart rate.	Vagal stimulation elicited through hypoxic brain tissues causes bradycardia and can increase intestinal motility, resulting in meconium release.
	3. Fetal hyperactivity.	Fetus may initially become hyperactive in an attempt to increase circulation.
	Initiate following interventions:	
	1. Administer O_2 to the mother with tight face mask at 6-7 liters/min, per physician order.	Administration of O_2 may increase amount of oxygen available for transport to fetus. Tight face mask is used because laboring mother tends to breathe through her mouth.
	2. Change maternal position.	Changed maternal position may relieve compression of the maternal vena cava and the cord, thereby facilitating O_2 exchange.
	3. Prepare equipment for fetal blood sampling.	Evaluate fetal acidotic state. Hypoxia causes increase in lactic acid and results in acidosis, which causes a drop in the pH of the fetal blood (normal pH is 7.25-7.30). Other tests that may be done on fetal blood sample are O_2 pressure (normal 18-22 mm Hg), CO_2 pressure (normal 48-50 mm Hg), base deficit (normal 0-10 mg/liter).
	4. Prepare patient for immediate delivery (may be vaginal or cesarean section).	
	5. Correct maternal hypotension if present: a. Administer IV fluids. b. Assess any maternal bleeding; if present, replace circulatory fluids.	Lowered maternal blood pressure or circulating blood volume affects O_2 exchange gradient of maternal-placental-fetal unit.
	6. Decrease uterine contractions. If oxytocin is infusing, decrease infusion rate or discontinue oxytocin.	Increased uterine tone decreases exchange at placental site and decreases fetal recovery time following contractions.
Impaired blood flow through umbilical cord		
Cord compression	Observe and note variable decelerations of fetal heart rate. If bradycardia lasts longer than 30 sec, change maternal position. If necessary, follow interventions listed under fetal asphyxia.	Umbilical vessels may be partially or completely occluded by compression of the cord. Cord may prolapse through cervix and vagina, or compression may occur when the cord is trapped between a fetal part and the bony pelvis. Transient episodes of compression are reflected by variable decelerations (decelerations that are unrelated to uterine contractions).

NURSING CARE PLAN Cont'd

Fetal Distress

Problem	Nursing interventions and actions	Rationale
Prolapsed cord	Evaluate each patient for predisposing factors: 1. Abnormalities in presentation: breech, shoulder, transverse lie. 2. Rupture of membranes. 3. Multiple gestation. Observe for prolapse of the cord externally through vaginal introitus. While doing vaginal exam, evaluate for presence of cord, which feels like rope and pulsates.	Occult or obvious prolapse of the cord may cause complete depletion of fetal oxygen within 2½ min if compression is not relieved.
	Institute emergency measures for prolapse of cord: 1. Manually exert pressure on the presenting part. This must be done continuously. Mother may be maintained in supine position, knee-chest position, or on her side with a pillow to elevate her hips. 2. If occult prolapse is suspected, change maternal position to side-lying position. 3. Notify physician immediately.	Emergency measures for a prolapsed cord are aimed at immediately relieving compression and reestablishing fetal-neonatal blood/oxygen circulation.
Impaired transplacental gas exchange	Assess mother for conditions that produce maternal hypoxia: 1. Severe pneumonia, maternal hypotension of any cause, congestive heart failure with diminished blood flow to maternal organs. 2. Disturbed O_2 carrying ability of hemoglobin.	Antepartal hypoxic insults influence the fetal response to labor and delivery by affecting O_2 exchange at placental site. Severe maternal disorders, such as abruptio placentae, seriously jeopardize the fetus, but the effects may be more pronounced in a fetus who has had antepartal stress such as toxemia, because O_2 exchange has been compromised and fetal reserve has decreased.
	3. Low environmental oxygen tension at high altitudes, preeclampsia-eclampsia, apnea with convulsions, vena caval syndrome.	Maternal hypoxia reduces O_2 tension in the blood that perfuses the placenta. Fetal O_2 deprivation follows as the maternal-fetal Po_2 gradient is reduced or eliminated.
	Assess mother for placental problems (placenta previa, abruptio placentae). Maintain maternal blood pressure. Maintain adequate maternal oxygenation by positioning (avoid supine position to prevent vena caval syndrome) and administration of O_2 as necessary.	These maternal conditions reduce placental gas exchange by reducing surface area available for oxygen diffusion.
	Replace circulating blood volume in presence of hemorrhage.	Maternal blood loss may cause hypotension and impair perfusion of the intact portion of the placenta.

Nursing Care Evaluation

Maternal conditions that produced maternal hypoxia are corrected or controlled.

A live birth is accomplished with no signs of permanent damage from fetal asphyxia.

Maternal blood volume is restored.

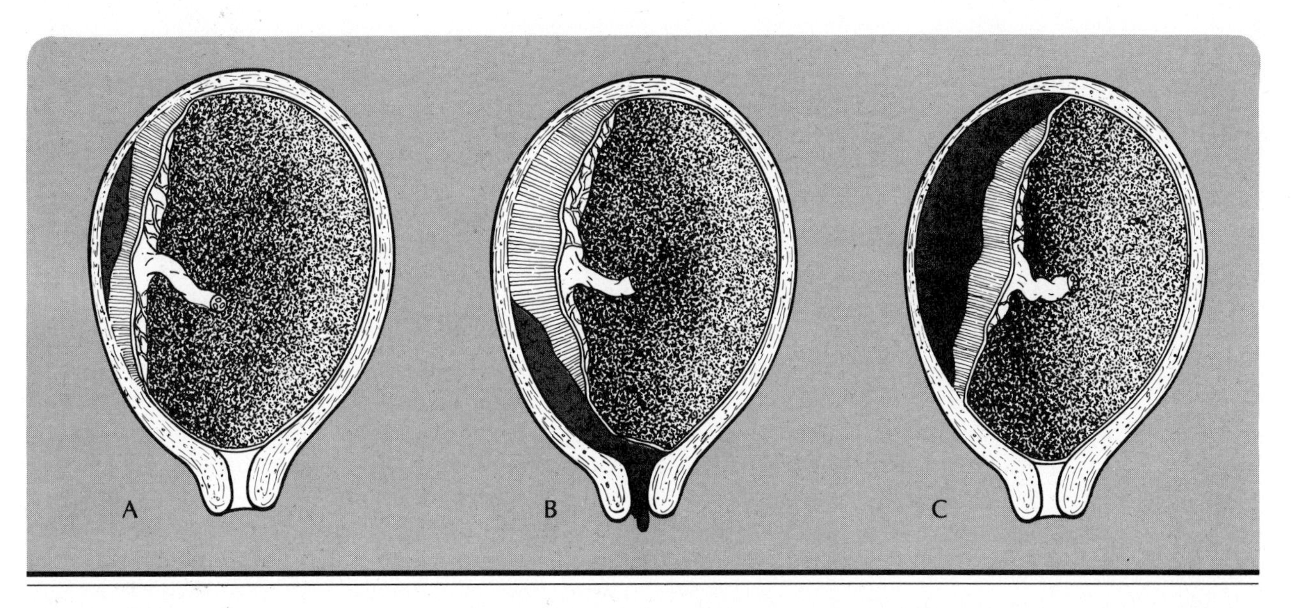

Figure 19–15. Abruptio placentae. **A,** Internal or concealed hemorrhage. **B,** External hemorrhage. **C,** Complete separation. (From Abnormalities of the Placenta, Clinical Educational Aid No. 12, Ross Laboratories, Columbus, Ohio.)

Placental Problems

Abruptio Placentae

Abruptio placentae is the premature separation of the placenta from the uterine wall. Premature separation is considered a catastrophic event because of the severity of the hemorrhage that occurs. The incidence is about one in 150-200 pregnancies. In 10% of the cases, the separation is severe, and maternal death occurs from hemorrhagic shock. In the other 90%, there is a less severe separation, and the results are not so serious. Increased risk of abruptio placentae occurs in women with a parity of five or more or who are over 30 years of age. It is also a greater risk for women with preeclampsia-eclampsia and renal or vascular disease.

The cause of abruptio placentae is largely unknown. Theories have been proposed relating its occurrence to decreased blood flow to the placenta through the sinuses during the last trimester. Excessive intrauterine pressure caused by hydramnios or multiple pregnancy may also be contributing factors.

Clinical Manifestations. Premature separation is subdivided into three types (Figure 19–15):

1. *Covert (severe).* In this situation, the placenta separates centrally and the blood is trapped between the placenta and the uterine wall.

2. *Overt (partial).* In this case, the blood passes between the fetal membranes and the uterine wall and escapes vaginally.

3. *Placental prolapse.* Massive vaginal bleeding is seen in the presence of almost total separation.

The signs and symptoms of these types of placental abruption are given in Table 19–3. In severe cases of covert abruptio placentae, a blood clot forms behind the placenta. With no place to escape, the blood invades the myometrial tissues between the muscle fibers. This occurrence accounts for the uterine irritability that is a significant sign of premature separation of the placenta. If hemorrhage continues, eventually the uterus turns entirely blue in color. Following delivery of the baby, the uterus contracts only with difficulty. This syndrome is known as a *Couvelaire uterus* and frequently necessitates hysterectomy.

As a result of the damage to the uterus wall and the retroplacental clotting, large amounts of thromboplastin are released into the maternal blood supply, which in turn triggers the formation of multiple tiny blood clots. This disorder is

Table 19–3. Differential Signs and Symptoms of Abruptio Placentae

Covert (severe)	Overt (partial)	Placental prolapse
No overt bleeding from vagina	Vaginal bleeding	Massive vaginal bleeding
Rigid abdomen	Rigid abdomen	Rigid abdomen
Acute abdominal pain	Acute abdominal pain	Acute abdominal pain
Decreased blood pressure, increased pulse	Decreased blood pressure, increased pulse	Shock
Uteroplacental insufficiency	Uteroplacental insufficiency	Marked uteroplacental insufficiency

referred to as *disseminated intravascular coagulation* (DIC), which results in hypofibrinogenemia. Fibrinogen levels, which are ordinarily elevated in pregnancy, may drop to incoagulable amounts within a matter of minutes as a result of rapidly developing premature separation of the placenta.

Maternal Implications. Maternal mortality is approximately 6%. Problems following delivery depend in large part on the severity of the intrapartal bleeding, coagulation defects (DIC), hypofibrinogenemia, and length of time between separation and delivery. In the postpartal period, mothers who have suffered this disorder are at risk for hemorrhage and renal failure due to shock, vascular spasm, intravascular clotting, or a combination of the three. Another cause of renal failure is incompatible emergency blood transfusion. Failure is directly proportional to the number of units transfused.

Fetal-neonatal Implications. Perinatal mortality associated with premature separation of the placenta is about 15%. In severe cases in which separation is almost complete, infant mortality is 100%. In less severe separation, fetal outcome depends on the level of maturity. The most serious complications in the neonate arise from prematurity, anemia, and hypoxia. With thorough assessment and prompt action on the part of the health team, fetal and maternal outcome can be optimized.

Interventions. Upon admission, the nursing assessment begins. Any sudden change in behavior, such as an aching pain in the abdomen, may signal the separation of the placenta during labor. Other important signs that should be noted include irritability of the uterus, faint or absent FHTs, fetal hyperactivity, increase in fundal height, any increase in bleeding, and symptoms of shock. Frequently, shock symptoms appear disproportionate to blood loss.

The psychologic aspects of the nursing care of this patient cannot be overestimated. Maternal apprehension increases as the clinical picture changes. Factual reassurance and an explanation of the procedures and what is happening are essential for the emotional well-being of the expectant parents. The nurse can reinforce positive aspects of the woman's condition, such as normal FHTs, normal vital signs, and decreased evidence of bleeding.

If the separation is mild and gestation is near term, labor may be induced and the baby delivered vaginally with as little trauma as possible. If the induction of labor by rupture of membranes and oxytocin infusion by pump does not initiate labor within eight hours, a cesarean section is usually done. A longer delay would increase the risk of increased hemorrhage, with resulting hypofibrinogenemia. Supportive treatment to decrease risk of DIC includes typing and crossmatching for blood transfusions (at least three units), clotting mechanism evaluation (fibrinogen on hand), and intravenous fluids.

In cases of moderate to severe placental separation, a cesarean section is done after hypofibrinogenemia has been treated by intravenous infusion of fibrinogen. Vaginal delivery is impossible in the event of a Couvelaire uterus, because it would not contract properly in labor. Cesarean section is necessary in the face of severe hemorrhage to allow an immediate hysterectomy to save both mother and fetus.

Medical and nursing management of complications of severe abruptio placentae is as follows. Hypovolemia is life-threatening and must be combated with whole blood. If the fetus is alive but in distress, emergency cesarean section is the method of choice for delivery. With a stillborn fetus, vaginal delivery is preferable unless shock from hemorrhage is uncontrollable. The hematocrit should be maintained at 30%. Pritchard and MacDonald (1976) recommend a balanced salt solution of Ringer's lactate intravenously. CVP monitoring may be needed to check fluid replacement. The nurse monitors fluid intake and output closely and accurately. Hourly recordings are suggested. Oliguria of less than 30 ml/hr should be reported to the physician. Intake may be increased or decreased depending on the output.

If a CVP line is inserted, elevations should be reported. The nurse should also look for signs of cough, rales, and shortness of breath, which might mean fluid overload and pulmonary edema.

Hourly bedside clotting times may be ordered and can be performed by the nurse. A stable clot that forms in less than 6 minutes indicates a good fibrinogen level. Blood that fails to clot within 30 minutes indicates a critically low clotting factor level. The time it takes the blood to clot plus retraction should be noted.

In the past, heparin was used in the treatment of DIC. It was thought to block the clotting cycle by inactivating thrombin, thus preventing the draining of the liver's fibrinogen stores. Pritchard and MacDonald (1976) advocate fibrinogen replacement instead of heparin; however, there is a risk of hepatitis with fibrinogen administration. A current method of monitoring the development of DIC is to do frequent laboratory testing for fibrin split products.

Measures should be taken to empty the uterus to prevent DIC from occurring. An amniotomy may be performed to decrease damage from the Couvelaire uterus, which in turn may lessen the possibility of DIC. Oxytocin stimulation is advocated to hasten delivery. The nurse will find it difficult to palpate contractions because of the hypertonic state of the uterus. However, the mother may complain with regularity, which signals increased uterine tone. Progressive dilatation and effacement usually occur (Pritchard and MacDonald, 1976).

Postpartally the nurse should continue close monitoring of the mother's fluid intake and output and her vital signs. The uterus must be palpated frequently for atony. In addition, the nurse must be alert for signs of postpartal hemorrhage.

If lactation occurs at the expected time, it is evidence that the pituitary has escaped serious damage from ischemia and that the threat of Sheehan's syndrome is reduced. The mother should be followed to determine whether menses returns. Tests of thyroid and adrenal function four to six months after delivery are part of proper follow-up care for patients who have suffered a severe placental abruption. (See the Nursing Care Plan for hemorrhage on p. 563.)

Placenta Previa

In placenta previa, the placenta is improperly implanted in the lower uterine segment. This implantation may be on a portion of the lower segment or over the internal os. As the lower uterine segment contracts and dilates in the later weeks of pregnancy, the placental villi are torn from the uterine wall, thus exposing the uterine sinuses at the placental site. Bleeding begins, but because its amount depends on the number of sinuses exposed, initially it may be either scanty or profuse.

The cause of placenta previa is unknown. Statistically it occurs in about one in every 200 deliveries and is more common in multiparas. Women with a previous history of placenta previa as well as those who have undergone a low cervical cesarean section appear to be at greater risk for its occurrence.

The types of placenta previa are as follows (Figure 19–16):

1. *Complete or total placenta previa.* The placenta totally covers the internal os.
2. *Partial placenta previa.* A small portion of the placenta covers the internal os.
3. *Low-lying or marginal placenta previa.* The placental edge is attached very close to but does not cover the internal os.

Clinical Manifestations. Painless, bright red vaginal bleeding is the best diagnostic sign of placenta previa. If this sign should develop during the last three months of a pregnancy, placenta previa should always be considered until ruled out by examination. Generally, the first bleeding episode is scanty. If no rectal or vaginal exams are performed, it often subsides spontaneously. However, each subsequent hemorrhage is more profuse.

The uterus remains soft, and if labor begins, it relaxes fully between contractions. The fetal heart rate usually remains stable unless profuse hemor-

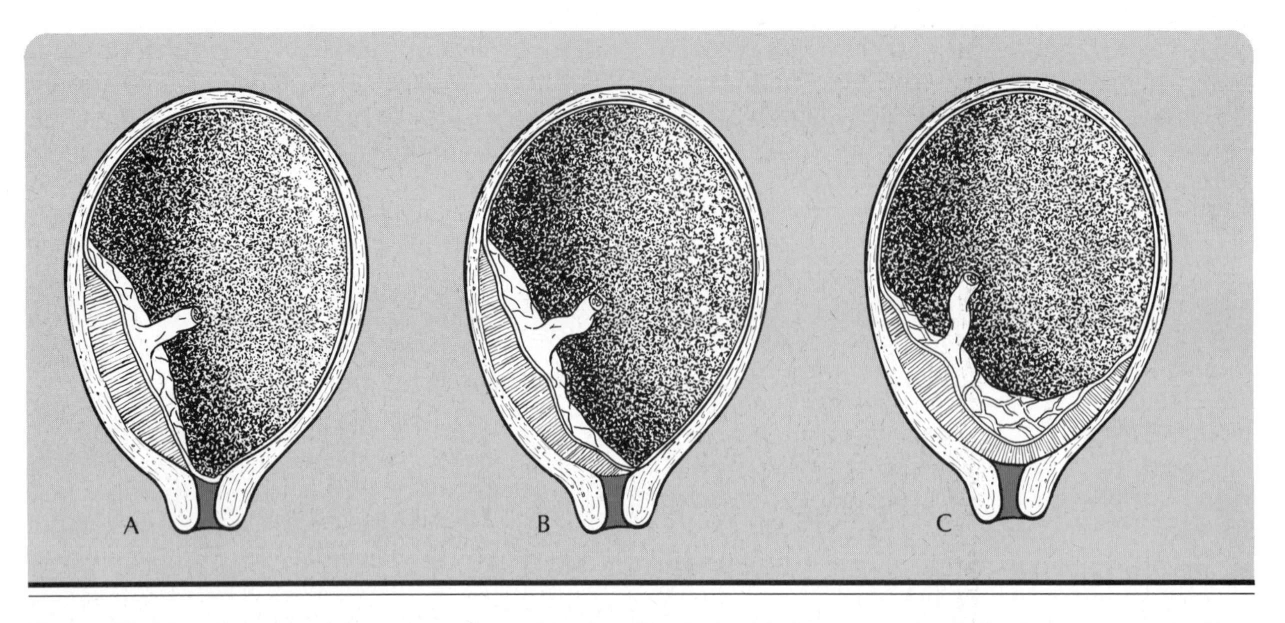

Figure 19–16. Placenta previa. **A,** Low placental implantation. **B,** Partial placenta previa. **C,** Total placenta previa. (From Abnormalities of the Placenta, Clinical Education Aid No. 12, Ross Laboratories, Columbus, Ohio.)

rhage and maternal shock occur. As a result of the placement of the placenta, the fetal presenting part is often unengaged, and abnormal lies can result.

Diagnosis. Direct diagnosis of placenta previa can only be made by feeling the placenta inside the os. However, profuse bleeding can result from this examination, so it should only be performed under two specific circumstances: (a) when the pregnancy is beyond 37 weeks' gestation and the fetus is mature enough to be born, and (b) when recurring hemorrhages make it imperative that delivery take place immediately to save both the mother and fetus. This examination is called the *double setup procedure* (see Procedure 19-1), and it requires that everything be at hand to perform an immediate cesarean section should profuse bleeding ensue.

Indirect diagnosis is made by localizing the placenta through tests that require no vaginal exam. The most commonly employed test is the ultrasound scan (Chapter 14). Many labor and delivery departments have a real time scanner that may be used for diagnosis. It is simple to use and highly accurate. Other techniques include radioisotopes localization, femoral arteriography, and x-ray placentography.

Differential Diagnosis. The differential diagnosis of cervical or uterine bleeding requires careful inspection and palpation. Suspicious areas should be biopsied. Partial separation of a normally implanted placenta may also exhibit painless bleeding, and a true placenta previa may not demonstrate overt bleeding until labor begins, thus confusing the diagnosis. Another important fact to note is that the causes of slight to moderate antepartal bleeding episodes in 20%–25% of patients are never accurately diagnosed.

Maternal Implications. The presence of placenta previa increases maternal risks in the postpartal period. Hemorrhage that may occur when the placental site is located in the lower uterine segment is a primary danger. This is the passive section of the uterus, and the contractility of this section of muscle fiber is poor. Uterine rupture could occur as a result of the weakening of the uterine musculature by the ingrowth of the placenta and the presence of its blood sinuses. Uterine infection from prolonged rupture of membranes, retained placental fragments, and possible anemia are also risks.

Fetal-neonatal Implications. The prognosis for the fetus depends on the extent of placenta

Procedure 19–1. Double Setup Examination

Objective	Nursing action	Rationale
Prepare patient	Explain procedure thoroughly. Consent form for a cesarean section is signed (in case it is needed).	Decreases anxiety. Informed consent is for legal purposes.
Assemble and prepare equipment	Set up delivery room for a vaginal delivery: 1. Assemble equipment on instrument table. 2. Warm infant crib. 3. Set out resuscitation equipment for newborn. 4. Obtain monitoring equipment: a. Sphygmomanometer and stethoscope. b. Ultrasound fetal monitoring system or fetoscope. Set up equipment for cesarean section if needed.	Sterile vaginal examination is done in the delivery room so that, if immediate delivery is required, a vaginal delivery or cesarean section may be done.
Position patient	Assist patient to delivery table. Place legs in stirrups, raising both legs at same time.	Reduces muscle strain.
Maintain adequate fluids	If IV infusion has not already been started, begin one with a large-bore needle. Administer fluids at a keep-open rate. Administer oxygen and suction as needed.	Patient is likely to develop excessive bleeding; IV is started so fluids may be administered quickly if needed.
Assemble personnel	Required personnel include scrub nurse, circulating nurse, physician, physician's assistant, anesthesiologist, pediatrician, and nursery nurse.	
Monitor procedure	Physician carefully performs vaginal examination. Dependent on findings, interventions may be as follows: 1. Rupture of membranes. 2. Vaginal delivery. 3. Cesarean section.	Method of treatment depends on presence and degree of placenta previa.

previa. In a profuse bleeding episode, the fetus is compromised and does suffer some hypoxia. Fetal heart rate monitoring is imperative on admission to the hospital, particularly if a vaginal delivery is anticipated. This is important, because the presenting part of the fetus may obstruct the flow of blood from the placenta or umbilical cord. If fetal distress occurs, delivery is by cesarean section.

After delivery of the infant, blood sampling should be done to determine whether any infant anemia has been caused by intrauterine bleeding episodes of the mother.

Interventions. Care of the patient with painless late gestational bleeding depends on (a) the week of gestation during which the first bleeding episode occurs and (b) the amount of bleeding. If the pregnancy is less than 37 weeks' gestation and if bleeding is scanty or has stopped, the placenta should be localized by indirect methods, such as real time scanning. If placenta previa is ruled out, a vaginal exam may be performed with a speculum to assess the cause of bleeding. If placenta previa is diagnosed, then *expectant management* is employed to delay delivery until about 37 weeks' gestation to allow the fetus to mature. Expectant management involves stringent regulation of nursing care as follows:

1. Bed rest with only bathroom privileges as long as the patient is not bleeding.
2. No rectal or vaginal exams.
3. Assessment of blood loss, pain, and uterine contractility.
4. Assessment of FHTs with external fetal monitor.
5. Monitoring of vital signs.
6. Complete laboratory evaluation: hemoglobin, hematocrit, Rh factor, and urinalysis.
7. Intravenous fluid (Ringer's lactate) with drip rate monitored.
8. Two units of cross-matched blood available for transfusion.
9. Communication with patient and family about what is happening and encouragement of their questions.

If frequent, recurrent, or profuse bleeding persists, a cesarean section is performed.

At 37 weeks, delivery is performed either by the vaginal route or by cesarean section. This decision is based on knowledge of the degree of previa and of the feasibility of labor induction. The double setup examination provides this information (see Procedure 19–1). If the placenta does not cover the os, membranes are ruptured and a vaginal delivery is anticipated. If bleeding becomes profuse, a cesarean section is done.

Before a double setup procedure is performed, the laboring couple should be physiologically and psychologically prepared for possible surgery (Chapter 20). A whole-blood setup should be readied for intravenous infusion and a patent intravenous line established before any intrusive procedures are undertaken. The maternal vital signs should be monitored every 15 minutes in the absence of hemorrhage and every 5 minutes with active hemorrhage. The external tocodynamometer should be connected to the maternal abdomen to continuously monitor uterine activity.

The precautions of a double setup are taken because the vaginal examination can cause overt bleeding. The medical and nursing team scrub and prepare for surgery. The newborn nursery is alerted, and adequate infant resuscitation equipment is readied. An anesthesiologist is also present. The mother is prepared for a cesarean section in the usual manner. She is then taken to the delivery room (or operating room) and examined in the lithotomy position. A speculum examination confirms the presence or absence of placenta previa. If previa is found, a cesarean section is performed without delay. The fetus should be continuously monitored until the pregnancy is terminated.

The newborn's hemoglobin, cell volume, and erythrocyte count should be checked immediately and then monitored closely. The infant may require oxygen and administration of blood.

Other Placental Problems

Other problems of the placenta can be divided into those that are developmental and those that are generative. Developmental problems of the placenta include placental lesions, placental succenturiata, circumvallate placenta, and battledore placenta. Degenerative changes include infarcts and placental calcification.

Placental Lesions. Angiomatous tumors, metastatic tumors, and cysts are classified as placental lesions. Cysts are the most common and occur in the chorionic membrane (Pritchard and MacDonald, 1976). About one-third of placental tumors are associated with maternal hydramnios. Maternal complications can result from hydramnios (see p. 594). Perinatal mortality is high because of the high rate of prematurity. These infants also have an increased incidence of metastatic lesions (Greenhill and Friedman, 1974).

Succenturiate Placenta. In succenturiate placenta, one or more accessory lobes of fetal villi have developed on the placenta, with vascular connections of fetal origin (Figure 19–17,*A*). The gravest maternal danger is postpartal hemorrhage if this lobe is severed from the placenta and is retained in the uterus. All placentas should be examined closely for intactness. If vessels appear to be severed at the margin of the placenta, the uterus should be explored for retained placental tissue. This condition usually is not diagnosed until after the delivery of the placenta (Pritchard and MacDonald, 1976). If the vascular connections rupture between the lobes, life-threatening fetal hemorrhage can result. At birth the infant should be inspected for pallor, cyanosis, retractions, tachypnea, tachycardia, and feeble pulse. The infant's cry will be weak and the muscle tone flaccid (Korones, 1976).

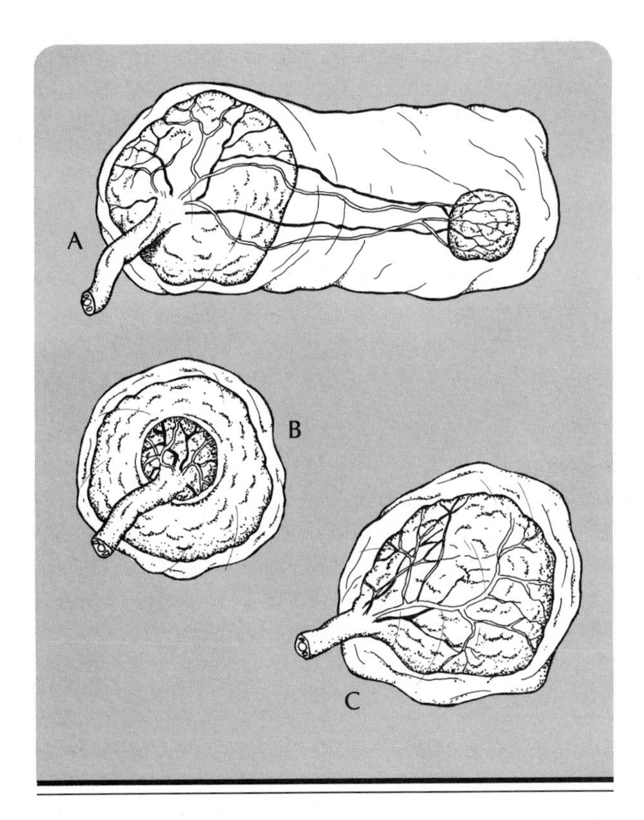

Figure 19–17. Placental variations. **A,** Succenturiate placenta. **B,** Circumvallate placenta. **C,** Battledore placenta. (From Abnormalities of the Placenta, Clinical Education Aid No. 12, Ross Laboratories, Columbus, Ohio.)

Circumvallate Placenta. In this condition the fetal surface of the placenta is exposed through a ring opening around the umbilical cord (Figure 19–17,*B*). The vessels descend from the cord and end at the margin of the ring instead of coursing through the entire surface area of the placenta. The ring is composed of a double fold of amnion and chorion with some degenerative decidua and fibrin between. The cause of this condition is unknown. Maternal-fetal problems include an increased incidence of late abortion or fetal death, antepartal hemorrhage, prematurity, and abnormal maternal bleeding during or following the third stage of labor, resulting from improper placental separation or shearing of membranes from the placenta.

Battledore Placenta. In this case the umbilical cord is inserted at or near the placental margin (Figure 19–17,*C*). As a result, all fetal vessels transverse the placental surface in the same direction. The chances of premature labor are high because of interference with fetal circulation and nutrition. Fetal distress or bleeding during labor is also likely because of cord compression or vessel rupture.

Placental Infarcts and Calcifications. In the aging process the placenta may develop infarcts and calcifications. They become significant if they cover a large enough area to interfere with the uterine-placental-fetal exchange. Altered exchange can also occur with certain maternal disease processes, such as hypertension.

Problems Associated with the Umbilical Cord

Prolapsed Umbilical Cord

Conditions associated with a prolapsed cord include breech presentation, transverse lies, contracted inlets, small fetus, extra long cord, low-lying placenta, hydramnios, and twin gestations. Any time the inlet is not occluded and the membranes rupture, the cord can be washed down (Figure 19–18) into the birth canal in front of the presenting part.

Maternal Implications. When predisposing factors to cord prolapse exist, the patient should be considered high risk and should be monitored closely. If prolapse occurs prior to complete cervical dilatation, cesarean section is the treatment of choice.

Fetal-neonatal Implications. Because with each contraction the umbilical cord becomes compressed between the maternal pelvis and the presenting part, fetal distress is common. If the cord ceases to pulsate, it is generally indicative of fetal demise.

Interventions. Bed rest is indicated for all laboring mothers with a history of ruptured membranes, until engagement with no cord prolapse has been documented. Furthermore, at the time of spontaneous rupture of membranes or amniotomy, the fetal heart rate should be auscultated for at least a full minute. During labor, if fetal bradycardia is detected on auscultation, the mother should be examined to rule out a cord prolapse. Electronic monitor tracings in the presence of cord prolapse show severe, moderate, or

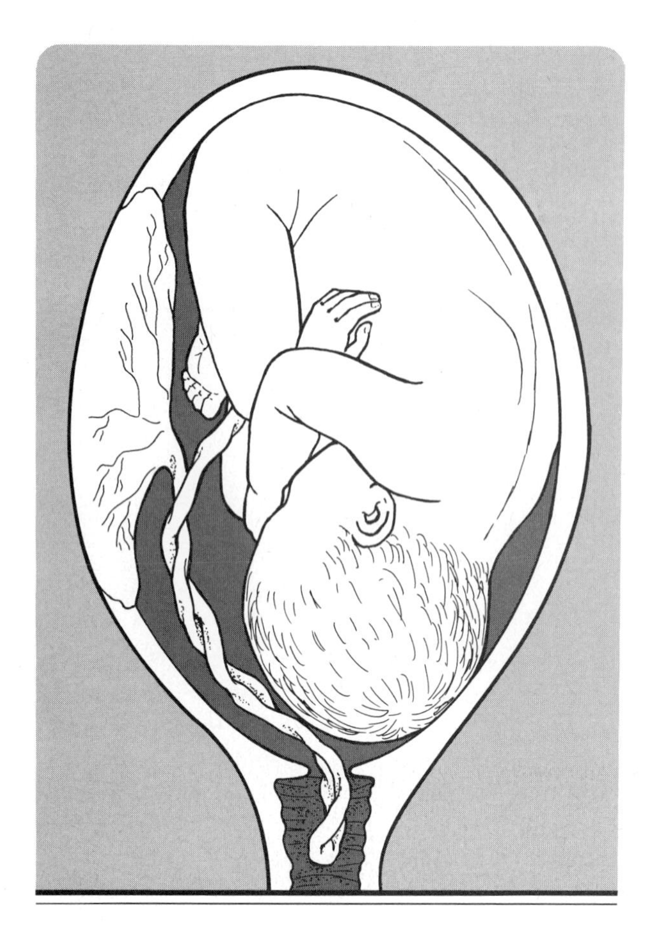

Figure 19–18. Prolapse of cord.

prolonged variable decelerations with baseline bradycardia. If these patterns are found, the nurse should examine the mother vaginally.

If a loop of cord is discovered, the gloved fingers are left in the vagina, and attempts are made to lift the fetal head off the cord to relieve the compression until the physician arrives. *This is a life-saving measure.*

The force of gravity can be employed to relieve the compression. The mother assumes the knee-chest position or the bed is adjusted to the Trendelenburg position. The nurse must remember that the cord may be occultly prolapsed with an actual loop extending into the vagina or lying alongside the presenting part. It may be pulsating strongly or so weakly that it is difficult to determine on palpation of the cord whether the fetus is alive. Greenhill and Friedman (1974) advocate that a Doppler device be used for auscultation before a fetal death is confirmed.

Occasionally a cord prolapses out the introitus. If this condition is identified in a home situation, some of the previously discussed life-saving actions can be implemented by the nurse. The lateral Sims position may be more feasible for the mother if the position is to be assumed for any extended period of time. The pelvis should be elevated on pillows. Compression on the cord can be relieved in the vagina as in the hospital situation, and wet dressings soaked in a mild salt solution should be wrapped around the protruding cord. The mother should be transported to the hospital immediately. If the cord is pale, limp, and obviously not pulsating, no action is necessary other than transport. At no time should attempts be made to replace the cord into the uterus, because this could cause devastating trauma to the cord and could greatly increase the possibility of intrauterine infection. Vaginal delivery (with or without forceps) is possible if the following criteria are met:

1. Cervix is completely dilated.
2. A vertex is presenting at least at zero station.
3. Membranes are ruptured.
4. Pelvic measurements are adequate.

If these conditions are not present, cesarean section is the method of choice for delivery. The mother is taken to the delivery room while the nurse vaginally relieves the pressure on the cord until the infant has been delivered. The medical and nursing team must work together quickly to facilitate delivery in this obstetric emergency.

Umbilical Cord Abnormalities

Umbilical cord abnormalities include congenital absence of an umbilical artery, insertion variations, cord length variations, and knots and loops of the cord. Insertion variations include velamentous insertion and vasa previa, and cord length problems include long and short cords.

Congenital Absence of Umbilical Artery

Absence of an umbilical artery has serious fetal implications. This condition usually is associated with life-threatening congenital anomalies, prematurity, and IUGR.

Immediately after the umbilical cord is cut, it should be inspected to determine whether the correct number of vessels is present. If an artery is absent, the nurse should examine the newborn more closely for anomalies and gestational age problems.

Velamentous Insertion

In this condition the vessels of the umbilical cord divide some distance from the placenta in the placental membranes (Figure 19–19). According to Pritchard and MacDonald (1976):

> The body stalk, which later becomes the umbilical cord, attaches the inner cell mass to the chorionic shell. Since the human egg implants with the inner cell mass down toward the endometrium, the placenta and body stalk are adjacent. According to one theory minor degrees of rotation give rise to the usual eccentric location of the cord. The more marked the rotation of the egg, the farther the umbilical cord will be from the center of the placenta. In that way, progressive rotation produces marginal and velamentous insertions. . . . when the egg implants with the inner cell mass 180 degrees from the endometrium, the umbilical cord and placenta come to lie at opposite poles and the fetal vessels will be located in the membranes.*

Velamentous insertions occur more frequently in multiple gestations than in singletons. Other placental anomalies often accompany this condition, such as succenturiate placenta. If the vessels become torn during labor, fetal hemorrhage can occur. Gabbe et al. (1977) state:

> The onset of fetal bleeding is marked by a tachycardia followed by a bradycardia with intermittent accelerations or decelerations. Small amounts of vaginal bleeding associated with fetal heart rate abnormalities should raise suspicion of fetal hemorrhage.†

Vasa Previa

When the vessels of a velamentous insertion transverse the internal os and appear in front of the fetus, a vasa previa has occurred. Fetal hemorrhage with asphyxia is likely to result because the hemorrhage will probably be diagnosed as maternal. There is a 60% fetal mortality with vasa previa (Greenhill and Friedman, 1974).

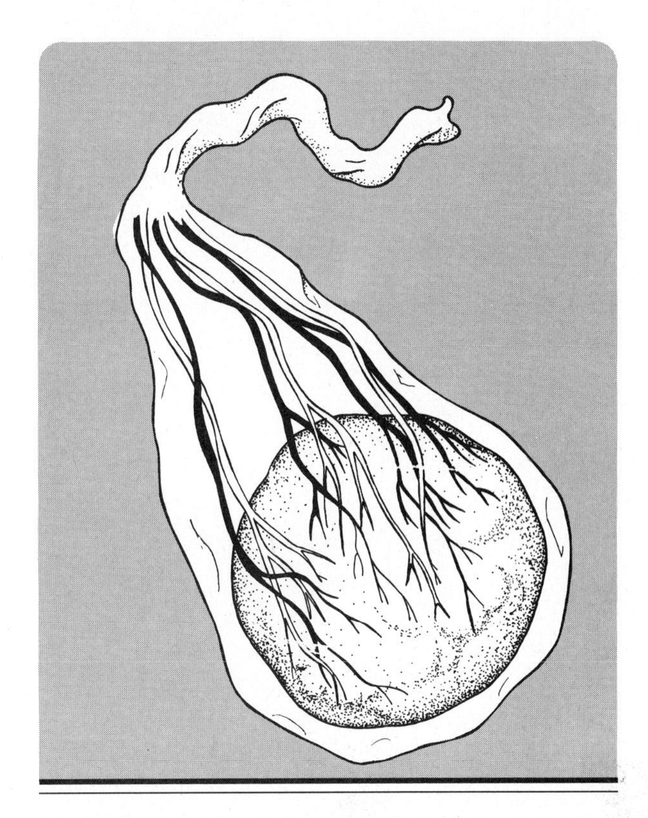

Figure 19–19. Placenta with a velamentous umbilical cord insertion.

Interventions. In the presence of any vaginal bleeding during labor, continuous monitoring of the fetus is imperative. Monitoring is best done with the aid of the external electronic monitor. Any signs of fetal distress should be reported immediately. Fetal hemorrhage is resolved by termination of the pregnancy vaginally or through cesarean section and by correction of neonatal anemia.

Cord Length Variations

The average length of the umbilical cord is 55 cm. Although short cords rarely cause complications directly, they have been associated with umbilical hernias in the fetus, abruptio placentae, and cord rupture. Long cords tend to twist and tangle around the fetus, causing transient variable decelerations. A long cord rarely causes fetal death,

---

*From Pritchard, J. A., and MacDonald, P. C. 1976. *Williams obstetrics.* 15th ed. New York: Appleton-Century-Crofts, p. 473.

†From Gabbe, S. G., et al. 1977. Fetal heart rate response to acute hemorrhage. *Obstet. Gynecol.* 49(2):247.

however, because it is generally not pulled tight until descent at the time of delivery. With a long cord and an active fetus, one or more true knots can result. Again, these knots usually are not pulled tight enough to cause fetal distress until the infant has been delivered, and the cord may then be clamped and cut.

Interventions. Any mild or moderate variable deceleration can be managed by the nurse, frequently with success. Repositioning of the mother often alleviates pressure on the cord if this is the reason for the deceleration.

Problems Associated with the Amniotic Fluid

Amniotic Fluid Embolism

Amniotic fluid embolism can occur naturally after a tumultuous labor or from oxytocin induction. In the presence of a tear in the amnion or chorion, the fluid may leak into the chorionic plate and enter the maternal circulation through the gaping venous system. The fluid can also enter at areas of placental separation or cervical tears. Under pressure from the contracting uterus, the fluid is driven into the maternal system.

Maternal Implications. This condition frequently occurs during or after the delivery when the mother has had a difficult, rapid labor. Suddenly the mother experiences respiratory distress, circulatory collapse, acute hemorrhage, and cor pulmonale, as the embolism blocks the vessels of the lungs. The more debris in the amniotic fluid (such as meconium), the greater the maternal problems. The acute hemorrhage is a result of DIC (p. 585), which is caused by the thromboplastin-like material found in amniotic fluid, in which factor VII is not essential. It has been demonstrated in vitro and in vivo that mucus, which is also found in amniotic fluid, induces coagulation by activation of factor X.

Maternal mortality is extremely high. In suspected cases in which the patients survive, it is difficult to determine whether an amniotic fluid embolism actually occurred.

Fetal-neonatal Implications. Delivery must be facilitated immediately to obtain a live birth. In many cases the delivery has already occurred or the fetus can be delivered vaginally with forceps. If labor has been tumultuous, the fetus may suffer problems associated with dysfunctional labor.

Interventions. Any mother exhibiting chest pain, dyspnea, cyanosis, frothy sputum, tachycardia, hypotension, and massive hemorrhage needs the cooperation of every member of the health team if her life is to be saved. Medical and nursing interventions are supportive.

Every delivery room should be equipped with a working oxygen unit. In the absence of the physician, the nurse administers oxygen under positive pressure until medical help arrives.

The nurse readies the equipment necessary for blood transfusion and for the insertion of the central venous pressure line. As the blood volume is replaced, using fresh blood to provide clotting factors, the CVP is monitored frequently. In the presence of cor pulmonale, fluid overload could easily occur.

DIC is controlled with fibrinogen replacement. The nurse is responsible for obtaining fibrinogen and other medications needed.

As one nurse assists the physician to maintain maternal homeostasis, another nurse intervenes as necessary to maintain the well-being of the fetus in utero and the newborn after delivery.

Hydramnios (Polyhydramnios)

Hydramnios occurs when there is over 2000 ml of amniotic fluid in utero. The exact cause of hydramnios is unknown. It is postulated that a major source of amniotic fluid is found in special amnion cells that lie over the placenta (Danforth, 1977). During the second half of the pregnancy, the fetus begins to swallow and inspire amniotic fluid and to urinate, which contributes to the amount present. In cases of hydramnios, no pathology has been found in the amniotic epithelium. However, hydramnios is associated with fetal malformations that affect the fetal swallowing mechanism and neurologic disorders in which the fetal meninges are exposed in the amniotic cavity. This condition is also found in cases of anencephaly in which the fetus is thought to urinate excessively due to overstimulation of the cerebrospinal centers. When a monozygotic twin manifests hydramnios, it is possible that the twin with the increased blood volume urinates excessively. The weight of the placenta has been found to be increased in some cases of hydramnios, indicating that an increased functioning of the placental tissue may be contributory.

There are two types of hydramnios: chronic and acute. In the chronic type, there is a gradual increase in the fluid volume. Most cases are of this variety. In acute cases, the volume increases rapidly over a period of a few days.

Maternal Implications. When the amount of amniotic fluid is over 3000 ml, the mother experiences shortness of breath and edema in the lower extremities from compression of the vena cava. If hydramnios is severe enough, she can experience intense pain. The acute form of hydramnios tends to be more severe. Milder forms of hydramnios occur more frequently and are associated with minimal symptoms. Hydramnios is associated with such maternal disorders as diabetes and Rh sensitization. As mentioned earlier, it may be found in multiple gestations.

Antepartally, if the amniotic fluid is removed too rapidly, abruptio placentae can result from a decreased attachment area. Because the uterine musculature is overstretched, the mother runs a risk of postpartal hemorrhage. Because of these overstretched fibers, uterine dysfunction can occur intrapartally, and there is increased incidence of postpartal hemorrhage.

Fetal-neonatal Implications. Fetal malformations and premature delivery are common with hydramnios; thus perinatal mortality is high. Prolapsed cord can occur when the membranes rupture, which adds a further complication for the fetus. The incidence of malpresentations is also increased.

Interventions. Hydramnios should be suspected when the fundal height increases out of proportion to the gestational age. As the amount of fluid increases, the nurse may have difficulty palpating the fetus and auscultating the FHTs. In the more severe cases, the maternal abdomen appears extremely tense and tight on inspection. On sonography, large spaces can be identified between the fetus and the uterine wall. Also at this time, an anencephalic infant or a dilated fetal stomach resulting from esophageal atresia may be identified, and multiple gestations may be confirmed. An x-ray fetogram will also show a radiolucent area of space and fetal skeletal defects if present.

If the accumulation of amniotic fluid has become severe enough to cause maternal dyspnea and pain, hospitalization and removal of the excessive fluid are required. This can be done vaginally or by amniocentesis. The dangers of performing the technique vaginally are prolapsed cord and the inability to remove the fluid slowly. If amniocentesis is performed, it should be done with the aid of sonography to prevent inadvertent damage to the fetus and placenta. The fluid should be removed slowly to prevent abruption (Pritchard and MacDonald, 1976).

When performing amniocentesis, it is vital to maintain sterile technique. The nurse can support the parents by explaining the procedure to them and can assist the physician in interpreting sonographic or x-ray findings.

Oligohydramnios

Oligohydramnios, in which the amount of amniotic fluid is severely reduced and concentrated, is a rare maternal finding. The exact cause of this condition is unknown. It is found in cases of postmaturity and in fetal conditions associated with renal and urinary malfunction. If oligohydramnios occurs in the first part of pregnancy, there is a danger of fetal adhesions (one part of the fetus may adhere to another part). Pulmonary hypoplasia has been found, theoretically due to lack of fluid inhaled in the terminal air sacs (Pritchard and MacDonald, 1976).

Maternal Implications. Labor can be dysfunctional and can begin before term. It is usually extremely painful for the mother, and progress is protracted.

Fetal-neonatal Implications. Fetal hypoxia may occur due to umbilical cord compression (Greenhill and Friedman, 1974). At birth these infants appear wrinkled and leathery, and serious skeletal deformities are often found (Pritchard and MacDonald, 1976).

COMPLICATIONS INVOLVING THE PASSAGE

The passage includes the maternal bony pelvis, beginning at the pelvic inlet and ending at the pelvic outlet, and the maternal soft tissues within these anatomic areas. A contracture in any of the described areas can result in cephalopelvic disproportion (CPD). Abnormal fetal presentations and positions occur in CPD as the fetus attempts to accommodate to its passage.

The gynecoid and anthropoid pelvis types usually are adequate for vertex delivery, but the android and platypelloid types predispose to CPD. Certain combinations of types also can result in pelvic diameters inadequate for vertex delivery. (See Chapter 15 for an in-depth description of the types of pelves and their implications for childbirth.)

Maternal Implications. Labor is prolonged and protracted in the presence of CPD, and premature rupture of membranes can result from the force of the unequally distributed contractions being exerted on the fetal membranes. In obstructed labor, uterine rupture can occur. With protracted descent, necrosis of maternal soft tissues can result from pressure exerted by the fetal head. Eventually necrosis can cause fistulas from the vagina to other nearby structures. Difficult forceps deliveries can also result in damage to maternal soft tissue.

Fetal-neonatal Implications. If the membranes rupture and the fetal head has not entered the inlet, there is a grave danger of cord prolapse. Extreme molding of the fetal head can result in skull fracture or intracranial hemorrhage. Traumatic forceps deliveries can cause damage to the fetal skull and central nervous system.

Interventions. The adequacy of the maternal pelvis for a vaginal delivery should be assessed intrapartally as well as antepartally. During the intrapartal assessment, the size of the fetus and its presentation, position, and lie must also be considered. (See Chapter 16 for intrapartal assessment techniques.)

The nurse should suspect CPD when labor is prolonged, cervical dilatation and effacement is slow, and engagement of the presenting part is delayed. Contractions should be monitored continuously, and the labor progress should be charted on the Friedman graph. The fetus should also be monitored continuously.

If the obstetrician is uncertain whether the infant will be delivered vaginally, a trial of labor may be given. If contractions are not strong enough, oxytocin is administered to stimulate uterine activity. The trial of labor is allowed to continue only as long as dilatation and descent is progressive (Friedman and Sachtleben, 1976). Nursing actions during the labor trial are the same as during any procedure in which oxytocin is being administered. The mother and fetus must be monitored continuously.

The couple may need support coping with the stresses of this complicated labor. The nurse should keep the couple informed of what is transpiring and explain the procedures that are being utilized. This knowledge can reassure the couple that measures are being taken to resolve the problem.

COMPLICATED CHILDBIRTH: EFFECTS ON THE FAMILY

A complicated pregnancy and difficult labor and delivery are crisis situations that can test the coping mechanisms of every individual involved. The family may respond to the crisis in relatively typical ways or may respond dysfunctionally.

During the antepartal period, the family may have ambivalent feelings toward a complicated pregnancy. Fear and anxiety about the mother's health and the health and welfare of the fetus may be exhibited as hostile behaviors and guilt feelings. The mother may have feelings of inadequacy with regard to her womanhood and her ability to reproduce (Cabela, 1977). The father may blame himself for impregnating his wife, or the family may accuse the health care team of poor management.

Simultaneously, the parents, especially the mother, are emotionally investing themselves in the child. The mother perceives the child as part of herself. With birth, the child becomes a person in his own right and the process of attachment occurs.

When a child is stillborn or dies following delivery, the parents must mourn and deal with the pain of detaching themselves. This process involves anger, guilt, pain, and sadness. However, because they have had little or no time to know the child as a person, the soothing part of the mourning process—"identification" built on memories, shared experiences, and mutual living—is absent (Furman, 1978).

Parents of an ill or deformed infant must not only resolve their feelings of guilt and grief, but they must also prepare themselves to care for that child. This couple may be unable to face the possibility that their infant may not survive. They may doubt their ability to properly care for the child. The costs of caring for the high-risk child are great, perhaps creating financial difficulties for the family. In addition, the emotional toll of caring for such a child may be extreme.

Nursing Management

The birth of an ill, abnormal, or stillborn infant presents the couple with the reality that they may have feared throughout pregnancy. It is imperative that the medical and nursing staff respond in supportive and sympathetic ways. Typically, however, health care personnel avoid eye contact and communication with the mother. Another common reaction on the part of the nursing staff is the use of cliches (Saylor, 1977). Comments such as "The poor thing is better off" or "You can have other children" are offered as comfort. However, the bereaved parents perceive the loss not only as the death of their child but also as a loss of a portion of themselves, and such comments seem to negate the child's very existence.

When a malformed infant is born, powerful reactions, even among caregivers, are not unusual. Kennell (1978) points out that initially the staff may be fascinated to hear about a malformed baby and be eager to see him. Frequently, such a child is the focus of a great deal of staff attention in the nursery. After they have seen him, they feel shock and sadness similar to that experienced by the parents. This reaction is especially likely for those who have had little experience with congenital anomalies. Finally, in an effort to deal with their reactions, they have a tendency to wish to avoid the parents. In such instances it is frequently helpful to provide the staff with occasions to talk through their feelings so that they can be more supportive of the family in its grief. In some centers with intensive care nurseries, this practice has been formalized through regular staff meetings and has been of great benefit to staff and, indirectly, to families.

Basic actions the nurse can take to provide emotional support are often of real help to a family. When a labor is complicated or when the fetus has died, it is imperative that the patient have consistent support and not be left alone. The husband should be encouraged to remain, and the nurse should also be present to observe the patient and provide support. Thoughtful comfort measures such as ice chips, clean chux, and judicious use of analgesics also demonstrate caring (Kowalski and Osborn, 1977).

In the event of a stillborn delivery or infant death, the parents are given the opportunity to see and hold their child, regardless of condition or abnormality. Parents should not be forced, but if they are uncertain, the nurse can explain that fantasy is often worse than fact and that seeing the infant frequently facilitates the grieving process. The father must not make this decision for his wife. The parents should, of course, be prepared for what they will see. Simple explanations of the baby's appearance—including a description of color, skin, any abnormalities or bruises, and body temperature—will prepare the parents. The nurse should wipe off any blood or feces before showing the infant to his parents. At this time the nurse may tactfully point out attractive aspects of the infant's appearance so that he becomes more of an individual to the parents. Some agencies are even showing parents infants stillborn before the age of viability and report positive results (Kowalski and Osborn, 1977).

When a malformed baby is born, the parents must deal with their mourning and with the future needs of their child. Kennell (1978) points out that whenever possible the parents and their infant should be kept together following delivery. Frequently, the child can be returned to the parents after a brief physical assessment in the nursery. The contact between the parents and child may ultimately be a source of great satisfaction to the parents if successfully accomplished.

The decision to permit the siblings to view the dead baby should be based on the child's age and personality. Adolescents may be offered a choice. School-aged children are not helped by seeing the infant but may benefit by attending the funeral service. Some preschool children may benefit from attending the service with their parents, but they especially are *not* helped by seeing their dead sibling (Furman, 1978).

Any time a complication occurs during pregnancy, financial difficulties may occur, even in families that are not classified as low income. Financial strain may be embarrassing for the family, and they may be hesitant to voice their concerns. The nurse must be familiar with hospital, federal, and local resources in her community so that she can make them known to high-risk clients.

The parents of a child born with a disability require time to work through their feelings of grief. They then need and desire factual information about their child's disability, his special needs, and the care he requires. Using a collaborative approach, members of the health team can provide the necessary teaching and information. They can also refer the parents to community groups and resources that are directed toward providing financial assistance and helping the child develop to his fullest potential. Community groups also exist that provide support to the parents and can be a source of great benefit to them.

SUMMARY

Childbirth is traditionally viewed as normal, happy, and uneventful, and usually it is. However, a wide variety of complications may develop that represent a hazard to the mother and her unborn child. It is essential that the labor and delivery patient be assessed carefully and provided with appropriate care to prevent problems when possible or to treat them to facilitate satisfactory outcome.

SUGGESTED ACTIVITIES

1. Given a patient situation involving a complication of labor or delivery, role-play the actions you would take in assessing the situation. Then verbally describe an appropriate plan of care, including emotional support, and return to role playing to implement the plan.

2. Arrange an "on call" situation with your instructor and agency whereby you will be called in the event that a patient with suspected complications is admitted to labor and delivery.

REFERENCES

Assali, N. S. 1972. *Pathophysiology of gestation: maternal disorders.* New York: Academic Press.

Bonica, J. J. 1967. *Principles and practices of obstetric analgesia and anesthesia.* Philadelphia: F. A. Davis Co.

Brazy, J. E., and Pupkin, M. J. 1979. Effects of maternal isoxsuprine administration on pre-term infants. *J. Pediatr.* 94:444.

Cabela, B. 1977. Complications of childbearing: psychological and socioeconomic implications. In *Maternity nursing today,* eds. J. P. Clausen et al. New York: McGraw-Hill Book Co.

Cohen, W. 1977. Influence of the duration of second stage labor on perinatal outcome and puerperal morbidity. *Obstet. Gynecol.* 49:266.

Csapo, A. I., and Herczeg, J. Nov. 1977. Arrest of premature labor by isoxsuprine. *Am. J. Obstet. Gynecol.* 129:482.

Danforth, D., ed. 1977. *Obstetrics and gynecology.* Hagerstown, Md.: Harper & Row Publishers, Inc.

Dick-Read, G. 1972. *Childbirth without fear.* 4th ed. New York: Harper & Row Publishers, Inc.

Epstein, M. F., et al. 1979. Neonatal hypoglycemia after beta-sympathomimetic tocolytic therapy. *J. Pediatr.* 94:449.

Erickson, M. 1976. The relationship between psychological variables and specific complications of pregnancy, labor and delivery. *J. Psychosom. Res.* 20:21.

Friedman, E. A., and Sachtleben, M. R. 1976. Station of the fetal presenting part, VI. Arrest of descent in nulliparas. *Obstet. Gynecol.* 47:129.

Friedman, E. A., et al. 1977. Dysfunctional labor, XII. Long-term effects on infant. *Am. J. Obstet. Gynecol.* 127:779.

Furman, E. Winter 1978. The death of a newborn: care of the parents. *Birth Fam. J.* 5:214.

Gabbe, S. G., et al. 1977. Fetal heart rate response to acute hemorrhage. *Obstet. Gynecol.* 49:247.

Greenhill, J. P., and Friedman, E. 1974. *Biological principles and modern practice of obstetrics.* Philadelphia: W. B. Saunders Co.

Kauppila, A., et al. March 1978. Effects of ritodrine and isoxsuprine with or without dexamethasone during late pregnancy. *Obstet. Gynecol.* 51(3):288.

Kennell, J. H. Winter 1978. Birth of a malformed baby: helping the family. *Birth Fam. J.* 5:219.

Kochenour, N. 1977. The management of breech presentations. *PCC News.* 3:32.

Korones, S. 1976. *The high risk newborn infant: the basis for intensive care.* St. Louis: The C. V. Mosby Co.

Kowalski, K., and Osborn, M. Jan.–Feb. 1977. Helping mothers of stillborn infants to grieve. *Am. J. Mat. Child Nurs.* 2:29.

Paul, R. H., and Petrie, R. H. 1973. *Fetal intensive care: current concepts.* Los Angeles: University of Southern California School of Medicine.

Pritchard, J. A., and MacDonald, P. C. 1976. *Williams obstetrics.* 15th ed. New York: Appleton-Century-Crofts.

Reid, D. E., et al. 1972. *Principles and management of human reproduction.* Philadelphia: W. B. Saunders Co.

Saylor, R. D. 1977. Nursing response to mothers of stillborn infants. *J. Obstet. Gynecol. Neonatal Nurs.* 6:39.

Spellacy, W. N., et al. July 15, 1978. The acute effects of ritodrine infusion on maternal metabolism: measurements of levels of glucose, insulin, glucagon, triglycerides, cholesterol, placental lactogen and chorionic gonadotrophin. *Am. J. Obstet. Gynecol.* 131(6):637.

Stubblefield, P. G. Oct. 1978. Pulmonary edema occurring after therapy with dexamethasone and terbutaline for premature labor: a case report. *Am. J. Obstet. Gynecol.* 132:341.

Thornfeldt, R. E., et al. May 1978. The effect of glucocorticoids on the maturation of premature lung membranes. *Am. J. Obstet. Gynecol.* 131:143.

ADDITIONAL READINGS

Berkowitz, R. L., et al. July 1978. The relationship between premature rupture of the membranes and the respiratory distress syndrome. *Am. J. Obstet. Gynecol.* 131:503.

Brodicks, K. 1965. *Patterns of shock: implications for nursing care.* New York: The Macmillan Co.

Freeman, R. K. 1974. Management of acute fetal distress. In *A clinical approach to fetal monitoring.* San Leandro, Calif.: Berkeley BioEngineering, Inc.

Freeman, R. K. 1974. Monitoring records from selected clinical cases. In *A clinical approach to fetal monitoring.* San Leandro, Calif.: Berkeley BioEngineering, Inc.

Friedman, E. A. 1974. Management of difficult labor. Med-Com slide presentation.

Guyton, A. 1976. *Textbook of medical physiology.* Philadelphia: W. B. Saunders Co.

Klaus, M. H., and Fanaroff, A. A. 1973. *Care of the high risk neonate.* Philadelphia: W. B. Saunders Co.

Kübler-Ross, E. 1969. *On death and dying.* New York: The Macmillan Co.

Miller, J. M., et al. Sept. 1978. Premature labor and premature rupture of the membranes. *Am. J. Obstet. Gynecol.* 132:1.

Rubin, R. 1961. Puerperal change. *Nurs. Outlook.* 9:753.

CHAPTER 20

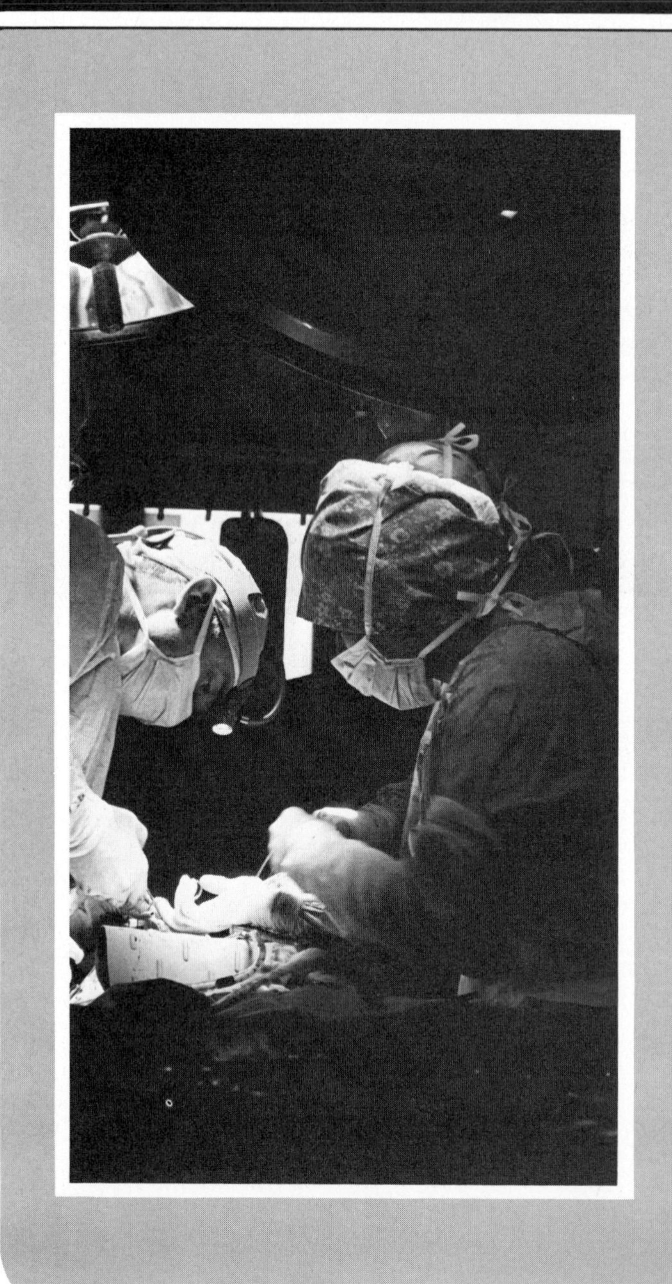

COMMON ELECTIVE AND OPERATIVE OBSTETRICS

OBJECTIVES

- Explain why amniotomy is the most common operative procedure in obstetrics.
- Compare the methods for inducing labor, explaining their advantages and disadvantages.
- Describe the types of episiotomies performed, the rationale for each, and the nursing interventions for caring for a patient with an episiotomy.
- List the indications for forceps delivery, the type of forceps that would be used, and the complications that may occur.
- Discuss the various methods for version and the nursing interventions for each method.
- List the indications for cesarean section and the type of procedure that would be performed.

The use of operative or other obstetric procedures has increased in recent years. More childbearing women are being identified as high risk, and the birth experience must be facilitated whenever possible in these cases to ameliorate the possible dangers to the mother and infant. In addition, certain obstetric procedures are performed to accommodate the wishes of the expectant family or the physician.

Obstetric procedures discussed in this chapter are amniotomy, induction of labor, episiotomy, repair of lacerations, forceps delivery, vacuum extraction, versions, and cesarean section.

AMNIOTOMY

Amniotomy, the artificial rupturing of membranes to shorten labor, is probably the most common operative procedure in obstetrics. In a study conducted by Martell et al. (1976), it was noted that 66% of all laboring women reach full dilatation with intact membranes. Of these women, 12% have intact membranes at the time of delivery. Martell et al. demonstrated that labor is shortened after an amniotomy if it is performed when the cervix is dilated 4–5 cm, probably because the hard fetal head comes in contact with the cervix and hastens cervical dilatation. However, Martell found that infants born following artificial rupture of the membranes at 4–5 cm cervical dilatation had a slightly lower pH and an increased incidence of type I decelerations. These side effects could be deleterious in the case of a high-risk pregnancy, in which the fetus may already be compromised.

Before an amniotomy is performed, the fetus is assessed for presentation, position, and station. Unless the head is well engaged in the pelvis, most physicians do not advocate an amniotomy because of the danger of prolapsed cord and a potential transverse lie.

The nurse explains the procedure to the laboring woman, who is draped in preparation for a vaginal examination and whose perineum is prepared according to hospital procedure. The nurse may apply fundal pressure. When performing the sterile vaginal examination, the physician introduces an amnihook (or other rupturing device) into the vagina. A small tear is made in the amniotic membrane. Explanation of the sensations the laboring woman will feel helps decrease anxiety. She can expect to feel the draining of amniotic fluid onto her perineum but no increase in discomfort. It is imperative that the FHTs be auscultated before and immediately after the procedure so that any changes from the previous FHR pattern can be noted. If there are marked changes, the nurse should check for prolapse of the cord. The amniotic fluid should be inspected for amount, color, odor, and presence of meconium or blood. The perineal area is cleaned and dried after the procedure. There is now an open pathway for organisms to ascend into the uterus, so strict sterile precautions must be taken when doing vaginal examinations, the number of vaginal exams must be kept to a minimum, and the woman's temperature should be monitored every two hours.

INDUCTION OF LABOR

The American College of Obstetricians and Gynecologists defines *induction of labor* as the deliberate initiation of uterine contractions prior to their spontaneous onset (Hughes, 1972). Induction of labor is one of the most controversial issues facing obstetric medicine because of the possible risks.

When, why, and *how* to electively induce labor (initiate uterine contractions) are questions frequently asked by the medical team as well as by the expectant couple. Labor induction should be considered for women with vascular diseases that are life-threatening to them or to their infants in the second and third trimesters. In addition, preeclampsia, Rh incompatibility, diabetes, and such conditions as premature rupture of the membranes, postmaturity, and antenatal death are frequent medical indications for inducing labor.

Elective inductions—those for which there is no medical indication—may be performed for rea-

---

The chapter opening photograph is from Kozier, B., and Erb, G. L. 1979. *Fundamentals of nursing: concepts and procedures.* Menlo Park, Calif.: Addison-Wesley Publishing Co.

sons of physician or patient convenience. Patients who reside some distance from the hospital and who have a history of rapid labor are candidates for elective inductions.

Induction of labor is generally a safe procedure today and is used more frequently because of improved synthetic oxytocic drugs, improved methods of drug administration, availability of fetal and maternal electronic monitoring devices, new diagnostic techniques, and better insight into the psychologic needs of the patient.

Negative feelings about induced labor can be reduced when good clinical judgment prevails. Expected outcomes of a successful induction should be discussed with the mother and family. She should be told that labor should begin in four to eight hours with well-established and effective contractions and that the first stage of labor tends to be slightly shorter than in unassisted labors. Since some mothers report that the contractions are more intense or sharper, the laboring woman should be told that this may result from having contractions of good intensity and duration early in the labor process and not having the slower progressive buildup of intensity as in an average labor process. Also, since oxytocin is externally introduced, the woman may have more oxytocin working on the uterine muscle than usual. All laboring women need to be assured of the normalcy of the contractions in order to decrease their tendency to tense up. The woman should be encouraged to use her childbirth education breathing exercises, which can be effective in induced labor situations.

The nurse should also explore and discuss with the couple the reason for the induction, especially if it is for medical reasons. Feelings of failure may develop if the mother perceives that most women go into labor on their own.

Obstetricians and family practitioners should seek all available data to support their decision to intervene in both indicated and elective cases. Ancillary services such as clinical and radiology laboratories should be utilized to this end.

Advantages and Disadvantages

Induction of labor allows the patient to better prepare herself for the labor process. For example, the patient can be well rested and can limit her food intake before admission. If the patient has had a previous precipitous labor, a scheduled induction may give her peace of mind with regard to the possibilities of delivery at home or en route to the hospital. Another advantage to planned labor is the more effective utilization of hospital and ancillary services, such as the laboratory and x-ray facilities and health care personnel (for example, additional nursing staff is more readily available during the day, thus assuring more comprehensive management of each patient). In addition, the primary physician's presence at delivery is virtually ensured, and his or her time can be scheduled more effectively.

Induction of labor can result in complications, however. Fetal distress, prematurity, cervical lacerations, midforceps delivery, and cesarean section occur at a much higher rate if the pregnancy is interrupted by elective induction before the end of the full 40-week gestation period.

In screening patients, any error in judgment that predisposes to prematurity or to undesirable fetal outcome from prolapsed cord, uterine infection, prolonged labor, or uterine rupture is the responsibility of the obstetrician.

Patient Consent

Elective inductions for the convenience of the physician should have the full cooperation and consent of the patient. All inductions require a written consent form explaining the risks of induction and listing the most frequent complications, with the percentage of occurrence. Prematurity is the most frequent complication, followed by an increased risk of infection and postpartal hemorrhage. Fetal distress should be mentioned in case a cesarean section is required. The possibility of a failed induction must be discussed with the patient and her partner.

Induction of labor for medical reasons is discussed in detail with the couple. The elective plan deserves the same consideration. This joint decision-making and sharing of information between the expectant couple and the health care team promotes better understanding and more participation on the part of the family.

Labor Readiness

Fetal Maturity

Early diagnosis of pregnancy with adequate recorded data during the early months of pregnancy is helpful in determining the EDC. Ex-

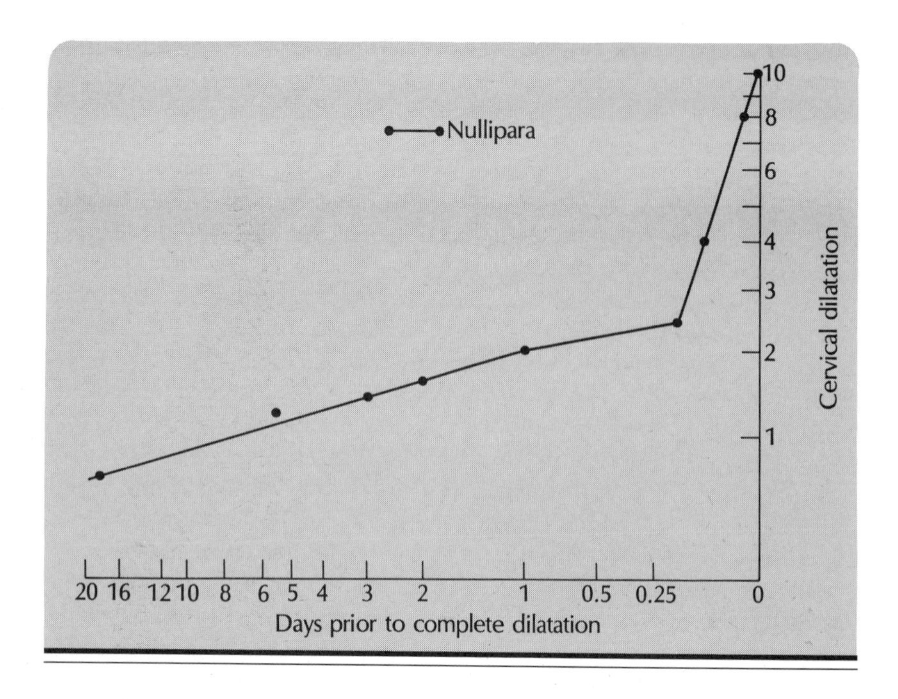

Figure 20–1. Cervical dilatation in late pregnancy. (From Hendricks, C. H., et al. 1970. Normal cervical dilatation pattern in late pregnancy and labor. *Am. J. Obstet. Gynecol.* 106:1065.)

ternal abdominal examination of the growing uterus also aids in determining fetal growth. Rapid changes in uterine growth may indicate a large-for-gestational-age infant, multiple pregnancy, or perhaps polyhydramnios. The lack of uterine growth suggests a small-for-gestational-age infant.

Amniotic fluid studies to determine the L/S ratio and the creatinine concentration are beneficial in assessing fetal maturity. Serial sonographic examinations measuring the fetal head (biparietal diameter) and the chest wall thickness are helpful, provided that the tests are performed early in the second trimester (20–22 weeks) and again prior to the 38th week. It is difficult to estimate fetal age from one examination performed between 39 and 40 weeks' gestation. One needs to compare findings with those from earlier examinations. A biparietal diameter of 9.5 cm could occur at 39 weeks or at 43 weeks (Quennan, 1977).

Maternal Readiness

Weekly vaginal examinations, beginning at 36 weeks, are useful in recognizing the progressive cervical changes (ripening of the cervix) as gestation advances. Hendricks et al. (1970) have provided useful information regarding cervical dilatation during late pregnancy that is beneficial in determining the delivery date (Figure 20–1). The mean cervical dilatation during the last three days prior to the onset of labor is 1.8 cm in nulliparas and 2.2 cm in multiparas. When admitted to the hospital in active labor, average dilatation is 2.5 cm for nulliparas and 3.5 cm for multiparas. With this information and evaluation of cervical softening, one can better predict a woman's readiness for labor.

Bishop (1964) developed a prelabor scoring system that has proved to be helpful in predicting the inducibility of patients (Table 20–1). Components evaluated are cervical dilatation, effacement, consistency, and position, as well as the station of the fetal presenting part. The higher the total score for all the criteria, the more likely it is that labor will ensue. The lower the total score, the higher the failure rate. A favorable cervix is the most important criterion for a successful induction. A cervix that is soft, anterior, more than 50% effaced, and dilated more than 2 cm (with the fetal head flexed and fixed in the pelvis) is a positive sign of labor readiness (Tricomi, 1973).

The least important item for consideration is the location or station of the fetal head. If it were a significant factor, the multipara with a history of precipitous labors would not meet the criteria and therefore would not benefit from the procedure.

In a study of multiparous women, Bishop (1964) found that inductions were successful in patients with a total score of 9 or more. There was a 5% failure rate in women with total scores of 5–8, and a 20% failure rate in women with scores below 4.

Bishop's scoring system is useful in determining cervical readiness but is not a guarantee against prematurity. Therefore, the previously discussed parameters for determining fetal maturity are necessary.

It is essential that the nurse and physician carefully assess the readiness of each patient prior to beginning the induction procedure. The methods discussed in this section serve as screening tools, providing means to select patients for whom induction of labor will be most effective and safest. For nursing management of induction of labor, see the accompanying Nursing Care Plan.

Contraindications

All contraindications to spontaneous labor and vaginal delivery are contraindications to the induction of labor (Cibils, 1972). Absolute contraindications are as follows:

1. Cephalopelvic disproportion (CPD).
2. Previous cesarean section for CPD.
3. Previous uterine surgery (for example, hysterotomy).
4. Severe fetal distress.
5. Placenta previa centrally located.
6. Abruptio placentae, severe or complete.
7. Invasive carcinoma of the cervix.
8. Soft tissue masses (for example, myomas, ovarian cysts, pelvic kidneys).
9. Lack of patient acceptance.
10. Herpesvirus type 2.

Relative contraindications include the following:

1. An unfavorable cervix.
2. Estimated fetal weight under 2500 gm.
3. Vertex not engaged in the pelvis
4. Abnormal presentations (for example, breech or transverse lie).
5. No past pregnancies.
6. Parity of four or more (grandmultiparity).
7. Multiple pregnancy or polyhydramnios.

Methods

The most frequently used methods of induction are amniotomy, intravenous oxytocin (Pitocin) infusion, or both.

Amniotomy

Amniotomy is the most potent single means of inducing labor (Theobald, 1968). Under favorable conditions, which include cervical readiness and position of the fetal head against the lower segment and dipping into the pelvis, about 80% of the patients go into active labor within 24 hours after amniotomy (Cibils, 1972). In elective induction procedures, if the cervix is favorable, 84% of the patients will deliver within 12 hours of amniotomy (Keettel, 1969).

Table 20–1. Prelabor Status Evaluation Scoring System*

	Assigned value			
Factor	**0**	**1**	**2**	**3**
Cervical dilatation	Closed	1–2 cm	3–4 cm	5 cm or more
Cervical effacement	0%–30%	40%–50%	60%–70%	80% or more
Fetal station	−3	−2	−1, 0	+1 or lower
Cervical consistency	Firm	Moderate	Soft	
Cervical position	Posterior	Midposition	Anterior	

*Modified from Bishop, E. H. 1964. Pelvic scoring for elective induction. *Obstet. Gynecol.* 24:266.

NURSING CARE PLAN

Induction of Labor

Patient Data Base

History

Previous pregnancies

Past mothering experience

Marital status

Race

Religious beliefs

Financial status

Preparation for childbirth

EDC

See the Nursing Care Plan on labor and delivery, Chapter 17, for other information

Physical examination

1. Examination of pregnant uterus (Leopold's maneuvers to determine fetal size and position, p. 460)
2. Vaginal examination to evaluate cervical readiness
   a. Ripe cervix: feels soft to the examining finger, is located in a medial to anterior position, is more than 50% effaced, and is 2-3 cm dilated
   b. Unripe cervix: feels firm to the examining finger, is long and thick, perhaps in a posterior position, with little or no dilatation
3. Presence of contractions
4. Membranes intact or ruptured
5. Fetal size (Leopold's maneuvers, ultrasound)
6. Fetal readiness
7. CPD evaluation

Laboratory evaluation

Fetal maturity tests (L/S ratio, creatinine concentrations, estriol levels, ultrasonography)

Maternal blood studies (CBC, hemoglobin, hematocrit, blood type, Rh factor)

Urinalysis

Nursing Priorities

1. Monitor and evaluate status of mother and fetus continuously throughout the induction.
2. Provide continuous physical and emotional support.
3. Evaluate and monitor uterine response to induction.
4. Evaluate and monitor fetal response to induction.
5. Continously evaluate patient for complications associated with induction (abruptio placentae, fetal distress, any rise or decrease in maternal BP, hemorrhage, shock, uterine rupture, tetanic contractions).

Problem	Nursing interventions and actions	Rationale
Hypotension	Observe and record vital signs and FHTs every 15 min. Position patient on her side.	Patient is frequently on her back at beginning of induction while monitors are attached and IV is started. Vena cava is obstructed, causing maternal hypotension, which may lead to fetal bradycardia. Initial hypotension is secondary to peripheral vasodilation induced by oxytocin, which causes diminished blood supply to placenta and resultant decrease in O_2 supply to fetus. May be responsible for severe cases of palsy or fetal death.
Inadequate labor response	Increase IV rate of flow 2-5 mU every 15-20 min until adequate uterine contractility is achieved. Maintain by keeping infusion at acquired rate or by reducing oxytocin rate by 30%. Decrease rate if contractions are more frequent than every 2½ min, or increase if frequency of contractions is	Adequate uterine contractility is three contractions in a 10-min period with uterine resting tone at 12-15 mm Hg. Fetal heart baseline should be between 120-160 beats/min with good variability range.

Problem	Nursing interventions and actions	Rationale
	less than every 3½ min. When cervix is 6-8 cm dilated and fetal head is descending adequately, oxytocin infusion may be stopped. Oxytocin regulation and administration is by physician order and supervision.	
Tetanic contractions	Observe contraction rate and length. In presence of contractions lasting over 90 sec: 1. Discontinue oxytocin infusion. 2. Assess maternal status. 3. Assess fetal status.	Contractions last over 90 sec with decreased resting tone may result in fetal hypoxia. Ruptured uterus or abruptio placentae can result from drug-induced tumultuous labor.
Cervical dilatation	Evaluate cervical dilatation by vaginal examination with each oxytocin dosage increase after labor is established.	When cervix responds by stretching or pulling, *do not* increase oxytocin dosage because overdosage may occur, causing rapid labor with possible cervical lacerations and fetal damage. When there is no change in cervix, additional oxytocin is needed.
Prolapsed cord	Monitor FHTs continuously. Look for cord immediately after membranes rupture. Evaluate for prolapsed cord when doing each vaginal examination.	Premature rupture of membranes with presenting part high in pelvis may allow cord to prolapse.
Rapid delivery	Assist with rapid delivery. Observe and record the following intrapartally: 1. Laceration of tissues in the birth canal. 2. FHR for signs of distress (FHR >160 or <120 beats/min or loss of baseline variability). Evaluate postpartally: 1. Check mother for lacerations and contractility of fundus. 2. Check neonate for birth injuries.	Overstimulation or overdosage of oxytocin may occur as additional endogenous oxytocin is produced by maternal system. Rapid delivery increases risk of maternal laceration of tissues in birth canal. Pressure within fetal head changes rapidly with precipitous, rapid delivery. Infant is prone to cerebral edema and hemorrhage.
Prematurity	Calculate EDC. Notify nursery personnel and pediatrician if infant is premature. Have extra personnel available in delivery room to care for neonate should resuscitation measures be needed.	Incidence of prematurity is high in presence of maternal vascular diseases. Prematurity can occur in elective inductions due to poor patient selection.
Failed induction	Explain procedure to patient and spouse. Assess presence of favorable cervical conditions. Observe and record presence or absence of contractions.	Oxytocin may have been improperly administered. Vascular disease will not allow a favorable cervix.
Fetal hypoxia – asphyxia	Monitor FHR continuously (normal range is 120-160/min). In episodes of bradycardia (<120 beats/min) lasting for more than 30 sec, administer O_2 by face mask at 4-7 liters/min. Stop oxytocin infusion. Position mother on left side if quick recovery of FHR does not happen. Carefully evaluate fetal tachycardia (>160/min).	O_2 deficiency may occur over a long period of time. In cases of placental insufficiency or cord compression, compensated tachycardia may be evoked. Persistent fetal tachycardia causes more prominent

NURSING CARE PLAN Cont'd

Induction of Labor

Problem	Nursing interventions and actions	Rationale
	Sustained tachycardia may necessitate discontinuation of oxytocin infusion.	O_2 deficiency (hypoxia) and CO_2 increase in fetal blood. Vasoconstriction occurs, with increased fetal blood flow through coronary arteries, brain, and placenta. This increased demand on myocardial performance leads to cardiac decompensation if oxygen exchange is impaired and hypoxia continues. Fetal hypoxia may also cause central vasomotor center to release adrenal catecholamines. At term, this enhances depolarization of cardiac pacemaker cells, which will result in direct bradycardia. Bradycardia or subsequent reflex tachycardia temporarily remedies the O_2 deficiency.
Water intoxication	Monitor and record amount of fluid intake, oxytocin dosage, and urinary output. Administer oxytocin in a physiologic saline solution or Ringer's lactate per physician order.	Oxytocin has antidiuretic effect when large amounts are administered in electrolyte-free solution.
Infection	Prevent exposure to infections. Maintain sterile technique when doing vaginal examinations.	Organisms may be introduced during vaginal examinations, especially when bag of waters is ruptured.

Nursing Care Evaluation

Normal sterile vaginal delivery is accomplished without complications (lacerations, precipitous delivery).

Postpartally the maternal fundus is firm; blood flow is moderate; blood pressure, pulse, and respirations are stable and within normal limits.

Neonate's respirations, color, and temperature are within normal limits.

Maternal bonding is begun by allowing interactions among mother, baby, and father in delivery room.

There does not appear to be any greater risk in artificial rupture of the membranes than in their spontaneous rupture as long as the fetal head is engaged and there is no evidence of a presenting cord. Variable or late deceleration FHR patterns have been noted during amniotomy, but other factors could have caused the deceleration, such as cord compression, small placenta, oxytocin infusion, and CPD (Gabert and Stenchever, 1973).

Fetal bradycardia and tachycardia have been noted following amniotomy and are probably related to a decrease in uterine blood flow from the relative decrease in uterine size (Brotanek and Hodr, 1968). Prior to membrane rupture, the osmotic pressure above and below the presenting part is equal. After amniotomy, the downward pressure is greater, causing closer contact of the fetal head with the lower uterine wall. This position causes more intense mechanical irritation and stimulates contractions (Vorherr, 1974).

The decrease in myometrial oxygen saturation, or uterine hypoxia, may trigger uterine irritability, alter the progesterone content, and change tissue electrolyte concentrations to levels associated with the onset of the labor cycle.

The advantages of amniotomy as a method of labor induction are as follows:

1. The contractions elicited are similar to those of spontaneous labor.
2. There is usually no risk of hypertonus or rupture of the uterus.
3. The patient does not require close surveillance as in oxytocin infusion.
4. Fetal monitoring is facilitated because amniotomy does not interfere with the following:
   a. Scalp blood sampling for pH determinations.
   b. Scalp electrode application.
   c. Intrauterine catheter placement.
5. The color and composition of amniotic fluid can be evaluated.

The following are disadvantages of amniotomy:

1. The danger of a prolapsed cord is increased.
2. There is a risk of infection from ascending organisms.
3. Compression and molding of the fetal head are increased.
4. Labor may not be induced, resulting in cesarean delivery.

Oxytocin Infusion

Oxytocin is one of the hormones produced by cells of the hypothalamic nuclei, and it is stored in the neurohypophysis of the pituitary. Its release is influenced by the presence of neurogenic stimuli (Cibils, 1972). This hormone and the other neurohypophysial hormone, vasopressin, are closely related and share certain antidiuretic properties. Both hormones stimulate the contraction of specific musculature. Vasopressin primarily affects the intestinal musculature, the muscular tissue of the capillaries and arterioles, and the nonpregnant uterine musculature; oxytocin stimulates contractions of the pregnant uterus (Fuchs, 1976).

Du Vigneaud et al. (1954, 1958) identified the chemical structures of vasopressin and oxytocin and were then able to prepare these substances synthetically. When synthetic oxytocin replaced the poorly standardized impure extracts clinically, the incidence of hypertensive vascular and allergic reactions was reduced drastically. The use of oxytocin increased.

The exact mechanism by which oxytocin stimulates the smooth muscle cells of the myometrium is still not known. The response of the myometrial cell to exogenous oxytocin varies, depending on the reactivity of the cells, which may be affected by placental steroids (Fuchs, 1976). The sensitivity of the uterus to oxytocin increases steadily throughout pregnancy.

Most patients at term or close to term respond to 2–5 mU/min intravenous oxytocin; others require as much as 10 mU/min. Labor is usually well established by dosages of less than 20 mU/min when the cervix is ripe. Rarely does a patient need a dose of 20 mU/min. When the patient is 32–36 weeks pregnant, 20–30 mU/min are necessary to induce a laborlike contractility pattern (Cibils, 1972). Cervical readiness influences the dosage amount.

Oxytocin should be administered by means of an angiocatheter in the radial vein, and an infusion pump should be used to assure a constant flow rate. A two-bottle system is necessary (one without oxytocin) to maintain adequate control if the oxytocin needs to be terminated and the vein kept open. An initial dosage of 1–2 mU/min is advisable. Dosages of 2 mU/min of oxytocin successfully induce labor in approximately 75% of patients at term (Hendricks and Brenner, 1964).

Many obstetricians and induction teams use a more aggressive approach by starting with an infusion rate at the recommended 1–2 mU/min and increasing the amount to 4, 8, and 16 mU/min as needed for adequate contractions. Constant observation is mandatory to provide optimal care to both mother and fetus, because uterine and fetal response may vary as labor is established. Cervical changes are slow initially, and perseverance is necessary to prevent a failed induction. When cervical changes are noted, the rate of infusion must be redetermined. Many practitioners elect to keep the concentration at the established level until delivery, whereas others prefer to gradually decrease the concentration, provided the contractions persist.

Approximately 20 minutes of infusion at a given dose per minute is necessary to achieve steady blood levels of oxytocin. Pitocin is rapidly excreted by the kidney and inactivated by placental oxytocinase. Two or three minutes after the infusion is stopped, uterine activity ceases. Therefore, continuous dosage is required to maintain contractions. Increasing the dosage rate at intervals of less than 20 minutes may lead to overdose and thus elicit uterine hypertonus, contracture, and possible rupture of the uterus, with added hazards to mother and baby (Theobald, 1968).

To reduce the risk of such complications as uterine rupture and maternal and infant morbidity and mortality, it is imperative that clinicians be aware of the amount of oxytocin in the body of the patient, not just the amount placed in the intravenous bottle. Oxytocin should be considered a potentially dangerous drug to be administered only when indicated and under close observation (Pauerstein, 1973).

When exogenous oxytocin produces excessive uterine contractions, the oxytocin infusion should be diminished or perhaps discontinued. The uterus appears to be tolerant of oxytocin abuse but can be overdosed should the myometrium be hypersensitive, which may cause interference in the uterine blood supply (Theobald, 1968).

Internal or external fetal monitoring and uterine contraction monitoring are indicated with all inductions of labor. It must be remembered that each uterine contraction is a repetitive stress on the fetus (equivalent to apnea when viewed from a respiration standpoint). In uncomplicated pregnancies in which the margin of fetal oxygen reserve is normal, this apnea presents no problem. In cases of complicated and chronic uteroplacental insufficiency, in which the margin of fetal oxygen reserve is diminished, the repetitive uterine contractions could damage the fetus (Hon, 1976).

The resting pressure or relaxation period between contractions is of utmost importance. An elevated resting tonus from tetanic contractions over an extended period causes fetal bradycardia, fetal hypoxia, and fetal acidosis and may eventually lead to fetal death from diminished uterine blood flow. Abruptio placentae and uterine rupture are additional complications that may occur, resulting in possible fetal and maternal death.

Monitoring equipment, well-defined procedures, and knowledgeable clinical personnel are necessary for a well-managed oxytocin infusion. Continuous monitoring has shown that with oxytocin-induced labor the fetal heart remains relatively stable when contractions last 40–60 seconds, tonus does not exceed 60–70 mm Hg, and there is no occurrence of polysystole (more than five contractions in a ten-minute period). See the accompanying box for guidelines for oxytocin induction of labor.

Amniotomy Accompanied by Oxytocin Infusion

This method is preferred in North America because of its success rate. Oxytocin infusion prior to amniotomy provides a safety feature in case the uterus fails to respond to the attempts at induction. Amniotomy can be justified after labor is established, with cervical dilatation in progress. When the fetal head is too high to perform the initial amniotomy, the induction should be by oxytocin infusion alone.

Amniotomy with simultaneous administration of an oxytocin infusion results in shorter labors than if amniotomy alone is performed. Added benefits include less dehydration, fewer indications for forceps delivery, and less puerperal blood loss (Barham, 1973). The failure rate of induction is higher in the oxytocin infusion group when not accompanied by amniotomy (Vorherr, 1974). If the latent period extends to six to eight hours after amniotomy, oxytocin infusion should be supplemented.

Other Methods

Buccal and nasal administration of oxytocin, stripping of the membranes, acupuncture, electrical stimulation, fat emulsions, and prostaglandin infusion are infrequently used methods of labor induction. Intramuscular injection of oxytocin is not an approved method because of the inability to control the dosage effect. It is obsolete for the modern obstetrician because of the unpredictable results and the prolonged hypertonus factor.

Buccal oxytocin and prostaglandin infusion are discussed below. The other methods have been documented, but more research is needed before they become widely accepted.

Buccal Oxytocin

Buccal oxytocin (Pitocin) is sometimes used because of its convenience and its easy method of administration. It must be remembered that the rate of oxytocin absorption is variable from patient to patient; thus dosage is difficult to monitor, and control of hypersensitivity is difficult. If adverse reaction occurs, the tablets must be removed immediately and thorough washing of the

GUIDELINES FOR THE OXYTOCIN INDUCTION OF LABOR

To prevent serious complications resulting from the exogenous use of oxytocin, the following guidelines—adopted by both the American College of Obstetricians and Gynecologists (ACOG) and the Nurses Association of the American College of Obstetricians and Gynecologists (NAACOG)—are recommended:

> Oxytocic agents should be used for induction or stimulation of labor only when qualified personnel, determined by the hospital staff and administration, can attend the patient closely. Written policies and procedures should be available to the team member assuming this responsibility. It is recommended that the following be included in these policies:

- The attending physician should evaluate the patient for induction or stimulation, especially with regard to indications.
- The physician or other individual starting the oxytocin should be familiar with its effects and complications, and be qualified to identify both maternal and fetal complications.
- A qualified physician should be as immediately available as is necessary to manage any complications effectively.
- The intravenous route is preferable. It is recommended that an infusion pump, or other device for accurate control of the rate of flow, and a two-bottle system, one of which contains no oxytocic substance, be used. The administration of oxytocin by other means, or the use of other oxytocic preparations for induction or stimulation of labor, should be discouraged. If another drug or method of administration is used, a physician should be present for the duration of the pharmacologic effect.
- During oxytocin administration, the following should be recorded at least every 15 minutes: fetal heart rate, frequency and character of contractions, rate of oxytocin flow, and blood pressure. Continuous fetal monitoring should be encouraged.
- A maximum concentration of solution and maximum rate of administration should be established.*

mouth must be done to prevent partially dissolved particles from remaining in the mouth. The demand for close observation when using this drug is just as great as with any means of induction.

Prostaglandin Administration

Use of prostaglandins to induce labor is being researched and has not yet been approved as a routine means of induction. There is an open question as to the role they will play in inducing labor.

A study comparing the efficacy and safety of prostaglandin $F_{2\alpha}$ and oxytocin in induction of labor showed that the success rate depended on cervical conditions. The patients to whom prostaglandin $F_{2\alpha}$ was administered had an increased incidence of uterine hypertonus, hot flashes, and vein phlebitis. The incidence of cesarean section was higher in the prostaglandin-induction group. Indication for the sections in all cases was fetal distress. There was no significant difference between the prostaglandin-induced and oxytocin-induced groups in the incidence of fetal bradycardia, nausea, vomiting, or diarrhea. Laboratory toxicity studies before and after the infusions were similar, except that the postinfusion hemoglobin levels were significantly higher in the oxytocin group. There were more failures in the prostaglandin group in obese patients. Caution should be used before prostaglandins are used in inductions of labor at term (Spellacy et al., 1973).

*From Nurses Association of the American College of Obstetricians and Gynecologists. 1974. *Obstetric, gynecologic and neonatal nursing functions and standards.* Chicago: The Association, p. 55.

EPISIOTOMY

An *episiotomy* is a surgical incision of the perineum. This procedure is performed more commonly in primigravidas than multigravidas for the following reasons:

1. A primigravida is likely to suffer lacerations during delivery. A surgical incision is easier to repair, heals faster, and can be controlled directionally.
2. Trauma to the fetal head is decreased.
3. The second stage of labor is shortened.
4. Stretching and tissue necrosis of the vaginal mucosa, which can result in a fistula, are prevented.

In addition, many physicians routinely perform episiotomies on women in premature labor to decrease the incidence of cerebral trauma to the infant during the birth process.

The routine use of episiotomies is becoming an increasingly controversial issue. Cogan and Edmunds (1977) have found no evidence to support the reasons for episiotomies just listed. However, most medical textbooks still advocate the prophylactic use of this procedure in cases in which it appears that second- and third-degree lacerations are likely to occur.

The episiotomy is performed just prior to delivery, when the presenting part is crowning. The incision begins at the midline and may be extended down the midline through the perineal body, or it may extend at a 45 degree angle in a mediolateral direction to the right or left (Figure 20-2). A midline episiotomy is preferred if the perineum is of adequate length and no difficulty during delivery is anticipated, as it is easy to repair and heals with less discomfort for the mother. In the presence of a short perineum or a difficult delivery, a mediolateral episiotomy provides more room and decreases the possibility of a traumatic extension into the rectum. The mediolateral episiotomy may be complicated by greater blood loss, a longer healing period, and more discomfort postpartally for the mother.

The episiotomy is usually performed with the patient under a regional or light general anesthesia but may be performed without anesthesia in emergency situations. (As crowning occurs, the distention of the tissues causes numbing.) Adequate anesthesia must be given for the repair.

The nurse ensures that there are at least two suture packs on the delivery table. Extra sponges also may be required. Chromic 00 or 000 suture on a general closure needle is frequently used for the repair of an episiotomy.

To alleviate pain and swelling after the repair, ice packs are beneficial for the first eight hours. Hot sitz baths are recommended to increase the circulation to the area and to promote healing. The episiotomy site should be inspected every 15 minutes during the first hour after delivery and thereafter daily for redness, swelling, tenderness, and hematomas. Mild analgesic sprays and oral analgesics are ordered as needed. The mother will need instruction in perineal hygiene care and may need instructions about use of the analgesic spray.

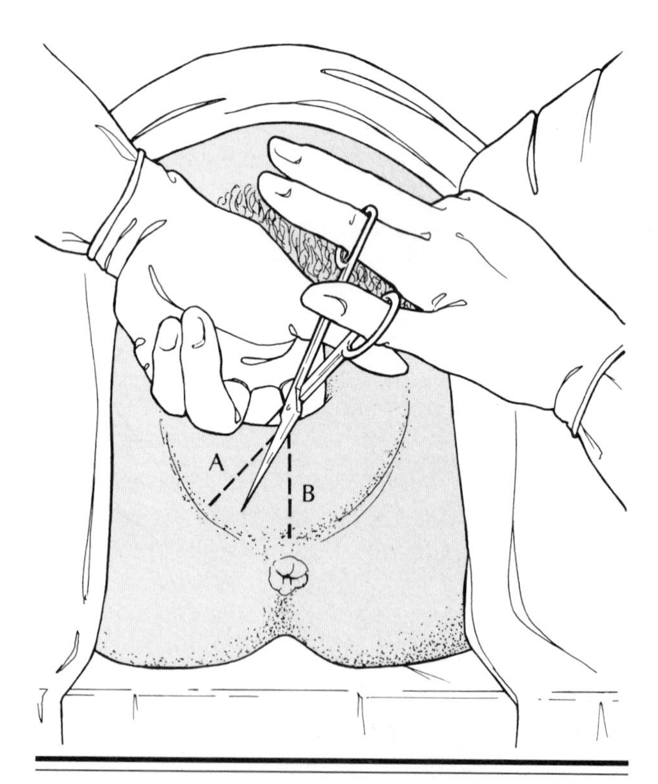

Figure 20–2. The two most common types of episiotomies are mediolateral (**A**) and midline (**B**).

REPAIR OF LACERATIONS

Perineal lacerations may occur when the physician elects not to do an episiotomy. The lacerations that may occur are classified according to tissue and muscle involvement.

A *first-degree laceration* is a tear that begins at the fourchette and involves the perineal skin and vaginal mucosa. A *second-degree laceration* involves the perineal skin, vaginal mucosa, and muscles and fascia of the perineal body. A *third-degree laceration* involves the perineal skin, vaginal mucosa, and perineal muscles and fascia and extends into the anal sphincter. A *fourth-degree laceration*, a classification that has not been universally adopted by all clinicians, extends through the rectal mucosa, exposing the rectal lumen.

The repair of perineal lacerations is similar to the repair of an episiotomy. Patients with fourth-degree lacerations should be given stool softeners to facilitate the first bowel movement. The patient may be afraid to move her bowels because of discomfort and fear that the "stitches will come loose." The nurse can educate the patient to avoid use of rectal medications and enemas and encourage good nutrition and adequate fluid intake, as these measures can decrease the woman's discomfort.

FORCEPS DELIVERIES

Forceps may be used to provide traction, to rotate, or both. The forceps used in obstetrics have four parts: a blade, handle, shank, and lock. The blades are designated as right and left and are either fenestrated or solid. Most blades have a pelvic and cephalic curve and articulate at the lock. Fenestrated blades are lighter, grip the fetal head better, and are less likely to slip than solid blades.

There are two types of forceps deliveries. The delivery is termed a *low* or *outlet forceps delivery* when the fetal head is visible on the perineum without spreading the labias apart. When the fetal head is higher than the level of the ischial spines, delivery is termed a *midforceps delivery*. The lower part of the fetal head must be at the level of the ischial spines and the biparietal diameter must have entered the inlet in order to perform a midforceps delivery. Most midforceps deliveries are rotations of the fetus from an occiput-posterior or occiput-transverse position to an occiput-anterior position. *High forceps deliveries* are no longer used because they are extremely dangerous for the mother and the fetus.

Types of Forceps

The following forceps are depicted in Figure 20–3.

Simpson forceps are outlet forceps. They have a fenestrated blade and an English lock and are separated at the shanks to allow for cutting of the episiotomy after the application. These forceps can be used successfully on infants with well-molded heads.

Tucker-McLean forceps have a solid blade and closed shanks. They are also outlet forceps but may be used for midforceps rotations of fetuses in the occiput-posterior position. Due to the shape of the Tucker-McLean cephalic curve, they work well with premature infants with little molding.

The *Kjelland forceps* have a sliding lock with no pelvic curve. They are designed for occiput-posterior and occiput-transverse midforceps rotations.

The *Barton forceps* have one hinged blade and are used for midforceps rotation of the fetus from an occiput-transverse position to an occiput-anterior position.

Elliot forceps have a fenestrated blade and an English lock and are closed at the shanks. They are used as outlet forceps.

Piper forceps have long shanks that curve down. The handle is lower than the blades. The blades are fenestrated. The forceps are used for the aftercoming head of a fetus in a breech presentation.

Indications

Indications for the use of forceps include any condition that threatens the life of the mother or fetus. Maternal conditions include heart disease,

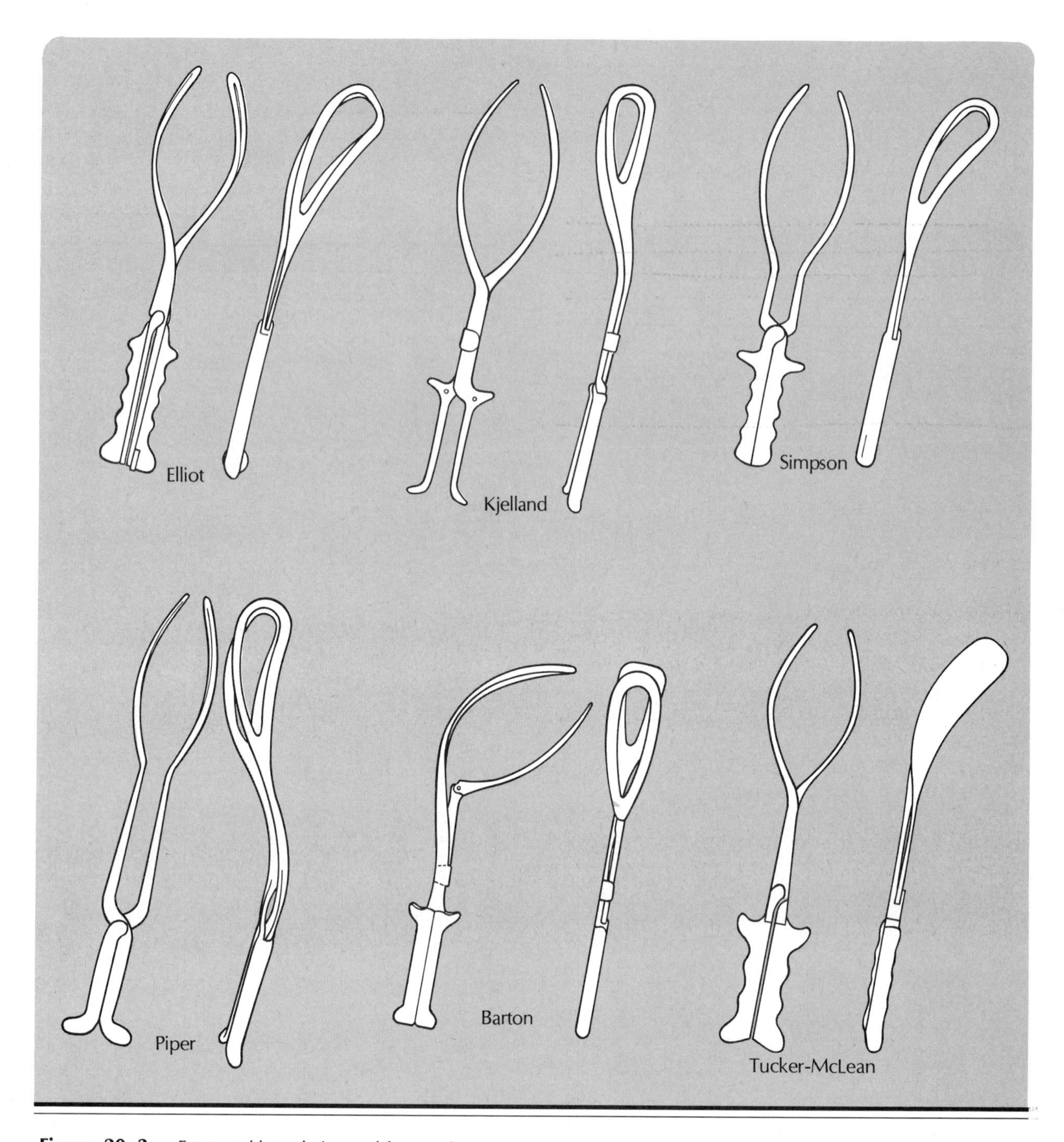

Figure 20–3. Front and lateral views of forceps in common use.

acute pulmonary edema, intrapartal infection, or exhaustion. Fetal conditions include prolapsed cord, premature placental separation, and fetal distress. Forceps may be used electively to shorten the second stage of labor, sparing the mother the pushing effort, or when regional or general anesthesia has affected the mother's motor innervation. They are advocated in a premature infant delivery (Pritchard and MacDonald, 1976), as discussed in Chapter 19.

Complications

Perinatal morbidity and mortality are increased with midforceps deliveries. Neonatal depression and birth trauma have been closely correlated with the use of midforceps, especially if a rotation is done (Friedman and Sachtleben, 1976). The incidence of postpartal hemorrhage is increased with midforceps deliveries if the second stage lasts over three hours. No such increase is found in cases in which operative techniques are not used but in which the second stage of labor is prolonged (Cohen, 1977). Friedman et al. (1977) also found a lower IQ score in children 3–4 years old who were delivered by midforceps as compared to those delivered by low forceps or spontaneously.

Prerequisites for Forceps Application

Use of forceps requires complete dilatation of the cervix and knowledge of the exact position of the fetal head. The membranes must be ruptured to get a firm grasp on the fetal head. The presentation must be vertex or face with the chin anterior, and the head must be engaged, preferably on the perineum. Under no circumstances should there be any CPD.

Trial or Failed Forceps Delivery

In a trial forceps procedure, the physician attempts to use forceps with the knowledge that there is a degree of CPD. If a good application cannot be obtained or if no descent occurs with the application, then cesarean section is the method of choice for the delivery. A failed forceps procedure is an attempt to deliver with forceps without success (Pritchard and MacDonald, 1976).

Nursing Interventions

It is the nurse's responsibility to provide the physician with the type of forceps requested. Frequently this request can be anticipated, as with outlet forceps or a premature delivery. The Piper forceps should always be available on the delivery table with a breech delivery in case they are needed.

The nurse can explain the procedure briefly to the patient if she is awake. With adequate regional anesthesia, the mother should feel some pressure but no pain. Encourage the mother to maintain her breathing techniques to prevent her from pushing. When directly assisting the physician with the delivery, the nurse should provide the left blade first and support it after it is applied to the fetal head while the physician is applying the right blade (Figure 20–4). The fetal heart rate should be monitored continuously by the circulating nurse until the delivery. It is not uncommon to observe bradycardia as traction is being applied to the forceps. This bradycardia results from head compression and is transient in nature. With midforceps rotations, pediatric assistance may be needed. Adequate resuscitation equipment should be readied.

Occasionally the infant will have a forceps bruise from the application. The couple should be informed what it looks like and that it will disappear in a few days.

Neonates who have had a forceps delivery should be inspected for cerebral trauma and Erb's palsy.

VACUUM EXTRACTION

The vacuum extractor has been used widely in Europe since the early 1950s and has, in fact, completely replaced forceps in some European countries (Ott, 1975). The vacuum extractor is composed of a suction cup attached to a suction bottle (pump) by tubing. The suction cup comes in four sizes. It is attached to the infant's head, and with gradual negative pressure and traction, the head is delivered. An artificial caput is created while the physician applies traction on a short chain, which is attached to the cup. Traction should not be exerted for longer than 30 minutes or three "pull-offs" (Chukwedebelu, 1977).

The vacuum extractor may be used in a patient whose cervix is dilated at least 4 cm. The infant's head does not have to be engaged, as with forceps. Advantages to its use are that the head can rotate according to the shape of the bony pelvis and that no greater traction than 8–10 psi can be exerted on the fetus because the cup will separate from the fetal head (Ott, 1975).

The major risks to the fetus when the vacuum extractor is used are possible tissue necrosis of the fetal head at the cup attachment, cephalhematoma, and cerebral trauma. If the cup is misapplied or slips off the fetal head, vaginal and cervical damage can result.

The most common indication for use of the vacuum extractor is prolonged labor. Other indications for its use include (a) fetal distress,

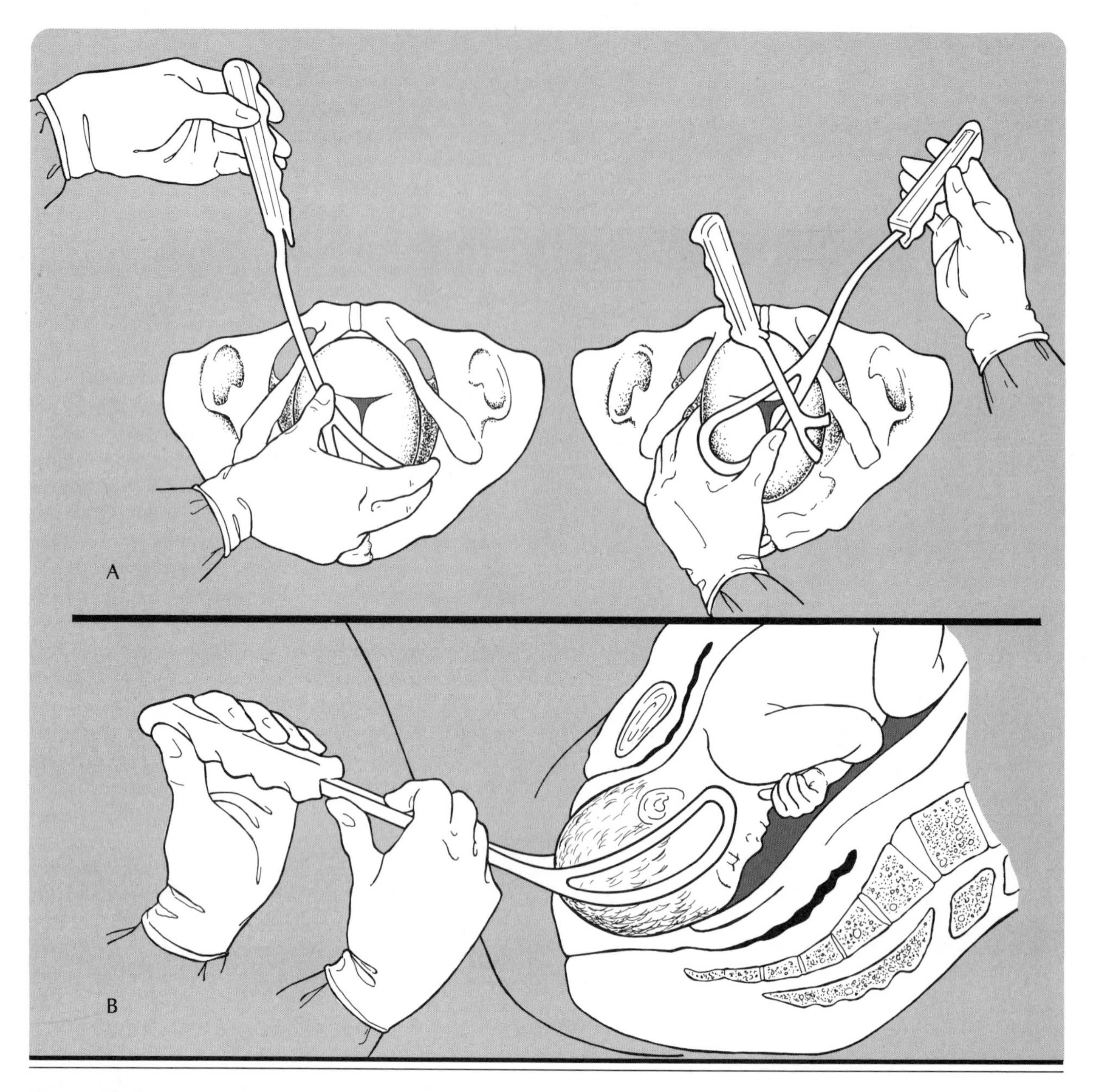

Figure 20–4. **A,** Application of foreceps. **B,** Placement of forceps on fetal head. Traction on forceps is downward and outward.

(b) malpositions, (c) delivery of a second twin, and (d) such maternal complications as cardiopulmonary disease, shock, pregnancy-induced hypertension, and abruptio placentae.

Perinatal mortality and morbidity are less in vacuum extractor deliveries than in midforceps deliveries. The use of a vacuum extractor is contraindicated in cases of premature deliveries, because perinatal mortality is increased (Ott, 1975).

The nurse is responsible for gathering the equipment and providing the physician with the size of cup requested. Sterile tubing should be provided along with the cup. After the physician assembles the cup and tubing, he or she hands the distal end to the nurse to connect to the suction bottle. When the cup is applied to the fetal head, the nurse is directed to pump the suction according to one of the following methods:

1. 0.2 kg/cm every two minutes, up to 0.8 kg/cm.

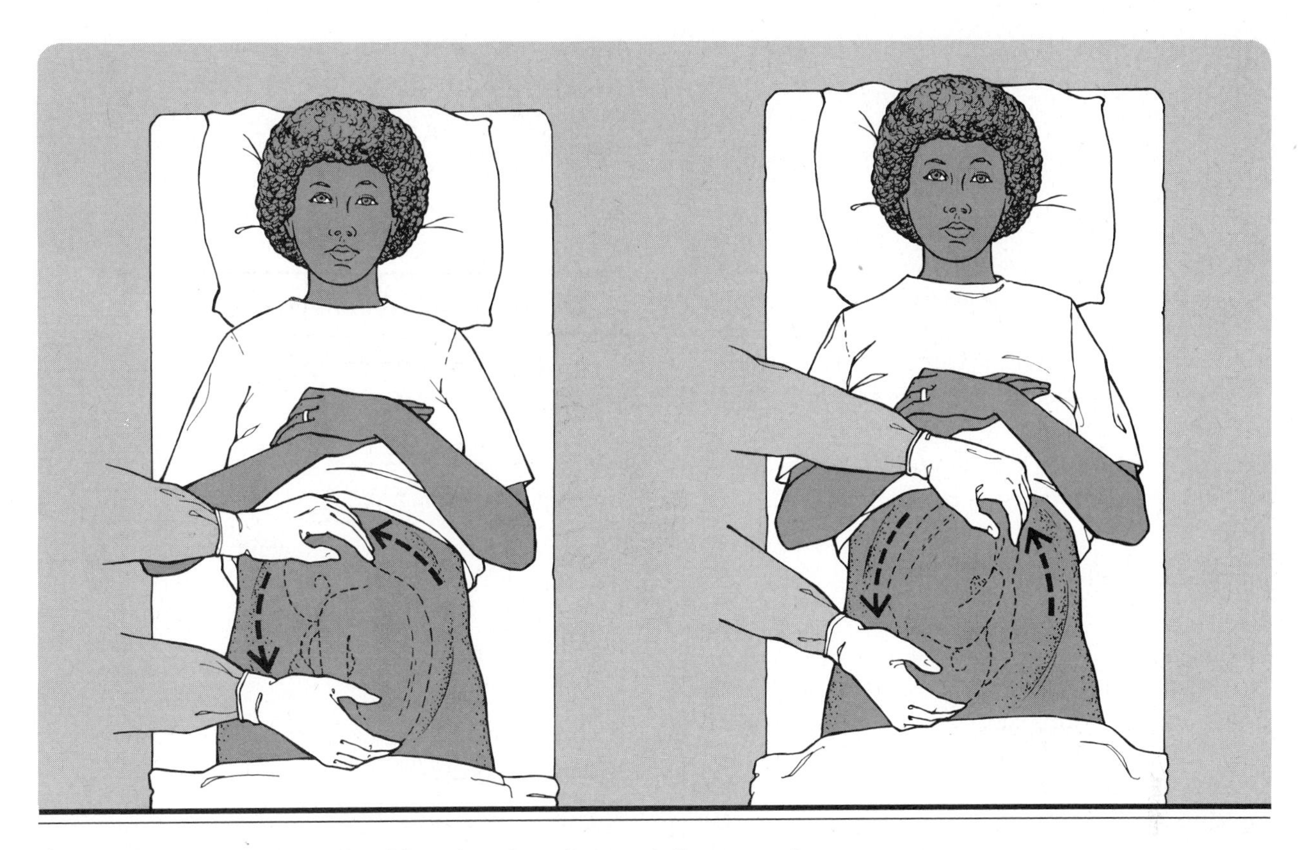

Figure 20–5. External version of fetus from breech to cephalic presentation.

2. 0.2 kg/cm for two minutes, then up to 0.8 kg/cm.

The nurse should be ready to quickly release the suction in the event that the cup accidentally slips off during traction, in order to prevent damage to the maternal tissues.

During the procedure, the mother should be informed about what is transpiring. If adequate regional anesthesia has been administered, the mother feels only pressure during the procedure. The fetus should be auscultated every five minutes or more frequently, and proper infant resuscitation equipment should be readied. The nurse must explain to the mother that the caput will disappear in a few days.

Assessment of the newborn should include inspection and continued observation for cerebral trauma. Postpartally the mother needs to be assessed closely for hemorrhage.

VERSION

Version is the alteration of fetal position by abdominal or intrauterine manipulation to accomplish a more favorable fetal position for delivery. Three types of version are recognized. *External* or *cephalic version* (Figure 20–5) is externally accomplished; *podalic version* is an internal procedure; and *combined version* includes a simultaneous external and internal procedure.

External or Cephalic Version

The infant is rotated from a breech or transverse position to cephalic position by abdominal manipulation. This version may be done before term in the physician's office or in the clinic, but the infant often returns to the original presentation.

The prerequisites for cephalic version are as follows:

1. The presenting part must not be engaged (an unengaged breech presentation).
2. The abdominal wall must be thin enough to permit good palpation, because a contracting or tight uterus will prevent cephalic version.
3. The uterine wall must not be irritable.
4. There must be a sufficient quantity of amniotic fluid in the uterus, and the membranes must be intact. Oligohydramnios or rupture of the membranes prevents adequate amniotic fluid from being present for unrestricted turning of the fetus.
5. There must be no fetopelvic disproportion that would prevent a vaginal delivery.

Internal or Podalic Version

Internal or podalic version is used to rotate a fetus in a vertex or transverse position to a breech position. It is usually attempted near the end of the first stage or in the second stage of labor in the case of delivery of a second twin. The membranes should be intact. General anesthesia is used to provide uterine relaxation. The physician then ruptures the membranes and brings the baby down as a double footling breech. This procedure should not be performed if the cervix is not completely dilated or if the membranes are ruptured before the beginning of the procedure. If the membranes are ruptured, the uterus will be too tight around the fetus to allow manipulation.

The fetus, regardless of gestational size, is in danger during a podalic version. This emergency procedure should be utilized with prolapsed cord resulting in fetal distress, with eclampsia resulting in maternal difficulty, or when immediate delivery is required. If time permits, cesarean section is a more desirable procedure than podalic version.

There is a danger of uterine rupture in the presence of a stretched lower uterine segment, or prolapse of the umbilical cord may occur with a fully dilated cervix and an unengaged fetal part. Podalic version is contraindicated with a partially dilated cervix, a contracted pelvis, or an abnormally contracted uterus and after uterine operations such as cesarean section or hysterotomy.

Combined Version

Combined version includes a simultaneous external and internal rotation of the fetus. All of the advantages and disadvantages of cephalic and podalic version are applicable to a combined version.

Nursing Interventions

Nursing care during a version should include close monitoring of the fetus. The physician may request an elbow-length version glove for internal rotation, which is worn over a regular sterile glove.

Postpartally, the mother should be observed closely for hemorrhage (see the Nursing Care Plan for hemorrhage in Chapter 19). General anesthesia can cause atony postpartally. The intrauterine manipulation may also cause trauma to the uterine musculature, thus preventing it from contracting properly.

CESAREAN SECTION

Cesarean section is the delivery of the infant through an abdominal incision. The word *cesarean* is derived from the Latin word *caedere,* meaning "to cut."

The first cesarean sections were probably performed for the purpose of baptizing unborn children of women who had died before giving birth. The first reliable reports of cesarean sections performed on living women were published about 1668 by Francois Mauriceau. The operation was only performed as a last measure, and in the majority of cases the mother died.

Maternal mortality continued to be extremely high until late in the nineteenth century. An American physician, Max Sanger, documented the value of suturing the uterus. This procedure reduced maternal death from hemorrhage, but peritonitis continued to cause maternal mortality.

In 1907 F. Frank, a physician, introduced the extraperitoneal technique, which was modified by B. Kronig in 1912. In 1926 the transverse uterine incision was recommended, which is the most commonly used method today.

Deliveries by cesarean section have almost

doubled since the 1940s. This increase in abdominal deliveries is probably a result of the greater use and sophistication of assessment tools, such as electronic monitors, which have permitted the detection of a greater number of cases in which maternal or fetal well-being is at risk.

Cesarean sections are performed in cases of breech presentation, fetal distress, dysfunctional labor, and uteroplacental insufficiency from maternal disease conditions (Hibbard, 1976; Jones, 1976). The most commonly occurring indication for cesarean section is dystocia caused by CPD. Other indications for this procedure include prolapsed cord, placenta previa, abruptio placentae, and occasionally tumors blocking the vagina. Primary cesarean sections are increasingly done for breech presentations in primigravidas.

A cesarean section is contraindicated in the presence of a dead fetus or a fetus too small to survive outside of the uterus.

Elective Repeats

In North America elective repeat cesarean sections are popular after a primary section has been done. However, because most incisions are in the lower uterine segment, where the least uterine activity occurs during labor, it is becoming more common to allow a mother to deliver vaginally if the first cesarean section was not performed for CPD, if the postoperative course was uncomplicated, and if there is no overdistention of the uterus or possibility of dystocia.

Timing of elective repeat sections is of utmost importance. In the past, the occurrence of respiratory distress syndrome with cesarean sections was attributed to the lack of the squeezing action on the infant's chest wall during the birth process. The current theory attributes this complication to poor timing and immature fetal lungs. If one waits for labor to occur, there is the disadvantage of doing the cesarean section as an emergency procedure.

To assure that the infant is mature, the physician should consider the due date, fundal height, fetal weight by palpation, the date when the fetal heart could be auscultated, and the date when the mother first felt fetal movement. Some hospitals are equipped to do sonography to measure the biparietal diameter of the fetal head. Amniocentesis can also be done for L/S determinations to determine fetal lung maturity.

Types of Cesarean Section

The types of cesarean sections performed are (a) the low-segment transverse or low cervical transverse, (b) the classic, (c) the cesarean section–hysterectomy, (d) the postmortem cesarean section, and (e) the peritoneal exclusion cesarean section.

Low-Segment, Transverse, or Low-Cervical Method

This method is the most common and most preferred for the following reasons:

1. The lower segment is the thinnest portion of the uterus. Therefore, an incision here results in a minimal blood loss.

2. The concentration of the contractile proteins actin and myosin is least in the lower uterine segment. Thus the chance of uterine rupture is decreased with subsequent pregnancies.

3. The chance of peritonitis is decreased.

4. Because of the location of the incision, there is less postoperative distention. With the low-segment transverse incision, the abdomen may be opened with a vertical Pfannenstiel incision, in which the skin and tissue are incised transversely at the level of the mons pubis. The vertical incision is the incision of choice when (a) there is a need for a rapid delivery, (b) the woman is obese, or (c) a large operating field is needed, as with a large baby.

Classic Cesarean Section

The classic incision (Figure 20-6) is used in the presence of adhesions from previous cesarean sections, when the fetal position is the transverse lie, or with an anteriorly implanted placenta. Because large blood vessels in the myometrium are cut, there is more blood loss with this incision than with others and a slight increase in rupture of the uterine scar in subsequent labors.

Cesarean Section–Hysterectomy

In cesarean section–hysterectomy the uterus is removed at the time of delivery. Indications for this procedure include pathologic conditions, an intrauterine infection, a hypotonic uterus, an inadvertent laceration into the hypogastric artery, and

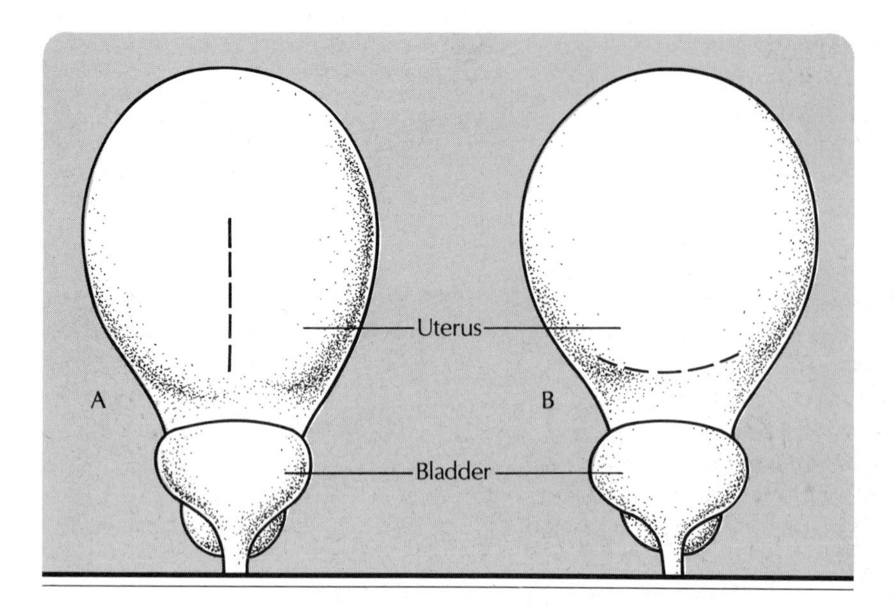

Figure 20–6. Types of uterine incisions for cesarean section. **A,** Classic. **B,** Lower uterine transverse.

uterine fibroids. Occasionally a hysterectomy may be performed at the time of a cesarean section for sterilization reasons (Pritchard and MacDonald, 1976).

Postmortem Cesarean Section

A postmortem section may be performed after the death of the mother to save the fetus. According to Weber (1970), a satisfactory outcome for the fetus depends on six factors:

1. Anticipation of the death of the mother.
2. Fetal age of more than 28 weeks.
3. Personnel and appropriate equipment immediately available.
4. Continued postmortem ventilation and cardiac massage for the mother.
5. Prompt delivery.
6. Effective resuscitation of the fetus.

Peritoneal Exclusion Cesarean Section

This method is used when it is desirable to prevent the intraperitoneal spill of infected fluid and blood. A low-cervical cesarean section is performed, with suture of the parietal peritoneum to the transversely incised visceral peritoneum prior to incision through the lower uterine segment. An outside passageway is established for drainage fluid. This procedure has become less common with increased administration of intensive antibiotic therapy.

Nursing Interventions

If the cesarean section is scheduled and not an emergency, the nurse has ample time for preoperative teaching, which should include assessing the couple's knowledge about the procedure and supplying information as needed. Ideally, someone whom the mother knows (her husband) should be available to reassure her and explain events to her. The mother needs to practice her turning, coughing, and deep breathing. It is helpful if she is taught to splint her abdominal muscles when she coughs. The nurse should determine whether the mother wants to breast-feed or bottle-feed, so that medication to inhibit lactation can be sent to surgery as needed.

To prepare the mother for the surgery, she is kept NPO, an abdominal and perineal prep is done (from below breasts to the pubic region), and an indwelling catheter is inserted to dependent drainage, to prevent bladder distention and obstructed delivery. An operative permit must be signed by the mother. At least two units of whole blood are readied for administration. An IV is started, with an adequate size needle to permit blood administration, and preoperative medication is ordered. The pediatrician should be notified and adequate preparation made to receive the infant. The nurse should make sure that the Krieselman crib (or infant warmer) is functional and that appropriate resuscitation equipment is available. The circulating nurse assists in positioning the mother on the operating table. Fetal heart rate should be ascertained before surgery and during preparation, since fetal hypoxia can result from supine maternal hypotension. The operating table may be adjusted so it slants slightly to one side. This helps relieve the pressure of the gravid uterus on the vena cava and lessens the incidence of supine maternal hypotension. The circulating nurse assists the scrub nurse in setting up the equipment and assists the physicians by tying their gowns. The suction should be in working order, and the urine collection bag should be positioned under the operating table to ensure proper urinary drainage.

As with any surgery, the sponge count is very important. The circulating nurse must count the sponges with the scrub nurse and the surgeon and correctly record the number on a designated chart. The nurse should stand by to connect the suction when the operating team is ready and should record the actual time the incision is made and the infant is delivered. An oxytocin preparation is administered intravenously just as the baby is born. A sterile blanket is draped over the circulating nurse's arms in preparation to receive the baby.

After delivery, the nurse assists the pediatrician with physiologic support of the neonate and clamps the umbilical cord. As with any delivery, the mother and infant should be properly identified according to hospital procedure. After the infant's condition is stable, he should be shown to the mother if she is awake, as occurs with spinal anesthesia, then he should be taken to the nursery for observation and continued care. In addition, the woman's family should be shown the infant if his condition permits.

It is mandatory that the second and last sponge counts be recorded and correct and that this information be reported to the surgeon. Repeat administration of oxytocin during surgery may be necessary to control uterine bleeding. The circulating nurse assists with the application of the dressing to the incision and, with the aid of other staff, helps the mother back into bed.

The postpartal recovery room must be equipped with suction and oxygen to adequately ensure a patent airway and to protect from respiratory obstruction resulting from secretions. The recovery room nurse should check the mother's vital signs every 5 minutes until they are stable, then every 15 minutes for an hour, then every 30 minutes until she is discharged to the postpartal floor. The nurse should remain with the patient until she is stable.

The dressing and perineal pad must be checked every 15 minutes for at least an hour, and the fundus should be gently palpated to determine whether it is remaining firm. The fundus may be palpated by placing a hand to the side of the incision. Direct pressure on the incision increases the patient's discomfort. If the mother has been under general anesthesia, she should be positioned on her side to facilitate drainage of secretions, turned, and assisted with coughing and deep breathing every two hours. If the mother has received a spinal anesthetic, the level of anesthesia should be checked every 30 minutes until sensation has fully returned. It is important to monitor intake and output and to observe the urine for bloody tinge, which could mean surgical trauma to the bladder. The physician prescribes medication to relieve the mother's pain and nausea, and this should be administered as needed.

The mother should be informed about her infant's condition as soon as possible if she has had general anesthesia. The infant and his family should be brought together as soon as possible to facilitate bonding. The husband can be very supportive to the mother in her early postoperative period and can give her information about their baby. Before bringing the infant to the mother, it is important that she be comfortable. The nurse should ensure that the mother has received the ordered analgesia and that the analgesic agent is not harmful to the infant if she is nursing.

Psychologic Support

When the birth entails a variation in the delivery method, it is imperative that the nurse assess how the woman and her family perceive and react to the experience. Ann Clark and Dyanne Affonso (1979) have described some of the concerns of women who have undergone a cesarean birth. Some expressed feelings of inadequacy, of loss of their sense of womanliness and loss of control over their ability to have a vaginal delivery (viewed as an extension of the self). They expressed disappointment about being unable to fully participate in the birth process and not having mates participate in or witness the event as planned. Many expressed concerns about themselves and their babies as a result of the surgical procedure. They were concerned about the effects of cesarean section on their body image, including the presence of a scar and the ability to return to their previous shape. They also worried about their ability to fulfill the mothering role.

The nurse's key role is to listen, clarify, and provide information to help the woman deal with these concerns and integrate the experience. Careful explanation of all procedures preoperatively is important, and continued verbal interactions and human contact help decrease the mother's feelings of exposure, abandonment, and isolation. Availability of the husband for as long as possible and preferably having the husband view the birth assists in making the delivery appear more "normal" and facilitates bonding.

Immediately after delivery, the nurse must ascertain and meet the mother's dependency and comfort needs so that the woman can tune in to her mothering activities and her baby. In many areas, prenatal classes for prospective cesarean mothers are being conducted so they can be better informed and perhaps deal better with their concerns.

For further nursing care of the patient with cesarean section, see the accompanying Nursing Care Plan.

SUMMARY

Elective and operative procedures are widely utilized in obstetrics. Amniotomy, the most common operative procedure, is performed to shorten labor. Labor can be induced when the fetus is mature and the cervix is ripe. Episiotomies reduce tearing of perineal tissues and promote their healing. Forceps were developed to assist in difficult delivery situations. Other alternatives to difficult deliveries include version procedures and cesarean section. Operative obstetrics provides a means for health care practitioners to promote the safety, health, and comfort of the laboring patient.

NURSING CARE PLAN
Cesarean Section

Patient Data Base

History

Course of recovery from previous cesarean sections

Past mothering experience

EDC

Preparation for childbirth

Sensitivity to medications and anesthetic agents

Past bleeding problems

Physical examination

1. Fetal size, fetal status (FHR), and fetal maturity
2. Lung and cardiac status
3. Complete physical examination prior to administration of anesthetic

Laboratory evaluation

CBC

Hemoglobin and hematocrit

Type and cross-match for two units whole blood

Rh

Pro-time

VDRL

Urinalysis

Nursing Priorities

1. Preoperatively, educate patient about procedures and need for turning, coughing, and deep breathing.
2. Postoperatively:
   a. Promote optimum recovery.
   b. Maintain fluid and nutrition status.
   c. Prevent complications.
   d. Promote bonding.

NURSING CARE PLAN Cont'd
Cesarean Section

Problem	Nursing interventions and actions	Rationale
Recovery from surgery	Assess vital signs every 5 min until stable, then every 15 min for an hour, then every 30 min for 8 hours.	Vital signs may vary in response to medications or anesthetic.
Fluids and nutrition	Maintain intravenous infusion flow rate. Check patency and inspect IV site for redness or swelling.	IV fluids are maintained for 24-48 hours, or until bowel sounds are present. Oxytocic agent is usually added to the IV infusion for a few hours after surgery to enhance contraction of uterine muscles.
	Administer ice chips for first 24 hours, then advance diet as bowel sounds return.	
Bladder drainage	Connect indwelling bladder catheter to dependent drainage. Catheter is usually removed 1-2 hours after IV fluids are discontinued.	Enhances bladder emptying.
	Measure urine output on first two voidings and check bladder for distention.	Measuring urine provides information regarding adequate output and indicates whether the bladder is being emptied.
Blood loss	Check hemoglobin and hematocrit a few hours after surgery and on first postoperative day.	Identifies existence of anemia related to blood loss.
Nausea and vomiting	Administer antiemetic as needed. Check vital signs before administering.	Establishes baseline vital signs. Some antiemetics lower blood pressure.
Pain	Administer pain medication as needed. Assess vital signs before administering.	Controls or alleviates pain at incision site and gas pains. Establishes baseline vital signs, because pain medications may lower blood pressure.
	Monitor maternal drug use if she is nursing.	Many drugs taken by the mother are passed into in the breast milk.
	Place patient in comfortable position and splint incision when coughing or deep breathing.	Provides support and relief of pain.
Healing of incision	Inspect incision for redness, swelling, drainage, bruising, and separation of tissues.	Healing of incision is facilitated when infection is absent. If signs of infection are present, antibiotic therapy is indicated.
Bowel function	Auscultate bowel sounds.	Bowel sounds are absent for 24-36 hours as a result of anesthetic and pain medication.
	Progressive ambulation after 24 hours. Discuss rationale for early ambulation and assist in the ambulation process. Offer positive reinforcement for all attempts and steps in ambulation process.	Ambulation enhances return of bowel function.
Pulmonary status	Turn patient and have her cough and deep breathe every 2 hours for 24 hours.	Provides aeration of lungs and assists in preventing pulmonary complications.
	Splint incision while patient is coughing or deep breathing.	Promotes comfort.
Hemorrhage	Evaluate firmness and position of fundus.	Monitor involution.
	Palpate fundus after pain medication is administered to promote patient comfort.	Palpation of fundus causes discomfort to the patient and is frequently neglected and therefore becomes increasingly important.
	Fundus may be palpated from side of abdomen to avoid discomfort.	Tenderness at incisional site.
	Evaluate lochia.	Lochia progresses from rubra to serosa to alba. Increase in flow indicates inefficient contraction of uterus and/or subinvolution.

NURSING CARE PLAN Cont'd

Cesarean Section

Problem	Nursing interventions and actions	Rationale
Bonding	Enhance bonding by maintaining patient comfort. Provide information about the baby as soon as possible (such as sex, condition and normalcy). Provide early opportunities for mother-infant interaction.	Interaction may be delayed because of recovery from anesthesia and discomfort in first few hours after delivery.
	Discuss her feelings about the cesarean section and her self-image as a mother.	Emergency cesarean sections may cause feelings of inadequacy and sense of failure to have a "normal" birthing process.

Nursing Care Evaluation

No sign of infection is present.

Involution proceeds normally.

Patient is discharged in good physical state.

Education is provided for self-care and infant care.

SUGGESTED ACTIVITIES

1. Obtain the protocols for induction of labor from several hospitals within your area, and list their similarities and differences.
2. Draw a picture to illustrate the location of each type of episiotomy.
3. Observe a forceps delivery, and explain the reasons for forceps application and the types of complications that can be expected to occur.
4. Mrs. Jones is to have a repeat cesarean section. Her husband expresses a desire to be in the operating room during the cesarean section. Discuss the pros and cons of fathers in attendance at cesarean sections and draft a protocol for use in such situations.
5. List some priorities of nursing interventions for common elective and operative obstetrical procedures.

REFERENCES

Barham, K. 1973. Amnioscopy amniotomy: a look at surgical induction of labor. *Am. J. Obstet. Gynecol.* 117:35.

Bishop, E. H. 1964. Pelvic scoring for elective inductions. *Obstet. Gynecol.* 24:266.

Brotanek, V., and Hodr, J. 1968. Fetal distress after artificial rupture of membranes. *Am. J. Obstet. Gynecol.* 101:502.

Chukwedebelu, W. O. 1977. The vacuum extractor in difficult labor. *Internatl. Surg.* 62:89.

Cibils, L. A. 1972. Enhancement and induction of labor. In *Risks in the practice of modern obstetrics*, ed. S. Aladjem. St. Louis: The C. V. Mosby Co.

Clark, A. L., and Affonso, D. D. 1979. *Childbearing: a nursing perspective.* 2nd ed. Philadelphia: F. A. Davis Co.

Cogan, R., and Edmunds, E. P. 1977. The unkindest cut. *Contemp. OB/Gyn.* 9:55.

Cohen, W. 1977. Influence of the duration of second stage labor on perinatal outcome and puerperal morbidity. *Obstet. Gynecol.* 49:266.

du Vigneaud, V., et al. 1954. The synthesis of an octopeptide amide with the hormonal activity of oxytocin. *J. Am. Chem. Soc.* 75:4879.

du Vigneaud, V., et al. 1958. Synthesis of the pressor antidiuretic hormone, arginine vasopressin. *J. Am. Chem. Soc.* 80:3355.

Friedman, E., and Sachtleben, M. R. 1976. Station of the fetal presenting part. VI. Arrest of descent in nulliparas. *Obstet. Gynecol.* 47:129.

Friedman, E., et al. 1977. Dysfunctional labor. XII. Long term effects on infant. *Am. J. Obstet. Gynecol.* 127:779.

Fuchs, F. 1976. The sensitivity of the uterus to oxytocin. In *Oxytocin induced labor,* ed. Parke-Davis Company. Greenwich, Conn.: CPC Communications, Inc.

Fuchs, F., and Klopper, A., eds. 1977. *Endocrinology of pregnancy.* 2nd ed. Scranton, Pa.: Harper & Row Publishers, Inc.

Gabert, H. A., and Stenchever, M. A. 1973. Effect of ruptured membranes on fetal heart patterns. *Obstet. Gynecol.* 41:279.

Hendricks, C. H., and Brenner, W. E. Oct. 1964. Patterns of increasing uterine activity in late pregnancy and the development of uterine responsiveness to oxytocin. *Am. J. Obstet. Gynecol.* 90:485.

Hendricks, et al. 1970. Normal cervical dilatation in late pregnancy and labor. *Am. J. Obstet. Gynecol.* 106:1065.

Hibbard, L. 1976. Changing trends in cesarean sections. *Am. J. Obstet. Gynecol.* 75:798.

Hon, E. A. 1976. Fetal monitoring during induction of labor. In *Oxytocin induced labor,* ed. Parke-Davis Company. Greenwich, Conn.: CPC Communications, Inc.

Hughes, E. C., ed. 1972. *Obstetrics-gynecology terminology.* Philadelphia: F. A. Davis Co.

Jones, O. H. 1976. Cesarean section in present-day obstetrics. *Am. J. Obstet. Gynecol.* 76:798.

Keettel, W. C. No. 1969. Inducing labor by rupturing membranes. *Postgrad. Med.* 44:199.

Martell, M., et al. 1976. Blood acid-base balance at birth in neonates from labors with early and late rupture of membranes. *J. Pediatr.* 89:693.

Nurses Association of the American College of Obstetricians and Gynecologists. 1974. *Obstetric, gynecologic and neonatal nursing functions and standards.* Chicago: The Association.

Ott, W. 1975. Vacuum extraction. *Obstet. Gynecol. Survey.* 30:643.

Pauerstein, C. J. 1973. Use and abuse of oxytocic agents. *Clin. Obstet. Gynecol.* 16:262.

Pritchard, J. A., and MacDonald, P. C. 1976. *Williams obstetrics.* New York: Appleton-Century-Crofts.

Quennan, J. S. 1977. Ultrasound: diagnostic applications in obstetrics (symposium). *Contemp. OB/Gyn.* 9:119.

Spellacy, W. N., et al. 1973. The induction of labor at term: comparisons between prostaglandin $F_{2\alpha}$ and oxytocin infusions. *Obstet. Gynecol.* 41:14.

Theobald, G. W. 1968. Oxytocin reassessed. *Obstet. Gynecol.* 23:109.

Tricomi, V. 1973. Induction of labor: a contemporary view. *Clin. Obstet. Gynecol.* 16:226.

Vorherr, H. 1974. Induction and stimulation of labor. *Obstet. Gynecol.* 3:283.

Weber, C. W. 1970. Postmortem caesarean section: review of the literature and case reports. *Am. J. Obstet. Gynecol.* 60:158.

ADDITIONAL READINGS

Aladjem, S., ed. 1972. *Risks in the practice of modern obstetrics.* St. Louis: The C. V. Mosby Co.

Barter, R. H. 1968. Induction of labor: helpful or harmful? *Postgrad. Med.* 43:141.

Cardano, A., and Kraus, V. 1972. Clinical experience with oxytocin. *Obstet. Gynecol.* 39:247.

Cibils, L. A. Dec. 1970. Effect of intrauterine contraceptive devices upon human uterine contractility. *J. Reprod. Med.* 5:242.

Cibils, L. A. Sept. 1971. Effect of mesuprine hydischloride upon nonpregnant uterine contractility and the cardiovascular system. *Am. J. Obstet. Gynecol.* 111:187.

Fields, H., et al. 1959. Intravenous Pitocin in induction and stimulation of labor. *Obstet. Gynecol.* 13:353.

Friedman, E. A., et al. 1966. Relation of pre-labor evaluation to inducibility and the course of labor. *Obstet. Gynecol.* 28:495.

Granat, M. 1976. Oxytocin contraindication in the presence of uterine scar. *Lancet.* 2:1411.

Hellman, L. M., and Pritchard, J. A., eds. 1971. *Williams obstetrics.* 14th ed. New York: Appleton-Century-Crofts.

Hess, O. W., and Hon, E. H. 1960. The electronic evaluation of fetal heart rate. III. The effect of an oxytocic agent used for the induction of labor. *Am. J. Obstet. Gynecol.* 80:558.

McNay, M. B., et al. 1977. Perinatal deaths: analysis by clinical cause to assess value of inductions of labour. *Br. Med. J.* 1:347.

Murphey, H. 1976. Delivery following cesarean section. *J. Irish Med. Assoc.* 69:533.

Niswander, K. R., et al. 1967. Prelabor pelvic score as a predictor of birth weight. *Obstet. Gynecol.* 29:256.

Patterson, W. 1971. Amniotomy, with or without simultaneous oxytocin infusion. *J. Obstet. Gynaecol. Br. Commonw.* 78:310.

Pawson, M. D., and Simmons, S. C. 1970. Routine induction of labour by amniotomy and simultaneous syntocinon (synthetic oxytocin) infusion. *Br. Med. J.* 3:243.

Tafeen, C. H., et al. 1956. Elective induction of labor. *Obstet. Gynecol.* 8:700.

Zuckerman, M. B. et al., eds. 1969. *Quick references to OB-Gyn procedures.* Philadelphia: J. P. Lippincott Co.

Zuspan, F. P., coordinator. 1971. Induction of labor—part I (symposium). *J. Reprod. Med.* 6(1):18.

Zuspan, F. P., coordinator. 1971. Induction of labor—part II (symposium). *J. Reprod. Med.* 6(2):17.

CHAPTER 21

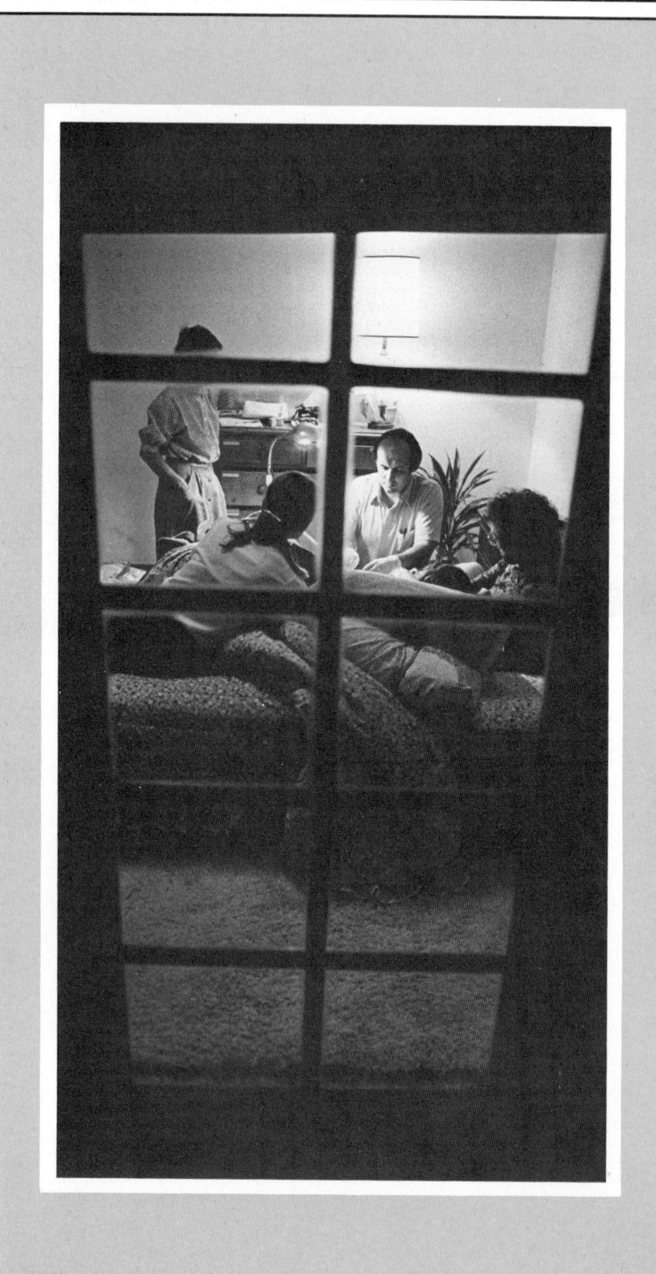

BIRTH ALTERNATIVES AND EMERGENCY DELIVERIES

BIRTH ALTERNATIVES

- **The Leboyer Method**
- **Birth Centers**
- **Home Births**

EMERGENCY DELIVERIES

- **Hospital Births**
- **Out-of-Hospital Births**

OBJECTIVES

- Discuss alternative birth methods.
- Describe the procedure for managing a delivery in an emergency situation.
- Describe possible adaptations that may be used in out-of-hospital deliveries.

BIRTH ALTERNATIVES

Increasing numbers of expectant parents are dissatisfied with what they consider the intrusive, inflexible, and arbitrary rules and regulations of maternity wards and the inability or unwillingness of the hospital's medical and nursing staff to pay heed to the family's desires. Following are common requests of expectant parents:

1. That labor and delivery be performed in a supportive, quiet, and relaxed environment.
2. That an enema and perineal shave not be given at admission.
3. That the father be allowed to participate as much as the couple desires.
4. That medications and treatments be administered only with the couple's permission and only after a complete explanation about their actions and possible side effects has been given.
5. That invasive fetal monitoring be avoided.
6. That forceps and anesthesia not be used unless medically indicated.
7. That the mother may labor and deliver in the same room and bed.
8. That an episiotomy not be performed.
9. That the baby be delivered in a dimly lighted room and gently handled.
10. That the parents be allowed maximal interaction with their child or that the infant be allowed to nurse immediately after delivery.
11. That the baby be allowed to remain with his parents.

Some hospitals are not equipped to meet some of these demands. Others refuse because they believe that certain of the procedures are necessary to maintain maternal and fetal well-being. Others refuse because of resistance to change to new ideas and methods. In any case, many expectant families are frustrated in their attempt to make decisions about the kind of child-bearing experience they want. As a result, they are seeking alternate modes of maternity care and individuals who are more responsive to their desires.

The Leboyer Method

The Leboyer method is directed toward easing the birth trauma for the newborn infant. In a conventional delivery the newborn is subjected to bright lights, voices, and new sensations as he is dried and placed in blankets. The Leboyer method provides soothing, comforting measures to use in handling the newborn at delivery. The lights in the delivery room are kept low, and talking is kept to a minimum. As the baby is delivered, the physician avoids touching the infant's head, in order to further reduce trauma. The newborn is placed on his stomach on the mother's abdomen, and while handling the newborn, care is taken to keep his spine in a curved position as it was in utero. The mother is encouraged to touch and stroke her infant. The umbilical cord is cut after all pulsations have ceased. Leboyer (1976) believes that this delay helps the respiratory effort of the newborn as he adjusts to his new extrauterine breathing. After the umbilical cord is clamped, the infant is gently placed in water that has been warmed to 98–99°F. The newborn remains in the tub until he shows complete relaxation. The warm water simulates the intrauterine environment in consistency and temperature. He is then carefully dried and wrapped in soft blankets, but his head and hands remain free to move. The newborn is placed on his side to avoid stress on his spine, and then he is left alone to quietly take in his new environment.

Couples may request that the Leboyer method be followed in its entirety or may make some adaptations, depending on their beliefs and available facilities. It is necessary to talk with the physician to ascertain his or her willingness to use this birth method.

Birth Centers

Birth centers, or birth rooms, are located in a hospital or close to a health care facility. They may be staffed with nurse-midwives, labor and delivery nurses, or physicians. In these birth centers, parents take more responsibility for the birth experience.

The hospital birthing room or birth center is usually furnished in a homelike style, similar to a bedroom. The room is furnished with a bed that can be used during labor and the actual delivery. Comfortable chairs are available for the father and other relatives or friends who may be in attendance. In some birth centers, children are also welcome.

Couples who intend to use the birth center are screened during pregnancy for such high-risk factors as the following:

Social factors

- Fewer than five prenatal visits
- Primipara more than 35 years of age
- Multipara more than 40 years of age

Preexisting maternal disease

- Chronic hypertension
- Renal, cardiac, or respiratory disease
- Diabetes
- Preeclampsia-eclampsia
- Anemia

Previous pregnancy history

- Previous stillbirth, cesarean section, or infant born with respiratory distress syndrome

Present pregnancy

- Preeclampsia-eclampsia
- Gestation less than 37 weeks or greater than 42 weeks
- Multiple pregnancy
- Abnormal fetal presentation
- Third trimester bleeding or known placenta previa
- Multiparity greater than five
- Ruptured membranes for longer than 24 hours
- Estimated fetal weight of less than 5 lb or more than 9 lb
- Contracted pelvis or cephalopelvic disproportion

The presence of any one factor may not automatically exclude the mother from a birth room experience, but it does necessitate careful and continuous assessment.

The eligible couple is usually encouraged or in some instances required to attend prenatal classes. In some areas, a class that provides orientation to the birthing room is also required. Couples are encouraged to meet birthing room personnel and discuss the couple's desires and preferences for their birth experience.

The expectant mother is admitted directly to the birth room after labor has begun. She is encouraged to utilize breathing and relaxation techniques during the labor. She is supported and coached by those present. The prevailing mood is quiet and unhurried. The delivery occurs in the birth room, which eliminates the need for changing rooms as delivery becomes imminent. This in itself adds to the unhurried atmosphere. After delivery, physical contact between the parents and newborn is encouraged. The mother may breastfeed her infant immediately after delivery.

The mother and newborn are monitored for a minimum of 2–24 hours after delivery and then are discharged from the hospital to home or from labor and delivery to the postpartum unit. Nursing staff may be involved in postpartal visits in the patient's home.

A home visit is scheduled within one to two days after delivery. Continuation of home visits may vary, depending on each hospital or birth center's established routines. In some centers, weekly visits are made through the first six weeks following delivery. The home visit provides an opportunity to see the family in their home setting, to make assessments of the mother and infant, to answer questions, and to provide information and support. The accompanying Postpartal Home Visit Assessment Guide provides assessments that may be made. Detailed information on postpartum and newborn assessment is presented in Chapters 22 and 27.

Case Study

Allison and Scott Jones are expecting their first child. During the pregnancy they have attended prenatal classes and have made special preparation in anticipation of using the birthing room at their local hospital. The pregnancy has proceeded without difficulty or problems.

POSTPARTAL HOME VISIT ASSESSMENT GUIDE (24 hours after delivery)

Assess	Normal findings	Deviations and possible causes*	Nursing interventions†
Mother			
Vital signs	BP between 90/60 and 140/90	BP below 90/60 (reduction in blood volume)	For deviations in BP, refer to physician.
		BP above 140/90 (hypertensive disorder)	If BP is elevated, assess patient for edema. Obtain urinalysis for protein.
	Pulse 70-100	Pulse below 70 or above 100 (cardiac disorder)	Refer to physician.
	Oral temperature 98-99F	Temperature above 100F (infectious process)	Assess for signs of infection. Refer to physician.
Breasts	Presence of colostrum, engorgement may be beginning	Absence of colostrum (inadequate letdown)	Assess mother's feeding practices.
	Nipples smooth, no evidence of cracking	Cracking of nipples (prolonged breast-feeding)	Assess mother's feeding practices. Counsel her in cleansing of the breast and exposing the nipples to air.
	Absence of localized swelling or redness	Localized swelling or redness (infectious process)	Refer to physician. Instruct mother in breast massage. Depending on severity of infection, mother may need to be counseled about alternate feeding methods.
Fundus	Firm and in the midline	Boggy (inadequate uterine contractions) Out of midline (bladder distention)	Instruct mother in fundal massage. May need to refer to physician. Assess lochia for amount and presence of clots.
	2-3 finger-breadths below the umbilicus	At or above umbilicus (inadequate uterine contractions)	Assess lochia for amount and presence of clots. Assess bladder for distention. Instruct mother in fundal massage. May need to refer to physician.
	Progressive decrease in size	Subinvolution (inadequate contractions)	Assess lochia for amount and presence of clots. Assess temperature. Instruct mother in fundal massage. Encourage frequent rest periods. Refer to physician.
Lochia	Lochia rubra for first 2-3 days; small clots	Excessive lochia—one pad saturated in 2 hours; large	Assess fundus. If uterus is firm, assess for perineal

*Possible causes of deviations are placed in parentheses.
†Nursing interventions are primarily directed toward deviations.

POSTPARTAL HOME VISIT ASSESSMENT GUIDE Cont'd

Assess	Normal findings	Deviations and possible causes*	Nursing interventions[†]
		clots (inadequate uterine contractions, subinvolution, vaginal lacerations)	laceration. Refer to physician.
	Odor similar to menstrual flow	Foul odor (infection)	Refer to physician.
Episiotomy	Close approximation of skin edges; small amount of bruising	Separation of skin edges, excessive bruising, presence of indurated area at episiotomy site	Refer to physician.
Bladder	No distention	Distention (loss of muscle tone)	Refer to physician.
	Absence of frequency, urgency, and dysuria	Frequency, urgency, dysuria (bladder infection)	Assess temperature. Refer to physician. Assess fluid intake.
Bowels	Bowel movement by 3rd postpartum day	Constipation (inadequate fluid intake or nutritional intake; fear of pain if episiotomy is present)	Assess fluid and nutritional intake. Encourage mother to force fluids. Stool softener may be needed. Provide counseling and support if mother indicates fear of defecation because of episiotomy.
Newborn			
Vital signs	Axillary temperature 97-98F	Axillary temperature below 97 (inadequate temperature control, lack of subcutaneous fat)	Provide external means of warming newborn.
	Apical pulse 110-160 beats/min	Apical pulse <110 or >160 (cardiac disorder)	Assess respirations and general color. Refer to physician.
	Respirations 30-60/min (count for one full minute)	Respirations above 60/min (respiratory problems)	Assess apical pulse, temperature, and general color. Refer to physician.
Skin color	Pinkish	Jaundice (hemolytic disease, physiologic jaundice)	Draw bilirubin. Refer to physician.
Umbilical cord	Dry	Moist, oozing, odor, exudate (infection); bleeding	Culture exudate. Instruct mother in cleansing of cord and allowing exposure to air. Refer to physician if needed.
Feedings	6-8 per day	<6 or >8 (inadequate knowledge of feeding needs, disinterest of the newborn)	Assess mother's feeding practices and knowledge base. Provide counseling. Assess newborn's weight.

*Possible causes of deviations are placed in parentheses.
[†]Nursing interventions are primarily directed toward deviations.

POSTPARTAL HOME VISIT ASSESSMENT GUIDE Cont'd

Assess	Normal findings	Deviations and possible causes*	Nursing interventions†
Alertness	Awake for 1-4 hr per day	Excessive wakefulness or sleeping	Assess sleep habits, number and amount of feedings. Counsel as necessary. Instruct in expected newborn behavior.
Education			
Self-care	Mother has adequate knowledge of the following self-care measures: breast care, perineal care, sitz baths, fundal massage, adequate fluid intake, optimum nutrition, Kegel exercises	Inadequate knowledge	Assess knowledge base. Provide counseling and information as needed.
Baby care	Mother has adequate knowledge of the following baby care measures: bathing, feeding, sleeping habits, clothes, temperature (axillary, rectal), safety (home and car), quieting techniques	Inadequate knowledge	Assess knowledge base. Provide counseling and information as needed.

*Possible causes of deviations are placed in parentheses.
†Nursing interventions are primarily directed toward deviations.

When labor begins, they proceed to the hospital and are greeted by Marie Carlson, a nurse in the labor and delivery department. Ms. Carlson helps Allison and Scott get settled and completes the admission process. Allison is having contractions every two to three minutes lasting 45 seconds, and cervical dilatation is 5 cm. She is breathing with the contractions and is excited that the delivery day is at hand.

Ms. Carlson works to provide a comfortable, unhurried atmosphere. She is already acquainted with the Joneses because they have attended the prenatal classes that she teaches. She is familiar with their level of knowledge and will now work to support them as labor progresses. She notes that Allison and Scott are working well together in timing contractions and utilizing relaxation techniques and breathing methods. Ms. Carlson completes her physical assessment, then talks with the couple about the progress. Ms. Carlson leaves, letting the Joneses know she is available whenever they need her. She has found that parents who use the birthing room are well prepared and that she may not need to stay quite so close. She is able to go in and assess progress and how the Joneses are coping with the labor, and as long as all is going well she allows the couple privacy. She has notified the obstetrician of Allison's admission and labor status, and he is on his way to the hospital.

As Allison proceeds into transition, Ms. Carlson notes that the Joneses are needing more encouragement and support, so she stays in constant attendance. She assesses maternal, fetal, and labor status and keeps the Joneses informed of their progress.

Dr. J. G. Grey comes in to see the Joneses and stays close by because the labor is progressing rapidly. Toward the end of the transition, Ms. Carlson prepares the equipment to be used during delivery. She assists Allison in her pushing efforts when the cervix has completely dilated. During the delivery, she assists Allison, Scott, and Dr. Grey. The delivery is managed in the same unhurried manner. Ms. Carlson assesses physical parameters and offers continuing support as Allison delivers a healthy appearing baby girl. Ms. Carlson assesses the newborn quickly and then places her in her mother's arms.

The postdelivery recovery period is monitored closely so that any problems can be identified. Allison is recovering without problems and is eager to learn more about her new daughter. Ms. Carlson talks to the Joneses to assess their level of knowledge and provides information that is needed. She does a physical assessment of the newborn and explains the findings to the Joneses. She assists Allison as she breast-feeds her baby for the first time. After the feeding, the nurse assists Scott in giving the baby her first bath. Ms. Carlson has found that the bath time provides opportunities to talk and share information.

During the recovery period, she provides quiet time for the new family to be together and get acquainted.

A few hours after delivery, Ms. Carlson assists the Joneses as they prepare for dismissal. She will be making a visit to the Joneses' home the next morning and then weekly, to assess the mother and infant and to provide information and continued support.

Home Births

Another alternative to the traditional hospital delivery is home birth. Parents who have participated in home delivery find that it is a warm, close, loving experience for which they have responsibility and control. The newborn infant is immediately incorporated into the family, and the continuous contact between the newborn and his family facilitates the bonding process and establishment of a family unit. Siblings present during delivery are able to welcome the newborn into the family and are participants in an exciting and beautiful experience. A home birth may be accompanied by unexpected complications, such as prolonged labor, malpresentation of the fetus, or bleeding problems. Adequate medical backup is an important part of a successful home birth.

Assessment

Families who choose home birth should be screened and counseled extensively throughout the pregnancy. A number of different criteria must be met for a successful home birth experience. The following questions can be asked to determine the feasibilty or desirability of home birth for a particular couple.

1. *Why does the couple desire a home birth?*

2. *Are they choosing home birth to challenge authority or to "get back" at the system?* The couple who perceives home birth as a political act may not have the mother's or infant's best interests at heart. The couple may have had what they perceive as "bad" experiences with the health care system.

3. *What is the family's financial status?* The couple who chooses home birth for financial reasons may be a risk if their income is such that it precludes adequate nutrition.

4. *Is the woman able to adequately care for herself?* The woman who is unable to take proper care of herself because of psychologic or physical factors may not be in optimal condition to cope with the stresses of labor and delivery and therefore may be classified as high risk.

The expectant mother should undergo a thorough physical examination, including laboratory studies, to assess her health status. The amount of information and understanding about birth and related processes held by the family must also be evaluated so that counseling can be directed toward filling the gaps in their knowledge.

The presence of the following factors may preclude the possibility of home birth:

1. Age under 16 years or over 40 years.
2. Weight under 100 lb or over 200 lb.
3. History of long labors.

The following photographs were taken at a birth center. We wish to express our appreciation to the delivering couple for sharing their unique and moving childbirth experience.

There were two nurses and a physician in attendance. Unexpectedly the mother chose a standing delivery position, and the father helped support her body during the birth.

We do not advocate this particular delivery position. We do believe that every maternity nurse should be aware that there is no one "correct" way to have a baby. Each birth is special.

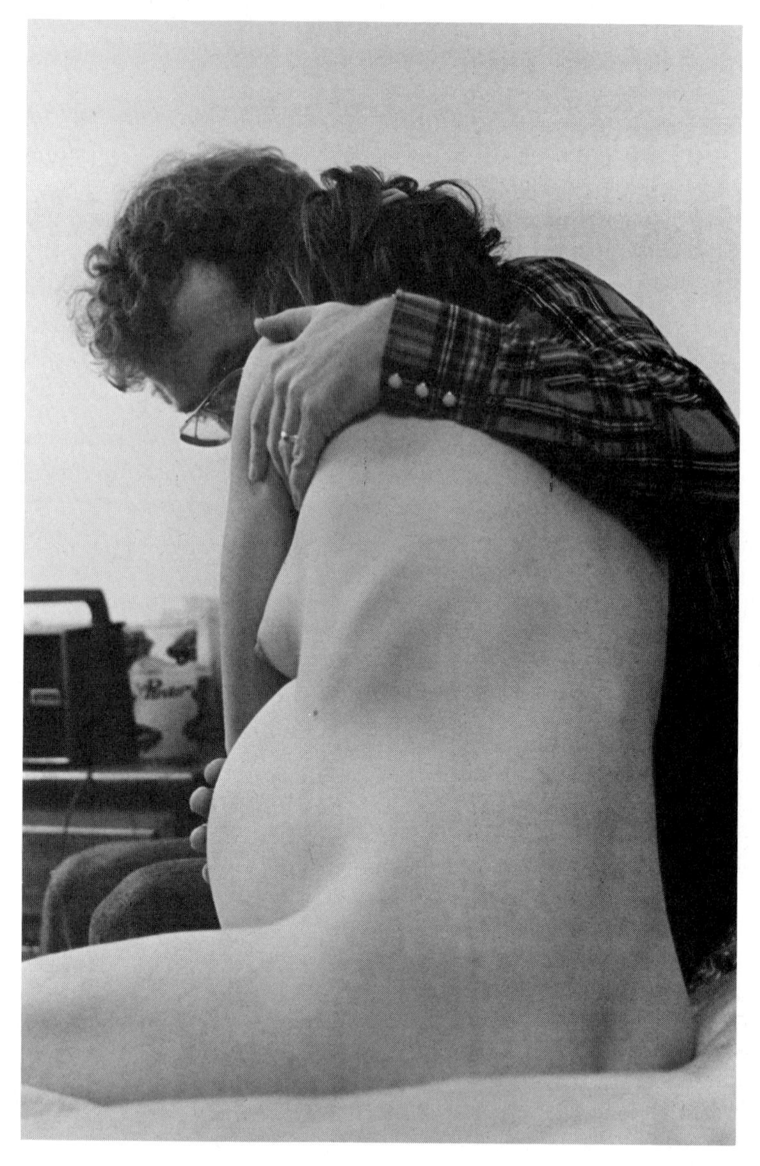

The woman is in labor. She has just taken a shower, and is now resting.

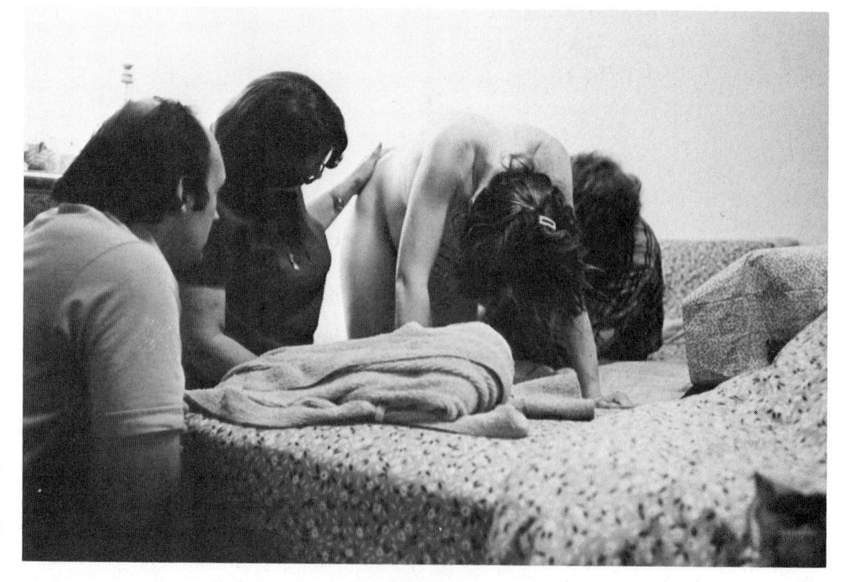

The woman walks around the room. Moments later she feels the urge to begin pushing. The nurse and her husband support her body as she begins to push.

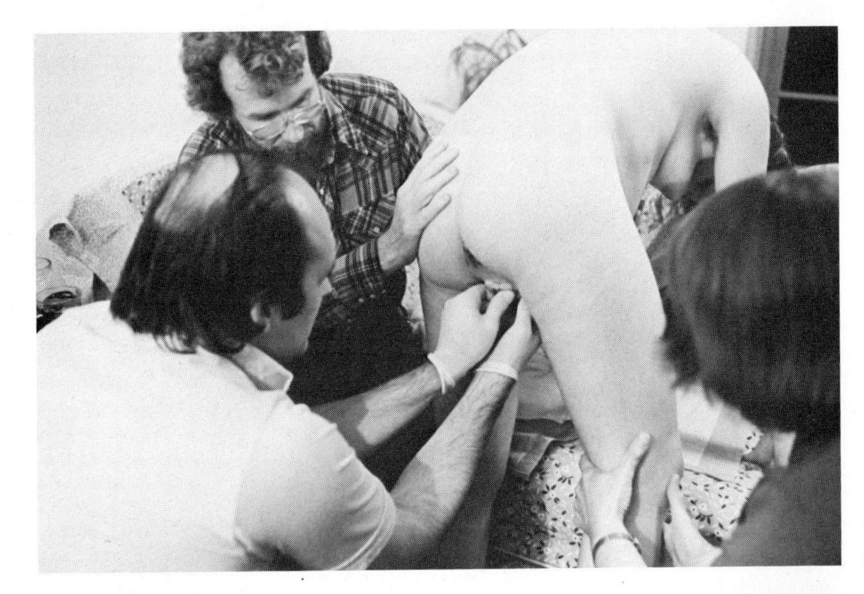

Within one minute the head has crowned, and rapid delivery ensues.

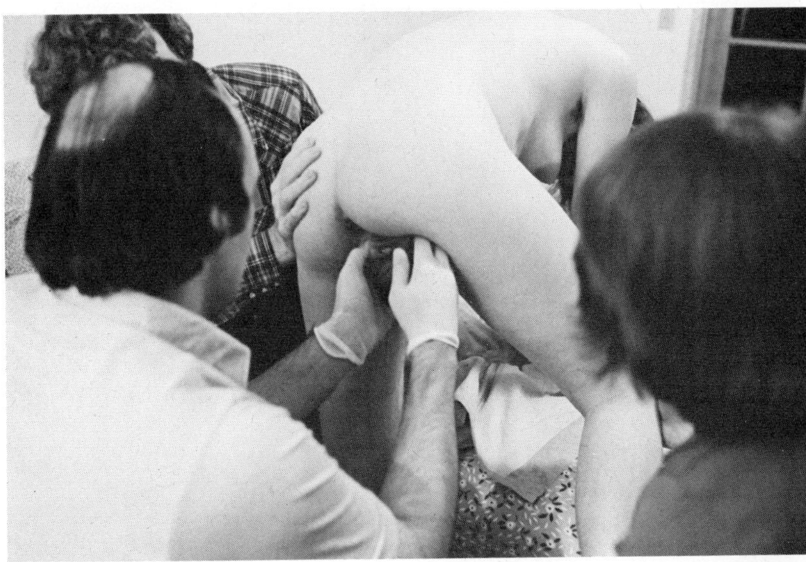

Delivery of the head is beginning.

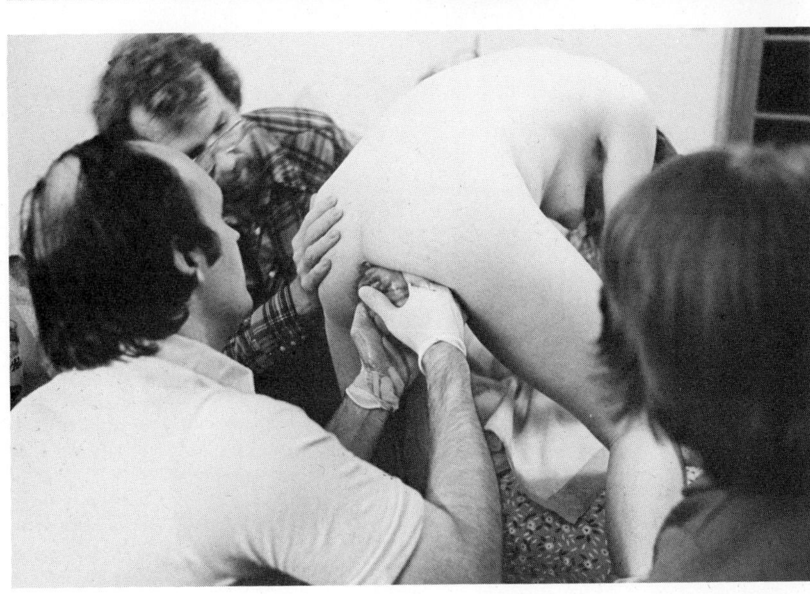

Complete delivery of the head.

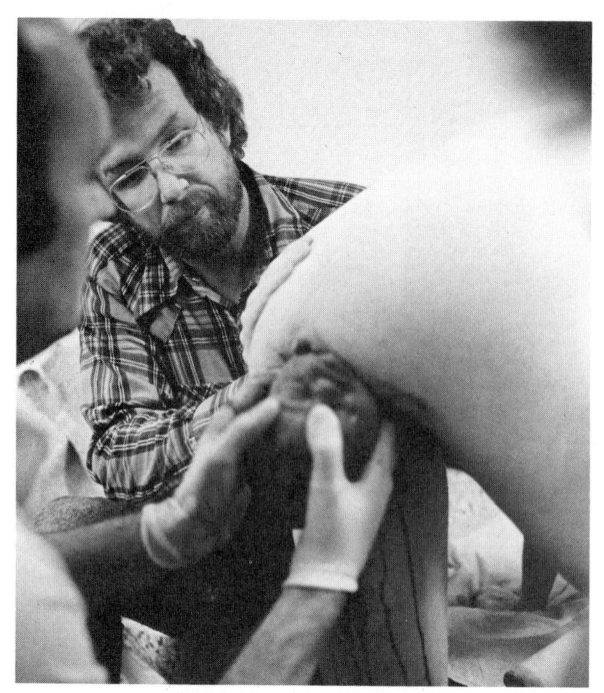

External rotation and restitution have occurred.

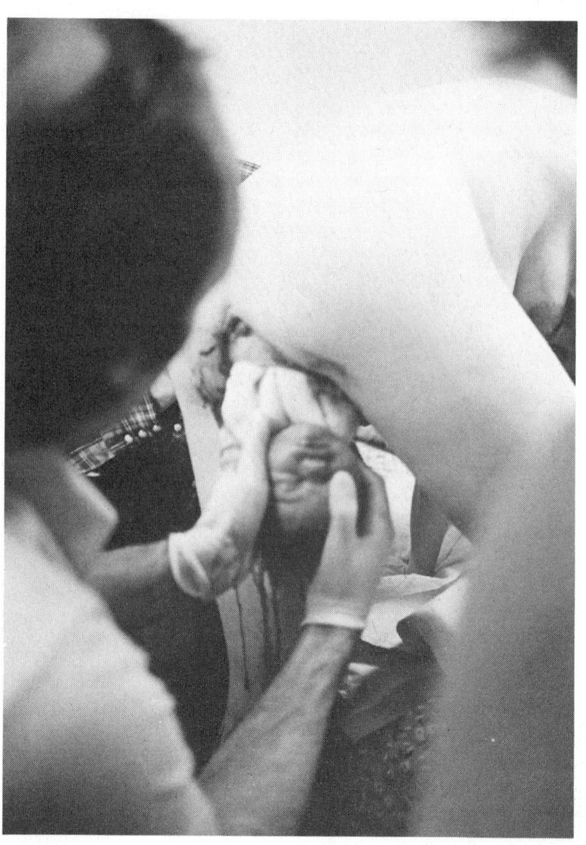

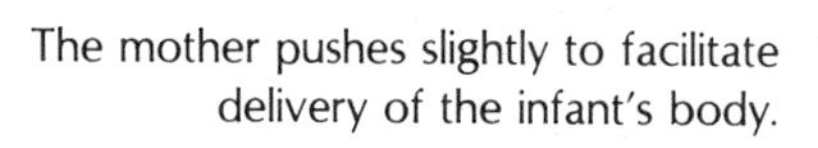

The mother pushes slightly to facilitate delivery of the infant's body.

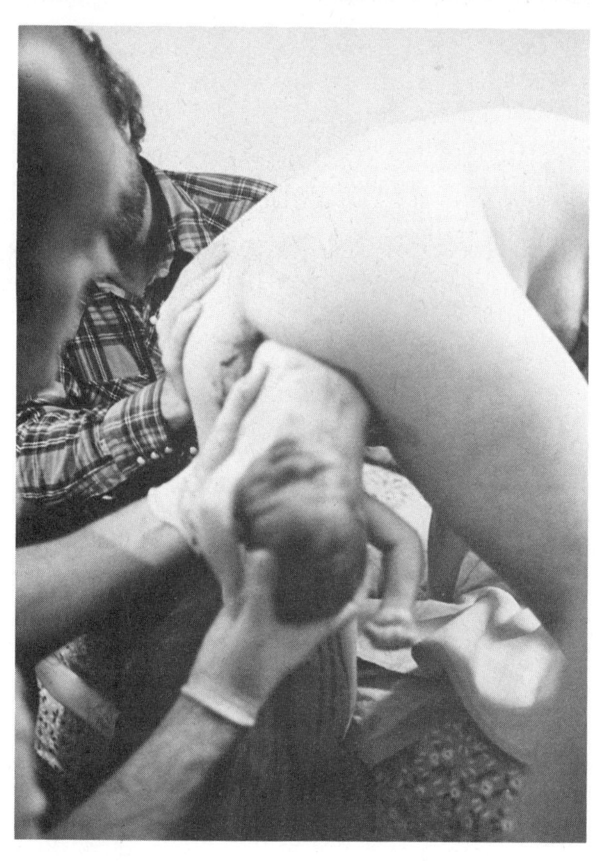

Delivery of the infant's body.

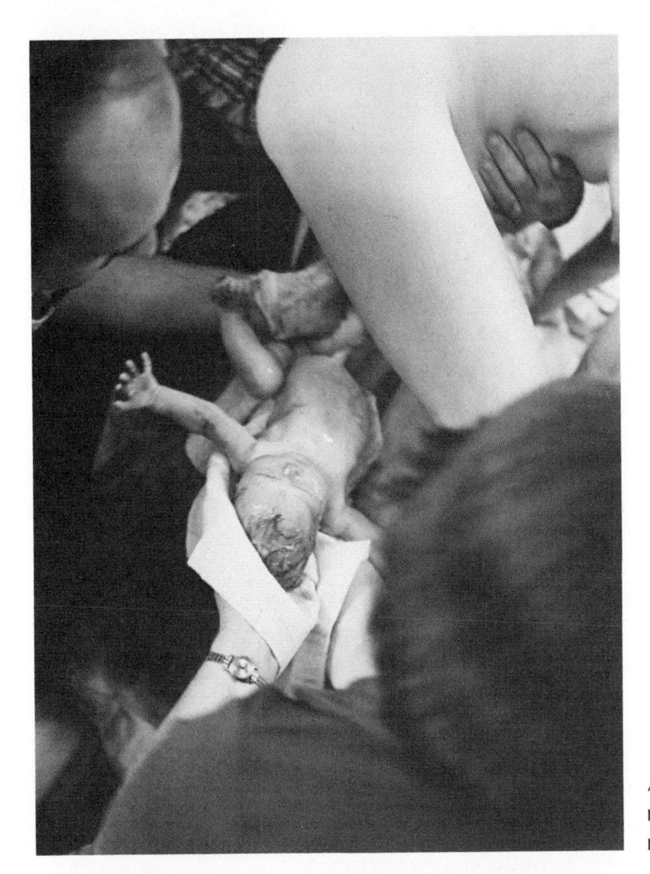

A little girl has been born. Note the nurse's position as she handles the newborn with a warm towel.

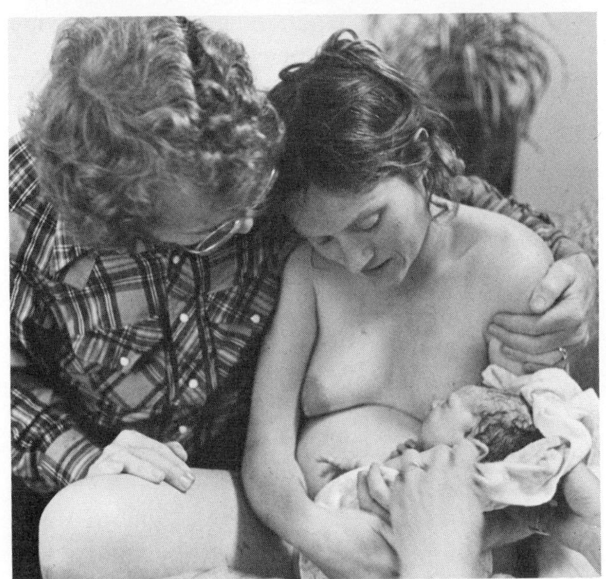

The nurse hands the baby to the mother. In this photograph the baby is two minutes old.

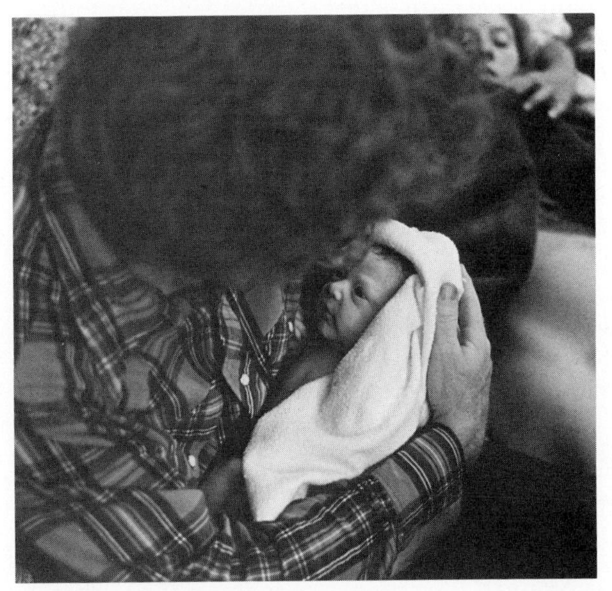

The father holds his baby five minutes after the delivery. The nurse is standing behind the mother, covering her with warm blankets as the mother awaits delivery of the placenta.

4. Previous cesarean sections.
5. Repeated miscarriages.
6. Previous Rh incompatibility.
7. Parity greater than six.
8. Malpresentation of fetus.
9. Previous delivery of premature infant (under 38 weeks) or postmature infant (over 42 weeks).
10. Presence of maternal disease (preeclampsia-eclampsia, diabetes, cardiac disease, respiratory disease, polyhydramnios, vaginal bleeding, herpesvirus type 2 infection).
11. Psychologic risk factors.
12. Multiple pregnancy.

If any of these high-risk factors are found during the assessment process, the family should be advised that home birth may not be in the mother's or infant's best interests.

Antepartal Interventions

One of the most important prerequisites for a successful home birth is that the pregnant woman be in excellent health. The nurse can help the woman achieve this end by giving her and her family quality health care throughout the prenatal period. Education and counseling of the family are important aspects of this care, and these can be effectively accomplished through a series of childbirth classes. Classes begin in midpregnancy. It is emphasized throughout these classes that the parents are ultimately responsible for the successful outcome of the planned home birth. The following subjects are stressed because they may affect the kind of birth and childrearing experiences the family has:

1. Nutrition.
2. Exercise.
3. Breathing and relaxation techniques.
4. Normal physiologic changes during pregnancy.
5. Normal labor and delivery processes.

The couple is encouraged to ask their physician for information about laboratory results, blood pressure, general physical condition of the expectant mother, and the status of the fetus as evaluated by fetal heart rate. They are told to request information about possible complications and typical obstetric procedures. Nurses should encourage class members to cooperate with the physician and other members of the health care team should a hospital delivery become necessary.

Participants in these prenatal classes receive explanations about bonding and parenting. They are urged to read and study independently about the birth process as well as to participate in group learning experiences. In addition, parents are taught how to recognize problems that might need further attention.

Delivery

Home deliveries may be attended by a lay midwife, certified nurse-midwife (contingent upon the laws of respective states), or physician. The attendant should have the following supplies:

- Disposable underpads.
- Sterilized cord tie and scissors.
- Bulb syringe.
- Four to six receiving blankets (to be warmed in the oven at 100F when labor begins so they will be warm for the newborn).
- Six towels.
- Two sets of sheets.
- Plastic sheet.
- Sterile sheet (may be sterilized by placing in paper bag and putting it in the oven).
- Perineal pads and belt.
- Large bowl for placenta and small bowl for placing solutions.
- Cotton balls and bottle of alcohol.
- Betadine scrub solution.

When labor begins, the nurse-midwife or midwife is summoned to the home. She monitors the labor and provides support to the family. Maternal vital signs are monitored frequently, and the fetal heart rate is assessed every 15 minutes. A vaginal examination is performed at the beginning of labor to ascertain position, presentation, dilatation, and effacement of the cervix, and this examination is repeated infrequently unless a problem arises.

If a physician is attending the birth, he or she arrives at the end of the first stage, attends the delivery, performs a neonatal assessment, and remains for at least one hour after delivery to assess maternal bleeding and the newborn status.

If a midwife or nurse-midwife assists the parents during delivery, she remains with the family until maternal bleeding has been assessed, the mother has urinated, and the baby has begun nursing. She returns to the home 24 and 48 hours after delivery to check maternal bleeding and temperature and to assess the neonate's skin for jaundice. The midwife or nurse-midwife also assists the mother if she is having difficulty breastfeeding the infant. The attendant is available by telephone or during home visits to answer questions and to provide information and support to the new family concerning problems as they arise. The mother and infant are examined by the physician one week and six weeks after birth.

EMERGENCY DELIVERIES

Emergency delivery occurs in a variety of physical settings and during a variety of climatic disturbances. The two areas that are addressed in this chapter are hospital births unattended by a physician and other unattended out-of-hospital births.

Hospital Births

Occasionally labor progresses so rapidly that the maternity nurse is faced with the task of delivering the baby. The attending maternity nurse has the primary responsibility for providing a physically and psychologically safe experience for the mother and her baby.

A mother whose physician or nurse-midwife is not present may feel disappointed, frightened, and abandoned, especially if she is not prepared through childbirth education. Fear is an inhibiting factor in birth rooms; therefore, the nurse can support the mother by keeping her informed about the labor progress and assuring the patient that the nurse will stay with her. If delivery is imminent, the nurse must not leave the patient alone. Auxiliary personnel can be directed to contact the physician and to retrieve the emergency delivery pack ("precip pack"). An emergency delivery pack should be readily accessible to the labor rooms. A typical pack contains the following items:

1. A small drape that can be placed under the mother's buttocks to provide a sterile field.
2. Several 4 × 4 gauze pads for wiping off the baby's face and removing secretions from the mouth.
3. A bulb syringe to be used to clear mucus from the baby's mouth.
4. Two sterile clamps (Kelly or Rochester) to clamp the umbilical cord.
5. Sterile scissors to cut the umbilical cord.
6. A sterile umbilical cord clamp, either Hesseltine or Hollister.
7. A baby blanket to wrap the baby in after delivery.
8. A package of sterile gloves.

As the materials are being gathered, the nurse must remain calm. The patient is reassured by the composure of the nurse and feels that the nurse is competent.

Delivery of Infant in Vertex Presentation

The nurse who manages an emergency in-hospital delivery conducts it as follows: The mother is allowed to assume a comfortable position. If time permits, the nurse scrubs her hands with soap and water and puts on sterile gloves. Sterile drapes are placed under the patient's buttocks.

At all times during the delivery, the nurse gives clear instructions to the woman, supports her efforts, and praises her for doing a good job.

When the head crowns, the nurse instructs the mother to pant, which decreases the urge to push. The nurse checks whether the amniotic sac is intact. If it is, the sac is torn so the baby will not breathe in amniotic fluid with is first breath.

As the head descends, the nurse may place her index finger inside the lower portion of the vagina and the thumb on the outer portion of the perineum and gently massage the tissues to aid in stretching of perineal tissues. This is called "ironing the perineum."

With one hand, the nurse applies gentle pressure against the fetal head to prevent it from popping out rapidly. *She does not hold the head back forcibly.* Rapid delivery of the head may result in tears in the mother's perineal tissues; in the fetus the rapid change in pressure within the fetal head may cause subdural or dural tears. The nurse supports the perineum and allows the head to be delivered between contractions.

As the mother continues to pant with contractions, the nurse inserts one or two fingers along the back of the fetal head to check for the umbilical cord. If the cord is around the neck, the nurse bends her fingers like a fish hook, grasps the cord, and pulls it over the baby's head. It is important to check that the cord is not wrapped around more than one time. If the cord is tightly looped and cannot be slipped over the infant's head, two clamps are placed on the cord, the cord is cut between the clamps, and the cord is unwound.

Immediately after delivery of the head, the infant's hair and face are checked for meconium. The mouth, throat, and nasal passages are suctioned to prevent the baby from aspirating meconium during breathing. The nurse places one hand on each side of the head and exerts gentle downward pressure until the anterior shoulder passes under the symphysis pubis. At this time, gentle upward pressure facilitates delivery of the posterior shoulder. The nurse then instructs the mother to push gently so that the rest of the body can be delivered quickly.

The baby is held at the level of the uterus to facilitate blood flow through the umbilical cord. The nurse must be careful to avoid dropping the infant, as the combination of amniotic fluid and vernix makes the baby slippery. The nose and mouth of the infant are cleared immediately, using a bulb syringe. The nurse then dries the baby to prevent heat loss.

As soon as the nurse determines that the infant's respirations are adequate, he can be placed on his mother's abdomen. The weight of the infant on her abdomen stimulates uterine contractions, which aids in placental separation. The umbilical cord should not be pulled.

The nurse is alert for signs of placental separation (slight gush of dark blood from the vagina, lengthening of the cord, or a change in uterine shape from discoid to globular). When these signs are present, the mother is instructed to push so that the placenta can be delivered. The nurse inspects the placenta to determine whether it is intact.

The umbilical cord may now be cut. Two sterile clamps are placed approximately 4–6 in. from the baby's abdomen. The cord is cut between them with sterile scissors. A sterile cord clamp (Hollister or Hesseltine) can be placed adjacent to the clamp on the baby's cord, between the clamp and the infant's abdomen. The clamp *must not* be placed snugly against the baby's abdomen, because the cord will dry and shrink.

The nurse checks the firmness of the uterus. The fundus may be gently massaged to stimulate contractions and to decrease bleeding. Putting the baby to breast also stimulates uterine contractions through release of oxytocin from the pituitary gland.

The area under the mother's buttocks is cleaned, and the perineum is inspected for lacerations. Bleeding from lacerations may be controlled by pressing a clean perineal pad against the perineum and instructing the mother to keep her thighs together.

Record-keeping

The following information is included in the patient's chart:

1. Position of fetus.
2. Presence of cord around neck or shoulder.
3. Time of delivery.
4. Apgar scores at one and five minutes after birth.
5. Sex of infant.
6. Time of delivery of placenta.
7. Method of placental expulsion.
8. Appearance and intactness of placenta.
9. Mother's condition.
10. Any medications that were given to mother or newborn.

Postdelivery Interventions

If the physician arrives soon after delivery, the nurse assists him or her in the examination of the mother, infant, and placenta. Other nursing interventions directed toward the infant include the following:

1. Keep the airway clear.
2. Maintain warmth.
3. Note and record a meconium stool or voiding.
4. Inspect the cord for the number of vessels and record this information.
5. Instill erythromycin (Ilotycin) or another ap-

propriate prophylactic agent into the infant's eyes.

6. Place an identification bracelet on the infant's wrist or ankle.
7. Transfer the infant to the nursery.

If the infant is premature, a careful evaluation of his respiratory status should also be made. (See Chapter 17 for more complete assessment of the newborn following delivery.)

Nursing interventions directed toward the mother are as follows:

1. Monitor vital signs every 5–15 minutes.
2. Assess firmness and position of uterus.
3. Evaluate amount of lochia and presence of clots.
4. Assess bladder fullness (a distended bladder can exert pressure on the uterus and increase the amount of bleeding).
5. Ensure her warmth.

Additional interventions include those that will enhance maternal-infant bonding, which are as follows:

1. Encourge the mother to look at and touch her baby.
2. Praise the mother for her accomplishments during labor and delivery.
3. If the mother desires, assist her in assuming a position of comfort to breast-feed the infant.

The nurse should include the father in the bonding process. If he was present at the delivery, he should be praised for any support that he offered. If the father was not present, he is permitted to be with the mother and baby as soon as possible after the birth. He should be encouraged to hold and touch the baby.

If the physician's arrival is delayed or if the infant is having respiratory distress, the infant should be transported immediately to the nursery. *Be sure the infant is properly identified before he leaves the delivery area.*

Delivery of Infant in Breech Presentation

A significant factor in a breech delivery is that the smallest part of the fetus presents first; succeeding parts are progressively larger. The cervix is not as effectively dilated when the fetus is in breech presentation as when it is in the vertex position. Therefore, descent is usually slow and may not occur until the cervix is fully dilated and the membranes rupture.

The emergency delivery of an infant in breech position is conducted similarly to that of an infant in vertex presentation. However, when the breech crowns, the nurse instructs the mother to pant so that the part is delivered between contractions. The nurse supports the breech in her hands. The infant's body is lifted slightly upward for delivery of the posterior shoulder and arm. The baby may then be lowered, and the anterior shoulder and arm will pass under the symphysis.

Flexion of the head occurs as with other presentations. It is important to maintain the flexion. The nape of the neck pivots under the symphysis, and the rest of the head is borne over the perineum by a movement of flexion.

The remaining delivery and postdelivery interventions are described in the above section on emergency delivery of an infant in vertex presentation.

Out-of-Hospital Births

Every woman who is in labor should be transported to a care facility as soon as possible. However, this is not always possible. Emergency deliveries may be necessary in various locations, such as in cars, ambulances, airplanes, and ships; out of doors; and at shelters during natural disasters such as earthquakes and floods. Home delivery is considered an emergency only if it is unexpected and unplanned.

If a hospital or birth center is not accessible and birth is imminent, the following are important considerations:

1. Privacy for the delivering mother (or couple).
2. A clean place to deliver.
3. Protection from infection.
4. Safeguard against hemorrhage.

Nursing Management of the Mother

The woman who is laboring under such unusual circumstances will need a great deal of psychologic support. The beautiful experience that she had planned is now impossible, and she may react with hostility, bitterness, and resentment. In addition, she may be extremely frightened and alarmed by the lack of equipment and skilled personnel. An attitude of calm and confidence helps both the nurse and the mother.

The nurse must communicate to the mother that her needs are understood. In addition, the nurse must let the mother know that she is willing to work with the mother (and the mother's support persons) to provide the best experience under the circumstances.

Do not separate the woman from her partner or other persons whom the woman chooses to be present. However, the expectant mother should be screened from curious strangers. The less exposure the mother and newborn have to strangers, the less chance they have of contracting infections. If the woman is inside a shelter, folding chairs or carts draped with blankets or coats make an efficient screen, as do sleeping bags tied to low-hanging branches of trees if one is outdoors. A private room is desirable if available. Women in labor take precedence over any other individual or group when it comes to the use of space and transportation.

A clean surface should be provided for the woman. Unread newspapers, clean towels, blankets, garment bags turned inside out, the inside of a coat, or even a shirt or pair of slacks turned inside out can be placed under the mother's hips to cover a floor, a carpet, or the ground.

If the room or car temperature can be regulated, a warm environment 26.7-28.9C (80-84F) degrees is preferred. Two roaring fires, one on each side of the mother, provide warmth if the delivery is outside.

If one is attending a birth in a shelter, one should obtain the following supplies if possible:

- Bulb syringe.
- Cord clamp.
- Scissors.
- Basin.
- Four bath blankets.
- Four sheets.
- Four towels.
- Two pillows.
- Two baby shirts.
- A dozen diapers (cloth or disposable).
- Ophthalmic silver nitrate solution (to instill in eyes).
- Sterile water and eyedropper to rinse eyes.
- Two dozen peripads.
- A sanitary belt.

The delivery can proceed as described for an in-hospital emergency birth (p. 641). Substitution may need to be made in equipment. Cord ties or new shoestrings may be used to tie the umbilical cord. A clean soft cloth may be used to wipe off the baby's face and the inside of his mouth. A new razor or scissors (clean or boiled) may be used to cut the cord. If necessary, the cord may be left intact and the placenta may be wrapped in a blanket with the baby. Care must be taken to keep the baby and placenta close together so that no unnecessary traction is put on the umbilical cord.

Nursing Management of the Newborn

The care of the newborn under these circumstances is directed toward the same considerations as those born in a hospital or maternity center: protection from overstimulation, infection, and heat loss; adequate resuscitation; and facilitation of parent-infant bonding.

Protection from Overstimulation and Infection

Loud music, spotlights, and large numbers of extraneous personnel are usually not in evidence in hospitals, and they are contraindicated during any birth. Overstimulation can occur in the presence of a great deal of noise and activity. The chances of infection are increased by the number of people the newborn is exposed to.

At sites designated as shelters during natural disasters, such as schools or church basements, these forms of overstimulation are very much in evidence. Under these circumstances, the nurse attempts to provide to the mother in labor a quiet, screened, and restricted area that has some soundproofing and indirect lighting. If this is not possible, the nurse should request that the noise level be lowered. If spotlights or lanterns are used, the newborn's eyes must be shielded, or the light should be adjusted so that it does not shine directly into his eyes. The number of people in the immediate area should be restricted to care givers, the woman's family, and other support persons chosen by the mother.

Protection from Heat Loss

Protecting the newborn from heat loss without a radiant warmer is a challenge to the nurse attending the family under emergency conditions. Any of several methods may be available. If the environment is unheated, that is, below 27.8C (82F), the nurse dries the infant thoroughly, especially the hair. She instructs the mother to roll onto her side (even if the placenta has not separated) and places the baby on its side against the mother, skin-to-skin, so they face each other. The mother and infant are then wrapped up together or covered by one of the following methods:

1. Wrap the pair with unused plastic food wrap. Do not cover the baby's face.

2. Wrap them with a garment bag turned inside out. The baby should be wrapped as if in a blanket, but his face must not be covered. If the temperature is very low, a cap should be fashioned for the infant and taped or tied in place, because the majority of the newborn's heat loss is from the head.

3. Place layers of unread newspapers over the mother and baby. The nurse must ensure that the infant's feet are well covered and that there are no gaps in the paper where the heat can be lost. It is better to provide too many newspapers than too few.

4. Drape the mother and baby with clothing and cover with blankets, coats, and so on.

When the mother and baby are wrapped together, the nurse need not disturb the ambient environment to check the temperature. The mother can check the baby's body temperature by feeling his stomach with the back of her fingers.

Even if the environment is warmer than 27.8C (82°F), it is necessary to dry the infant thoroughly and to protect him from heat loss. Wrapping the baby up with the mother in a blanket, coat, or other materials is recommended.

Ensuring Adequate Resuscitation

During an emergency situation outside of the hospital, resuscitation equipment may not be available. If the infant is mildly depressed, institute the following measures:

1. Position the infant on his side, with his head slightly lower than the trunk. This position facilitates drainage of mucus by gravity.

2. Wipe mucus from the infant's face and mouth with a soft rag or your finger.

3. Keep the infant dry and warm to avoid cold stress.

4. *Do not* hold the baby by the ankles and slap his buttocks because these actions cause excessive stimulation of the newborn. *Do* rub the infant's back and stimulate the bottom of his feet by stroking with your fingers.

5. If these measures are not effective and there is no respiratory effort, give mouth-to-mouth resuscitation.

6. Evaluate for the presence of a heartbeat by placing fingers over the sternum. If a heartbeat is absent, initiate cardiopulmonary massage.

Facilitation of Parent-Infant Bonding

The mother and infant are encouraged to get to know each other. The nurse can point out the newborn's behavior and how the mother can deal with this behavior. For example, if the newborn is looking at the mother's face, the nurse can encourage the mother to make eye-to-eye contact and to smile at the infant. When the baby puts its fist or fingers in its mouth, the mother can offer to breast-feed. When the infant no longer wants to nurse and shows signs of sleepiness, the mother can stroke him gently, hum or sing to him, and rock him to sleep. This give-and-take behavior helps alleviate much of the mother's fear that her delivery under these unusual circumstances has adversely affected her ability to mother the baby.

SUMMARY

Expectant parents are requesting and in some instances demanding alternative birthing methods. Many hospitals are now providing alternative birthing experiences through birthing rooms and inclusion of Leboyer methods when requested. The obstetric nurse needs to be informed of alternative birthing methods, their advantages and disadvantages. The role of assessment and teaching takes on an even more important aspect as contact with the patient may be possible only over a short period of time.

Emergency childbirth challenges the nurse's ability to organize, improvise, teach, and provide emotional support for the family. Providing and ensuring a safe, clean environment for the mother and infant is of extreme importance. Facilitating the bonding process is possible even in emergency situations.

SUGGESTED ACTIVITIES

1. Interview parents who have participated in a conventional delivery, birthing room, and home delivery. Compare their prenatal education and birth experience.
2. In the classroom laboratory, use a teaching model to practice delivering an infant in a vertex presentation. Practice delivery of an infant in a breech presentation.
3. Make a list of equipment that would be needed in an emergency delivery pack.
4. Plan prenatal classes for parents who are planning a traditional delivery and parents who are planning a home birth. How will the classes be similar? How will they be different?

REFERENCES

Leboyer, F. 1976. *Birth without violence.* New York: Alfred A. Knopf, Inc.

ADDITIONAL READINGS

Arms, S. 1975. *Immaculate deception.* Boston: Houghton Mifflin Co.

Brazelton, T. B. 1969. *Infants and mothers: differences in development.* New York: Delacorte Press.

Davis, A. 1959. *Let's have healthy children.* New York: Harcourt Brace Jovanovich.

Enlien, M. Fall–Winter 1975–1976. The family in labour. *Birth Fam. J.* 2:133.

Haire, D. 1972. *The cultural warping of childbirth.* Seattle: International Childbirth Education Association.

Klaus, M., and Kennell, J. H. 1972. Maternal attachment: importance of the first postpartum days. *N. Engl. J. Med.* 256:460.

Klaus, M. H., and Kennell, J. H. 1976. *Maternal-infant bonding: the impact of early separation or loss on family development.* St. Louis: The C. V. Mosby Co.

Klaus, M., et al. 1970. Human maternal behavior at the first contact with her young. *Pediatrics.* 46:187.

Lange, R. 1972. *The birth book.* Ben Lomond, Calif.: Genesis Press.

Lewis, M., and Rosenblum, L. A., eds. 1974. *The effect of the infant on its caregiver.* New York: John Wiley & Sons, Inc.

May, I. M. 1978. *Spiritual midwifery.* Summertown, Tenn.: The Book Publishing Company. Printed on the Farm.

Myles, M. 1975. *Textbook for midwives.* Baltimore: The Williams & Wilkins Co.

Ritche, C. A. 1976. Childbirth outside the hospital—the resurgence of home and clinic deliveries. *MCN.* 1:372.

White, G. 1968. *Emergency childbirth: a manual.* Franklin Park, Ill.: Police Training Foundation.

UNIT V

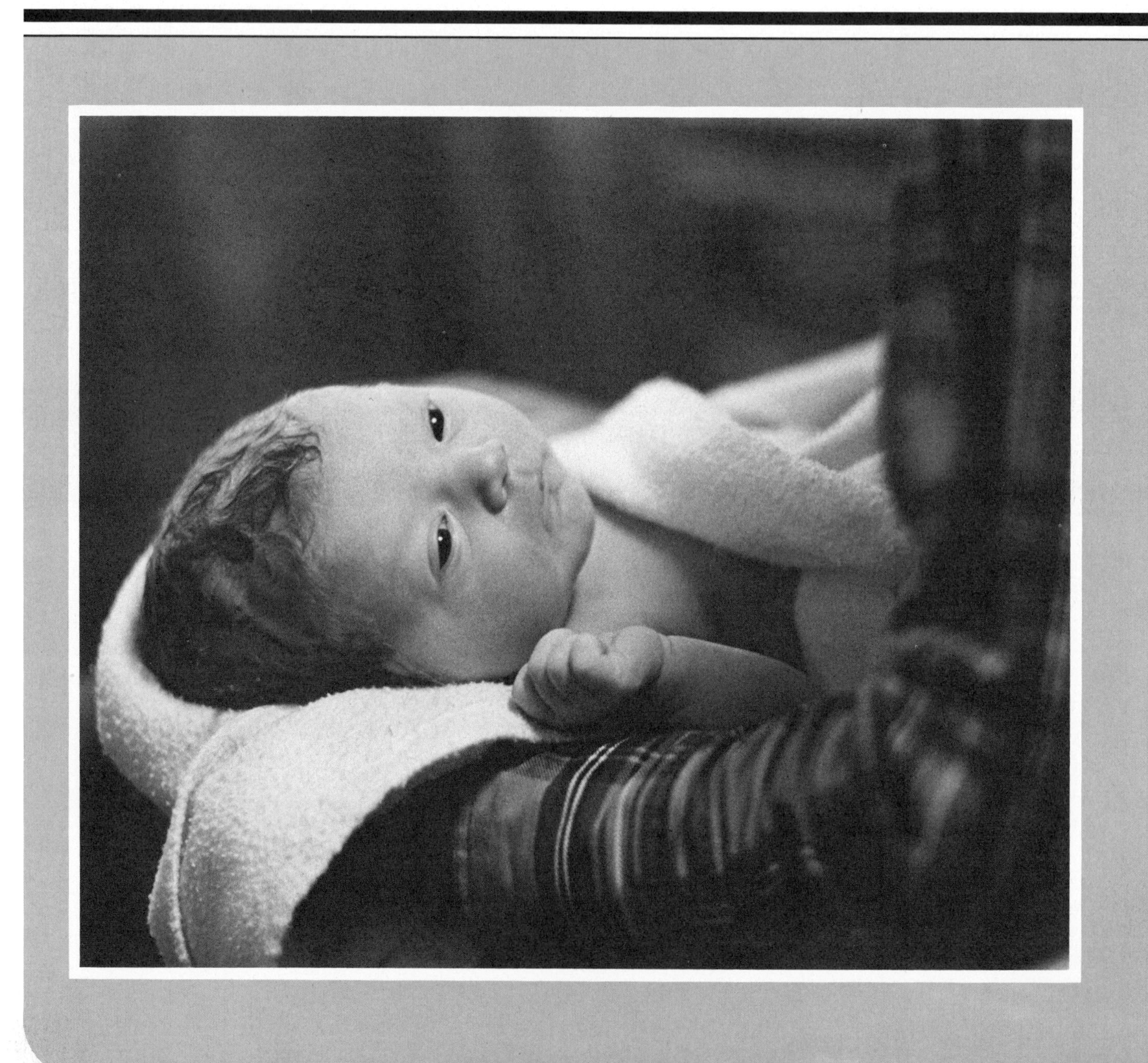

THE NEONATE

CHAPTER 22

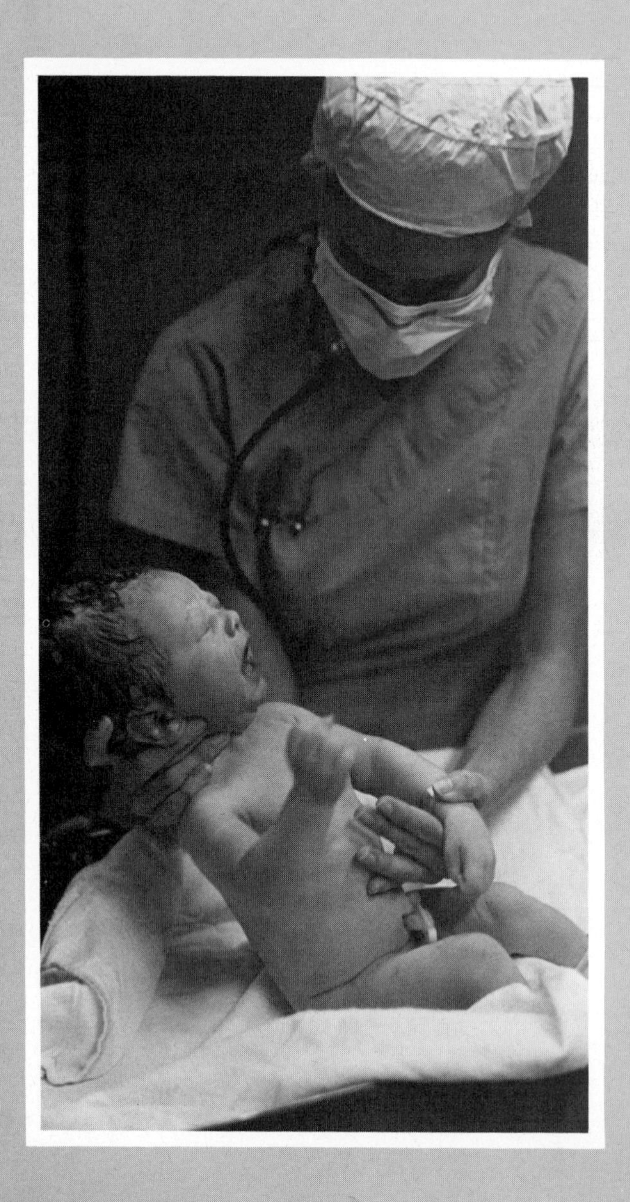

NURSING ASSESSMENT OF THE NEWBORN

OBJECTIVES

- Describe the normal physical characteristics of the newborn.
- Identify the various methods of determining gestational age.
- Describe the neurologic characteristics of the newborn and the reflexes that may be present at birth.
- Describe the components of the neonatal behavioral assessment.

The nurse is the only member of the health team who is a 24-hour observer of the infant. In many hospitals there is no full-time medical staff to provide constant medical care to the newborn. Because the pediatrician is present in the nursery for only a brief period of time, signs and symptoms of disease or injury of the newborn usually appear when the pediatrician is absent. Unlike the verbalizing adult patient, the neonate communicates his needs primarily by his behavior. The nurse, through objective observations and evaluations, must be able to interpret this behavior into information about the infant's condition and to respond with appropriate nursing interventions. This chapter focuses on the assessment of the neonate and on interpretations of the findings.

Assessment of the newborn is a continuous process designed to evaluate his development and adjustments to extrauterine life. In the delivery room, the Apgar scoring procedure and careful observation of the neonate form the basis of assessment and are correlated with information such as the duration of labor, maternal analgesia and anesthesia, and any complications of labor or delivery that have occurred.

Although an initial assessment of the newborn is done in the delivery room, the first thorough examination occurs in the nursery within 24 hours after delivery. A nursing information profile, such as the one shown in Figure 22-1, assimilates the information forming the data base:

- Maternal history.
- Features of labor and delivery.
- Apgar score.
- Treatment instituted in the delivery room, in conjunction with determination of clinical gestational age.
- Consideration of the infant's mortality risk, based on the classification of newborns by their weight and gestational age and by neonatal mortality risk.
- Physical examination of the newborn.

When data from these various sources are incorporated with the findings of the assessment of the newborn in the nursery, a plan for nursing intervention is formulated.

The first 24 hours of life are significant because this is the critical period of transition from intrauterine to extrauterine life. Statistically, the risk of mortality and morbidity is high within this period. Nurses must establish the infant's gestational age and status on admission to the nursery so that careful attention can be given to problems associated with gestational age.

ESTIMATION OF GESTATIONAL AGE

Traditionally, the gestational age of an infant was determined on the basis of the dates that the mother gave her physician as to when she last menstruated. This method was accurate only 75% to 85% of the time. Because of the problems that develop with the infant who is premature or whose weight is inappropriate for his gestational age, a more accurate system was developed to evaluate each infant. Once learned, these observations can be made in a few minutes. Every neonatal nurse should be familiar with the methods for evaluating gestational age.

The clinical approach to the estimation of gestational age has two components: the neurologic evaluation and the evaluation of physical characteristics. The neurologic evaluation is most effectively used after the first 24 hours of life. During the first 24 hours, the nervous system of the newborn is unstable as he adjusts to extrauterine life; thus findings from the neurologic assessment are of limited accuracy during this period. Physical characteristics include such features as sole creases, amount of breast tissue, nature of the hair, cartilaginous development of the ear, testicular descent, and scrotal rugae or labial development. These objective clinical criteria are not altered in the first 24 hours of life.

Three forms are frequently used by nurses in assessing the gestational age of infants. Figure 22-2,*A* lists the physical features assessed immediately on admission to the nursery. The neurologic criteria that are evaluated after the infant has stabilized are shown in Figure 22-2,*B*. Figure 22-3 illustrates Dubowitz and Dubowitz's (1977) alternate scoring method for determining gestational age, which may be used independently or in conjunction with other criteria.

Name: ______

Nursing admission: ______ (Time and date) Duration of labor: ______

Complications

Pregnancy: ______

Labor and/or delivery: ______

PHYSICAL EXAMINATION

General Condition

Color ______
Cry ______
Activity ______
Anomalies ______
Resting ______
Recoil ______

Head and neck

Head circumference ______ cm
Hair ______
Scalp and skull ______
Fontanelles ______
Sutures ______
Eyes ______
Ears ______
Nose ______
Mouth ______
Neck ______ cm

Thorax conformation

Chest circumference ______ cm
Respirations ______

Abdomen conformation ______

Umbilical cord ______ Vessels: ______

Genitals ______
Rectum ______
Extremities ______

Upper ______
Lower ______
Sole creases ______

Vernix ______
Skin ______
Length ______ cm
Breasts ______
Clavicles ______
Heart ______
Lungs ______

Newborn classification

Gestational age (GA) ______
Birth weight (BW) ______

Neonatal Mortality Risk (NMR) ______

Nursing Evaluation:

Signature ______

Figure 22–1. Nursing information profile.

Examination First Hours

CLINICAL ESTIMATION OF GESTATIONAL AGE

An Approximation Based on Published Data*

PHYSICAL FINDINGS		WEEKS GESTATION	
VERNIX		20–23	APPEARS
		24–37	COVERS BODY, THICK LAYER
		38–39	ON BACK, SCALP, IN CREASES
		40–41	SCANT, IN CREASES
		42–48	NO VERNIX
BREAST TISSUE AND AREOLA		20–33	AREOLA & NIPPLE BARELY VISIBLE NO PALPABLE BREAST TISSUE
		34–35	AREOLA RAISED
		36–37	1-2 MM NODULE
		38	3-5 MM
		39	5-6 MM
		40–43	7-10 MM
		44–48	?12 MM
EAR	FORM	20–33	FLAT, SHAPELESS
		34–35	BEGINNING INCURVING SUPERIOR
		36–38	INCURVING UPPER 2/3 PINNAE
		39–48	WELL-DEFINED INCURVING TO LOBE
	CARTILAGE	20–31	PINNA SOFT, STAYS FOLDED
		32–35	CARTILAGE SCANT RETURNS SLOWLY FROM FOLDING
		36–39	THIN CARTILAGE SPRINGS BACK FROM FOLDING
		40–48	PINNA FIRM, REMAINS ERECT FROM HEAD
SOLE CREASES		20–31	SMOOTH SOLES $\bar{s}$ CREASES
		32–34	1-2 ANTERIOR CREASES
		35	2-3 ANTERIOR CREASES
		36–37	CREASES ANTERIOR 2/3 SOLE
		38–41	CREASES INVOLVING HEEL
		42–48	DEEPER CREASES OVER ENTIRE SOLE
SKIN	THICKNESS & APPEARANCE	20–31	THIN, TRANSLUCENT SKIN, PLETHORIC, VENULES OVER ABDOMEN EDEMA
		32–35	SMOOTH THICKER NO EDEMA
		36–37	PINK
		38–39	FEW VESSELS
		40–41	SOME DESQUAMATION PALE PINK
		42–48	THICK, PALE, DESQUAMATION OVER ENTIRE BODY
	NAIL PLATES	20	APPEAR
		32–41	NAILS TO FINGER TIPS
		42–48	NAILS EXTEND WELL BEYOND FINGER TIPS
HAIR		20–22	APPEARS ON HEAD
		23–27	EYE BROWS & LASHES
		28–36	FINE, WOOLLY, BUNCHES OUT FROM HEAD
		37–41	SILKY, SINGLE STRANDS LAYS FLAT
		42–48	?RECEDING HAIRLINE OR LOSS OF BABY HAIR SHORT, FINE UNDERNEATH
LANUGO		20	APPEARS
		21–32	COVERS ENTIRE BODY
		33–37	VANISHES FROM FACE
		38–41	PRESENT ON SHOULDERS
		42–48	NO LANUGO
GENITALIA	TESTES	28–35	TESTES PALPABLE IN INGUINAL CANAL
		36–39	IN UPPER SCROTUM
		40–48	IN LOWER SCROTUM
	SCROTUM	28–35	FEW RUGAE
		36–39	RUGAE, ANTERIOR PORTION
		40–41	RUGAE COVER
		42–48	PENDULOUS
	LABIA & CLITORIS	30–35	PROMINENT CLITORIS LABIA MAJORA SMALL WIDELY SEPARATED
		36–39	LABIA MAJORA LARGER NEARLY COVERED CLITORIS
		40–48	LABIA MINORA & CLITORIS COVERED
SKULL FIRMNESS		20–27	BONES ARE SOFT
		28–34	SOFT TO 1" FROM ANTERIOR FONTANELLE
		35–37	SPONGY AT EDGES OF FONTANELLE CENTER FIRM
		38–41	BONES HARD SUTURES EASILY DISPLACED
		42–48	BONES HARD, CANNOT BE DISPLACED
POSTURE	RESTING	20–25	HYPOTONIC LATERAL DECUBITUS
		26–29	HYPOTONIC
		30–31	BEGINNING FLEXION THIGH
		32–33	STRONGER HIP FLEXION
		34–35	FROG-LIKE
		36–37	FLEXION ALL LIMBS
		38–41	HYPERTONIC
		42–48	VERY HYPERTONIC
	RECOIL - LEG	20–31	NO RECOIL
		32–37	PARTIAL RECOIL
		38–48	PROMPT RECOIL
	ARM	20–33	NO RECOIL
		34–35	BEGIN FLEXION NO RECOIL
		36–39	PROMPT RECOIL MAY BE INHIBITED
		40–48	PROMPT RECOIL AFTER 30" INHIBITION

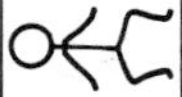

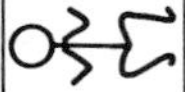

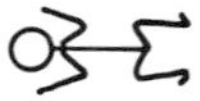

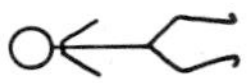

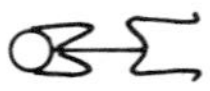

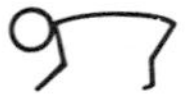

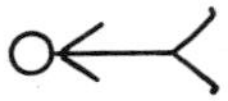

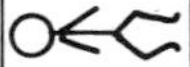

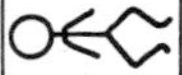

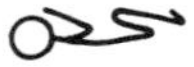

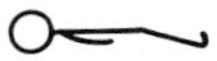

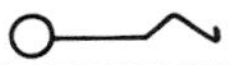

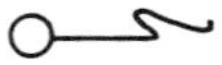

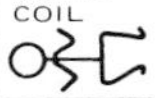

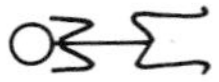

A

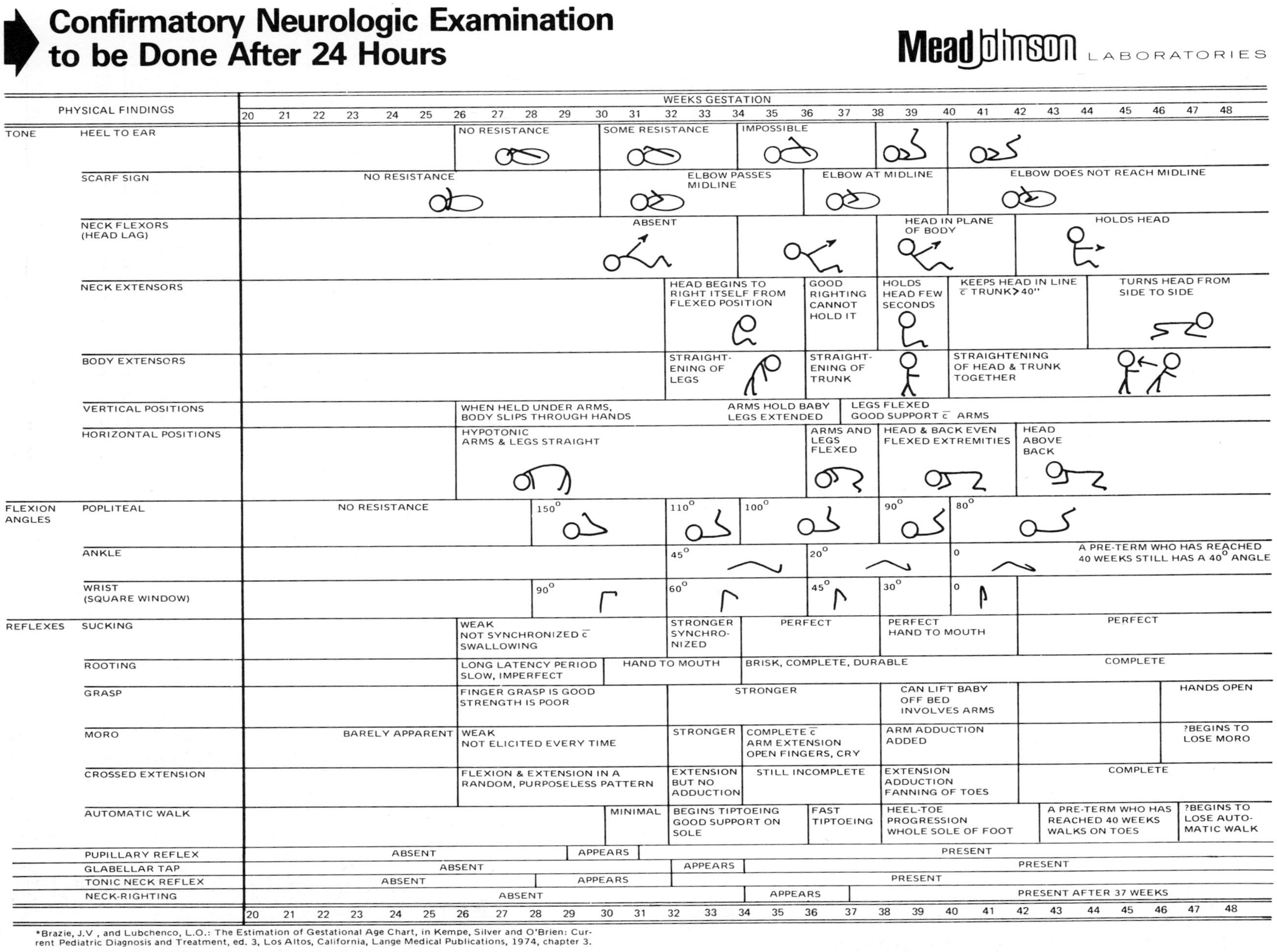

Confirmatory Neurologic Examination to be Done After 24 Hours

Mead Johnson LABORATORIES

	PHYSICAL FINDINGS	WEEKS GESTATION (20 21 22 23 24 25 26 27 28 29 30 31 32 33 34 35 36 37 38 39 40 41 42 43 44 45 46 47 48)
TONE	HEEL TO EAR	NO RESISTANCE | SOME RESISTANCE | IMPOSSIBLE
	SCARF SIGN	NO RESISTANCE | ELBOW PASSES MIDLINE | ELBOW AT MIDLINE | ELBOW DOES NOT REACH MIDLINE
	NECK FLEXORS (HEAD LAG)	ABSENT | HEAD IN PLANE OF BODY | HOLDS HEAD
	NECK EXTENSORS	HEAD BEGINS TO RIGHT ITSELF FROM FLEXED POSITION | GOOD RIGHTING CANNOT HOLD IT | HOLDS HEAD FEW SECONDS | KEEPS HEAD IN LINE c̄ TRUNK>40° | TURNS HEAD FROM SIDE TO SIDE
	BODY EXTENSORS	STRAIGHTENING OF LEGS | STRAIGHTENING OF TRUNK | STRAIGHTENING OF HEAD & TRUNK TOGETHER
	VERTICAL POSITIONS	WHEN HELD UNDER ARMS, BODY SLIPS THROUGH HANDS | ARMS HOLD BABY LEGS EXTENDED | LEGS FLEXED GOOD SUPPORT c̄ ARMS
	HORIZONTAL POSITIONS	HYPOTONIC ARMS & LEGS STRAIGHT | ARMS AND LEGS FLEXED | HEAD & BACK EVEN FLEXED EXTREMITIES | HEAD ABOVE BACK
FLEXION ANGLES	POPLITEAL	NO RESISTANCE | 150° | 110° | 100° | 90° | 80°
	ANKLE	45° | 20° | 0 | A PRE-TERM WHO HAS REACHED 40 WEEKS STILL HAS A 40° ANGLE
	WRIST (SQUARE WINDOW)	90° | 60° | 45° | 30° | 0
REFLEXES	SUCKING	WEAK NOT SYNCHRONIZED c̄ SWALLOWING | STRONGER SYNCHRONIZED | PERFECT | PERFECT HAND TO MOUTH | PERFECT
	ROOTING	LONG LATENCY PERIOD SLOW, IMPERFECT | HAND TO MOUTH | BRISK, COMPLETE, DURABLE | COMPLETE
	GRASP	FINGER GRASP IS GOOD STRENGTH IS POOR | STRONGER | CAN LIFT BABY OFF BED INVOLVES ARMS | HANDS OPEN
	MORO	BARELY APPARENT | WEAK NOT ELICITED EVERY TIME | STRONGER | COMPLETE c̄ ARM EXTENSION OPEN FINGERS, CRY | ARM ADDUCTION ADDED | ?BEGINS TO LOSE MORO
	CROSSED EXTENSION	FLEXION & EXTENSION IN A RANDOM, PURPOSELESS PATTERN | EXTENSION BUT NO ADDUCTION | STILL INCOMPLETE | EXTENSION ADDUCTION FANNING OF TOES | COMPLETE
	AUTOMATIC WALK	MINIMAL | BEGINS TIPTOEING GOOD SUPPORT ON SOLE | FAST TIPTOEING | HEEL-TOE PROGRESSION WHOLE SOLE OF FOOT | A PRE-TERM WHO HAS REACHED 40 WEEKS WALKS ON TOES | ?BEGINS TO LOSE AUTOMATIC WALK
	PUPILLARY REFLEX	ABSENT | APPEARS | PRESENT
	GLABELLAR TAP	ABSENT | APPEARS | PRESENT
	TONIC NECK REFLEX	ABSENT | APPEARS | PRESENT
	NECK-RIGHTING	ABSENT | APPEARS | PRESENT AFTER 37 WEEKS

B

*Brazie, J.V., and Lubchenco, L.O.: The Estimation of Gestational Age Chart, in Kempe, Silver and O'Brien: Current Pediatric Diagnosis and Treatment, ed. 3, Los Altos, California, Lange Medical Publications, 1974, chapter 3.

Figure 22–2. Clinical estimation of gestational age. **A,** Physical examination. **B,** Neurologic examination. (Courtesy Mead Johnson Laboratories, Evansville, Ind.)

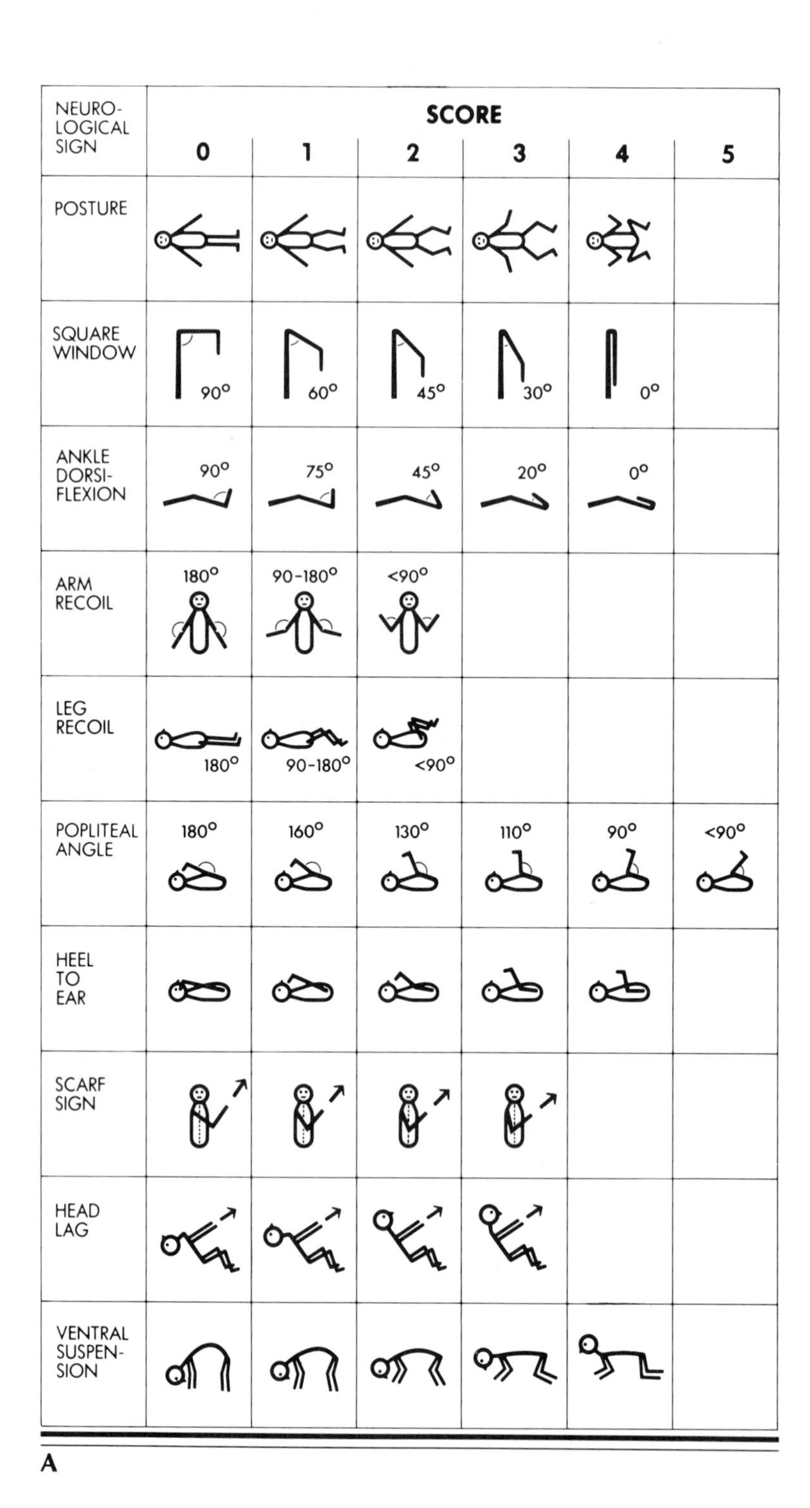

Assessment of Physical Characteristics

Physical characteristics can be assessed according to the Clinical Estimation of Gestational Age chart. When observations are recorded on the chart, a pattern indicating gestational age quickly becomes apparent (Figure 22-4). To accurately assess the neonate, one first evaluates the characteristics that can be observed without disturbing the infant and then evaluates those that may disturb him. The physical characteristics are presented here in the order in which they might be evaluated most effectively:

1. *Resting posture* is observed as the infant lies undisturbed on a flat surface (Figure 22-5).

EXTERNAL SIGN	SCORE 0	1	2	3	4
OEDEMA	Obvious oedema hands and feet; pitting over tibia	No obvious oedema hands and feet; pitting over tibia	No oedema		
SKIN TEXTURE	Very thin, gelatinous	Thin and smooth	Smooth; medium thickness. Rash or superficial peeling	Slight thickening. Superficial cracking and peeling esp. hands and feet	Thick and parchment-like; superficial or deep cracking
SKIN COLOUR (Infant not crying)	Dark red	Uniformly pink	Pale pink: variable over body	Pale. Only pink over ears, lips, palms or soles	
SKIN OPACITY (trunk)	Numerous veins and venules clearly seen, especially over abdomen	Veins and tributaries seen	A few large vessels clearly seen over abdomen	A few large vessels seen indistinctly over abdomen	No blood vessels seen
LANUGO (over back)	No lanugo	Abundant; long and thick over whole back	Hair thinning especially over lower back	Small amount of lanugo and bald areas	At least half of back devoid of lanugo
PLANTAR CREASES	No skin creases	Faint red marks over anterior half of sole	Definite red marks over more than anterior half; indentations over less than anterior third	Indentations over more than anterior third	Definite deep indentations over more than anterior third
NIPPLE FORMATION	Nipple barely visible; no areola	Nipple well defined; areola smooth and flat diameter <0.75 cm.	Areola stippled, edge not raised; diameter <0.75 cm.	Areola stippled, edge raised diameter >0.75 cm.	
BREAST SIZE	No breast tissue palpable	Breast tissue on one or both sides < 0.5 cm. diameter	Breast tissue both sides; one or both 0.5–1.0 cm.	Breast tissue both sides; one or both > 1 cm.	
EAR FORM	Pinna flat and shapeless, little or no incurving of edge	Incurving of part of edge of pinna	Partial incurving whole of upper pinna	Well-defined incurving whole of upper pinna	
EAR FIRMNESS	Pinna soft, easily folded, no recoil	Pinna soft, easily folded, slow recoil	Cartilage to edge of pinna, but soft in places, ready recoil	Pinna firm, cartilage to edge, instant recoil	
GENITALIA MALE	Neither testis in scrotum	At least one testis high in scrotum	At least one testis right down		
FEMALES (With hips half abducted)	Labia majora widely separated, labia minora protruding	Labia majora almost cover labia minora	Labia majora completely cover labia minora		

B

Figure 22–3. Estimation of gestational age. **A,** Neurologic criteria. **B,** External (superficial) criteria. (From Dubowitz, L., and Dubowitz, V. 1977. *Gestational age of the newborn.* Menlo Park, Calif.: Addison-Wesley Publishing Co.)

2. *Vernix distribution* (and protection) decreases as term approaches. As a result, the preterm infant is covered with vernix, and the postterm infant has no vernix. After noting vernix distribution, the delivery room nurse dries the infant to prevent evaporative heat loss. Thus vernix distribution is disturbed by the time the infant enters the nursery. The delivery room nurse must communicate to the neonatal nurse the amount and areas of vernix coverage.

3. *Skin* appears transparent in the preterm infant and more opaque with increased deposition of subcutaneous tissue as term approaches. Disappearance of protective vernix promotes skin desquamation.

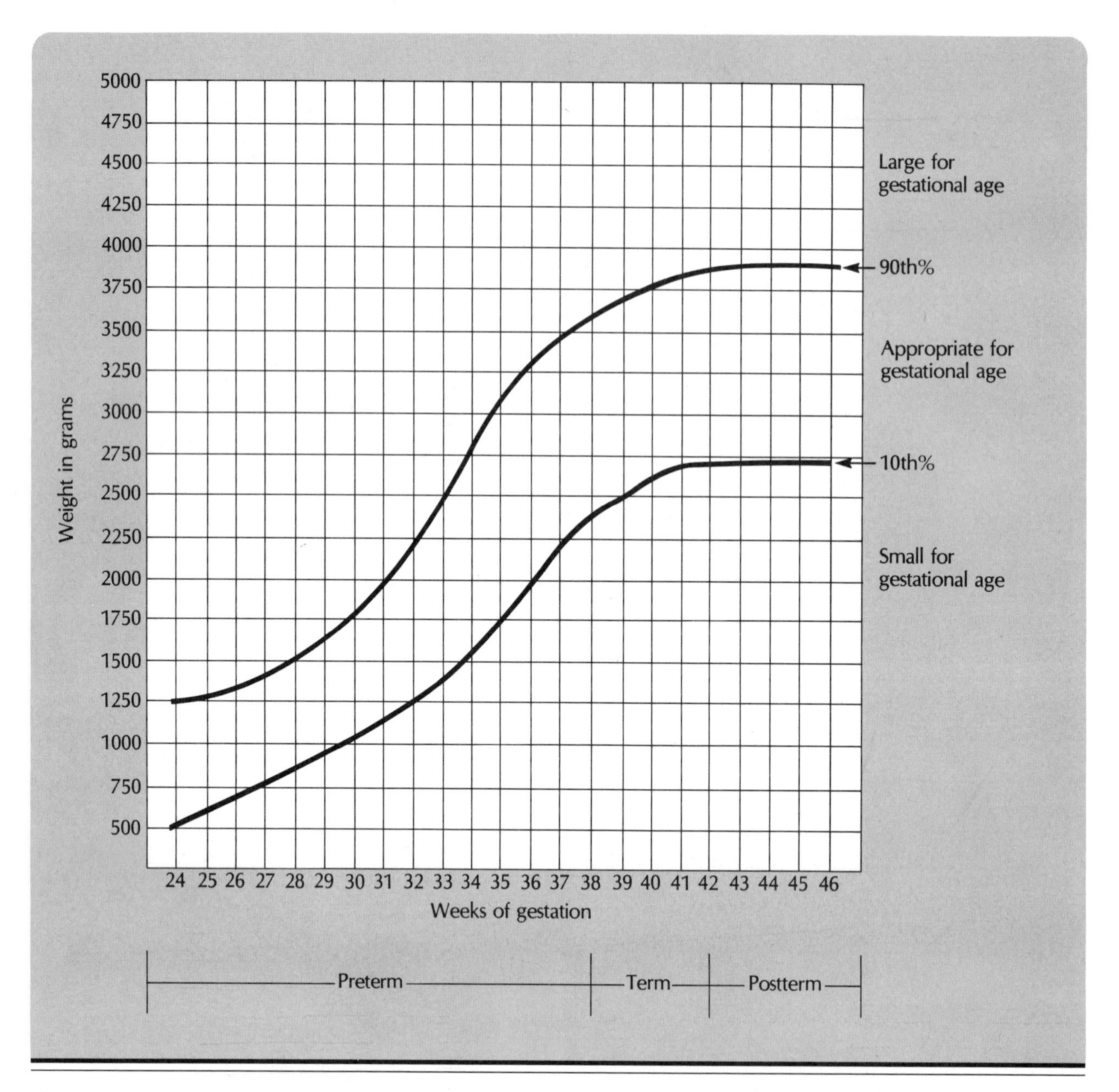

Figure 22–4. Classification of newborns by birth weight and gestational age and by neonatal mortality risk. The newborn's birth weight and gestational age are plotted on the graph. The newborn is then classified as large for gestational age, appropriate for gestational age, or small for gestational age. (From Battaglia, F. C., and Lubchenco, L. O. 1967. A practical classification of newborn infants by weight and gestational age. *J. Pediatr.* 71:161.)

4. *Nails* develop as the gestational age increases.

5. *Lanugo*, a fine hair covering, decreases as gestational age increases. *Hair* of the preterm infant has the consistency of matted wool or fur and lies in bunches rather than in the silky, single strands of the term infant's hair.

6. *Sole creases* are reliable indicators of gestational age in the first 12 hours of life. After this, the skin of the foot begins drying, and creases appear. Development of sole creases is systematic, beginning at the anterior portion of the foot and, as gestation progresses, proceeding to the heel (Figure 22–6).

7. *Skull firmness* increases as the infant matures.

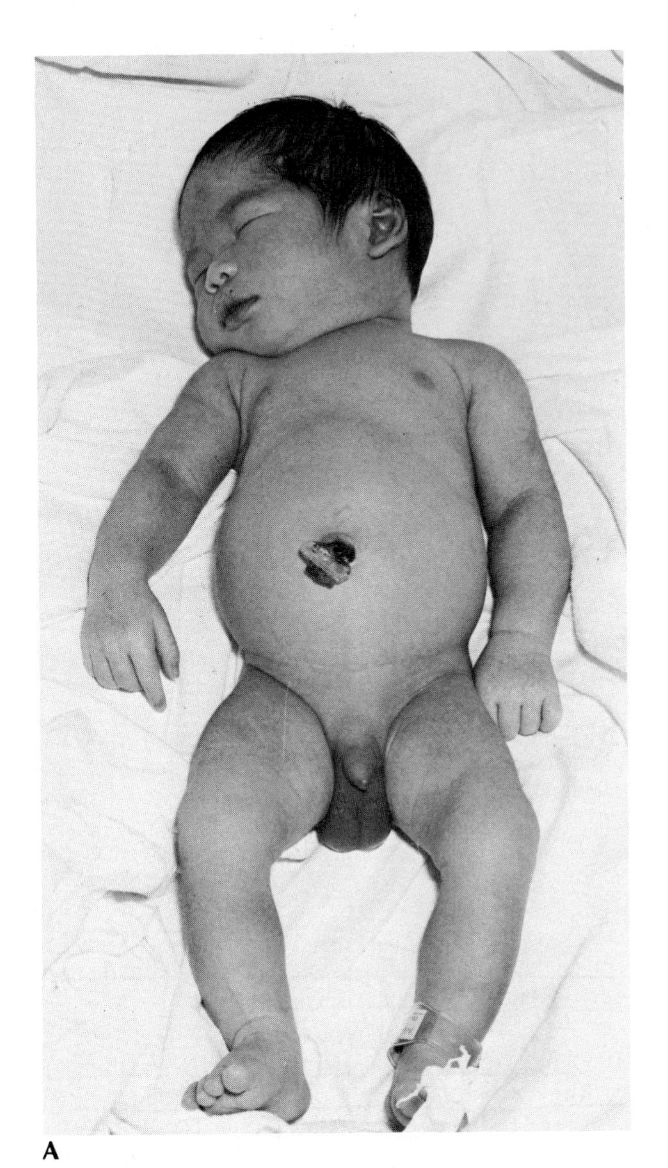

A

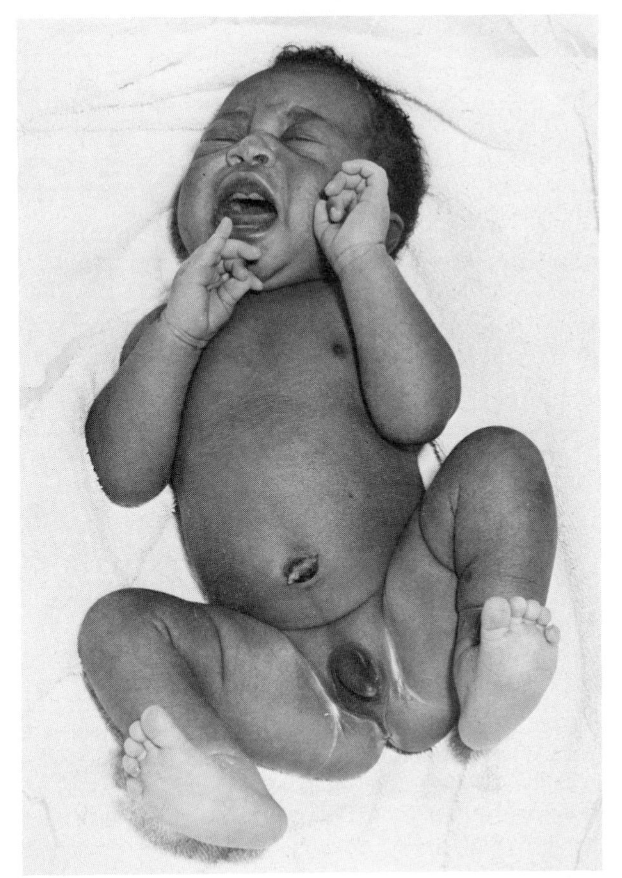

B

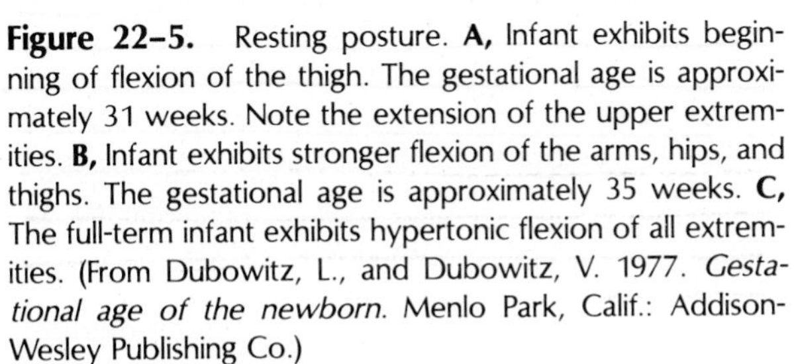

Figure 22–5. Resting posture. **A,** Infant exhibits beginning of flexion of the thigh. The gestational age is approximately 31 weeks. Note the extension of the upper extremities. **B,** Infant exhibits stronger flexion of the arms, hips, and thighs. The gestational age is approximately 35 weeks. **C,** The full-term infant exhibits hypertonic flexion of all extremities. (From Dubowitz, L., and Dubowitz, V. 1977. *Gestational age of the newborn.* Menlo Park, Calif.: Addison-Wesley Publishing Co.)

In a term infant the bones are hard, and the sutures are not easily displaced.

8. *Breast tissue and areola* are palpated by application of the forefinger and middle finger to the breast area. The nipple should not be grasped with thumb and forefinger, as skin and subcutaneous tissue will prevent accurate estimation of

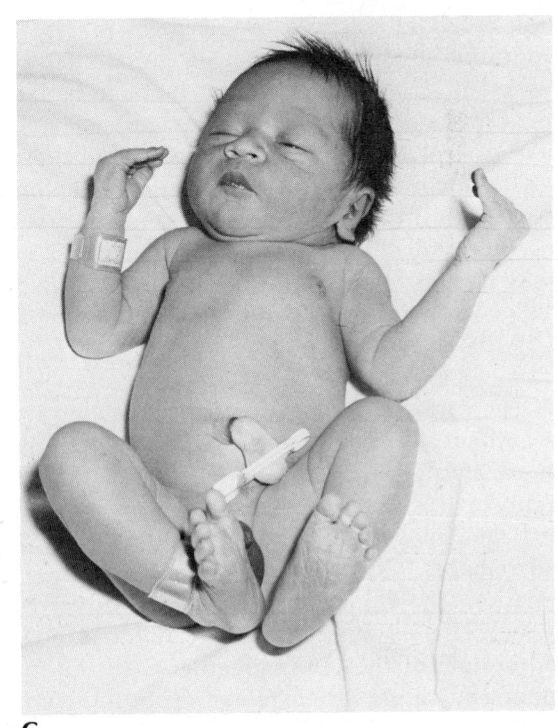

C

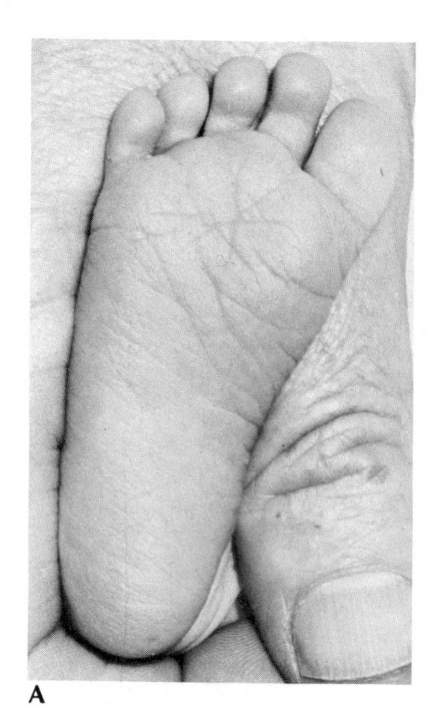
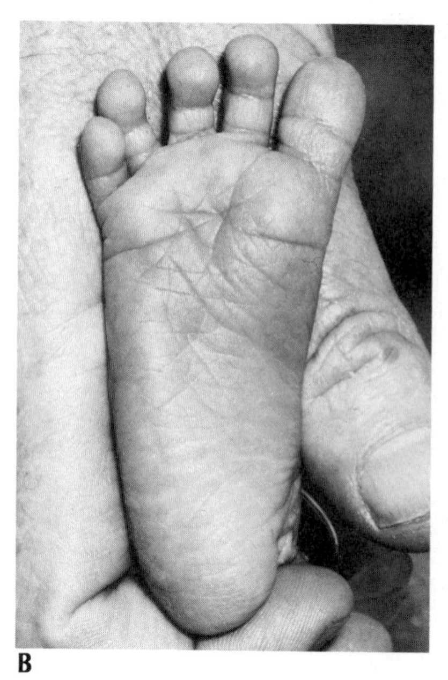
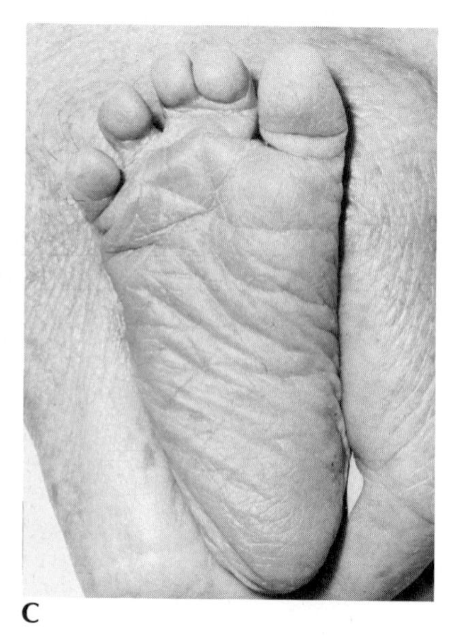

Figure 22–6. Sole creases. **A,** Infant has a few sole creases on the anterior portion of the foot. Note the slick heel. The gestation age is approximately 35 weeks. **B,** Infant has a deeper network of sole creases on the anterior two-thirds of the sole. Note the slick heel. The gestational age is approximately 37 weeks, **C,** The full-term infant has deep sole creases down to and including the heel. (From Dubowitz, L., and Dubowitz, V. 1977. *Gestational age of the newborn.* Menlo Park, Calif.: Addison-Wesley Publishing Co.)

size. As gestation progresses, the breast tissue mass and areola enlarge (Figure 22–7). However, a large breast tissue mass can occur as a result of conditions other than advanced gestational age. The infant of a diabetic mother tends to be large for gestational age, and the premature development of breast tissue is a reflection of subcutaneous fat deposits. A small-for-gestational-age term or postterm infant may have utilized subcutaneous fat (which would have been deposited as breast tissue) to survive in utero; as a result, his lack of breast tissue may indicate a gestational age of 34 to 35 weeks.

9. *Ear form and cartilage distribution* develop with gestational age. The deposition of cartilage gives the ear its shape and substance (Figure 22–8). An infant of less than 34 weeks' gestation has little cartilage deposition, so the ear folds over on itself and remains folded. By approximately 36 weeks' gestation, the pinna springs back slowly when folded. (This response is tested by holding the top and bottom of the pinna together with the forefinger and thumb, then releasing the pinna and observing the response.) By term the infant's pinna is firm, stands away from the head, and springs back quickly from folding.

10. *Male genitals* are evaluated in terms of the size of the scrotal sac, the presence of rugae, and whether the testes have descended (Figure 22–9). Prior to 36 weeks the male has a small scrotum with few rugae, and the testes are palpable in the inguinal canal. By 36 to 38 weeks, the testes are found in the upper scrotum and rugae have developed over the anterior portion of the scrotum. By term the testes are generally located in the lower scrotum, which is pendulous and covered with rugae.

The appearance of the *female genitals* depends in part on subcutaneous fat deposition and therefore relates to fetal nutritional status. At 30 to 32 weeks, the clitoris is prominent and the labia majora are small and widely separated. As gestational age increases, the labia majora increase in size. At 36 to 40 weeks, they nearly cover the clitoris. At 40 weeks and beyond, the labia majora cover the labia minora and clitoris.

The clitoris varies in size and occasionally is so large that it is difficult to identify the sex of the

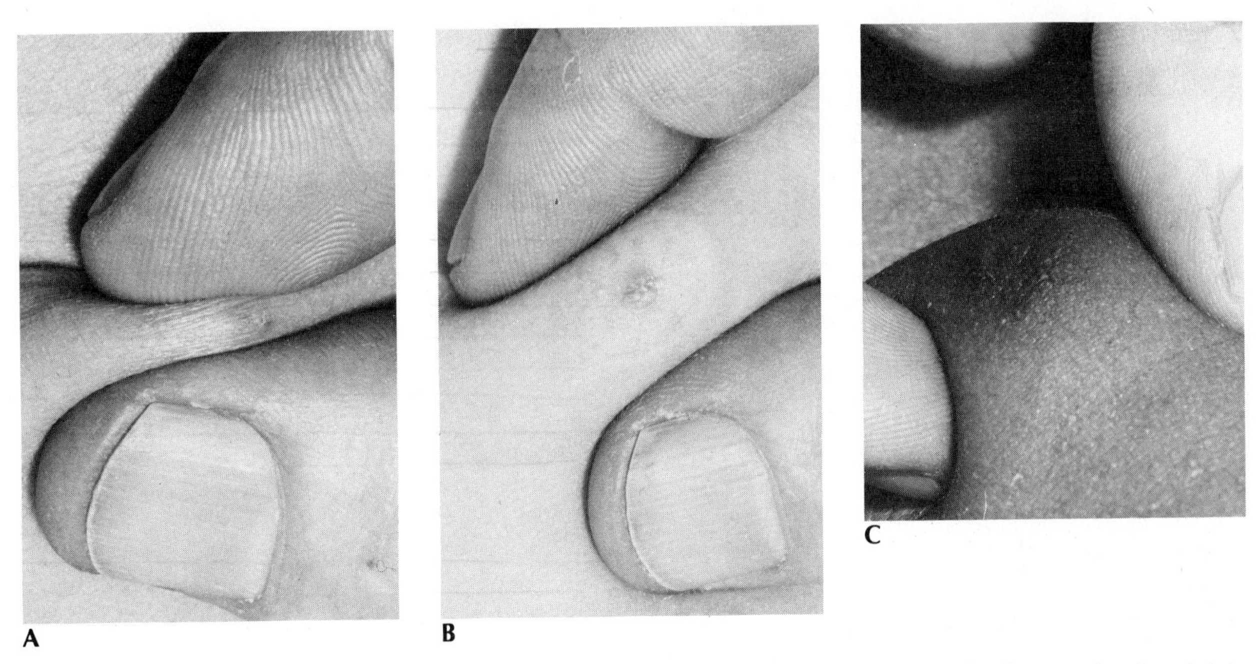

Figure 22-7. Breast tissue. **A,** Infant has a barely visible areola and nipple. No tissue is palpable. The gestational age is less than 33 weeks. **B,** Infant has a visible raised area. On palpation the area is 4 mm. The gestational age is 38 weeks. **C,** Infant has a 10 mm breast tissue area. The gestational age is 40–44 weeks. (From Dubowitz, L., and Dubowitz, V. 1977. *Gestational age of the newborn*. Menlo Park, Calif.: Addison-Wesley Publishing Co.)

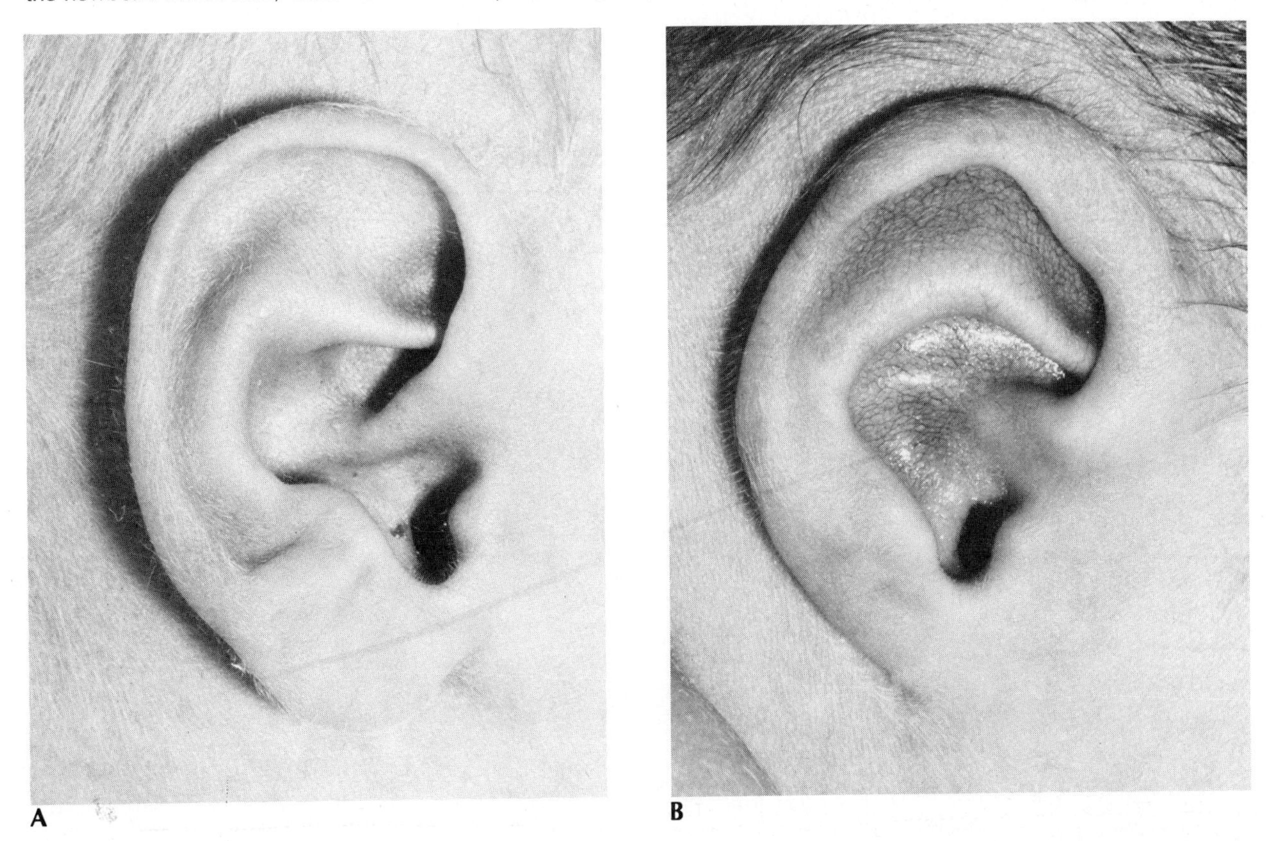

Figure 22-8. Ear form and cartilage. **A,** The ear of the infant at approximately 36 weeks' gestation shows incurving of the upper two-thirds of the pinna. **B,** Infant at term shows well-defined incurving of the entire pinna. (From Dubowitz, L., and Dubowitz, V. 1977. *Gestational age of the newborn*. Menlo Park, Calif.: Addison-Wesley Publishing Co.)

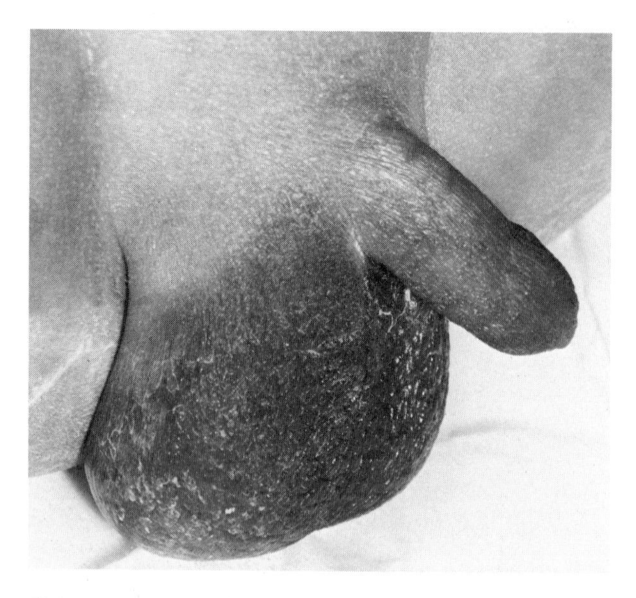

Figure 22–9. Male genitals. A term infant's testes are generally fully descended. The entire surface of the scrotum is covered by rugae. (From Dubowitz, L., and Dubowitz, V. 1977. *Gestational age of the newborn.* Menlo Park, Calif.: Addison-Wesley Publishing Co.)

infant. This may be caused by adrenogenital syndrome, which causes excessive secretions of androgen and other hormones from the adrenals.

In the full-term female infant there may be some tissue that protrudes from the floor of the vagina. This tissue, the hymenal tag, is a normal segment of the hymen and disappears in several weeks (Korones, 1976) (Figure 22–10).

11. *Recoil* is the final characteristic that is evaluated, because it is the most disturbing to the quiet infant. Recoil is a test of flexion development. There is about a two-week delay between the development of resting flexion and recoil (in the flexed position) in response to extension. Because flexion first develops in the lower extremities, recoil is first tested in the legs. The infant is placed on his back on a flat surface. With her hand on the infant's knees and while manipulating the hip joint, the nurse places the infant's legs in flexion, then extends them parallel to each other and flat on the surface. The response to this maneuver is recoil of the infant's legs. According to gestational age, they may not move or they may return slowly or quickly to the flexed position. Recoil in the upper extremities is tested by flexion at the elbow and extension of the arms at the infant's side.

Assessment of Neurologic Status

The central nervous system of the human fetus matures at a fairly constant rate. Specific neurologic parameters correlated to gestational age have been established. Tests have been designed to evaluate neurologic status as manifested by neuromuscular tone development. In the fetus, neuromuscular tone develops from the lower to the upper extremities. The neurologic evaluation requires more manipulation and disturbances than the physical evaluation of the infant and

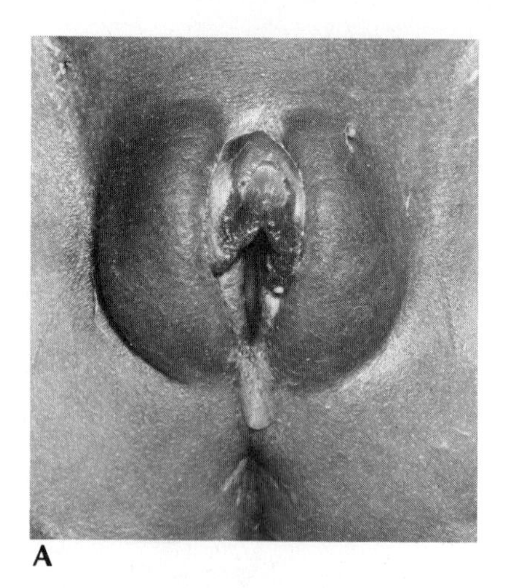

A

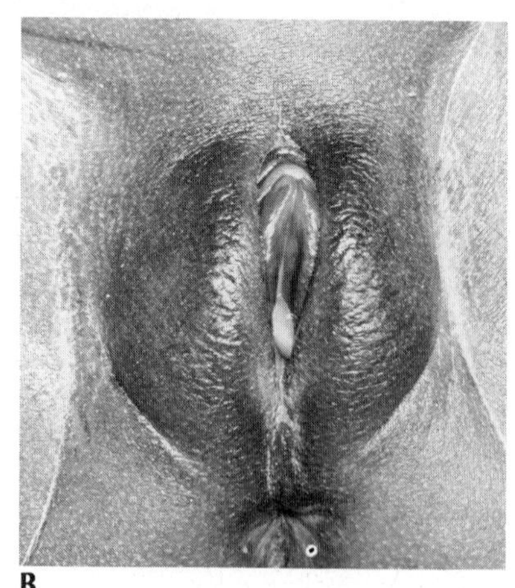

B

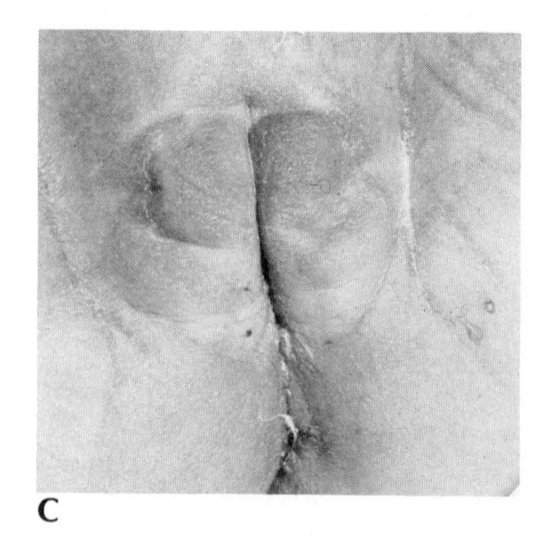

C

Figure 22–10. Female genitals. **A,** Infant has a prominent clitoris. The labia majora are widely separated, and the labia minora, viewed laterally, would protrude beyond the labia majora. The gestational age is 30–36 weeks. **B,** The clitoris is still visible; the labia minora are now covered by the larger labia majora. The gestational age is 36–40 weeks. **C,** The term infant has well-developed, large labia majora that cover both the clitoris and labia minora. (From Dubowitz, L., and Dubowitz, V. 1977. *Gestational age of the newborn.* Menlo Park, Calif.: Addison-Wesley Publishing Co.)

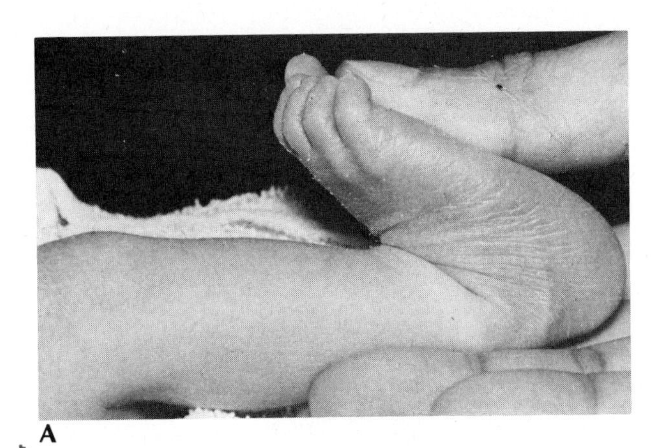

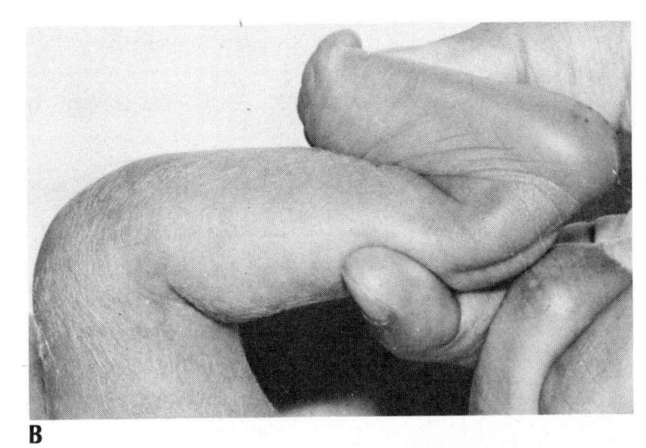

A B

Figure 22-11. Ankle dorsiflexion. **A,** A 45° angle is indicative of 32-36 weeks' gestation. A 20° angle is indicative of 36-40 weeks' gestation. **B,** An angle of 0° is common at a gestational age of 40 weeks or more. (From Dubowitz, L., and Dubowitz, V. 1977. *Gestational age of the newborn.* Menlo Park, Calif.: Addison-Wesley Publishing Co.)

therefore is difficult to administer if the newborn is ill and requires supportive therapies, which tend to immobilize the infant.

The neurologic evaluation (see Figure 22-3,*B*) is best performed and interpreted after the first 24 hours of life or when the infant has stabilized. The following characteristics are evaluated:

1. *Ankle dorsiflexion* is determined by flexing the ankle on the calf. The sole of the infant's foot is pushed with the examiner's thumb while her fingers support the back of the infant's leg. Then the angle formed between the foot and the interior leg is measured (Figure 22-11).

2. The *square window sign* is elicited by flexing the infant's hand toward the ventral forearm. The angle formed at the wrist is measured (Figure 22-12).

3. The *popliteal angle* is determined with the infant supine and flat. His thigh is flexed on his chest, and the examiner places her index finger behind the infant's ankle to extend the lower leg. The angle formed is then measured. Results vary from no resistance in the very immature infant to an 80° angle in the term infant.

4. The *heel-to-ear maneuver* is performed by placing the infant supine and then gently drawing his foot toward his ear on the same side until resistance is felt. Both the popliteal angle and the

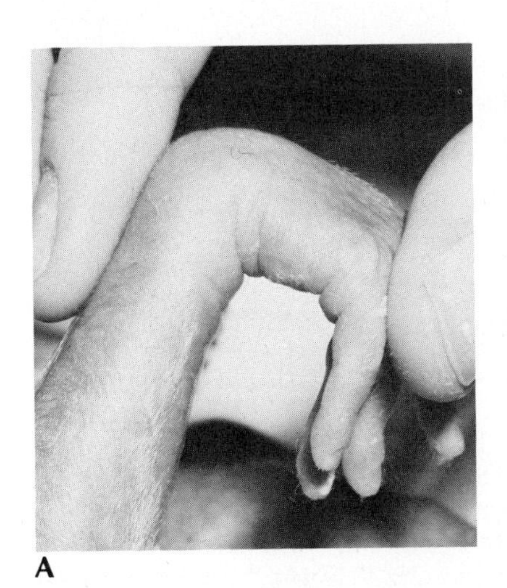

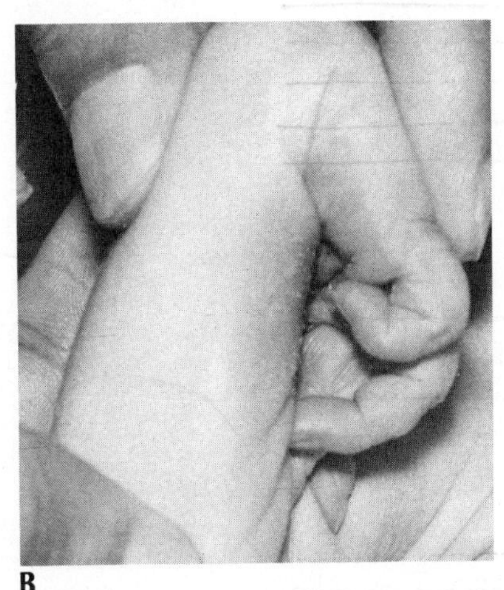

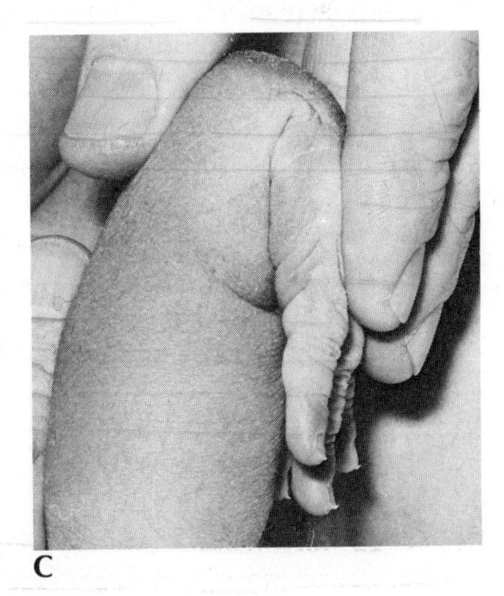

A B C

Figure 22-12. Square window sign. **A,** This angle is 90° and suggests an immature infant of 28-32 weeks' gestation. **B,** A 30° angle is commonly found from 38 to 40 weeks' gestation. **C,** A 0° angle occurs from 40 to 42 weeks. (From Dubowitz, L., and Dubowitz, V. 1977. *Gestational age of the newborn.* Menlo Park, Calif.: Addison-Wesley Publishing Co.)

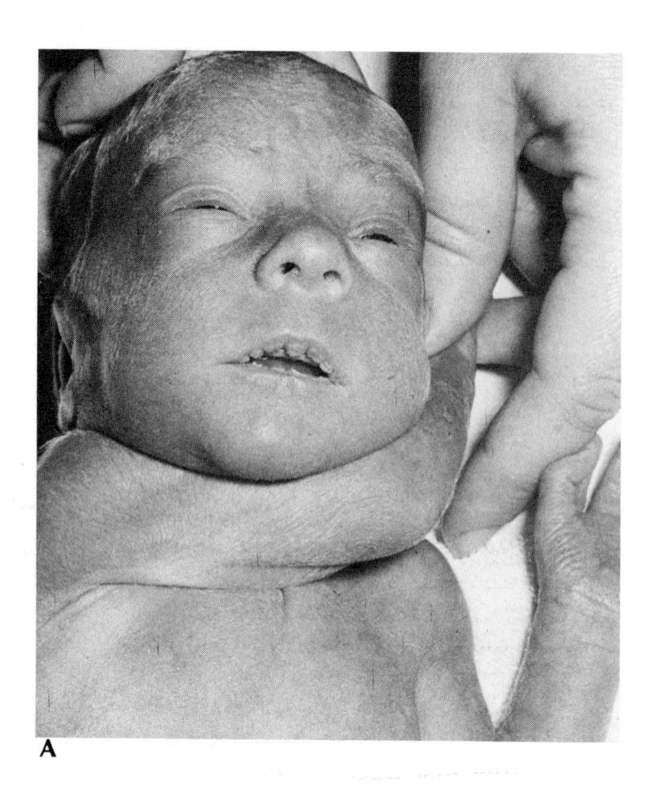

A

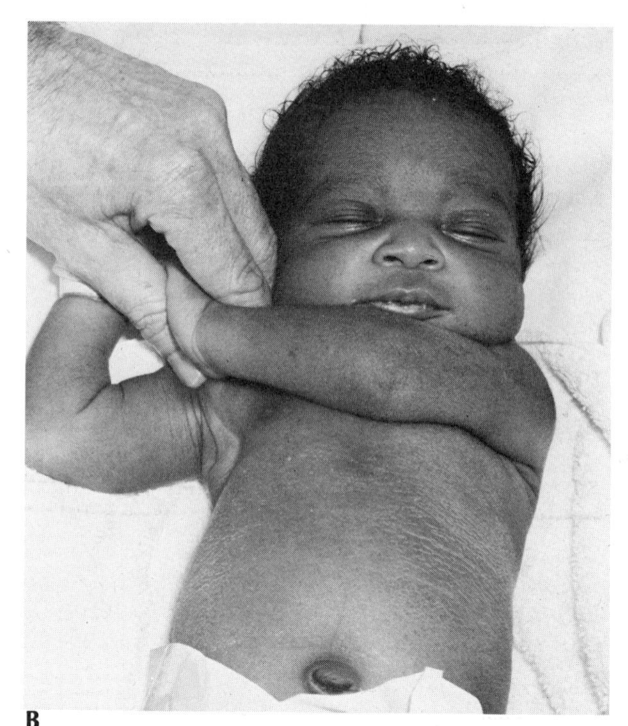

B

proximity of foot to ear are assessed. In a very immature infant, the leg will remain straight and the foot will go to the ear or beyond.

5. The *scarf sign* is elicited by placing the infant supine and drawing his arm across his chest toward his opposite shoulder until resistance is met. The location of the elbow is then noted (Figure 22–13).

6. *Neck extensors* are measured with the infant in a sitting position, head flexed on his chest. At 32 to 36 weeks' gestation, an infant begins to extend his head. A term infant is able to hold his head erect and in line with his trunk for more than 40 seconds.

7. *Neck flexors* are measured by pulling the infant to a sitting position and noting the degree of head lag. Total lag is common in infants up to 34 weeks' gestation, whereas the postmature infant (42 weeks) will hold his head in front of his body line.

8. *Horizontal position* is evaluated by holding the infant prone on the examiner's hand. The position of head and back and degree of flexion in the arms and legs are then noted. Some flexion of arms and legs indicates 36 to 38 weeks' gestation;

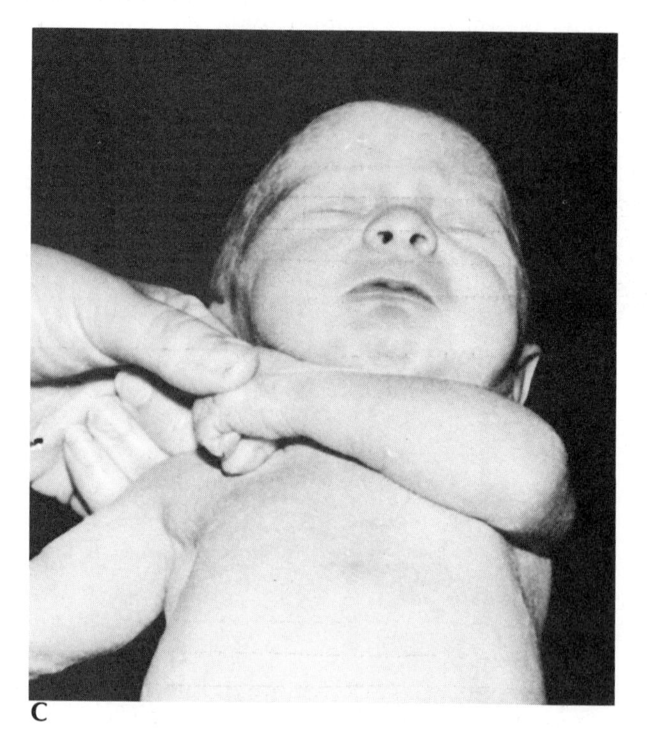

C

Figure 22–13. Scarf sign. **A,** No resistance is noted until after 30 weeks' gestation. The elbow can be readily moved past the midline. **B,** The elbow is at the midline at 36–40 weeks' gestation. **C,** Beyond 40 weeks' gestation, the elbow will not reach the midline. (From Dubowitz, L., and Dubowitz, V. 1977. *Gestational age of the newborn.* Menlo Park, Calif.: Addison-Wesley Publishing Co.)

fully flexed extremities, with head and back even, are characteristic of a term infant.

9. *Major reflexes* such as sucking, rooting, grasping, Moro, tonic neck, and others are evaluated and scored according to the description in Figure 22-3,*B*.

Determination of gestational age and correlation with birth weight enables the nurse to assess the infant more accurately and to anticipate possible physiologic problems. This information is then used in conjunction with a complete physical examination to determine priorities and to establish a plan of care appropriate to the individual infant.

PHYSICAL EXAMINATION

After the initial determination of gestational age and related potential problems, a more detailed physical examination is conducted. The nurse should choose a warm, well-lighted area that is free of drafts. She should perform the examination systematically and record her findings. When assessing the physical and neurologic status of the newborn, the nurse should first consider his general appearance and then proceed to specific areas.

General Appearance

The newborn's head is disproportionately large for his body. The center of the baby's body is the umbilicus rather than the symphysis pubis, as in the adult. The torso appears long and the extremities short. The flexed position that the neonate maintains contributes to the apparent shortness of the extremities. The hands are tightly clenched. The neck is short because the chin rests on the chest. The baby has a prominent abdomen, sloping shoulders, narrow hips, and a rounded chest. He tends to stay in a flexed position similar to the one maintained in utero.

Posture

Although the newborn's posture is influenced by intrauterine position and type of delivery, a full-term infant is usually flexed and will offer resistance when the extremities are straightened. With a breech presentation, the feet are usually dorsiflexed and may take several weeks to assume typical neonatal posture.

Weight and Measurements

The normal full-term white infant has an average birth weight of 3405 gm (7 lb 8 oz), whereas others (black, Oriental, American Indian) are usually somewhat smaller. Other factors that influence weight are age and size of parents, health of mother, and the interval between pregnancies. Half of all infants weigh between 2950 gm (6 lb 8 oz) and 3515 gm (7 lb 12 oz). After the first week and for the first six months, the infant's weight will increase about 227 gm (8 oz) weekly.

Approximately 70%–75% of the infant's body weight is water. During the initial newborn period (the first three or four days), there is a normal physiologic weight loss of about 5%–10% because of fluid shifts. Larger babies may tend to lose more weight because of greater fluid loss in proportion to birth weight. If weight loss is greater than expected, clinical reappraisal is indicated. Factors contributing to weight loss include small fluid intake, adjustment to formula, loss of meconium, and urination. Weight loss may be marked in the presence of temperature elevation because of associated dehydration.

The length of the normal newborn is difficult to measure, because the legs are flexed and tensed. To measure length, the infant should be flat on his back with legs extended as much as possible. The average length is 49.4 cm (19½ in.), with the range being 45.8–52.3 cm (18–20.5 in.). The newborn will grow approximately an inch a month for the next six months. This is the period of most rapid growth.

At birth the newborn's head is one-third the size of the adult head. The ratio of the face to cranium is 1:8 in the infant and 1:2 in the adult. The circumference of the newborn's head is 33–35 cm (13–14 in.). For accurate measurement, the tape is placed over the most prominent part of the occiput and brought to just above the eyebrows (Figure 22–14). The circumference of the infant's head is approximately 2 cm greater than the circumference of the infant's chest at birth and will remain this way for the next few months.

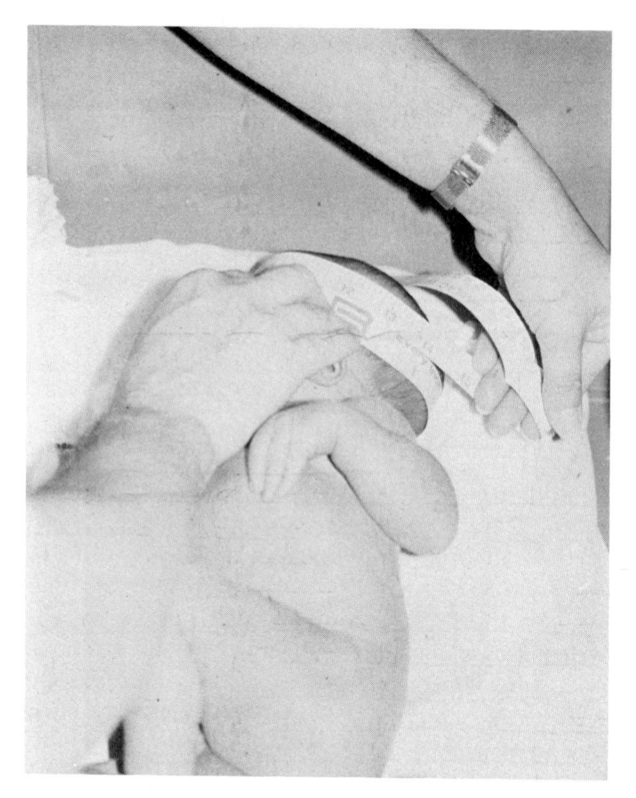

Figure 22–14. Measuring the head circumference of the newborn.

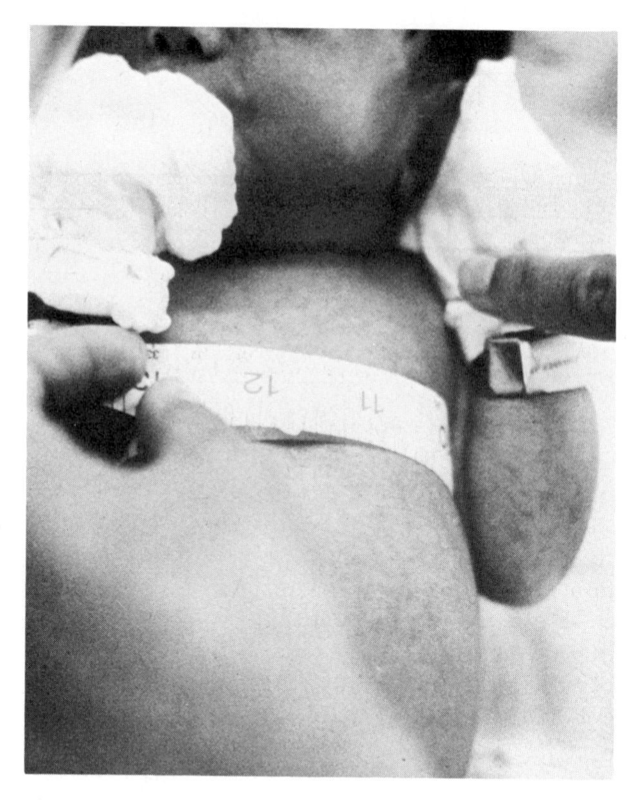

Figure 22–15. Measuring the chest circumference of the newborn.

The chest is circular at birth, becoming more rectangular as the infant grows older. The average circumference of the chest at birth is 32 cm (12.5 in.). Chest measurements should be taken with the tape measure at the lower edge of the scapulae and brought around anteriorly directly over the nipple line (Figure 22–15). The abdominal circumference is also measured at this time by placing the tape around the infant's abdomen at the level of the umbilicus.

Temperature

Initial assessment of the newborn's temperature is critical. In utero, the temperature of the fetus approximates or is slightly higher than its mother's. With exposure to the outside world, the infant's temperature can suddenly drop as a result of adaptation to the extrauterine environment, exposure to cold drafts, and the skin's heat-loss mechanisms. Upon arrival in the nursery, a newborn's temperature may be as low as 36C (96.8F), but it should stabilize at around 36.7C (98F) within 8 to 12 hours. The temperature should be monitored every hour until stable, then every four hours for 24 hours. (See Chapter 23 for a discussion of the physiology of temperature regulation.)

The temperature may be taken either by axilla or rectally (Figure 22–16). If the axillary method is used, the thermometer must remain in place at least ten minutes (unless an electronic thermometer is used). If taken rectally, the thermometer should be held by the nurse for a period of five minutes. Care must be taken to avoid inserting the thermometer too far. It is not unusual for an imperforate anus to be diagnosed initially when the nurse is unable to take the temperature rectally.

Temperature instability, a deviation of more than 1C (2F) from one reading to the next, or a subnormal temperature may indicate an infection. In contrast to an elevated temperature in older children, an increased temperature in a newborn may indicate reactions to too much covering, too hot a room, or dehydration. Dehydration, which tends to increase body temperature, occurs in newborns whose feedings have been delayed for any reason. Infants respond to overheating (temperature greater than 37.5C [99.5F]) by increased restlessness and eventually by perspiration.

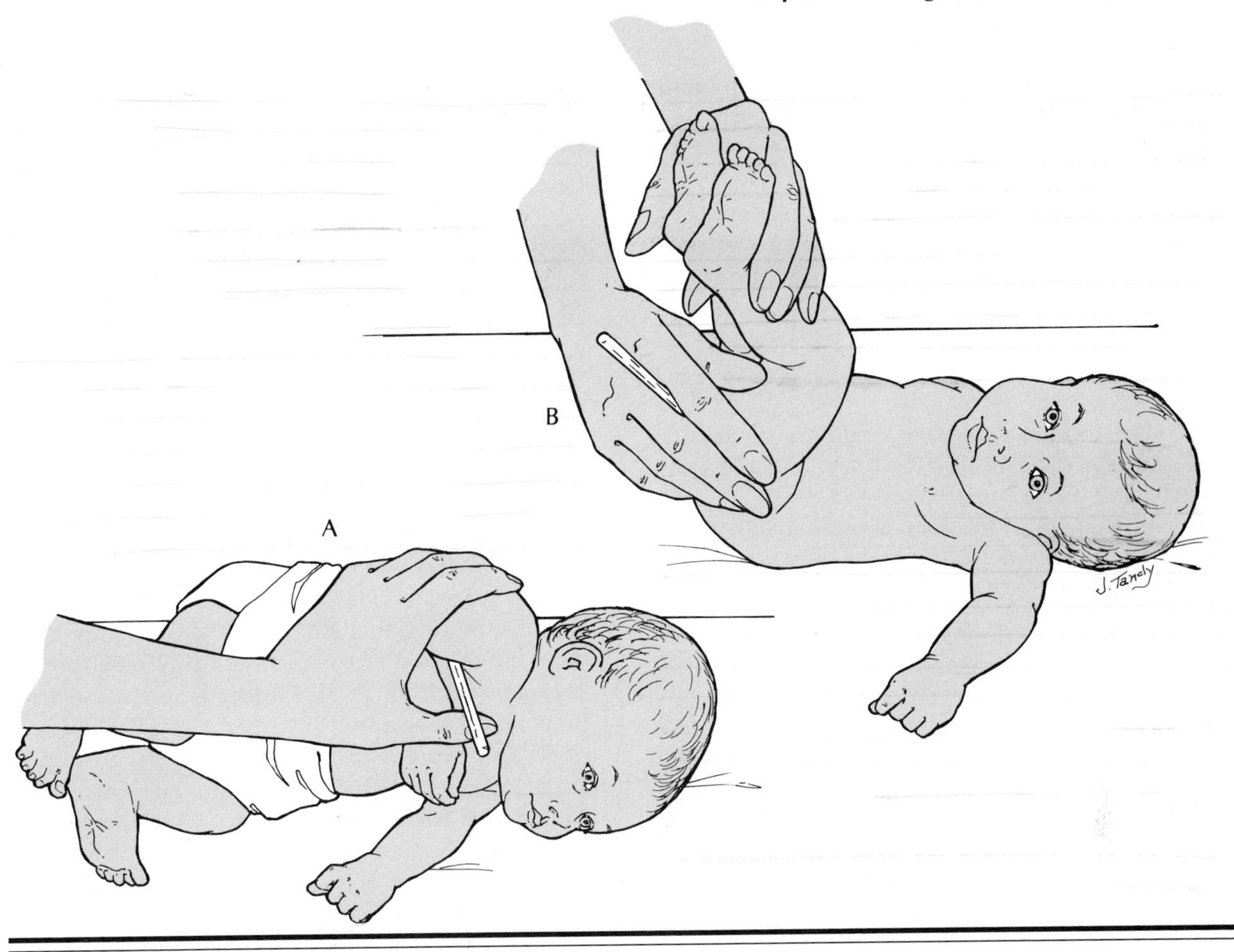

Figure 22–16. **A,** The axillary temperature must be taken for 10 minutes. **B,** The rectal thermometer must be held in place for 5 minutes and the legs supported.

Skin

The skin of the newborn should be pink-tinged or ruddy in color and warm to the touch. The ruddy color results from increased concentration of red blood cells in the blood vessels and from limited subcutaneous fat deposits. *Acrocyanosis* (bluish discoloration of the hands and feet) or *circumoral cyanosis* (blue or pale color around the mouth) may be present, due to poor peripheral circulation with resultant vasomotor instability and capillary stasis, especially when the infant is exposed to cold. This condition is transient and usually disappears within ten days. If the central circulation is adequate, the blood supply should return quickly when the skin is blanched with a finger. Occasionally a *harlequin* (clown) color change will be noted: A deep red color develops over one side of the infant's body while the other side remains a pale pink, so that the skin resembles a clown's suit. This color aberration results from a vasomotor disturbance in which blood vessels on one side dilate while the vessels on the other side constrict. It usually disappears in a few hours or a day.

Suspected jaundice is evaluated by blanching the tip of the nose or the gum line. If jaundice is present, the area will appear yellowish immediately after blanching. This test determines the existence and, to a limited extent, the degree of jaundice. Evaluation and determination of the cause of jaundice must be initiated immediately to prevent possible serious sequelae. The jaundice may be related to breast-feeding (small incidence), hematomas, or immature liver function, or may be caused by blood incompatibility or severe hemolytic process.

Erythema neonatorum toxicum is a perifollicular eruption that may be seen in 30 to 70 percent of full-term infants. The peak incidence is 24 to 48 hours of life. The lesions are firm, vary in size from 1 mm to 3 mm, and consist of a white or pale yellow papule or pustule with an erythematous base. The rash may appear suddenly, usually over the trunk and diaper area, and is frequently widespread. The lesions do not appear on the palms of the hands or the soles of the feet. Diagnosis may be confirmed by obtaining a smear of aspirated pustule, which after staining shows numerous eosinophils and no bacteria culture. The etiology is unknown and no treatment is necessary. The lesions disappear in one to two weeks (Avery, 1975).

Skin turgor is evaluated to determine hydration status, the timing of feedings, and the presence of any infectious processes.

Vernix caseosa, a whitish cheeselike substance, covers the infant while in utero and serves as a skin lubricant for the newborn. It is generally more pronounced on preterm infants. The skin of the term or postterm infant is frequently dry, and peeling is common, especially on the hands and feet. *Milia*, which are plugged sebaceous glands, appear as raised white spots on the face, especially across the nose. *Mongolian spots*, which are macular areas of bluish black pigmentation found on the lumbar dorsal area and the buttocks, are common in Oriental and black infants and newborns of other dark-skinned races. They gradually fade during the first or second year of life.

After a difficult forceps delivery, the infant may have reddened areas over the cheeks and jaws. It is important to reassure the mother that these will disappear, usually within one or two days. Transient facial paralysis resulting from the forceps pressure is a rare complication.

Telangiectatic nevi, or "stork bites," are thought to be superficial telangiectatic areas as opposed to new growth of tissue. They appear as pale pink or red spots and are frequently found on the eyelids, nose, lower occipital bone, and nape of the neck. These lesions are common in light-complexioned neonates and are more noticeable during periods of crying. These areas blanch easily, have no clinical significance, and usually fade by the second birthday. *Nevus flammeus*, or port-wine stain, is a capillary angioma directly below the epidermis. It is a nonelevated, sharply demarcated, red to purple birthmark. The size and shape is variable but it commonly appears on the face. It does not grow in size, does not fade with time, and does not blanch. In the black infant, the nevus flammeus appears jet black in color. The birthmark may be concealed by using an opaque cosmetic cream such as "covermark." If convulsions, contralateral hemiplegia, or intracortical calcification accompanies the nevus flammeus, it is suggestive of Sturge-Weber syndrome (Avery, 1975). It will not fade and does not blanch with pressure (Figure 22–17). *Nevus vasculosus*, or "strawberry mark," is a capillary hemangioma. It consists of newly formed and enlarged capillaries in the dermal and subdermal layers (Mead Johnson, 1978). It is a raised, clearly delineated, dark red, rough-surfaced birthmark commonly found in the head region. Such marks usually grow (often rapidly) for several months and become fixed in size by eight months of age. They then begin to regress in size and, except in rare cases, are completely gone by the time the child is 7 years old.

Birthmarks are frequently a cause of concern for the parents. The mother may be especially anxious, fearing that she is to blame ("Is my baby 'marked' because of something I did?"). Guilt feelings are common in the presence of misconceptions about the cause. Birthmarks should be identified and explained to the parents. By providing appropriate information about the cause and course of birthmarks, the nurse frequently allays the fears and anxieties of the family.

Head

General Appearance

The infant's head is large (approximately one-fourth of his body size), with soft, pliable skull bones. The head may appear asymmetrical in the infant of a vertex delivery. This asymmetry, called *molding*, is caused by overriding of the cranial bones during delivery. The degree of molding varies with the degree and length of the pressure exerted. Within a few days after delivery, the overriding usually diminishes and the suture lines become palpable. Because head measurements are affected by molding, a second measurement is indicated a few days after delivery. The heads of breech-born babies and those delivered by caesarean section are characteristically round and well shaped, because pressure was not exerted on them during birth. Any extreme differences in head size may indicate microencephaly or hydrocephaly. Variations in the shape, size, or appearance of the head may be due to craniostenosis (premature closure of the cranial sutures) and plagiocephaly (asymmetry caused by pressure on the fetal head during gestation).

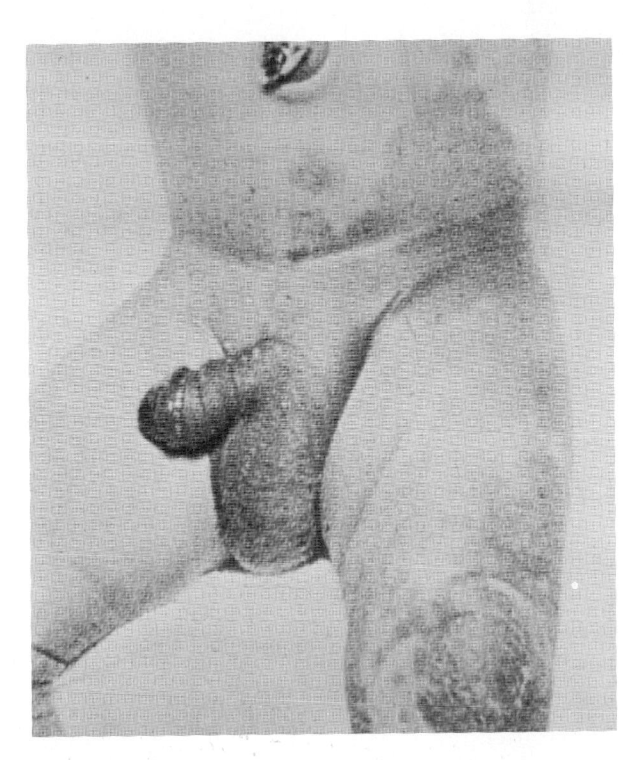

Figure 22–17. Port wine stain, or nevus flammeus. (Courtesy Mead Johnson Laboratories, Evansville, Ind.)

Two *fontanelles* ("soft spots") may be palpated on the infant's head. Fontanelles, which are openings at the juncture of the cranial bones, can be measured with the fingers. Accurate measurement necessitates that the examiner's finger be measured in centimeters. The diamond-shaped *anterior fontanelle* is approximately 3–4 cm long by 2–3 cm wide. It is located at the juncture of the frontal and parietal bones. The *posterior fontanelle*, smaller and triangular, is formed by the parietal bones and the occipital bone. The fontanelles will be smaller immediately after birth than several days later because of molding. The anterior fontanelle closes within 18 months, whereas the posterior fontanelle closes within 8 to 12 weeks.

The fontanelles are a useful indicator of the infant's condition. The anterior fontanelle may swell when the infant cries or may pulsate with the heartbeat, which is normal. However, a bulging fontanelle usually signifies increased intracranial pressure, and a depressed fontanelle indicates dehydration. An overlapping of the anterior fontanelle occasionally occurs in malnourished or premature infants. The sutures between the cranial bones should be palpated for amount of overlapping.

In addition to being inspected for degree of molding and size, the head should be evaluated for soft tissue edema and bruising.

Cephalhematoma. Cephalhematoma is a collection of blood resulting from ruptured blood vessels between the surface of a cranial bone and the periosteal membrane. The scalp in these areas feels loose and slightly edematous. These areas emerge as defined hematomas between the first and second day. Although external pressure may cause the mass to fluctuate, it does not increase in size with crying. Cephalhematomas may be unilateral or bilateral, do not cross over suture lines, are relatively common in vertex deliveries, and disappear within 2 to 3 weeks. (Figure 22–18). They are often associated with increased bilirubin levels with the increased breakdown of red blood cells as the cephalhematoma absorbs.

Caput Succedaneum. Caput succedaneum is a localized, easily identifiable soft area of the scalp, generally resulting from a long and difficult labor. The sustained pressure of the presenting part against the cervix results in compression of local vessels, and venous return is slowed (Korones, 1976). This causes an increase in tissue fluids and an edematous swelling results. The caput may vary from a small area to a severely elongated head. The fluid of the caput is reabsorbed within 12 hours or a few days after birth. It is possible to distinguish between a cephalhematoma and the caput because the caput overrides suture lines whereas the cephalhematoma, because of its location, never crosses a suture line (Figure 22–19) (Avery, 1975).

Face

The infant's face is well designed for sucking. Sucking (fat) pads are located in the cheeks, and a labial tubercle is frequently found in the center of the upper lip. The chin is recessed, and the nose is flattened. The lips are sensitive to touch, and the sucking reflex is easily initiated. Symmetry of the eyes, nose, and ears is evaluated. See Assessment Guide pg. 683 for deviations in symmetry and variations in size, shape, and spacing of facial features.

Eyes

The eyes of the neonate are a blue or slate blue-gray in color. Scleral color tends to be bluish

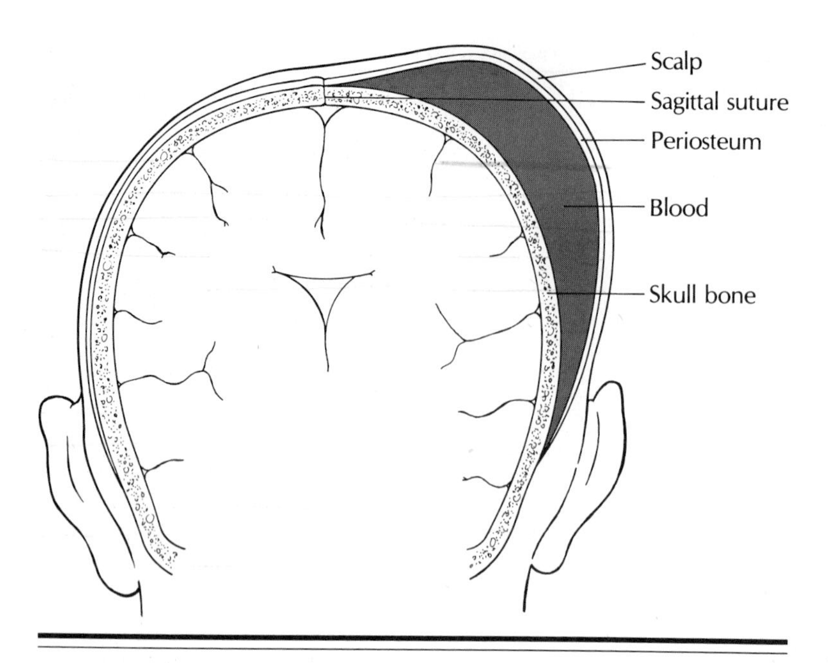

Figure 22–18. Cephalhematoma is a collection of blood between the surface of a cranial bone and the periosteal membrane.

because of its relative thinness. The infant's eye color usually is established at approximately 3 months of age, although it may change anytime up to 1 year. Dark-pigmented babies tend to have dark eyes at birth.

The eyes should be checked for size, equality of pupil size, reaction of pupils to light, blink reflex to light, and edema and inflammation of the eyelids. The eyelids are usually edematous during the first few days of life because of the delivery and the instillation of silver nitrate drops in the baby's eyes. Chemical conjunctivitis appears a few hours after the instillation of the silver nitrate drops but disappears without treatment in one to two days. In infectious conjunctivitis the infant has the same purulent exudate as in chemical conjunctivitis, but it is caused by staphylococci or a variety of gram negative rods and requires treatment with ophthalmic antibiotics. Onset is usually after the second day. Edema of the orbits or eyelids may persist for several days until the neonate's kidneys can evacuate the fluid.

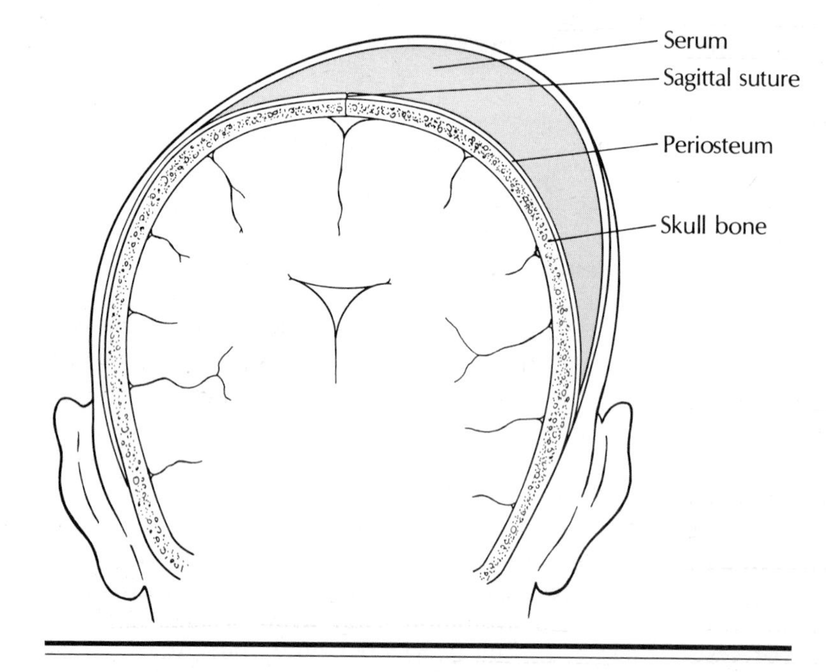

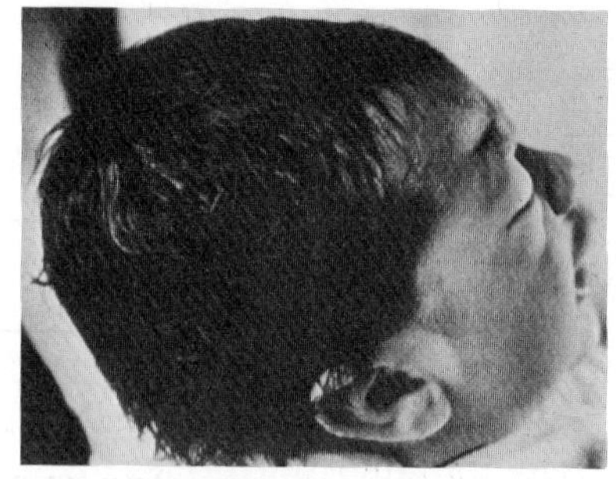

Figure 22–19. Caput succedaneum is a collection of fluid (serum) under the scalp. (Photo courtesy Mead Johnson Laboratories, Evansville, Ind.)

Small subconjunctival hemorrhages appear in about 10% of newborns and are commonly found on the inner aspect of the sclera. These are caused by the changes in vascular tension during birth. They will remain for a few weeks and are of no pathologic significance, but mothers need reassurance that this bleeding is unimportant, that the infant is not bleeding from within the eye, and that his vision will not be impaired.

The neonate may demonstrate transient strabismus due to poor neuromuscular control of eye muscles (Figure 22-20). It gradually regresses in three to four months.

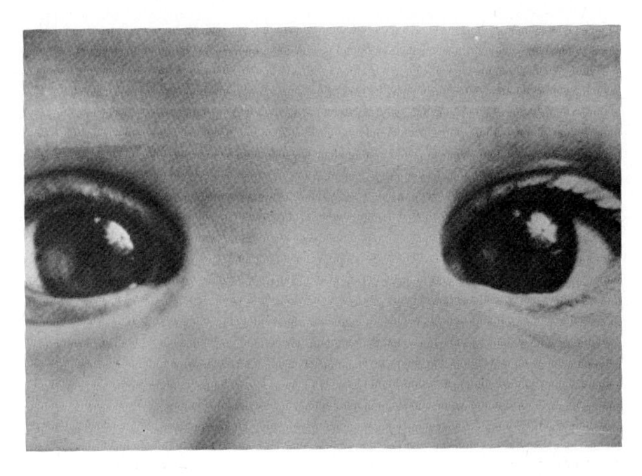

Figure 22-20. Transient strabismus may be present in the newborn due to poor neuromuscular control. (Courtesy Mead Johnson Laboratories, Evansville, Ind.)

The nurse should observe the neonate's pupils for opacities or whiteness and for the absence of a normal red reflex. These are signs of congenital cataracts, which should be suspected in infants of mothers with a history of rubella or cytomegalic inclusion disease.

The cry of the neonate is commonly tearless, because the lacrimal structures are immature at birth and do not usually become fully functional until the second month of life, although on occasion there are infants who do produce tears during the neonatal period.

Although the newborn's vision is not so acute as that of an adult, newborn infants do see. Poor oculomotor coordination and absence of accommodation limit visual abilities, but the infant does have peripheral vision and can fixate on near objects (3-30 inches) for short periods of time (Kempe, 1978). The infant can perceive faces, shapes, and colors and begins to show visual preferences early. He blinks in response to bright lights, to a tap on the bridge of the nose, or to a light touch on the eyelids. Pupillary light reflex is also present. Examination of the eye is best accomplished by rocking the infant from an upright position to the horizontal a few times or by other methods that will alert him and elicit an opened-eye response.

Nose

The neonate's nose is small and narrow. Infants are characteristically nose breathers for the first few months of life and the reason for nose breathing is not clear (Avery, 1975). A clear passage must be maintained, free of mucus, or the neonate will suffer respiratory distress. The newborn generally removes the obstruction by sneezing. The nose may also be cleansed by gentle suction with a bulb syringe or catheter. Nasal patency is assured if the neonate breathes easily with his mouth closed. If respiratory difficulty occurs, the nurse should check for choanal atresia (see pg. 850).

The newborn has the ability to smell after the nasal passages are cleared of amniotic fluid and mucus. This ability is demonstrated by his search for milk. The infant will turn his head toward the milk source, whether bottle or breast. It has also been demonstrated that the neonates can distinguish their mother's breast pad from other mothers' by 2-4 days of age.

Mouth

The lips of the newborn should be pink, and touching the lips should produce sucking motions. Saliva is normally scant. The taste buds are developed prior to birth, and the newborn can easily discriminate between sweet and bitter.

The easiest way to completely examine the mouth of the newborn infant is to gently stimulate the infant to cry by depressing his tongue, thereby causing him to open his mouth fully. It is extremely important to observe the entire mouth to look for a *cleft palate,* which can be present even in the absence of a cleft lip. The examiner places a clean index finger along the hard and soft palate to feel for any openings.

Occasionally an examination of the gums will reveal *precocious teeth* on the lower central incisor. If they appear loose, they should be removed to prevent aspiration. Gray-white lesions *(inclusion cysts)* on the gums may be confused with teeth.

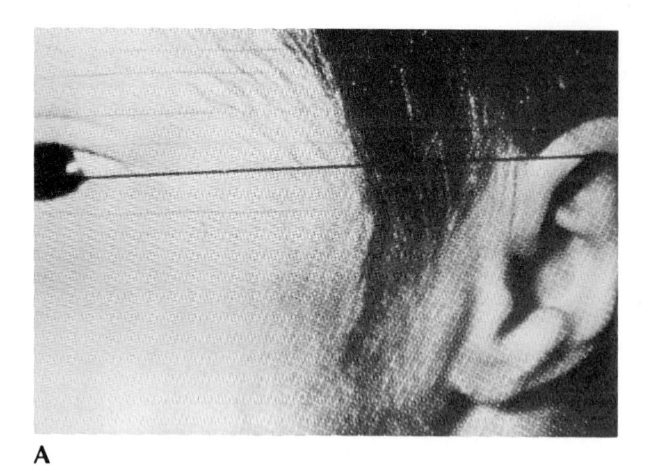

A

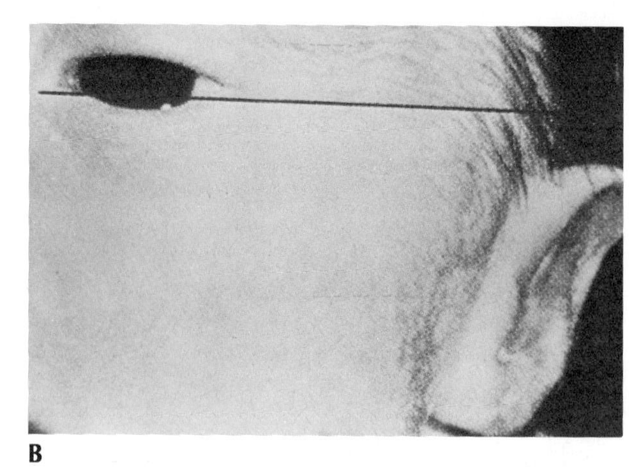

B

Figure 22–21. The position of the external ear may be assessed by drawing a line across the inner and outer canthus of the eye to the insertion of the ear. **A,** Normal position. **B,** True low-set. (Courtesy Mead Johnson Laboratories, Evansville, Ind.)

On the hard palate and gum margins, *Epstein's pearls,* small glistening white specks (keratin-containing cysts) that feel hard to the touch are often present. These usually disappear in a few weeks and are of no significance. Thrush may appear as white patches that look like milk curds adhering to the mucous membranes and that cause bleeding when removed. Thrush is caused by *Candida albicans,* often acquired from infected vaginal tract during birth, and is treated with a preparation of Mystatin.

An infant who is *tongue-tied* has a ridge of frenulum tissue attached to the underside of the tongue at varying lengths from its base, causing a heart shape at the tip of the tongue. "Clipping the tongue," or cutting the ridge of tissue, is not recommended. This ridge does not affect speech or eating, but cutting does create an entry for infection.

Transient nerve paralysis resulting from birth trauma may be seen by asymmetrical mouth movements when the neonate cries or may be seen as difficulty with sucking and feeding.

Ears

The ears of the newborn may be crumpled or flattened against the skull and should have well-formed cartilage (one determinant of gestational age). In the normal newborn, the top of the ear should be parallel to the outer and inner canthus of the eye. The ears should be inspected for shape, size, and position. Low-set ears are characteristic of many syndromes and may indicate chromosomal abnormalities (especially trisomies 13 and 18), mental retardation, and/or internal organ abnormalities, especially bilateral renal agenesis as a result of embryologic developmental deviations (Figure 22–21). Preauricular skin tags may be present. They are ligated at the base and allowed to slough off.

Following the first cry, the newborn can hear. His hearing becomes acute as mucus from the middle ear is absorbed and the eustachian tube becomes aerated.

Downs and Silver (1972) have identified the following risk factors associated with potential hearing loss:

1. The presence of hearing loss in any family member prior to the age of 50 years.
2. Serum bilirubin level greater than 20 mg/100 ml in the newborn period.
3. Suspected maternal rubella infection during pregnancy, resulting in congenital rubella syndrome.
4. Defects of the ear, nose, or throat.
5. Small neonatal size, particularly less than 1500 gm at birth.

The newborn's hearing is evaluated by his response to loud or moderately loud noises unaccompanied by vibrations. He should stir or awaken in response to the nearby sounds while he is asleep.

Neck

A short neck, creased with skin folds, is characteristic of the normal newborn. Because muscle tone is not well-developed, the neck cannot support the full weight of the head, which rotates freely. The head lags considerably when the child is pulled from a supine to a sitting position, but the prone infant is able to raise his head slightly. The neck should be palpated for masses and for the presence of lymph nodes and should be inspected for webbing. Adequacy of range of motion and neck muscle function is determined by fully extending the head in all directions. Injury to the sternocleidomastoid muscle (congenital torticollis) must be considered in the presence of neck rigidity.

The clavicles should be evaluated for evidence of fractures, which occasionally occur during difficult deliveries or in infants with broad shoulders. The normal clavicle is straight. If fractured, a lump may be palpated along the course of the side of the break. The Moro reflex should also be elicited. If the clavicle is fractured, the response will be demonstrated only on the unaffected side.

Chest

The thorax is cylindrical at birth, and the ribs are flexible. Chest circumference is less than head circumference and remains so until the child is about 2 years old. The general appearance of the chest should be assessed. A protrusion at the lower end of the sternum, called the *xiphoid cartilage*, is frequently seen. It is under the skin and will become less apparent after several weeks because of accumulation of adipose tissue.

Engorged breasts occur frequently in male and female newborns. This condition, which occurs by the third day, is a result of maternal hormonal influences and may last up to two weeks. Sometimes the breast secretes "witches' milk," a liquid discharge. The infant's breast should not be massaged or squeezed, because this practice may cause a breast abscess. Extra or *supernumerary nipples* are occasionally noted below and medial to the true nipples (Figure 22–22). These harmless pink spots vary in size and do not contain glandular tissue (Korones, 1976). At puberty, the accessory nipple may darken. Assessment and differentiation from a pigmented nevi (mole) is facilitated by placing the fingertips alongside the accessory nipple and pulling the adjacent tissue laterally. The accessory nipple will appear dimpled (Mead Johnson, 1978).

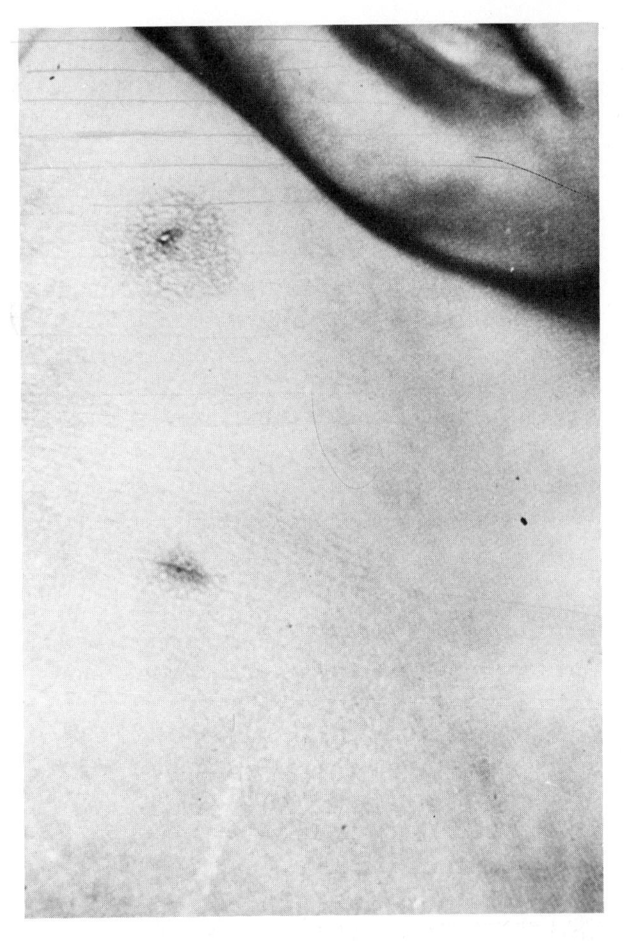

Figure 22–22. Extra or supernumerary nipples may appear below and medial to the true nipples. (Courtesy Mead Johnson Laboratories, Evansville, Ind.)

Cry

The infant's cry should be strong, lusty, and of medium pitch. A high-pitched, shrill cry is abnormal and may indicate neurologic disorders. The infant's cry is an important method of communication and alerts his caretakers to changes in his condition and needs.

Respiration

Normal breathing for a newborn is between 30 and 50 respirations per minute. It is predominantly diaphragmatic, with associated rising and falling of the abdomen with inspiration and expiration. Any signs of respiratory distress, nasal flaring, intercostal or xiphoid retraction, expiratory grunt or sigh, or tachypnea should be noted. Hyperextension (chest appears high) or hypoextension (chest appears low) of the anteroposterior diameter of the chest should also be noted. Auscultation should be done over both the anterior and posterior chest. Some breath sounds are heard better when the infant is crying, but localization and identification of breath sounds are difficult in the newborn. Because sounds may be transmitted from the unaffected lung to the affected lung, the absence of breath sounds cannot be diagnosed.

Heart

Heart rates are rapid (100–180 beats per minute) in neonates but fluctuate a great deal. Auscultation provides the nurse with valuable assessment data. The heart is examined for rate and rhythm, position of apical impulse, and heart sound intensity.

The pulse rate is labile and follows the trend of respirations in the neonatal period. The pulse rate is influenced by physical activity, crying, state of wakefulness, and body temperature. The usual rate is 120–150 beats per minute. If the neonate is sleeping, the rate can be as low as 70–90 beats per minute. If the infant is crying, the pulse rate may be as high as 180 beats per minute. Auscultation should be performed over the entire precordium, below the left axilla, and posteriorly below the scapula.

The placement of the heart in the chest should be determined when the infant is in a quiet state. The heart is relatively large at birth and is located high in the chest, with its apex somewhere between the fourth and fifth intercostal space.

A shift in the mediastinum to either side may indicate pneumothorax, dextrocardia (heart placement on the right side of the chest), or a diaphragmatic hernia. These and many other problems can be diagnosed early with a stethoscope and a trained ear. Normally the heart beat has a "toc tic" sound. A slur or slushing sound (usually after the first sound) may indicate a *murmur*. Although 90% of all murmurs are transient and are considered normal (Korones, 1976), they should be observed closely by a physician. Some murmurs are evidence of a delay in closure of the fetal circulatory passages. Conversely, significant murmurs may not appear immediately after birth.

Neonatal peripheral circulation is sluggish initially, resulting in cyanosis of the extremities (acrocyanosis) for several hours after delivery. *Mottling* also occurs as a result of general circulatory lability. It may last several hours to several weeks or may come and go periodically.

Brachial pulses should be palpated bilaterally for equality and should be compared with the femoral pulses. Femoral pulses are palpated by applying gentle pressure with the middle finger over the femoral canal. Decreased or absent femoral pulses indicate coarctation of the aorta, and require additional investigation. A wide difference in blood pressure between the upper and lower extremities also indicates coarctation. Blood pressure is usually 80/40 mm Hg at birth, and by the tenth day of life, 100/50 mm Hg. It may be difficult to obtain the diastolic pressure or to hear the blood pressure with a standard sphygmomanometer. Blood pressures may not routinely be measured on the newborn unless he is having distress, is premature, or is suspected of some anomaly.

Abdomen

Without disturbing the infant, one can learn a great deal about the newborn's abdomen. The shape should be cylindrical, with some protrusion. A certain amount of laxness of the abdominal muscles can be seen. The absence of abdominal contents is suggested if the abdomen has a scaphoid appearance. No cyanosis should be present, and few if any blood vessels should be apparent to the eye. There should be no gross distention or bulging. The more distended the abdomen, the tighter the skin becomes, with engorged vessels appearing. Distention is the first sign of many of the abnormalities found in the gastrointestinal tract.

Abdominal palpation should be done in a systematic manner. The nurse palpates each of the four abdominal quadrants and moves in a clockwise direction until all four quadrants have been palpated for softness or tenderness and the presence of masses.

When palpating the abdomen, one should feel the liver and both kidneys. The newborn's liver is large in proportion to the rest of the body and can usually be felt between 1 and 2 cm below the right costal margin. Kidneys are more difficult to feel, but examination is facilitated if done within 4–6 hours after birth, before the intestines become distended with air and feedings are initiated. By placing a finger at the posterior flank and pushing upward while pressing downward with the opposite hand, each kidney may be palpated as a firm oval mass between the examiner's finger and hand (Korones, 1976). The lower pole of the kidney is usually found about 1–2 cm above the umbilicus. The spleen tip is palpated in the lateral aspect of the left upper quadrant in the normal newborn.

Initially the umbilical cord is white and gelatinous in appearance, with the two umbilical arteries and one umbilical vein readily apparent. Because a single umbilical artery is frequently associated with congenital anomalies, the vessels should be counted as part of the newborn assessment. The cord begins drying within one to two hours after delivery and is shriveled and blackened by the second or third day. Within a week to ten days, it sloughs off, although a granulating area may be evident for a few days longer.

Cord bleeding is abnormal and may result because the cord was inadvertently pulled or because the cord clamp loosened. Foul-smelling drainage is also abnormal and is generally caused by infection. This infection requires immediate treatment to prevent the development of septicemia. If the infant has a patent urachus (abnormal connection between the umbilicus and bladder), moistness or draining urine may be apparent at the base of the cord.

Genitals

Male Infants

The penis should be inspected to determine whether the urinary orifice is correctly positioned. *Hypospadias* occurs when the urinary meatus is located on the ventral surface of the penis. It occurs most commonly in whites in the United States (Holmes, 1976). *Phimosis* is a condition commonly occurring in newborn males in which the opening of the prepuce is narrowed and the foreskin cannot be retracted over the glans. This condition may interfere with urination, so the adequacy of the urinary stream should be evaluated.

The scrotum should be inspected for size and symmetry and should be palpated to verify the presence of both testes. Scrotal edema and discoloration are common in breech deliveries. Hydroceles are common in newborns and should be identified. The testes should be palpated separately between the thumb and forefinger, with the thumb and forefinger of the other hand placed together over the inguinal canal.

Female Infants

The labia majora, labia minora, and clitoris should be examined, and the nurse should note the size of each as appropriate for gestational age. A vaginal tag or hymenal tag is often evident and will usually disappear in a few weeks. During the first week of life, the infant may have a vaginal discharge composed of thick whitish mucus. This discharge, which can become tinged with blood, is referred to as *pseudomenstruation* and is caused by the withdrawal of maternal hormones. Smegma, a white cheeselike substance, is often present under the labia.

Anus

The anal area should be inspected to verify that it is patent and has no fissure. Imperforate anus and rectal atresia may be ruled out by a digital examination. The passage of the first meconium stool should also be noted. Atresia of the gastrointestinal tract or meconium ileus with resultant obstruction must be considered if no meconium has been passed in the first 24 hours of life.

Extremities

Extremities are examined for gross deformities, extra digits or webbing, clubfoot, and range of motion. The infant's extremities appear short, are generally flexible, and move symmetrically.

Arms and Hands

Nails are present and extend beyond the fingertips in term infants. Fingers and toes should be counted. *Polydactyly* occurs when there are extra digits on either the hands or feet. Polydactyly is more common in blacks (Holmes, 1976). It can be seen with a dominant disorder. If the child has polydactyly and his parents do not, a dominant disorder can be ruled out. *Syndactyly* refers to fusion (webbing) of fingers or toes. Hands should be inspected for normal palmar creases. A single palmar crease, called a *simian line,* is frequently present in children with Down's syndrome.

Brachial palsy, which is partial or complete paralysis of portions of the arm, results from trauma to the brachial plexus during a difficult delivery. It occurs most commonly when strong traction is exerted on the head of the neonate in an attempt to deliver a shoulder lodged behind the symphysis pubis in the presence of shoulder dystocia. Brachial palsy may also occur during a breech delivery if an arm becomes trapped over the head and traction is exerted.

The portion of the arm affected is determined by the nerves damaged. *Erb-Duchenne paralysis* involves damage to the upper arm (fifth and sixth cervical nerves) and is the most common type. Injury to the eighth cervical and first thoracic nerve roots and the lower portion of the plexus produces the relatively rare *lower arm injury,* whereas the *whole arm type* results from damage to the entire plexus.

With Erb-Duchenne paralysis, the infant's arm lies limply at his side. The elbow is held in extension, with the forearm pronated. The infant is unable to elevate the arm, and the Moro reflex cannot be elicited on the affected side. When lower arm injury occurs, paralysis of the hand and wrist results; complete paralysis of the limb occurs with the whole arm type.

Treatment involves passive range-of-motion exercises to prevent muscle contractures and to restore function. The nurse should carefully instruct the parents in the correct method of performing the exercises and provide for supervised practice sessions. In more severe cases, splinting of the arm is indicated until the edema decreases. The arm is held in a position of abduction and external rotation with the elbow flexed 90°. The "Statue of Liberty" splint is commonly used, although similar results are obtained by attaching a strip of muslin to the head of the crib and tying the other end around the wrist, thereby holding the arm up.

Prognosis is related to the degree of nerve damage resulting from trauma and hemorrhage within the nerve sheath. Complete recovery occurs within a few months with minimal trauma. Moderate trauma may result in some partial paralysis. Recovery is unlikely with severe trauma, and muscle wasting may develop.

Legs and Feet

The legs of the infant should be of equal length, with symmetrical skin folds. *Ortolani's maneuver* is performed to rule out the possibility of congenital hip dysplasia. With the infant supine, the nurse places her thumbs on the inner thighs and her fingers on the outer aspect of the infant's leg from the knee to the head of the femur. The legs are flexed, then abducted and pressed downward. If a click is felt under the index finger, a dislocation exists.

The feet are then examined for evidence of a talipes deformity (clubfoot). Intrauterine position frequently causes the feet to appear to turn inward. If the feet can easily be returned to the midline by manipulation, no treatment is indicated. Further investigation is indicated when the foot will not turn to a midline position or align readily.

The femoral and pedal pulses should be palpated. Absence of pulses in the lower extremities is a classic sign of coarctation of the aorta and requires additional investigation.

Back

With the infant prone, the nurse should examine his back. The spine should appear straight and flat, because the lumbar and sacral curves do not develop until the child begins to sit. The base of the spine is then examined for a dermal sinus. The nevus pilosus ("hairy nerve") is only occasionally found at the base of the spine in newborns, but it is significant because it is frequently associated with spina bifida.

Laboratory Data

Blood values in the infant are different from those in the adult in many respects. Both the hemoglobin and erythrocyte counts are higher because of the nature of fetal circulation. These levels gradually decrease during the first three months after birth, then begin to increase slowly as the child grows to adulthood. Leukocytosis is normal, because the trauma of birth stimulates the production of high levels of neutrophils during the first week of life. Eventually lymphocytes become the predominant type, and the total white blood count decreases. Normal blood values for a full-term infant are as follows:

Hemoglobin	13.7–24 gm/100 ml
RBC	5–7.5 million/mm^3
Hematocrit	43%–65%
WBC	9000–38,000/mm^3
Neutrophils	40%–80%
Eosinophils	2%–3%

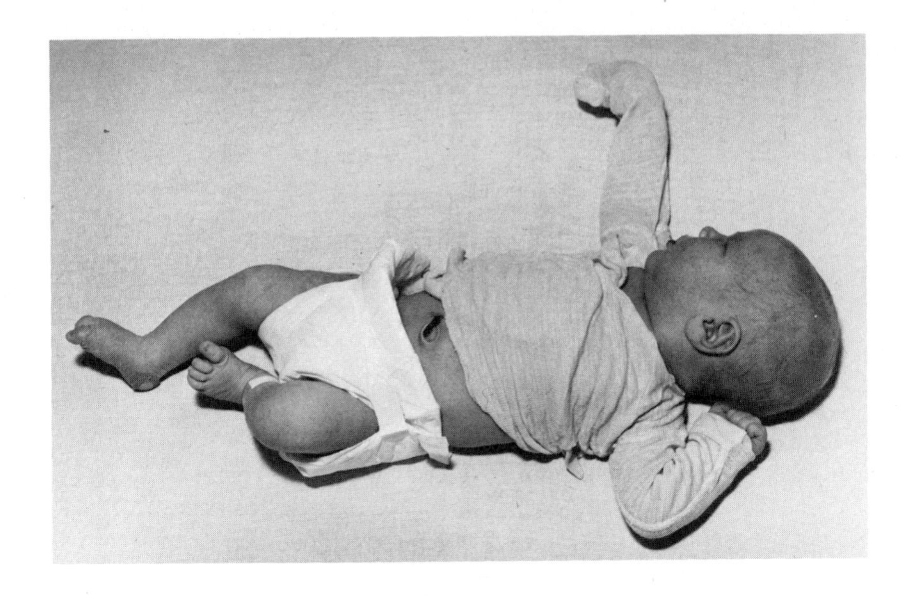

Figure 22–23. Tonic neck reflex.

Lymphocytes	30%–31%
Monocytes	6%–12%
Immature WBC	3%–10%
Platelets	100,000–350,000/mm^3
Reticulocytes	4%–6%

Neurologic Status

Neonatal tremors are common in the full-term infant and must be evaluated to differentiate them from a convulsion. A fine jumping of the muscle is likely to be a central nervous system disorder and requires further evaluation. Tremors may also be related to hypoglycemia or hypocalcemia. Neonatal seizures may consist of no more than chewing or swallowing movements, deviations of the eyes, rigidity, or flaccidity because of central nervous system immaturity.

The central nervous system of the newborn is immature and characterized by a variety of reflexes. Because the newborn's movements are uncoordinated, his methods of communication are limited, and his control of bodily functions drastically limited, the reflexes serve a variety of purposes. Some are protective (blink, gag, sneeze), some aid in feeding (rooting, sucking), and some stimulate human interaction (grasping). His reflexes and general neurologic activity should be carefully assessed.

The most common reflexes found in the normal neonate are the following:

- *Tonic neck reflex (fencer position):* When the infant is in the supine position, if the head is turned to one side, the extremities on the same side straighten, whereas on the opposite side they flex (Figure 22–23). This reflex may not be seen during the early neonatal period, but once it appears it persists until about the third month.
- *Moro reflex:* When the infant is startled by a loud noise or by being lifted slightly above the crib and then suddenly lowered, he straightens his arms and hands outward while his knees flex. Slowly his arms return to his chest, as in an embrace. His fingers spread, forming a C.
- *Grasp reflex:* If the palm is stimulated with a finger or object, the infant grasps and holds it firmly enough to be lifted momentarily from the crib.
- *Rooting reflex:* When the side of the infant's mouth or cheek is touched, he turns toward that side and open his lips to suck (Figure 22–24).
- *Sucking reflex:* When an object is placed in the infant's mouth, a sucking motion begins.

In addition to these reflexes, the infant can blink, yawn, cough, sneeze, and draw back from pain (protective reflexes). The infant can even move a little on his own. When placed on his stomach, he pushes up and tries to crawl *(prone crawl).* When he is held upright with one foot touching a flat surface, he puts one foot in front of the other and walks *(stepping reflex)* (Figure 22–25). This reflex is more pronounced at birth and is lost in one to two months.

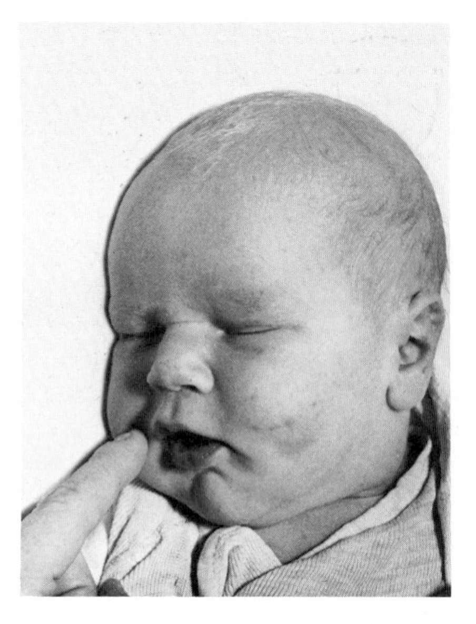

Figure 22-24. Rooting reflex.

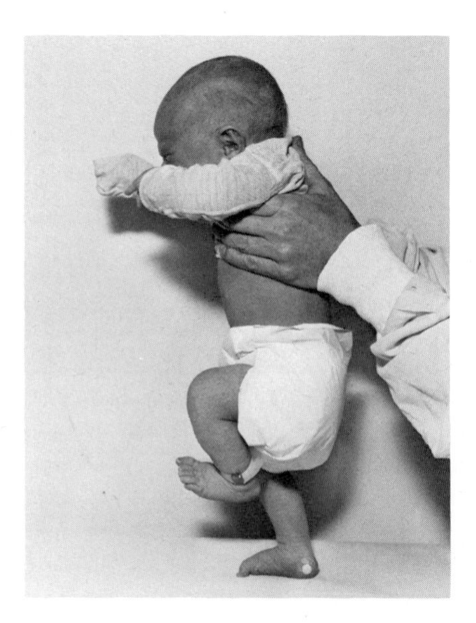

Figure 22-25. Stepping reflex disappears after about one month.

NEONATAL PHYSICAL ASSESSMENT

Following is a guide for systematically assessing the newborn. Normal findings, deviations, and related causes are presented, in correlation with suggested nursing interventions. The findings are based on a full-term neonate.

NEONATAL PHYSICAL ASSESSMENT GUIDE

Assess	Normal findings	Deviations and possible causes*	Nursing interventions[†]
Vital signs			
Blood pressure	At birth: 80-70/40-30 mm Hg Day 10: 100/50 mm Hg (may be unable to measure diastolic pressure with standard sphygmomanometer)	Low BP (hypovolemia, shock)	Monitor BP in all cases of distress, prematurity, or suspected anomaly. With low BP, refer immediately to support adequacy of circulation.
Pulse	120-150 beats/min (if asleep, 70-90/min; if crying, up to 180/min)	Weak pulse (decreased cardiac output) Bradycardia (severe asphyxia)	

*Possible causes of deviations are placed in parentheses.
[†]Nursing interventions are primarily directed toward identified deviations.

NEONATAL PHYSICAL ASSESSMENT GUIDE Cont'd

Assess	Normal findings	Deviations and possible causes*	Nursing interventions†
		Tachycardia (over 160/min at rest) (Infection, CNS)	
Respirations	30-50 respirations/min Synchronization of chest and abdominal movements Diaphragmatic and abdominal breathing Transient tachypnea	Tachypnea (pneumonia, RDS) Rapid, shallow breathing (hypermagnesemia due to large doses given toxemic mothers) Grunting expiratory, subcostal, and substernal retractions, flaring of nares (respiratory distress) Apnea (cold stress, respiratory disorder) Respirations below 30/min (maternal anesthesia or analgesia)	Evaluate for all signs of respiratory distress; confer with physician regarding findings.
Crying	Strong and lusty Moderate tone and pitch Alternate periods of excitability and quietness Cries vary in length from 3-7 min after consoling measures are used	High-pitched, shrill (neurologic disorder) Weak or absent (central nervous system disorder, laryngeal problem)	Discuss infant's use of cry for communication. Assess and record abnormal cries.
Temperature	Rectal: 36.7-37C (98-98.6F) Axilla: 35.5-37.2C (96-99F); 36.8C (98.8F) desired Heavier infants tend to have higher body temperatures	Elevated temperature (room too warm, too much clothing or covers, dehydration, sepsis, brain damage) Subnormal temperature (infection, brain stem involvement, cold) Swings of more than 2F from one reading to next or subnormal temperature (infection)	Attempt to identify cause; notify physician of elevation. Counsel parents on possible causes of elevated or low temperatures, appropriate home care measures, when to call their physician. Teach parents how to take rectal temperature. Assess ability to read thermometer. Provide information as needed.
Weight	2950-3515 gm (6½-7¾ lb)	<2748 gm (6 lb) = SGA or premature infant >4050 gm (9 lb) = LGA (infants of diabetic mothers)	Plot weight and gestational age to identify high-risk infants. Ascertain genetic predisposition for body build. Counsel parents regarding appropriate caloric intake.

*Possible causes of deviations are placed in parentheses.
†Nursing interventions are primarily directed toward identified deviations.

NEONATAL PHYSICAL ASSESSMENT GUIDE Cont'd

Assess	Normal findings	Deviations and possible causes*	Nursing interventions†
	Within first 3-4 days, normal weight loss of 5-10% Larger babies tend to lose more due to greater fluid loss in proportion to birth weight	Loss greater than 5%-10% (small fluid intake, loss of meconium and urine, feeding difficulties)	
Length	45 cm (18 in.) to 52.3 cm (20.5 in.) Grow 10 cm (4 in.) during first 3 months or approximately 2.5 cm (1 in.)/month for next 6 months	Too short (congenital dwarf) Too long Short long bones proximally (achondroplasia) Short long bones distally (Ellis-Van Creveld)	Assess for other signs of dwarfism. Determine other signs of skeletal system adequacy. Plot progress at subsequent well-baby visits.
Posture	Body usually flexed, hands tightly clenched, neck appears short as chin rests on chest	Only extension noted, inability to move from midline (trauma, hypoxia, immaturity) Constant motion	Record spontaneity of motor activity and symmetry of movements. Further evaluate if parents express concern about infant's movement patterns. Describe and accurately record parents' report. Reassure parents about the appropriateness of their observations and concerns.
	Appearance: prominent abdomen with sloping shoulders, narrow hips, rounded chest In breech deliveries, feet are usually dorsiflexed		
Skin			
Color	Color consistent with racial background Pink-tinged or ruddy color over face, trunk, extremities Common variations: acrocyanosis, periorbital cyanosis, circumoral cyanosis, or harlequin color change	Pallor of face, conjunctiva (anemia, hypothermia, anoxia) Beefy red (hypoglycemia, immature vasomotor reflexes) Meconium staining (fetal distress) Icterus (hemolytic reaction from blood incompatibility, sepsis)	Discuss with parents common skin color variations to allay fears. Document extent and time of occurrence of color change. Obtain Hgb and HCT values. Perform differential diagnosis to determine whether deviation is physiologic or pathologic jaundice or carotenemia.

*Possible causes of deviations are placed in parentheses.
†Nursing interventions are primarily directed toward identified deviations.

NEONATAL PHYSICAL ASSESSMENT GUIDE Cont'd

Assess	Normal findings	Deviations and possible causes*	Nursing interventions†
	Mottled when undressed	Cyanosis (choanal atresia, central nervous system damage or trauma, respiratory or cardiac problem)	Determine degree of cyanosis and causative condition. Refer to physician.
	Minor bruising over buttock in breech presentation and over eyes and forehead in facial presentations		
Texture	Smooth, soft, flexible; may have dry and peeling hands and feet	Generalized cracked or peeling skin (SGA or postmaturity, blood incompatibility, metabolic kidney dysfunction) Scalines (eczema on cheeks, behind ears, on popliteal and antecubital areas)	Perform differential diagnosis.
		Seborrhea-dermatitis (cradle cap) Large amount of lanugo (prematurity) Rough or dry (frequent bathing) Absence of vernix Yellow vernix (bilirubin staining)	Instruct parents to shampoo the scalp and anterior fontanelle area daily. Soap should be used and oil avoided.
Turgor: pinch skin (lower abdomen) in "tent shape"	Elastic, returns to normal shape after pinching	Maintains tent shape (dehydration)	Assess for other signs and symptoms of dehydration.
Pigmentation	Clear; milia are located across bridge of nose or on chin and disappear within a few weeks		Advise parents not to pinch or prick these pimplelike areas.
	Café-au-lait spots (1-2)	6 or more (neurologic disorder such as Recklinghausen's disease, cutaneous neurofibramatosis)	
	Mongolian spots or macular bluish black pigmentation over lumbar dorsal area and buttocks; common in ethnic infants of color	Xanthoma (benign or may be associated with abnormal metabolism of lipids)	Assure parents of normalcy of this pigmentation. Reassure parents that plaques will disappear in a few weeks.

*Possible causes of deviations are placed in parentheses.
†Nursing interventions are primarily directed toward identified deviations.

NEONATAL PHYSICAL ASSESSMENT GUIDE Cont'd

Assess	Normal findings	Deviations and possible causes*	Nursing interventions[†]
	Erythema neonatorum toxicum	Impetigo (group A β-hemolytic streptococcus or *Staphylococcus aureus* infection)	If impetigo occurs, instruct parents about hand-washing and linen precautions during home care.
	Telangiectatic nevi		
	Birthmarks	Hemangiomas: Nevus flammeus (port-wine stain) Nevus vascularus (strawberry hemangioma) Cavernous hemangiomas	Collaborate with physician. Counsel parents about birthmark's progression to allay misconceptions. Record size and shape of hemangiomas. Refer for follow-up at well-baby clinic.
	Moles	Any mole or growth that changes in color or character	Refer to physician.
		Rashes (infection)	Assess location and type of rash (macular, papular, vesicular). Obtain history of onset, prenatal history, and related signs and symptoms.
	Petechiae of head or neck (breech presentation)	Generalized petechiae (clotting abnormalities)	Refer to physician.
Head			
General appearance, size, movement	Round, symmetrical, and moves easily from left to right and up and down; soft, pliable	Asymmetrical, flattened occiput on either side of head (plagiocephaly)	Instruct parents to change infant's sleeping positions frequently.
		Head held at angle (torticollis)	
		Unable to move head side-to-side (neurologic trauma)	Determine adequacy of all neurologic signs.
	Circumference: 33-35 cm (13-14 in.); 2 cm greater than chest circumference	Extreme differences in size may be: microencephaly (Cornelia DeLange syndrome, CID, rubella, toxoplasmosis, chromosome abnormalities), hydrocephaly (meningomyelocele, achondroplasia), anencephaly (neural tube defect) Head is 3 cm or more larger than chest circumference (prematurity, hydrocephaly)	Measure circumference from occiput to frontal area, using metal or paper tape. Measure chest circumference using metal or paper tape and compare to head circumference.

*Possible causes of deviations are placed in parentheses.
[†]Nursing interventions are primarily directed toward identified deviations.

NEONATAL PHYSICAL ASSESSMENT GUIDE Cont'd

Assess	Normal findings	Deviations and possible causes*	Nursing interventions[†]
	One-fourth of body size		Record measurements on growth chart.
	Size increases 2 in. during first 4 months of life		Reevaluate at well-baby visits.
	Common variations: Molding—overriding of cranial bones during delivery Breech and cesarean section babies—heads are round and well shaped	Cephalhematomas (trauma during delivery, persists up to 3 weeks) Caput succedaneum (long labor and delivery, disappears in 1 week)	Reassure parents regarding common manifestations due to birth process and when they should disappear.
Fontanelles Palpation of juncture of cranial bones	Anterior fontanelle: 3-4 cm long by 2-3 cm wide, diamond shaped, closes within 18 months	Overlapping of anterior fontanelle (malnourished or premature infant)	Discuss normal closure times with parents and care of "soft spots" to allay misconceptions.
	Posterior fontanelle: 1-2 cm at birth, triangle shaped, closes in 8-12 weeks	Premature closure of sutures (craniostenosis) Late closure (hydrocephaly)	Refer to physician. Observe for signs and symptoms of hydrocephaly.
Pulsation	Slight pulsation	Moderate to severe pulsation (vascular problems)	Refer to physician.
	Moderate bulging noted with crying or pulsations with heartbeat	Bulging (increased intracranial pressure, meningitis) Sunken (dehydration)	Evaluate hydration status.
Hair			
Texture	Smooth with fine texture variations (Note: variations dependent on ethnic background)	Coarse, brittle, dry hair (hypothyroidism) White forelock (Waardenburg's syndrome)	Instruct parents regarding routine care of hair and scalp.
Distribution	Scalp hair high over eyebrows (Spanish-Mexican hairline begins midforehead and extends down back of neck)	Low forehead and posterior hairlines may indicate chromosomal disorders	Assess for other signs of chromosomal aberrations. Refer to physician.
Face	Symmetrical, normal hairline, eyebrows and eyelashes present; symmetry of facial movement; chin recessed and nose flattened; milia present on nose and forehead		Assess and record symmetry of all parts, shape, regularity of features, sameness or differences in features.
Spacing of features	Eyes at same level; nostrils equal size; fullness of cheeks and sucking pads present	Eyes wide apart—ocular hypertelorism (Aperts syndrome, cri-du-chat, Turner's syndrome)	Observe for other signs and symptoms indicative of disease states or chromosomal aberrations.

*Possible causes of deviations are placed in parentheses.
[†]Nursing interventions are primarily directed toward identified deviations.

NEONATAL PHYSICAL ASSESSMENT GUIDE Cont'd

Assess	Normal findings	Deviations and possible causes*	Nursing interventions†
	Lips equal on both sides of midline	Abnormal face (Down's syndrome, cretinism, gargoylism)	
	Chin recedes when compared to other bones of face	Abnormally small jaw—micrognathia (Pierre Robin syndrome, Treacher Collins syndrome)	Initiate surgical consultation and referral.
	Face sensitive to light, touch, warmth, cold	Lack of facial sensation (fifth and seventh cranial nerve damage)	Initiate neurologic assessment and consultations.
Movement	Makes facial grimaces	Inability to suck, grimace, and close eyelids (cranial nerve injury)	
	Symmetrical when resting and crying	Asymmetry (paralysis of facial cranial nerve)	
Frontal and maxillary sinuses	Frontal—absent at birth Maxillary—nontender		
Eyes			
General placement and appearance	Bright and clear; even placement; slight nystagmus	Gross nystagmus (damage to third, fourth, and sixth cranial nerves)	
	Concomitant strabismus	Constant and fixed strabismus	Reassure parents that strabismus is considered normal up to 6 months.
	Moves in all directions		
	Blue or slate blue-gray (permanent color established by age 3 months)	Lack of pigmentation (albinism)	Refer to physician.
		Brushfield spots (may indicate Down's syndrome)	Assess for other signs of Down's syndrome.
	Brown color at birth in ethnic babies of color		
Eyelids			
Position	Above pupils but within iris, no drooping	Elevation or retraction of upper lid (hyperthyroidism) "Setting sun" (hydrocephaly)	Assess for signs of hydrocephaly and hypothyroidism.
		Ptosis (congenital or paralysis of oculomotor muscle)	Evaluate interference with vision in subsequent well-baby visits.
	Eyes on parallel plane	Upward slant in non-Orientals (Down's syndrome)	Assess for other signs of Down's syndrome.
	Epicanthal folds in Oriental babies and 20% of white newborns	Epicanthal folds (Down's syndrome, cri-du-chat)	
Movement	Blink reflex in response to light stimulus		

*Possible causes of deviations are placed in parentheses.
†Nursing interventions are primarily directed toward identified deviations.

NEONATAL PHYSICAL ASSESSMENT GUIDE Cont'd

Assess	Normal findings	Deviations and possible causes*	Nursing interventions†
Palpation and inspection for infection	Edematous for first few days of life, resulting from delivery and instillation of silver nitrate (chemical conjunctivitis)	Purulent drainage (infection) Infectious conjunctivitis (staphylococcus or gram-negative organisms)	Refer to physician.
	No lumps or redness	Marginal blepharitis (lid edges red, crusted, scaly)	Evaluate infant for seborrheic dermatitis; scales can be removed easily.
Cornea and retina	Clear Circular red reflex Corneal reflex present	Ulceration (herpes infection) Large cornea or corneas of unequal size (congenital glaucoma) Clouding, opacity of lens (cataract)	Refer to ophthalmologist.
Sclera	May appear bluish in newborn, then white; slightly brownish color frequent in blacks	True blue sclera (osteogenesis imperfecta)	Refer to physician.
Pupils	Pupils are equal in size, round, and react to light by accommodation	Anisocoria—unequal pupils (CNS damage) Dilatation or constriction (intercranial damage, retinoblastoma glaucoma) Pupils nonreactive to light or accommodation (brain injury)	Refer for neurologic examination.
	Slight nystagmus in infant who has not learned to focus Pupil light reflex demonstrated at birth or by 3 weeks of age	Nystagmus (labyrinthine disturbance, CNS disorder)	
Conjunctiva	Chemical conjunctivitis (subsides in 2–7 days)	Pale color (anemia)	Obtain hematocrit and hemoglobin.
	Palpebral conjunctiva (red but not hyperemic)	Inflammation or edema (infection, blocked tear duct)	Perform differential diagnosis.
	Subconjunctival hemorrhage common in newborns (disappears within 10 days)		
Vision	20/150 plus some degree of color discrimination and pattern Tracks moving object to midline	Cataracts (congenital infection)	Record any questions about visual acuity and initiate follow-up evaluation at first well-baby checkup.

*Possible causes of deviations are placed in parentheses.
†Nursing interventions are primarily directed toward identified deviations.

NEONATAL PHYSICAL ASSESSMENT GUIDE Cont'd

Assess	Normal findings	Deviations and possible causes*	Nursing interventions†
	Fixes focus on objects at a distance of about 7½ in.; may be difficult to evaluate in newborn		
Lashes and lacrimal glands	Presence of lashes (lashes may be absent in premature infants)	No lashes on inner two-thirds of lid (Treacher Collins syndrome) Bushy lashes (Hurler's syndrome) Long lashes (Cornelia DeLange syndrome)	
	Cry commonly tearless because duct not functional until 2-4 weeks of age	Excessive tearing (plugged lacrimal duct, natal narcotic abstinence syndrome)	Refer to ophthalmologist if tearing is excessive before third month of life.
Nose			
Appearance			
External nasal aspects	May appear flattened as a result of delivery process	Continued flat or broad bridge of nose (Down's syndrome)	Arrange consultation with specialist.
	Small and narrow in midline; even placement in relationship to eyes and mouth	Low bridge of nose, beaklike nose (Apert's, Treacher Collins syndrome) Upturned (Cornelia DeLange syndrome)	Initiate evaluation of chromosomal abnormalities.
	Patent nares bilaterally (nose breathers)	Blockage of nares (mucus and/or secretions) Flaring nares (respiratory distress) Choanal atresia	
Internal nasal aspects	Pink and firm mucous membranes		
	Septum midline and without polyps or tumors	Deviated or perforated septum; tumors or polyps of septum	Collaborate with physician.
	No swelling or nasal discharge	Swelling and erythema (infection)	Note and record characteristics of nasal discharge.
Smelling and breathing abilities	Identifies odors; appears to smell breast milk Breathes through nose (does not open mouth to breathe) Sneezing common to clear nasal passages	No response to stimulating odors	Inspect for obstructions of nares.

*Possible causes of deviations are placed in parentheses.
†Nursing interventions are primarily directed toward identified deviations.

NEONATAL PHYSICAL ASSESSMENT GUIDE Cont'd

Assess	Normal findings	Deviations and possible causes*	Nursing interventions[†]
Mouth			
Function of facial, hypoglossal, glossopharyngeal, and vagus nerves	Symmetry of movement and strength	Mouth draws to one side (transient seventh cranial nerve paralysis due to pressure in utero or trauma during delivery, congenital paralysis)	Initiate neurologic consultation. Administer eye care if eye on affected side is unable to close.
		Fishlike shape	
	Adequate salivation	(Treacher Collins syndrome)	
	Presence of gag and swallowing and sucking reflexes	Suppressed or absent reflexes	Evaluate other neurologic functions of these nerves.
	Tongue midline	Deviations from midline (cranial nerve damage)	
Palate (soft and hard)	Hard palate dome-shaped	High-steepled palate (Treacher Collins syndrome)	
	Uvula midline with symmetrical movement of soft palate		
	Palate intact, sucks well when stimulated	Clefts in either hard or soft palate (polygenic disorder)	Initiate a surgical consultation referral.
	Epithelial (Epstein's) pearls appear on mucosa		Assure parents that these are normal in newborn and will disappear at 2 or 3 months of age.
Pharynx	Unobstructed, with no drainage in back of throat		
	No exudate on tonsils	Exudate present (infection)	Examine for other signs of infection.
	Esophagus patent; some drooling common in newborn	Excessive drooling or bubbling (esophageal atresia)	Test for patency of esophagus.
Tongue	Free-moving in all directions, midline	Lack of movement or asymmetrical movement	Further assess neurologic functions.
		Tongue-tied	Test reflex elevation of tongue when depressed with tongue blade. Check for signs of weakness or deviation.
	Pink color, smooth to rough texture, noncoated	White cheesy coating (thrush)	Differentiate between thrush and milk curds.
		Tongue has deep ridges	Reassure parents that tongue pattern may change from day to day.
	Tongue proportional to mouth	Large tongue with short frenulum (cretinism, Down's and other syndromes)	

*Possible causes of deviations are placed in parentheses.
[†]Nursing interventions are primarily directed toward identified deviations.

NEONATAL PHYSICAL ASSESSMENT GUIDE Cont'd

Assess	Normal findings	Deviations and possible causes*	Nursing interventions†
	Sucking and rooting reflexes present		
	Discriminates pleasant from unpleasant tastes	Absence of reaction of tongue to various stimuli (seventh cranial nerve damage)	Initiate neurologic collaboration.
Gums	Dark pink, firm, smooth	Inflamed (infection) Pallor (anemia) Precocious teeth	Obtain Hgb and HCT.
	Dark (melanotic) line along gums in blacks		
Cheeks	Fat pads in cheeks for sucking		
Lips	Labial tubercle (pink, sucking blisters) Mucosa of lips well demarcated from surrounding skin Saliva scant		
	Lips fused in midline	Cleft lip (polygenic disorder)	Counsel parents on special feeding techniques that may be necessary.
Ears			
Appearance	May be crumpled or flattened against skull Well-formed cartilage Firm pinna and incurving of upper pinna Rapid recoil of both ears	Preauricular skin tags and sinuses Decreased length (Down's syndrome) Unilateral abnormality accompanied by microsomia (Goldenhar syndrome) Bilateral abnormalities (Treacher Collins syndrome)	Assess for other abnormalities.
	Normal size in comparison to head	Large, protruding ears	Reassure parents about protruding ears.
Placement	Ears set at same level on both sides of head		
	Pinna inserted on head on horizontal plane to outer canthus of eye	Low-set (chromosomal abnormalities such as trisomy 13 or 18, bilateral renal agenesis)	Determine other signs of congenital malformations, particularly renal abnormalities. Embryologically the ear is formed at the same time as the kidney so it is important to assess kidney function.

*Possible causes of deviations are placed in parentheses.
†Nursing interventions are primarily directed toward identified deviations.

NEONATAL PHYSICAL ASSESSMENT GUIDE Cont'd

Assess	Normal findings	Deviations and possible causes*	Nursing interventions†
			Evaluate in well-baby clinic to assess developmental delays. Refer to physician.
External ear	Without lesions, cysts, or nodules	Nodules, cysts, or sinus tracts in front of ear Adherent earlobes	Evaluate characteristics of lesions. Counsel parents to clean external ear with washcloth only; discourage use of cotton-tip applicators.
		Preauricular skin tags	Refer to physician for ligation.
Inner canal and tympanic membrane	Bony landmarks present (may not be visible)	Bulging (infection) Discharge, disagreeable odor (infection)	Consult with physician.
	Tympanic membrane light color, pearly gray Translucent, intact	Ruptured tympanic membrane	Remove wax and vernix debris with wire loop or curette under constant visualization.
Hearing	With first cry, eustachian tubes are cleared		
	Absence of all risk factors	Presence of one or more risk factors	Assess history of risk factors for hearing loss.
	Attends to sounds; sudden or loud noise elicits Moro reflex	No response to sound stimuli (deafness)	Test for Moro reflex.
Neck			
Appearance	Short, straight, creased with skin folds	Abnormally short neck (Turner's syndrome) Arching or inability to flex neck (meningitis, congenital anomaly)	Complete differential diagnosis in collaboration with physician.
	Posterior neck lacks loose extra folds of skin	Webbing of neck (Turner's syndrome, Down's syndrome, trisomy (18))	Collect more data indicative of chromosomal aberrations.
	Head moves freely from side to side	Neck rigidity (congenital torticollis, eleventh cranial nerve damage)	
	Sternocleidomastoid muscle should be symmetrical on both sides If infant is held upright and body tilted, head returns to upright position		
Thyroid	Thyroid not usually palpable in newborn No masses		Palpate for lymph nodes and masses.

*Possible causes of deviations are placed in parentheses.
†Nursing interventions are primarily directed toward identified deviations.

NEONATAL PHYSICAL ASSESSMENT GUIDE Cont'd

Assess	Normal findings	Deviations and possible causes*	Nursing interventions†
Clavicles	Straight and intact	Knot or lump on clavicle (fracture during difficult delivery)	Obtain detailed labor and delivery history. Apply figure-8 bandage.
	Moro reflex elicitable	Unilaternal Moro reflex reponse on unaffected side (fracture of clavicle, brachial palsy, Erb-Duchenne syndrome)	Collaborate with physician.
	Bilateral movement of both shoulders	Hypoplasia	
Chest			
Appearance and size	Circumference: 32.5 cm, 1-2 cm less than head Wider than it is long		Measure at level of nipples after exhalation.
	Normal shape without depressed or prominent sternum	Funnel chest (congenital or associated with Marfan's syndrome)	Determine adequacy of other respiratory and circulatory signs.
	Lower end of sternum (xiphoid cartilage) may be protruding, is less apparent after several weeks	Continued protrusion of xiphoid cartilage (Marfan's syndrome, "pigeon chest")	Assess for other signs and symptoms of various syndromes.
	Sternum 8 cm long	Barrel chest	
Expansion and retraction	Bilateral expansion	Unequal chest expansion (pneumonia, pheumothorax respiratory distress)	Collect more data regarding respiratory effort if chest expansion is unequal (regularity, flaring of nares, difficulty on both inspiration and expiration).
	No intracostal, subcostal, or suprasternal retraction	Retractions (respiratory distress)	Record and consult physician.
Percussion	Decreased percussion, note of dullness found over liver, diaphragm, heart, with these areas well demarcated	Dullness in lung fields (consolidation of lungs, atelectasis)	Examine chest thoroughly using techniques of inspection, palpation, and auscultation.
		Hyperresonance of chest (pneumonia, pneumothorax, distended stomach)	Report positive findings to physician.
Auscultation	Breath sounds are louder in infants Heard bilaterally	Decreased breath sounds (decreased respiratory activity, atelectasis, pneumothorax)	Perform complete physical exam and collaborate with physician regarding positive findings.
	Chest and axilla clear on crying	Increased breath sounds are heard with resolving pneumonia	

*Possible causes of deviations are placed in parentheses.
†Nursing interventions are primarily directed toward identified deviations.

NEONATAL PHYSICAL ASSESSMENT GUIDE Cont'd

Assess	Normal findings	Deviations and possible causes*	Nursing interventions†
Bronchial breath sounds (heard where trachea and bronchi closest to chest wall, above sternum and between scapulae)	Bronchial sounds bilaterally Air entry clear Rales may indicate normal newborn atelectasis Cough reflex absent at birth, appears in 2 or more days	Adventitious or abnormal sounds (respiratory diseases or distress)	
Determination of point of maximal impulse (PMI)	Difficult to assess exact PMI in infant up to 2 years old, but usually lateral to midclavicular line at third or fourth interspace	Malpositioning (enlargement, abnormal placement, pneumothorax, dextrocardia, diaphragmatic hernia)	Initiate cardiac evaluation.
Heart			
Auscultation and palpation	Location: lies horizontally, with left border extending to left of midclavicle		
	Regular rhythm and rate	Arrhythmia (anoxia) Tachycardia, bradycardia	All arrhythmia and gallop rhythms should be referred to physician.
	Functional murmurs No thrills	Location of murmurs (possible congenital cardiac anomaly)	Evaluate murmur: location, timing, and duration; observe for accompanying cardiac pathology symptoms, and ascertain any family history.
Trachea (palpate from top to bottom with thumb and index fingers)	Slightly right of midline	Deviated left or right (pneumothorax, tumor of chest or neck)	
Rib cage and diaphragm	Horizontal groove at diaphragm shows flaring of rib cage to mild degree	Harrison's groove with marked flaring (vitamin D deficiency) Inadequacy of respiration movement	Initiate cardiopulmonary evaluation.
Breasts	Breasts flat with symmetrical nipple Breast tissue diameter 5 cm or more at term Distance between nipples 8 cm	Lack of breast tissue (prematurity or SGA)	
	Breast engorgement occurs on third day of life, liquid discharge may be expressed in term infants	Breast abscesses	Reassure parents of normalcy of breast engorgement.
	Nipples	Supernumerary nipple 5-6 cm below and	

*Possible causes of deviations are placed in parentheses.
†Nursing interventions are primarily directed toward identified deviations.

NEONATAL PHYSICAL ASSESSMENT GUIDE Cont'd

Assess	Normal findings	Deviations and possible causes*	Nursing interventions†
		medial to true nipples Dark-colored nipples	
Abdomen			
Appearance	Cylindrical with some protrusion; appears large in relation to pelvis; some laxness of abdominal muscles No cyanosis, few vessels seen Observe for synchronous movement with breathing	Distention, shiny abdomen with engorged vessels (gastrointestinal abnormalities, infection, congenital megacolon) Scaphoid appearance (diaphragmatic hernia) Increased or decreased peristalsis (duodenal stenosis, small bowel obstruction)	Examine abdomen thoroughly for mass or organomegaly. Collaborate with physician; assess other signs and symptoms of obstruction.
	Diastasis recti—common in black infants	Localized flank bulging (enlarged kidneys, ascites, or absent abdominal muscles)	
Palpation	Nontender	Tense abdomen with marked rigidity or resistance to pressure (infection)	Take temperature and assess other signs and symptoms. Consult with surgeon.
	No palpable masses	Solid masses (Wilm's tumor)	
Umbilicus	No protrusion of umbilicus and no umbilical hernia Protrusion of umbilicus common in black infants Bluish white color Cutis navel (umbilical cord projects); granulation tissue in navel	Umbilical hernia Patent urachus (congenital malformation) Omphalocele Gastroschisis Redness or exudate around cord (infection) Yellow discoloration (hemolytic disease, meconium staining)	Measure umbilical hernia by palpating the opening and record. It should close by 1 year of age. If not, refer to physician. Instruct parents on cord care and hygiene.
	Two arteries and one vein apparent Begins drying 1–2 hours after birth, blackens by 3–5 days, sloughs off by 7–9 days No bleeding	Single umbilical artery (congenital anomalies)	
Liver	Liver 1–2 cm below right costal margin	Enlarged liver (sepsis, erythroblastosis)	Note and record size, consistency, and tenderness.
Spleen	Tip under left costal margin	Enlarged spleen (trauma)	
Kidney	Posterior flank firm, oval mass, not enlarged, less	Displaced kidney (Wilm's tumor, neuroblastoma,	Initiate nephrologic consultation.

*Possible causes of deviations are placed in parentheses.
†Nursing interventions are primarily directed toward identified deviations.

NEONATAL PHYSICAL ASSESSMENT GUIDE Cont'd

Assess	Normal findings	Deviations and possible causes*	Nursing interventions[†]
	commonly palpable	polycryptic kidney, agenesis)	
Auscultation and percussion	Soft bowel sounds heard shoftly after birth; heard every 10-30 sec	Bowel sounds in chest (diaphragmatic hernia)	Collaborate with physician.
		Absence of bowel sounds	
	Normal peristalsis	Hyperperistalsis (intestinal obstruction)	Assess for other signs of dehydration and/or infection.
	Abdomen has tympanic sound except over liver and spleen (dull sound)	Increased dull sound (mass or organomegaly)	Examine abdomen thoroughly by light and deep palpation.
Femoral pulses	Palpable, equal, bilateral	Absent or diminished femoral pulses (coarctation of aorta)	Monitor blood pressure in upper and lower extremities.
Inguinal area	No bulges along inguinal area	Inguinal hernia	Collaborate with physician.
	No inguinal lymph nodes felt		
Bladder	Percusses 1-4 cm above symphysis	Failure to void within 24 hours after birth	
	Emptied about 3 hours after birth; if not, at time of birth	Exposure of bladder mucosa (extrophy of bladder)	
	Urine—nonoffensive, mild odor	Foul odor (infection)	
Genitals	Gender clearly delineated	Ambiguous genitals	Refer for genetic consultation.
Male			
Penis	Slender in appearance, 2.5 cm long, 1 cm wide at birth	Micropenis (congenital anomaly)	
	Normal urinary orifice, urethral meatus at tip of penis	Meatal atresia	Observe and record first voiding.
		Hypospadius, epispadius	Collaborate with physician in presence of abnormality.
	Noninflamed urethral opening	Urethritis (infection)	Palpate for enlarged inguinal lymph nodes and record painful micturition.
	Foreskin adheres to glans, prepuce can be retracted beyond urethral opening	Ulceration of meatal opening	Evaluate whether ulcer is due to diaper rash. Counsel regarding care.
		Infection, inflammation	
	Uncircumcised foreskin tight for 2-3 months	Phimosis—if still tight after 3 months	Instruct parents to retract foreskin gently for cleaning at monthly intervals after 4 months of age.

*Possible causes of deviations are placed in parentheses.
[†]Nursing interventions are primarily directed toward identified deviations.

NEONATAL PHYSICAL ASSESSMENT GUIDE Cont'd

Assess	Normal findings	Deviations and possible causes*	Nursing interventions[†]
	Circumcised Erectile tissue present		Teach parents how to care for circumcision.
Scrotum	Skin loose and hanging or tight and small; extensive rugae		
	Scrotum of normal size	Large scrotum containing fluid (hydrocele)	Shine a light through scrotum (transilluminate) to verify diagnosis.
	Normal skin color	Red, shiny scrotal skin (orchitis)	
	Scrotal discoloration common in breech		
Testes	Descended by birth; not consistently found in scrotum	Undescended testes (cryptorchidism)	If testes cannot be felt in scrotum, gently palpate femoral, inguinal, perineal, and abdominal areas for presence.
	Testes size 1.5-2 cm at birth	Enlarged testes (tumor) Small testes (Klinefelter's syndrome or adrenal hyperplasia)	Refer and collaborate with physician for further diagnostic studies.
Female			
Mons	Normal skin color; area pigmented in dark-skinned races		
	Labia majora cover labia minora, symmetrical size appropriate for gestational age	Hematoma, lesions	Evaluate recent trauma.
Clitoris	Normally large in newborn Edema and bruising in breech delivery	Hypertrophy (hermaphroditism)	
Vagina	Urinary meatus and vaginal orifice visible (0.5 cm circumference)	Inflammation; erythema and discharge (urethritis)	Collect urine specimen for laboratory examination.
	Vaginal tag or hymenal tag, which disappears in a few weeks	Congenital absence of vagina	Refer to physician.
	Discharge: smegma under labia	Foul-smelling discharge (infection)	Collect data and further evaluate reason for discharge.
	Bloody or mucoid discharge	Excessive vaginal bleeding (blood coagulation defect)	
Buttocks and anus	Buttocks symmetrical	Pilonidal dimple	Examine for possible sinus. Instruct parents about cleansing this area.

*Possible causes of deviations are placed in parentheses.
[†]Nursing interventions are primarily directed toward identified deviations.

NEONATAL PHYSICAL ASSESSMENT GUIDE Cont'd

Assess	Normal findings	Deviations and possible causes*	Nursing interventions†
	Anus patent and passage of meconium within 24-48 hours after birth	Imperforate anus, rectal atresia (congenital gastrointestinal defect)	Evaluate extent of problems. Initiate surgical consultation. Perform digital examination to ascertain patency.
	No fissures, tears, or skin tags	Fissures	
Extremities and trunk	Short and generally flexed; extremities move symmetrically through range of motion but lack full extension	Unilateral or absence of movement (spinal cord involvement) Fetal position continued or limp (anoxia, central nervous system problems, hypoglycemia)	
	All joints move spontaneously; good muscle tone, of flexor type, birth to 2 months	Spasticity when infant begins using extensors (cerebral palsy, lack of muscle tone, "floppy baby" syndrome)	Collaborate with physician.
Arms	Equal in length Bilateral movement Flexed when quiet	Brachial palsy (difficult delivery) Erb-Duchenne paralysis Muscle weakness Absence of limb or change of size (phocomelia, amelia)	
Hands	Normal number of fingers and size of hands	Polydactyly (Ellis-Van Creveld syndrome) Syndactyly – one limb (developmental anomaly) Syndactyly – both limbs (genetic component)	Collect data to rule out possible syndromes.
	Normal palmar crease	Simian line on palm (Down's syndrome)	
	Nails present and extend beyond fingertips in term infant	Short fingers and broad hand (Hurler's syndrome) Cyanosis and clubbing (cardiac anomalies) Nails long (postmature)	
Spine	C-shaped spine Flat and straight when prone Slight lumbar lordosis Easily flexed and intact when palpated At least half of back devoid of lanugo	Spina bifida occulta (nevus pitosus) Dermal sinus Myelomeningocele Head lag, limp, floppy trunk (neurologic problems)	Evaluate extent of neurologic damage; initiate care of spinal opening.

*Possible causes of deviations are placed in parentheses.
†Nursing interventions are primarily directed toward identified deviations.

NEONATAL PHYSICAL ASSESSMENT GUIDE Cont'd

Assess	Normal findings	Deviations and possible causes*	Nursing interventions†
	Full-term infant in ventral suspension should hold head 45°, back straight		
Hips	No signs of instability No resistance to hip abduction Hips abduct to more than 60° Iliac crests are equal	Sensation of abnormal movement, jerk, or snap of hip dislocation	Examine all newborn infants for dislocated hip prior to discharge from hospital. If this is suspected, refer to orthopedist for further evaluation. Reassess at well-baby visits.
Legs	Both legs equal in length Legs shorter than arms at birth Legs one-third overall length of body when infant supine with legs flexed at knees	Shortened leg (dislocated hips)	Refer to orthopedist for evaluation. Counsel parents regarding symptoms of concern and discuss therapy.
Inguinal and buttock skin creases	Symmetrical inguinal and buttock creases	Asymmetry	Refer to orthopedist for evaluation; counsel parents regarding symptoms of concern and therapy.
Feet	Foot is in straight line Postional clubfoot—based on position in utero Fat pads and creases on soles of feet	Talipes equinovarus (true clubfoot)	Discuss differences between positional and true clubfoot with parents. Teach parents passive manipulation of foot. Refer to orthopedist if not corrected by 3 months of age.
Arches	Pes planus (flatfoot) normal under 3 years of age		Reassure parents that flatfeet are normal in infant.
Neurologic—muscular			
Motor function	Symmetrical movement and strength in all extremities	Limp, flaccid, or hypertonic (central nervous system disorders, infection, dehydration)	Appraise infant's posture and motor functions by observing activities and motor characteristics.
	May be jerky or have brief twitchings	Tremors (hypoglycemia, hypocalcemia, infection, neurologic damage)	Evaluate electrolyte imbalance and neurologic functioning.
	Head lag not over 45°	Delayed or abnormal development (prematurity, neurologic involvement)	
	Neck control adequate to maintain head erect briefly	Asymmetry of tone or strength	

*Possible causes of deviations are placed in parentheses.
†Nursing interventions are primarily directed toward identified deviations.

NEONATAL PHYSICAL ASSESSMENT GUIDE Cont'd

Assess	Normal findings	Deviations and possible causes*	Nursing interventions†
Reflexes			
Moro	Response to sudden movement or loud noise should be one of symmetrical extension and abduction of arms with fingers extended; then return to normal relaxed flexion Fingers form a C Present at birth, disappears at 1–4 months of age	Asymmetry of body response (fractured clavicle, injury to brachial plexus) Consistent absence (brain damage)	Discuss normalcy of this reflex in response to loud noises and/or sudden movements.
Sucking and rooting	Turns in direction of stimulus to cheek or mouth; opens mouth and begins to suck; difficult to elicit after feeding; disappears by 7 months of age Sucking is adequate for nutritional intake and meeting oral stimulation needs; disappears by 12 months	Poor sucking or easily fatiguable (prematurity, breast-fed infants of barbiturate-addicted mothers) Absence of response (prematurity, neurologic involvement, depressed infants)	Observe infant during feeding and counsel parents about mutuality of feeding experience and infant's responses.
Palmar grasp	Fingers grasp adult finger when palm is stimulated and hold momentarily; lessens at 3–4 months of age	Asymmetry of response (neurologic problems)	Evaluate other reflexes and general neurologic functioning.
Plantar grasp	Toes curl downward when sole of foot is stimulated; lessens by 8 months	Absent (defects of lower spinal column)	
Stepping	When held upright and one foot touching a flat surface, will step alternately; disappears at 7–8 months of age	Asymmetry of stepping (neurologic abnormality)	Evaluate muscle tone and function on each side of body. Refer to specialist.
Babinski	Hyperextension of all toes when one side of sole is stroked from heel upward across ball of foot	Absence of response (lower spinal cord defects)	Refer for further neurologic evaluation.
Tonic neck	Fencer position—when head is turned to one side, extremities on same side extend and on opposite side flex; this reflex may	Absent after 1 month of age or persistent asymmetry (cerebral lesion)	

*Possible causes of deviations are placed in parentheses.
†Nursing interventions are primarily directed toward identified deviations.

NEONATAL PHYSICAL ASSESSMENT GUIDE Cont'd

Assess	Normal findings	Deviations and possible causes*	Nursing interventions[†]
	not be evident during early neonatal period; disappears at 3-4 months of age Response often more dominant in leg than in arm		
Prone crawl	While on abdomen, infant pushes up and tries to crawl	Absence or variance of response (prematurity, weak or depressed infants)	Evaluate motor functioning. Refer to specialist.
Trunk incurvation	In prone position, stroking of spine causes pelvis to turn to stimulated side	Failure to rotate to stimulated side (neurologic damage)	

*Possible causes of deviations are placed in parentheses.
[†]Nursing interventions are primarily directed toward identified deviations.

NEONATAL BEHAVIORAL ASSESSMENT

Two conflicting forces influence parents' perceptions of their infant. One is the parents' preconceptions, based on hopes and fears, of what their infant will be like. The other is their initial reaction to the infant's temperament, behaviors, and physical appearance.

Brazelton (1973) has developed a tool that has revolutionized our understanding and perception of the newborn's capabilities and responses, permitting us to recognize each infant's individuality. This assessment tool provides valuable guidelines for assessing the newborn's state changes, temperament, and individual behavior patterns. It provides a means by which the health care provider, in conjunction with the parents (primary caregivers), can identify and understand the individual newborn's states. Parents learn which responses, interventions, or activities best meet the special needs of their infant, and this understanding fosters positive bonding experiences.

The assessment tool attempts to identify the infant's repertoire of behavioral responses to his environment and also documents the infant's neurologic adequacy. The examination usually takes 20 to 30 minutes and involves about 30 different tests and maneuvers.* The scale includes 27 behavioral items, each scored on a 9-point scale, and 20 elicited reflexes, which are scored on a 3-point scale. The behavioral items are as follows:

- Response decrement to light
- Response decrement to rattle
- Response decrement to bell
- Response decrement to pinprick
- Inanimate visual orientation
- Inanimate auditory orientation
- Animate visual orientation
- Animate auditory orientation
- Animate visual and auditory orientation
- Alertness
- General tonus
- Motor maturity
- Pull to sit
- Cuddliness
- Defensive movements

*For a complete discussion of all test items and maneuvers, the student is referred to the original scale.

- Consolability
- Peak of excitement
- Rapidity of buildup
- Irritability
- Activity
- Tremulousness
- Startles
- Lability of skin color
- Lability of states
- Self-quieting activity
- Hand-mouth facility
- Smiles

Some items are scored according to the infant's response to specific stimuli; others, such as consolability and alertness, are scored as a result of continuous behavioral observations throughout the assessment.

Generally, the scales are set up so that the midpoint is the norm for most items. The Brazelton scale differs from most assessment tools in that, for all but a few items, the infant's score is determined not on his average performance but on his best. In the case of the infant who is uncoordinated for 48 hours after delivery, the behavior of the third day must be taken as the expected mean. Every effort should be made to elicit the best response. This may be accomplished by repeating tests at different times or by testing during situations that facilitate the best possible response, such as when parents are alerting their infants by holding, cuddling, rocking, and singing to them.

The assessment of the infant should be carried out initially in a quiet, dimly or softly lit room, if possible. The infant's state of consciousness should be determined, because scoring and introduction of the test items are correlated with the sleep or awake state. The newborn's state depends on physiologic variables, such as the amount of time from the last feeding, positioning, environmental temperature, and health status; presence of such external stimuli as noises and bright lights; and the wake-sleep cycle of the infant. An important characteristic of the neonatal period is the *pattern of states,* as well as the transitions from one state to another. The pattern of states is a predictor of the infant's receptivity and his ability to respond to stimuli in a cognitive manner. Infants learn best in a quiet, alert state and in an environment that is supportive and protective and that provides appropriate stimuli.

The sleep-wake states are as follows (Prechtl and Beintema, 1964; Brazelton, 1973):

Sleep States

1. Deep sleep with regular breathing, eyes closed, no spontaneous activity except startles or jerky movements at quite regular intervals; external stimuli produce startles with some delay; suppression of startles is rapid, and state changes are less likely than from other states. No eye movements. . . .

2. Light sleep with eyes closed; rapid eye movements can be observed under closed lids; low activity level, with random movements and startles or startle equivalents; movements are likely to be smoother and more monitored than in state #1; responds to internal and external stimuli with startle equivalents, often with a resulting change of state. Respirations are jagged or irregular sucking movements off and on. . . .

Awake States

3. Drowsy or semidozing; eyes may be open or closed; eyelids fluttering; activity level variable, with interspersed, mild startles from time to time; reactive to sensory stimuli, but response often delayed; state change after stimulation frequently noted. Movements are usually smooth. . . .

4. Alert, with bright look; seems to focus attention on source of stimulation, such as an object to be sucked, or a visual or auditory stimulus; impinging stimuli may break through, but with some delay in response. Motor activity is at a minimum. . . .

5. Eyes open; considerable motor activity, with thrusting movements of the extremities, and even a few spontaneous startles; reactive to external stimulation with increase in startles or motor activity, but discrete reactions difficult to distinguish because of general high activity level.

6. Crying; characterized by intense crying, which is difficult to break through with stimulation.*

---

*From Brazelton, T. 1973. *The neonatal behavioral assessment scale.* Philadelphia: J. B. Lippincott Co., pp. 7–8.

The nurse should observe the infant's state patterns, the rapidity with which he moves from one state to another, his ability to be consoled, and his ability to diminish the impact of disturbing stimuli. The following questions may provide the nurse with a framework for assessment:

Does the infant's response style and ability to adapt to stimuli indicate a need for parental interventions that will alert him to his environment so that he can grow socially and cognitively?

Are parental interventions necessary to lessen the outside stimuli, as in the case of the infant who responds to sensory input with intensity?

Can the infant control the amount of sensory input that he must deal with?

The scale items and maneuvers and the sleep-awake states in which they are assessed are categorized as follows:

1. *Habituation* (state 1, 2, or 3). The infant's ability to diminish or shut down his innate responses to specific repeated stimuli, such as a rattle, bell, light, or pinprick to his heel, is assessed. The tests are continued until the infant effectively blocks out or becomes unresponsive to three consecutive stimuli. Normal newborns can filter out stimulation and stop responding, demonstrating the infant's ability to control himself by his responses to the external environment. Inability to habituate to these stimuli may be related to transient problems, such as medication given to the mother during labor or possible central nervous system damage, and warrants further evaluation. The immature or central nervous system–damaged infant demonstrates a failure to habituate to the pinprick stimulus by withdrawing the opposite foot from the pinprick, and the whole body responds as quickly as the stimulated foot.

2. *Orientation to inanimate and animate visual and auditory assessment stimuli* (state 4 or 5). How often and where he attends to auditory and visual stimuli are observed. The infant's orientation to the environment is determined by his ability to respond to clues given by others and by his natural ability to fix on and to follow a visual object horizontally and vertically. This capacity and parental appreciation of it are important for positive communication between infant and parents; the parents' visual *(en face)* and auditory (soft, continuous voice) presence stimulate their infant to orient to them. Inability or lack of response may indicate visual or auditory problems. It is important for parents to know that their infant can turn to voices by 3 days of age and can become alert at different times with a varying degree or intensity of response to sounds.

3. *Motor activity (maturity)*. Several components are evaluated. Motor tone (state 4; not to be assessed in state 6) of the baby is assessed in his most characteristic state of responsiveness. This summary assessment includes overall use of tone as he responds to being handled—whether during spontaneous activity, prone placement, or holding him horizontally—and overall assessment of body tone as he reacts to all stimuli.

Smooth movement of extremities and free, wide range of movement (states 4 and 5) demonstrate motor maturity. One assesses smoothness of movement versus jerkiness. In the premature or central nervous system–irritated infant, an unbalanced cogwheel movement appears. One assesses freedom of arcs of movements versus restricted arcs. Premature infants demonstrate unlimited freedom of movement (floppy) in lateral, sagittal, and cephalad areas, but the movements are jerky and coglike, overshooting the marks. The average newborn is somewhat limited in arcs of movement, especially in those above the head and some in the lateral plane. Very mature infants exhibit freedom of movement in all directions and smooth, balanced performance (not floppy).

Other items used to assess motor maturity are the ability to pull to sit (states 3 and 5) and the ability to coordinate hand-to-mouth movements. The nurse should discuss with the parents normalcy of hand-to-mouth movements as a self-control and comforting device and not necessarily an expression of hunger. Degree and frequency of startling (states 3 to 6), tremulousness (all states), and defensive movements (state 4), such as a baby's attempts to remove a cloth placed over his head, are items that evaluate motor activity.

4. *Variations*. Frequency of alert states (state 4 only), state changes, color changes (throughout all states as examination progresses), activity, and peaks of excitement (state 6) are assessed. Periods of alertness can occur at any time during the examination period and are often best elicited while the examiner holds the infant. Infants are alert for only short periods. *Alerting* is defined as a brightening and widening of the eyes, and *orienting* is identified as the response of turning toward the direction of stimulation (Brazelton, 1973). Color

changes reflect the autonomic nervous system's responses to stress, whereas rapidity of state changes reflect the newborn's ability to control himself in the presence of increasing aversive stimulation.

5. *Self-quieting activity* (states 6 and 5 to 4, 3, 2, and 1). Assessment is based on how often, how quickly, and how effectively the newborn can utilize his resources to quiet and console himself when upset or distressed. Considered in this assessment are such self-consolatory activities as putting hand to mouth, sucking on a fist or the tongue, and attuning to an object or sound. One must also consider the infant's need for outside consolation, for example, visualizing a face, rocking, holding, dressing, using a pacifier, and restraining extremities.

6. *Cuddliness or social behaviors* (states 4 and 5). This area encompasses the infant's need for and response to being held. Also considered is how often the newborn smiles. These behaviors influence the parents' self-esteem and feelings of acceptance or rejection. Schaeffer and Emerson's (1964) study indicated that cuddling also appears to be an indicator of personality. Cuddlers appear to enjoy, accept, and seek physical contact; are easier to placate; sleep more; and form earlier and more intense attachments. Noncuddlers are active, restless, have accelerated motor development, and are intolerant of physical restraint. Smiling, even as a grimace reflex, greatly influences the parent-infant feedback system. Parents identify this response as positive.

SUMMARY

The various neonatal assessments and the data obtained from them are only as effective as the degree to which the findings are shared with the parents and incorporated into the interaction between parents and infant. Parents must be included in the assessment process from the moment of their child's birth. The Apgar score and its meaning should be explained immediately to the parents. As soon as possible, the parents should be a part of the physical and behavioral assessments. The examiner should emphasize the uniqueness of their infant.

The nurse can encourage the parents to identify the unique behavioral characteristics of their infant and to learn nurturing activities. Bonding is facilitated when parents are allowed to explore their infant in private, identifying individual physical and behavioral characteristics.

The nurse's supportive responses to the parents' questions and observations are essential throughout the assessment process. With her help, bonding is facilitated, and the beginning interactions between family members are established.

SUGGESTED ACTIVITIES

1. With the help of your instructor, assess a newborn to determine gestational age.
2. In a role-playing situation with a classmate, assume the role of a nurse explaining normal newborn reflexes to a new mother.

REFERENCES

Avery, G. B., ed. 1975. *Neonatology.* Philadelphia: J. B. Lippincott Co.

Battaglia, F. C., and Lubchenco, L. O. 1967. A practical classification of newborn infants by weight and gestational age. *J. Pediatr.* 71:159.

Brazelton, T. 1973. *The neonatal behavioral assessment scale.* Philadelphia: J. B. Lippincott Co.

Downs, M. P., and Silver, H. K. Oct. 1972. The A,B,C,D's to H.E.A.R. Early identification in nursery, office and clinic of the infant who is deaf. *Clin. Pediatr.* 11:563.

Dubowitz, L., and Dubowitz, V. 1977. *Gestational age of the newborn.* Menlo Park, Calif.: Addison-Wesley Publishing Co.

Holmes, L. B. 1976. Congenital malformations: incidence, racial differences and recognized etiologies. In *Biological and clinical aspects of malformations.* Mead Johnson Symposium on Perinatal and Developmental Medicine, No. 7. Evansville, Ind.

Kempe, C. H., et al. 1978. *Current pediatric diagnosis and treatment.* Los Altos: Lange Medical Publications.

Korones, S. B. 1976. *High-risk newborn infants.* St. Louis: The C. V. Mosby Co.

Lubchenco, L. O. 1970. Assessment of gestational age and development at birth. *Pediatr. Clin. N. Am.* 17:125.

Mead Johnson series. 1978. The skin. In *Variations and minor departures in infants.* Evansville, Ind.: Mead Johnson.

Prechtl, H. F. R., and Beintema, D. L. 1964. *The neurological examination of the full-term newborn infant.* London: Spastics Society International Medical Publications in association with William Heinemann Ltd.

Schaeffer, H., and Emerson, P. 1964. Patterns of response to physical contact in early human development. *J. Child Psychol. Psychiatry.* 5:1.

ADDITIONAL READINGS

Affonso, D. Nov.-Dec. 1976. The newborn's potential for interaction. *J. Obstet. Gynecol. Nurs.* 5:9.

Aladjem, S., and Brown, A. 1977. *Prenatal intensive care.* St. Louis: The C. V. Mosby Co.

Arturo, H. 1967. Nursery evaluation of the newborn. *Am. J. Nurs.* 67:1671.

Brann, A. Oct. 1977. Determining gestational age. *Emergency Med.* 9:51.

Clark, A. L., and Affonso, D. 1976. Infant behavior and maternal attachment: two sides to the coin. *Mat.-Child Nurs.* 1:94.

Chinn, P. 1974. *Child health maintenance: concepts in family-centered care.* St. Louis: The C. V. Mosby Co.

Erickson, M. 1976. *Assessment and management of developmental changes in children.* St. Louis: The C. V. Mosby Co.

Jensen, M., et al. 1977. *Maternity care: the nurse and the family.* St. Louis: The C. V. Mosby Co.

Marcil, V. March 1976. Physical assessment of the newborn. *Canadian Nurse.* 72:21.

Maurer, D. M., et al. Oct. 1976. Newborn babies see better than you think. *Psych. Today.* 10:85.

Moore, M. L. 1978. *Realities in childbearing.* Philadelphia: W. B. Saunders Co.

Sullivan, R., et al. Jan.-Feb. 1979. Determining a newborn's gestational age. *MCN.* 4:38.

Usher, R., et al. 1966. Judgment of fetal age. II. Clinical significance of gestational age and an objective method for its assessment. *Pediatr. Clin. N. Am.* 13:835.

Ziegel, E., and Cranley, M. 1978. *Obstetric nursing.* 7th ed. New York: The Macmillan Co.

CHAPTER 23

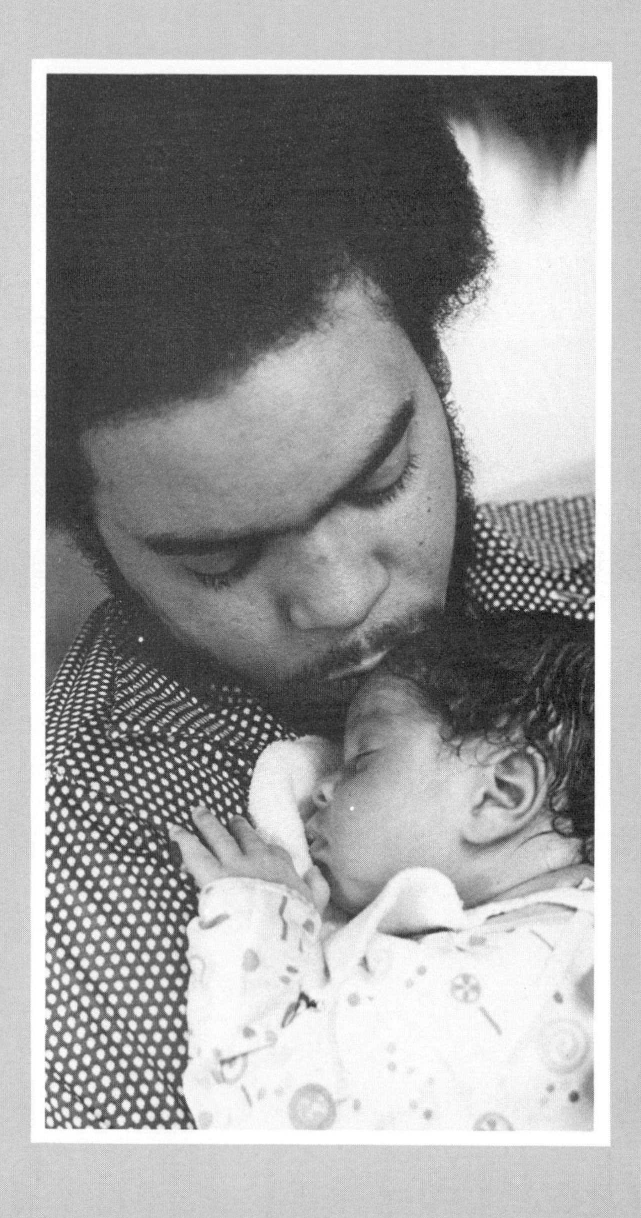

RESPONSE TO BIRTH

- Respiratory Adaptations
- Cardiovascular Adaptations
- Hepatic Adaptations
- Gastrointestinal Adaptations
- Renal Adaptations
- Immunologic Adaptations

PERIODS OF REACTIVITY

IMMEDIATE NURSING CARE

THE NORMAL NEWBORN: NEEDS AND CARE

OBJECTIVES

- Describe the newborn's physiologic adaptations to the birth process.
- Discuss periods of reactivity after birth.
- Discuss nursing care of the newborn.
- Compare various feeding preparations and feeding techniques.
- Identify common parental concerns regarding infants.
- Describe a model for parent education with new infants.

The neonatal period includes the time from birth through the 28th day of life. It involves the adjustments from intrauterine to extrauterine life that the infant must make in order to effectively function as a unique individual. The initial examination of the newborn reveals how this adaptation process is proceeding and includes assessment and evaluation of the general characteristics, variations, and responses of the neonate. The nursery nurse must be a skilled observer, because subtle symptoms or changes may herald significant developments in the newborn. Consequently, the nurse must be totally cognizant of the normal in order to recognize deviations from it.

Birth marks the beginning of the expansion of the family unit, and care of the neonate must include his family, too. As a result, today's nurse should be knowledgeable about the family adjustments that need to be made as well as the health care needs of the newborn. With such a background, the nurse can provide comprehensive care and promote the establishment of a positive family unit.

RESPONSE TO BIRTH

Birth propels the infant from a warm, weightless, fluid environment to a cold, dry, pressurized environment within a short time. Separation from the placenta requires that the infant assume responsibility for major body functions.

To begin life as an independent being, the neonate must first and foremost establish his pulmonary ventilation, and marked circulatory changes must occur. These changes are rapid and radical. All other body systems can change their functions or establish themselves at a much slower pace.

Respiratory Adaptations

The respiratory system is in a continuous state of development from fetal life to early childhood. By the 26th week of fetal life, the lungs might be sufficient to maintain life if the infant were born at this time. Between the 30th and 36th week of fetal life, the lungs have grown enough to give more expansion, thereby increasing the infant's ability to survive in extrauterine life. After the 36th week, the lungs are structurally developed enough to permit maintenance of good lung expansion and adequate exchange of gases (Avery, 1975).

Initiation of Breathing

To maintain life, the lungs must function immediately after birth. Two radical changes must take place for the lungs to function: (a) pulmonary ventilation must be established through lung expansion following birth, and (b) a marked increase in the pulmonary circulation must occur.

Several factors apparently serve as stimulators to assist in the initiation of respiratory movement. Recent research has demonstrated that the fetus does indeed demonstrate breathing movements in utero as early as the fourth month of gestation, with an average rate of 30–70 respirations per minute. These breathing episodes are sometimes decreased in high-risk pregnancies and may be a significant parameter for monitoring to detect fetal distress (Platt et al., 1978). How significant these respirations are in establishing respiratory activity following birth remains to be seen (see p. 386).

Transitory asphyxia, with its resultant elevation in PCO_2 and decrease in pH and PO_2, occurs when the umbilical cord is cut and stops pulsing and is a significant stimulator for the initiation of breathing. These changes, which are present in all newborns to some degree, stimulate the aortic and carotid chemoreceptors, initiating impulses that trigger the medulla's respiratory center. Although brief periods of asphyxia are a significant stimulator, prolonged asphyxia is abnormal.

The significant decrease in ambient temperature that follows delivery (from 98.6F to 70–75F) is another significant stimulus for initiation of breathing. Nerve endings in the skin are stimulated and transmit impulses to the medulla. Excessive cooling may result in profound depression and evidence of cold stress, but the normal temperature changes that occur are apparently within physiologic limits.

The tactile stimulation involved in slapping the buttocks or heels and in normal handling of the infant is no longer considered especially beneficial. Although it may have minor significance, other resuscitative measures are of far greater value (Korones, 1976).

Two major forces may oppose the initiation of respiratory activity: (a) surface tension in the alveoli and (b) the viscosity of pulmonary fluid within the respiratory tract. Because of surface tension within the alveoli, the small airways and alveoli would collapse between each inspiration if it were not for the presence of *surfactant*, which reduces the cohesive force between the moist surfaces of the alveoli. Surfactant is necessary for good lung expansion and prevents the alveoli from completely collapsing with each expiration. There should always be some residual air left in the lungs after each expiration so that there will not be a need to completely reopen each alveolus with each breath.

Fetal lungs continuously produce fluid during the latter half of intrauterine development. This secretion fills the lung almost completely, expanding the air spaces. Some of the fluid drains out of the lungs into the amniotic fluid and is soon swallowed by the fetus. The respiratory passages of a normal term baby contain approximately 80–110 ml of fluid, which must be removed at the time of delivery to provide for adequate movement of air. As the baby's chest is compressed through the birth canal during a normal delivery, approximately one-third of the fluid is squeezed out of the lungs. The subsequent recoil of the chest wall after the birth of the newborn's trunk is thought to produce a small passive inspiration of air that is drawn into the lungs to replace the fluid that was squeezed out. The fluid that has been left in the lungs is drawn back farther with the breath and is later absorbed into the bloodstream through the pulmonary capillaries and pulmonary lymphatics. Some of the air is also forced into the proximal airways. An air-liquid interface is established in the smaller airways and alveoli. It is not definitely known how quickly the remaining alveolar fluid is reabsorbed, but under normal circumstances it is reabsorbed after a few breaths or within the first hour after birth (Korones, 1976).

Although the initial expiration should clear the airways of accumulated fluid and should permit inspiration, it is wise to suction mucus and fluid from the infant's mouth with a bulb syringe as the head and shoulders are delivered. Respirations should be monitored every 15 minutes for 1 hour and then every 30 minutes for 2 hours after birth. An aspiration bulb should be with the baby in the nursery, and respiratory function should be observed closely, especially during the second reactive phase, when there is an increase in mucus secretion.

Normal respirations are 30–50 per minute, may initially be largely diaphragmatic, and are shallow and irregular in depth and rhythm. Respirations are primarily abdominal and synchronous with the chest. Short periods of apnea are normal. The neonate is an obligatory nose breather, and any obstruction will cause respiratory distress, so it is important to keep the throat and nose clear. If respirations drop below 35 or exceed 60 per minute when the infant is at rest, or if dyspnea or cyanosis occurs, the physician should be notified. (Some initial dyspnea or cyanosis may be normal.) Any increased use of the intercostal muscles may also indicate respiratory distress.

Delay in clearing the lungs may result from (a) underdeveloped lymphatics, which decrease the rate at which the fluid is absorbed from the lungs, or (b) complications antenatally or during labor and delivery that interfere with adequate lung expansion and result in increased pulmonary vascular resistance and decreased blood flow. These complications may include inadequate compression of the chest wall in a very small infant, the absence of chest wall compression in the infant delivered by cesarean section, or severe asphyxia at birth. Spontaneous movements after birth also contribute to minute ventilation and influence the other physical and sensory factors.

Neonatal Pulmonary Physiology

The first breath of life—a gasp in response to tactile, thermal, and chemical changes associated with birth—initiates the serial opening of the alveoli. Thus begins the transition from a fluid-filled environment to an air-breathing existence and from a dependent existence to an independent extrauterine life. Resistive forces of the fluid-filled lungs and the small radii of the respiratory airways require the generation of pressures of 80–100 cm H_2O for the initial inflation of the lung. Indeed, the first breath of life may be the most difficult.

The function of the lungs, to maintain oxygen and carbon dioxide exchange, is influenced by many factors. Chemical, pharmacologic, pulmonary reflex, pressoreceptor, and thermal factors

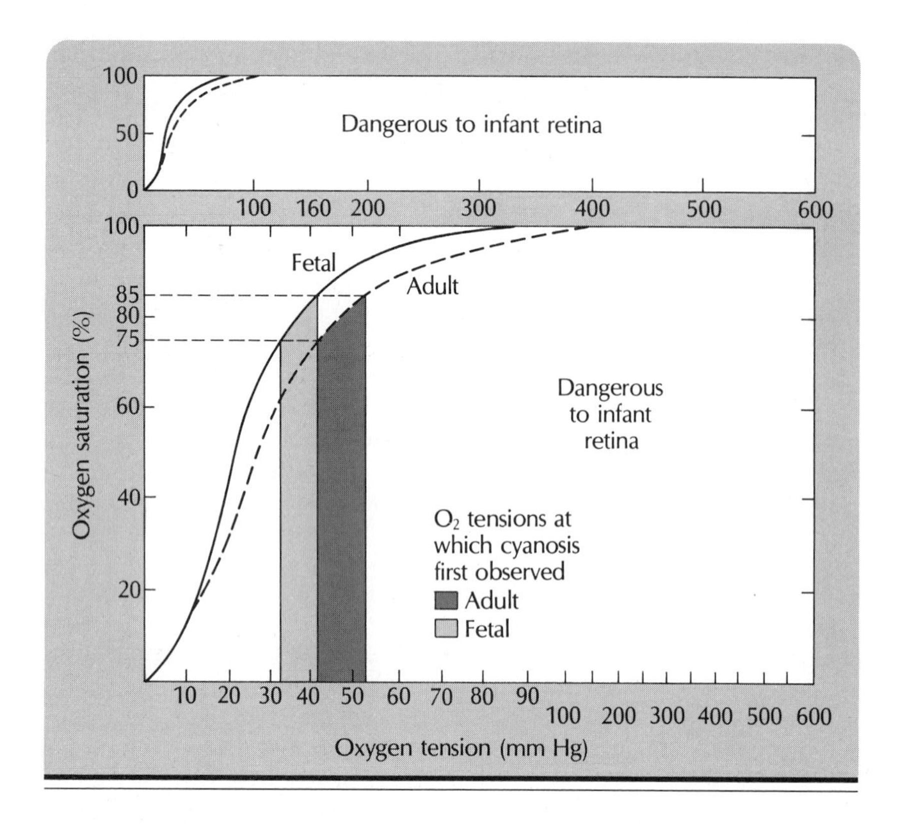

Figure 23–1. Fetal oxygen dissociation curve. (From Klaus, M., and Fanaroff, A. A. 1973. *Care of the high-risk infant.* Philadelphia: W. B. Saunders Co., p. 122.)

influential in adult respiratory regulation have not been extensively evaluated in the neonate. Chemical stimuli (P_{CO_2} and P_{O_2} concentrations) have been studied, and in response to hypercarbia (increased P_{CO_2}), the newborn increases his respiratory rate to remove the retained carbon dioxide. The effects of hypoxia (decreased P_{O_2}) as a ventilatory stimulus depend on temperature, hemoglobin content, and shunting of blood.

Adequate oxygenation at the cellular level depends on the physical solution of oxyhemoglobin. The fetal oxygen dissociation curve (quantity of oxygen bound to hemoglobin and partial pressure of oxygen) (Figure 23–1) shifts to the left. This leftward shift indicates the ability of fetal blood to bind more oxygen at any level of P_{O_2} less than 100 mm Hg. The ability of fetal hemoglobin to carry more oxygen is an advantage for the infant. Clinical manifestation of cyanosis as an indicator of hypoxia is more difficult because cyanosis can be observed at lower oxygen tension. Maintenance of oxygen tension depends on several factors: (a) the ventilation and diffusion capacity of the lungs, (b) the ventilation-perfusion ratio within the lungs, and (c) the amount of shunting (right-to-left) within the cardiovascular system.

Right-to-left shunting in normal neonates is the bidirectional flow of blood through the ductus arteriosus. This bidirectional flow of blood, which may divert a significant amount of blood away from the lungs, depends on the pressure changes of respiration, crying, and the cardiac cycle. Thus adequate amounts of blood must be delivered by the heart to the lungs for adequate oxygenation to occur.

From a physiologic standpoint, the movement of air into and out of the lungs (for oxygenation of the blood delivered by the heart) is accomplished by pressure differences, resistances to gas flow, and gaseous exhange. Pressure gradients within the respiratory system account for the flow of gas: (a) at inspiration there is decreased alveolar pressure, so that gas flows into the lungs; and (b) at expiration there is an increase in alveolar pressure, so that gas flows out of the lungs.

Gas flow into the lungs is opposed by two forces—lung compliance and airway resistance. *Compliance,* a measure of lung distensibility, is influenced by the elastic recoil of lung tissue and by anatomical variations. The anatomical differences between the neonate and the adult influence lung compliance. The infant has a relatively large heart and mediastinal structures that reduce available lung space. The protuberant abdomen further encroaches on the high diaphragm to decrease lung space. Anatomically, the neonatal chest is equipped with weak intercostal muscles, a rigid rib cage with horizontal ribs, and a high diaphragm that inhibits available space for lung expansion.

Impedance to ventilation is also offered by airway resistance, which depends on the radii, length, and number of airways as well as on lung compliance. A reduction in size of the airway, as in the anatomical size of an infant's airway as opposed to an adult airway, or continued retention of secretions within the airway will greatly increase resistance to gaseous flow.

Surface forces also affect lung compliance, as pressures are utilized to overcome surface-tension forces at the air-liquid interface of the alveoli. With respiration, the alveoli undergo changes: inspiration (the radius of the alveolus is greatest) and expiration (the radius of the alveolus is smaller).

The alveoli are lined with surfactant. This lining-layer functions to (a) lower surface tension as the radius of the alveolus is reduced in expiration (less pressure is required to hold the alveolus open); and (b) maintain alveolar stability by variance of the surface tension as the size of the alveolus changes.

The surfactant system develops systematically as gestation progresses. Recently, estimation of fetal pulmonary maturity by examination of amniotic fluid for phospholipids and lecithin/sphingomyelin ratio (L/S ratio) has become an accepted tool (see Chapter 14). The ratio of the surface-active phospholipids, lecithin and sphingomyelin, is an indication of lung maturity.

These concentrations of lecithin and sphingomyelin are established in a definite changing relationship as pregnancy and gestation advance. In the immature fetal lung, the L/S ratio is less than 1:1; transitional ratios are about 1.5:1.0; and the mature ratio is greater than 2:1. Lecithin is produced via two major enzymatic pathways, the methyl-transferase system and the phosphocholine-transferase system (Figure 23-2). The methyl-transferase system is first detectable at 22–24 weeks' gestation, appears to contribute little to maturing surfactant, and increases gradually toward term. It is very susceptible to damage by acidosis, hypothermia, and hypoxia. The second enzymatic pathway, the phosphocholine-transferase system, becomes active at about 35 weeks' gestation and rises rapidly toward term, paralleling late fetal lung development. It is a fairly stable system, relatively resistant to the insults of hypothermia. Clinically, the occurrence of the second pathway closely corresponds with the marked decrease in incidence of idiopathic respiratory distress syndrome after the 35th week of gestation. Production of sphingomyelin remains constant throughout gestation.

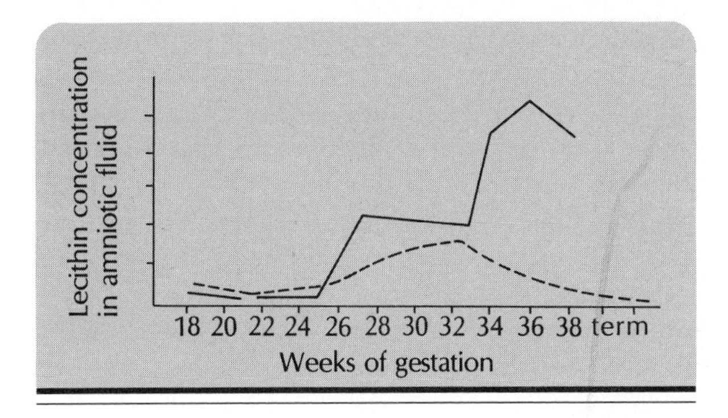

Figure 23–2. Development of lecithin in the fetal lung. The broken line represents the methylation pathway, and the solid line represents the phosphocholine transferase pathway. (From Gluck, L., and Kulovich, M. V. 1973. Fetal lung development. *Pediatr. Clin. North Am.* 20:373.)

The infant delivered before the L/S ratio is 2:1 will have varying degrees of respiratory distress.

Adequate oxygenation also depends on gaseous exchange at the cellular level. Within lung tissue this gas exchange depends on two principles: (a) diffusion, which is responsible for gas exchange between capillary blood and the alveoli and which depends on the substance (the gas and its pressure) crossing the membrane and the properties of the membrane (such as thickness and available surface area for exchange); and (b) the ventilation-perfusion ratio within the alveolar space, which is necessary for adequate gaseous exchange. A delicate balance exists between blood flow (perfusion) and alveolar ventilation. Lung tissue that is ventilated poorly (decreased PO_2) promotes airway constriction. Alveolar ventilation is thus regulated to maintain constant alveolar and arterial carbon dioxide tension.

Cardiovascular Adaptations

Changes in the cardiovascular system occur at the same time as the pulmonary changes. They involve five major areas of change (see Figure 6–14):

1. *Increased aortic pressure and decreased venous pressure.* With severing of the cord, the placental vascular bed is eliminated and the intravascular space is reduced. Consequently, aortic blood pressure is increased. At the same time, placental separation results in decreased blood return via the inferior vena cava, resulting in a small decrease in pressure within the venous circulation.

2. *Increased systemic pressure and decreased pulmonary artery pressure.* Pressure increases in the systemic circulation because severing the placenta produces greater resistance. At the same time, adequate lung expansion produces increased pulmonary blood flow, while the increased blood Po_2 associated with initiation of respirations produces vasodilatation. The combination of increased pulmonary blood flow and vasodilatation results in decreased pulmonary artery resistance.

3. *Closure of the foramen ovale.* Closure of the foramen ovale is a function of atrial pressures. In utero, pressure is greater in the right atrium, and the foramen ovale is open. Decreased pulmonary resistance and increased pulmonary blood flow result in increased pulmonary venous return into the left atrium, thereby increasing left atrial pressure slightly. The decreased pulmonary vascular resistance also causes a decrease in right atrial pressure. The pressure gradients are now reversed, left atrial pressure is greater, and the foramen ovale is functionally closed. It requires several months for it to become permanently closed.

4. *Closure of the ductus arteriosus.* The presence of oxygen causes the pulmonary arterioles to dilate, but an increase in blood Po_2 triggers the opposite response in the ductus arteriosus—it constricts. If the lungs fail to expand or if Po_2 levels drop, the ductus remains patent. Fibrosis of the ductus usually occurs within three weeks, but functional closure is accomplished within 15 hours.

5. *Closure of the ductus venosus.* The mechanism initiating closure of the ductus venosus is not known. Fibrosis occurs within three to seven days (Korones, 1976).

Hepatic Adaptations

In the newborn the liver is frequently palpable 2 to 3 cm below the right costal margin, because it is relatively large and occupies approximately 40% of the abdominal cavity. The liver plays an important part in blood coagulation during fetal life, and it continues this function to a degree during the first few months following birth. Substances necessary for blood coagulation are also synthesized in the liver when vitamin K is present. The absence of normal intestinal flora in the newborn gut results in low levels of vitamin K, resulting in a transient blood coagulation deficiency, usually between the second and fifth day of life. To combat this situation, an injection of vitamin K (aquamephyton) is given prophylactically on the day of birth.

The infant's liver also stores iron for use in hemoglobin production during the early months of life. If the mother's iron intake has been adequate, enough iron will be stored to last until the fifth month of life. At this time iron-containing foods or iron supplements must be given to prevent anemia.

Gastrointestinal Adaptations

The newborn's stomach has a capacity of 50–60 ml and will empty in about three hours. The cardiac sphincter is still immature, and the nervous control of the stomach is incomplete at birth, so some regurgitation may be noted in the neonatal period. Avoiding overfeeding and bubbling the infant well during and following feedings can lessen this problem.

The salivary glands are immature at birth, and little saliva is manufactured until the infant is about three months old. The majority of digestive enzymes are available in adequate quantities, with the exception of pancreatic amylase and lipase. They are deficient for several months, and as a result the infant has difficulty digesting the more complex carbohydrates. Fat absorption is also poor, but simple carbohydrates and protein are absorbed without difficulty. Although the gastrointestinal tract is sterile at birth, bacteria can be cultured within five hours after delivery in most infants. These bacteria are essential for normal digestion and for the synthesis of vitamin K.

Renal Adaptations

In the newborn the kidneys are relatively large and may extend below the iliac crests. They are easily palpable through the abdominal wall. Because the infant pelvis is small and unable to contain it, the bladder is also an abdominal organ.

In utero the fetal kidneys are functional, and they begin producing urine about the ninth week of gestation. By four months' gestation, urine is found in the bladder, and amniotic fluid analysis indicates that the fetus does void in utero. It is not unusual for the infant to void at delivery, but the initial voiding may be delayed 12 to 24 hours. This and subsequent voidings should be recorded. If the neonate has not voided after 24 hours, he should be assessed for adequacy of fluid intake and symptoms of distention, pain, and restlessness, and the physician should then be notified.

Unless edema is present, urinary output is often limited, and the voidings are scanty until fluid intake increases. (The fluid of edema is eliminated by the kidneys, so infants with edema have a much higher urinary output.) Initially the infant may void 2 to 6 times per day, with an average daily output of 60 ml. The number of voidings and amount of urine both gradually increase. By the end of the first week, the infant may void 10 to 30 times per day and have a daily output of approximately 225 ml.

Following the first voiding, the newborn's urine frequently appears cloudy (due to mucus content) and has a high specific gravity, which decreases as fluid intake increases. Occasionally pink stains ("brick dust spots") appear on the diaper. These are caused by urates and are innocuous. Blood may occasionally be observed on the diapers of female infants. This *pseudomenstruation* is related to the withdrawal of maternal hormones. Males may have bloody spotting from a circumcision. In the absence of apparent causes for bleeding, the physician should be notified. Normal urine during early infancy is straw-colored and almost odorless, although odor occurs when certain drugs are given or when infection is present.

Immunologic Adaptations

The immunoglobulins are a type of antibody secreted by lymphocytes and plasma cells into body fluids. The three major types of immunoglobulins—IgG, IgA, and IgM—are primarily involved in immunity. Of these three, only IgG crosses the placenta by a process as yet not clearly understood. The mother forms antibodies in response to illness or immunization. This process is called *active acquired immunity.* When IgG antibodies are transferred to the fetus in utero, *passive acquired immunity* results, because the fetus does not produce the antibodies itself.

Because this transfer of maternal immunoglobin occurs primarily during the third trimester, premature infants (especially those born prior to 34 weeks) may be more susceptible to infection. In general, infants receive immunity to tetanus, diphtheria, smallpox, measles, mumps, poliomyelitis, and a variety of other bacterial and viral diseases. The period of resistance varies: Immunity against common viral infections such as measles may last four to eight months, whereas immunity to certain bacteria may disappear within four to eight weeks.

The normal newborn does produce antibodies in response to an antigen, but not as effectively as an older child would. It is customary to begin immunization at 2 months of age, and then the child develops actively acquired immunity.

IgM immunoglobulins are primarily antibodies to blood group antigens, gram negative enteric organisms, and some viruses in the mother, although IgM production in the neonate occurs as part of the initial antigen-antibody response to practically all infectious agents. Because IgM does not normally cross the placenta, most or all is produced by the fetus beginning at 10–15 weeks' gestation. Elevated levels of IgM at birth (greater than 20 mg/100 ml) may be indicative of placental leaks or, more commonly, of antigenic stimulation in utero. Consequently, elevations suggest that the infant was exposed to an intrauterine infection such as rubella, syphilis, toxoplasmosis, herpes virus, or cytomegalovirus. The lack of available maternal IgM in the newborn also accounts for the infant's increased susceptibility to gram negative enteric organisms such as *E. coli* (Schaffer and Avery, 1977).

The functions of IgA immunoglobulins are not fully understood, although they appear to provide protection mainly on secreting surfaces such as the respiratory tract, gastrointestinal tract, and eyes. IgA does not cross the placenta and is not normally produced by the fetus in utero. Unlike the other immunoglobulins, IgA is not affected by gastric action. Colostrum, the forerunner of breast milk, is very high in IgA. Consequently, it may be of significance in providing some passive immunity to the infant of a breastfeeding mother (Schaffer and Avery, 1977).

PERIODS OF REACTIVITY

Newborn infants are rather unstable at birth but demonstrate predictable behavior patterns during the first several hours after birth (Figure 23–3). The *first period of reactivity* lasts approximately 30 minutes after birth. During this phase, the infant is awake and active. He may appear hungry and demonstrate a strong sucking reflex. There may be bursts of random, diffuse movements alternating with relative immobility. Respirations are rapid, as high as 80 per minute, and there may be retraction of the chest, transient flaring of the alae nasi, and grunting. Bowel sounds are absent. The heart rate is rapid and irregular.

Gradually this activity diminishes, heart rate and respiration decrease, and the infant enters the sleep phase. First sleep usually occurs an average of three hours after birth. This sleep may last from a few minutes to two to four hours. During this period, bowel sounds become audible, cardiac and respiratory rates return to baseline values, and the cord ceases pulsating.

The infant is again awake and alert during the *second period of reactivity.* Heart rate accelerates in response to stimulation, the first meconium stool is frequently passed, and the baby's color may become mildly cyanotic at times. Gagging, choking, and regurgitation of mucus frequently occur during this period, and careful observation of the infant is indicated. Because the second period of reactivity is variable, the nurse must be particularly alert for the first 12–18 hours.

Some authors discuss another period, called the *stability phase,* which lasts 6–24 hours. During this time, physiologic parameters normalize and abnormal clinical manifestations are detected, particularly those associated with blood incompatibility, infection, cerebral trauma, and congenital abnormalities.

IMMEDIATE NURSING CARE

When the newborn is admitted to the nursery from labor and delivery, identification is checked and confirmed. A concise report is made of significant information. This report includes:

1. *Prenatal history.* Any physical problems existing during pregnancy, such as spotting, maternal illness, toxemia, and so on, are noted. Also included should be information on maternal age, estimated day of confinement (EDC), previous pregnancies, and resulting children.

2. *Labor and delivery record.* Information regarding the length and difficulty of labor, use of forceps, use of medications, and symptoms of fetal distress are recorded. Anesthesia and analgesia prior to and during delivery should be reported, as well as the type of delivery and any variations, such as a cord around the neck or a precipitous delivery.

3. *Condition of the infant.* This item includes the infant's Apgar score, respirations, number of cord vessels, cry, voiding, and any complications such as excessive mucus, bones fractured during delivery, and delayed respirations or responsiveness.

4. *Immediate care of the newborn.* A record is kept of such measures as footprinting, eye prophylaxis, and resuscitative measures.

If no distress is apparent, the infant is weighed and measured (length and head and chest circumference). Temperature, pulse (apical), and respirations (some institutions include blood pressure) are measured, and a rapid appraisal is made of the infant's color, muscle tone, alertness, and general state. A prophylactic injection of vitamin K is given intramuscularly. The instillation of silver nitrate or antibiotic ointment in the eyes

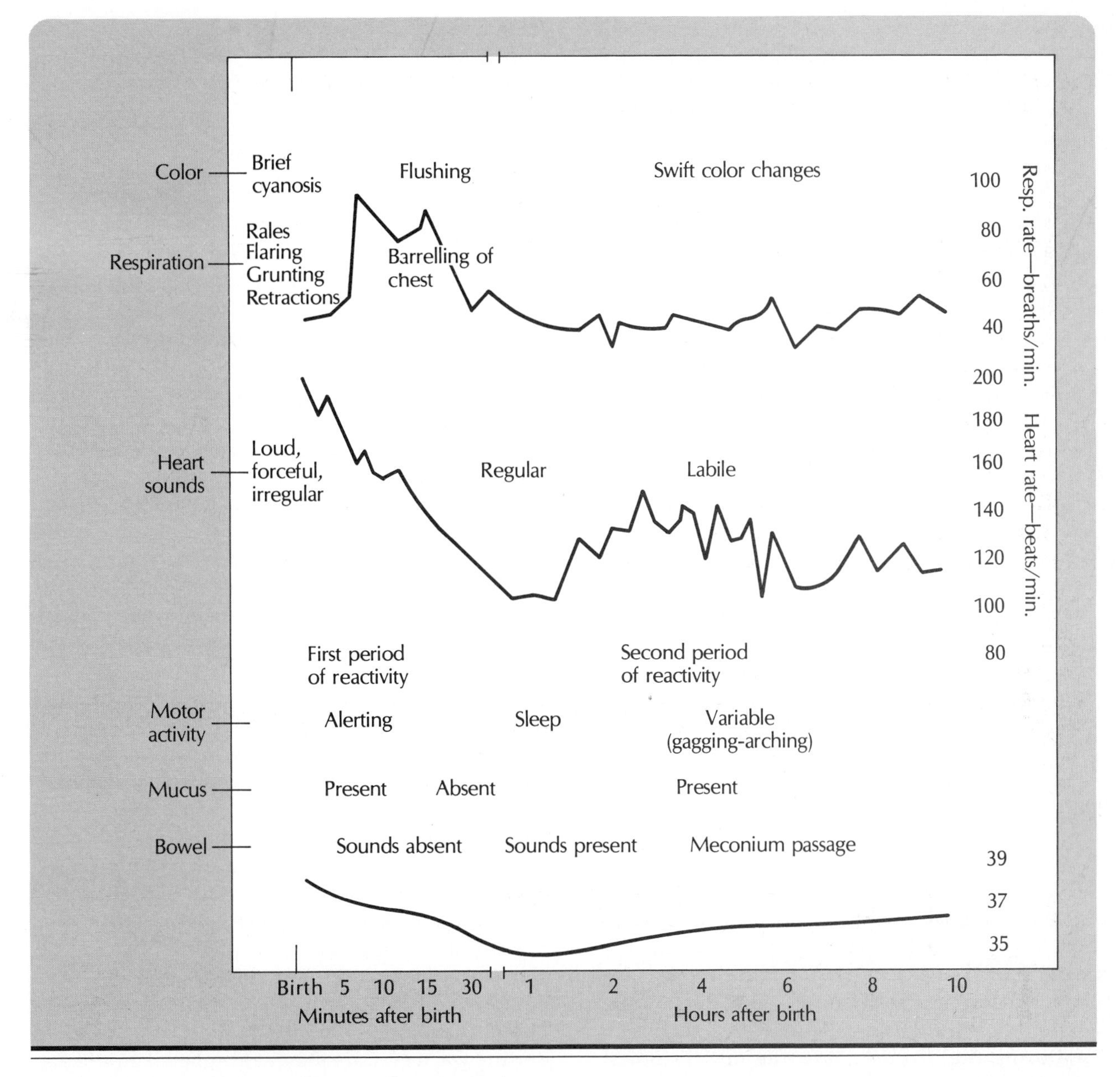

Figure 23–3. Example of periods of reactivity in normal newborn. (From Desmond, M. M. et al. 1966. The transitional nursery: a mechanism for preventive medicine. *Pediatr. Clin. North Am.* 13:656.)

often results in lid edema. To facilitate eye contact and to promote maternal bonding, eye prophylaxis is frequently done in the nursery rather than in delivery. The infant is then placed on his side in a warmer until his temperature stabilizes. A gooseneck lamp may also be used to provide additional heat.

NURSING OBSERVATION AND ACTIONS

It is customary to place the infant in an observation nursery for several hours following birth. This procedure allows the nurse to carefully assess the infant and to institute nursing care measures as indicated. The observation nursery is staffed at all times and must be equipped with necessary emergency care equipment. In alternative birth situations during this early time, close observation is essential to the well-being of the neonate. During this time, respirations are checked frequently.

Close observation of the newborn for signs of distress is vital. The nurse's responsibility in the care of the newborn requires that she be able to appraise accurately what is normal behavior versus the abnormal. In order to do so, the nurse must be knowledgeable in the characteristics of neonates and have experience in their care.

The most common signs of distress in the newborn are (Marlow, 1977):

1. Increased rate (more than 50/min) or difficulty of respirations.
2. Sternal retractions.
3. Excessive mucus.
4. Facial grimacing.
5. Cyanosis (generalized).
6. Abdominal distention or mass.
7. Lack of meconium elimination within 24 hours after birth.
8. Lack of or inadequate urine elimination.
9. Vomiting of bile-stained material.
10. Unusual jaundice of the skin.
11. Convulsions.

Gagging, vomiting, cyanosis, and restlessness may indicate the presence of mucus in the esophagus. This is not unusual, especially during the second period of reactivity, and appropriate measures, including positioning and suctioning, should be instituted.

During the first 24 hours, the infant's apical pulse should be taken every four hours. It is assessed for rate, regularity, and the presence of murmurs. Within the first 24 hours a complete physical examination and estimation of gestational age is done by the physician or pediatric nurse practitioner (see Chapter 22). The physical is repeated on the day of discharge.

The infant is transferred to the normal newborn nursery when his behavior is normal, his vital signs have been stabilized, and he has tolerated the first feeding—usually within 5 to 10 hours after birth. Some breast-feeding mothers request that they begin breast-feeding as soon as possible after delivery. Some agencies permit rooming-in to begin at this time. Others prefer to wait until after the first 24 hours. By this time mucus has decreased and the initial voiding and defecation have occurred.

Temperature

In utero the infant's temperature is approximately the same as or slightly higher than the mother's. Following birth, the infant must adapt to a heat-losing environment, and his temperature may drop one or two degrees despite the initiation of warming measures. The infant is especially susceptible to heat loss because (a) his temperature-regulating mechanism is immature and (b) his larger body surface in relation to weight promotes more exposure to environmental factors. Low-birth-weight infants are also affected by the absence of subcutaneous fat, which functions as an insulator. (The infant attempts to maintain his temperature by increasing his metabolic rate, which results in increased oxygen consumption, increased caloric requirements, and the use of brown fat stores. See the discussion on nonshivering thermogenesis in Chapter 24.)

Because the infant may lose heat through *evaporation* (the conversion of liquid to a vapor), it is important to keep the infant dry and covered. He is especially susceptible to cooling by evaporation immediately following delivery, when he is wet with amniotic fluid. Therefore, quickly drying the infant, especially his head, and wrapping him in warm blankets is very important. In some hospitals the infant may be placed with the mother, and temperature can be maintained by skin-to-skin contact and wrapping both the mother and newborn in a warm blanket. After his parents have held him, he can then be placed under the warmer. Care should also be taken during the bath and during diaper changes to prevent prolonged exposure and chilling.

Conductive heat loss occurs through direct skin contact with a cooler solid object. Thus the infant should not be placed on a cold counter or come in contact with cold equipment. Blankets and clothing should be stored in a warm place.

Convective heat loss, related to air currents, occurs when heat flows from the body surface to the cooler surrounding air. Thus infants should be protected from drafts from open windows or doors, from air conditioning units, and so on.

Radiant heat loss involves loss of body heat to solid surfaces not in direct contact with the body and is independent of the ambient temperature.

This process involves heat loss to windows, an outside wall, and so on.

Because a normal newborn requires about 8 hours to stabilize his body temperature, infants are initially placed in a warmer following delivery to allow the temperature to return to normal (about 2 to 4 hours). The infant is then bathed. Temperature should be rechecked after the bath, and if stable, the infant is dressed, wrapped, placed in a crib, and given a trial period at room temperature. If he does not successfully maintain his temperature at 36.5C (97.6F), he is returned to the warmer. The temperature should be recorded every hour until stable, then every 4 hours for the remaining 24 hours. When stable, it may be recorded twice daily.

A newborn's temperature may be as low as 36C (96.8F), but it should stabilize at 36.5C (97.6F) within 8 to 12 hours.

Weight

The neonate is weighed daily at the same time (Figure 23-4). The scales are covered to prevent cross-infection and heat loss by conduction. A weight loss of up to 10% is expected and is caused by limited initial intake and the loss of excess fluid. Parents should be informed about this expected weight loss and the reason for it.

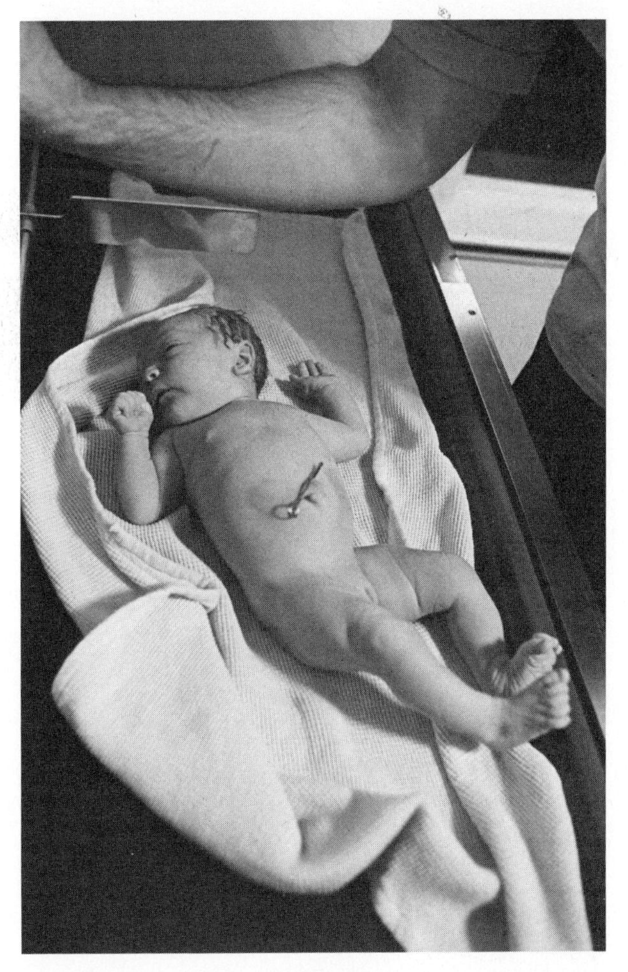

Figure 23-4. The scale is balanced before each weight, with the protective pad in place. The caretaker's hand is poised above the infant as a safety measure.

Feeding and Voiding

A sterile water feeding is given in the nursery 4 to 6 hours after birth. This feeding allows the nurse to assess the infant's suck, gag, and swallow reflexes and to observe for symptoms of esophageal atresia. (See discussion on feeding later in this chapter.) Some breast-feeding mothers request that their infant not receive water feedings and choose to begin breast-feeding as soon as possible after delivery. In this instance, the nurse should observe the newborn during the first feeding so that assessments of feeding can be made.

The initial voiding is noted, and all voidings should be recorded. The passage of meconium is recorded, as are all subsequent stools. Notation is made as to the type (meconium, transitional, and so on) and the amount.

The first stools, called *meconium,* are sticky, black, and odorless and are actually amniotic fluid swallowed in fetal life. Often a mucous plug will precede the first meconium. A stool should be passed within 24-36 hours after birth. If not, the infant should be checked for patency of the anus, bowel sounds, and abdominal distention. Fluid intake should also be noted. A digital examination of the rectum will frequently initiate stooling. If not, a piece of glycerin suppository may be utilized. It is not unheard of for a healthy infant to go 48 hours before stooling. However, delays beyond this require further investigation.

During the next three to six days, the stool will change to a greenish black, called *transitional,* to a greenish brown, then to a brownish yellow and a bright yellow. Stools of bottle-fed versus breast-fed infants vary. The stools of the infant fed on cow's milk or formula are yellow and more solid, and one or more per day is normal. The breast-fed infant has several stools a day that are loose and spongy and that may contain mucus. They have an aromatic odor. The number of stools varies. One a day is considered normal, but it is common to see four to eight a day. It is not uncommon to also see a breast-fed baby who has a bowel movement every third or fourth day. Minute spots of blood from bowel irritation are often seen in the first few days. The infant's stools should be assessed for frequency, color, and consistency and compared with the infant's age and the kind of feeding he is receiving. The addition of solid foods changes the characteristics of the stool, and parents need to be aware of this.

CIRCUMCISION

Circumcision is a surgical procedure in which the prepuce of the penis is separated from the glans and a portion is excised. This permits exposure of the glans and easier retraction of the foreskin for cleansing purposes.

Opinion varies as to the value of circumcision. It is a rite of the Jewish religion, and proponents of the procedure cite studies indicating that the incidence of cervical cancer is lower in women married to circumcised men. The incidence of cancer of the penis is also lower in circumcised men (Jensen et al., 1977). In addition, some believe circumcision allows for improved cleanliness and individual comfort. Those opposed to circumcision maintain that continued retraction and good hygienic practice result in equal

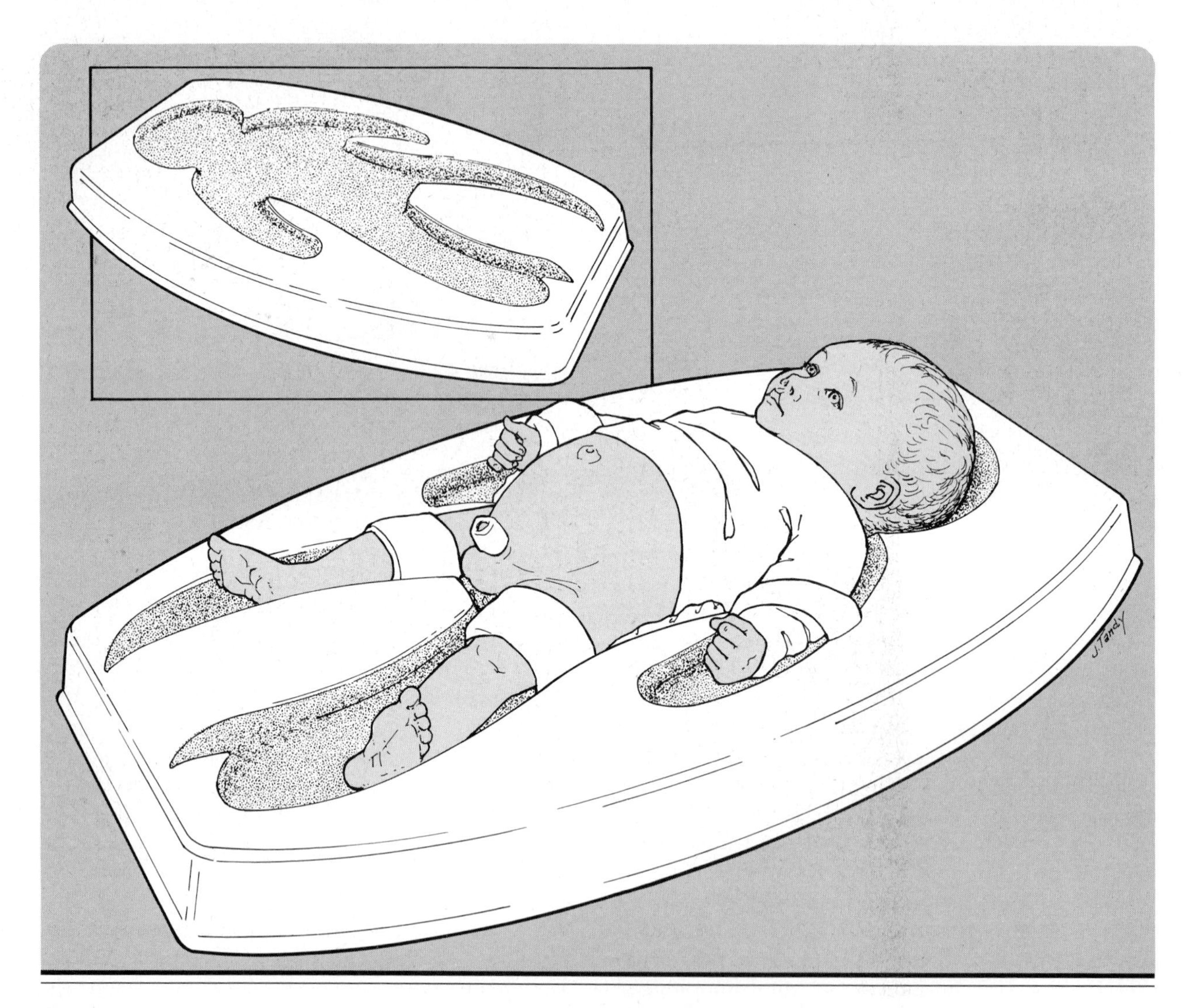

Figure 23–5. Proper positioning of the infant on a restraining board for circumcision.

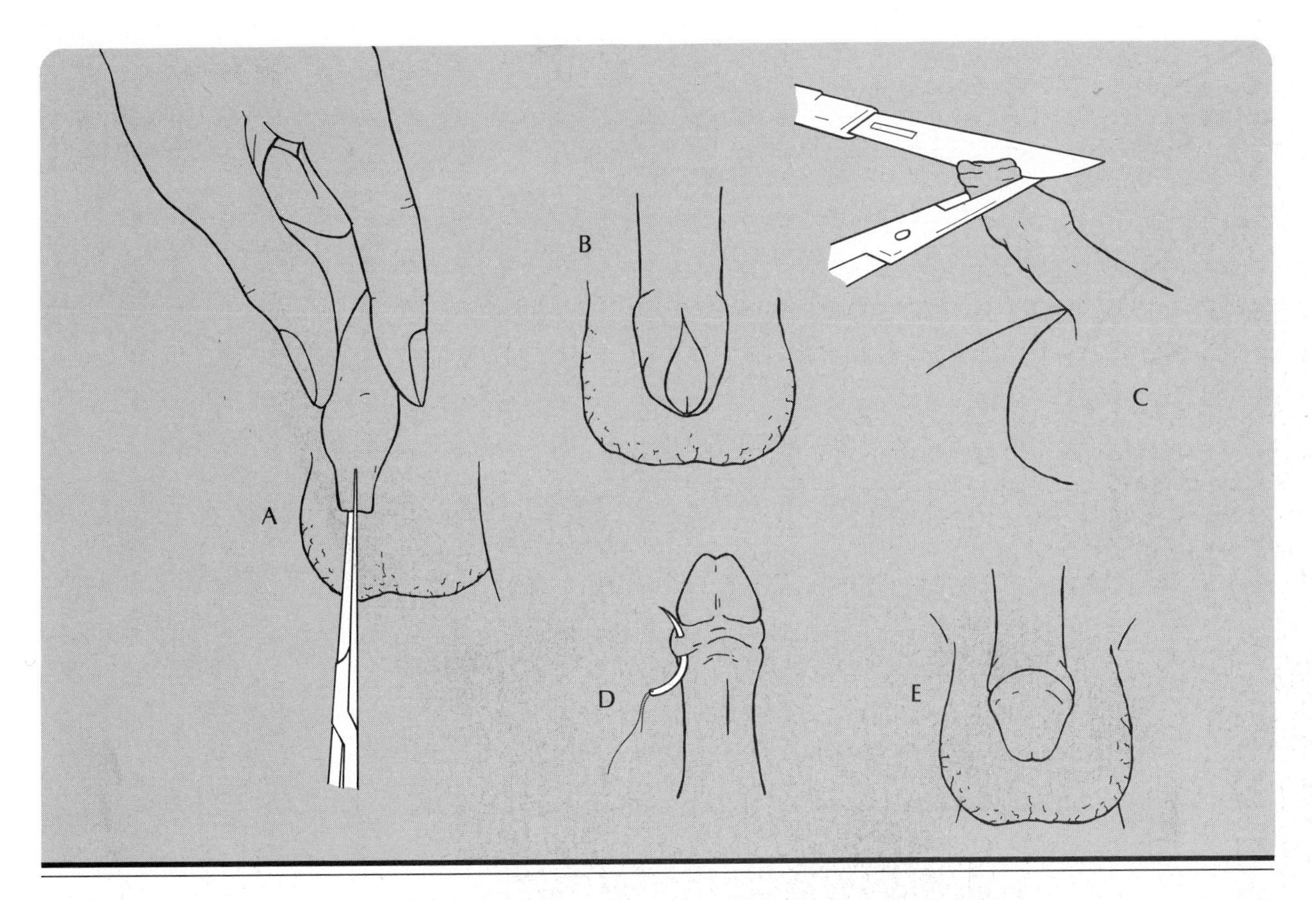

Figure 23–6. **A and B,** In this circumcision procedure, the prepuce is slit and retracted. **C,** Excess prepuce is then cut off. **D,** The prepuce is sutured in place. **E,** Circumcised penis.

cleanliness and comfort. Opponents question the statistical data about cervical carcinoma and feel that, following circumcision, the penis may become ulcerated and eventually develop meatal stenosis. Considerable controversy exists regarding the pros and cons of circumcision.

To decrease the incidence of cold stress, the procedure is usually not done until the day prior to discharge, when the infant is well stabilized. The nurse's responsibilities during a circumcision begin with checking to see that the circumcision permit is signed. Equipment is prepared, and then the infant is prepared by removing the diaper and placing him on a circumcision board or some other type of restraint (Figure 23–5). During the procedure, the nurse assesses the newborn's response. A variety of techniques for circumcision are available (Figures 23–6, 23–7, and 23–8), and all produce minimal bleeding. A small Vaseline gauze strip may be applied following surgery to keep the diaper from adhering to the operative site. The infant's voiding should be assessed for amount, adequacy of the stream, and the presence

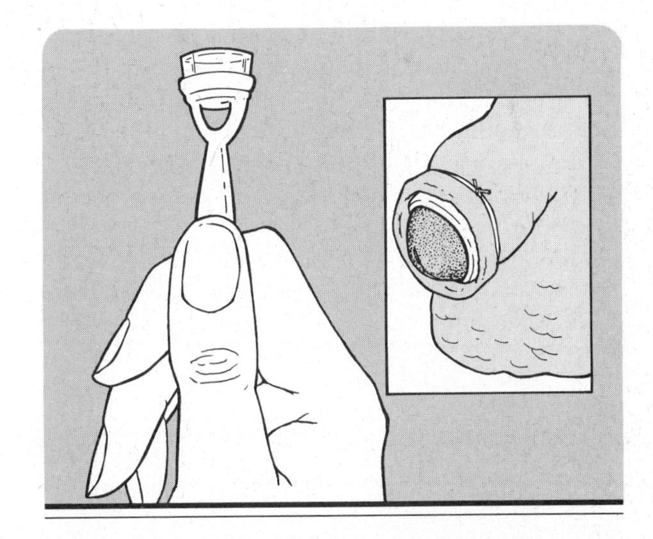

Figure 23–7. When the Plastibell is used, the bell is fitted over the glans. Suture is tied around the rim of the bell and the excess prepuce is cut away. The plastic rim remains in place for 3–4 days until healing takes place. The bell may be removed or allowed to fall off.

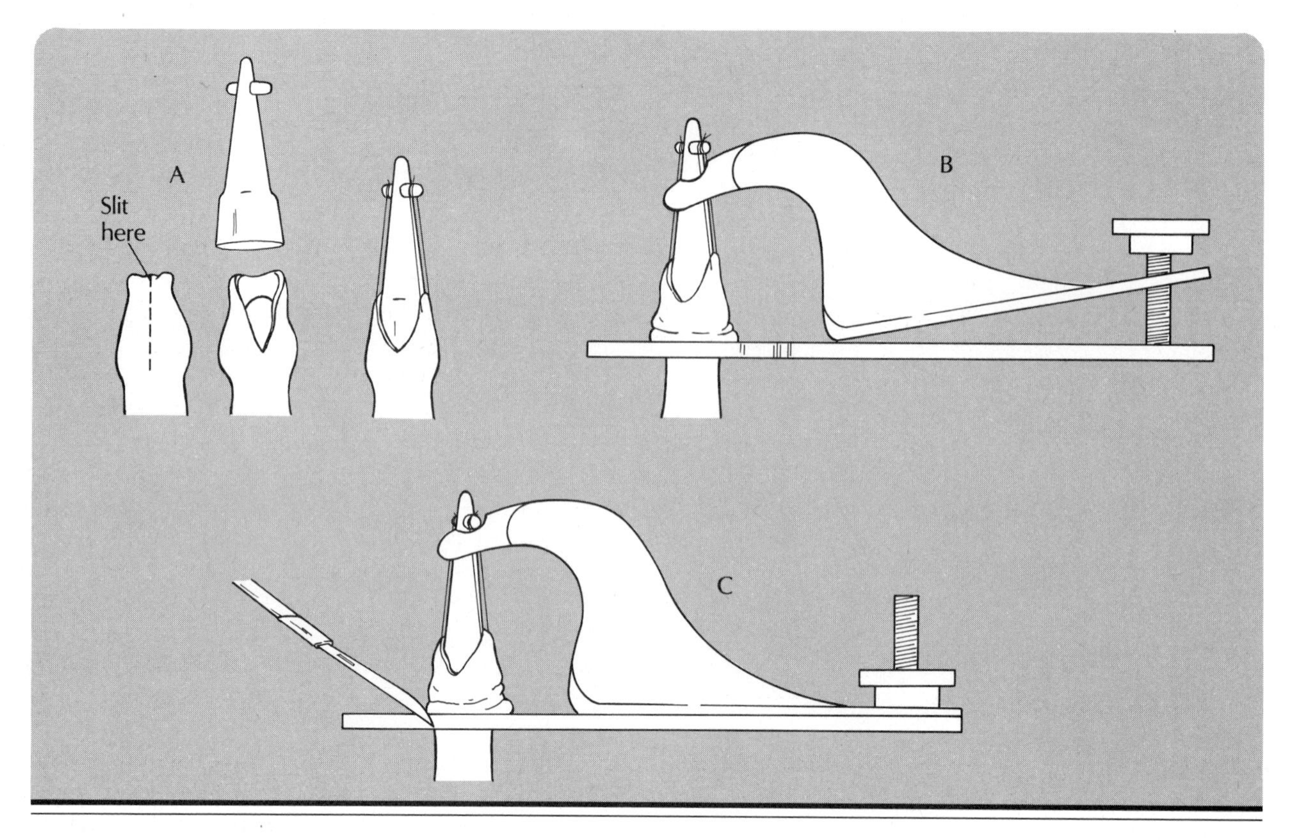

Figure 23-8. When the Yellen clamp is used for circumcision, the prepuce is drawn over the cone (**A**), and the clamp is applied (**B**). Pressure is maintained for 3-5 minutes, and then the excess prepuce is cut away (**C**).

of blood. The Vaseline gauze frequently controls any bleeding. If bleeding does occur, pressure is applied to the surgical site with a sterile gauze, and the physician is then notified.

The infant may be fussy for a few hours after the procedure but generally shows no other signs of distress. He should be positioned on his side with the diaper pinned loosely to prevent undue pressure.

Before dismissal, the parents should be instructed to observe the penis for bleeding or possible signs of infection. There may be a whitish yellow exudate around the glans, which is normal and not a part of the infection process. The parents may be instructed to gently wash the penis and pat it dry. The diaper needs to be pinned loosely for two to three days, because the glans remains tender for this length of time.

Circumcision requires the written consent of the parents. They should be given information for and against the surgery. In most cases, if the father is circumcised, the parents prefer that the son be, too.

PHENYLKETONURIA

Phenylketonuria (PKU) is an uncommon inborn error of metabolism caused by an autosomal recessive gene. There is a deficiency in the liver enzyme phenylalanine hydroxylase, which is necessary to convert the amino acid phenylalanine to tyrosine. Phenylalanine is an essential amino acid used by the body for growth. Any excess is changed to tyrosine in the normal individual. The infant with PKU lacks this ability, however, resulting in an accumulation of phenylalanine in the blood, which eventually spills into the urine. Excessive accumulation in the tissues leads to progressive mental retardation.

Incidence of this disorder is one for every 10,000 to 20,000 births. The highest incidence is noted in the white population (from northern Europe and the United States). It is rarely observed in African, Jewish, or Japanese peoples.

The clinical picture involves a normal-appearing newborn, most often with blond hair, blue eyes, and fair complexion. Without treatment, the infant develops vomiting, failure to thrive, and eczematous rashes. By about 6 months of age, the infant exhibits behaviors indicative of mental retardation and other central nervous system (CNS) involvement (seizures, abnormal EEG).

Testing for PKU is mandatory in many states. The Guthrie test is done in many nurseries prior to discharge and is a simple screening tool. This test uses blood obtained by a heel stick, usually on the day of discharge. A second test may be run four to six weeks later to determine the results after milk feedings have been well established. Phenylalanine is found in milk, so its metabolites begin to build up in the infant with PKU once milk feedings are initiated. In order for the screening tests to be accurate, the infant should receive milk feedings for at least 24 hours. This is especially significant for breast-fed infants. It is important to verify that the mother's milk is indeed "in" before performing the test. Hospitals and birth centers frequently discharge mother and infant 24–48 hours after delivery. It is vital that the parents understand the need for the screening procedure, and follow-up is necessary to confirm that the test was done.

Some physicians have the parents do a diaper test for PKU. At about 6 weeks of age, they should take a freshly wet diaper and press the prepared Phenistix against the wet area. They should note the color of the test stick, record the color on the prepared sheet, and mail the form back to the hospital nursery. A green color reaction is positive and indicates probable PKU.

Once identified, an afflicted infant can be treated by a special diet that limits ingestion of phenylalanine. Special formulas such as Lofenalac, which is low in phenylalanine, are available. Special food lists are also available for parents of a PKU child. If treatment is begun before three months of age, CNS damage can be minimized. The diet should be continued through adolescence.

Female children with PKU are now living longer and may bear children. There is a 95% risk of producing a child with mental retardation if the mother with PKU is not on a low-phenylalanine diet during pregnancy. It is recommended that the woman reinstate her low phenylalanine diet a few months before becoming pregnant (Mathews and Smith, 1979).

PARENT EDUCATION

Nursing Management

The birth of the infant produces a definite change in the family unit. The presence of the child results in changed relationships, increased responsibilities, modified life-style, and, it is hoped, pleasure and satisfaction. To be effective, the nurse must assess the family and approach interactions with a family with a clear understanding of their goals and needs. A nonjudgmental approach is a requirement for effective communication.

Before beginning teaching, the nurse must assess the mother's knowledge base: How much does she know, how much does she need to know, and how much can she absorb at one time? Assessment involves both discussion with the mother and observation of her responses and approaches when with her baby.

Demonstration, discussion, film strips, and literature are all effective teaching approaches. Many maternity units offer classes for mothers. These classes provide basic information about physical characteristics, feeding, bathing, dressing, and cord care and answer any questions the mothers may have. Often the group atmosphere and relaxed approach is very beneficial to anxious mothers and provides an ideal opportunity for questions. The new mother may also be anxious about her ability to be a successful parent, and occasions for supervised practice may be especially helpful. In these instances rooming-in provides an opportunity for parents to become acquainted with their child in a controlled environment.

Throughout the hospital stay, care, support, and health teaching of the new family unit should take place. In a brief three or four days, the care of the newborn will be primarily the parents' responsibility. The nursing focus should be on instruction and practice in care of the newborn and preparation for discharge. Follow-up assistance may be needed. Resources such as Visiting Nurse, the La Leche League, and numerous childbirth groups are now offering "after baby is born" classes to assist new parents in the adjustment to a baby. These resources might be shared with couples as part of the discharge planning. In summary, caring for the infant is caring for the family.

Basic Care Information

Prior to discharge, the nursery nurse should discuss basic infant care with the new parents. Information should be provided about the following areas of concern.

Skin Care and Bathing

The newborn is bathed in a warm, draft-free area, and only a portion of the body should be exposed at one time. An infant should *never* be held under a faucet of running water, because rapid water temperature changes may occur. The scalp and genital area should be washed daily. The scalp is lathered using a mild soap and using a soft-bristled brush the lather is then brushed across the scalp. This procedure loosens any scalp desquamation and is beneficial in preventing *cradle cap*. The head is then rinsed well. If cradle cap develops, the use of a dandruff shampoo may be prescribed or an ointment may be ordered to be massaged into the scalp. Manual removal of cradle cap with a comb is an alternative method.

In bathing the infant, one should progress from the cleanest area to the dirtiest. Thus the eyes are bathed first, the genitals last. In cleansing the eyes, care should be taken to wash from the inner canthus to the outer, using a separate area of the washcloth for each eye. Soap is not used on the face, but a mild, nonperfumed soap is used on the remainder of the body. In cases of skin infection, physicians may occasionally order the use of dilute pHisoHex, which should be rinsed thoroughly off the skin. Because pHisoHex has neurotoxic effects, its use is generally restricted, and it is never used routinely. Special care is taken to bathe the body creases. Excessive rubbing may cause skin irritation and should be avoided.

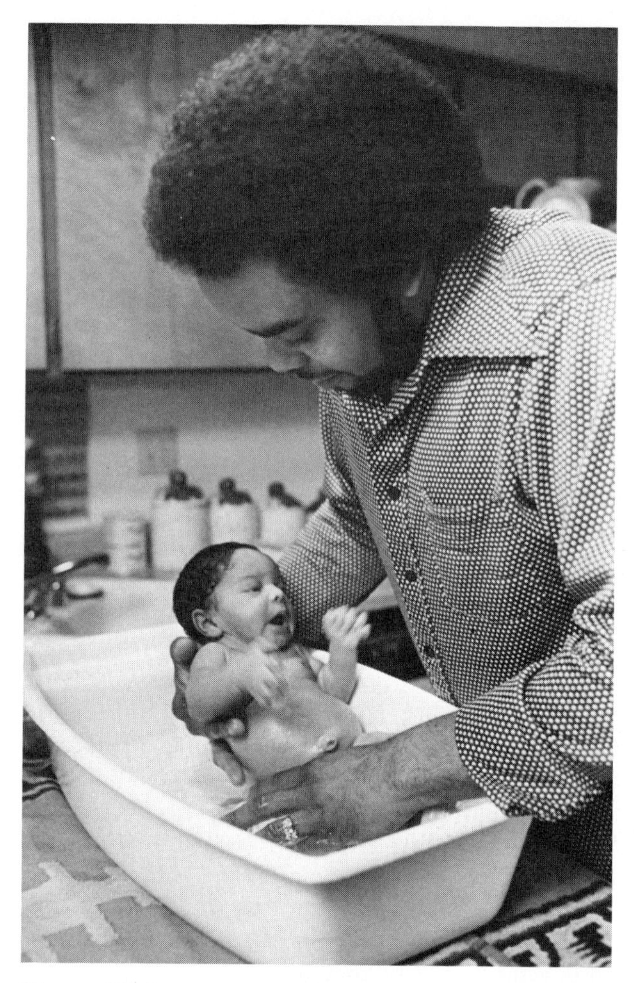

Figure 23–9. When bathing the infant, it is important to support her head. Note that the cord site has healed on this 2-week-old baby.

Cord care is given during the bath and daily as required. The infant is not submerged in water until the cord has separated, which occurs in one to two weeks (Figure 23–9). Until then, the cord is cleansed with alcohol or betadine, which promotes drying and helps prevent infection. The diaper should be attached below the cord so that the cord may be exposed to the air. Foul-smelling discharge or redness around the umbilical area may indicate infection, and the mother is advised

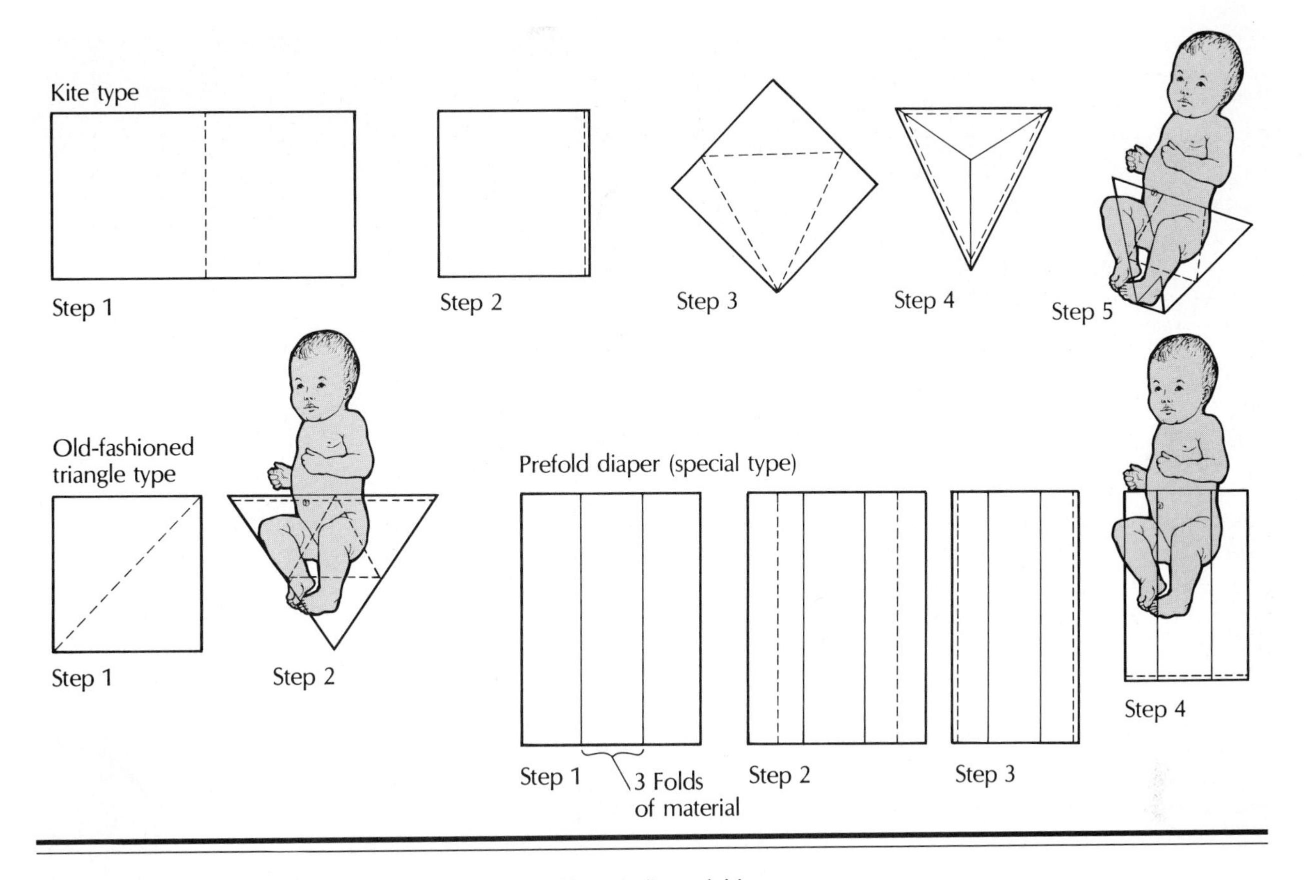

Figure 23–10. Three basic diaper shapes. Dotted lines indicate folds.

to report this to her pediatrician or nurse practitioner.

The genital area is bathed daily and as necessary. The labia in girls are separated and the area washed from front to back. Parents of circumcised boys should be instructed that tub baths are contraindicated until the site heals. The area may be cleansed by moistening a cotton ball and gently squeezing clear water over the site. Practice varies as to the continued use of petroleum jelly or a bactericidal ointment, although excessive quantities should be avoided because they may obstruct the meatal opening. After three to four days, the mother may begin gently retracting the foreskin for cleaning. She should be instructed to observe for bleeding or signs of infection.

Uncircumcised boys should have the foreskin retracted so the glans may be cleansed to remove smegma and accumulated urine. The foreskin is then replaced to prevent edema. A tight foreskin with adhesions should not be forced to retract but may respond to gentle pressure over a period of days or weeks. *Phimosis,* or extremely narrowed opening of the prepuce, may require surgical release by circumcision. Powder is not used, because it may accumulate in the creases and become a source of infection. In very dry climates, a light application of a mild lotion is permitted. Unless otherwise indicated, the mother should limit full baths to three times per week to avoid excessive drying and removal of protective body oils. The face, genitals, and scalp may be washed daily, however.

Diaper rash is caused by the reaction of urea with bacteria and may occur even with good care. Although meconium and breast-milk stools are not irritating, the stools of bottle-fed babies are and may contribute to the development of diaper rash. Prompt diaper changes, cleansing of the area with each change, and the prophylactic use of vitamin A and D ointment help prevent the development of rash. Additional interventions may include leaving the diaper off and exposing the area to air, refraining from use of rubber pants, and use of cloth diapers.

Diaper rash may appear as reddened, chafed,

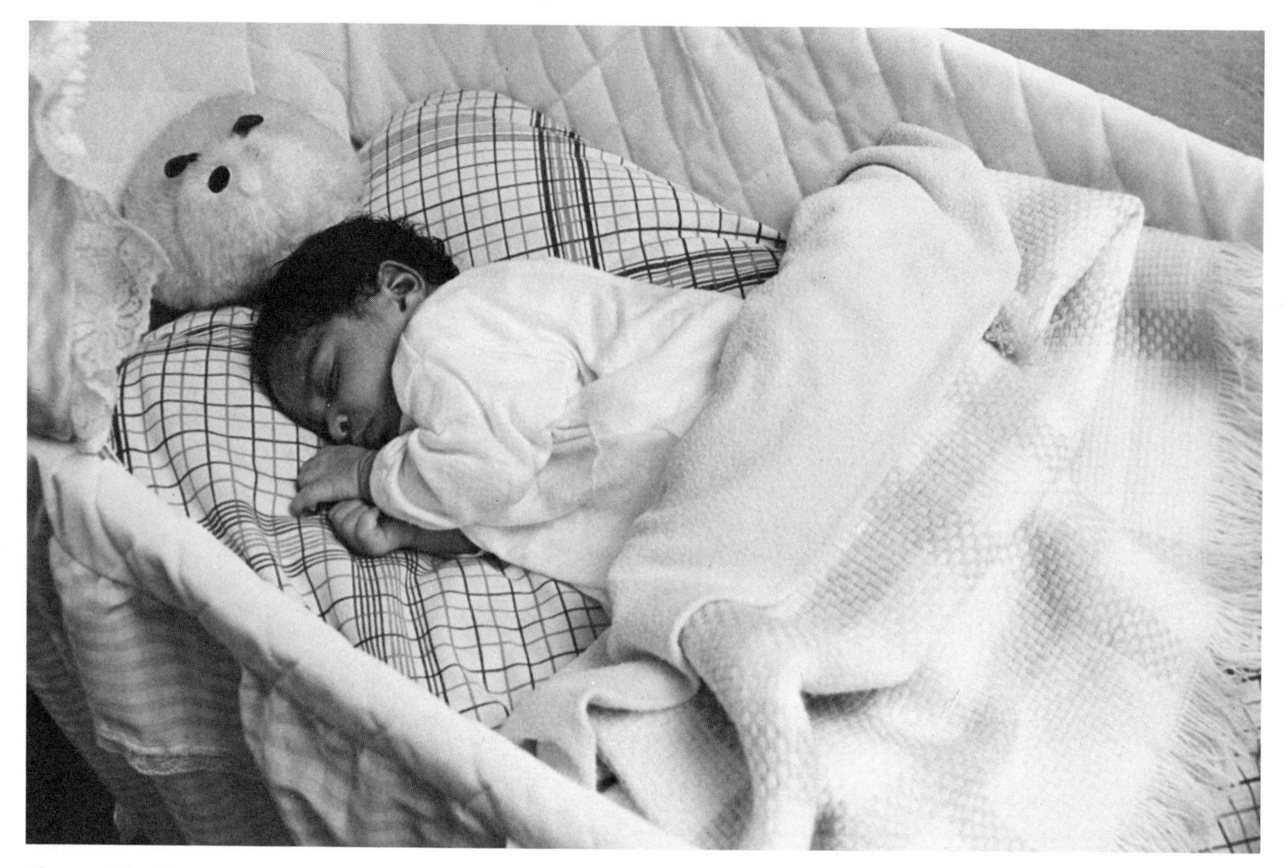

Figure 23-11. The most common sleeping position of the newborn is on the side. The little girl shown here does not need the additional support provided by a rolled blanket.

nonraised areas. In its more severe form, red papules may appear that form craterlike ulcers. Treatment for mild rashes includes cleanliness, exposure to air, and the prescription of specific medications, usually in the form of ointments.

Nail Care

The nails of the newborn are seldom cut in the hospital. During the first days of life, the nails may adhere to the skin of the fingers, and cutting is contraindicated. Within a week the nails separate from the skin and frequently break off. If the nails are long or if the infant is scratching himself, the nails may be trimmed. This is most easily done while the infant sleeps. They should be cut straight across using adult cuticle scissors.

Clothing

In the hospital the infant is dressed in a shirt and diaper and covered with a blanket. A fussy baby frequently quiets if firmly bundled in a blanket, because this seems to promote a sense of security and to help maintain body temperature.

At home the amount of clothing the infant wears is determined by the temperature. Families who maintain the home at 60–65F will dress the infant more warmly than those who maintain the temperature at 70–75F. Diaper shapes vary and are subject to personal preference (Figure 23-10). Prefolded and disposable diapers are generally rectangular. Diapers may also be kite-folded or triangular. The extra material is placed in the front for boys and toward the back for girls to aid in absorbency.

Infant clothing should be laundered separately using a mild soap or detergent. Diapers may be presoaked prior to washing. All clothing should be rinsed twice to remove soap and residue and to decrease the possibility of rash. Some infants may not tolerate the use of clothing treated with fabric softeners; in this case softeners should be avoided.

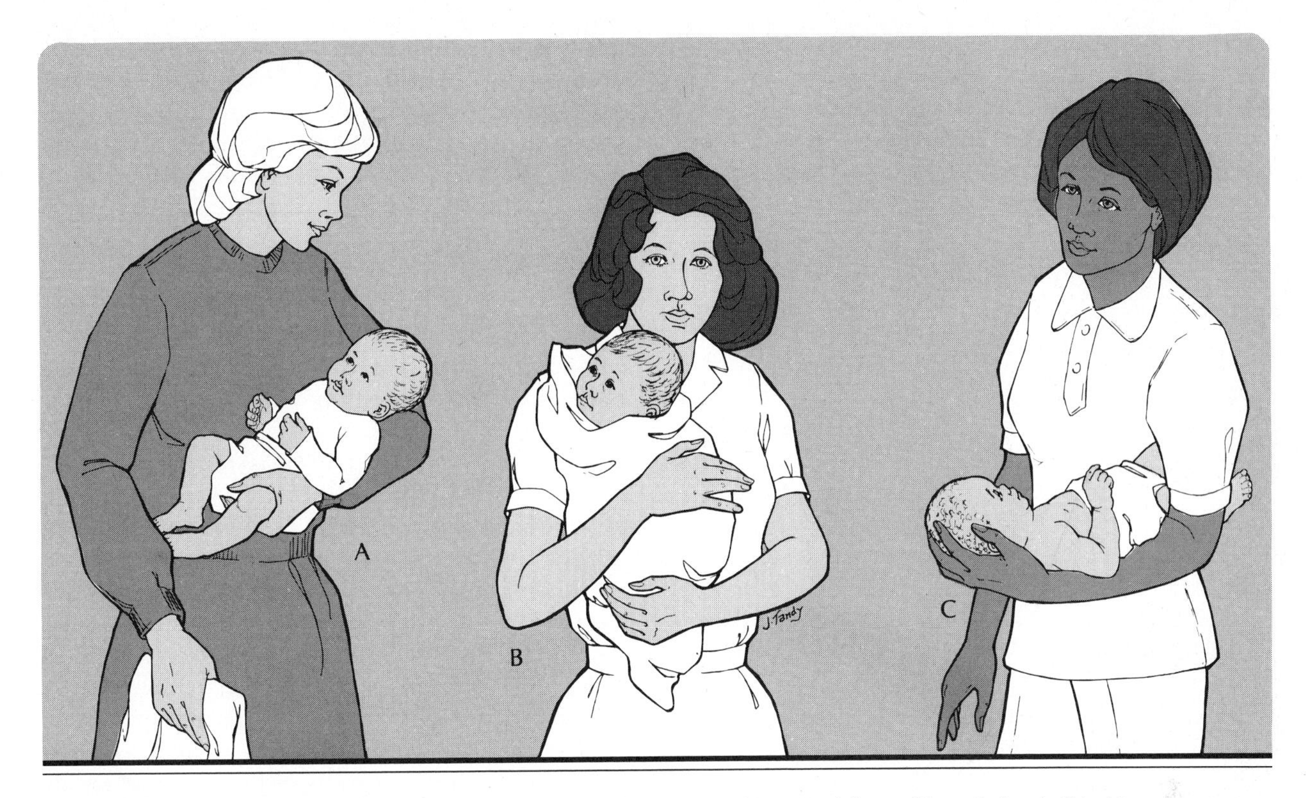

Figure 23–12. Various positions for holding an infant. **A,** Cradle hold. **B,** Upright position, **C,** Football hold.

Positioning the Newborn

The newborn infant is most frequently positioned on his side with a rolled blanket or diaper behind him for support (Figure 23–11). This position facilitates the drainage of mucus and allows air to circulate around the cord. It is also more comfortable for the newly circumcised male. After feeding, the infant is placed on his right side to aid digestion and to prevent aspiration. Once the cord has healed, many infants prefer to lie prone. Care should be taken to periodically change the infant's position during the early months of life, because his skull bones are soft, and flattened areas may develop if the child consistently lies in one position.

Handling the Newborn

The neck muscles of the newborn are weak, and care must be taken to support the head when carrying the baby. He will be able to support his head himself by about the third month.

The *cradle hold* is frequently used with babies, especially during feeding (Figure 23–12,*A*). It provides a sense of warmth and closeness, permits eye contact, frees one of the mother's hands, and provides security because the mother's arm protects the infant's body. The *upright position* provides a sense of closeness and is ideal for burping the baby (Figure 23–12,*B*). In very small infants, the mother's second hand must be used to support the head. The *football hold* frees one of the mother's hands and permits eye contact, although bodily closeness is decreased (Figure 23–12,*C*). It is ideal for shampooing the infant or for carrying him.

Even a newborn infant must be protected from falling, and he should never be left unattended on an unguarded surface.

Nasal Suctioning

The infant generally maintains the patency of his air passages by coughing or sneezing. During the first few days of life, the infant has increased mucus, and gentle suctioning with a bulb syringe may be indicated. The bulb is compressed, then the tip is placed in the nostril and the bulb is permitted to reexpand. The drainage is then compressed out of the bulb onto gauze or a tissue. The bulb may be rinsed in water or normal saline solution. A bulb syringe should always be kept with the infant, and the mother should be familiar with its use.

Infant Feeding

It is the practice in most institutions to offer the infant an initial feeding of sterile water approximately four hours after birth. Parents of breast-fed infants need to be informed of this practice, of the rationale for it, and of the fact that it will not hinder the baby's intake of breast milk. If aspiration should occur, the water is readily absorbed by the lung tissue. Previously glucose water was used, but recent research suggests that glucose may be as damaging to the infant's lung as milk is if aspirated (Avery, 1975). The sterile water provides an opportunity for the nurse to assess the effectiveness of the infant's suck, swallow, and gag reflexes. A softer nipple, often called a "preemie" nipple, may be used if the infant appears to tire easily. Extreme fatigue coupled with rapid respiration and circumoral cyanosis may indicate cardiovascular complications and should be reported. This initial feeding also provides an opportunity to assess the infant for symptoms of tracheoesophageal fistula or esophageal atresia. In cases of atresia, the esophagus ends in a blind pouch. Consequently the feeding is taken well initially, but as the esophageal pouch fills, the feeding is quickly regurgitated unchanged by stomach contents. When a fistula is present, the infant gags, chokes, regurgitates mucus, and may become cyanotic as fluid passes through the fistula into the lungs.

It is not unusual for the neonate to regurgitate some mucus and water following a feeding even though it was taken without difficulty. Consequently the infant should be positioned on his side to facilitate drainage and should be observed carefully. To decrease this mucus, some nurseries routinely aspirate the stomach contents and do gastric lavage when the neonate is admitted from labor and delivery. Inability to successfully pass the stomach tube suggests the possibility of atresia and should be reported immediately.

Some mothers who plan to breast-feed will ask to nurse their infants immediately following birth, while on the delivery table. This practice provides stimulation for milk production and aids in maternal-infant bonding. If the infant appears to have difficulty nursing, the sterile water feeding by the nurse allows an opportunity for assessment. If the water feeding is taken without difficulty and retained, the mother may resume breast-feeding.

Establishing a Feeding Pattern

Following the initial feeding, hospitals frequently establish artificial four-hour time frames for feedings. This scheduling may present difficulties for the new mother. Breast milk is rapidly digested by the infant, and he may desire to nurse every 2 to 3 hours initially, with one to two feedings during the night.

Rooming-in permits the mother to feed as needed. When rooming-in is not available, a supportive nursing staff and flexible nursery policies will allow the mother to feed when the baby is hungry. Nothing is more frustrating to a new mother than attempting to nurse a baby who is sound asleep because he is either not hungry or worn out from crying. Once lactation is established and the family is home, a general feeding pattern, agreeable to both mother and child, is usually established.

Formula-fed infants may waken for feedings every 2 to 5 hours but are frequently satisfied with feedings every 3 to 4 hours. Because formula is digested more slowly, the bottle-fed baby may go longer between feedings and may begin skipping the night feeding within about six weeks.

Both breast-fed and bottle-fed babies may experience growth spurts at certain times during infancy and require increased feeding. These spurts occur at about 10–14 days, at 5–6 weeks, and at around 3 months. The mother of a breast-fed infant may meet these increased demands by nursing more frequently to increase her milk supply, and a slight increase in feedings will meet the needs of the formula-fed infant.

Providing nourishment for her infant is a major concern of the new mother, and her feelings of success or failure may influence her self-concept as she assumes her maternal role. With proper instruction, support, and encouragement, feeding may become a source of pleasure and satisfaction to both parents and child. (See Chapter 27 for a discussion of methods of assisting a mother to breast-feed or bottle-feed her infant.)

Breast Milk and Formula: Nutritional Aspects

Numerous types of commercially prepared formulas meet the nutritional needs of the infant. Bottle-fed babies gain weight a little faster than breast-fed babies because of the higher protein content (as much as 50%–75% more) in cow's milk or commercially prepared formula than in human milk (Table 23–1).

Commercial formulas are fortified with essential nutrients, even iron if specified. According to the Recommended Dietary Allowances, infants from birth to five months of age require 117 cal/kg/day, with a slight reduction in calories required during the second half of infancy (Slattery, 1977). With the standard 20 cal/oz formulas, a 7½-lb infant would need to take 19 oz per day, or 3–4 oz every four hours. Until feedings are established, this intake may help account for the initial weight loss expected. Allergies to artificial formulas may develop, necessitating the use of special formula, whereas breast-fed babies rarely develop milk-associated allergies.

Skim milk does not provide an acceptable alternative for infant feeding, because it provides excessive protein but inadequate calories, fat, and fatty acids. It also causes problems as a result of altered osmolarity. Nutritionists advise against its use for children under 2 years old.

Table 23–1. A Comparison of the Nutritive Content of One Quart of Various Types of Milk*

Nutrient	Cow's milk, whole (3.75) fluid†	Human milk	Ready-prepared infant formula†	Goat's milk, whole fluid	Cow's milk, low fat, 2% fluid‡	Cow's milk, skim fluid‡	1974 NAS-NRC RDA 0–6 mo	6–12 mo
Calories	626.0	684.0	640.0	672.0	485.0	342.0	702.0	972.0
Protein (gm)	32.0	10.12	14.2	34.75	32.50	33.42	—	—
Carbohydrate (gm)	45.4	67.82	66.2	43.43	46.85	47.53	—	—
Lipid (gm)	35.7	43.12	35.0	40.41	18.74	1.76	—	—
Vitamin A (IU)	1347.0	2370.0	1600.0	1806.0	2000.0	2000.0	1400.0	2000.0
Vitamin D (IU)	400.0	4.0**	400.0	23.0	400.0	400.0	400.0	400.0
Vitamin E (IU)**	(1.4)	6.0	12.0	—	—	—	4.0	5.0
Vitamin C (mg)	14.0	49.2	50.0	12.59	9.3	4.6	35.0	35.0
Folic acid (mcg)	49.0	52.0	100.0	6.0	50.0	51.0	50.0	50.0
Thiamine (mg)	0.37	0.136	0.5	0.468	0.381	0.353	0.3	0.5
Riboflavin (mg)	1.57	0.356	0.6	1.347	1.610	1.372	0.4	0.6
Niacin (mg)	0.820	1.740	8.0	2.704	0.839	0.862	5.0	8.0
Vitamin B_6 (mg)	49.0	0.108	0.4	0.449	0.420	0.392	0.3	0.4
Vitamin B_{12} (mcg)	3.475	0.444	2.0	0.634	3.553	3.704	0.3	0.3
Pantothenic acid (mg)	3.05	1.74	3.0	3.026	3.123	3.224	—	—
Calcium (mg)	1161.0	316.0	520.0	1303.0	1187.0	1209.0	360.0	540.0
Potassium (mg)	1474.0	504.0	660.0	1995.0	1507.0	1623.0	—	—
Phosphorus (mg)	909.0	132.0	440.0	1080.0	928.0	989.0	240.0	400.0
Iodine (mcg)	200.0	30.0	65.0	—	—	—	35.0	45.0
Iron (mg)	trace	0.28	1.4/12.0	0.49	0.49	0.39	10.0	15.0
Magnesium (mg)	120.0	32.0	45.0	63.0	133.0	111.0	60.0	70.0
Zinc (mg)	3.71	168.0	4.0	2.93	3.81	3.92	3.0	5.0
Sodium (mg)	496.0	168.0	265.0	486.0	487.0	505.0	—	—

*Modified from *Composition of foods.* 1976. Agricultural Handbook No. 8–1.

†Cow's milk is fortified.

‡Enfamil, values from Mead-Johnson.

**Values taken from Fomon, S. 1974. *Infant nutrition.* 2nd ed. Philadelphia: W. B. Saunders Co.

There is a tendency toward overfeeding with bottle-fed infants. Mothers tend to establish artificial goals and encourage the infant to finish his bottle every time he feeds. This approach does not permit the infant to determine his own requirements. Overfeeding coupled with the higher protein levels of cow's milk and formula may result in rapid weight gain. The formula-fed infant generally doubles his weight within 3½–4 months, whereas nursing infants double theirs at about 5 months (Slattery, 1977).

Opinion as to the use of vitamin supplements for newborns varies. Recommended amounts of vitamins A, D, and C, thiamine, niacin, riboflavin, and ascorbic acid may be obtained from commercially prepared cow's milk or soy-based formulas (see Table 23–1). Human milk does not provide sufficient amounts of vitamin D, iron, or fluoride, and enriched cow's milk has inadequate amounts of vitamin C (Slattery, 1977). Some pediatricians prescribe multivitamins for bottle-fed infants, but this is not a universal practice. If a nursing mother is taking a daily multivitamin, no vitamins will be prescribed for the infant. If she is not taking daily vitamins, a vitamin supplement may be prescribed for her baby.

In 1971 the Committee on Nutrition of the American Academy of Pediatrics recommended that all bottle-fed infants receive an iron-fortified formula for the first year of life. Breast-fed infants should be given an iron supplement in the form of soluble dissociated ferrous salts (Fomon, 1979). Parents need to be informed about the constipation that sometimes results from iron-enriched formula and about various methods to alleviate the constipation.

Effects of Drugs in Human Milk

Drugs in the maternal circulation are frequently found in the breast milk and are then ingested by the infant. Some produce definite adverse effects, whereas others do not. For instance, bromides may produce drowsiness and a rash; heroin appears in breast milk, and withdrawal symptoms may occur in the infant if the feeding is withheld or if his mother is deprived of the drug; anticoagulants administered to treat maternal phlebitis may result in the alteration of infant prothrombin times (Bergersen, 1979).

SUMMARY

At the moment of birth, numerous adaptations must take place in the newborn's system. Immediate initiation of respiration and changes in the circulatory patterns are essential for extrauterine life. Other systemic changes occur at a slower rate. An understanding of the normal adaptations is necessary to provide a basis for nursing assessment and intervention. Comprehensive nursing care of the newborn must be given over the short period of time that the newborn remains hospitalized. An important component is the instruction and counseling of parents so they will be better able to care for their infant.

SUGGESTED ACTIVITIES

1. Prepare a care plan for a newborn during his first day of life.
2. Write out the response you would make if a parent were to ask: Should I breast-feed my baby? Isn't formula just as good? Why should I have my baby circumcised?
3. Assist with a parent education class. Demonstrate infant care techniques, such as bathing and formula preparation.
4. Develop an instruction sheet that can be used to give parents information for care of the newborn after discharge from the hospital.

REFERENCES

Avery, G. B. 1975. *Neonatology.* Philadelphia: J. B. Lippincott Co.

Bergersen, B. S. 1979. *Pharmacology in nursing.* St. Louis: The C. V. Mosby Co.

Desmond, M. M., et al. 1966. The transitional nursery: a mechanism for preventive medicine. *Pediatr. Clin. N. Am.* 13:656.

Fomon, S. 1974. *Infant nutrition.* 2nd ed. Philadelphia: W. B. Saunders Co.

Fomon, S. J., et al. Jan. 1979. Recommendation for feeding normal infants. *Pediatrics.* 63:52.

Gluck, L., and Kulovich, M. V. 1973. Fetal lung development. *Pediatr. Clin. North Am.* 20:373.

Jensen, M., et al. 1977. *Maternity care: the nurse and the family.* St. Louis: The C. V. Mosby Co.

Klaus, M., and Fanaroff, A. A. 1973. *Care of the high-risk infant.* Philadelphia: W. B. Saunders Co.

Korones, S. 1976. *High-risk newborn infants.* 2nd ed. St. Louis: The C. V. Mosby Co.

Marlow, D. R. 1977. *Pediatric nursing.* Philadelphia: W. B. Saunders Co.

Mathews, A., and Smith, A. Oct. 1979. NAACOG Conference on Genetics. Colorado Springs, Colo.

Platt, L. D., et al. 1978. Human fetal breathing: relationship to fetal condition. *Am. J. Obstet. Gynecol.* 132:514.

Schaffer, A., and Avery, M. E. 1977. *Diseases of the newborn.* 4th ed. Philadelphia: W. B. Saunders Co.

Slattery, J. D. March–April 1977. Nutrition for the normal healthy infant. *MCN.* 2:105.

ADDITIONAL READINGS

Acosta, P. B. 1964. Nutritional aspects of phenylketonuria. In *The clinical team looks at phenylketonuria.* Rev. ed. Washington, D.C.: Children's Bureau, U.S. Department of Health, Education, and Welfare.

Affonso, D. Nov.–Dec. 1976. The newborn's potential for interaction. *J. Obstet. Gynecol. Nurs.* 5:9.

Aladjem, S., and Brown, A. 1977. *Perinatal intensive care.* St. Louis: The C. V. Mosby Co.

Cahill, B. Jan.–Feb. 1974. The neonatal nurse specialist: new techniques for asymptomatic newborns. *J. Obstet. Gynecol. Nurs.* 3:34.

Chalmers, I. July 15, 1976. Neonatal jaundice: cause not known. *Nurs. Times.* 72:1084.

Marcil, V. March 1976. Physical assessment of the newborn. *Canadian Nurse.* 72:21.

Maurer, D. M., et al. Oct. 1976. Newborn babies see better than you think. *Psych. Today.* 10:35.

Miller, G. T., et al. 1965. Phenylalanine content of fruit. *J. Am. Diet. Assoc.* 46:43.

Ounstad, M. May 6, 1976. Infant feeding. *Nurs. Times.* 72:700.

Overback, A. M. Dec. 1974. Drugs used with neonates and during pregnancy: drugs that may cause fetal damage or cross into breast milk, part 3. *RN.* 37:39.

Reeder, S., et al. 1976. *Maternity nursing.* New York: J. B. Lippincott Co.

Scipien, G., et al. 1975. *Comprehensive pediatric nursing.* New York: McGraw-Hill Book Co.

Stokan, R. E. Mar.–Apr. 1977. The right formula for the right infant: making sense of infant nutrition. *MCN.* 2:101.

Wier, R., et al. Spring 1975. A study of infant feeding practices. *Birth Fam. J.* 2:63.

Williams, J. K., et al. Nov.–Dec. 1976. Thermoregulation of the newborn. *MCN.* 1:355.

Wood, C. S. July–Aug. 1976. Immunology related to the newborn. *Nurse Pract.* 1:37.

Worthington, P. Jan.–Feb. 1977. Infant nutrition and feeding techniques. *Pediatr. Nurs.* 3:8.

Ziejel, E., and Van Blarcom, C. 1972. *Obstetric nursing.* 6th ed. New York: The Macmillan Co.

CHAPTER 24

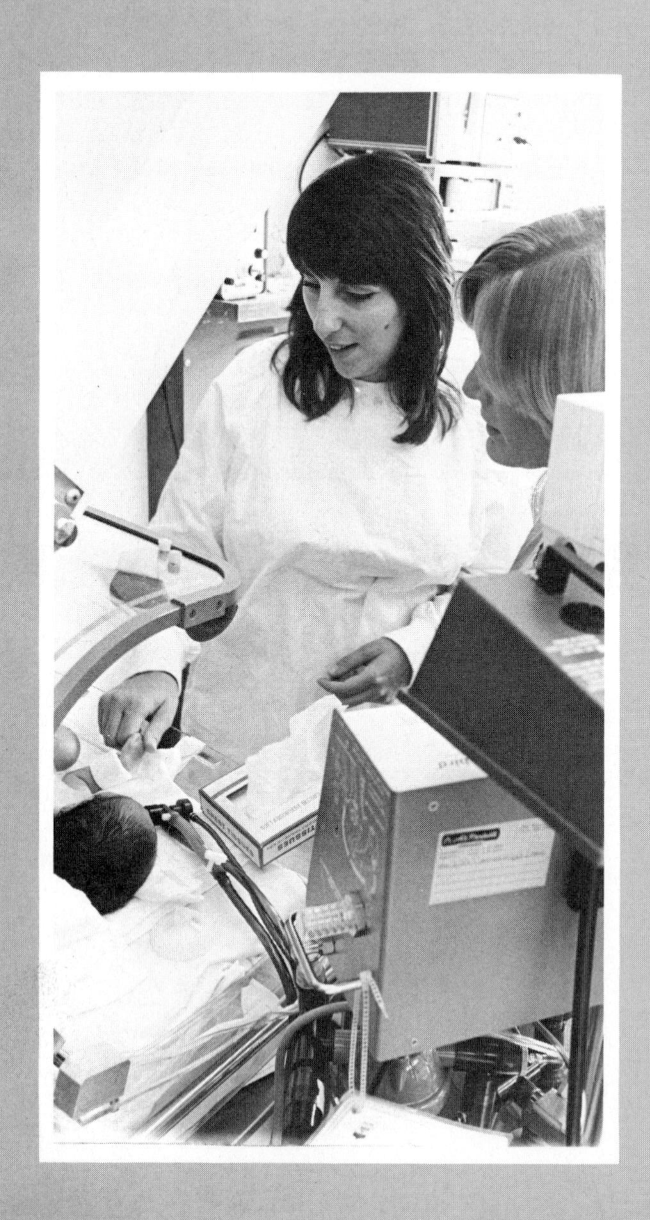

THE HIGH-RISK NEWBORN: NEEDS AND CARE

OBJECTIVES

- Discuss the physical and psychologic handicaps associated with premature, small-for-gestational-age, and large-for-gestational-age infants.
- Describe the methods used to feed a premature infant, the criteria used to determine which method should be used, and the special nursing factors considered when feeding a premature infant.
- Differentiate between postmaturity and placental insufficiency syndrome and explain why infants with these conditions sometimes require care similar to that for a premature infant.
- Identify the needs and nursing support necessary for family members to deal with the crisis of premature birth.
- Discuss reasons why parents are now encouraged to visit and to have early contact with their premature infant and how the nurse can best support the parents in the "mothering" process.
- Identify the clinical manifestations of a newborn in narcotic withdrawal and describe appropriate nursing interventions.
- Relate why hypoglycemia is a nursing problem when caring for the infant of a diabetic and explain its cause and subsequent nursing care.

Within the last 20 years, the field of neonatology has broadened greatly as the findings of its research have become utilized in clinical situations. This process has led to a similar evolution in the hospital care of the neonate, so that today there are many levels of nursery care: special care, transitional care, and low-, medium-, and high-risk care. The nurse is an important caregiver in all types of nurseries. Nursing responsibilities are expanding, and the nurse is the vital link in the multidisciplinary health care communication system. The collaborative efforts of nurses, physicians, specialists, audiologists, nutritionists, inhalation therapists, laboratory personnel, physical therapists, pharmacists, social service personnel, parents, and clergy contribute to the high level of perinatal care available today.

Neonatal care has benefited from such advances in technology as monitoring devices, neonatal respirators, and microscopic laboratory techniques. Nursing and medical management stress the importance of the quality of life for high-risk survivors. Consequently, the incidence of severe sequelae such as neurologic impairment, spasticity, blindness, and hearing loss has decreased. The majority of neonates (85%–95%) surviving current intensive care units are normal; only 5%–10% show definite abnormalities.

Other factors besides the availability of high-level neonatal care influence the outcome. These factors include birth weight, gestational age, type and length of neonatal illness, and environmental and maternal factors.

RISK FACTORS

A high-risk infant is one whose health status renders him susceptible to increased morbidity or mortality because of dysmaturity, immaturity, physical disorders, or complications of birth. In the vast majority of instances the infant is the product of a pregnancy involving one or more predictable risk factors. These risk factors include low socioeconomic level of the mother, preexisting maternal conditions such as heart disease, obstetric factors such as age or parity, medical conditions related to pregnancy such as prenatal maternal infection, and obstetric complications such as abruptio placentae. Tables 24–1, 24–2, and 24–3 list various risk factors and their specific effects on the pregnancy outcome. High-risk factors are also discussed in Chapter 10.

Because these factors and the perinatal risks associated with them are known, the birth of a high-risk neonate can be anticipated and prepared for through adequate prenatal care. The pregnancy can be closely monitored, treatment can be instituted as necessary, and arrangements can be made for delivery to occur at a facility with appropriate equipment and personnel to care for both mother and child.

Identification of High-Risk Infants

Identification of a high-risk pregnancy is usually made during prenatal visits and is based on the history and on laboratory data such as serology, blood type, Rh factor determination (father and mother, if mother is Rh negative), and serum antibody tests for rubella and other infections. Amniocentesis may be indicated to determine the presence of chromosomal disorders or of certain inherited metabolic disorders. Bilirubin pigment tests may be required to estimate Rh isoimmunization, and the L/S ratio may be determined to evaluate fetal lung maturity (Chapter 14). Proper follow-up of high-risk conditions is in order to give optimal care (medical, nursing, and psychologic) to the mother and fetus.

Intrapartally, a valuable tool in identifying the high-risk neonate is the Apgar score. As discussed in Chapter 17, a normal infant will receive a score of 7–10, a moderately depressed infant will have a score of 3–6, and a severely depressed infant will have a score of 0–2. Infants with scores of 0–6 receive resuscitative treatment as necessary (see p. 783). It has been demonstrated that the lower the Apgar score at five minutes after birth, the higher the percentage of neurologic abnormalities after one year. This percentage also increases significantly as birth weight decreases (Korones, 1976).

The newborn classification and neonatal mortality risk chart is another useful tool in identifying newborns at risk (Figure 24–1). Prior to construction of this classification tool, birth weight of

Table 24–1. Risk Factors—Preconception*

Factor	Risk	Factor	Risk
Social			
Low income level	Poor antenatal care Multiparity Eclampsia	Hereditary disease	Cystic fibrosis Meconium ileus
Heavy work during pregnancy	Placental insufficiency Antepartum hemorrhage	Renal and cardiac disease	Toxemia Maternal cardiac decompensation Increased maternal death rate and perinatal mortality
Poor diet	Fetal malnutrition Prematurity		
Lack of cooperation with physician	Undetected hypertension Anemia Albuminuria	Obesity	Hypertension Pelvic disproportion
Illegitimacy	Poor antenatal care Increased birth risks	Living at high altitude	Low birth weight
Medical		*Obstetric*	
Anemia due to iron or vitamin B_{12} deficiency	Prematurity Malnourished babies	<16 or >40 years	Abortion Toxemia Congenital abnormalities
Diabetes mellitus	Hypertension Preeclampsia Toxemia Large-for-gestational-age babies Congenital abnormalities Increased cesarean section rate	Older primipara	Increased risks to baby
		Multiparity >3	Ante- and postpartum hemorrhage
		Previous history of fetal loss	
		Low-birth-weight infant	
		Multiple pregnancy	Fetal risk

*From Avery, G. B., ed. 1975. *Neonatology.* Philadelphia: J. B. Lippincott Co., p. 24.

Table 24–2. Medical Risk Factors—Pregnancy*

Factor	Risk	Factor	Risk
Infective		Herpes simplex	Neonatal hepatitis
Viral		Cytomegalovirus	Neonatal hepatitis Encephalopathy
Rubella, first trimester	Congenital heart disease Cataracts Nerve deafness Bone lesions Prolonged virus shedding	Vaccinia (especially first trimester)	Congenital vaccinia
		Maternal varicella	Congenital varicella
		Bacterial	
Rubella, second and third trimesters	Hepatitis Thrombocytopenia	Syphilis	Abortion Congenital syphilis

Table 24–2. Cont'd

Factor	Risk	Factor	Risk
Tuberculosis	Neonatal transplacental transmission	Hyperthyroidism	Neonatal goiter from antithyroid drugs Neonatal thyrotoxicosis (LATS)
Coliform urinary tract infection	Premature delivery Neonatal infection		
		Myasthenia gravis	Exacerbation and resistance to drug therapy
Protozoal		Preeclampsia, nephritis, hypertension, excessive smoking by mother	Premature births Intrauterine growth retardation with small-for-gestational-age babies
Toxoplasmosis	Retinal, CNS lesions Hepatitis Microcephaly Thrombocytopenia		
		Unusual maternal medication or addictive drug abuse	Congenital abnormalities Neonatal withdrawal symptoms
Malaria	Transplacental spread		
Noninfective		Falling urinary estriol levels	Failing placental (placental insufficiency) function, fetal risk
Hypertension and other cardiovascular disease	Premature birth Fetal embarrassment		

*From Avery, G. B., ed. 1975. *Neonatology.* Philadelphia: J. B. Lippincott Co., p. 25.

less than 2500 gm was the sole criterion for the determination of maturity. It was eventually recognized that an infant could weigh more than 2500 gm but be immature. Conversely, an infant less than 2500 gm might be functionally at term or beyond. Thus, birth weight and gestational age became the criteria used to assess neonatal maturity and mortality risk.

According to the newborn classification and neonatal mortality risk chart, *gestation* is divided as follows:

- Preterm = 0–37 (completed) weeks
- Term = 38–41 (completed) weeks
- Postterm = 42+ weeks

In Figure 24–1, intrauterine growth curves are represented for the 10th and 90th percentiles. Large-for-gestational-age (LGA) infants are those above the 90th percentile. Appropriate-for-gestational-age (AGA) infants are those between the 10th and 90th percentiles. Small-for-gestational-age (SGA) infants are those below the 10th percentile.

A newborn is assigned to one of the following nine categories depending on birth weight and gestational age:

- (Pr LGA) Preterm, large for gestational age
- (Pr AGA) Preterm, appropriate for gestational age
- (Pr SGA) Preterm, small for gestational age
- (F LGA) Term, large for gestational age
- (F AGA) Term, appropriate for gestational age
- (F SGA) Term, small for gestational age
- (Po LGA) Postterm, large for gestational age
- (Po AGA) Postterm, appropriate for gestational age
- (Po SGA) Postterm, small for gestational age

Neonatal mortality risk is the chance of death within the neonatal period (see Chapter 2). As in-

Table 24-3. Obstetric Risk Factors—Labor*

Factor	Risk
Abnormal presentation	Prematurity Malformation Cesarean section
Abruptio placentae	Fetal asphyxia Fetal exsanguination Perinatal mortality
Eclampsia, preeclampsia	Fetal morbidity, mortality
Fetal heart aberrations	Fetal distress Paroxysmal tachycardia
Multiple births	Small-for-gestational-age babies Prematurity Feto-fetal transfusion Failure to recognize increased perinatal mortality
Oligohydramnios	Postmaturity Congenital malformation Renal lesions
Hydramnios	Esophageal or other high alimentary tract atresias CNS anomalies Myelocele Hydrops
Precipitate delivery	Tentorial tears Neonatal asphyxia
Prolonged labor	Fetal asphyxia Intracranial birth injury
Rhesus or blood group sensitization	Hydrops Icterus gravis Neonatal anemia Kernicterus Hypoglycemia
Uterine rupture	Fetal asphyxia
Early rupture of the membranes (>48 hours before delivery)	Infection
Postcontraction fetal bradycardia	Fetal asphyxia
Fever	Premature delivery Neonatal infection
Meconium staining of amniotic fluid	Fetal asphyxia indicated by fetal scalp sample of blood pH <7.2

*From Avery, G. B., ed. 1975. *Neonatology.* Philadelphia: J. B. Lippincott Co., p. 26.

dicated in Figure 24-1, the neonatal mortality risk decreases as both gestational age and birth weight increase. Infants with less maturity (small for gestational age) and smaller birth weight have the highest neonatal mortality risk. Examination of the figure also reveals that two infants of the same birth weight with different gestational ages may have very different neonatal mortality risks. For example, infant A may have a birth weight of 3250 gm and a gestational age of 34 weeks. If two lines are drawn from these values on the chart, one horizontal and one vertical, the point at which the two meet gives the risk—in this case 1%. Infant B, on the other hand, may also have a birth weight of 3250 gm but a gestational age of 40 weeks. The graph indicates that his risk is only 0.1%. Infant A thus has a mortality risk ten times as great as infant B has, although they are of the same birth weight.

Neonatal mortality risk can be used to anticipate complications. In Figure 24-2 the infant's birth weight is located in the vertical column and his gestational age in weeks is found horizontally. The area where the two meet on the graph identifies commonly occurring problems and assists in the identification of the needs of particular infants for special observation and care. For example, an infant of 2000 gm at 40 weeks' gestation should be carefully assessed for evidence of fetal distress, hypoglycemia, congenital anomalies, congenital infection, and polycythemia.

Nursing Management of High-Risk Infants

The assessment of the at-risk newborn is an ongoing process beginning with the history of the infant, which considers family and maternal history and other factors that may influence in utero development. Family history provides useful information about the parents and close relatives and has been correlated with neonatal disease. The maternal history contains information about elements of the prenatal environment, including medications and any complications of pregnancy, that can influence the infant's adaptation to extrauterine life. This historical information about the newborn enables the nurse to assess existing or potential nursing care needs and to utilize them as a basis for planning and giving individual nursing care.

In the delivery room, the Apgar score and careful observation form the basis of assessment and are correlated with information such as the

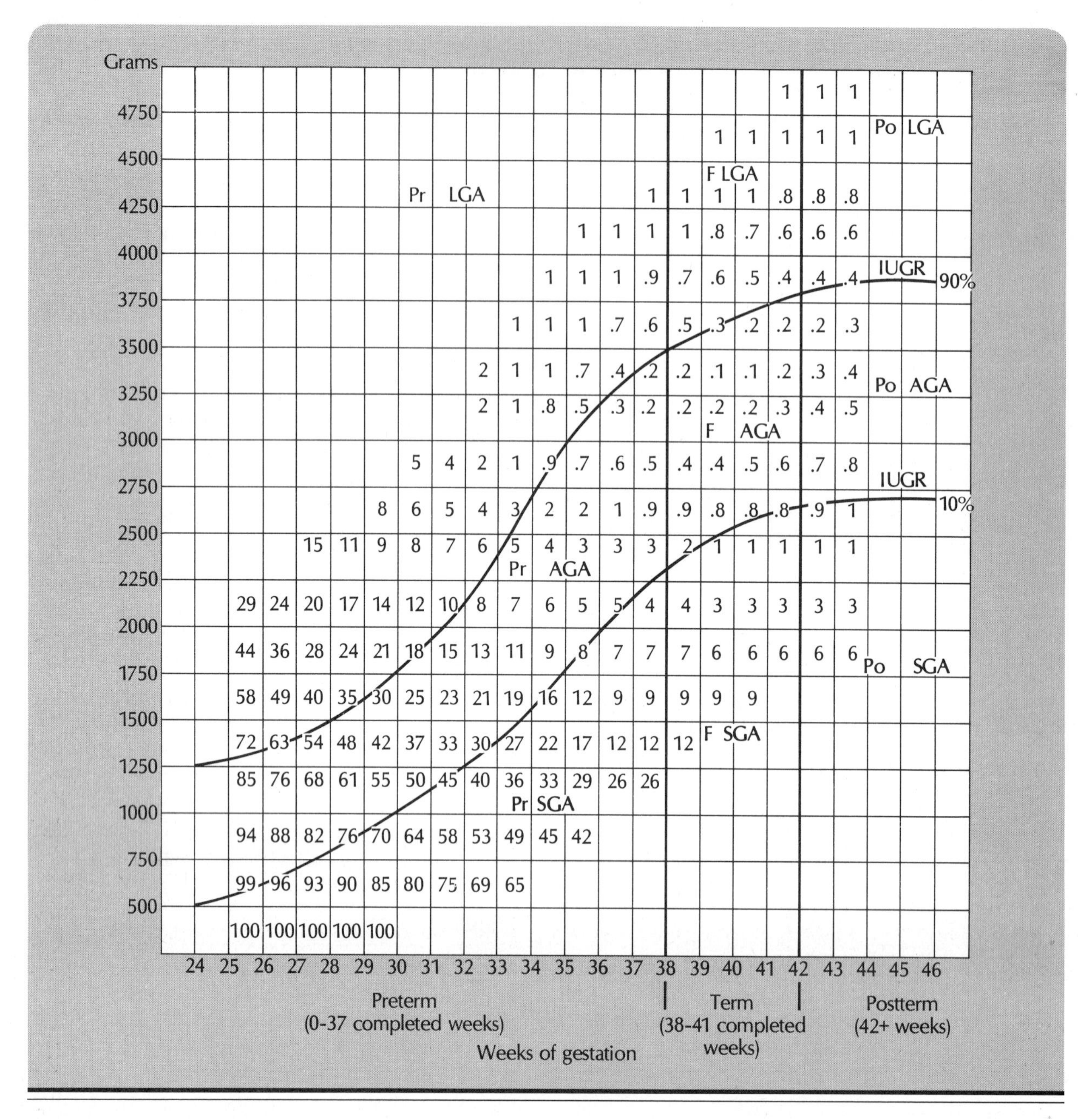

Figure 24–1. Newborn classification and neonatal mortality risk. (Modified from Lubchenco, L. O., et al. 1972. Neonatal mortality rate: relationship to birth weight and gestational age. *J. Pediatr.* 81:814.)

duration of labor, maternal analgesia and anesthesia, and any complications of labor or delivery that may have occurred.

Assessment continues when the newborn is admitted to the nursery. The family history, maternal history, information about the labor and delivery, Apgar score, and treatments instituted in the delivery room are evaluated in conjunction with the physical examination of the newborn. As discussed in Chapter 22, the physical examination includes all of the following:

1. Completion of a nursing information profile (see Figure 22–1).
2. Consideration of the newborn's classification as AGA, SGA, or LGA, based on the newborn classification and neonatal mortality risk chart (see Figure 22–4).

PARENT-INFANT INTERACTION	COMMUNICATIONS:		
	Date	Information to Parents	Parental Reactions/Attitudes
NURSING HISTORY			

Figure 24–4. Kardex 2.

4. *36–38 weeks' gestation.* These infants have been called borderline or intermediate in their prematurity. They have characteristics of both term and preterm infants and may need minimal supportive therapy.

The incidence of premature births in the United States ranges from 7% in white infants to 14%–15% for nonwhites. The mortality and morbidity of preterm infants is higher than for those reaching term. As the gestational age and the birth weight decrease, the neonatal mortality risk increases.

The major problem of the preterm infant is (variable) immaturity of all systems. The degree of immaturity depends on the length of gestation. Thus infants of 27 weeks' gestation can be expected to exhibit more immaturity than infants of 38 weeks' gestation. The degree of immaturity also presents problems of management. Maintenance of the preterm infant falls within narrow physiologic parameters. "Catch-up care" is usually not possible if ground is lost in initial management. Improper physiologic management or lack of it adds stress and feeds the vicious cycle of physiologic deterioration. Care of the high-risk neonate depends on minute-to-minute observations and changes based on physiologic parameters.

Improved outcome of survivors has been traced to measures of physiologic management and support. It is essential to infant survival that the neonatal nurse understand the principles of physiologic management for her tiny patients (Figure 24–5). The organization of nursing care must be directed toward:

1. Decreasing physiologically stressful situations.
2. Constantly observing for subtle signs of change in clinical condition.
3. Interpreting laboratory data and coordinating interventions.
4. Conserving the infant's energy, especially in frail, debilitated prematures.
5. Providing for developmental stimulation and sleep cycle.
6. Assisting the family in attachment behaviors.

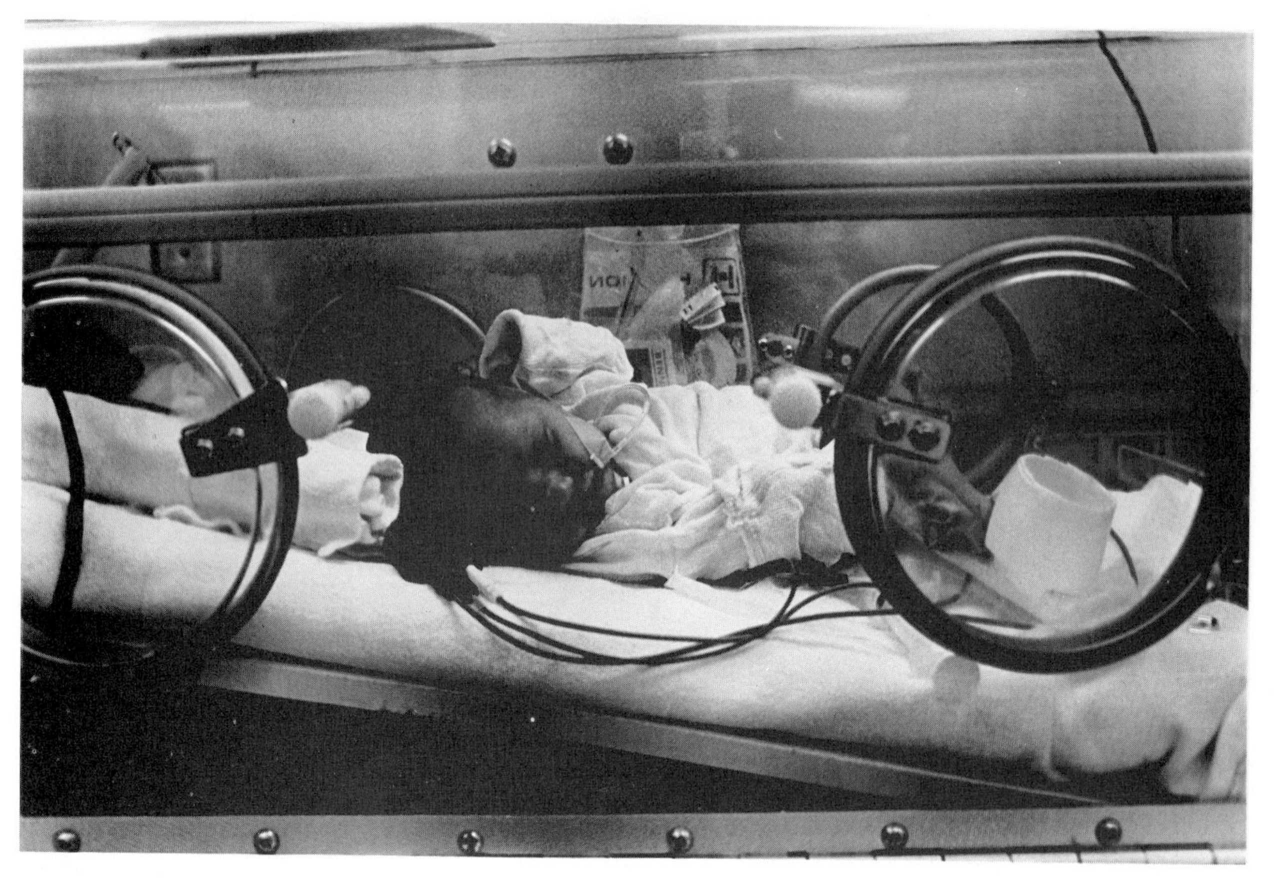

Figure 24–5. Premature infant.

Reactivity Periods

The newborn infant's response to extrauterine life is characterized by two periods of reactivity, as discussed in Chapter 23. Because of the immaturity of all systems in comparison to those of the full-term neonate, the preterm infant's periods of reactivity are delayed. The first period of reactivity, which is characterized by activity and tachycardia, is delayed in the premature infant. The nonreactive period that follows is also delayed. The infant is usually hypotonic and unreactive. The nurse should observe the infant closely for the development of respiratory distress, as indicated by cyanosis and tachypnea. The second period of reactivity is delayed in onset until approximately 12–18 hours of age. Premature infants should be observed closely with monitoring systems for onset of apnea and bradycardia, as the onset is insidious.

Nutrition and Fluid Requirements

Providing adequate nutrition and fluids for the premature infant is a major concern of the health care team. It is now recognized that early feedings are extremely valuable in maintaining normal metabolism and decreasing the possibility of such complications as hypoglycemia, hyperbilirubinemia, hyperkalemia, and azotemia.

Because of the preterm infant's general immaturity, certain problems are inherent in the feeding process:

1. There is marked danger of aspiration and its associated complications because of the infant's poorly developed gag reflex and incompetent esophageal cardiac sphincter.
2. Sucking and swallowing reflexes are poor.
3. Stomach capacity may be small, yet the caloric requirements are fairly high.

4. Absorption of essential nutrients is decreased because of malabsorption and nutritional loss associated with vomiting and diarrhea.
5. Fatigue associated with sucking may lead to increased basal metabolic rate, increased oxygen requirements, and its sequelae of complications.

Schedule of Feedings

Sterile water is the fluid of choice for the first few feedings, because fewer severe tissue reactions develop should aspiration occur. Feeding regimens are then established based on the weight and estimated stomach capacity of the infant (see Table 24-4). In many instances it is necessary to supplement the oral feedings with parenteral fluids in order to maintain adequate hydration and caloric intake.

Caloric intake necessary for growth is 110-125 cal/kg/day. In addition to the relatively high caloric needs, the preterm infant requires more protein (3-4 gm/kg, as opposed to 2.0-2.5 gm/kg/day for the full-term infant). To meet these needs, a number of higher calorie-higher protein formulas are available (Table 24-5) that meet the premature's nutritional demands yet do not overtax the concentration abilities of his immature kidneys. It is customary to begin feedings with concentrations of 20 cal/oz (although less concentrated formulas are available) and gradually increase to 24 or 27 cal/oz formulas as the infant tolerates them.

Parameters indicative of adequate nutritional state include:

1. Continued weight gain (there may be no gain for several days, but weight loss should not exceed 15% of the total body weight)
2. Normal blood pH (no metabolic acidosis)
3. Urine output
   a. Volume at 1-3 ml/kg/hr
   b. Specific gravity at 1.004-1.010
   c. Absence of glycosuria when checked by Dipstix/Clinitest
4. Normoglycemic state
   a. Observe for hypoglycemia—Dextrostix value below 45 mg/100 ml or clinical symptoms
   b. Observe for hyperglycemia—Dextrostix value above 130 mg/100 ml

Gavage Feeding

When the neonate is very immature, has a poorly developed gag reflex, and has CNS depression or

Table 24-4. Oral Feeding Schedule for the Low-Birth-Weight Infant*

Time and substance[†]	Less than 1000 gm Amount	Less than 1000 gm Frequency	1001-1500 gm Amount	1001-1500 gm Frequency	1501-2000 gm Amount	1501-2000 gm Frequency	More than 2000 gm Amount	More than 2000 gm Frequency
First "drink": sterile H_2O, 0.45% saline, 5% glucose	1-2 ml	1 hr	3-4 ml	2 hr	4-5 ml	2-3 hr	10 ml	3 hr
Formula: Subsequent feedings, 12-72 hr	Increase 1 ml every other feeding to maximum 5 ml	1 hr	Increase 1 ml every other feeding to maximum 10 ml	2 hr	Increase 2 ml every other feeding to maximum 15 ml	2-3 hr	Increase 5 ml every other feeding to maximum 20 ml	3 hr
Formula: Final feeding schedule, 150 ml/kg	10-15 ml	2 hr	20-28 ml	2-3 hr	28-37 ml	3 hr	37-50 ml	3-4 hr

*Modified from Avery, G. B., ed. 1975. *Neonatology.* Philadelphia: J. B. Lippincott Co., p. 863.
[†]Supplemental IV fluids should be given to fulfill fluid requirements of 150-200 ml/kg or to give urine specific gravities of 1.005-1.008.

Table 24-5. Commonly Used Premature Formulas*

Formula	Caloric content	Contents per 100 ml usual dilution: CHO		Protein		Fat	
		Gm %	Approx. cal distrib. %	Gm %	Approx. cal distrib. %	Gm %	Approx. cal distrib. %
Enfamil 24 premature formula†	79	9.1	45.0	2.8	14	3.7	41.0
Enfamil 24 w/iron†	80	8.3	41.0	1.8	9	4.5	50.0
Similac 27‡	93	9.4	41.0	2.5	11	4.9	48.0
Similac 24 w/iron‡	81	8.3	41.0	2.2	11	4.3	48.0
Similac PM 60/40‡	68	7.5	44.5	1.6	9	3.5	46.9
SMA 24**	79	8.4	43.0	1.8	9	4.2	48.0

*From Avery, G. B., ed. 1975. *Neonatology.* Philadelphia: J. B. Lippincott Co., p. 865.
†Trademark, Mead Johnson.
‡Trademark, Ross.
**Trademark, Wyeth.

associated complications, gavage feeding may be indicated. This is accomplished by passing an orogastric or nasogastric tube. It is imperative that the correct placement of the tube be verified prior to each feeding. When correctly placed, there is little danger, and nutritional requirements can be provided without exhausting the infant. See Procedure 24-1 for nursing management of gavage feeding.

A variation that has become popular is the use of the nasojejunal tube for gavage feeding. Its main advantage is that it decreases the danger of regurgitation and aspiration because the tube is passed directly into the jejunum. More skill, time, and effort are required to pass the tube, but it can be left in place for prolonged periods (up to several weeks) without harmful sequelae. A nasogastric tube may be placed to check for gastric residual fluid related to regurgitation through the pyloric sphincter (Avery, 1975).

Complications

The premature infant is susceptible to various conditions. The following occur most frequently:

1. Preterm LGA:
   Respiratory distress syndrome
   Hypoglycemia
   Hypocalcemia
   Polycythemia
   Birth trauma
   Hyperbilirubinemia
   Infection
   Congenital malformations
2. Preterm AGA:
   Respiratory distress syndrome
   Apnea

Procedure 24–1. Gavage Feeding

Objective	Nursing action	Rationale
Ensure smooth accomplishment of the procedure	Gather necessary equipment, including: 1. No. 8 to No. 12 Fr. feeding tube. 2. Small cup of sterile water. 3. 30–60 ml syringe. 4. ¼-in. paper tape. 5. Stethoscope. 6. Appropriate formula. 7. Blanket for restraint. Explain procedure to parents.	Gavage feeding is used when something interferes with infant's or small child's ability to take feedings by mouth. Size of feeding tube depends on size of infant and viscosity of formula. Sterile water is used to lubricate the feeding tube as well as to flush tubing after feeding. Syringe is used to inject air into stomach for testing tube placement as well as for holding measured amount of formula. Tape is used to mark tube for insertion depth as well as for securing tube during feeding. Stethoscope is needed to auscultate rush of air into stomach when testing tube placement.
Insert tube accurately into stomach	Immobilize the infant in a mummy restraint, and position on his back with the head elevated.	Such immobilization and positioning ensures maximum freedom of nurse's hands for feeding as well as optimal positioning for infant.
	Take tube from package and measure the distance from the tip of the ear to the nose to the xiphoid process, and mark the point with a small piece of paper tape (Figure 24-6).	This measuring technique ensures enough tubing to enter stomach when tube is passed through nose.

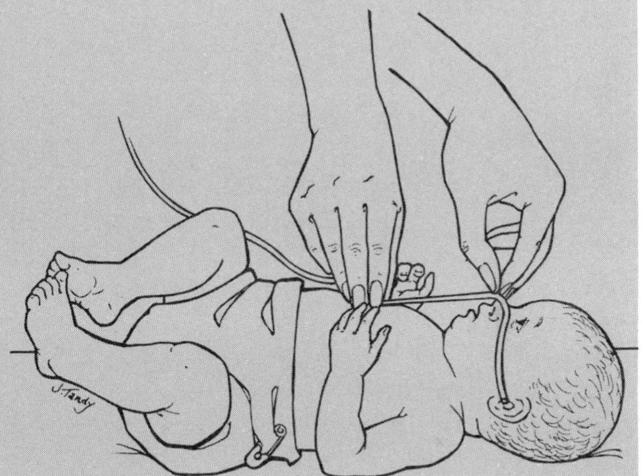

Figure 24–6.

Objective	Nursing action	Rationale
	Lubricate tube by inserting tip in sterile water.	Water should be used, as opposed to an oil-based lubricant, in the event tube is inadvertently passed into lung.
	Stabilize infant's head with one hand, and pass the tube via the nose into the stomach, to the point previously marked. If the infant begins coughing or choking or becomes cyanotic or aphonic, remove the tube immediately.	Any signs of respiratory distress signal likelihood that tube has entered trachea.
	If no respiratory distress is apparent, lightly tape tube in position, draw up 3 ml of air in syringe, and connect it to tubing. Place	Nurse should hear a sudden rush of air as it enters stomach.

Procedure 24-1. Cont'd

Objective	Nursing action	Rationale
	stethoscope over the epigastrium and briskly inject the air (Figure 24-7).	
	Aspirate stomach contents with syringe, and note amount, color, and consistency. Return residual to stomach unless otherwise ordered to discard it.	Residual formula should be evaluated as part of the assessment of infant's tolerance of gavage feedings. It is not discarded, unless particularly large in volume or mucoid in nature, because of the potential for causing an electrolyte imbalance.
	If only a clear fluid or mucus is found upon aspiration and if any question exists as to whether the tube is in the stomach, the aspirate can be tested for pH.	Stomach aspirate tests in the 1-3 range for pH.
Introduce formula into stomach without complication	Separate syringe from tube, remove plunger from barrel, reconnect barrel to tube, and pour formula into syringe.	Feeding should be allowed to flow in by gravity. It should not be pushed in under pressure with syringe.
	Elevate syringe 6-8 in. over infant's head. Allow formula to flow at slow, even rate.	Raising column of fluid increases force of gravity. Nurse may need to initiate flow of

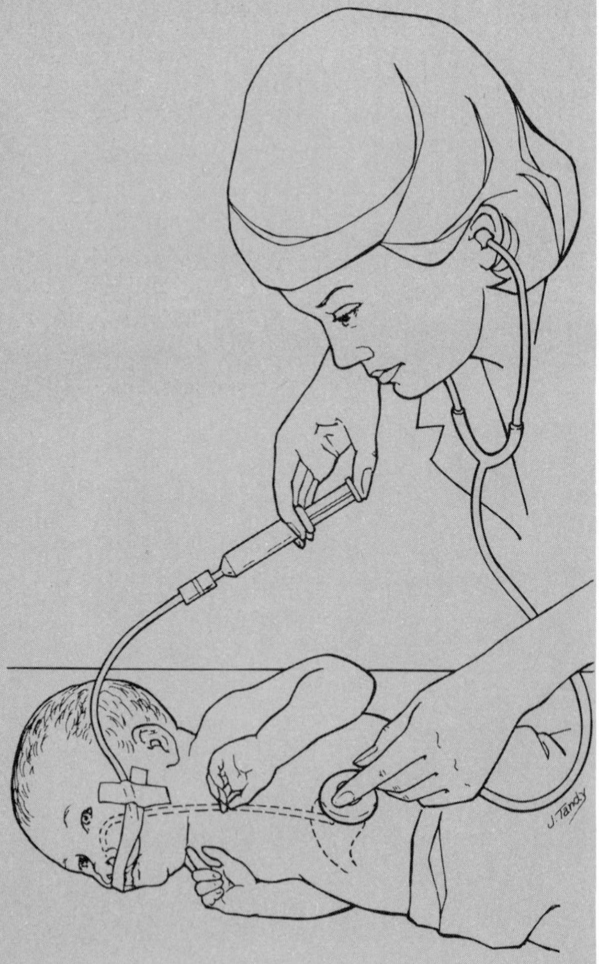

Figure 24-7.

Procedure 24–1. Cont'd

Objective	Nursing action	Rationale
		formula by inserting plunger of syringe into barrel just until formula is seen to enter feeding tube. Rate should be regulated to prevent sudden stomach distention, with possibility of vomiting and aspiration.
	Continue adding formula to syringe until desired volume has been absorbed. Then rinse tubing with 2–3 ml sterile water.	Rinsing tube ensures that infant receives all of formula. It is especially important to rinse tube if it is going to be in place, because this decreases risk of clogging and bacterial growth in tube.
	Remove tube by loosening tape, folding it over on itself, and quickly withdrawing it in one smooth motion. If tube is to be left in, clamp it and position it so that infant is unable to remove it.	Folding tube over on itself minimizes potential for aspiration of fluid, which would otherwise flow from tubing as it passes epiglottis. A tube left in place should be replaced at least every 72 hours.
Maximize feeding pleasure of infant	Whenever possible, hold infant during gavage feeding. If it is too awkward to hold infant during feeding, be sure to take time for holding afterward.	Feeding time is important to infant's tactile sensory input.
	Offer a pacifier to infant during feeding.	Infants fed for long periods by gavage can lose their sucking reflex. Sucking during feeding comforts and relaxes infant, making formula flow more easily.

Hypothermia
Hypoglycemia
Central nervous system hemorrhage
Infection
Malnutrition

3. Preterm SGA:
   Congenital anomalies
   Discordant twin
   Hypoglycemia
   Hypothermia

Hypoglycemia and hypothermia are discussed in this section. The respiratory distress syndrome and other complications are considered in Chapter 25.

Hypoglycemia

Hypoglycemia is the most common metabolic disorder occurring in both AGA and LGA preterm infants. The pathophysiology of hypoglycemia differs for each classification.

AGA preterm infants have not been in utero a sufficient time to store glycogen and fat. Therefore, they have decreased glycogen and fat stores and a decreased ability to carry out gluconeogenesis. This situation is further aggravated as a result of increased utilization of glucose by the tissues (especially the brain and heart) during stress and illness (chilling, asphyxia, and RDS).

LGA preterm infants, on the other hand, are often infants of diabetic mothers (diagnosed, suspected, or gestational diabetics). These infants have increased stores of glycogen and fat. However, there is also increased circulating insulin and insulin responsiveness compared to other newborns. Because of the cessation of high in utero glucose loads at birth, the neonate experiences rapid and profound hypoglycemia.

Hypoglycemia in a preterm infant is defined as a blood glucose below 20 mg/100 ml whole blood (below 25 mg in plasma or serum) in the first three days of life and below 40 mg/100 ml after the first three days.

There may be no clinical symptoms, or some or all of the following may occur:

1. Lethargy, irritability.
2. Poor feeding.
3. Vomiting.
4. Pallor.
5. Apnea, irregular respirations, respiratory distress.
6. Hypotonia.
7. Tremors, jerkiness, seizure activity.
8. High-pitched cry.

The prognosis for untreated hypoglycemia is poor. It may result in permanent, nontreatable central nervous system damage or death.

Differential diagnosis of an infant with nonspecific hypoglycemic symptoms includes:

1. Central nervous system disease.
2. Sepsis.
3. Metabolic aberrations.
4. Polycythemia.
5. Congenital heart disease.
6. Drug withdrawal.
7. Temperature instability.

Interventions are based on knowledge of those at risk, observation for symptoms, screening for asymptomatic occurrence, and provision of adequate caloric intake. Early formula feeding is one of the major preventive approaches. It should be remembered that, if early feedings or IV glucose are started to meet the recommended fluid and caloric needs, the blood glucose is likely to remain above the hypoglycemic level. When hypoglycemia is diagnosed, early feeding is often initiated, along with the administration of intravenous glucose solutions as adjunct therapy. In more severe cases corticosteroids may be administered. It is thought that steroids enhance gluconeogenesis from noncarbohydrate protein sources (Avery, 1975).

Hypothermia and Cold Stress

Several physiologic and anatomic factors predispose the premature infant to heat loss:

1. Because the premature infant tends to be in a position of extension rather than flexion, there is a large surface area for cooling in relation to his body mass.
2. There is inadequate insulation due to lack of or small amount of subcutaneous tissue.
3. There is poor temperature control because of his immature central nervous system.
4. There are decreased stores of brown fat and glycogen for chemical thermogenesis.

Thermogenesis is the term used to describe heat production in response to cold stress. The adult achieves thermogenesis through either involuntary muscle activity (shivering) or an increased metabolic rate (nonshivering thermogenesis). Except in instances of very low environmental temperatures (15C), the infant does not shiver, although he does demonstrate increased muscular activity and restlessness in response to cold (Avery, 1975). Thus the newborn infant's major source of heat production in nonshivering thermogenesis is brown fat. Brown fat (so-called because in gross appearance it is easily distinguishable from regular, white fat) is located between the scapulae, at the axillae, along the vertebral column, around the kidneys and adrenals, and in small deposits around the blood vessels and muscles of the neck. Approximately 2%–6% of the infant's weight is composed of brown fat (Korones, 1976). Generally it is depleted and disappears several weeks after birth.

Nonshivering thermogenesis in the infant occurs as follows:

Cold
↓ triggers
Release of norepinephrine from sympathetic nerve endings
↓ stimulates
Brown fat metabolism
↓ results in
Heat production

Cold stress refers to excessive heat loss resulting in utilization of compensatory mechanisms (increased respirations and nonshivering thermogenesis) to maintain (core) body temperature. Metabolic effects of cold stress include:

1. Increase in nonesterified fatty acids (NEFA) (as a result of anaerobic metabolism), which compete for albumin binding sites with bilirubin.

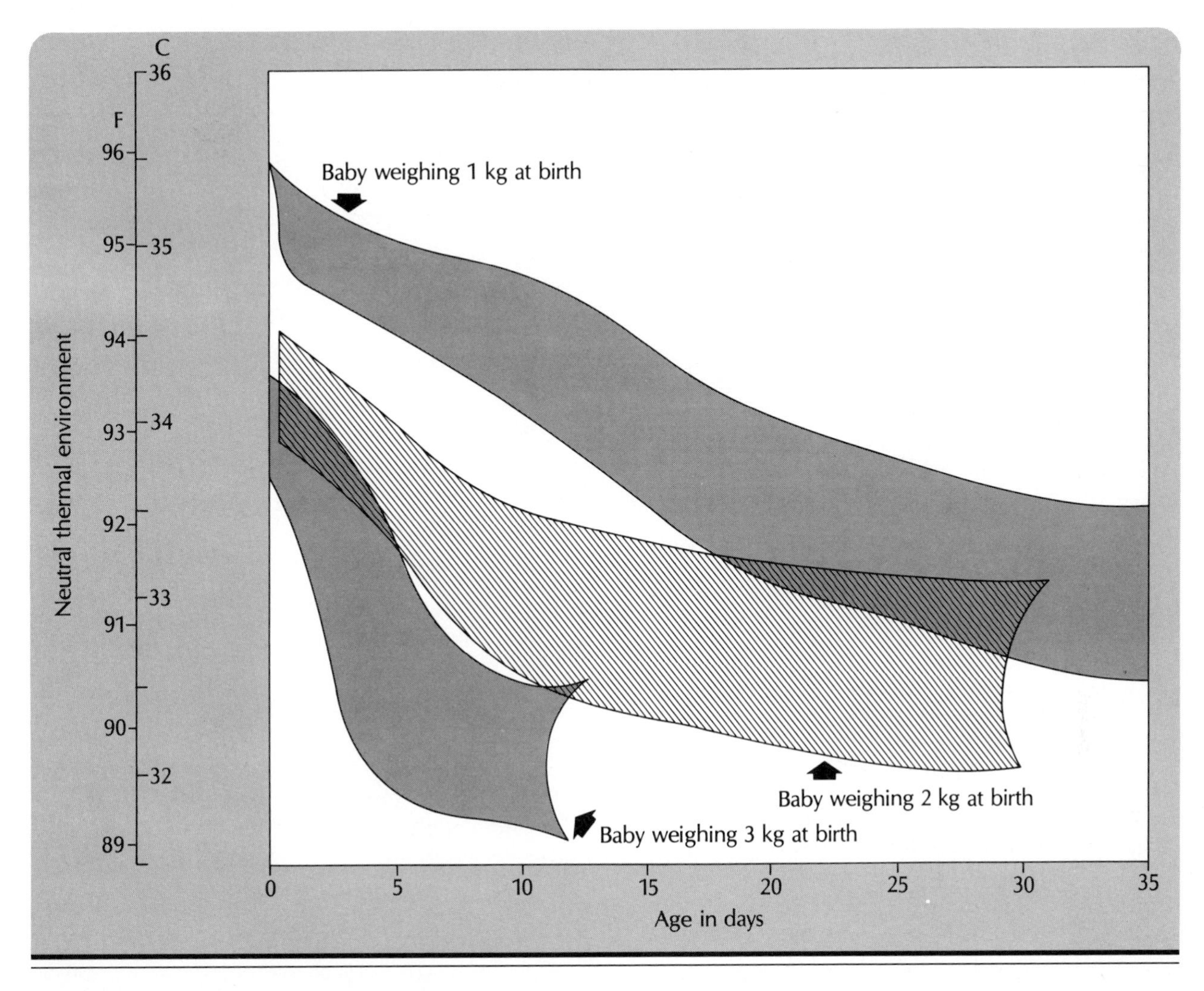

Figure 24–8. Thermal environment of newborn infants. Smaller infants have a higher neutral thermal environment. (Modified from Lubechenco, L. 1976. *The high-risk infant.* Philadelphia: W. B. Saunders Co., p. 133.)

2. Release of norepinephrine to stimulate brown fat metabolism, causing pulmonary vasoconstriction.
3. Occurrence of hypoglycemia as available glucose is utilized for thermogenesis.
4. Increase in oxygen consumption, lactic acid, and metabolic acidosis as body attempts to burn brown fat.

LGA preterm infants, as well as AGA preterms, have difficulty with thermal stability (Figure 24–8). Although LGA preterms have more subcutaneous insulation and glycogen stores than AGA preterms, their system development is immature. They, too, may be ill and stressed and thus need physiologic maintenance and support to prevent additional stress.

Prolonged cold stress can deplete brown fat stores, interfere with normal temperature control, and result in infant death. Because conditions such as hypoxia, hypoglycemia, and intracranial hemorrhage can interfere with the infant's ability to respond to cold stress, it is important that the nurse recognize these conditions and treat than when possible. Prevention is of the utmost importance and is facilitated by careful temperature monitoring and maintenance of neutral thermal environment. For specific nursing interventions in the event of cold stress, see the Nursing Care Plan for AGA and LGA preterm infants.

NURSING CARE PLAN

AGA and LGA Preterm Infants

Patient Data Base

History

1. Maternal history, including general, obstetric, and events of labor and delivery. Factors frequently associated with preterm delivery include:
   a. Age – very young mothers
   b. Closely spaced pregnancies
   c. Low socioeconomic group
   d. Previous history of preterm pregnancy
   e. Abnormalities of reproductive system: uterine malformations, incompetent cervix, infections (both urinary tract and systemic)
   f. Elective cesarean section
   g. Obstetric complications such as abruptio placentae, placenta previa, premature rupture of membranes, amnionitis
2. Fetal conditions associated with preterm delivery include:
   a. Blood incompatability, with resultant erythroblastosis fetalis
   b. Multiple gestations

Physical examination

1. Physical characteristics vary according to gestational age, but certain characteristics are frequently present:
   a. Skin – reddened, translucent, blood vessels readily apparent, lack of subcutaneous fat
   b. Nails – soft, short
   c. Lanugo – plentiful, widely distributed
   d. Small genitals (testes may not be descended)
   e. Head size – appears large in relation to body
   f. Ears – minimal cartilage, pliable, folded over
   g. Resting position – flaccid, froglike position
   h. Cry – weak, feeble
   i. Reflexes – poor sucking, swallowing, and gag
   j. General appearance – emaciated, "wizened old man" look
2. Gestational age determined by utilizing either clinical estimation of gestational age soon after birth with confirmatory neurologic examination to be done after 24 hours or Dubowitz's criteria soon after birth
3. Temperature fluctuates easily – maintenance at 97F ± 1F (36C)
4. Pulse taken apically – often rapid and irregular, normal range 120-160
5. Respirations – 40-60 per minute, shallow, irregular, usually diaphragmatic with intermittent periodic breathing
6. Blood pressure – determine BP for low-weight newborns using normograms (Table 24-6)
7. Color usually pink but may be acrocyanotic; observe for cyanosis, jaundice, or pallor
8. Activity – jerky, generalized movements (Note: Seizure activity is abnormal)
9. Elimination – observe for patency of anus
10. Stool – first stool meconium: stool volume may be decreased because of hypomotility of intestine
11. Voiding – first voiding within 24 hours of birth: output scanty and infrequent for 1-3 days
12. Skull – bones pliable, fontanelle smooth and flat; presence of bulging may indicate central nervous system problem, depressed fontanelle suggests dehydration; observe for cephalhematoma or caput succedaneum
13. Evaluate for common preterm infant morbidities

Laboratory evaluation

Chest x-ray (PA and left lateral) – clear with no infiltration

Complete blood count (CBC) (Table 24-7, p. 755)

Rh determination if mother Rh negative and father Rh positive

Urinalysis on second voided specimen

Specific gravity every voiding – normal range 1.003-1.010

Hematest all stools (if positive, consider necrotizing enterocolitis)

Dextrostix every 4-6 hours – normal 90-120 mg/ml

Blood glucose level drawn if Dextrostix below 45 mg/ml

NURSING CARE PLAN Cont'd

AGA and LGA Preterm Infants

Nursing Priorities

1. Enhance respiratory efforts.
2. Promote homeostasis through provision of neutral thermal environment and through meeting nutrition and fluid needs.
3. Protect from infections.
4. Support psychologic well-being of parents and infant by facilitating positive parent-child bonding and sensory stimulation of infant.
5. Evaluate possible complications with appropriate interventions.

Table 24–6. Blood Pressure of Newborns with Low Weight*

	Gestational age (weeks)													
Body weight (kg)	27	28	29	30	31	32	33	34	35	36	37	38	39	40
0.80	43	44	44	45	45	46	46	47	47	48	48	49	49	50
0.90	44	45	45	46	46	47	47	48	48	49	49	50	50	51
1.00	45	45	46	46	47	47	48	48	49	49	50	50	51	51
1.10	46	46	47	47	48	48	49	49	50	50	51	51	52	52
1.20	46	47	47	48	48	49	49	50	51	51	52	52	53	53
1.30	47	48	48	49	49	50	50	51	51	52	52	53	53	54
1.40	48	49	49	50	50	51	51	52	52	53	53	54	54	55
1.50	49	49	50	50	51	51	52	52	53	53	54	54	55	55
1.60	50	50	51	51	52	52	53	53	54	54	55	55	56	56
1.70	51	51	52	52	53	53	54	54	55	55	56	56	57	57
1.80	51	52	52	53	53	54	54	55	55	56	56	57	57	58
1.90	52	53	53	54	54	55	55	56	56	57	57	58	58	59
2.00	53	53	54	54	55	56	56	57	57	58	58	59	59	60
2.10	54	54	55	55	56	56	57	57	58	58	59	59	60	60
2.20	55	55	56	56	57	57	58	58	59	59	60	60	61	61
2.30	55	56	56	57	57	58	58	59	59	60	60	61	61	62
2.40	56	57	57	58	58	59	59	60	60	61	61	62	62	63

Add for a postnatal age of[†]

Hours	3–7	8–12	13–18	19–24	25–32	33–40	41–54	55–89	90–96
mm Hg	1	2	3	4	5	6	7	8	7

*From Bucci, G., et al. 1972. The systemic systolic blood pressure of newborns with low weight. *Acta Paediatr. Scand.* (Supp.). 229:1.
[†]Systolic blood pressure is determined based on body weight and gestational age. Additional points are added according to postnatal age in hours.

NURSING CARE PLAN Cont'd
AGA and LGA Preterm Infants

Problem	Nursing interventions and actions	Rationale
Respiratory distress	Maintain airway patency through judicious suctioning. Position with head slightly elevated and neck extended. Avoid increased oxygen consumption by maintaining adequate body temperature (97F ± 1F). Observe, record, and report signs of respiratory distress, including: 1. Cyanosis – serious sign when generalized. 2. Tachypnea – sustained respiratory rate greater than 60/min after first 4 hr of life. 3. Retractions. 4. Respiratory grunting. 5. Flaring nostrils. 6. Episodes of apnea. 7. Presence of rales or ronchi on auscultation. Implement treatment plan for respiratory distress, if indicated. Administer oxygen per physician order for relief of symptoms of respiratory distress.	Anatomic and physiological characteristics predispose preterm infant to respiratory distress because: 1. Increased danger of obstruction results from small diameter of bronchi and trachea. 2. Newborn is nose breather and prone to nasal obstruction. 3. Chest wall musculature is weak and efficiency of cough reflex is decreased. 4. Cough and gag reflexes may be absent due to immaturity. 5. Lung surfactant necessary to maintain alveolar stability and prevent collapse is inadequate (Avery, 1975).
Heat losses and cold stress	Increase environmental temperature to maintain thermal neutrality (see Figure 24-8). Reflect principles of anatomy and physiology of temperature control and thermogenesis in planning of care. Minimize heat losses and prevent cold stress by: 1. Warming and humidifying oxygen without blowing over face in order to avoid increasing oxygen consumption. 2. Maintaining skin in dry condition. 3. Keeping isolettes, radiant warmers, and cribs away from windows and cold external walls and out of drafts; utilizing heat shields with small infants. 4. Warming blood for exchange transfusions. 5. Utilizing skin probe to monitor infant skin temperature at 36-37C. 6. Avoiding placing infant on cold surfaces such as metal treatment tables, cold x-ray plates. 7. Padding cold surfaces with diapers and using radiant warmers during procedures.	A neutral thermal environment requires minimal oxygen consumption to maintain a normal core temperature. Body temperature fluctuates because: 1. Assuming a position of extension exposes a relatively large body surface in relation to body mass. 2. Infant lacks subcutaneous fat for adequate insulation. 3. Immature central nervous system provides poor temperature control. 4. Stores of brown fat for chemical thermogenesis are decreased; a small infant (less than 1200 gm) can lose 80 cal/kg/day through radiation of body heat. Physical principles of heat loss effects include: 1. Evaporation – lungs and skin when cooling occurs as a result of water evaporation. 2. Convection – air currents. 3. Conduction – skin contact with cooler object. 4. Radiation – loss of warmth to cooler surrounding objects.
	Implement measures to counteract cold stress by:	Prolonged cold stress depletes brown fat stores, increases oxygen consumption, and results in infant's demise.
	1. Warming slowly to prevent apnea. 2. Observing and recording skin temperature every 15 minutes.	Rapid temperature elevation may cause apnea. Initial response to cold stress is

NURSING CARE PLAN Cont'd
AGA and LGA Preterm Infants

Problem	Nursing interventions and actions	Rationale
	3. Observing, recording, and reporting presence of hypoglycemia, including Dextrostix values below 45 mg/ml, tremors, irritability or lethargy, apnea or seizure activity. Observe, record, and report presence of anaerobic metabolism and initiate interventions for metabolic acidosis.	vasoconstriction and decrease in skin temperature; therefore, monitoring rectal temperature is not satisfactory. A decrease in rectal temperature represents long-standing cold stress with decompensation in infant's ability to maintain core temperature. Attempts to burn brown fat increase oxygen consumption, lactic acid, and metabolic acidosis.
Caloric and fluid intake necessary for growth	Initiate feeding of sterile water at 2-4 hr of age in well preterm infant. Promote growth by providing caloric intake of 110-125 cal/kg/day in small amounts; increased slowly in small amounts (1-2 ml) given more frequently (every 2-3 hr). Supplement oral feedings with intravenous intake per physician orders. Utilize concentrated formulas that supply more calories in less volume, such as Similac 24 calorie or Enfamil 27 calorie. Feed with soft "premie" nipple and burp frequently. Observe, record, and report signs of respiratory distress or fatigue occurring during feedings. Evaluate for signs of dehydration, including depressed fontanelle, poor skin turgor, decreased urine output, sunken eyeballs, and dry mucous membranes. Monitor daily weight, blood pH, normal urine output of 1-3 ml/kg/hour, specific gravity, Dipstix/Clinitest for evidence of glycosuria.	Sterile water is desirable for first feedings because, in the presence of gastrointestinal tract abnormalities and/or aspiration of feeding, fewer pulmonary complications will result. Adequate nutritional and fluid intake promotes growth and prevents such complications as metabolic catabolism, hypoglycemia, and dehydration. Small, frequent feedings of high caloric formula are utilized because of limited gastric capacity and decreased gastric emptying. Growth is evaluated by increase in weight, length, and body measurements.
Fatigue during feedings	Utilize an orogastric or nasogastric tube or nasojejunal gavage feedings in small premature infants not tolerating intermittent volumes of feeding. Facilitate continuous feedings and prevent vomiting by placing nasojejunal tube past pylorus. Initiate safety factors with gavage feedings: 1. Evaluate proper tube placement by aspiration of gastric contents; inject a small amount of air into stomach and auscultate with a stethoscope; place end of catheter in water and watch for continuous bubbling. 2. Allow gravity flow for feedings and never push a tube feeding. Determine presence of residual formula in stomach prior to initiating feeding by aspirating from gastric tube and replacing amount before remainder of feeding is given.	Suck, swallow, and gag reflexes are immature at birth of preterm infant. Nipple feeding, an active rather than passive intake of nutrition, requires energy expenditure and burning of calories by infant. Gavage feedings require less energy expenditure on the part of the preterm infant. Decrease in exhaustion is an important consideration in feeding an infant who is ill, has poorly developed suck reflex, or is less than 32 weeks' gestation. Presence of residual formula in stomach is indication of intolerance to amount of feeding or to increase in amount of feeding or is indicative of obstruction, paralytic ileus, or necrotizing enterocolitis. Residual feeding is calculated by: 1. Feeding order – 24 ml every 2 hours. 2. Residual – 3 ml. 3. Formula this feeding – 21 ml plus 3 ml residual.

NURSING CARE PLAN Cont'd

AGA and LGA Preterm Infants

Problem	Nursing interventions and actions	Rationale
	Observe, record, and report complications of nasojejunal tube including misplacement, perforation, plugging, vomiting due to excessive volume, or sepsis. Establish a nipple feeding program that is begun slowly and progresses slowly, such as nipple feed once per day, nipple feed once per shift, and then nipple feed every other feeding. Monitor daily weight with anticipation of small amount of weight loss when nipple feedings start. Supplement gavage or nipple feedings with intravenous therapy per physician order until oral intake is sufficient to support growth. Develop a plan of care that involves parents in feeding of infant. Observe, record, and report presence of complications such as hypoglycemia or hypocalcemia.	Residual formula is readministered because digestive processes have already been initiated. As infant matures, gavage feedings should be replaced with nipple feedings to assist in strengthening sucking reflexes and meeting psychologic needs. Involvement of parents in feeding of preterm infant is essential to development of attachment and expansion of parental knowledge and coping mechanisms. Preterm infant requires delicate balance for homeostasis and prevention of complications.
Susceptibility to infection	Initiate a plan of care to prevent exposure to infection. Implement treatment per physician orders in presence of infection (refer to section on sepsis neonatorum, p. 830, for review of nursing care).	Infection is common occurrence due to immaturity of immunologic system, increased use of invasive procedures and techniques, and more prolonged hospitalization.
Prolonged separation of infant and mother	Support emotionally the psychologic well-being of family, including positive maternal-child bonding and sensory stimulation of infant. Include parents in determining infant's plan of care and encourage their participation. Encourage parents to visit frequently. Provide opportunities for parents to touch, hold, talk to, and care for infant. Determine type and amount of sensory stimulation appropriate and implement sensory stimulation program. Prepare for discharge by instructing parent in such areas as feeding techniques, formula preparation (including bottle sterilization), and breast-feeding; bathing, diapering, and hygiene; rectal temperature monitoring; administration of vitamins; sibling rivalry; care of complications and preventing exposure to infections; normal elimination patterns, normal reflexes and activity, and how to permit normal growth and development without being overprotective; returning for continued medical care per physician schedule; and availability of community resources if indicated.	Maternal bonding occurs in first few hours or days following birth of an infant. Preterm infants experience prolonged periods of separation from their mothers, which necessitates intervention to insure maternal-child bonding. Related to prolonged separation of preterm infants from their mothers following delivery is increased incidence of child neglect and child abuse. Parents should receive same postpartum teaching as any mother taking a new infant home. Mothers with preterm infants desiring to breast feed will pump their breasts to keep milk flowing and in some situations to provide milk for their infant. This activity allows breast-feeding after discharge from hospital. Mothers need to understand changes to expect in color of stool and number of bowel movements plus odor from bottle or breast-feeding in order to avoid unnecessary concern on mother's part. Preterm infants usually do not require referral to community agencies such as visiting nurse associations unless there is a specific problem

NURSING CARE PLAN Cont'd

AGA and LGA Preterm Infants

Problem	Nursing interventions and actions	Rationale
		requiring assistance. Infants with congenital abnormalities, feeding problems, or resolving complications with infections or mothers unable to cope with defective infants are examples of conditions requiring referral to community resources.
Possible complications Apnea	Identify cause of apnea. Recognize and document frequency and severity of apneic episodes. Implement treatment based on severity of apneic episode, including: 1. Respiratory stimulation if color pink, not hypotonic, and heart rate above 100 beats/min. 2. Utilize bag and mask for apnea if infant has pallor, duskiness, cyanosis, and a rapid fall in heart rate. 3. Apply respirator if frequent apneic attacks have required bag and mask resuscitation. Administer oxygen and warm humidified air per physician order to control dyspnea and cyanosis. Monitor and record concentration of oxygen every two hours. Evaluate and report variations in blood gases and electrolyte reports. Administer theophylline per physician order for intractable neonatal apnea. Modify care plan to reduce or prevent apnea, including: 1. Gentle handling. 2. Indwelling orogastric or nasogastric tube rather than intermittent passage of feeding tube. 3. Nonstimulating nasopharyngeal suction when necessary. 4. Maintenance of thermal neutrality.	Immature central nervous system of premature infant, especially those under 36 weeks, results in periodic breathing (apnea lasting up to 10 seconds followed by briefly increased ventilatory rate) or apnea (cessation of respirations for more than 25 seconds). Apnea is result of immaturity, sepsis, hypoglycemia, acidosis, hypothermia, respiratory distress syndrome, patent ductus arteriosis, seizure activity, anemia, hyponatremia, or hypernatremia. Apneic onset is often insidious; however, with cardiorespiratory monitoring, early recognition and intervention prevents the need for resuscitative efforts. There is increased possibility of apnea during vagal stimulation, including distention of stomach with feeding, rectal stimulation, nasopharyngeal stimulation (as during suctioning), or with temperature instability. Severe apnea may preclude, for a time, oral feeding, requiring nutritional maintenance with intravenous therapy. Adequate nutrition prevents catabolism of body tissues as well as biochemical aberrations such as hypoglycemia, hyperglycemia, acidosis, or electrolyte imbalance.
Hypoglycemia	Screen and monitor for hypoglycemia: 1. Complete Dextrostix or laboratory blood sugar on admission (see Procedure 24-2). 2. On LGA infants complete Dextrostix every 30 min six times, then every hour three times, then every 2 hr six times until stable. 3. On AGA infants complete Dextrostix every 4 hr six times until stable. 4. Continue Dextrostix measurements after glucose therapy (IV or oral) is started. 5. Complete urine Dipstix and monitor urine volume to evaluate osmotic diuresis and glycosuria (above 1-3 ml/kg/hour). Observe, record, and report clinical	Hypoglycemia develops in preterm AGA infants because of decreased glycogen and fat stores related to premature delivery. Preterm LGA infants have increased stores of glycogen and fat with increased circulating insulin and insulin responsiveness. Untreated hypoglycemia may result in irreversible brain damage. Hypoglycemia is defined as Dextrostix below 45 mg/100 ml when corroborated with laboratory blood sugar value. LGA infants may require large doses of glucagon to promote conversion of glycogen from liver to glucose. Corticosteroids may be administered to

NURSING CARE PLAN Cont'd

AGA and LGA Preterm Infants

Problem	Nursing interventions and actions	Rationale
	symptoms including lethargy, irritability, poor feeding, vomiting, pallor, apnea, hypotonia, tremors, seizures, high-pitched cry, possible loss of swallowing reflex. Implement per physician orders early formula feeding, IV glucose, or corticosteroids.	stimulate gluconeogenesis from noncarbohydrate sources (Avery, 1975).
Hypocalcemia and neonatal tetany	Evaluate and report variations in laboratory reports of serum calcium levels below 7–7.5 mg/100 ml. Observe, record and report signs and symptoms of hypocalcemia, including neonatal tetany, twitching, jerking tremors, or focal or generalized seizure. Administer per physician order 10% calcium gluconate IV in bolus or continuous IV drip. Initiate safety factors with calcium administration to include: 1. Constant observation and monitoring during bolus with injection given slowly (no faster than 1 ml/min). 2. Utilize cardiac monitor during calcium administration. 3. Determine patency of peripheral IV before administration of calcium in order to prevent tissue sloughs. 4. When oral maintenance is utilized for 2–4 weeks, calcium should be slowly tapered off before discontinuing.	Hypocalcemia is common occurrence in sick neonate due to delay in oral feedings, resulting in less intestinal absorption of calcium, increased excretion by kidney, and low-calcium or calcium-free intravenous therapy management. Calcium deposition in fetus occurs primarily after 28 weeks' gestation, so that preterm infant "pushed out" of his intrauterine environment is born with calcium deficit. Neonatal tetany commonly occurs about 5–10 days after birth and is related to administration of milk formulas with relatively high levels of phosphorus in relation to calcium. High levels of phosphorus depress parathyroid gland, which results in decreased serum calcium (Korones, 1976). Rapid administration of calcium produces bradycardia and causes cardiac arrest. Calcium is extremely necrotic to tissues and may cause disastrous tissue sloughing.
Birth trauma	Screen and monitor all LGA infants for birth injury, including: 1. Presence of cry that is high-pitched, weak, absent or constant, and irritable. 2. Note activity such as flaccidity, floppiness, poor muscle tone, spasticity, hyperactivity, opisthotonos, twitching, hypertonicity, tremors, or frank convulsions. 3. Observe resting posture for asymmetry resulting from intrauterine pressure or birth trauma. 4. Evaluate fontanelles for bulging, tenseness, or fullness. 5. Observe eyes for constricted pupil, unilateral, dilated fixed pupils, nystagmus, or strabismus. 6. Asymmetry of chest may indicate diaphragmatic paralysis. 7. Evaluate for fracture of clavicle, which is detected by palpable mass, crepitus, and tenderness at fracture site or by limited movements of arm such as unilateral decrease in Moro response. 8. Assess movement of extremities for palsies due to injury to brachial plexus, for	Disproportion between birth canal and size of LGA infant results in birth trauma and an increased rate of cesarean section. LGA infants are in at-risk grouping. Physical examination of LGA infant may reveal symptoms of increased intracranial pressure—with high-pitched cry—or presence of brain injury—with weak cry, absent cry, or constant, irritable crying. Central nervous system damage may be indicated by spasticity, hyperactivity, opisthotonos, twitching, hypertonicity, tremors, or convulsion. Birth trauma may result in brain damage or injury, diaphragmatic paralysis, fracture of clavicle, palsies, and/or paralysis.

NURSING CARE PLAN Cont'd

AGA and LGA Preterm Infants

Problem	Nursing interventions and actions	Rationale
	fractures or dislocation. 9. Note paralysis of lower extremities.	Paralysis of both legs is due to pressure or severe trauma to spinal cord.
Polycythemia	Initiate screening of hematocrit on admission to nursery. Observe, record, and report symptoms, including: 1. Decrease in peripheral pulses, discoloration of extremity, alteration in activity or neurologic depression, renal vein thrombosis with decreased urine output, hematuria, or proteinuria in thromboembolic conditions. 2. Tachycardia or congestive heart failure. 3. Respiratory distress syndrome, cyanosis, tachypnea, increased oxygen need, labored respirations, or hemorrhage in respiratory system. Implement therapy per physician order to reduce central venous hematocrit to 60% or less by using partial exchange of plasma rather than phlebotomy without volume replacement.	Polycythemia is defined as a central venous hematocrit above 65%-70% in the first week of life. Hyperviscosity is resultant "thickness" of red-cell rich blood so that its ability to perfuse the tissues is disturbed due to thickness and decrease in deformability of cells. Hyperviscosity is more common in LGA infants, especially of diabetic mothers. Pathophysiologic mechanism is unknown. Symptoms are caused by poor perfusion of tissues.
Congenital malformation	Complete and record results of physical examination on LGA infants of diabetic mothers for presence of congenital anomalies including: 1. Cardiac anomalies, which usually are ventricular septal defects or transposition of great vessels resulting in murmur; cardiorespiratory distress with tachypnea, tachycardia, cyanosis, or labored respiration; and/or congestive heart failure. 2. Spinal anomalies, simple or extensive, resulting in missing vertebras on palpation, pilonidal dimple or sinus, spina bifida, or myelomeningocele.	Congenital malformations in LGA infants of diabetic mothers are more frequent due to increased incidence of: 1. Abnormal intrauterine environment due to diabetes and vascular complications. 2. Genetic predisposition. 3. Drugs taken by mother during pregnancy.
Central nervous system hemorrhage	Observe, record, and report clinical manifestations of central nervous system hemorrhage, including: 1. Sudden "crash" characterized by pallor and shocklike appearance. 2. Presence of cyanosis. 3. Apnea, bradycardia, or hypotension. 4. Neurologic symptoms such as seizure activity, rigidity, tremors, nystagmus, hypotonia, bulging fontanelle, or hypothermia. Monitor laboratory findings for drop in hematocrit, metabolic acidosis, hypoxia, or decreased partial arterial oxygen pressure (Pa_{O_2}).	Central nervous system hemorrhage is common occurrence in preterm infants due to capillary fragility, hypoxic insult, or birth trauma. Premature infants with respiratory distress syndrome or who have been given sodium bicarbonate may be especially prone to development of hemorrhage. Clinical diagnosis depends on results of spinal fluid analysis, including red blood cells, xanthochromia, or elevated protein content.

NURSING CARE PLAN Cont'd
AGA and LGA Preterm Infants

Problem	Nursing interventions and actions	Rationale
	Prepare infant and assist with lumbar puncture for spinal fluid analysis.	
	Maintain adequate oxygenation per physician order by increasing ambient oxygen concentration or placing on continuous positive airway pressure (CPAP) or respirator.	
	Administer replacement whole blood or albumin per physician order while closely monitoring blood pressure.	
	Provide continuous observation and monitoring of clinical condition and report variations.	
	Maintain thermal neutrality.	
	Administer medications per physician order for seizure control.	
Pulmonary problems, including RDS, wet lung, or atelectasis Sepsis neonatorum Retrolental fibroplasia Necrotizing enterocolitis Hyperbilirubinemia or kernicterus Anemia	These additional possible complications are covered in depth in following chapters.	

Nursing Care Evaluation

Respirations are 30-50 per minute, regular, with no episodes of apnea.

Temperature is stable.

Infant is gaining weight.

Infant takes nipple feedings without developing fatigue.

Complications are controlled or absent.

Infant is active without jerky generalized movement.

Infant is free from infection or infection is controlled.

Parent-child bonding is completed.

Infant responds to sensory stimulation.

Parents understand and can demonstrate knowledge of infant care, feeding, growth projections, prevention of exposure to infections, treatment of complications, and when to return for medical care.

Long-Term Needs

Discharge planning with the parents begins at admission of the infant. The parents must not receive hurriedly given instructions at the time of discharge. Throughout the hospitalization, it is the responsibility of the nurse to prepare the parents for discharge of the infant. Use of any special treatments or medications must be taught to the parents, practiced while in the hospital, and reevaluated for understanding by the parents. If the infant is discharged without special needs, it is important for the parents to realize that their previously sick newborn is now healthy and should be treated as "normal." His previous special needs have given way to normal needs.

It is important for parents to understand that the developmental level of their infant cannot be evaluated from the infant's chronologic age. Developmental progress must be evaluated from the expected date of birth and not from the actual date of (premature) birth.

During the first year of life, there is increased incidence of respiratory infection in "graduating"

Table 24–7. Selected Normal Laboratory Values in Newborn Premature Infants*

Laboratory test	Normal values	Laboratory test	Normal values
Hematologic		Total protein	4.3–7.6 gm
Red blood cells (RBC)	4–6 million/mm^3	Osmolality	270–285 milliosmols/liter
White blood cells (WBC)	10,000–15,000/mm^3	pH	7.35–7.42
Platelets	100,000–150,000/mm^3	Total CO_2 content	18–23 meq/liter
Reticulocytes	2–4/100 RBC	P_{CO_2}	33–38 mm Hg in Denver
Hematocrit	55%–70%	Urea nitrogen (BUN)	Less than 20 mg/100 ml
Hemoglobin	14–24; mean 17–19 gm/100 ml	Transaminase (SGOT)	Up to 100 units in first week of life
Fetal Hbg	55%–85% of total Hbg	Creatinine	0.4–1.4 mg/100 ml
Adult Hbg	15%–45% of total Hbg	*Serum glucose (fasting)*	40–100 mg/100 ml
		Total blood volume	80–90 ml/kg
Plasma electrolyte		*Total body water*	69%–83% of body weight
Chloride	97–104 meq/liter	*Extracellular body water*	42% of body weight
Sodium	136–143 meq/liter	*Intracellular body water*	35% of body weight
Potassium	4.1–5.6 meq/liter	*Urine osmolarity*	216–792
Calcium	8.5–11 mg/100 ml	*Total protein for term*	5.1–5.7
Phosphorus (first week)	4.2–8.5 mg/100 ml		

*Modified from University of Colorado School of Nursing. Adapted from Silverman, W. A. 1961. *Dunham's premature infants.* 3rd ed. New York: Paul B. Hoeber, Inc.; and from O'Brien, D., and Abbott, F. 1962. *Laboratory manual of pediatric microbiochemical techniques.* New York: Paul B. Hoeber, Inc.

prematures (especially if they had lung disease in the hospital). Parents should be counseled on how to prevent respiratory infections and should be advised to seek early treatment if they do occur.

LARGE-FOR-GESTATIONAL-AGE (LGA) INFANT

A large-for-gestational-age (LGA) neonate is one whose birth weight is at or above the 90th percentile on the intrauterine growth curve (at any week of gestation). Careful gestational age assessment is essential in identifying potential needs and problems of such infants.

An LGA infant is usually thought of as a term infant of 4000 gm, but an infant of 3000 gm at 34 weeks' gestation, although premature, also meets the criteria. The majority of infants categorized as LGA have been found to be so categorized because of miscalculation of dates due to postconceptual bleeding (Korones, 1976). Infants of diabetic mothers constitute only a minority of all LGA infants.

The etiology of the majority of LGA infants is unclear, but certain factors or situations have been found to be true:

1. Genetic predisposition is correlated proportionally to the pregnancy weight and to weight gain during pregnancy.
2. Multiparous women have three times the number of LGA infants as primigravidas.
3. Male infants are traditionally larger than female infants.

4. Infants born of diabetic mothers or with erythroblastosis fetalis or with transposition of the great vessels are usually large.

Characteristically the increase in the LGA infant's body size is proportional, although head circumference and body length are in the upper limits of intrauterine growth. The exception to this rule is the infant of the diabetic mother, whose body weight increases only in proportion to his length.

Common disorders of the LGA infant include:

1. Birth trauma because of cephalopelvic disproportion. Often these infants have a biparietal diameter greater than 10 cm or a fundal height measurement greater than 42 cm without the presence of polyhydramnios. Because of their excessive size, there are more breech and shoulder dystocias, with resultant potential asphyxia, fractured clavicles, brachial palsy, facial paralysis, depressed skull fractures, and intracranial bleeding.

2. Hypoglycemia (the development in LGA infants of nondiabetic mothers is unclear).

3. Polycythemia and hyperviscosity (pathophysiologic mechanisms are unknown, but symptomatology is caused by poor perfusion of tissues).

The perinatal history, in conjunction with ultrasonic measurement of fetal skull and gestational age testing, is important in identifying an at-risk newborn. Nursing management is directed toward early identification of the common disorders and appropriate immediate treatment. Essential components of the nursing assessment are monitoring vital signs and screening for hypoglycemia and polycythemia. For specific nursing interventions for common disorders of the LGA infant, see the Nursing Care Plan for AGA and LGA preterm infants.

SMALL-FOR-GESTATIONAL-AGE (SGA) INFANT

A small-for-gestational-age (SGA) infant is any infant who at birth is at or below the 10th percentile (intrauterine growth curve). This growth retardation is possible for infants of any gestational age—preterm SGA, term SGA, or postterm SGA. Other terms used to designate a growth-retarded neonate include intrauterine-growth-retarded (IUGR), small-for-dates (SFD), and dysmature.

After premature infants, SGA infants have the highest rate of perinatal mortality. Increased disorders in the SGA infant are due to hypoglycemia/nutritional deprivation, hypothermia, meconium aspiration, congenital infections, polycythemia, and congenital malformations.

The etiology of growth retardation in the fetus suggests placental or fetal causes. Intrauterine growth is linear from approximately 28 to 38 weeks of gestation. After 38 weeks, growth is variable, depending on the growth potential of the fetus and the functioning of the placenta. The most commonly occurring causes of growth retardation and their pathophysiology are as follows:

1. *Malnutrition.* In animal research, malnutrition or undernutrition has produced a reduction in weight of offspring, but this correlation has not been conclusively demonstrated in humans. The parasitic existence of the fetus enables him to live off the nutrient stores of the mother (even if her nutritional intake is poor). Chronic malnutrition may predispose to a reduction in cell number and growth retardation in the fetus.

2. *Vascular complications.* Complications associated with preeclampsia, eclampsia, chronic hypertensive vascular disease, and advanced diabetes mellitus cause a decrease in blood flow to the uterus. These conditions, resulting in decreased uterine blood flow, have been associated with SGA infants.

3. *Maternal disease.* Heart disease, alcoholism, narcotic addiction, sickle cell anemia, and phenylketonuria are associated with SGA.

4. *Maternal factors.* SGA is associated with such maternal factors as smoking, lack of prenatal care, low socioeconomic class—which usually results in poor health care, poor nutritional intake, poor education, and poor living conditions—and age (very young or older).

5. *Environmental factors.* Such factors include high altitude and maternal use of drugs and x-rays that have teratogenic effects.

6. *Placental factors.* Placental conditions such as infarcted areas, placenta previa, or thrombosis may affect vascular delivery to the fetus, which becomes more deficient with increasing gestational age.

7. *Fetal factors.* Congenital infections, congenital malformations, multiple pregnancy (twins, triplets) can predispose to intrauterine growth retardation.

Identification of infants at risk for IUGR is the first step in the identification and observation of common disorders. Again, the perinatal history of maternal conditions is important in identifying an at-risk newborn. Other avenues of data collection include an examination of the placenta and examination of the newborn.

Patterns of Intrauterine Growth Retardation

The clinical manifestations of intrauterine growth retardation are related to length, severity, and time of onset (critical period in organ development). Two patterns of IUGR have been described: proportional IUGR and disproportional IUGR (Avery, 1975).

Proportional IUGR is a pattern in which there has been chronic, prolonged retardation of growth in weight, length, and, in severe cases, head circumference. All body proportions are below normal for the gestational age (Figure 24-9).

Disproportional IUGR is an acute occurrence of placental insufficiency. Weight is decreased, yet length and head circumference remain normal for the gestational age. These infants appear wasted, with a loss of subcutaneous tissue and muscle mass; loose skin folds; wide-eyed faces; dry, desquamating skin; and a thin and often meconium-stained cord.

As previously mentioned, intrauterine growth retardation is possible at any gestational age. Despite growth retardation, physiologic maturity develops according to gestational age. Given infants of the same weight, one preterm and one SGA, the SGA infant will be more mature in development than the preterm infant. Because the SGA infant may have more physiologic maturity than the preterm AGA he is less predisposed to the development of respiratory distress, hyperbilirubinemia, and so on. His chances for survival will be better because of his organ maturity, although he still has many other potential difficulties.

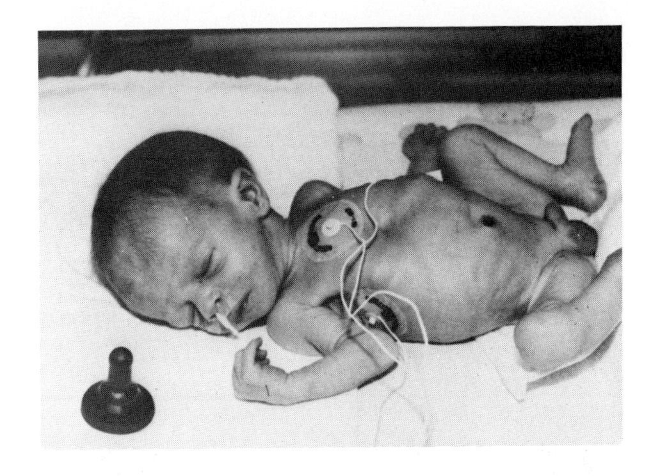

Figure 24-9. The infant with IUGR appears long, thin, and emaciated. The gestational age of the infant shown here is 41 weeks. He weighed approximately 1560 gm at birth.

Long-Term Effects

Growth occurs in two ways—an increase in cell number and an increase in cell size. If the fetal insult occurs during the critical period of cell number increase, the effects may last a lifetime. It is probable that subsequent nutritional supplementation will not overcome a deficit of cells in vital organs. The result is permanent growth retardation. Indeed, follow-up data show a persistence of growth retardation in stature and in weight percentiles. However, intrauterine growth retardation at birth is not predictive of ultimate growth. Normal postnatal growth may be achieved if the duration and magnitude of the insult is limited and if the infant's growth potential has not been affected.

In addition to somatic sequelae, developmental sequelae may occur, such as minimal brain dysfunction, learning problems, and some hearing loss. There is an overall deficit in the performance of SGA infants as compared to other children. As in growth sequelae, the severity of growth retardation at birth does not correlate with future developmental outcomes.

Other physiologic aberrations of the SGA infant may contribute to long-term sequelae. Aberrations of insulin secretion and glucose tolerance have implications for postnatal management.

Hypoglycemia, a most common metabolic aberration, has been shown to produce such sequelae as central nervous system abnormalities and mental retardation. In addition to hypoglycemia, conditions such as asphyxia, hyperviscosity, and chronic deprivation also may affect the outcome.

Therefore, as with the preterm infant, meticulous attention to physiologic parameters is essential in immediate management and for reduction of long-term disorders (see the Nursing Care Plan for SGA infants).

NURSING CARE PLAN

SGA Infants

Patient Data Base

History

1. Maternal history including general health, obstetric history, and events of labor and delivery; factors frequently associated with SGA infants include:
   a. Chronic maternal malnutrition
   b. Vascular complications
   c. Maternal disease, including heart disease, drug addiction, alcoholism
   d. Smoking
   e. Low socioeconomic class
   f. Environmental factors, including high altitude, drugs, x-ray procedures
   g. Placental factors
   h. Congenital infections, including rubella, cytomegalic inclusion disease, toxoplasmosis, syphilis
2. Fetal-neonatal factors, including:
   a. Congenital malformations
   b. Discordant twin
3. Parents' understanding of SGA and its significance

Physical examination

1. Disproportionate intrauterine growth rate:
   a. Head appears relatively large (although it approaches normal) because chest and abdominal size are decreased
   b. Loose dry skin
   c. Scarcity of subcutaneous fat, with emaciated appearance
   d. Long, thin in appearance
   e. Sunken abdomen
   f. Sparse scalp hair (may be more plentiful in postmature infants)
   g. Anterior fontanelle may be depressed
   h. May have vigorous cry and appear deceptively alert (this is related to chronic marginal hypoxia in utero)
2. Proportional intrauterine growth rate:
   a. Sizes of all body parts are decreased but are in proportion, so head does not appear overly large or length excessive
   b. Generally vigorous (Korones, 1976)
3. Utilize clinical estimation of gestational age soon after birth and confirmatory neurologic examination to be done after 24 hours or Dubowitz's criteria soon after birth to determine gestational age
4. Physical examination findings related to gestational age include:
   a. Increased tendency to respiratory distress related to aspiration syndrome
   b. Monitor temperature for increased problems of thermogenesis
   c. Monitor neurologic status for presence of cerebral edema that may occur, resulting in increased intracranial pressure, bulging fontanelles, or seizure activity

Laboratory evaluation

Dextrostix done frequently (every 2 hours initially); blood glucose levels may be less than 20 mg/100 ml because of tendency toward hypoglycemia

Hematocrit may be greater than 60%, which is indicative of polycythemia

NURSING CARE PLAN Cont'd

SGA Infants

Nursing Priorities

1. Maintain respirations.
2. Maintain homeostasis with neutral thermal environment and meeting nutrition and fluid requirements.
3. Protect from infection.
4. Support psychologic well-being of parents and infant by facilitating positive parent-child bonding and sensory stimulation of infant.
5. Evaluate possible complications and initiate appropriate interventions.

Problem	Nursing Interventions and Actions	Rationale
Respiratory distress	Nursing interventions and actions are same as for preterm LGA and AGA infants (see p. 748). (See Chapter 25 for detailed nursing care and treatment on respiratory distress and infant resuscitation.)	Respiratory distress in SGA infants is not due to lung immaturity as is respiratory distress in preterm infants. Pulmonary conditions of SGA include: 1. Neonatal asphyxia. 2. Aspiration of meconium. 3. Aspiration pneumonia and pneumothorax.
Heat losses and cold stress	Maintain skin temperature between 36-36.5C. Adjust and monitor incubator or radiant warmer to maintain skin temperature. Implement all other nursing care measures same as for temperature regulation in Nursing Care Plan for preterm LGA and AGA infants.	Neutral thermal environment charts utilized for preterm infant are not reliable for weight of SGA. Hypothermia is problem for SGA infant whose pathophysiology of thermal instability differs from that of preterm infant in the following manner: 1. Small in size, yet SGA can assume flexion position and thus decrease surface area available for heat loss. 2. Like preterm, SGA has decreased stores of brown fat available for thermogenesis, because SGA infant has utilized these stores in utero for survival. 3. Like preterm, SGA has poor insulation due to utilization of subcutaneous tissue in utero for survival. 4. SGA has mature central nervous system for temperature regulation. 5. SGA has ability to sweat and vasodilate in response to overheating, whereas this mechanism is unavailable to preterm infant. Other pathophysiology same as for temperature regulation and cold stress in preterm infant.
Caloric and fluid intake necessary for growth	Nursing interventions and actions are same as for preterm LGA and AGA infants.	Rationale same as for preterm infant.
Fatigue during feedings	Nursing interventions and actions are same as for preterm LGA and AGA infants.	Rationale same as for preterm infant.
Susceptibility to infection	Nursing interventions and actions are same as for preterm LGA and AGA infants.	Rationale same as for preterm infant.
Prolonged separation of infant and mother	Nursing interventions and actions are same as for preterm LGA and AGA infants.	Rationale same as for preterm infant.
Possible complications		
Hypoglycemia	Nursing interventions and actions are same as for preterm infants.	Hypoglycemia in SGA is indicated by blood sugar less than 20 mg/100 ml. Pathophysiology of

NURSING CARE PLAN Cont'd

SGA Infants

Problem	Nursing interventions and actions	Rationale
		hypoglycemia in SGA is due to a depletion of glycogen stores, especially hepatic glycogen stores. Combined with inhibited gluconeogenesis, this predisposes SGA infants to profound hypoglycemia within first two days of life.
Congenital malformations	Complete and record results of physical examination on SGA infants for presence of congenital anomalies including: 1. Autosomal anomalies such as Down's syndrome (trisomy 21), trisomy E (16-18), trisomy D (13-15). 2. Primordial short stature. 3. Inborn errors of metabolism such as Hurler's syndrome, Niemann-Pick disease, Gaucher's disease, maple syrup urine disease. Implement appropriate therapeutic actions.	Congenital malformations are statistically more common in SGA infants, because an anomaly of the fetus prevents normal growth (cell size and number), which results in small size of the neonate.
Congenital infections	Complete examination and identification of infected infants with clinical manifestations, including: 1. Rubella. 2. Cytomegalic inclusion disease. 3. Toxoplasmosis. 4. Syphilis. Monitor and report laboratory findings and radiographic surveys that aid in diagnosis. Institute protective measures to prevent spread of disease to other newborns, staff, or mothers. Isolate secretions and contaminated fomites. Enforce meticulous hand-washing.	Infants exposed to rubella, cytomegalic inclusion disease, toxoplasmosis, and syphilis are known to be small for their gestational age. Clinical manifestations of congenital infections include: 1. Rubella – cardiac anomalies; cataracts, retinopathy, cloudy cornea; gross anatomical abnormalities such as bone deformities and malformations, micrognathia, genitourinary anomalies, bony radiolucencies; central nervous system anomalies including encephalocele, microcephaly; hepatosplenomegaly, encephalitis; hearing loss; or "blueberry muffin" syndrome such as dermal erythropoiesis, and thrombocytopenia. 2. Cytomegalic inclusion disease: hepatosplenomegaly; jaundice with elevation of direct bilirubin level; thrombocytopenia with or without petechiae, or DIC (disseminated intravascular coagulopathy); microcephaly; or encephalitis. 3. Toxoplasmosis – hepatosplenomegaly; jaundice; meningoencephalitis with CSF changes (increased protein level); chorioretinitis; nervous system dysfunction including convulsions or calcifications. 4. Syphilis – bone deformities; hepatosplenomegaly; jaundice with elevated direct serum bilirubin; hepatitis; or anemias. Precaution: No pregnant women should care for or collect specimens for infected infants because they could infect their fetus in utero.
Polycythemia	Nursing interventions and actions are same as for preterm LGA infants.	Polycythemia may occur in half of all SGA infants. Exact etiology of polycythemia in SGA is not known yet is thought to be a physiologic response to chronic hypoxia.

NURSING CARE PLAN Cont'd

SGA Infants

Nursing Care Evaluation

Respirations are 30-50/min with no periods of apnea.

Temperature is stable.

Infant is gaining weight.

Infant takes nipple feedings without developing fatigue.

Complications are controlled or absent.

Infant is free from infection.

Infant shows no jerky generalized movement or other neurologic problems.

Infant responds to sensory stimulation.

Parent-child bonding is completed.

Parents understand and can demonstrate knowledge of infant care, feeding, growth projections, prevention of exposure to infections, treatment of complications, and when to return for medical care.

POSTMATURE INFANT

The postmature (or postterm) infant is any infant delivered after 42 weeks' gestation. The majority of infants delivered after 42 weeks have inaccurate obstetric dates, and most have no clinical manifestations of postmaturity. But because of increasing placental insufficiency with prolonged gestational age, true postmature infants are at risk for intrapartal death as a result of the stresses and distresses of labor.

Clifford (1957) has devised clinical criteria for the assessment of postmaturity:

Stage I. Long, thin infant. Loose skin (around thighs and buttocks) giving the appearance of recent weight loss. Peeling, parchmentlike skin. Decrease in or lack of vernix. Alert expression. Behavior of 1-to-3-week-old infant more mature than term newborn. Long nails—staining of nails and skin. No lanugo.

Stage II. Stage I symptoms plus meconium-stained amniotic fluid, skin, vernix, umbilical cord, and placental membranes—a manifestation of fetal anoxic insult.

Stage III. Stages I and II (survived acute anoxic phase of stage II) plus nails and skin are stained a bright yellow and the umbilical cord is yellow green.*

*Clifford, S. 1957. Postmaturity. *Advances Pediatr.* 9:13.

Prolonged gestation exposes the infant to progressive inability of the placenta to provide adequate nutrition. The nutritional deprivation is manifested in the thin, wasted appearance. Because of the nutritionally deprived environment, these infants need (and usually demand) early feedings. Hypoglycemia, caused by decreased glycogen stores (as in the SGA), is a common disorder of postterm infants. The postterm infant may be AGA if the placenta has continued to support linear growth. More often, the postmature infant is a victim of intrauterine growth retardation and is SGA.

Common disorders of the postterm infant (whether AGA or SGA) include:

1. Hypoglycemia.

2. Postmaturity syndrome with intrauterine asphyxia and fetal distress. Physiologic response to hypoxia in the fetus is a relaxation of the anal sphincter and passage of meconium into the amniotic fluid. Hence, the postterm infant is meconium-stained and is at risk for meconium aspiration. It is important that a postterm newborn with meconium-stained amniotic fluid be appropriately resuscitated and supported in the delivery room. Suctioning of the naso-oropharynx (while the infant is on the perineum) will prevent meconium aspiration (see Chapter 25).

3. Polycythemia. Same pathophysiology and nursing interventions as for the SGA infant with polycythemia.

4. Congenital anomalies (see Chapter 26).

5. Seizure activity due to hypoxic insult. Because of chronic hypoxia, possible fetal distress in labor, and birth asphyxia, these infants have a delayed transition to extrauterine life.

6. Cold stress because of loss or poor development of subcutaneous fat. Prevention of heat loss should be initiated during the resuscitative process.

Nursing interventions are primarily supportive measures, including (a) provision of warmth to balance muted response to cold stress and decreased liver glycogen and brown fat stores; (b) frequent monitoring of blood glucose and initiation of early feeding (at 1 or 2 hours of age) or IV glucose per physician order; (c) observation of cardiopulmonary parameters, as the stresses of labor are poorly tolerated and severe depression can ensue at birth; and (d) observation for disorders and appropriate management when possible. Nursing should be directed toward facilitation of parental expression of feelings and fears regarding the infant's condition and long-term needs.

INFANT OF DIABETIC MOTHER

Infants of diabetic mothers (IDMs) are considered at risk. They are often large for gestational age, and the chances of congenital abnormalities are great. The infants appear red-faced and fat (usually weighing 9 or 10 lb), and they seldom cry or move but just lie quietly. The cord and placenta are large. Infants of mothers in diabetic classes D through F are often small for gestational age as a result of maternal vascular involvement. Others may be large in size but immature in development, exhibiting many of the problems of prematurity.

The most common problem for these infants is hypoglycemia, resulting from loss of high maternal blood glucose supply and continued hyperinsulinism and depleted blood glucose 2 to 4 hours after birth.

Other major potential problems during the first hours and days of life are (Avery, 1975):

1. Hypocalcemia, with tremors the obvious clinical sign. This may be due to the IDM's increased incidence of prematurity and to the stresses of difficult pregnancies, labor, and delivery, which predispose any infant to hypocalcemia. Also, diabetic mothers tend to have higher calcium levels at term, causing possible secondary hypoparathyroidism in their infants (Tsang et al., 1972).

2. Hyperbilirubinemia, which may be seen at 48 to 72 hours, possibly due to a slightly decreased extracellular fluid volume, resulting in increased hematocrit and increased incidence of complicated vaginal deliveries, predisposing to enclosed hemorrhages.

3. Birth trauma, as discussed in the section on LGA infants.

4. Polycythemia, due to presence of increased hematocrit.

5. Respiratory distress syndrome, especially in babies of classes A through C of diabetic mothers. It is theorized that the high levels of fetal insulin interfere with the synthesis of the lecithin necessary for lung maturation. This does not appear to be a problem for infants born of mothers in classes D through F; for them the stresses of poor uterine blood supply may lead to increased production of steroids, resulting in acceleration of lung maturation.

6. Congenital heart defects, neurologic defects, small left colon syndrome, and caudal regression syndrome, possibly due to some intrauterine environmental factor.

Because the onset of hypoglycemia occurs at 2 to 4 hours of age, blood glucose determinations should be done on cord blood and at 1, 2, 4, and 6 hours of age. The normal blood sugar level for a full-term infant is 30–125 mg/100 ml. The test used by nurses to determine hypoglycemia in newborns is Dextrostix (Procedure 24–2), an extremely sensitive laboratory test. A color change occurs if the level is below 45 mg/100 ml. Hypoglycemia is suspected if two low readings are obtained. Distressed infants and infants of diabetic mothers of classes C through F should be given 10% dextrose immediately after birth at a rate of 65–70 ml/kg of body weight (Korones, 1976).

Procedure 24–2. Dextrostix

Objective	Nursing action	Rationale
Ensure quick, efficient completion of procedure	Gather the following equipment: 1. Lancet (do not use needles). 2. Alcohol swabs. 3. 2 × 2 sterile gauze squares. 4. Small Band-Aid. 5. Dextrostix and bottle.	All necessary equipment must be ready to ensure that blood sample is collected at time and in manner necessary. Do not use needles because of danger of nicking periosteum.
	Select clear, previously unpunctured site. Cleanse site by rubbing vigorously with 70% isopropyl alcohol swab, followed by dry gauze square. Grasp lower leg and heel so as to impede venous return slightly.	Selection of previously unpunctured site minimizes risk of infection and excessive scar formation. Friction produces local heat, which aids vasodilatation. Impeding venous return facilitates extraction of blood sample from puncture site.
Minimize trauma at puncture site	Dry site completely before lancing.	Alcohol is irritating to injured tissue and may also produce hemolysis.
	With quick piercing motion, puncture lateral heel with blade, being careful not to puncture too deeply. Avoid the darkened areas in Figure 24–10. Toes are acceptable sites.	Lateral heel is site of choice because it precludes damaging posterior tibial nerve and artery, plantar artery, and important longitudinally oriented fat pad of the heel, which in later years could impede walking.

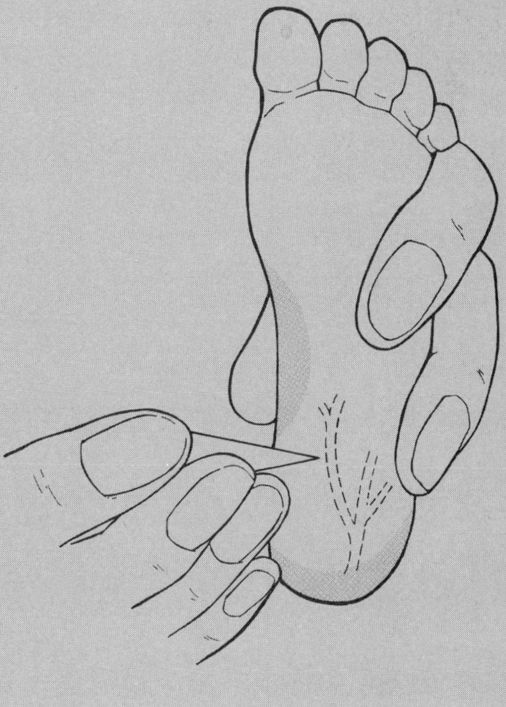

Figure 24–10.

Procedure 24–2. Cont'd

Objective	Nursing action	Rationale
		This is especially important for infant undergoing multiple Dextrostix procedures. Optimal penetration is 4 mm.
Ensure accurate blood sampling	After puncture has been made, remove first drop of blood with sterile gauze square and proceed to collect subsequent drops of blood onto Dextrostix, ensuring that it is a stand-up drop of blood on Dextrostix (Figure 24–11).	First drop is usually discarded because it tends to be minutely diluted with tissue fluid from puncture.

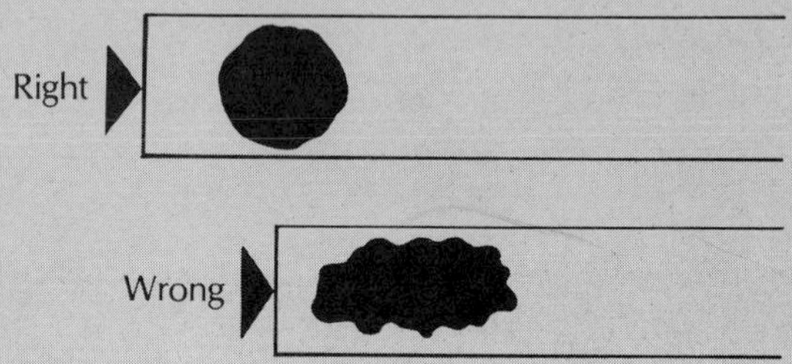

Right

Wrong

Figure 24–11.

Objective	Nursing action	Rationale
	Wait one minute (apply Band-Aid while waiting), then rinse blood gently from stick under a steady stream of running water (Figure 24–12). Compare immediately against color chart on side of bottle. Record results on vital signs sheet or on back of graph. Report immediately any findings under 45 mg/100 ml or over 175 mg/100 ml.	For accurate results, directions must be followed closely, and reagent strips must be fresh. False low readings may be caused by: 1. Timing. 2. Washing (chemical reaction can be washed off). 3. Squeezing foot, causing tissue fluid dilution.

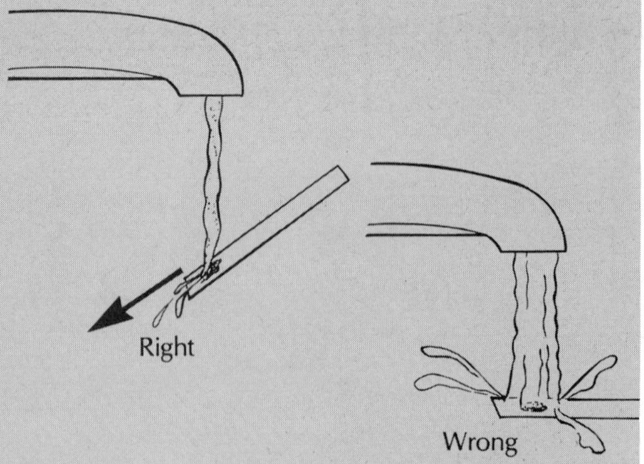

Right

Wrong

Figure 24–12.

Objective	Nursing action	Rationale
Prevent excessive bleeding	Apply folded gauze square to puncture site and secure firmly with bandage.	A pressure dressing should be applied to puncture site to stop bleeding.
	Check puncture site frequently for first hour after sample.	Active infants sometimes kick or rub their dressings off and can bleed profusely from puncture site, especially if bandage becomes moist or is rubbed excessively against crib sheet.

Nursing management is based on early attention to the prenatal history and assessment of maternal diabetes throughout pregnancy to identify the infant at risk. The infant of the diabetic mother should be treated as a premature or high-risk infant, and close observation in an intensive care nursery should be instituted immediately after birth. See the Nursing Care Plan for AGA and LGA premature infants for specific nursing interventions for infants of diabetic mothers with problems of polycythemia and birth trauma. Chapter 25 provides nursing interventions for respiratory distress syndrome.

INFANT OF MOTHER WITH CARDIAC DISEASE

The antepartal presence of cardiac disease increases the risk of perinatal mortality, prematurity, asphyxia, and intrauterine growth retardation. Thus the infant of a mother with cardiac disease must receive special attention to avoid possible complications. Maternal congestive heart failure decreases maternal cardiac output and thus the available circulating blood exchange through the placenta. Hypertensive cardiovascular disease can cause asphyxia and intrauterine growth retardation. The long-term vasoconstriction results in uteroplacental vascular insufficiency (decreased uterine and placental blood flow impairs placental function). It is often recommended that the delivery be facilitated by low or outlet forceps and conduction anesthesia.

Initiation of the first breath should be noted, and normal resuscitative procedures—including oxygen therapy, nasotracheal suctioning, and warmth—should follow immediately. After transfer from the delivery room, the infant should be monitored carefully in the special care nursery. Respirations, heart rate, temperature, color, and activity level should be assessed on admission and continuously thereafter. Long-term needs and management should be individualized and based on the assessment of the infant for asphyxia, prematurity, and intrauterine growth retardation.

ALCOHOL- OR DRUG-ADDICTED INFANT

The infant of an alcoholic or drug-addicted woman will also be alcohol- or drug-dependent. After birth, when his connection with the maternal blood supply is severed, he will suffer withdrawal. In addition, the drugs ingested by the mother may be teratogenic, resulting in congenital anomalies.

Alcohol Dependency

The fetal alcohol syndrome described by Jones et al. (1973) and Jones and Smith (1973) refers to a series of malformations frequently found in infants born to women who have been chronic, severe alcoholics. Characteristics of these infants include severe IUGR, microcephaly, short palpebral fissures, altered palmar dermatoglyphics, micrognathia, epicanthal folds, cardiac anomalies, joint limitations, external genital abnormalities, and a relatively short length for birth weight. These infants are frequently mentally retarded and demonstrate postnatal growth retardation (Lubchenco, 1976). The withdrawal symptoms of the alcohol-dependent neonate are similar to those exhibited by the mother, including abdominal distention, tremors, agitation, arching of the back, sweating, and seizures. They often appear within 6 to 12 hours and at least within the first 24 hours. Alcohol dependence in the infant is physiologic, not psychologic. Care of the alcohol-addicted newborn includes warmth, protection from injury during seizure, intravenous fluid therapy, reduction of environmental stimuli, and medication such as phenobarbital to reduce convulsions. With the establishment of a healthy maternal-infant bonding and supportive physical care, the prognosis for the neonate is favorable.

Drug Dependency

Heroin-addicted infants often weigh less than 2500 gm at birth, as a result of poor maternal nutrition and placental circulation, and often are premature. Withdrawal symptoms in the newborn may be seen early, usually within 72 hours after birth, or as late as the seventh day of life. It has been reported that infants of mothers on methadone (addicted infants) appear more ill than their heroin-addicted counterparts. The number of withdrawal symptoms and the severity of the symptoms are greater, and duration is prolonged.

Withdrawal symptoms include the following:

1. Tremors.
2. Hyperactivity and hypertonicity.
3. Marked perspiration, possibly due to central neurogenic stimulation of sweat glands (Glass, 1975).
4. Persistent shrill cry.
5. Respiratory symptoms including tachypnea, sneezing, and nasal stuffiness.
6. Increased tendon reflexes.
7. Decreased Moro reflex.
8. Vomiting.
9. Frantic sucking on the fists.
10. Convulsions (more common in methadone and barbiturate withdrawal).
11. Sleep disturbances.
12. Disturbance in sucking, feeding behavior, and gastrointestinal function.

Care of the newborn is based on reducing withdrawal symptoms and promoting adequate respiration, temperature, and nutrition. Specific nursery care measures include:

1. Temperature regulation.
2. Continuous monitoring of pulse and respirations every 15 minutes until stable; stimulation if apnea occurs.
3. Small frequent feedings, especially in the presence of vomiting, regurgitation, and diarrhea.
4. Intravenous therapy as needed.
5. Medications as ordered, such as phenobarbital, paregoric, diazepam (Valium), or chlorpromazine hydrochloride (Thorazine). Methadone should not be given because of possible addiction.
6. Proper positioning on side to avoid possible aspiration of vomitus or secretions.
7. Observation for problems of SGA infants.
8. Protection from injury.
9. Fostering positive mother-infant interaction in the presence of potential negative feedback from infant because of abnormal sleep and nutrition patterns, inability to cuddle, and continuous crying.

PARENTING THE HIGH-RISK NEONATE

Attachment

The process by which maternal-infant attachment and bonding occurs has been the focus of intense study, because the work of earlier researchers clearly demonstrated the devastating effects of prolonged maternal-infant separation. Added impetus was provided as caregivers became increasingly aware that a disproportionately high number of battered or neglected children had been born prematurely and had required care in an intensive nursery for prolonged periods following birth. The question naturally arose as to whether interruptions in maternal contact and caregiving were significant factors in the disruption of the bonding process.

Historically, parents have been physically excluded from nurseries and isolated from care and contact with their infants. These practices are traceable to the high rate of morbidity and mortality in hospitalized patients (circa 1900), which led to strict isolation procedures and visitor restrictions. The "incubator doctor," Dr. Martin Couney, also set an example of better newborn survival rates with parental exclusion, which served to reinforce total exclusion.

Only recently have behaviors been established as specific for development of maternal attachment, bonding, and effective mothering. Animal studies demonstrate species-specific behavior patterns in maternal behavior. Interruption of instinctive behaviors results in rejection of the offspring, inability to recognize one's own offspring, and indiscriminate feeding of other young.

Studies of mother-infant interactions in other cultures have found that mother and infant remain together, usually for three to seven days after birth, without separation. Only in the high-risk and premature nurseries of the Western world are mothers and infants separated after birth.

Researchers have designated the period immediately following birth as the *maternal sensitive period*, during which the parents begin attachment to their infant. Research suggests that interference with this process during the early postpartum period (such as separation because of necessary phototherapy or the need for incubator care for 24 hours or so) can disturb the developing relationship between a mother and her newborn. It has become obvious that early maternal anxieties about the infant may have long-lasting effects (Klaus and Kennell, 1976). See Chapter 30 for a discussion of problems in attachment.

Adjustment

The events of premature labor and delivery abruptly terminate the normal adaptive processes to pregnancy. Feelings of increased concern over the labor and delivery and over survival of the infant and feelings of separation, helplessness, and failure plague the mother of the premature infant.

Mothers harbor guilt and failure feelings regarding the onset of premature labor and delivery of a preterm infant. They search for why: "Why did labor start? What did I do (or not do)?" Guilt fantasies include "Was it because I had sexual intercourse with my husband (a week, three days, a day) ago?" "Was it because I carried three loads of wash up from the basement?" "Am I being punished for . . . (something done in the past—even in childhood)?"

Birth of a defective child also engenders feelings of guilt and failure. As in the birth of a preterm infant, there are ideas of causation: "What did I do (or not do) to cause this?" "Am I being punished for . . . ?"

Parental reactions and steps of attachment are altered by the birth of a premature infant or of one with a congenital anomaly. A variety of new feelings, reactions, and stresses must be recognized and dealt with before the family can work toward the establishment of a healthy parent-infant relationship.

Kaplan and Mason (1974) view maternal reactions to premature births as an acute emotional disorder. They have identified four psychologic tasks as essential for coping with the stress and for providing a basis for the maternal-infant relationship:

1. Anticipatory grief as a psychologic preparation for possible loss of the child, while still hoping for its survival.

2. Acknowledgment of maternal failure to produce a term infant, expressed as anticipatory grief and depression and lasting until the chances of survival seem secure.

3. Resumption of the process of relating to the infant, which had been interrupted by the threat of nonsurvival. This task may be impaired by continuous threat of death or abnormality, and the mother may be slow in her response of hope for the infant's survival.

4. Understanding of the special needs and growth patterns of the premature infant, which are temporary and yield to normal patterns.

Klaus and Kennell (1976), on the other hand, feel that with extra, sustained support and early contact with her infant a mother need not necessarily become involved in anticipatory preparation for her child's possible death.

Most authorities agree that the birth of a premature infant or a less than perfect infant does require major adjustments as the parents are forced to surrender the image they had nurtured for so long of their ideal child.

Solnit and Stark (1961) postulate that grief and mourning of the loss of the loved object—the idealized child—mark parental reactions to a defective child. The parents must grieve the loss of the valued object—their wish for the perfect child. Simultaneously, they must adopt the defective child as the new love object. Parental responses to a defective child may also be viewed as a staged process (Klaus and Kennell, 1976):

1. *Shock* at the reality of the birth of a defective child. This stage may be characterized by forgetfulness, amnesia of the situation, and a feeling of desperation.

2. *Denial* of the reality of the situation, characterized by a refusal to believe the child is defective. Assertions that "It didn't really happen!" "It isn't real!" "There has been a mistake; it's someone else's baby."

3. *Depression* over the reality of the situation. There has been an acceptance of the situation and a corresponding grief reaction to its reality. This stage is characterized by much crying and sadness. Anger about the reality of the situation may also occur at this stage. A projection of blame on others or on self and feelings of "not me" are characteristic of this stage.

4. *Acceptance* and equilibrium are characteristic of a decrease in the emotional reactions of the parents. This stage is variable and may be prolonged because of a prolongation of the threat to the infant's survival. Some parents experience chronic sorrow in relation to their defective child.

5. *Reorganization* of the family to deal with the child's problems. Mutual support of the parents facilitates this process, but the crisis of the situation may precipitate husband-wife alienation.

These stages of parental adjustment are similar to the stages of dying and of grieving. Indeed, reorganization in the face of a crisis concerning a defective child is necessary for dealing with the crisis.

In the birth of either a defective child or a premature infant, the process of mourning is necessary for attachment to the "less than perfect child." *Grief work,* the emotional reaction to a significant loss, is necessary before adequate attachment to the actual child is possible. Parental detachment precedes parental attachment.

Seeing and touching the newborn appear to be species-specific behaviors for human maternal attachment. Immediate performance of these behaviors may be impossible if the infant is preterm or has a congenital anomaly. Such immediate care as resuscitation, incubation, correction of shock, and separation from the mother to an intensive care area may preclude these behaviors. It is essential that, as soon as possible after birth, the mother be reunited with her infant. It is important for the mother to see her infant so that:

1. She knows that her infant is alive.
2. She knows what the infant's real problems are. The fantasy of the infant's problem may be more devastating than the reality of the problem. Early acquaintance between mother and infant allows a realistic perspective on the infant's problems.
3. She can begin the grief work over the loss of the idealized child and begin the process of attachment to the actual child.
4. She can share the experience of the infant with the father, who may have already seen and touched the infant.

Nursing Interventions

Before parents see their child, the nurse must prepare them to view their preterm or defective baby. It is important that a positive realistic attitude regarding the infant be presented to the parents, rather than a pessimistic attitude. An overly negative, pessimistic attitude will further alienate the parents from their infant and retard attachment behaviors. Instead of allowing attachment feelings and bonding to develop, the mother will begin the process of anticipatory grieving, and once started, this process is difficult to reverse.

In preparing parents for the first view of their infant, it is important that the professional look at the child. The parents should be prepared to see the congenital anomaly and the normal aspects of their infant. All infants exhibit strengths as well as deficiencies: "Your baby is small, about the length of my two hands. She weighs 2 lb 3 oz but is very active and cries when we disturb her. She is having some difficulty breathing but is breathing without assistance and in only 35% oxygen."

Intensive Care

The equipment being used for the baby and its purpose should be described before the parents enter the intensive care unit. Upon entering the unit, the parents may be overwhelmed by the sounds of monitors, alarms, and respirators as well as by the unfamiliar language and "foreign" atmosphere. It is reassuring if the parents are prepared and accompanied to the unit by the same person(s). The primary physician and primary nurse caring for the infant should be with the parents while they initially visit their child, should describe the infant's abnormality, and should point out the normal characteristics of the infant. Parental reactions are varied, but as there is usually an element of initial shock, provision of chairs and time to regain composure will assist the parents. Slow, complete, and simple explanations—first of the infant and then of all the equipment—will allay fear and anxiety.

Misconceptions about equipment and its placement on the child and about its potential harm are common. Such statements as "Does the fluid go into the brain?" "Does the white wire on the abdomen go into the stomach?" and "Does the monitor make the baby's heart beat?" imply much fear for the infant's safety and misconceptions about usage. These worries are easily overcome by simple explanations of all equipment being used on the infant.

Concern about the infant's physical appearance is common yet may remain unvoiced. Parents may express such concerns as "He looks so small and red—like a drowned rat." "Why do her genitals look so abnormal?" "Will that awful looking mouth (cleft lip and palate) ever be normal?" Such questions need to be anticipated by the nurse and addressed. Utilization of pictures, such as of an infant after cleft lip repair, may be reassuring to doubting parents. Knowledge of the development of a "normal" preterm infant will allow the nurse to make such statements as "The baby's vagina may look very abnormal to you, but it is normal for her maturity. As she grows, the outer lips of the vagina will become larger and the clitoris will be covered and the genitals will then look as you expect them to. She is normal for her level of maturity."

The tone of the neonatal intensive care unit is set by the nursing staff. Generally, residents and interns remain for a short time, specialists also rotate, and the permanent medical staff is not available minute-to-minute. Development of a safe, trusting environment depends on viewing the parents as essential and not as "visitors" or "nuisances" in the unit. Pleasant, relaxed physical surroundings convey the message of hospitality and encourage parents to "be at home here." Provision of chairs, privacy when needed, and easy access to staff and facilities is important in developing an open environment for all. Uncrowded and welcoming surroundings convey the message "You are welcome here." However, even in crowded physical surroundings the attitude of openness and trust is conveyed by the nursing staff.

A trust relationship for collaborative efforts in caring for the infant is essential. The nurse must therapeutically use her "self" in relating on a one-to-one basis with the parents. Each individual has different needs, different ways of adaptation to crisis, and different ways of support. It is essential that the professional utilize those techniques that are real and spontaneous to her and not adopt words or actions that are "foreign" to her spontaneity. She must also gauge her interventions to the parents' pace and needs.

Smaller hospitals may be unable to care for sick infants; thus transport to a regional referral center may be necessary. These centers may be as much as 500 miles away from the parents' community. It is therefore important that the mother see (and touch) her infant before he is transported. Facilitation of this contact may be the responsibility of the community professionals as well as the transport team. Bringing the mother to the nursery or taking the infant in a warmed transport incubator to the mother's bedside will allow her to see the infant before he is transported.

Support of the parents with explanations from the professional staff is essential. Occasionally the mother may be unable to see the infant before transport (if she is still under general anesthesia or if she is experiencing complications such as shock, hemorrhage, or seizures). Before the infant is transported, a photograph of the infant should be given to the mother, along with an explanation of the infant's condition, problems, and so on. Personal description of the infant's characteristics is also helpful until the mother can visit the infant.

Touching and Caretaking

Klaus and Kennell (1976) have demonstrated a significant difference in the amount of eye contact and touching behavior of mothers of preterm infants. Whereas mothers of normal newborns progress within minutes to palm contact of the infant's trunk, the mother of a preterm infant is slower in her progression from fingertip to palm contact and from touching the extremities to the infant's trunk. The progression to palm contact with the infant's trunk may take several visits, as illustrated in Figure 24–13.

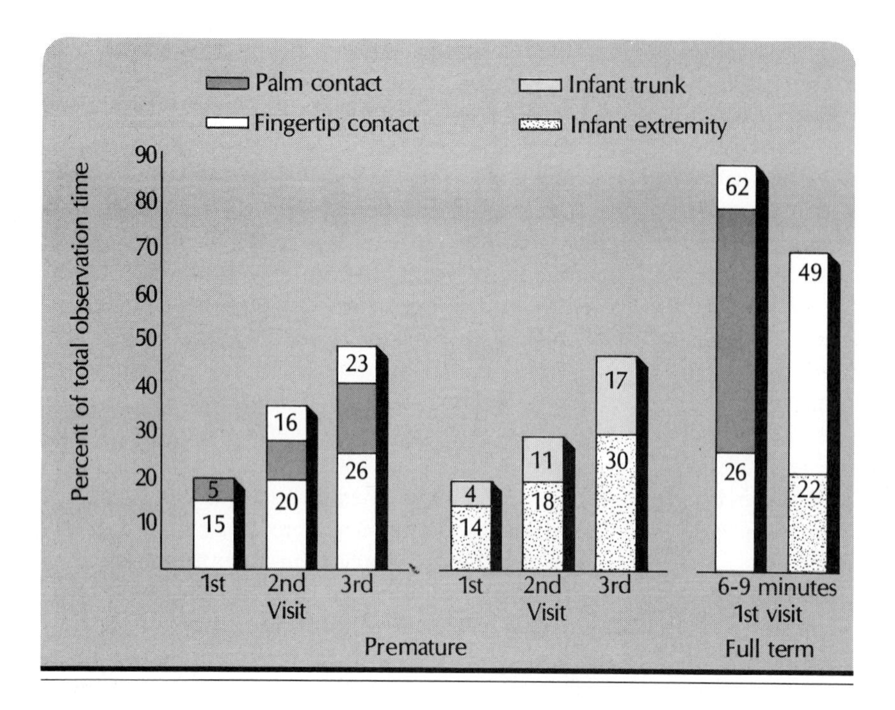

Figure 24–13. Fingertip and palm contact on the trunk and extremities at first of three postnatal visits in nine months of premature infants compared with the 6th to 9th minute of twelve mothers of full-term infants at their first visit. (From Klaus, M. H., and Kennell, J. H. 1976. *Maternal-infant bonding.* St. Louis: The C. V. Mosby Co.; modified from Klaus, M. H., et al. 1970. *Pediatrics.* 46:187.)

Mothers visiting a small or sick infant may need several visits to become comfortable and confident in their abilities to touch the infant without injuring him. Barriers such as incubators, incisions, monitor electrodes, and tubes may delay the mother's confidence. Knowledge of this "normal" delay in touching behavior will enable the nurse to understand parental behavior. Through support, reassurance, and encouragement, the nurse can facilitate the mother's positive feelings about her ability and her importance to her infant. Utilization of touching facilitates "getting to know" her infant and thus establishing a bond with the infant. Touching, as well as seeing the infant, helps the mother to realize the "normals" and potentials of her infant.

Caretaking may be delayed for the mother of a preterm, defective, or sick infant. The variety of equipment (warmers, monitors, respirators) needed for life support is hardly conducive to anxiety-free caretaking by the parents. However, even the sickest infant may be cared for, if even in a small way, by his parents. As a facilitator of parental caretaking, it is the responsibility of the nurse to promote the parents' success. Demonstration and explanation, followed by support of the parents in initial caretaking behaviors, positively reinforce this behavior. Asking the parents to give their infant skin care or oral care or to help the nurse turn the infant may at first be anxiety-provoking. The parents increasingly become more comfortable and confident in caretaking and receive satisfaction from the child's reactions and their ability "to do something." Complimenting the parents' competence in caretaking also serves to increase their self-esteem, which has received recent "blows" of guilt and failure. It is vitally important that the mother never be given a task if there is any possibility that she will not be able to accomplish it.

Nurse-Parent Interactions

Often mothers have ambivalent feelings toward the nurse, who for a time is the surrogate mother. Feeling inadequate in providing the sophisticated care needed by her infant, the mother watches the nurse competently perform the caretaking tasks. She feels both grateful to the nurse for her ability and expertise and jealous of the nurse's ability to care for her infant. These feelings may be acted out in criticism of the care being received by her infant, in manipulation of staff, or in personal guilt about such feelings. Instead of fostering (by silence) these inferiority feelings within mothers, nurses are in a special position to recognize these feelings and to intervene appropriately to facilitate mother-infant bonding.

If the nurse is understanding and secure, she will be able to support the parents' egos instead of collecting rewards for herself. In order to positively reinforce parenting behaviors, professionals must first believe in the importance of the parents. The nurse could hardly convince a doubting parent of her importance to the infant unless she really believes it. The attitude of the professionals communicates acceptance or rejection to the parents, regardless of what is said. During this crisis period, it is essential that attitudes and words say: "You are a good mother/father. You are a good person. You have an important contribution to make to the care of your infant." Unless equal care is taken in facilitating parental attachment as in providing physiologic care, the outcome will not be a healthy family.

Verbalizations by the nurse that improve parental self-esteem are essential and easily shared. Breast-feeding is possible and in many centers recommended for preterm or sick infants for nutrition as well as for defense against the development of necrotizing enterocolitis. In addition to physiologic use, breast milk is important because of the emotional investment of the mother. Pumping, storing, labeling, and delivering quantities of breast milk is time-consuming and a "labor of love" for mothers. Positive remarks regarding breast milk reinforce the maternal behavior of caretaking and providing for her infant: "Breast milk is something that only you can give your baby" or "You really have brought a lot of milk today" or "Look how rich this breast milk is" or "Even small amounts of milk are important, and look how rich it is."

If the infant begins to gain weight while being fed breast milk, it is important to point this out to the mother. At the same time, parents should be advised that initial weight loss with beginning nipple feeding is common because of the increased energy expended when the infant begins active rather than passive nutritional intake.

Within the past 20 years, increased attention has been given to the infant's need for sensory stimulation (Table 24-8). Evidence suggests that the infant who receives tactile, kinesthetic, and auditory stimulation has fewer apneic spells, decreased stooling, improved weight gain, and ad-

Table 24-8. Effects of Stimulation in the Newborn Period*

Number of patients	Premature or full term	Type of stimulation	Outcome	
			Experimental group	Control group
60	Premature	Sensory, tactile Kinesthetic (experimental handled 2.73 times more than controls for 14 days)	Greater incidence of disorders involving genital area Longer in state of quiescence Passed less feces	Greater incidence of disorders involving eye, mouth, body rash Cried more Cried more before feeding
10	Premature	Tactile, stroked 5 min/hr/day for 10 days	Regained birth weight in 10.8 days, active and healthy 7 to 8 months after discharge On Bayley developmental test 7 to 8 months after discharge, 1 infant showed poor gross and fine motor development	Regained birth weight in 15.4 days; 3 infants more than standard deviation below growth mean; 2 of 4 infants suspicious for cerebral palsy; 4 infants below mean for age in motor development

*From Klaus, M., and Kennell, J. 1976. *Maternal-infant bonding.* St. Louis: The C. V. Mosby Co., pp. 118-119.

Table 24–8. Cont'd

Number of patients	Premature or full term	Type of stimulation	Outcome: Experimental group	Outcome: Control group
32	Full term	Rockerbox	Faster rocking speed (60 times/min), less distress After rock, decreased activity level Distress declined	Slower rocking speed (30 times/min), less reduction in activity
18	8 premature 10 full term	Rockerbox White noise	Rockerbox quieted down infant Sound and rockerbox quieted down infant more than rockerbox alone	
62	Premature	Auditory – recorded mother's voice 6 times/day at 2-hr intervals until gestational age is 252 days	Higher motor score on general maturation scale of Rosenbüth test at 36 weeks Greater auditory response to bell or rattle Higher muscle tension responses	Lower tactile adaptive score Lower visual response to red rattle
15	Premature	Kinesthetic – rocker bed Auditory – recorded heartbeat 15 min/hr	Greater average daily weight gain Greater mental scale score and expressive language development	Less time in quiet sleep Less time in active sleep
60	Premature	Recorded female voice White noise 30 min/day	If quiet, increased heart rate at hearing white noise If crying, decreased heart rate at hearing recorded female voice	
36	Premature	Handled 20 min twice a day until 72 hr of age, then 20 min a day	4-month mental score 13.5 points higher 4-month motor score 16 points higher	Regained birth weight slower 6-month infant behavioral record lower
30	Premature	Visual – suspended nursery birds Tactile – extra play periods	Higher developmental status at 1 year	Lower IQ (10 points)
18	Premature	Rubbed extremities 5 min/15 min/3 hr	Decrease in frequency of apnea	
21	Premature	Gently oscillating waterbed	Decreased apneic episodes	
20	Premature	Waterbeds gently rocked Auditory stimuli	Increased weight gain Increased head circumference Increased biparietal diameter	

*From Klaus, M., and Kennell, J. 1976. *Maternal-infant bonding*. St. Louis: The C. V. Mosby Co., pp. 118–119.

vanced central nervous system functioning (Klaus and Kennell, 1976). Parents are ideally equipped to meet the need for stimulation. Stroking, rocking, cuddling, singing, and talking should be an integral part of the infant's care. Visual stimulation in the form of mobiles and *en face* interaction with the caretaker are also important. The nurse should work with the family to provide appropriate stimulation without sensory bombardment.

Provision of care by the parents is appropriate even for very sick or defective infants. It has been found that detachment is easier after attachment, because the parents are comforted by the knowledge that they did all they could have for their child while he was alive.

As parents attempt to deal with the initial stages of shock and grief at the birth of a premature or less than perfect child, they may fail to assimilate information and may require constant repetition by the nurse to accept the reality of the situation.

During crisis, maintenance of interpersonal relationships is difficult. Yet in a newborn intensive care area, the parents are expected to relate to many and varied care providers. It is important that parents have as few professionals as possible relaying information to them. A primary nurse should coordinate and provide continuity in information-giving to parents. Care providers are all individuals and thus will use different terms, inflections, and attitudes. These subtle differences are monumental to parents and only serve to confuse, confound, and produce anxiety. Several trusted relationships with professionals minimize unnecessary anxiety and concern and facilitate open communication. The nurse not only functions as a liaison between the parents and the wide variety of professionals interacting with the infant and parents; she also offers clarification, explanation, interpretation of information, and support to the parents.

Bonding can be facilitated by encouraging parents to visit and become involved in their child's care (Figure 24-14). When visiting is impossible, the parents should feel free to phone whenever they wish to receive information about their child. A warm, receptive attitude is very supportive. Nursing can also facilitate parenting by personalizing a child to his parents, by referring to him by name or by relating personal behavioral characteristics to the parents. Remarks such as "Jenny loves her pacifier" help make the infant more individual and unique.

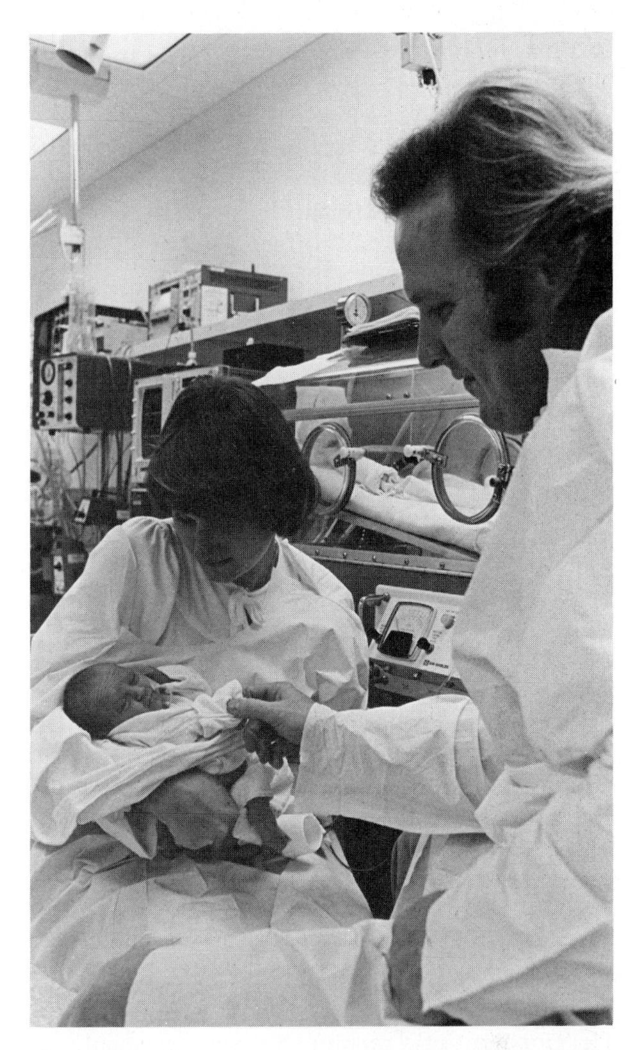

Figure 24-14. It is important that the parents of high-risk infants be given the opportunity to get acquainted with their children. Physical contact is extremely important in the bonding process and should be encouraged whenever possible.

Development of a professional-family relationship enables information-gathering into areas of concern. A concurrent illness of the mother or other family members or other concurrent stress (lack of hospitalization insurance, loss of job, age of parents) may alter the family response to the neonate. Feelings of apprehension, guilt, failure, and grief that are verbally or nonverbally expressed are important aspects of the nursing history. These observations enable all professionals to be aware of the parental state, coping behaviors, and readiness for attachment, bonding, and caretaking. Appropriate nursing observations during interviewing and relating to the family include:

1. *Level of understanding:* Observations concerning the ability to assimilate information given and to ask appropriate questions; the need for constant repetition of "the same" information.

2. *Behavioral responses:* Appropriateness of behavior in relation to information given; lack of response; "flat" affect.

3. *Difficulties with communication:* Deafness (reads lips only); blindness; dysphagia; understanding only of foreign language.

4. *Paternal and maternal education level:* Parents unable to read or write; only eighth grade completed; mother an M.D. or Ph.D.; and so on.

Documentation of such information, obtained by the nurse through continuing contact and development of a therapeutic family relationship, enables all professionals to understand and utilize the nursing history in providing continuous individual care.

The Role of the Family

Development of a relationship with the family is important because parenthood or the illness of a member affects the entire family. The parents should be encouraged to deal with the crisis while utilizing their support system. The extended family attempts to meet the emotional needs and provide support for family members in crisis and stress situations. In our mobile society of isolated, nuclear families, the extended family may be the next-door neighbor, the mother's best friend, or perhaps a school chum. Biologic kin is not the only valid criterion for a support system; an emotional kinship is the most important factor. The nurse must search out the significant others in the lives of the parents and assist them in understanding so that they are able to be a constant parental support.

The impact of the crisis on the family is individual and varied. In constructing a conceptual framework for family crisis, Hill (1974) has formulated an equation to show the relationship of all elements:

A (the event) ⟶ interacting with B (the family's crisis-meeting resources) ⟶ interacting with C (the definitions the family makes of the events) ⟶ produces X (the crisis).

The stressful event (A), a situation for which the family has little or no preparation, may be classified according to the source of trouble: *extra-family events,* which may solidify the family, and *intra-family events,* which may reflect negatively on the adequacy of the family.

Marked changes in the family configuration, such as accession of a new member (normal or premature infant, infant with congenital anomaly) may also be a stressful occasion for the family members. The ability of the family to adapt to changing situations is the basis of the crisis-meeting resource (B). This adaptability to events depends on the definition (C) ascribed to each event by the family. This "meaning aspect of the crisis" reflects the family. Thus, an interplay of an event, the crisis-meeting resources, and the family definition of the event produce the crisis situation.

Through the nurse-family relationship, information about the ability of the family to adapt to the situation is obtained. The event itself (normal newborn, premature infant, infant with congenital anomaly) can then be viewed as it is defined by the family, and appropriate intervention can be instituted.

Because the family as a unit composed of individuals must deal with the situation, it is important to encourage open interfamily communication. Secret-keeping should not be encouraged, especially between spouses, because secrets undermine the trust of their relationship. Well-meaning rationales such as "I want to protect her," "I don't want her to know," and so on can be destructive to open communication and to the basic element of a relationship—trust. The parents (and family) should be given information together. This practice helps to overcome misunderstandings and misinterpretations and helps to promote "working through" together.

The entire family—siblings as well as relatives—is encouraged to visit and receive information about the baby. Methods of intervention and assisting the family in coping with the situation include providing support, confronting the crisis, and understanding the reality. Extension of support, explanations, and the helping role must precede the kin network, as well as the nuclear family, in an attempt to aid them in communication and support ties with the nuclear family.

It is also essential to meet the needs of the individuals involved. Needs of the individuals must be respected and facilitated; differences are tolerable and able to exist side-by-side. Eliciting the parents' feelings is easily accomplished with the question: "How are you doing?" The emphasis is on *you*, and the interest must be sincere.

In the newborn care unit, the families become friends and support one another. Parent groups that discuss and "work through" feelings are helpful and supportive. Shared experience is a powerful tool in empathy and should be encouraged and facilitated.

Visiting and caregiving patterns give an indication of the level of (or lack of) parental attachment. A record of visits, caretaking procedures, affect (in relating to the newborn), and telephone calls is essential. Serial observations must be obtained, rather than an isolated instance of concern. If a pattern of distancing behaviors evolves, appropriate intervention should be instituted. A statistically significant number of preterm, sick, and congenitally defective infants have been found on follow-up to suffer failure to thrive, battering, or other disorders of mothering. Early detection and intervention will prevent these aberrations in mothering behaviors from leading to irreparable damage or death.

Predischarge

Reinforcement of positive parenting experiences must be continued into the home after discharge. From the time of admission to the nursery, the parents should be preparing for the discharge of their infant. It is totally inappropriate for the parents to receive a bombardment of discharge instructions about medicine, special formulas and feeding techniques, and special procedures on the day or hour before the discharge. From the beginning, the parents should be taught about and included in the care of their infant. The special needs and growth patterns of the infant must be understood by the parents. Predischarge care includes:

1. Long-term planning, beginning at admission and involving collaboration with the parents.

2. Utilization of teaching/learning methods in assessment of parental readiness to learn and in teaching them to caretake minimally and then expand their role.

3. Referrals to community agencies, such as visiting nurses and public health nurses, to assist parents in the traumatic transition from hospital to home. Normally the transition "from hospital to 24-hour home care" is anxiety-provoking, especially for the mother. Moral support is essential until the mother is comfortable with full-time mothering of her infant.

4. Home preparation of equipment, appliances, and clothes for the infant. Absence of home preparation is a sign for concern—the parents may not be ready or willing to accept the infant. Intervention is essential before and after discharge.

5. Home visit to reassure the parents and to visit the "new friends" of the professional.

Support cannot be given unless it can be received. Living in an emotional environment of "lots of living and lots of dying" takes its toll on staff. The emotional needs and feelings of the staff must be recognized and dealt with in order to support the parents. An environment of openness to feelings and dealing with their own humanness is essential for staff. Such techniques as group meetings, individual support, and primary care nursing may assist in maintaining staff mental health.

SUMMARY

Early identification of potential high-risk infants through assessment of prepregnant, prenatal, and intrapartal factors facilitates strategically timed nursing observations and interventions. High-risk infants, whether they are prematurely born, small or large for gestational age, postterm, or born of diabetic mothers, have many similar problems—although their problems are based on different physiologic processes. With early recognition and intervention, the potential long-term physiologic and emotional consequences of these problems can be avoided or at least lessened in severity.

SUGGESTED ACTIVITIES

1. During an observational experience in a neonatal high-risk nursery, correlate the specific problems of a premature infant, an SGA infant, or an infant of a diabetic mother with the physiologic rationale and resulting medical and nursing interventions.
2. Observe two or three premature infants being fed by various feeding techniques, and identify the rationale behind each method.
3. Develop a nursing plan of care that best facilitates the parent-infant bonding process for a premature infant.
4. Observe parent-infant interactions in a premature nursery.
5. Design a handout for home infant care.

REFERENCES

Avery, G. B., ed. 1975. *Neonatology.* Philadelphia: J. B. Lippincott Co.

Bucci, G., et al. 1972. The systemic systolic blood pressure of newborns with low weight. *Acta Paediat. Scand.* (Supp.). 229:1.

Clifford, S. 1957. Postmaturity. *Advances Pediatr.* 9:13.

Gardner, S. L. 1975. A systematic approach to assessment and nursing care planning for the newborn. Master's thesis, University of Colorado School of Nursing.

Glass, L. July 1975. The neonate in withdrawal: identification, diagnosis and treatment. *Pediatr. Ann.* 4:25.

Hill, R. 1974. Generic features of families under stress. In *Crisis interventions,* ed. H. J. Parad. New York: Family Services Association of America.

Jones, K. L., et al. 1973. Pattern of malformation in offspring of chronic alcoholic mothers. *Lancet.* 1:1267.

Jones, K. L., and Smith, D. W. 1973. Recognition of the fetal alcoholic syndrome in early infancy. *Lancet.* 2:999.

Kaplan, D. M., and Mason, E. A. 1974. Maternal reactions to premature birth viewed as an acute emotional disorder. In *Crisis interventions,* ed. H. J. Parad. New York: Family Services Association of America.

Klaus, M. H., and Kennell, J. H. 1976. *Maternal-infant bonding.* St. Louis: The C. V. Mosby Co.

Klaus, M. H., et al. 1970. Human maternal behavior at first contact with her young. *Pediatrics.* 46:187.

Korones, S. B. 1976. *High-risk newborn infants: the basis for intensive care nursing.* 2nd ed. St. Louis: The C. V. Mosby Co.

Lubchenco, L. O. 1970. Assessment of gestational age and development at birth. *Pediatr. Clin. N. Am.* 17:125.

Lubchenco, L. 1976. *The high risk infant.* Philadelphia: W. B. Saunders Co.

O'Brien, D., and Abbott, F. 1962. *Laboratory manual of pediatric microbiochemical techniques.* New York: Paul B. Hoeber, Inc.

Silverman, W. A. 1961. *Dunham's premature infants.* 3rd ed. New York: Paul B. Hoeber, Inc.

Solnit, A., and Stark, M. 1961. Mourning and the birth of a defective child. *Psychoan. Studies Children.* 16:505.

Tsang, R. C., et al. 1972. Hypocalcemia in infants of diabetic mothers. *J. Pediatr.* 80:384.

ADDITIONAL READINGS

Arturo, H. 1976. Nursery evaluation of the newborn. *Am. J. Nurs.* 67:1671.

Behrman, R. E., ed. 1973. *Neonatology: diseases of the fetus and infant.* St. Louis: The C. V. Mosby Co.

Brown, J. G., and Johnson, W. 1976. A fetal intensive care nursing program. *J. Obstet. Gynecol. Neonatal Nurs.* 5:23.

Christensen, A. 1977. Coping with the crisis of premature birth: one couple's story. *MCN.* 2:24.

Clark, A. L., and Affonso, D. 1976. Infant behavior and maternal attachment: two sides to the coin. *MCN.* 1:94.

Haynes, U. 1969. *A developmental approach to casefinding.* Maternal and Child Health Service Publication No. 2017. Washington, D.C.: U.S. Department of Health, Education, and Welfare.

Kantor, G. 1978. Addicted mother, addicted baby: a challenge to health care providers. *MCN.* 3:281.

Kennedy, J. C. 1973. The high risk maternal infant acquaintance process. *Nurs. Clin. N. Am.* 8:549.

Klaus, M. H., and Fanaroff, A. A. 1973. *Care of the high-risk neonate.* Philadelphia: W. B. Saunders Co.

Klaus, M. H., and Kennell, J. H. 1970. Mothers separated from their newborn infants. *Pediatr. Clin. N. Am.* 17:1016.

Miners, H. 1978. Problems and prognosis for the small-for-gestational-age and the premature infant. *MCN.* 3:221.

Olshansky, S. 1962. Chronic sorrow: a response to having a mentally defective child. *Soc. Casework.* 43:190.

Robert, M. F., et al. 1976. Maternal diabetes and the respiratory distress syndrome. *N. Eng. J. Med.* 294:357.

Rothstein, P., and Gould, J. 1974. Born with a habit: infants of drug-addicted mothers. *Pediatr. Clin. N. Am.* 2:307.

Seeds, A. E. 1970. Adverse effects on the fetus of acute events in labor. *Pediatr. Clin. N. Am.* 17:811.

Slade, C. I.; Reidl, C. J.; and Mangurten, H. H. 1977. Working with parents of high risk newborns. *J. Obstet. Gynecol. Neonatal Nurs.* 6:21.

Usher, R., et al. 1966. Judgment of fetal age. II. Clinical significance of gestational age and an objective method for its assessment. *Pediatr. Clin. N. Am.* 13:835.

Williams, J., and Lancaster, J. 1976. Thermo-regulation of the newborn. *MCN.* 1:355.

CHAPTER 25

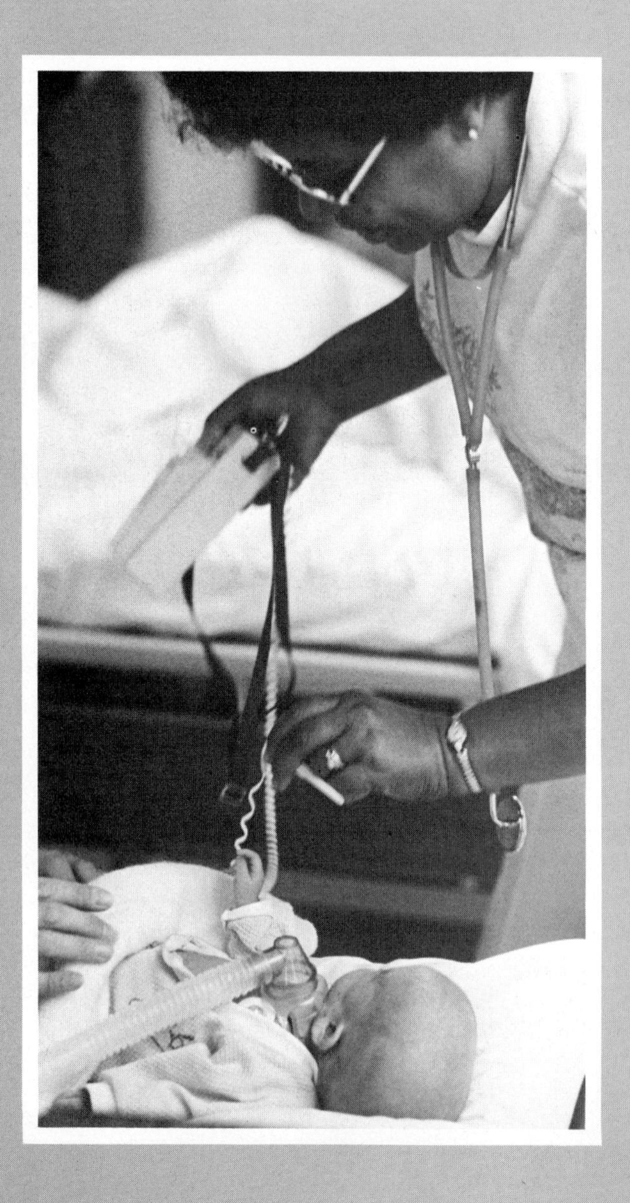

COMPLICATIONS OF THE NEONATE

OBJECTIVES

- Based on the labor record, Apgar score, and observable physiologic indicators, identify infants in need of resuscitation and the appropriate method of resuscitation.
- Based on clinical manifestations, differentiate the various types of respiratory distress (hyaline membrane disease, transient tachypnea, and type II respiratory distress) in the neonate.
- Identify the many components of nursing care of an infant with respiratory distress syndrome.
- Discuss the latest theory correlating the use of high concentrations of oxygen and positive pressure ventilation with development of the complications of respiratory distress.
- Differentiate between physiologic and pathologic jaundice based on onset, cause, possible sequelae, and specific management.
- Explain the set of circumstances that must be present for the development of erythroblastosis and ABO incompatibility and the nurse's role in the care of an infant with hemolytic disease.
- Discuss the process of candidate selection and current therapy employed to prevent Rh incompatibility in succeeding pregnancies.
- Identify the nursing responsibilities in phototherapy and exchange transfusion procedures.
- Describe the assessment of clinical manifestations that would make the nurse suspect neonatal sepsis.
- Relate the dangers of untreated syphilis, gonorrhea, or herpesvirus type 2 to management of the infant in the neonatal period.
- Explain the theories, clinical and diagnostic manifestations, nursing care, and medical treatment of necrotizing enterocolitis.

Marked homeostatic changes occur during the transition from fetal to neonatal life. Because the most rapid anatomic and physiologic changes of this period occur in the cardiopulmonary system, major problems of the newborn are usually related to this system. These problems include asphyxia, respiratory distress, jaundice, hemolytic disease, and anemia. Ideally, such problems are anticipated and identified prenatally and appropriate intervention measures are begun at such time.

ASPHYXIA

Consideration of neonatal asphyxia requires knowledge of the respiratory transition from intrauterine to extrauterine life, the pathophysiology of asphyxia, the effects on circulation and biochemical status, and sequelae. The prevention or treatment for asphyxia is resuscitation.

Fetal-Neonatal Transition

With the first breath of life and the cutting of the umbilical cord, the infant begins the transition from intrauterine to extrauterine life. During fetal life, better oxygenated blood is diverted to the heart and brain. Blood in the descending aorta is less oxygenated and supplies the kidney and intestinal tract. Some blood, pumped from the right ventricle toward the lungs, enters the pulmonary vessels. However, in the fetus there is increased pulmonary resistance, and most of the blood goes through the ductus arteriosus into the descending aorta (see Figure 6–14). Expansion of the lungs with the first breath decreases the pulmonary vascular resistance, as the clamping of the cord raises systemic vascular resistance and left atrial pressure. This physiologic mechanism marks the beginning of neonatal circulation. Elevation of left atrial pressure (above right atrial pressure) closes the foramen ovale and discontinues flow from right to left atrium. Elevation of systemic vascular pressure above pulmonary vascular pressure increases pulmonary blood flow by an alteration of flow through the ductus arteriosus (from right-to-left to left-to-right). Neonatal circulation now is established.

Pathophysiology

Research studies of various species have indicated species variability in response to asphyxial insults. These research studies are not easily extrapolated to the response of the human infant, since the length of asphyxia and the possibility of subsequent anoxic brain damage are not easily estimated in the human infant. Presentation of an apneic infant in the delivery room necessitates immediate resuscitative efforts. Circulatory patterns that accompany asphyxia represent an inability to make the transition to extrauterine circulation—in effect a return to fetallike circulatory patterns. Failure of lung expansion and establishment of respiration rapidly produces hypoxia (decreased PaO_2), acidosis (decreased pH), and hypercarbia (increased PCO_2). These biochemical changes result in pulmonary vasoconstriction, with retention of high pulmonary vascular resistance, hypoperfusion of the lungs, and a large right-to-left shunt through the ductus arteriosus. The foramen ovale opens (as right atrial pressure exceeds left atrial pressure), and blood flows from right to left.

Biochemical changes that occur in asphyxia contribute to these circulatory changes. The most profound biochemical aberration is a change from aerobic to anaerobic metabolism in the presence of hypoxia, with accumulation of lactate and the development of metabolic acidosis. There may also be a concomitant respiratory acidosis due to a rapid increase in PCO_2 during asphyxia. In response to hypoxia and anaerobic metabolism, there is an increase in free fatty acids (FFA) and glycerol in the blood. Glycogen stores are also mobilized to provide a continuous glucose source for the brain. Rapid utilization of hepatic and cardiac stores of glycogen may occur during an asphyxial attack.

Resuscitation

The neonate is supplied with protective mechanisms against hypoxial insults, yet prolonged hypoxia results in brain damage or death. The goal of resuscitation is to decrease PCO_2 by ventilating the alveoli and to increase oxygen concentration going to vital organs.

Identification of Infants in Need of Resuscitation

As discussed in Chapter 24, knowledge of the perinatal history enables caregivers to anticipate the birth of a high-risk infant who will need resuscitative efforts from appropriate personnel. Need for resuscitation may be anticipated in any of the following antepartal or intrapartal situations:

Antepartal Risk Factors for Resuscitation

1. Previous obstetric history of fetal or neonatal death; premature or growth-retarded infant; infant weighing 10 lb or more.
2. Maternal conditions that affect the placenta or fetus—preeclampsia-eclampsia (postterm 42 weeks, preexisting hypertension), diabetes (infection, chronic renal disease, maternal obesity, cardiac disease).
3. Maternal age—younger than 15 years or elderly primigravida.
4. Isoimmunization.
5. Abruptio placentae or placenta previa.
6. Multiple gestation.
7. Abnormal presentation.
8. Premature or prolonged rupture of the membranes.
9. Polyhydramnios or oligohydramnios.
10. Abnormal estriol.
11. Less than mature L/S ratio.
12. Maternal drug usage, especially alcohol.

Intrapartal Risk Factors for Resuscitation

1. Abnormal labor pattern—dystocia, precipitous delivery.
2. Meconium-stained amniotic fluid in cephalic presentation.
3. Fetal heart rate patterns—tachycardia (greater than 160/min without maternal temperature elevation); bradycardia (less than 120/min, particularly associated with smooth baseline, an ominous sign); irregular rate; lack of baseline variability of fetal heart rate (smooth or fixed); lack of significant variability with fetal movement; ominous patterns (moderate to severe variable deceleration and late deceleration of any magnitude).
4. Abnormal fetal presentation—breech, transverse lie, shoulder.
5. Prolapsed cord.
6. Abruptio placentae or placenta previa.
7. Indications for cesarean section.

Neonatal Risk Factors for Resuscitation

1. Difficult delivery.
2. Fetal blood loss.
3. Apneic episode unresponsive to tactile stimulation.
4. Cardiac arrest.
5. Inadequate ventilation.

Particular attention must be paid to these pregnancies during the intrapartal period, because labor and delivery are asphyxiating processes and often the high-risk fetus has less tolerance to the stress of labor and delivery.

Biophysical (uterine contractions, FHR, ECG) and biochemical (fetal and maternal pH and blood gases) monitoring during the intrapartal period may help to identify fetal distress so that appropriate measures can be taken to deliver the fetus immediately, before major damage occurs, and to treat the asphyxiated neonate. Fetal scalp blood sampling (p. 474), a valuable assessment tool, may indicate asphyxic insult and related degree of fetal acidosis if considered in relation to stage of labor, uterine contractions, and ominous fetal heart rate patterns. Normal fetal pH ranges from 7.3 to 7.35. The fall of pH is gradual during the first stage of labor but becomes more drastic during the second stage and delivery. The stress of labor causes an intermittent decrease in the exchange of gases in the intervillous space of the placenta and a fall in pH secondarily to the accumulation of pyruvic and lactic acid, resulting in an accumulation of hydrogen ions and the phenomenon of physiologic fetal acidosis. Physiologic fetal acidosis is metabolic rather than respiratory, because exchange of CO_2 at the placental level is more rapid than exchange of hydrogen ions. During labor, a fetal pH of 7.25 or higher is considered normal. A pH value of 7.21 to 7.24 is considered as "preacidosis." A pH value of 7.20 or less during first-stage labor is considered an ominous sign of fetal asphyxia (Modanlou, 1976); repeat samples should be obtained within 10–15 minutes to confirm the diagnosis, followed by immediate delivery of the fetus.

Nurse's Role

Communication between the obstetric office or clinic and the labor and delivery nurse facilitates the identification of potential infants in need of resuscitation.

Upon arrival of the mother in the labor area, the nurse should have the antepartal record and should note any contributory perinatal history factors and assess present fetal status. As labor progresses, nursing assessments include ongoing monitoring of fetal heartbeat and its response to contractions, assisting with fetal scalp blood sampling, and observing for expulsion of meconium, thereby identifying fetal asphyxia and hypoxia.

Equipment and Medications

Following anticipation, the next step in effective resuscitation is assembling the necessary equipment and ensuring proper functioning. Adequately trained personnel are a vital necessity in the delivery room for all high-risk and normal deliveries. Resuscitation is at least a two-person effort. Systematic assembly and checking of equipment is essential for efficient resuscitation and for preventing "flail" efforts. Provision for pH and blood gas determination is desirable.

Necessary equipment includes a radiant warmer, a device that should be in every delivery room. This equipment provides an overhead radiant heat source that is servocontrolled (a thermostatic mechanism that is taped to the infant's abdomen triggers the radiant warmer to turn on or off in order to maintain a level of thermoneutrality) and an open bed for easy access to the infant. It is essential that the nurse keep the infant warm. The infant is dried quickly to prevent evaporative heat loss and is placed under the radiant warmer.

The nurse calls for assistance. Adequate, well-trained personnel must always be available to assist the primary resuscitator.

Equipment needed is as follows (Jones, 1976):

1. Radiant warmer
2. Bag and mask (two mask sizes: one premature and one newborn)
3. Tubing and pressure gauges for bag
4. Suction equipment
   a. DeLee Trap
   b. Bulb syringe
   c. Mechanical suction apparatus
   d. Suction catheters (No. 5 or 6, No. 8 Fr.)
5. Intubation equipment
   a. Magill forceps (optional)
   b. Portex polyvinylchloride intubation tubes —sizes 2.5, 3, 3.5, 4 mm (fitted with adapter)
   c. Wire stylets for tubes (if desired)
   d. Laryngoscope handle with 2 blades—size 0 (premature), size 1 (newborn)
   e. Four extra batteries
   f. Two extra bulbs
6. Infant plastic airway (optional)
7. K-Y lubricating jelly
8. Benzoin
9. Adhesive tape
10. Scissors
11. Safety pins (for attachments)
12. Drugs
   a. Bicarbonate
   b. Insulin
   c. Epinephrine diluted to 1:10,000
   d. Narcan, Nalline
   e. Volume expanders
   f. Calcium gluconate 10%
   g. Glucose 10%

Resuscitative equipment in the delivery room must be sterilized after use on one infant and before use on another. In the high-risk nursery the need for resuscitation may occur at any time. Therefore, every infant should have his own bag and mask, available at the bedside. This equipment must be sterilized before use on another infant.

Equipment reliability must be maintained before an emergency arises. Inspect all equipment—bag and mask, laryngoscope, suction machines—for distorted or otherwise damaged or nonfunctioning parts before a delivery or assembly at the infant's bedside. A systematic check of the emergency cart and equipment should be a routine responsibility of each shift.

Initial Resuscitative Management

Initial resuscitative management of the infant is extremely important. The infant should be kept in a head-down position prior to the first gasp to avoid aspiration of the oropharyngeal secretions. The oropharynx and nasopharynx must be suctioned immediately. After the first few breaths, the infant is kept in a flat position under a radiant heat source and dried quickly to maintain skin temperature at about 36.5C. Drying is also a good

Table 25–1. Guidelines for Resuscitation of the Neonate

Apgar score	Heart rate	Arterial blood pH*	Appearance	Resuscitative measures
9 or 10	>100	7.30–7.40 (normal)	Regular respirations; flexed extremities; cries in response to flicking of soles of feet; may be dusky or show acrocyanosis	Gently suction airway; place under radiant heat source and dry immediately.
7 or 8	60–100	7.20–7.29 (slight acidosis)	Limp, cyanotic, or dusky and dyspneic; respirations may be shallow, irregular, or gasping; heart rate is normal; fair response to flicking of sole	Dry and place under warmers; give oxygen near face.
5 or 6	60–100	7.10–7.19 (moderate acidosis)	Same as for Apgar 7 or 8	Dry and place under warmers; clear airway and stimulate through drying process; if still not improved, place in "sniff" position, insert pharyngeal airway, and begin ventilation (100% O_2) with bag and mask, using pressure of 30 cm H_2O at rate of 30 per min. If difficulty persists, reevaluate maternal history of drug administration, especially if heart rate responds to ventilation but there is no spontaneous respiration. If tracheal aspiration reveals blood or meconium, directly visualize with laryngoscope and suction as needed before administering positive pressure.
3 or 4	<60	7.00–7.09 (marked acidosis)	Blue and limp, little or no respiratory effort	For Apgar 0 to 4: Dry under warmer; clear airway; consider immediate intubation. Ventilate after direct visualization with laryngoscope and appropriate suctioning. If heart rate remains low (0–40), immediately institute external cardiac massage. Correct hypotension. Obtain blood gas values (pH, P_{CO_2}, P_{O_2}) and BP.
0 to 2	<60	<7.00 (severe acidosis)	Same as for Apgar 3 or 4	

*Correlations of Apgar score and arterial blood pH adapted from Saling, E. 1972. Technical and theoretical problems in electronic monitoring of the human fetal heart. *Int. J. Gynecol. Obstet.* 10:211, and from Korones, S. 1976. *High-risk newborn infants: the basis for intensive nursing care.* 2nd ed. St. Louis: The C. V. Mosby Co.

stimulation to breathing. Heat loss through evaporation is tremendous during the first few minutes of life. The temperature of a 1500 gm baby wet in a 16C (62F) delivery room drops 1C every three minutes. Hypothermia increases oxygen consumption and in an asphyxiated infant increases the hypoxic insult and may lead to severe acidosis and development of respiratory distress.

Appraisal of the infant's need for resuscitation begins at the time of birth. The time of the first gasp, first cry, and onset of sustained respirations should be noted in order of occurrence. The Apgar score (p. 504) is important in determining the severity of neonatal depression and the immediate course of action that is necessary (Table 25-1).

Establish Airway

A patent airway is established by clearing the nasal and oral passages of fluid that may obstruct the airway. Suction is always performed before resuscitation so that mucus, blood, meconium, or formula is not aspirated into the lungs. If the infant is flaccid, the tongue may be lying against the posterior pharyngeal wall, thereby obstructing the airway. An infant pharyngeal airway, properly inserted in the oral cavity over the tongue, will correct this obstruction (usually optional for the neonate).

Establish Respirations

Begin with the simplest form of resuscitative measures and, if unsuccessful, proceed to more complicated methods.

1. Simple stimulation is provided by a slap on the soles of the feet.

2. If respirations have not been initiated or are inadequate (gasping or occasional respirations), the lungs must be inflated with positive pressure. Position mask securely on face (over nose and mouth; avoid covering eyes) with head in "sniffing" or neutral position (Figure 25-1). Hyperextension of the infant's neck will obstruct the trachea. Make an airtight connection between the infant's face and the mask (thus allowing the bag to inflate). Inflate the lungs rhythmically by squeezing the bag. (You should be familiar with the type of resuscitation bag your institution uses.

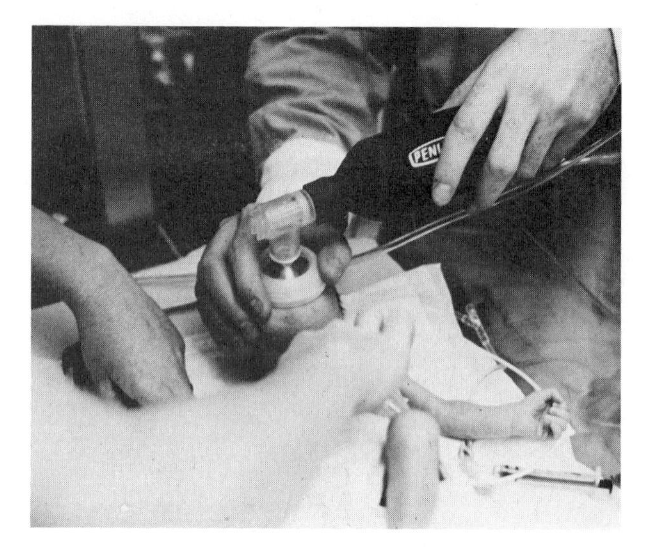

Figure 25-1. Rescusitation of infant with bag and mask. Note that the mask covers the nose and mouth and the head is in a neutral position.

An anesthesia bag will deliver 100% O_2 with adequate liter flow, whereas an Ambu or Hope bag will delivery only about 40% unless it has been adapted; in a crisis situation it is certainly preferable to deliver 100% O_2.) Observe the rise and fall of the chest for proper ventilation. Coordinate manual resuscitation with any voluntary efforts. The rate of ventilation should be between 30 and 50 per minute. Pressure should be less than 30 mm Hg. If ventilation is adequate, the chest moves with each inspiration, bilateral breath sounds are audible, and there is pinking of the lips and mucous membranes. If heart rate and color fail to respond, consider poor placement of the endotrachial tube, pneumothorax, diaphragmatic hernia, or hypoplastic lungs (Potter's syndrome). Control distention of the stomach by inserting a nasogastric tube for decompression.

3. Intubation (Figure 25-2, Procedure 25-1) is rarely needed, because most infants can be resuscitated by bag and mask.

Maintain Circulation

Once breathing has been established, the heart rate should increase to over 100 beats per minute. If the heart rate is less than 60 beats per minute, begin external cardiac massage:

1. Position infant properly on a firm surface.

Procedure 25–1. Tracheal Intubation

Objective	Nursing action	Rationale
Facilitate atraumatic insertion of endotracheal tube in support of adequate tissue oxygenation	Gather necessary equipment, ensuring that all possible variations are available: 1. Laryngoscope handle with extra batteries and bulbs.	Intubation is usually performed as an emergency measure. It is potentially hazardous to the patient. If confused or prolonged, the iatrogenic effects include local orotracheal tissue damage and/or generalized hypoxia. Necessary equipment is generally available on unit emergency cart.
	2. Detachable blades of curved and straight variety—infant and small child lengths.	Curved blades are used when unusual tongue and jaw formations make straight blades inadequate. Smallest internal diameter endotracheal tube (2.5 mm) is used in infants, with sizes increasing according to patient's weight and length.
	3. Variety of uncuffed endotracheal tubes. 4. Adaptors for oxygen hookup between endotracheal tube and ventilator or resuscitation bag. 5. Infant and pediatric masks and resuscitation bags. 6. Oxygen tubing and flow meter with wall outlet adapter. 7. Suction equipment (Procedure 25–2).	In pediatrics, uncuffed tubes can provide adequate seal.

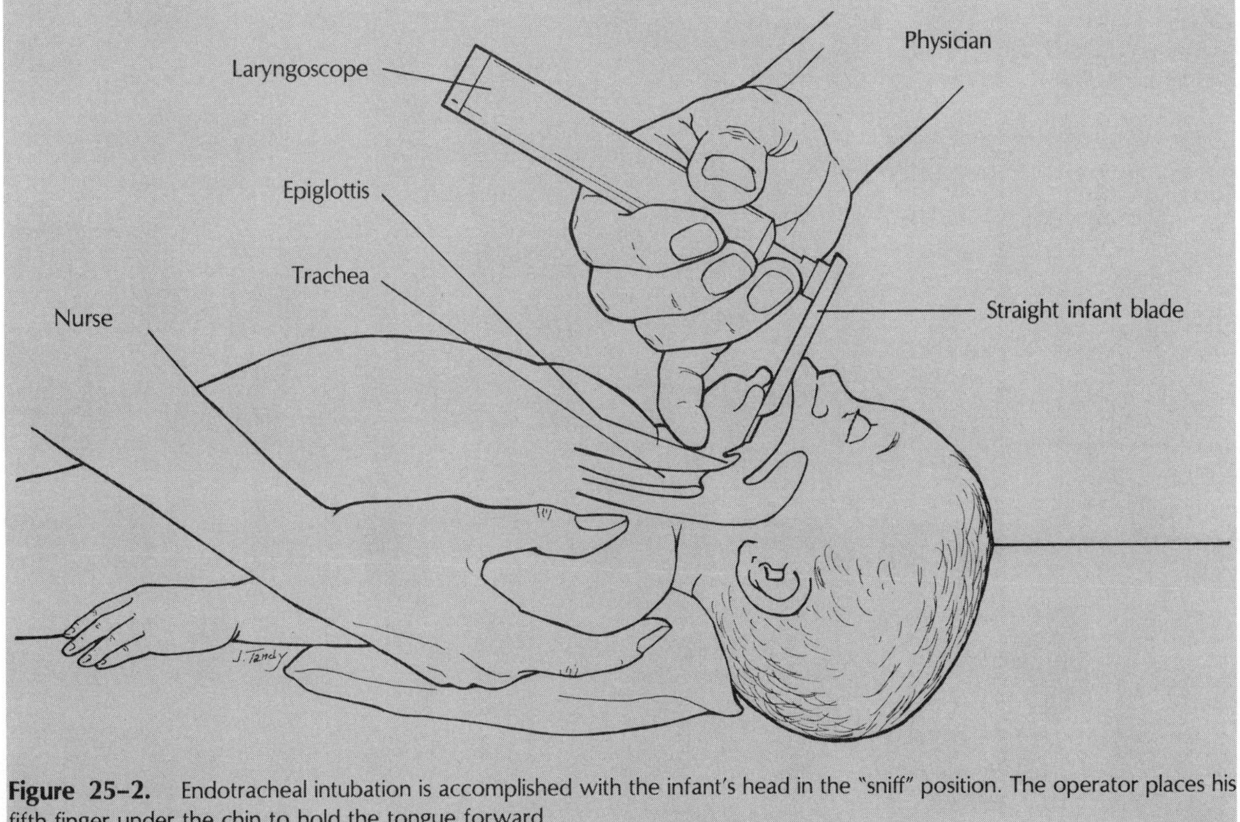

Figure 25–2. Endotracheal intubation is accomplished with the infant's head in the "sniff" position. The operator places his fifth finger under the chin to hold the tongue forward.

Procedure 25-1. Cont'd

Objective	Nursing action	Rationale
	Immediately set up oxygen supply system and suction equipment. Suction and preoxygenate patient by mask and bag as directed by physician.	Infant or child should be as well oxygenated as possible before intubation begins to delay onset of hypoxemia. Oropharyngeal suctioning prior to intubation can facilitate visualization of epiglottis.
	Position and immobilize patient as directed by physician during laryngoscopy and tube insertion (Figure 25-2). In the event of an unsuccessful intubation attempt, reoxygenate patient prior to next attempt.	Most frequently used position is supine with very slight extension of head. Physician stands at head of patient, nurse at side or foot.
	After physician has determined appropriate placement of tube (usually by portable x-ray), secure tube in that position by: 1. Applying tincture of benzoin to clean and dry upper lip and cheeks of the child. Allow it to dry. 2. Applying overlapping split 1-in. adhesive tape around tube and onto lips and cheeks (Figure 25-3).	Tube is inserted to a point just above the carina, which ensures effective ventilation of both lungs. With poor handling techniques, it is possible to dislodge tube, causing intubation of mainstem bronchus (usually on the right) with no ventilation of other lung or causing complete extubation. Taping tube minimizes possibility of dislodgement. Some physicians also suture tube to tape.

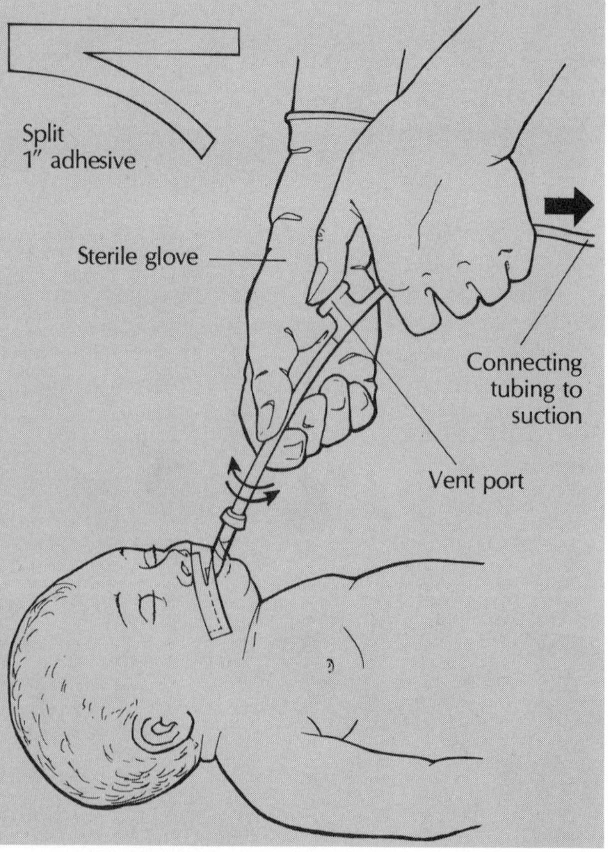

Figure 25-3.

Procedure 25-1. Cont'd

Objective	Nursing action	Rationale
	Measure length of tube from oral exit point to its connection point every 4 hr.	Frequent monitoring of tube length and respiratory status are measurable criteria for evaluation of tube placement.
	Assess bilateral breath sounds and chest excursion symmetry for equality every hour.	

Precautions: Only skilled practitioners should attempt to intubate patient in emergency situation. Intubation of unanesthetized children is usually carried out only in profoundly obtunded patient. Insertion and suctioning of endotracheal tubes call for use of sterile technique to minimize pulmonary infection. Assessment for signs and symptoms of tube obstruction and/or pneumothorax (especially with mechanical ventilation) should be of utmost priority for nurse caring for intubated patient.

2. Utilize two fingers (Figure 25-4).
3. Depress the midsternum at a rate of 80-100 beats/min.
4. Use a 3:1 ratio of heartbeat to assisted ventilation.

Drug Therapy

Drugs are not usually needed in the delivery room, except for shock, cardiac arrest, or narcosis. Oxygen, because of its effective use in ventilation, is the drug most often used.

Drugs that should be available in the delivery room include Narcan (used as a narcotic antagonist), whole blood (salt-poor albumin or plasmanate used for volume expansion), 10% dextrose in water (used for IV solution to prevent or treat hypoglycemia), sodium bicarbonate (used only for severe metabolic acidosis; not used routinely in the newborn), calcium gluconate (used for severe bradycardia or arrythmia despite adequate ventilation; used for severe hypocalcemia or hyperkalemia), atropine (used for severe bradycardia), and epinephrine (used after all else has failed—cardiac arrest).

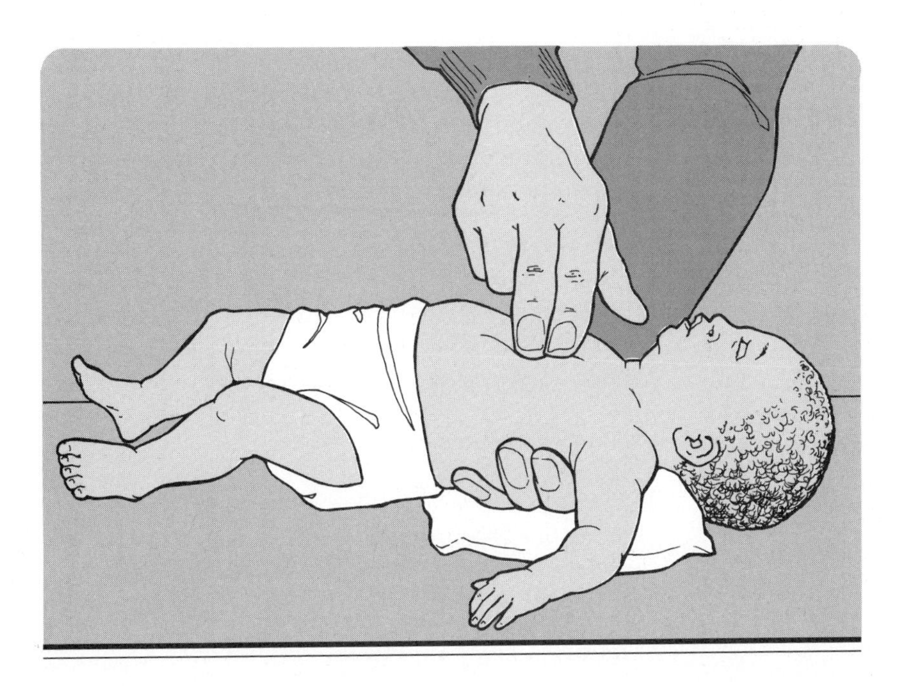

Figure 25-4. External cardiac massage. The midsternum is compressed with two fingertips at a rate of 80-100 beats/min.

RESPIRATORY DISTRESS

One of the prime aberrations to which the neonate is a victim is respiratory distress—an inappropriate respiratory adaptation to extrauterine life. The nursing care of a neonate with respiratory distress involves understanding of the normal pulmonary and circulatory physiology (Chapter 23), the pathophysiology of the disease process, clinical manifestations, and supportive and corrective therapies. Only with this knowledge can the nurse make appropriate observations concerning responses to therapy and development of complications. Unlike the verbalizing adult patient, the neonate communicates his needs only by his behavior. The neonatal nurse, through objective observations and evaluations, interprets this behavior into information about the individual infant's condition. Only with basic knowledge can the observations be recognized as meaningful interpretations of the neonate's condition.

Ideopathic Respiratory Distress Syndrome (Hyaline Membrane Disease)

The *respiratory distress syndrome* (RDS), also referred to as *hyaline membrane disease* (HMD), is a complex disease affecting primarily premature infants and accounts for 12,000–25,000 deaths per year in the United States alone. The factors precipitating the pathophysiologic changes of RDS have not been determined, but there are two main factors associated with the development of RDS:

1. *Prematurity.* All preterm infants, whether appropriate for gestational age (AGA), small for gestational age (SGA), or large for gestational age (LGA), and especially infants of diabetic mothers, are at risk for RDS. The maternal and fetal factors resulting in premature labor and delivery, complications of pregnancy, cesarean section (indications for cesarean section rather than the type of delivery), and familial tendency are all associated with RDS.

2. *Asphyxia.* Asphyxia, with a corresponding decrease in pulmonary blood flow, may interfere with surfactant production.

Pathophysiology

At birth, the neonate synthesizes surfactant at an increased rate to adjust to an air-breathing existence. Development of RDS by the preterm infant indicates a failure to synthesize lecithin at the rate required to maintain alveolar stability. Alveolar instability upon expiration with increasing atelectasis causes hypoxia and acidosis, which inhibit the surfactant system and cause pulmonary vasoconstriction. Thus the central pathophysiologic defect, lung instability due to this abnormality in the surfactant system, precipitates the biochemical aberrations of hypoxemia (decreased PO_2), hypercarbia (increased PCO_2), and acidemia (decreased pH), which further increases pulmonary vasoconstriction and hypoperfusion. The cycle of events of RDS leading to eventual respiratory failure are diagrammed in Figure 25–5 (Gluck and Kulovich, 1973).

Because of these pathophysiologic conditions, the neonate must expend increasing amounts of energy to reopen the collapsed alveoli with every breath, so that each breath becomes as difficult as the first. The progressive expiratory atelectasis upsets the physiologic homeostasis of the pulmonary and cardiovascular systems and prevents adequate gaseous exchange. There is a decrease in lung compliance and resultant stiff lungs, which account for the difficulty of inflation, labored respirations, and the increased work of breathing.

Adequate gaseous exchange dependent on diffusion and ventilation-perfusion ratio is upset with RDS. Hypoxia, the most critical determinant of survival, produces physiologic complications and consequences that increase hypoxia and decrease pulmonary perfusions:

1. Hypoxia causes vasoconstriction of the pulmonary vasculature, which increases pulmonary vascular resistance and further reduces pulmonary blood flow. Increased pulmonary vascular resistance may precipitate a reversal to fetal circulation as the ductus opens and blood flow is shunted around the lungs.

2. Hypoxia causes impairment or absence of metabolic response to cold, reversion to anaerobic metabolism, and lactate accumulation (acidosis).

Along with hypoxia, other biochemical aberrations accompany RDS:

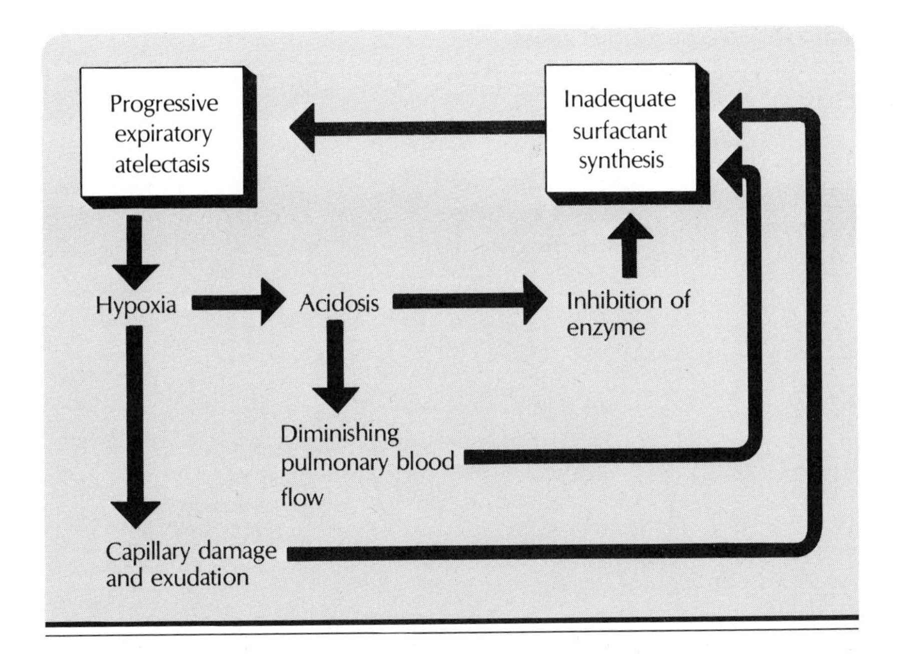

Figure 25-5. Cycle of events of RDS leading to eventual respiratory failure. (From Gluck, L. and Kulovich, M. V. 1973. Fetal lung development. 1973. *Pediatr. Clin. North Am.* 20:375.)

1. Respiratory acidosis (increased P_{CO_2}, decreased pH) is the result of alveolar hypoventilation. Carbon dioxide retention and resultant respiratory acidosis are the measure of ventilatory inadequacy, so that persistently rising P_{CO_2} and decrease in pH are poor prognostic signs of pulmonary function and adequacy.

2. Metabolic acidosis (decreased pH, decreased CO_2 tension) may be the result of impaired delivery of oxygen at the cellular level. Because of the lack of oxygen, the neonate begins an anaerobic pathway of metabolism, with an increase in lactate levels and a resultant base deficit. As the lactate levels increases, the pH becomes acidotic (decreased pH), and the buffer base decreases in an attempt to compensate and maintain acid-base homeostasis.

Clinical Manifestations

Myriad clinical manifestations are the result of the pathophysiology of the disease process and the efforts to compensate and maintain homeostasis. Clinical symptomatology for the neonate is often nonspecific for one particular disease entity, involves many systems, may be subjective, and is nonverbal. Table 25-2 provides a review of clinical findings associated with respiratory distress.

The classic radiologic picture of RDS is diffuse reticulogranular density (bilaterally), with the air-filled tracheobronchial tube outlined by the opaque lungs (air-bronchogram). Opacification of the lung fields may be due to massive atelectasis, diffuse alveolar infiltrate, or pulmonary edema. The progression of radiologic findings parallels the pattern of resolution (four to seven days in uncomplicated, mild-moderate RDS) and the time of surfactant reappearance.

The gross pathologic picture at autopsy reveals lungs that are dark red-purple, airless, and liverlike in consistency. There is widespread atelectasis, and the lungs are difficult to inflate. The presence of hyaline membranes in overdistended terminal bronchioles and alveoli are representative of destruction and damage to the basement membrane of the alveolar cells.

Interventions

The primary goal of management prenatally is the prevention of prematurity through aggressive treatment of premature labor and administration of glucocorticoids to enhance fetal lung development (see p. 562). Postnatally, supportive medical management consists of ventilatory therapy, correction of acid-base imbalance, environmental temperature regulation, adequate nutrition, and

Table 25–2. Clinical Findings Associated with Respiratory Distress

Clinical picture	Significance
SKIN	
Color	
Pallor or mottling	Represents poor peripheral circulation due to systemic hypotension and vasoconstriction and pooling of independent areas (usually in conjunction with severe hypoxia).
Cyanosis (bluish tint)	Depends on hemoglobin concentration, peripheral circulation, intensity and quality of viewing light, and acuity of observer's color vision; frankly visible in advanced hypoxia yet may be unobservable, because a large decrease in Pa_{O_2} may be tolerated without signs of cyanosis (see Figure 23–1).
Jaundice (yellow discoloration of skin and mucous membranes due to presence of unconjugated (indirect) bilirubin	Metabolic aberrations (acidosis, hypercarbia, asphyxia) of respiratory distress predispose to dissociation of bilirubin from albumin-binding sites and deposition in the skin and central nervous system.
Edema (presents as slick, shiny skin)	Characteristic of preterm infant because of low total protein concentration with decrease in colloidal osmotic pressure and transudation of fluid; edema of hands and feet frequently seen within first 24 hours and resolved by 5th day in infant with severe RDS.
RESPIRATORY SYSTEM	
Tachypnea (normal respiratory rate 40-60/min; elevated respiratory rate 60+/min)	Increased respiratory rate is most frequent and easily detectable sign of respiratory distress after birth; a compensatory mechanism that attempts to increase respiratory dead space to maintain alveolar ventilation and gaseous exchange in the face of an increase in mechanical resistance. As a decompensatory mechanism it increases work load and energy output (by increasing respiratory rate), which causes increased metabolic demand for oxygen and thus increase in alveolar ventilation (of already over-stressed system). During shallow, rapid respirations, there is increase in dead space ventilation, thus decreasing alveolar ventilation.
Apnea (episode of nonbreathing of more than 25 sec in duration; periodic breathing, a common "normal" occurrence in preterm infants, is defined as apnea of 5–10 sec alternating with 10–15 sec periods of ventilation)	Poor prognostic sign; indicative of cardiorespiratory disease, central nervous system disease, and immaturity; physiologic alterations include decreased oxygen saturation, respiratory acidosis, and bradycardia.
Chest	Inspection of thoracic cage and measurement of anteroposterior diameter of chest may reveal decreased thoracic gas volume.

Table 25–2. Cont'd

Clinical picture	Significance
Labored respirations (Silverman-Andersen chart — Figure 25-6 — indicates severity of retractions, grunting, and flaring, which are signs of labored respirations)	Indicative of marked increase in work of breathing.
Retractions (inward pulling of soft parts of chest cage — suprasternal, substernal, intercostal, subcostal — at inspiration)	Reflect significant increase in negative intrathoracic pressure necessary to inflate stiff, noncompliant lung; infants attempt to increase lung compliance by using accessory muscles; markedly decreases lung expansion; seesaw respirations are seen when chest flattens with inspiration and abdomen bulges; retractions increase work and O_2 need of breathing, so that assisted ventilation may be necessary due to exhaustion.
Flaring nares (inspiratory dilatation of nostrils)	Compensatory mechanism that attempts to lessen resistance of narrow nasal passage.
Expiratory grunt (Valsalva's maneuver in which infant exhales against closed glottis, thus producing audible moan)	Produces increase in transpulmonary pressure, which decreases or prevents atelectasis, thus improving oxygenation and alveolar ventilation; intubation should not be attempted unless infant's condition is rapidly deteriorating, because it prevents this maneuver and allows alveoli to collapse.
Rhythmic movement of body with labored respirations (chin tug, head bobbing, retractions of anal area)	Result of utilization of abdominal and other respiratory accessory muscles during prolonged forced respirations.
Auscultation of chest reveals decreased air exchange with harsh breath sounds and fine inspiratory rales, posterior lung base	Decrease in breath sounds and distant quality may indicate air or fluid occupying chest.
CARDIOVASCULAR SYSTEM	
Continuous systolic murmur may be audible	Patent ductus arteriosus is common occurrence with hypoxia, pulmonary vasoconstriction, right-to-left shunting, and congestive heart failure.
Heart rate usually within normal limits (fixed heart rate may occur with a rate of 110–120/min)	Fixed heart rate indicates decrease in vagal control.
HYPOTHERMIA	Inadequate functioning of metabolic processes that require oxygen to produce necessary body heat.
MUSCLE TONE	
Flaccid, hypotonic, unresponsive to stimuli Hypertonia and/or seizure activity	May indicate deterioration in neonate's condition and possible central nervous system damage, due to hypoxia, acidemia, or hemorrhage.

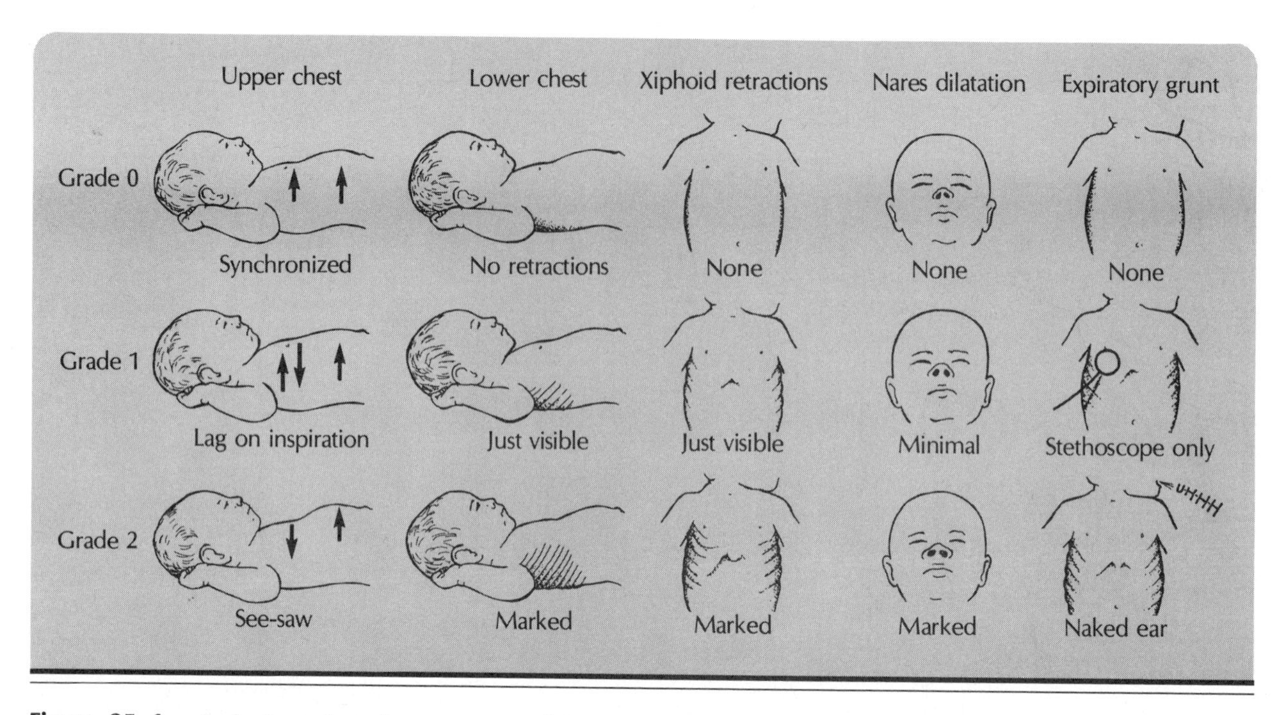

Figure 25–6. Evaluation of respiratory status utilizing the Silverman-Andersen index. (From Ross Laboratories, Nursing Inservice Aid No. 2, Columbus, Ohio; and Silverman, W. A., and Andersen, D. H. 1956. *Pediatrics.* 17:1. Copyright © American Academy of Pediatrics, 1956.)

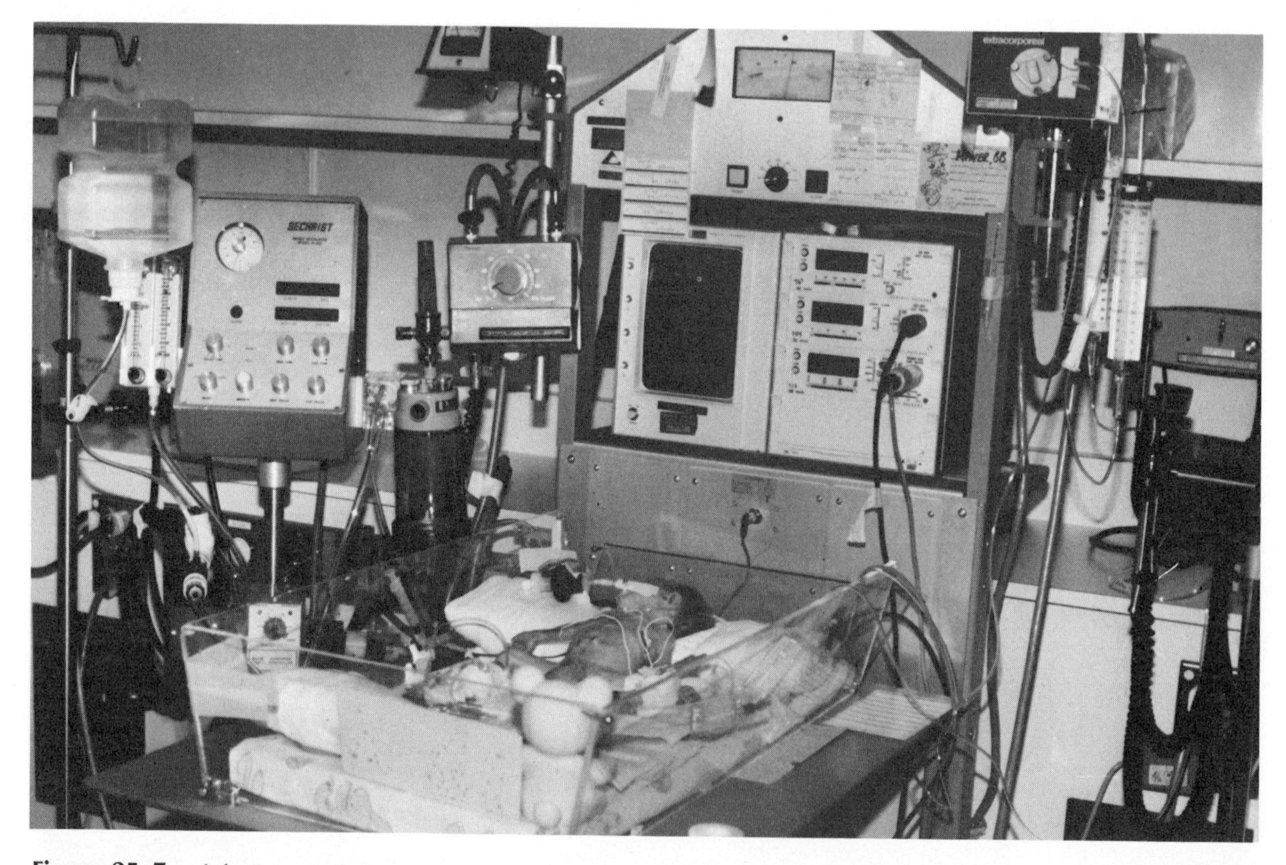

Figure 25–7. Infant on respirator.

protection from infection. Ventilatory therapy is directed toward prevention of hypoventilation and hypoxia. Mild cases of RDS may require only increased humidified oxygen concentrations. Use of continuous positive airway pressure (CPAP) or continuous negative pressure (CNP) methods may be required in moderately afflicted infants. Severe cases of RDS require mechanical ventilatory assistance (Table 25-3), with or without positive end-expiratory pressure (PEEP) (Figure 25-7).

The neonatal nurse can base the plan of care on the assessment of the clinical parameters, can implement therapeutic approaches to maintain physiologic homeostasis, and can provide supportive care to the neonate with respiratory distress syndrome (see the Nursing Care Plan on respiratory distress syndrome).

Table 25-3. Assisted Ventilatory Methods

Types	Functions and rationale	Nursing interventions
Transpulmonary pressure maintenance	Alveolar instability and collapse are prevented by continuous application of transpulmonary pressure.	Check infant for proper sealing at neck and attempt to prevent skin breakdown.
Continuous negative pressure (CNP)	Applied around chest wall while neonate is able to maintain spontaneous respirations; air leaks in system pull in cool room air and cool infant. Head compartment contains plastic neck sealing ring; place oxygen hood over head for deliverance of heated oxygen, easy access for suction, resuscitation, and feeding. Body compartment contains thorax and rest of body exposed to negative pressure. Utilization of CNP depends on deterioration in arterial blood gases and clinical condition. Disadvantages include cumbersome apparatus that makes provision of care logistically difficult; may also impede venous return to heart by negative pressure about chest wall. Advantages include decreased incidence of bronchopulmonary dysplasia; no increase in incidence of pneumothorax; no need for endotracheal intubation (unless positive ventilation is also used).	Maintain proper oxygen concentration by adequately sealing neck compartment and checking oxygenation concentration. Check neck seal, plastic sleeve parts, and end access part for air leaks. Check infant's skin temperature for indications of cold stress. Organize care to decrease number of accesses to body compartment in order to decrease cold stress and maintain constant pressure. Observe for alterations in cardiac functions with application or alteration of CNP: cardiac rate, rhythm, and regularity; alteration in blood pressure; peripheral circulation (color, capillary filling); metabolic acidosis.
Continuous positive airway pressure (CPAP)	Application of gas with greater than atmospheric pressure to airway during spontaneous respiratory effort. Infant must have spontaneous respirations, because apnea is absolute criterion for assisted	Maintain CPAP system through knowledge of elements of system and function of each.

Table 25-3. Cont'd

Types	Functions and rationale	Nursing interventions
	ventilation; persistently low PaO_2 (below 50 while breathing 80%-100% O_2) and repeated apneic episodes are criteria for CPAP application.	
Positive end-expiratory pressure (PEEP) (application of positive pressure to airway during expiratory phase of ventilatory assistance)	Utilization of CPAP or PEEP indicated by evaluation of arterial blood gases and clinical condition.	Record pressure being maintained by reading pressure gauge and filling anesthesia bag every 15 min and when necessary; monitor oxygen concentration as ordered; check patency of delivery system (orotracheal and nasotracheal tubes, nasal prongs, face mask, head hoods, etc.). Maintain water level in "pop-off" bottle at specified level. Evaluate response of infant to CPAP application or adjustment by arterial blood gases and by clinical condition (same as for evaluation under oxygen therapy). As a general rule, first decrease concentrations of oxygen, then slowly reduce pressure until neonate is able to maintain adequate arterial oxygenation with CPAP system at 2 cm.
Assisted ventilation ventilators		
Pressure-cycled respirators (operate by cessation of inspiratory phase when preset pressure has been reached) (see Figure 25-7)	Tidal volume and compliance of thorax and lungs is smaller in infants than adults; tidal volume is variable for newborn (15 ml) and preterm infant (5-12 ml).	Understand and maintain type of ventilatory support; check and record patency of system and respirator parameters (at least every hour), rate, volume, pressure, oxygen concentrations.
Volume-cycled respirators (deliver predetermined volume of air with each respiratory cycle; pressure is developed within system so that delivery of a known volume to a stiff lung increases pressure within system)	Pressures needed to inflate lungs of normal infant are 5-10 cm H_2O; conditions that decrease lung compliance, such as atelectasis, respiratory distress syndrome, and meconium aspiration syndrome, require higher pressures to acquire given tidal volume; with utilization of increased pressures, there is increased incidence of complications (see p. 806).	Maintain tight seal if face mask is used for artificial ventilation (as well as CPAP). Check around face mask for air leaks. Massage underlying skin every hour to prevent excoriation. Check integrity of skin and note any reddened areas, any blanched or cyanotic pressure points, and naso-oropharynx suctioning.
Time-cycled respirators (utilized by adjustment of inspiratory and expiratory phases of respiration)	Indications for use of mechanical ventilation are: 1. Apnea — absolute indication.	Keep bag breathing device and mask at bedside in the event of mechanical failure of ventilator or

Table 25-3. Cont'd

Types	Functions and rationale	Nursing interventions
	2. Hypoxia – evidenced by Pa_{O_2} less than 50 mm Hg when breathing 100% O_2 (on CPAP). 3. Hypercarbia – evidenced by Pa_{CO_2} greater than 65 mm Hg and respiratory acidosis (pH less than 7.20).	accidental or necessary extubation; if mechanical failure occurs, support neonate with bag and mask until corrections are made (an indispensable member of team is respiratory therapy department). For reintubation, keep proper size of tracheal tube at bedside. Evaluate response of infant to assisted ventilation or adjustments within system by arterial blood gas determinations and by clinical condition (same as for evaluations under oxygen therapy).

Transient Tachypnea of the Newborn (Wet Lung Syndrome)

Unexplained respiratory distress following an uneventful term pregnancy or a premature birth is detected in the transitional period. Tachypnea, mild cyanosis (some neonates require 30%–40% oxygen to remain pink), and increased perihilar density on x-ray (perhaps due to delayed reabsorption of amniotic fluid) are the major signs and symptoms. Unlike RDS, there are no expiratory grunts, rales, or biochemical aberrations. The respiratory distress is usually self-limiting and resolves with supportive care within 3–5 days. Wet lung x-ray results and course are similar to those for RDS. However, x-rays demonstrate hyperexpansion rather than miliary atelectasis. For treatment, see the Nursing Care Plan on respiratory distress syndrome.

Type II Respiratory Distress Syndrome (Aspiration Syndrome, Disseminated Atelectasis)

Some newborns, primarily AGA preterm and near-term infants, develop progressive respiratory distress that resembles classic RDS. Intrapartum or intrauterine asphyxia, with resultant biochemical changes and maternal oversedation, predispose to a mucus-clogged airway and inadequate removal of lung fluid by the lymphatics.

Clinical manifestations are expiratory grunting, flaring of the nares, cyanosis, and tachypnea, which occur during the first four days of life. (The expiratory grunting is an attempt to eject as much of the trapped alveolar air as possible; in true RDS the grunt is an attempt to retain as much air as possible in an effort to maintain alveolar expansion.) In six hours symptoms progressively improve.

Usually there is little or no difficulty at the onset of breathing. Cyanosis in room air may be noted but is usually cleared with relatively small amounts of ambient O_2 concentration. Unlike infants with RDS, whose oxygen requirements increase in the first 48 hours, Type II infants are easily oxygenated during the first 8 hours and the oxygen requirements may decrease during this time. The infants should be well by 24 hours, except for modest O_2 dependence (less than 30%). The duration of clinical course is approximately four days. Early acidosis, both respiratory and metabolic, is easily corrected. Ventilatory assistance is rarely needed, and most of these infants survive.

X-rays are characterized by generalized overexpansion of the lungs, which is identifiable principally by flattened contours of the diaphragm. Dense streaks radiate from the hilar region. Occasionally one or more dense patches indicate areas of collapse. X-rays are usually normal by 24 hours except in oxygen-dependent premature infants who develop chronic lung disease or in infants with patent ductus arteriosus who develop pulmonary edema. For nursing actions, see the Nursing Care Plan on respiratory distress syndrome.

NURSING CARE PLAN

Respiratory Distress Syndrome

Patient Data Base

History

Prematurity

Gestational history: recent episodes of fetal or intrapartum stress (that is, maternal hypotension, bleeding, maternal and resulting fetal oversedation)

Any event capable of severe fetal lung circulation compromise

Neonatal history: birth asphyxia resulting in acute hypoxia, exposure to extremes of hypothermia

Familial tendency

Physical examination

At birth or within 2 hours, rapid development initially of tachypnea (over 60 respirations/min), expiratory grunting (audible), or intercostal retractions

Followed by flaring of alae nasi on inspiration, cyanosis and pallor, signs of increased air hunger (apneic spells, hypotonus), rhythmic movement of body and labored respirations, chin tug

Auscultation: initially breath sounds may be normal; then there is decreased air exchange with harsh breath sounds and, upon deep inspiration, rales; later there is a low-pitched systolic murmur indicative of patent ductus in infants

Increasing oxygen concentration requirements to maintain adequate Po_2 levels

Laboratory evaluation

Arterial blood gases (indicating respiratory failure): Pao_2 less than 40 mm Hg while breathing 100% O_2 and Pco_2 above 80 mm Hg.

X-ray: Diffuse reticulogranular density bilaterally, with air-filled tracheobronchial tube outlined by opaque lungs on air bronchogram; miliary atelectasis/hypoexpansion is present; in severe cases, opacification of lung fields may be seen due to massive atelectasis, diffuse alveoli infiltrates, or pulmonary edema

Clinical course worsens first 24–48 hours after birth and persists for more than 24 hours

Nursing Priorities

1. Assure adequate oxygenation.
2. Provide for assisted ventilatory exchange.
3. Determine and correct acid-base imbalances.
4. Take supportive measures to maintain homeostasis—maintain neutral thermal environment, provide for adequate fluid and electrolyte and caloric requirements, prevent infection.
5. Provide for the emotional needs of the infant with respiratory distress without overstimulation and meet the needs of the family.
6. Observe possible complications of therapy and institute appropriate nursing interventions.

Problem	Nursing interventions and actions	Rationale
Oxygen concentration	Maintain on respiratory and cardiac monitors—note rates every 30–60 min and when necessary. Check and calibrate all monitoring and measuring devices every 8 hr. Calibrate oxygen devices to 21% and 100% O_2 concentrations. Control and monitor oxygen concentrations at least every hour.	Stable concentration of oxygen is necessary to maintain Pao_2 within normal limits (50–70 mm). Sudden increase or decrease in O_2 concentration may result in disproportionate increase or decrease in Pao_2 due to vasoconstriction in response to oxygen.
	Administer oxygen by: 1. Isolette or incubator (oxygen tubing is placed inside incubator).	Incubators may reach 70% or more concentration but fluctuates when portholes are opened for caregiving.

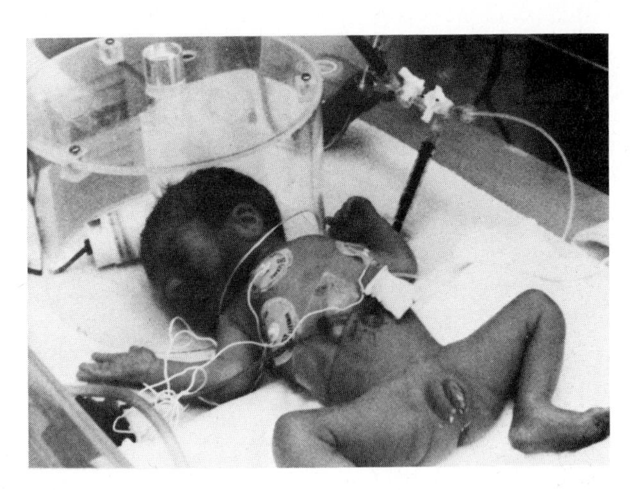

Figure 25-8. Infant in oxygen hood.

NURSING CARE PLAN Cont'd
Respiratory Distress Syndrome

Problem	Nursing interventions and actions	Rationale
	2. Oxygen hood – a small transparent head hood that contains an inlet and carbon dioxide outlet (Figure 25-8).	Used when high concentration of oxygen (over 35%) is needed or when observations indicate that infant is unable to tolerate oxygen fluctuations. Provides a constant oxygen environment.
	Maintain infant in stable oxygen concentration by increasing or decreasing by 5%-10% increments and then obtain arterial blood gases.	
Fluctuation in oxygen environment	Response of infant to therapy is evaluated by arterial blood gases and clinical assessment. Observe for: 1. Pink color, cyanosis (central or acrocyanosis), duskiness, pallor. 2. Respiratory effort (evaluation at rest), rate of respirations, patterns (apnea, periodic breathing), quality (easy, unlabored, abdominal, labored), auscultation (site of breath sounds – overall or part of lung fields – describe quality of breath sounds at 1-2 hr), accompanying sounds with respiratory effort (change from previous observations). 3. Activity – less active, flaccid, lethargic, unresponsive; increased activity, restless, irritable; inability to tolerate exertion, crying, sucking, or nursing care activity. 4. Circulatory response (evaluate at rest), rate, regularity and rhythm of heart rate, periods of bradycardia, alterations of blood pressure.	

NURSING CARE PLAN Cont'd

Respiratory Distress Syndrome

Problem	Nursing interventions and actions	Rationale
	Position infant with head slightly hyperextended. Observations of clinical condition are taken serially for comparison and for changes. Observations should be taken while infant is receiving oxygen and with any oxygen adjustment.	
	Return O_2 concentration to previous levels if there is deterioration in patient's condition. Repeat arterial blood gases (keep $Pa{O_2}$ 50-70 mm Hg). Gases should be done within 15-20 min after any change in ambient O_2 concentration or after inspiratory or expiratory pressure changes. Record and report clinical observations and action taken.	Any deterioration of clinical condition with oxygen adjustments (usually a decrease in ambient oxygen concentration) indicates inability of neonate to compensate for hypoxia.
Humidification of inspired oxygen	Provide humidified gas.	Oxygen is dry gas and therefore irritating to airways. Evaporative water losses from skin and lungs are also decreased in high humidity (50%-65%).
	Pay careful attention to infection control by cleaning and replacing nebulizers/humidifiers at least every 24 hr; use sterile tubing and replace every 24 hr; use sterile distilled water.	The warm, moist environment found in isolettes and with O_2 equipment promotes growth of microorganisms.
Warmed mist delivery	Provide heated mist (at the delivery site) 31-34C. Place a thermometer in the oxygen hood and monitor the temperature of the delivered gas. Observe infant for temperature instability and signs of increased oxygen consumption (need for increased O_2 concentration and metabolic acidosis).	Cold air/oxygenation blown in face of newborn is source of cold stress and is stimulus for increased consumption of oxygen and increased metabolic rate.
Monitoring of arterial blood gas values	Maintain stable environment prior to collection of arterial blood gas sample:	Values used to determine adequate oxygenation – normal $Pa{O_2}$ 50-70 mm Hg. Adequate ventilation – normal $Pa{CO_2}$ 30-45 mm. Acid-base balance – normal pH 7.35-7.45.
	1. Maintain constant O_2 concentration at least 5-10 min before sample.	Accurate arterial blood determinations are essential in management of any infant receiving oxygen, because presence or absence of cyanosis is unreliable.
	2. Avoid any disturbances of infant 10-15 min before gases are drawn. Do not suction; if suction is absolutely necessary, delay blood sample for 10-15 min. Maintain a warm temperature (pH should be	Crying or struggling may cause hyperventilation or breath holding and may increase shunting of blood.

NURSING CARE PLAN Cont'd

Respiratory Distress Syndrome

Problem	Nursing interventions and actions	Rationale
	measured at body temperature). Provide arterial blood gas set up (a 3 ml syringe with heparinized solution and a heparinized tuberculin syringe) for the physician and assist with obtained blood sample. After blood sample is taken, recheck flow through line to assure patency and prevent establishment of clot.	Utilization of temporal, radial, or brachial arteries takes skill and is time-consuming; therefore, most common technique for sampling is through umbilical artery catheter (Procedure 25-3, p. 809).
	Replace blood used to clear line.	Total blood volume of infant is small; blood removed to clear catheter must be returned to prevent hypovolemia, anemia.
Inadequate ventilation	Initial observation of respiratory effort, ventilatory adequacy – observation of chest wall movement, skin, mucous membranes, color; estimation of degree and equality of air entry by auscultation, arterial blood gases, and pH determination. Assess need for assisted ventilatory measures. Criteria for assisted ventilation: 1. Apnea. 2. Hypoxia (Pa_{O_2} 50 in Fi_{O_2} 100%) 3. Alert doctor if following criterion for assist is met: respiratory acidosis, pH 7.20. See Table 25-3 for specific nursing management.	Alveoli of normal infant remain stable during expiration due to presence of surfactant. Alveoli of infant with RDS lack surfactant and collapse with expiration. Grunting, a compensatory mechanism, increases transpulmonary pressure, overcomes high surface tension, forces and prevents atelectasis, and thus enables improved oxygenation and a rise in Pa_{O_2}. Application of CPAP or PEEP produces same stabilization force on alveoli as grunting does and produces same effect – improved oxygenation and rise in Pa_{O_2}.
Intubation (placement and patency of oral/nasal intubation tube)	Set up for endo/nasotracheal intubation and assist (see Procedure 25-1). Apply nasal prongs and set up with respiratory therapist. Set up CPAP or PEEP (see Table 25-3). Position infant in "sniffing" position. See Figure 25-2 for intubation. Attempts at intubation should not exceed 30 sec and should be terminated with evidence of hypoxia and bradycardia. Determine proper placement of tube by presence and quality of breath sounds. If breath sounds are better on one side, tube may be in main stem bronchus; slowly withdraw tube and auscultate chest for equal bilateral breath sounds.	Delivery of CPAP or PEEP can only be done by use of nasal prongs or intubation.
	Extubate if breath sounds are heard over stomach. Tube is properly placed if chest moves symmetrically, infant cannot cry, color and muscle tone improve with effective oxygenation. Improvement of heart rate and rhythm with effective oxygenation. Chest x-ray confirmation.	Tube is in esophagus.

NURSING CARE PLAN Cont'd

Respiratory Distress Syndrome

Problem	Nursing interventions and actions	Rationale
Production of and accumulation of secretion	Care of intubated neonate: 1. Observe type of secretions and ease of removal. 2. Because nasal passages are bypassed, provide humidity and moisture within system and better systemic hydration to avoid drying secretions and decreasing ciliary movement. 3. Change infant's position every 1-2 hr to maintain adequate ventilation, drain lung secretions, and promote skin integrity. 4. Secure and maintain with tape a properly positioned tube. 5. Observe nasal passage for position and deformity. Keep tube in neutral position without pulling on alae nasi. Observe for blanched area around nasal tube and reposition until blanching disappears. If oral tube is used, maintain neutral position within mouth. Observe color and integrity of gums; if blanched, reposition tube until blanching is relieved. 6. Auscultate breath sounds and observe arterial blood gas values and integrity of skin. 7. Suction to remove secretions (see Procedure 25-2). Check working order of each suction machine and pressure setting so that it will be in working order when needed.	Accumulation of secretions within tracheal tube decreases effective ventilation, increases PCO_2, and leads to clotted tube (airway). Maintenance of clear tube is especially important with pressure-cycled ventilators, because increased secretions decrease diameter of tube, increase resistance to gas flow, increase pressure within system (possibly to dangerous levels), and decrease tidal volume delivered.
	Tracheal tube suction should last no longer than 5-10 sec.	Apnea or bradycardia will occur if suction is longer than 15-20 sec.
	After each suction attempt, ventilate for a few breaths with pressures 25% above that routinely used for inspiration, to reinflate atelectatic areas. Observe and record: 1. Tolerance of neonate to suction procedure – color change, cyanosis or remains pink, cardiac changes, bradycardia, arrhythmia; evidence of spontaneous respiratory effort (or lack of) when off respirator for suction. 2. Time of suction. 3. Amount and type of secretions – thick, clear, bloody, green mucus. 4. Frequency of suction is determined by clinical assessment – amount and type of secretions in relation to frequency of suction. Observe for incidence of infection as noted by random culture and incidence of acquired	Hypoxia insult with drop in PaO_2 occurs during suction efforts. Suction, the application of negative pressure to the airway, decreases pulmonary compliance by 50% and tidal volume. Suction creates pulmonary atelectasis.

NURSING CARE PLAN Cont'd

Respiratory Distress Syndrome

Problem	Nursing interventions and actions	Rationale
	pulmonary infection.	
	Carry out percussion and postural drainage every 2 hr with frequent turning of patient.	Prevents stasis of secretions and promotes drainage.
Danger of extubation	Observe for symptoms of extubation (cyanosis, apnea, respiratory difficulty, bradycardia, no audible breath sounds). Whether accidental or symptomatic of a clogged tube, these conditions warrant *immediate* removal of ineffective tube and respiratory support with bag and mask until reintubation. Insert nasogastric tube (if not present) to decompress stomach.	
Weaning from assisted ventilation	Observe for signs of improvement in respiratory status and ability to have ventilatory support weaned and discontinued: 1. Evaluate blood gas determinations. 2. Observe toleration of lower O_2 concentrations and pressures. 3. Watch for evidence of spontaneous respirations—when ventilator is discontinued for suction; spontaneous respiratory effort against "set rate" of respirator; ability to assist ventilator by spontaneous respirations.	Criteria for weaning and ultimate discontinuance of ventilator: 1. Normal blood gas values—especially PaO_2, which is indicative of adequate oxygenation. 2. Decrease in ventilation pressures. 3. Decrease in O_2 concentrations. 4. Increased activity, muscle tone, and efforts at simultaneous respirations.
Maintenance of homeostasis Thermoregulation	See p. 748.	Increase in respiratory rate results in chemical thermogenesis (burning brown fat to maintain body temperature), which increases O_2 needs and insensible H_2O loss in already compromised infant.
Correction of acid-base imbalance Respiratory acidosis	Maintain adequate ventilation and excretion of returned CO_2 from the lungs by monitoring blood gases and regulating venitatory assistance mechanisms per physician's orders.	Correction of acidosis is essential to maintain homeostasis. Acidosis is powerful pulmonary vasoconstrictor, decreases pulmonary blood flow, and may upset surfactant synthesis. Acidosis dissociates bilirubin from albumin binding sites and predisposes to kernicterus at low bilirubin levels. Acidosis is central nervous system depressant that depresses respiratory center, which causes increase in CO_2 retention and hypoxia.
Metabolic acidosis	Treat with volume replacement and cautious administration of bicarbonate.	
Provision for adequate fluid, caloric, and electrolyte requirements	Maintain IV rate at prescribed level; record type and amount of fluid infused hourly. Use infusion pump. Observe vital signs for signs of too rapid infusion. Maintain normal urine output (1-3 ml/kg/hr). Maintain specific gravity of urine between 1.004 and 1.010. Take daily weights.	Fluids are provided to sick neonate by intravenous route and are calculated to replace sensible and insensible water losses as well as evaporative losses due to tachypnea. Overload of circulatory system by too much or too rapid administration of fluid causes pulmonary edema and cardiac

NURSING CARE PLAN Cont'd

Respiratory Distress Syndrome

Problem	Nursing interventions and actions	Rationale
	Manage route of IV administration. a. With umbilical catheter: Protect catheter from strain or tension (see Procedure 25-3). Restrain as necessary. Prevent dislodgement of catheter. Always keep catheter and stopcock on top of bed linens so they are easily visible. Observe for occlusion of vessels by clot and for vasospasm—discoloration of skin, discoloration of toes or feet (blanching or cyanosis). If discoloration occurs, wrap contralateral foot with warm cloth. Observe for signs of infection or sepsis: temperature instability, drainage, redness or foul odor from cord, lethargy, irritability, vomiting, poor feeding, hypotonia.	embarrassment that may be fatal. Greater nutritional fluid is required because of energy needed to cope with stress. Stressed infants are predisposed to hypoglycemia because of increased metabolic demands as well as reduced glycogen stores and decreased ability to convert fat and protein to glucose. Vasospasm in unwrapped foot will be relieved by treatment; discoloration will disappear and toes will be pink. If discoloration persists, clot may be occluding vessel—catheter must be removed, or loss of extremity is possible.
	b. Peripheral IV in scalp or extremity vein: Prepare equipment, insert IV in vein, and restrain infant (Procedure 25-4, p. 810). Vessel chosen is artery if it pulsates. Place peripheral IV in vein (which doesn't pulsate). Maintain proper placement of IV. Advance as soon as possible from intravenous to oral feedings. Gavage or nipple feedings are utilized, and IV is used as supplement (discontinued when oral intake is sufficient) (see Procedure 24-1).	Ability to aspirate blood and/or easily inject small amount of saline indicates patent IV. Infiltration is evaluated by area of edema and redness about site, inability to obtain blood on aspiration, or difficulty in injecting through IV line.
	Provide adequate caloric intake: amount of intake, type of formula, route of administration, and need for supplementation of intake by other routes. Take daily weight measurement. Blood pH remains normal (no metabolic acidosis). Measure urine output and specific gravity.	Calories are essential to prevent catabolism of body proteins and metabolic acidosis due to starvation or inadequate caloric intake.
	Observe for hypocalcemia. Observe for hypoglycemia: Dextrostix below 45 mg, urine screening. Observe for hyperglycemia: Dextrostix above 130 mg, urine screening, increased urine output (osmotic diuresis), sugar in urine with Dipstix and Clinitest. Treatment—glucose is highest priority (calcium is next). Usually 10% calcium gluconate is administered.	Hypocalcemia and hypoglycemia result from delayed or inadequate caloric intake and stress.
Prevention of infection	See section on sepsis nursing care, p. 832.	Decreased lung expansion predisposed to atelectasis and secondary superimposed infections.
Provision of stimulatory needs of infant	Plan care to allow for rest periods to avoid exhausting infant.	

NURSING CARE PLAN Cont'd

Respiratory Distress Syndrome

Problem	Nursing interventions and actions	Rationale
Support of family	Explain procedures to family. Facilitate parental participation in infant's care even when he is critically ill.	(See p. 766 for a discussion of parenting high-risk infants.)
Complications of respiratory therapy		
Retrolental fibroplasia	Maintain O_2 at prescribed levels, usually below 70-100 mm Hg PaO_2. Make arterial blood gas determinations 15-30 min after adjustment of settings. Monitor O_2 concentration every 4 hr minimum. If possible, periodically check fundi during O_2 therapy; definitely check at time of discharge. Perform frequent eye examination for at least 3 months.	Oxygen toxicity results in damage to retina.
Residual pulmonary disease	Observe for residual pulmonary disease (usually in recovery phase from initial disease): dependence on oxygen to overcome cyanosis and remain pink; low PaO_2 in room air; inability to tolerate exertion of care, sucking, or crying; and increase in cyanosis and respiratory distress.	Positive pressure ventilation and endotracheal intubation may result in additional respiratory distress.
	Obtain chest x-ray.	Confirms diagnosis.
Bronchopulmonary dysplasia	Prevent respiratory distress attack. Facilitate weight gain. Maintain minimal levels of ambient O_2 concentration. Organize nursing care to decrease disturbance, conserve energy, and prevent increased respiratory distress and O_2 requirements.	Positive pressure ventilation may result in pathologic condition of pulmonary epithelium.
	Practice caution when feeding neonate. Schedule frequent, small feedings.	Abdominal distention, which results in upward pressure on thoracic cavity, is prevented and thus respiratory embarrassment is prevented. Respiratory distress decreases after feeding.
	Naso-orogastric tube feeding may be utilized for respiratory distress of tachypnea associated with sucking; handle gently and maintain constant ambient oxygen concentrations.	Prevents aspiration and reduces energy output of feedings.
	Position properly to maintain open airway and to facilitate maximal chest expansion: elevate head of bed; a shoulder roll may prevent the neck from flexing on the chest and obstructing the trachea; turn head to either side; change and rotate position every 1-2 hr.	Gravitational downward position of diaphragm and abdominal contents allows for maximal lung expansion.
Interstitial pulmonary emphysema	Frequently auscultate breath sounds (presence and quality) to locate emphysema. Assemble appropriate equipment for air	Knowledge of location of pulmonary emphysema enables prediction and observation for impending catastrophe.

NURSING CARE PLAN Cont'd

Respiratory Distress Syndrome

Problem	Nursing interventions and actions	Rationale
	evacuation – needle aspiration syringe, needle, and stopcock – and for thoracotomy – tray, chest drainage, and suction apparatus. Assist with thoracentesis procedure and insertion of chest tubes.	
Pneumothorax	Be alert for symptoms: 1. Sudden, unexplained deterioration in clinical condition. 2. Cyanosis. 3. Cardiac abnormalities – bradycardia, arrhythmia, or decrease in height of ECG tracing. 4. Decrease in BP. 5. Mottling of skin and shocklike appearance. 6. Diminished or absent breath sounds on affected side. 7. Shift in apical cardiac sound. 8. Bulging of chest wall on affected side. 9. Hyperresponse of affected lung on percussion.	
	Obtain chest x-ray films.	Confirm diagnosis of pneumothorax.
	Assist resuscitative measures: 1. 100% O_2 by plastic oxygen hood. 2. Needle aspiration of pleural cavity. 3. Utilization of water-seal drainage. Assist with insertion of chest tubes.	Aids in resolution of air in pleural space and prevents further accumulation. Thoracentesis and chest tube insertion removes trapped air and fluid, returns negative pressure to thoracic cavity, removes tension, and facilitates expansion.
	Observe for oscillation of fluid level in chest tubes. Cessation of oscillation occurs if: 1. Lung has reexpanded. 2. Blood or fibrin clot occludes tube (before lung has reexpanded).	Water-seal drainage provides for escape of air and fluid into drainage bottle. Water acts as seal and keeps air from being drawn back into chest. Oscillation of water level in tubing shows that there is effective communication between pleural cavity and drainage bottle.
	Obtain serial x-rays.	Ascertains degree of lung involvement; visualizes effect of treatment.
	Observe for development of complications: 1. Hemorrhage – hourly observation of chest tube drainage for color, amount, and consistency. Observe for rapid increase in amount of drainage. Total and record amount of chest tube drainage every 8 hr. 2. Pneumothorax due to air leak into pleural cavity. Notify medical staff immediately of development of complication.	
Other pulmonary complications: pneumomediastinum, pneumopericardium, and pneumoperitoneum	Observe for signs of air dissection into the neck (pneumomediastinum); crepitus – a crackling feeling and noise of the skin when light pressure is applied; appearance of	Collection of air in the mediastinum either anterior to the heart or laterally compresses the mediastinal pleurae. Air may dissect into soft tissue of the neck.

NURSING CARE PLAN Cont'd

Respiratory Distress Syndrome

Problem	Nursing interventions and actions	Rationale
	fullness to the neck (looks like a bullfrog).	
	Observe for symptoms of compromised cardiac function.	Massive collection of air around the heart results in compression of vena cava, tachypnea, and cyanosis.
	Observe for abdominal distention and tenderness.	Collection of air in peritoneal cavity must be differentiated from perforated viscus.
Cardiac complication – patent ductus arteriosus	Observe for symptoms of alteration in cardiac output: alteration in blood pressure, peripheral circulation (color and capillary filling), metabolic acidosis.	Alteration in cardiac output is possible, because application of positive pressure may impede venous return to heart.
	Observe for clinical findings of patent ductus arteriosus: continuous murmur (most often audible in small prematures); bounding peripheral pulses; signs of congestive heart failure – tachypnea, tachycardia, cyanosis, edema (weight gain), intolerance of exertion, cardiomegaly. See Chapter 26 for care of infant with cardiac anomaly.	Failure of ductus arteriosus to close after birth, with resultant left-to-right shunting (if ductus is large enough) and hemodynamic changes, leads to congestive heart failure. Persistence of ductus may occur in preterm infants (due to musculature), in preterm infants with RDS (associated with hypoxemia), and as a complication of positive pressure therapy (period of improvement followed by deterioration).

Nursing Care Evaluation

Oxygen therapy is discontinued and no apnea, cyanosis, or other complications are evident.

Infant is afebrile and vital signs are stable.

Infant is gaining weight or stabilized at desired discharge weight and tolerating food and fluids.

Parent-infant bonding is appropriate.

Parents understand need for continued medical supervision.

Parents are aware of available parent groups for assistance after discharge.

Referral is completed to public health nurse and other community resources.

Meconium Aspiration Syndrome

The presence of meconium in amniotic fluid is a reflection of an asphyxial insult to the neonate. The physiologic response to asphyxia is relaxation of the anal sphincter and passage of meconium into the amniotic fluid. Meconium-stained neonates, the victims of intrauterine asphyxia, are often depressed at birth and require resuscitative efforts to establish adequate respiratory effort.

Clinical Manifestations

Clinical manifestations include: (a) fetal hypoxia in utero a few days or a few minutes prior to delivery, as indicated by a sudden increase in fetal activity followed by diminished activity and slowing of fetal heart or weak and irregular heartbeat; and (b) fetal distress signs present at delivery, including meconium staining of amniotic fluid in vertex position, pallor, cyanosis, apnea, and slow heartbeat.

The clinical course is as follows: Blood gases indicate varying degrees of mixed respiratory acidosis (shunting and alveolar hypoventilation); metabolic acidosis (due to cardiopulmonary shunting and hyperfusion); hypoxia (requiring 100% O_2 concentration and ventilatory assistance); and respiratory problems (usually subsiding in 48 hours, although they may persist for six to seven days).

Presence of meconium in the lungs produces a ball-valve action, so that alveoli rupture and pneumothorax is a common occurrence. The meconium also initiates a chemical pneumonitis in the lung, and secondary bacterial pneumonias are common. The chest x-ray reveals patchy densities and hyperinflation. These infants have massive biochemical aberrations: (a) extreme metabolic acidosis resulting from the cardiopulmonary shunting and hypoperfusion, (b) extreme respiratory acidosis due to shunting and alveolar hypoventilation, and (c) extreme hypoxia, even in 100% O_2 concentrations and with ventilatory assistance. The extreme hypoxia is also caused by the cardiopulmonary shunting.

Symptoms of respiratory distress are severe. Treatment includes pulmonary toilet (chest percussion, vibration, and postural drainage) to remove the debris, assisted ventilation, high ambient oxygen concentrations, steroids, and antibiotics. Alkali therapy may be necessary for severely ill neonates for several days. Mortality rates in term or postterm infants are very high, because they are so difficult to oxygenate.

Interventions

Recently a technique for preventing meconium aspiration has been utilized in several perinatal centers (Carson et al., 1976). This simple technique has significantly reduced the incidence and severity of this syndrome.

After the head of the infant is delivered and while the chest is still within the birth canal (so that the infant is unable to initiate respirations), the delivering physician passes a DeLee catheter into each nostril to the nasopharynx and suctions and then into the mouth to the oropharynx and suctions.

After the delivery is completed, the cords are visualized with a laryngoscope, and if meconium is present, direct suctioning of the trachea is performed (see Procedure 25-2). Failure to adequately suction on the perineum or before resuscitative efforts are begun pushes meconium into the airway and into the lungs.

Stimulation of the infant is avoided to minimize respiratory movements. Further resuscitative efforts follow the same principles mentioned earlier. Resuscitated neonates should be immediately transferred to the nursery for close observation and continuation of treatment. An umbilical arterial line may be used for direct monitoring of arterial blood pressure, blood sampling for pH and blood gases, and infusion of fluids, blood, or medications. Nursing interventions after a resuscitation should include temperature regulation at 37C, Dextrostix at 3–4 hours of age to observe for hypoglycemia, observation of intravenous fluids with calculation of necessary fluid and caloric requirements, and observation of renal output for fluid overload or damage due to anoxia. Hematocrit and blood pressure are determined to evaluate fluid requirements, possible hypotension, and need for volume expanders.

Complications of Respiratory Therapy

Oxygen is considered a drug whose dosage and duration of administration must be regulated to prevent complications and to provide maximum benefit—reduction of hypoxia, ischemia, and infarction of vital organs. The concentration of ambient oxygen administered to the neonate must be titrated according to oxygen tension within arterial blood. Oxygen is toxic to retinal blood vessels as a result of vasoconstriction, dilatation, hemorrhage, and detachment and also to lung tissue in prolonged hyperoxic exposure. Interventions for the following conditions are explained in the Nursing Care Plan on respiratory distress syndrome.

Retrolental Fibroplasia

Oxygen toxicity to the retinal vessels occurs in premature infants exposed to increased PaO_2 concentrations (over 70–100 mm Hg). Excess oxygen saturation produces vasoconstriction of retinal vessels, followed by vaso-obliteration and vasoproliferation of abnormal retinal vessels, and later produces retinal detachment and eventual blindness.

Procedure 25–2. Endotracheal Suctioning

Objective	Nursing action	Rationale
Minimize potential for pulmonary infection through cross-contamination	Assess respiratory status to determine necessity for suctioning.	Child should be suctioned only as often as necessary to maintain patent airways and adequate oxygenation.
	Gather all necessary equipment: catheters, suction machine, disposable sterile suction tubing, saline (no preservatives), sterile syringe/needle, and gloves (not powdered). Ensure that gloves, catheters, lubricants, and liquefying solutions are sterile. Maintain sterile technique throughout entire suctioning procedure.	In healthy individual, lower respiratory tract is free of pathogenic organisms.
	Discard catheter, glove, and lubricant after each procedure.	Once equipment is moistened and contaminated with body flora and mucus, it becomes a culture bed for noxious organism growth.
	Set wall suction for not more than 50 mm Hg.	Mucosal hemorrhages and tissue invagination occur more frequently when higher pressure is used.
Alleviate partial or total airway obstruction in support of cell oxygenation	Prior to suctioning, preoxygenate patient for at least 10 min with 100% O_2.	Suctioning physically removes oxygen from airways. In addition, it mechanically occludes airways and therefore diminishes potential for oxygenation. It usually stimulates coughing and increased work of breathing, thereby increasing tissue demand for oxygen. Presuction elevation of Pa_{O_2} mitigates intrasuction hypoxemia.
	Position and immobilize infant (see mummy restraint) according to desired suction site.	It is quite difficult to suction alert infant successfully without restraint. A full body restraint or an assistant should be employed to ensure effective, atraumatic suctioning in children. To suction right main bronchus, child's head should be turned to left. To suction left main bronchus, head should be turned to right with left shoulder slightly elevated.
	Using sterile technique, don sterile glove; hook up appropriate suction catheter; lubricate tip with single-use, water-soluble lubricating jelly; position catheter angle toward desired suction site.	"Whistle-tip" catheter should be used for respiratory tract suctioning, because it tends to be less traumatizing to tissues. Catheter size should be no more than ½ the size of lumen to be suctioned in order to minimize hypoxemia due to airway obstruction. Single-use, water-soluble lubricant should be used to ensure sterility and to prevent lipoid pneumonia. Sterile normal saline in a sterile specimen cup may be used if preferred. But prelubrication of catheter is essential to minimize tissue trauma with subsequent obstructive edema.
	If child is intubated:	
	1. Disconnect source of oxygenation from child.	Suction applied while entering airway increases removal of oxygen from airways

Procedure 25–2. Cont'd

Objective	Nursing action	Rationale
	2. Insert catheter without applied suction into tube the distance from tube opening to anatomic location of target bronchus (this can be predetermined by measuring distance externally prior to suctioning). 3. Apply suction by placing thumb of assistive hand over vent port or Y-connector (see Figure 25–3).	and increases potential for tissue invagination once catheter tip passes end of tube. Placing thumb over venting device closes negative pressure system, which allows atmospheric pressure to push secretions and debris into catheter, facilitating their removal.
	4. Slowly withdraw catheter in a pill-rolling rotation. 5. Clear catheter with sterile saline.	Rotating catheter in a slow, steady fashion maximizes catheter access to secretions while minimizing potential for tissue invagination.
	6. After each suction attempt, ventilate for a few breaths with pressures 25% above that routinely used for inspiration, to reinflate atelectatic areas. 7. Repeat procedure for opposite bronchus.	Hypoxia insult with a drop in Pa_{O_2} occurs during suction efforts. Suction, the application of negative pressure to the airway decreases by 50% the pulmonary compliance and tidal volume. Suction creates pulmonary atelectasis.
	8. If tenacious secretions are encountered, instill ½ ml of 5% sodium bicarbonate with syringe (needle-less) into tube prior to suctioning.	Instillation of sodium bicarbonate liquefies and loosens secretions by lowering surface tension of and alkalating respiratory secretions.
	If infant is not intubated: After having failed to get infant to cough voluntarily in effective manner, follow procedure for suctioning intubated infant with these exceptions:	Suctioning to clear airways should be employed only when infant is unable to clear his own airways effectively by use of cough reflex. It should be considered a last resort.
	1. Enter airway via nasopharynx, advancing catheter into trachea on inspiration. 2. Attempt to liquefy tenacious secretions by humidification via mist tent, face mask, or hand-held nebulizer.	Inspiration opens glottis and tends to entrain catheter along with inspired air. Achieving coordination with inspiration is often quite easy with pediatric patient, because he is frequently crying involuntarily during procedure. Instillation of liquefying agents directly into trachea in unintubated infant is not possible. Indirect means must be relied upon.
Minimize iatrogenic hypoxemia secondary to suctioning	Suction only when absolutely necessary.	Always assess need for suctioning. There should never be standing orders such as "Suction every hour."
	Limit each catheter insertion to no more than 10 sec. Reoxygenate infant with 100% O_2 between each insertion and at conclusion of procedure.	Limiting suction time and frequent reoxygenation counterbalance the mechanical obstruction of airway and removal of available oxygen.
	Remove catheter with suction applied as soon as infant begins to cough.	Holding catheter in airway while infant coughs can deprive infant of needed inspiratory volume at end of cough because of airway obstruction by catheter.
	During procedure, assess infant for signs of bradycardia.	Suctioning can cause vagal response in form of bradycardia, which, if unchecked, can lead to asystole.

Precautions: Never suction an infant with any type of bleeding disorder.

Procedure 25–3. Umbilical Catheterization
(Umbilical arterial catheter is used for monitoring arterial pressures, for obtaining arterial blood for blood gas studies, and for infusion in the absence of a venous line.)

Objective	Nursing action	Rationale
Assemble equipment	Obtain the following equipment:	
	1. IV solution and tubing.	
	2. Infusion pump.	Regulates infusion.
	3. Umbilical arterial catheter tray.	Contains equipment for insertion.
	4. Sterile stopcock.	
	5. Solution for skin preparation.	Removes bacteria that may be present.
	6. Sterile No. 4-Osille suture and umbilical tape.	Ties around umbilical stump.
	7. Sterile umbilical catheter – 3½–5.	Inserts in umbilical artery.
	8. Heparinized sterile saline in sterile syringe.	Used to flush tubing as necessary.
	9. Sterile gloves.	Maintain sterility.
	10. Nonallergic tape.	Tape is less irritating to skin.
Prepare infant	Place infant on restraining board or have another person hold infant's arms and legs.	Prevents sudden movement.
Prepare equipment	Attach tubing to solution and hang on IV standard. Remove all air from tubing and attach to infusion pump. Open umbilical catheter tray and add skin preparation solution, suture, cord ties. Prepare gloves for physician.	Prepares for infusion.
Monitor procedure	Physician drapes and preps patient and puts catheter in place.	Procedure is done only by physician.
	Syringe containing heparinized sterile saline is attached to catheter by stopcock. IV tubing is attached to stopcock. Catheter is secured by umbilical tape and suture. Secure catheter to infant with nonallergic tape. Set prescribed rate on infusion pump.	Catheter placement is checked by x-ray.
Assess infant	Observe the following: 1. Pulse. 2. Respiration. 3. Color of legs.	Evaluates infant's status.
	Notify physician immediately in case of: 1. Blanching. 2. Mottling. 3. Cyanosis. 4. Coolness of one or both legs.	Blood flow to extremities is disrupted.
Maintains patient records	Record the following: 1. IV – site, type of catheter, solution. 2. Infusion flow rate. 3. Time infusion was started. 4. Patient response.	Maintain patient's chart.

Procedure 25–4. Venipunctures

Objective	Nursing action	Rationale
Facilitate efficient completion of procedure	Gather necessary equipment: 1. Appropriate restraints. 2. IV tray containing assortment of syringes, needles, tourniquets, alcohol wipes, 2 × 2 in. gauze sponges, tapes, rubber bands, safety pins. 3. Specimen containers, such as blood culture tubes or serum collection tubes.	Regardless of whether venipuncture is transient specimen collection procedure or for purpose of establishing intravenous line, introduction of needle or catheter demands certain basic equipment. Selection from among equipment depends on site selection. Most commonly used sites are external jugular, femoral, or variety of peripheral veins, including scalp veins.
Facilitate atraumatic needle entry into selected vein	Ensure adequate supplemental lighting to illuminate puncture site.	Standard ceiling light is inadequate for visualization of underlying vessels.
1. Scalp venipuncture	Immobilize infant in mummy restraint.	Veins of scalp are very fragile; proper immobilization of head facilitates entry into vein.
	Place tourniquet or rubber band with small adhesive tag (for release) around forehead to distend scalp veins. Palpate desired vein.	Application of tourniquet facilitates distention of neonate's fragile and small scalp veins.
2. Peripheral venipuncture (hands or feet)	Restrain on armboards. Place tourniquet proximal to puncture site.	Same as for scalp venipuncture.
3. External jugular venipuncture	Immobilize child in mummy restraint. Place child's shoulders at edge of treatment table and hyperextend head with face contralateral to entry site.	It is crucial that child be held perfectly still during this procedure to avoid excessive trauma and hematoma formation in this highly mobile area. Mummy restraint allows nurse to use both hands in support of head and hyperextension of infant's neck. This position increases visibility in neck region and increases distention of external jugular by slightly impeding venous return.
4. Femoral venipuncture	Immobilize child in modified mummy restraint, with legs in frog position and nurse's hands on child's knees. Position child with his head toward nurse and feet toward physician.	Use of modified mummy restraint immobilizes child's arms, leaving nurse's hands free to immobilize legs. This position gives physician an unobstructed approach to puncture site and gives nurse a close vantage point for assessment and comforting of infant during procedure.
Prevent complications of venipuncture	When preparing for venipuncture, be sure to wash site thoroughly with soap and water first, then shave scalp aseptically (for scalp venipuncture).	Jugular and femoral sites on infants are often contaminated with food and saliva or excreta. Nurse should be sure sites are hygienic before antiseptic preparation of site.
	For scalp and peripheral venipuncture, palpate target vein with one hand and grasp plastic wings of needle with the other. Pierce skin slightly to one side and 0.5 cm distal to entry site. Reverse insertion directions for blood sample only.	Neonates' veins, especially of scalp, are usually superficial, and a deep thrust may cause distal wall penetration and hematoma.
	Following venipuncture, apply pressure over site with dry gauze square for 3 min, to prevent hematoma formation.	Jugular and femoral veins require longer application of direct pressure than peripheral sites because they are larger

Procedure 25-4. Cont'd

Objective	Nursing action	Rationale
		vessels with greater blood flow and are more prone to oozing.
	Place inverted paper cup over site with "door" cut in one side to permit passage of tube (Figure 25-9).	Inverted cup protects continuous infusion site from accidental dislodgement.
	Remove any bandage applied to puncture site within 4 hr.	Dressings over puncture sites on neck or groin are prone to moisture collection, which increases potential for bacterial growth and infection. If oozing persists after 4 hr, change dressing and notify physician.

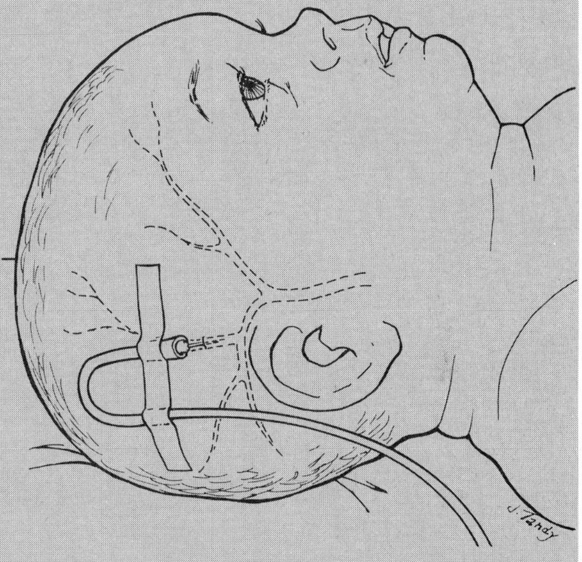

Figure 25-9.

Residual Pulmonary Disease

Oxygen toxicity of the lungs depends on a combination of factors: the concentrations of oxygen used, duration of exposure, and individual susceptibility; it is not correlated with the nature of the underlying disease.

The infant may manifest residual respiratory distress during the recovery phase of initial illness. Clinical signs and symptoms include rapid respiratory rate, abnormal respiratory patterns, periodic respirations, retention of retractions, and rales or wheezing on auscultation.

Residual pulmonary disease may result from treatment with positive pressure ventilation and (usually) endotracheal intubation. Infants so treated are more susceptible during the first year of life to respiratory illness requiring hospitalization.

Bronchopulmonary Dysplasia

Bronchopulmonary dysplasia is a result of positive ventilation. This condition is rarely found in the neonate treated with negative pressure devices or with high oxygen concentrations (60% or more) from endotracheal intubation.

A pathology of epithelial destruction with regeneration, accompanied by dysplasia and changes in lung fields, is similar to the Wilson-

Mikity syndrome (pulmonary dysmaturity). There is often difficulty in weaning the infant from the positive pressure ventilation and from long-term dependence on oxygen. Some infants may demonstrate this with recurrent lower respiratory tract infections during infancy. Most infants show slow clearing of the abnormal pulmonary characteristics and have normal x-rays at 6 months to 2 years of age. A few infants develop progressive pulmonary fibrosis or cardiac disease secondary to the pulmonary lesions (Avery, 1975).

Interstitial Pulmonary Emphysema

Pulmonary emphysema is the pathologic accumulation of air in the tissues of the lungs. Extra-alveolar air collections are most common with use of positive pressure ventilation. Air collections outside the lung are a function of compliance of the lung and utilization of increased pressures to ventilate. In interstitial pulmonary emphysema, there is air dissection along perivascular spaces but not yet into pleural space or mediastinum. This condition is a precursor of pneumothorax or pneumomediastinum.

Pneumothorax

Pneumothorax, a collection of air and/or fluid in the thoracic cavity, is a common complication of respiratory distress syndrome. It is a result of the stiff, noncompliant lungs and the use of assisted, positive pressure ventilation with high inspiratory pressure. Meconium aspiration with subsequent obstruction of the airways and a ball-valve phenomenon often produce pneumothorax as a complication. Pneumothorax results in several physiologic changes: collapse of the lung, development of tension in the pleural space, and cardiac and mediastinal shift to the contralateral side.

Symptoms of pneumothorax include a sudden unexplained deterioration in the neonate's condition, cyanosis, abnormal ECG findings, decrease in blood pressure, mottled and shocklike appearance, and others. X-ray examination of the chest is the only procedure that confirms the presence of suspected pneumothorax.

Other Pulmonary Complications

Pneumomediastinum is a massive collection of air in the mediastinum, either anterior to the heart or laterally, compressing mediastinal pleurae. This condition results in compression of venae cavae, tachypnea, cyanosis, and distant or barely audible heart sounds. Air may dissect into the soft tissues of the neck.

Pneumopericardium is a collection of air about the heart with resultant tamponade and diminution of cardiac size.

Pneumoperitoneum is a collection of air in the peritoneal cavity. This condition must be differentiated from a perforated viscus.

NEONATAL JAUNDICE

The most common abnormal physical finding in neonates is *jaundice* (icterus). Jaundice develops from deposit of the yellow pigment, *bilirubin,* in tissues. Unconjugated (indirect) bilirubin is a breakdown product derived from hemoglobin that is released from lysed red blood cells and heme pigments found in cell elements (nonerythrocyte bilirubin).

Fetal unconjugated bilirubin is normally cleared by the placenta in utero, so total bilirubin at birth is usually less than 3 mg/100 ml unless an abnormal hemolytic process has been present. Postnatally, the infant must conjugate bilirubin in his liver, producing a rise in serum bilirubin in the first few days of life. The bilirubin level at which an infant is harmed varies and depends on a number of factors; furthermore, many conditions can cause a more rapid rise in bilirubin and have the potential to produce permanent neurologic defects and even death. Management of the jaundiced infant presents unique problems that are not present in other periods of life.

Physiology and Pathophysiology

The neonate has a shorter erythrocyte (RBC) life span (88 days instead of 120) and a proportionately larger amount of nonerythrocyte bilirubin formed than the adult. Therefore, he has two to three times greater production or breakdown of bilirubin. Unconjugated bilirubin is normally transported in the plasma firmly bound to albumin, which makes it water soluble. Albumin-bound bilirubin cannot enter intracellular compartments or cross the blood-brain barrier, so it is nontoxic. However, if the bilirubin is not bound to albumin, it crosses the blood-brain barrier and damages the cells of the central nervous system and produces kernicterus. Unconjugated albumin-bound bilirubin is taken up by the liver cells via a still little-understood mechanism. Two intracellular proteins, labeled Y and Z, determine the amount of bilirubin held in a liver cell for processing and consequently the potential amount of bilirubin uptake into the liver. The clearance and conjugation of bilirubin depends on the enzyme glucuronyl transferase system, which results in the attachment of unconjugated bilirubin to glucuronic acid (product of liver glycogen), producing conjugated (excretable, direct, bound) bilirubin. It is excreted into the tiny bile ducts, then into the common duct and duodenum. It then progresses down the intestines, where bacteria transform it into urobilinogen, which is not reabsorbed, and it is excreted as a yellow-brown pigment in the stools.

When the amount of bilirubin in the vascular system overwhelms the clearing capabilities of the liver, jaundice develops. Conjugated bilirubin is cleared from the body after it is processed in the liver, excreted into the bile, and eliminated with the feces. Unconjugated bilirubin is not in excretable form and is a potential toxin. Total serum bilirubin is the sum of direct and indirect bilirubin.

The rate and amount of conjugation depends on the rate of hemolysis, on the maturity of the liver, and on albumin-binding sites. The rate of hemolysis of the excess number and kind of fetal red blood cells that are no longer needed by the neonate is such that physiologic jaundice does not occur until after 24 hours of age. A normal, healthy, full-term infant's liver is usually sufficiently mature and is producing enough glucuronyl transferase so that serum bilirubin levels do not reach pathologic levels (above 12 mg/100 ml blood). Too great a bilirubin level may result from polycythemia (twin-to-twin transfusion, large placental transfer of blood), enclosed hemorrhage (cephalhematoma, bleeding into internal organs, ecchymoses), or increased hemolyses (sepsis and hemolytic disease of the newborn).

Serum albumin-binding sites are usually sufficient to meet the usual demands. However, certain conditions tend to decrease the sites available. Fetal or neonatal asphyxia decreases the binding affinity of bilirubin to albumin; chilling, hypoglycemia, and maternal use of sulfa drugs or salicylates interfere with conjugation or interfere with serum albumin-binding sites by competing with bilirubin for these sites.

The liver of the newborn infant, particularly that of the premature infant, has relatively less glucuronyl transferase activity at birth and in the first few weeks of life than the adult. In 1% of breast-fed infants, a substance in breast milk (pregnanediol) can inhibit bilirubin conjugation. A number of bacterial and viral infections (cytomegalic inclusion disease, toxoplasmosis, herpes, syphilis) can also affect the liver and produce jaundice.

Even after the bilirubin has been conjugated, it can be converted back to unconjugated bilirubin via the "enterohepatic circulation." In the intestines a β-glucuronidase enzyme system acts to split off (or deconjugate) the bilirubin from glucuronic acid if it has not first been reduced by gut bacteria to urobilin, and the free bilirubin is reabsorbed through the intestinal wall and brought back to the liver via portal vein circulation. This recycling of the bilirubin and decreased ability to clear bilirubin from the system is prevalent in the newborn and particularly in premature infants, who have very high β-glucuronidase activity levels as well as delayed bacterial colonization of the gut.

Types of Jaundice

Physiologic Jaundice (Icterus Neonatorum)

About 50% of full-term neonates and 80% of premature neonates exhibit physiologic jaundice on about the second or third day. The characteristic icteric (yellow) color results from increased levels of serum bilirubin, which occur as a normal product of red blood cell hemolysis, and a temporary inability of the body to eliminate this bilirubin.

Expected serum bilirubin levels are as follows:

	Full-Term	Premature
1st 24 hours	2–6 mg/100 ml	1–6 mg/100 ml
Day 2	6–7 mg/100 ml	6–8 mg/100 ml
Days 3–5	4–12 mg/100 ml	10–15 mg/100 ml

Serum levels of bilirubin are about 5–7 mg/100 ml before yellow coloration of the skin and sclera appears.

Peak bilirubin levels in the premature infant are usually reached between days 6 and 8 and seldom exceed 15 mg/100 ml.

Nursery environment, including lighting and practices, affects the early detection of the degree and type of jaundice. Blue walls and artificial lights mask the beginning of jaundice. Daylight assists the observer in early recognition by eliminating many of the distortions caused by artificial lights.

Nursery procedures are designed to decrease the probability of high bilirubin levels. These actions are as follows:

1. The infant's body temperature is maintained at 97.6F or above because chilling results in acidosis, which in turn decreases available serum albumin binding sites and causes elevated bilirubin levels.
2. Passage of stool is monitored for amount and type. Bilirubin is eliminated via the feces, and inadequate stooling may result in reabsorption and recycling of bilirubin.
3. Early feedings are encouraged to promote intestinal elimination.

If jaundice is suspected, the nurse can quickly assess the neonate's coloring by pressing his skin with a finger. When blanching occurs, the nurse can observe the icterus. If jaundice becomes apparent, feedings of 5% dextrose in water or 10% dextrose in water may be started between milk feedings. This keeps the infant well hydrated and promotes intestinal elimination. Phototherapy is indicated in cases of hyperbilirubinemia (see p. 824).

Approximately 50% of the infants with physiologic jaundice show signs of improvement by day 7 and resolution of the problem by day 14.

Physiologic jaundice may be very upsetting to parents; they require emotional support and thorough explanation of the condition. If it is necessary for the baby to be hospitalized for a few additional days, this can be devastating to the parents. They should be encouraged to provide for the emotional needs of their child by continuing to feed, hold, and caress him. If the mother is discharged, the parents should be encouraged to return for feedings and should feel free to call or visit whenever possible. In many instances the mother, especially if she is breast-feeding, may elect to remain hospitalized with her infant; this decision should be supported.

Breast-feeding Jaundice

Breast-feeding is implicated in prolonged jaundice in some infants. The breast milk of some women contains an enzyme (pregnanediol) that inhibits glucuronyl transferase and, if in high enough concentration, inhibits the conjugation of bilirubin. The bilirubin level begins to rise about the fourth day, peaks at 2 to 3 weeks of age, and may reach 15 to 20 mg/100 ml. Infants do not seem to be damaged by these high levels of breast-feeding–induced hyperbilirubinemia. Within 48 hours after discontinuing breast-feeding, the infant's serum bilirubin levels begin to fall and return to within normal range by four to eight days.

Many physicians believe that breast-feeding may be resumed once the diagnosis has been made, because the bilirubin concentration may rise to 2–3 mg/100 ml but does not reach previous high levels. Nursing mothers need encouragement and support in their desire to nurse their infants, assistance and instruction regarding pumping and expressing milk during the interrupted nursing period, and reassurance that nothing is wrong with their milk or mothering abilities.

Pathologic Jaundice

High serum bilirubin levels, especially in the unconjugated state, are dangerous to the neonate. The more premature the neonate, the more susceptible he is to tissue damage. Since the cerebral cortex and thalamus are the last to be myelinated, the nuclei of these cells are more susceptible to being infiltrated by the unconjugated bilirubin, with subsequent brain damage (Kempe et al., 1978). Jaundice of any origin must be considered pathologic if it appears within the first 24 hours or persists beyond seven days in the full-term and ten days in the premature infant, if serum bilirubin levels rise by more than 5 mg/100 ml in 24 hours or exceed 12 mg/100 ml in the full-term and 15 mg/100 ml in the premature neonate, and if direct bilirubin is greater than 1.5 mg/100 ml. The most likely causes of jaundice are hemolytic disease of the newborn (Rh incompatibility and ABO incompatibility) and sepsis. In utero infections such as toxoplasmosis, rubella, herpes, and syphilis may produce jaundice in the first 24 hours. Such affected infants also have petechiae and an enlarged liver and spleen.

The nurse is aware of the infant's prenatal and natal history and assesses him several times each day for color and change in behavior. Behavior changes rarely occur prior to 36 hours of age, occurring most frequently between days 2 and 6.

Hyperbilirubinemia

During fetal life, bilirubin is cleared rapidly by the maternal-placental unit. In early neonatal life, the rate of bilirubin clearance depends on several factors: rate of red blood cell lysis, maturity of the liver, coexisting conditions that interfere with conjugation or compete for serum albumin binding sites, or coexisting conditions that interfere with the excretion of conjugated bilirubin.

Neonatal *hyperbilirubinemia* (level of serum bilirubin in excess of accepted norms) is partly preventable. During pregnancy, women are checked for conditions that may predispose to neonatal hyperbilirubinemia: hereditary spherocytosis, diabetes, infections (toxoplasmosis, cytomegalic inclusion disease, rubella, infections with gram-negative bacilli) that stimulate production of maternal isoimmune antibodies, and drug ingestion (sulfas, salicylates, novobiocin, some tranquilizers). The woman who is Rh-negative or who has blood type O is asked about outcomes of any previous pregnancies and her history of blood transfusion. Prenatal amniocentesis with spectrophotographic examination may be indicated in some cases. Cord blood from neonates is evaluated for bilirubin level, which should not exceed 5 mg/100 ml. Neonates of these mothers are carefully assessed for appearance of jaundice and levels of serum bilirubin.

Some neonatal conditions predispose to hyperbilirubinemia: polycythemia (hematocrit 60% or more), obstruction or atresia of the biliary duct or of the lower bowel, low-grade urinary tract infection, hypothyroidism, enclosed hemorrhage (cephalhematoma, large bruises), asphyxia neonatorum, hypothermia, acidemia, hypoglycemia. Hepatitis from an infectious or metabolic liver disease elevates the level of conjugated bilirubin. This type of hepatitis is associated with intrauterine infection such as rubella syndrome, cytomegalic inclusion disease, syphilis, herpesvirus type 2 ("genital herpes"), or cystic fibrosis. Neonatal hepatitis (giant cell hepatitis) is a disorder of unknown etiology that results in spontaneous cure in one-third of those affected, chronic liver disease in another one-third, and death for the remaining one-third. Neonates born with congenital biliary duct atresia have a poor prognosis; about 90% have an inoperable lesion and succumb during the first three years of life.

Livers of healthy term neonates are more mature than those of the premature infant. Efforts to prevent premature delivery must be directed toward improving the mother's social, economic, and nutritional status; implementing informed family planning; and providing acceptable and accessible prenatal care to diversified populations.

The goal of the management of hyperbilirubinemia is to treat the anemia, remove maternal antibodies and sensitized erythrocytes, increase serum albumin levels, and reduce the levels of serum bilirubin. Methods include phototherapy, exchange transfusion, infusion of albumin, and drug therapy. (These treatment techniques are discussed later in this chapter.)

Kernicterus

Unbound (unconjugated) bilirubin, although not soluble in body fluids, is capable of crossing cell membranes. *Kernicterus* (meaning "yellow nucleus") refers to the deposition of unconjugated bilirubin in the basal ganglia of the brain and to the symptoms of neurologic damage that follow untreated hyperbilirubinemia. Kernicterus is most commonly found with blood-group incompatibility.

Kernicterus is associated with bilirubin levels of over 20 mg/100 ml in normal term infants; safe levels for premature infants or sick infants are lower and vary considerably. Sick premature infants may develop kernicterus with serum bilirubin levels as low as 10 mg/100 ml. Severe brain cell damage may result in cerebral palsy, mental retardation, sensory difficulties, or death. Neurologic damage from lesser amounts of bilirubin may be expressed later in childhood as perceptual impairment, delayed development of speech, hyperactivity, and perhaps learning difficulties.

Nursing Management

The primary nursing priority is to identify jaundice as soon as it is apparent. If jaundice appears, careful observation of the increase in depth of color and of the infant's behavior is mandatory. Should the infant require phototherapy (discussed on p. 824), the nurse provides the necessary care. The nurse assists with the exchange transfusion (Procedure 25-5) and observes the infant carefully following the procedure. The nurse who is working with the mother administers RhoGAM if ordered and assists the parents in coping with the situation.

As the first step in identifying jaundice, the nurse reviews each neonate's prenatal and perinatal history for factors that predispose to hyperbilirubinemia. The neonate's blood type, Rh, and Coombs' test results (if done) are noted. The nurse assesses each neonate for gestational age, for cephalhematoma, and for whether he is breast-fed or bottle-fed.

In the presence of one or more predisposing factors, laboratory determination should be made of serum bilirubin levels and CO_2 combining power (decrease in CO_2 combining power is consistent with increased hemolysis). In addition, the nurse checks the neonate for jaundice about every two hours and records observations.

To check for jaundice, the nurse should blanch the skin over a bony prominence (forehead, sternum) by pressing firmly with the thumb. After pressure is released, the area appears yellow before normal color returns. The nurse should check oral mucosa and the posterior portion of the hard palate and conjunctival sacs for yellow pigmentation in darker-skinned neonates, because the underlying pigment of dark-skinned people normally appears yellow. Assessment in daylight gives best results, as pink colors may cause yellowish tints; yellow colors make differentiation of jaundice difficult. The time of onset of jaundice is recorded and reported.

The neonate's behavior is assessed for neurologic signs of kernicterus, especially between days 3 and 10. Kernicterus never appears before 36 hours of age, even in severe cases of hemolytic disease. Clinical features of encephalopathy appear in four stages. Kernicterus is initially evidenced by diminished response—hypotonia, poor rooting and sucking, lethargy. During the second stage, hyperreflexia, spasticity (with or without opisthotonus), high-pitched cry, and fever may be seen. After about 1 week of age, during the third stage, all clinical manifestations may disappear. The fourth stage, appearing after the neonatal period, reveals the extent of neurologic damage. Late sequelae may include cerebral palsy (spasticity, athetosis), impaired or absent hearing, learning difficulties, and mental retardation.

HEMOLYTIC DISEASE OF THE NEWBORN

Physiology and Pathophysiology

Isoimmune hemolytic disease, also known as *erythroblastosis fetalis,* occurs following transplacental passage of a maternal antibody that predisposes fetal and neonatal red blood cells to early destruction. Jaundice, anemia, and compensatory erythropoiesis result. Immature red blood cells—erythroblasts—are found in large numbers in the blood; hence the designation erythroblastosis fetalis.

Although there are more than 60 known red blood cell antigens, clinically significant hemolytic disease is associated with maternal-fetal incompatibility associated with the D factor in the Rh group and with the ABO blood types.

ABO incompatibility, although frequent (20% of pregnancies), rarely results in hemolytic disease severe enough to be clinically diagnosed and treated. The most common incompatibility occurs when the mother is type O and the fetus is type A_1. Types A_2 and B do not seem to have the same antigenicity as A_1. A type O person already has "natural" anti-A and anti-B antibodies, so that even a first pregnancy can be affected. The maternal anti-A or anti-B antibodies cross the placenta and produce hemolysis of the fetal red blood cells. In addition, incompatibility results when the mother is type A and the fetus is type B or the mother is type B and the fetus is type A.

The Rh incompatibility system is more complex. Those whose red blood cells contain the Rh factor (antigen) are said to be positive; those who do not are negative. Several variant forms of Rh antigen exist. The factors implicated in pathogenesis, in order of antigenic potential, are D, C,

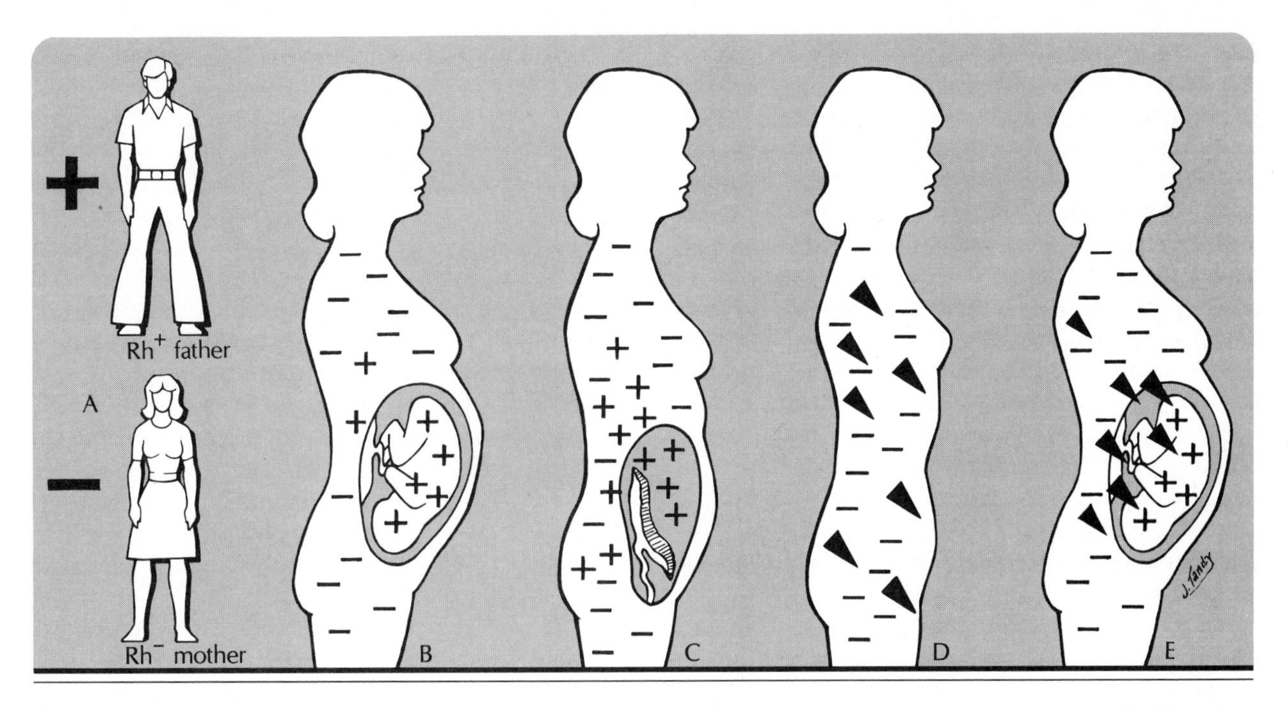

Figure 25–10. Rh isoimmunization sequence. **A,** Rh positive father and Rh negative mother. **B,** Pregnancy with Rh positive fetus. Some Rh positive blood enters the mother's blood. **C,** As placenta separates, further inoculation of mother by Rh positive blood. **D,** Mother sensitized to Rh positive blood; anti-Rh positive antibodies are formed. **E,** With subsequent pregnancies with Rh positive fetus, Rh positive red blood cells are attacked by the anti-Rh positive maternal antibodies causing hemolysis of red blood cells in the fetus.

E, c, e, and, hypothetically, d (d has never been demonstrated but is thought to exist). There are many genetic combinations (genotypes) possible, such as CDE, cDe, Cde, and so forth. The D antigen is most significant clinically in that it provides the strongest stimulus to antibody formation in Rh-negative people. Therefore, individuals who are homozygous for the D antigen (DD) or heterozygous (Dd) are Rh-positive; those whose genotype is dd are Rh-negative. Despite the antigenicity of the D factor, only 10% of pregnancies with Rh-positive fetuses result in immunization of Rh-negative women, even after five pregnancies. This phenomenon has been attributed to a rapid lysis of fetal cells entering the maternal bloodstream.

The distribution of the D factor is approximately 85% of white, 93% of black, and 99% of Chinese populations. The incidence of hemolytic disease from this cause is about three times as high among whites as among blacks and is rarely seen in Chinese.

Isoimmunization occurs when an Rh-negative woman carries an Rh-positive fetus. When fetal Rh antigens (an antigenic substance on the surface of the fetal red blood cell) leak in minute amounts into the maternal circulation, antibodies are produced, creating a sensitization reaction. In subsequent pregnancies the maternal antibodies cross the placenta and cause immediate or delayed destruction (hemolysis) of the fetal red blood cells (Figure 25–10). The leakage of fetal Rh antigens into the maternal circulation most commonly occurs at the time of delivery. Other obstetric factors known to increase the likelihood of maternal Rh sensitization are toxemia of pregnancy, amniocentesis, version procedure, cesarean section, breech deliveries, and manual removal of placentas.

Hydrops fetalis, the most severe form of erythroblastosis fetalis, results when maternal antibodies attach to the Rh antigen of the fetal red blood cells, making them susceptible to destruction by phagocytes. The fetal system responds by increased erythropoiesis within foci in the placenta, hyperplastic bone marrow, and extramedullary sites. Rapid and early destruction of erythrocytes results in a marked increase of immature red blood cells—erythroblasts—which do not have the functional capabilities of mature cells. If the anemia is severe, as seen in hydrops fetalis, cardiomegaly with severe cardiac decompensation and hepatosplenomegaly occur. Severe edema, ascites, and hydrothorax (anasarca) develop. Jaundice is not present, because the bili pigments are being excreted through the placenta into the maternal circulation.

Severe anemia is also responsible for hemorrhage in pulmonary and other tissues. The hydropic hemolytic disease process is also characterized by hyperplasia of the fetal zone of the adrenal cortex and pancreatic islets. Hyperplasia of the pancreatic islets predisposes the infant to neonatal hypoglycemia similar to that of infants of diabetic mothers. These infants also have increased bleeding tendencies due to associated thrombocytopenia and hypoxic damage to the capillaries. In addition, the grossly enlarged edemic fetal body and placenta may cause uterine rupture.

Laboratory Data

If the hemolytic process is due to Rh sensitization, laboratory findings reveal the following: (a) an Rh-positive neonate with a positive Coombs' test; (b) increased erythropoiesis with many immature circulating red blood cells (nucleated blastocysts); (c) anemia, in most cases; (d) elevated levels (5 mg/100 ml or more) of bilirubin in cord blood; and (e) a reduction in albumin-binding capacity. Maternal data may include an elevated anti-Rh titer and spectrophotometric evidence of fetal hemolytic process.

Prognosis

Prognosis depends on the extent of the hemolytic process and the underlying cause. Severe hemolytic disease results in fetal and early neonatal death from the effects of anemia—cardiac decompensation, edema, ascites, and hydrothorax. Hyperbilirubinemia that is not promptly treated or adequately treated leads to kernicterus. The resultant neurologic damage is responsible for death, cerebral palsy, mental retardation, sensory difficulties, or to a lesser degree, perceptual impairment, delayed speech development, hyperactivity, muscle incoordination, or learning difficulties (Klaus and Fanaroff, 1973). Another late consequence of hyperbilirubinemia is yellowish green tooth staining and enamel hypoplasia. The best treatment for hemolytic disease is prevention.

Nursing Management

Maternal Assessment

A careful health and obstetric history is essential in establishing a correct diagnosis. The gravida is asked (a) if she has had or is now suffering from infections such as tuberculosis, syphilis, or rubella; (b) whether she is on medication and the type of medication; (c) whether she has knowledge of familial blood dyscrasias; (d) the number and outcome of previous pregnancies; (e) the condition at birth and the current health status of other children.

Hematologic studies include determination of Rh and blood type, identification of genetic blood disorders such as spherocytosis, and presence of infection such as syphilis or cytomegalic inclusion disease. The gravida is asked whether she has a habit of eating raw meat (usually hamburger served at parties as appetizers) or has recently acquired a cat that roams freely out of doors. If she is the one who cleans the litter box and this is her first exposure to cats, she may be in danger of contracting toxoplasmosis.

The Rh-negative woman who has experienced one or more abortions (especially if she has not received Rh immunoglobulin after each) or who has had one pregnancy with an Rh-positive fetus is scheduled for a Hemantigen test (containing the common antigens) at about 20 weeks' gestation. If the test is negative, it is repeated at 28, 32, and 36 weeks and at 6 weeks postdelivery. If the test shows a maternal antibody titer of 1:16 or greater, amniocentesis is performed at 26 weeks.

Amniotic fluid, obtained by transabdominal amniocentesis, is separated from its cellular components by centrifuge. The amount of pigment from the degradation of red blood cells can be measured when in solution in amniotic fluid. The fluid is subjected to spectrophotometric studies to determine the severity of the fetal hemolytic process and the obstetric-pediatric management.

Paternal Assessment

If the woman is Rh-negative (dd), the father of the unborn child is asked to come into the clinic or physician's office to be assessed for his Rh factor and blood type. If he is homozygous for Rh-positive (DD), all of his offspring will be Rh-positive. If he is heterozygous (Dd), 50% of his offspring can be Rh-negative and 50% heterozygous for Rh-positive.

Neonatal Assessment

Hemolytic disease of the newborn is suspected if the placenta is enlarged (placental weight is usually only one-seventh of fetal weight), if the neonate is edematous with pleural and pericardial effusion plus ascites, if pallor or jaundice is noted during the first 24 to 36 hours, if hemolytic anemia is diagnosed, or if the spleen and liver are enlarged. Changes in the neonate's behavior or bleeding tendencies must be carefully assessed to determine the causative factor. Neonates who have received vitamin K or sulfonamides may have increased incidence of hyperbilirubinemia because these agents reduce the number of available binding sites by competing for them (Kempe et al., 1978).

Prenatal Interventions

Prenatal management includes identification and treatment for maternal conditions that predispose to hemolytic disease, identification and evaluation of the Rh-sensitized woman, coordinated obstetric-pediatric efforts for prenatal and/or postnatal treatment for the seriously affected neonate, and prevention of Rh sensitization if none is present. The following discussion is focused on management of the woman who is Rh-negative or has blood type O.

Maternal-Fetal Nursing Actions

At the first prenatal visit (a) a history is taken of previous sensitization, abortions, blood transfusions, or children who developed jaundice or anemia during the neonatal period; (b) typing is done for blood group, Rh, and type; and (c) antibody screening is done.

If the woman is Rh-negative and unsensitized, the husband is typed for ABO and Rh zygosity. Antibody screening is repeated at 28, 32, and 36 weeks and at 6 weeks postdelivery. Negative titers of antibodies are a good indicator to deliver this infant at term. Within 72 hours after delivery of an Rh-positive neonate, the woman is given an anti-D gamma globulin injection (which will be discussed later).

If antibody titers are high, management becomes more complex. Indirect Coombs' test, titers, and amniotic fluid analysis are scheduled. The indirect Coombs' test measures the amount of antibodies in the mother's blood. Rh-positive red blood cells are added to the maternal blood sample. If the mother's serum contains antibodies, the Rh-positive red blood cells will agglutinate (clump) when rabbit immune antiglobulin is added.

The direct Coombs' test reveals the presence of antibody-coated (sensitized) Rh-positive red blood cells in the fetus or neonate. Rabbit immune antiglobulin is added to the fetal-neonatal blood specimen. If the fetal-neonatal red blood cells agglutinate, they have been coated with maternal antibodies.

If the indirect Coombs' test is positive, tests are repeated and titers are scheduled at one-month intervals until 34 weeks and at two-week intervals thereafter.

Analysis of amniotic fluid obtained by transabdominal amniocentesis is scheduled for the sensitized woman (antibody titer greater than 1:16) after 26 weeks. If the spectrophotometric readings are in the A zone ΔOD at 450 mμ, a normal or mildly anemic infant may be anticipated and delivery at term may be permitted. Prognosis for this infant is good, but phototherapy or exchange transfusion may be necessary. A reading in the B zone ΔOD at 450 mμ indicates a moderately anemic fetus who may be hydropic or stillborn if delivered at term. Once the fetus reaches viability, induced vaginal or cesarean delivery is indicated. A fair prognosis and possible need for exchange transfusion can be anticipated. Readings within the C zone ΔOD at 450 mμ indicate a severely affected fetus who may require intrauterine transfusion every one to two weeks between 26 and 32 weeks until viability is reached, followed by delivery, usually by cesarean section. Neonatal exchange transfusion is anticipated. Prognosis is guarded (see Figure 14–12).

Intrauterine Transfusion

Intrauterine transfusion is done to correct the anemia produced by the red blood cell hemolysis (see Procedure 13–1). If intrauterine transfusion is considered, an amniogram using water-soluble contrast medium is performed to identify the hydropic fetus and to locate the placenta. It is inadvisable to transfuse a fetus diagnosed as hydropic. Several hours after injection of contrast medium, the fetal gastrointestinal tract may be seen with fluoroscopy. With the mother under local anesthesia, a plastic catheter threaded through an 18 cm, 16-gauge Tuohy needle is introduced through the abdomen into the intrauterine space and into the fetal peritoneal cavity. About 100 ml of packed red blood cells is selected for transfusion according to the following criteria: It must be less than 24 hours old (blood over 24 hours old has lost the enzyme 2,3-diphosphoglycerase, which is necessary before oxygen can be released from the red blood cells into the tissues), type O, Rh-negative, and cross-matched against the mother's serum. Diaphragmatic lymphatics absorb the red blood cells into fetal circulation within a week after transfusion. Repeat transfusions can be scheduled every ten days to three weeks.

About 50%–60% of transfused nonhydropic fetuses survive. The procedure is hazardous to the fetus, resulting in mortality in 6% of cases. Direct trauma to the fetus with the needles and catheter is possible. Maternal complications are few; those that occur are usually due to bleeding or infection. The neonate is usually delivered about the 34th week. In general, premature neonates are more susceptible to damage from hemolytic disease, often require exchange transfusion, and require intensive nursery care.

Postpartal Interventions

The goals of postpartal care are to prevent sensitization in the as-yet-unsensitized mother and to treat the isoimmune hemolytic disease in the neonate.

Treatment of the Mother

The Rh-negative mother who has no titer (Coombs' negative, nonsensitized) and who has delivered an Rh-positive fetus is given an intramuscular injection of anti-Rh_0 (D) gamma globulin such as RhoGAM within 72 hours so that she does not have time to produce antibodies to fetal cells that entered her bloodstream when the placenta separated. The anti-Rh_0 (D) gamma globulin works to destroy the fetal cells in the maternal circulation before sensitization occurs, thereby blocking maternal antibody production. The nurse must follow the instructions on the packet of RhoGAM carefully. The used packet containing the vial of drug cross-matched to the mother's serum is returned to the pharmacy, where it is saved. The mother is observed for possible symptoms of blood transfusion reaction (Behrman, 1973).

RhoGAM (1 ml or 300 mg) is also given after each abortion (especially if induced) or ectopic pregnancy. (By the 11th week of fetal life, the D-antigen is often present and can stimulate maternal isoimmunization, which would jeopardize the next Rh-positive fetus.) RhoGAM is never given to the neonate or the father.

Occasionally, the coating of maternal antibodies on fetal cells may block an accurate typing of cord blood; that is, an Rh-positive fetus may be erroneously typed as Rh-negative. Consequently, the RhoGAM will not be given, and the mother may become sensitized.

Treatment of the Neonate

The management of the neonate is directed toward preventing anemia and hyperbilirubinemia (Figure 25–11). Exchange transfusion, phototherapy, and drug therapy are utilized.

Exchange transfusion. Exchange transfusion is indicated in the presence of anti-Rh titer of greater than 1.6 in the mother, severe hemolytic disease in a previous newborn, clinical hemolytic disease of the newborn at birth or within the first 24 hours, positive direct Coombs' test, cord serum direct bilirubin levels greater than 3.5 mg/100 ml in the first week, serum bilirubin levels greater than 15 mg/100 ml in the first week, hemoglobin less than 12 gm/100 ml, or infants who are hydropic at birth. Infants who are at greater risk for developing kernicterus are exchanged at lower serum bilirubin levels. Withdrawal of neonate's blood and replacement with donor blood is used to (a) treat anemia with red blood cells that are not susceptible to maternal antibodies, (b) remove sensitized red blood cells that would be lysed soon (a two-volume exchange removes 85% of the infant's red blood cells), (c) remove serum bilirubin, and (d) provide bilirubin-free albumin and increase the binding sites for bilirubin. For more transfusions, fresh (under two days old) whole blood or packed red blood cells is chosen, group O, Rh-negative, with low anti-A and anti-B titers. Packed cells are used if the infant is anemic. CPD

<table>
<tr><th>Serum bilirubin mg/100 ml</th><th colspan="2">Birth weight</th><th><24 hrs</th><th>24-48 hrs</th><th>49-72 hrs</th><th>72 hrs</th></tr>
<tr><td><5</td><td colspan="2">All</td><td></td><td></td><td></td><td></td></tr>
<tr><td>5-9</td><td colspan="2">All</td><td>Phototherapy if hemolysis</td><td></td><td></td><td></td></tr>
<tr><td rowspan="2">10-14</td><td colspan="2"><2500 gm</td><td rowspan="2">Exchange if hemolysis</td><td colspan="3">Phototherapy</td></tr>
<tr><td colspan="2">>2500 gm</td><td></td><td colspan="2">Investigate bilirubin > 12 mg</td></tr>
<tr><td rowspan="2">15-19</td><td colspan="2"><2500 gm</td><td rowspan="2" colspan="2">Exchange</td><td colspan="2">Consider exchange</td></tr>
<tr><td colspan="2">>2500 gm</td><td colspan="2">Phototherapy</td></tr>
<tr><td>20 and +</td><td colspan="2">All</td><td colspan="4">Exchange</td></tr>
</table>

☐ Observe ▨ Investigate jaundice

Figure 25–11. Therapy for isoimmune hemolytic disease in the neonate. Phototherapy is used after any exchange transfusion. If the following conditions are present, treat the neonate as if he were in the next higher bilirubin category: perinatal asphyxia, respiratory distress, metabolic acidosis (pH 7.25 or below), hypothermia (temperature below 35C), low serum protein (5 gm/100 ml or less), birth weight less than 1500 gm, or signs of clinical or central nervous system deterioration. (From Avery, 1975. *Neonatology.* Philadelphia: J. B. Lippincott Co., p. 335.)

(citrate-phosphate-dextrose) blood is preferred, because it presents less of an acid load to the infant.

In case of ABO incompatibility, group O blood of the same Rh as the neonate's blood is appropriate. A 3 kg (6½ lb) infant has about 250 ml blood. By removing 10–20 ml of blood from the infant at a time and transfusing with 10–20 ml of donor blood, 85% of the neonate's blood may be exchanged if the total amount of donor blood used is 500 ml.

During this aseptic procedure, the infant is kept warm (even the blood is warmed by draping the tubing from the bottle through a warm bath before it reaches the infant), vital signs are monitored continuously, a syringe of 10% calcium gluconate is on hand, and a careful record is kept of each step. Every four to eight hours after the transfusion, bilirubin determinations are made. Repeat exchange may be necessary if the serum bilirubin level exceeds 20 mg/100 ml. Daily hemoglobin estimates should be obtained until stable, and hemoglobin determinations every two weeks for two months are valuable.

Salt-poor albumin (1 gm/kg body weight) given prior to the transfusion augments the neonate's albumin-binding capacity. Albumin is never given to the severely anemic neonate or to one who is edemic or in congestive heart failure, because of the hazard of hypervolemia.

The nurse's responsibilities during exchange transfusion are several: assemble equipment, prepare the neonate, assist the physician during the procedure, maintain a careful record of all events, and observe the neonate after the procedure for complications from the transfusion and clinical signs of hyperbilirubinemia and neurologic damage (Procedure 25-5).

Procedure 25-5. Exchange Transfusion
(Exchange transfusion is therapeutic procedure for hyperbilirubinemia of any etiology.)

Objective	Nursing action	Rationale
Assemble equipment	Obtain the following equipment:	
	1. Sterile gown and gloves for physician.	Maintains sterility.
	2. Disposable exchange transfusion tray.	Provides necessary equipment.
	3. Umbilical cut-down tray (if there is no umbilical catheter).	Provides equipment for starting umbilical IV.
	4. Sterile umbilical cord ties or sterile No. 4-Osille silk suture.	To tie around umbilical catheter.
	5. IV standard.	Hangs the blood.
	6. One unit Rh negative blood, type O or infant's own type.	Blood of choice.
	7. Blood tubing.	
	8. Blood warmer.	Decreases chilling.
	9. Oxygen mask and tubing hooked to O_2 source.	To use if infant is in distress.
	10. Suction tubing attached to wall outlet or DeLee trap or bulb syringe.	To use if infant is in distress.
	11. Pulse and respiration monitor.	Monitors pulse and respirations continuously.
	12. Umbilical catheter, 3½ or 5.	To place in umbilical vein.
	13. At least two red-topped tubes.	To obtain blood samples.
	14. Blood culture tube (optional).	To obtain culture if desired.
	15. Solution for preparing skin (Betadine or Merthiolate).	Cleanses skin and prepares site.
	16. Infant restraining board.	Positions infant.
	17. Spotlight.	To visualize the field.
	18. Laboratory slips.	
Prepare infant	Identify infant.	To prepare correct infant.
	Place infant on restraining board.	Infant may be left in open bed warmer to provide warmth.
	Cleanse abdomen by scrubbing.	Reduces number of bacteria present.
	Attach monitor to infant.	To assess pulse and respiration.
Prepare equipment	Obtain blood and check it with physician.	Ensures using correct blood.
	Attach blood tubing.	Allows infusion.
	Apply blood warmer.	Reduces chill.
	Open trays. Pour prep solution into basins.	
	Prepare gown and gloves for physician.	
Monitor infant status	Assess pulse, respirations, color, activity state.	To recognize possible problems.
Record blood exchange and medications used	Using blood exchange sheet, record time, amount of blood in, amount of blood out, and medications.	Donor blood is given at rate of 170 ml/kg of body weight. It replaces 85% of infant's own blood.
Assess infant response after exchange transfusion	Assess pulse, respiration, color, activity state, bleeding from umbilical catheter, and patency of IV tubing.	Umbilical venous IV is left in place after exchange in case another exchange is needed.
Prepare blood samples	Label tubes and send to laboratory with appropriate laboratory slips.	Follow routines of your institution.

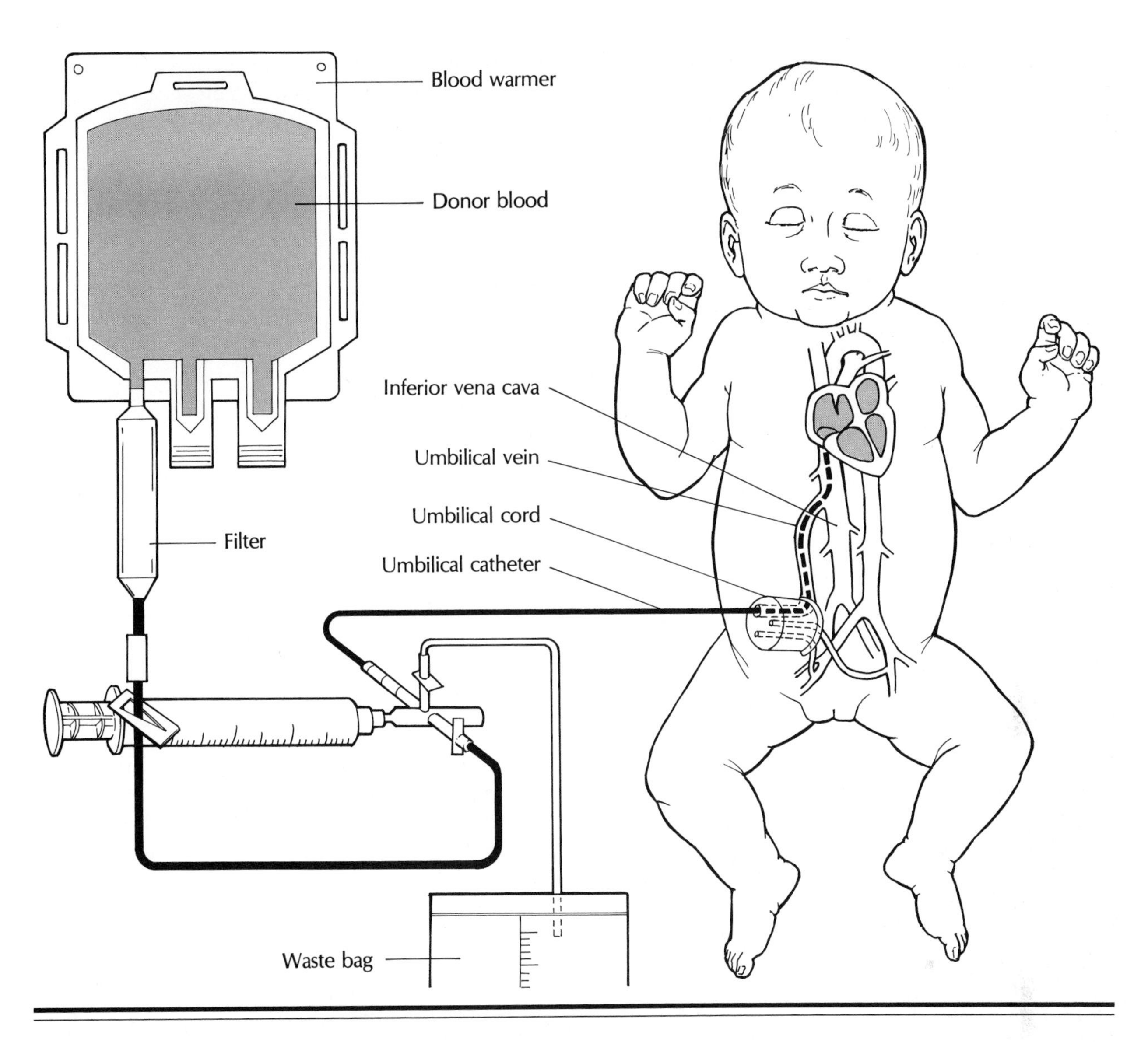

Figure 25–12. Infant receiving exchange transfusion.

Necessary equipment varies with the hospital. In general, equipment includes two units of donor's blood; exchange transfusion set and record; monitors; water bath (38C or 100F); medications drawn up in syringes with No. 24 needles (10% calcium gluconate, 50% glucose, sodium bicarbonate or trimethamine); sterile gowns, gloves, masks, drapes; method of keeping the neonate warm; lighting; restraints; resuscitation equipment.

The neonate should not ingest anything for four hours or should have his stomach aspirated prior to the procedure. The neonate is positioned supine, is restrained, and is kept warm (Figure 25–12). Resuscitation equipment is assembled in an easily accessible area near the neonate. Vital signs are taken and recorded. The catheter location should be verified by radiograph. Continuous monitoring equipment is used, if available. Both physician and nurse check donor blood for type, Rh, and age, to minimize error. Tubing from the blood bottle (or bag) is draped through the warm bath or a blood warmer.

The nurse assists the physician in cleansing the infusion site (usually the umbilical vein or the jugular or femoral artery) and in draping, gowning, and gloving. The physician measures the central venous pressure (CVP) prior to starting the exchange; the nurse records the time and the reading. The nurse records the time and amount of each withdrawal of fetal blood and infusion of donor blood and keeps a current tally of the total amount. The nurse alerts the physician when 100 ml have been exchanged. The physician usually administers calcium gluconate after each 100 ml is exchanged to minimize possible cardiac irritability. The nurse continues to monitor and record heart rate, respiratory rate, all medications (type, amount, time), infant response, and any other pertinent information.

Following the transfusion, the nurse observes the neonate closely for 24 to 48 hours for vital signs (temperature, pulse, respirations; bradycardia may result if calcium is injected too rapidly, pedal pulses if umbilical vein or femoral arteries were used for the exchange site), neurologic signs (lethargy, increased irritability, jitteriness, or convulsions), dark urine, and developing edema. Necrotizing enterocolitis may result from a misplaced catheter and compromised bowel circulation. Complications for which the nurse must be alert may arise from hemorrhage or infection at the infusion site or from the blood transfusion. Possible complications following any blood transfusion include heart failure, hypokalemia, hypoglycemia (result of continued anaerobic glycolysis within donor red blood cells), septicemia, shock, and thrombosis. The nurse remains observant for increasing jaundice and the appearance of neurologic signs that may signify kernicterus.

Phototherapy. Phototherapy may be used alone or in conjunction with exchange transfusion to reduce serum bilirubin levels. Exposure of the neonate to high-intensity light (a bank of fluorescent light bulbs or bulbs in the blue-light spectrum) decreases serum bilirubin levels in the skin. Unbound (unconjugated) bilirubin is thought to be photo-oxidized into nontoxic compounds that are excreted in the urine and feces (via bile) (Korones, 1976). The newborn's entire skin area is exposed to the light for 24 to 48 hours. Phototherapy success is measured by daily serum bilirubin levels. Phototherapy plays an important role in preventing a rise in bilirubin levels but does not alter the underlying cause of jaundice, and hemolysis may continue and produce anemia.

Currently under study is the possible effect that intensified light may have on other compounds or tissues and on biorhythms. Although it is not known whether this light injures the delicate eye structures, particularly the retina, eyes are padded while the neonate is receiving phototherapy. The nurse applies eye patches over the neonate's closed eyes while under the lights (Figure 25–13). Phototherapy is discontinued and the eyes are checked and patches reapplied at least once per shift to check the condition of the eyes and to allow eye contact during feeding (social stimulation) or when parents are visiting (parental attachment). Minimal covering is applied over the genitals and buttocks to expose maximum skin surface and to protect bedding.

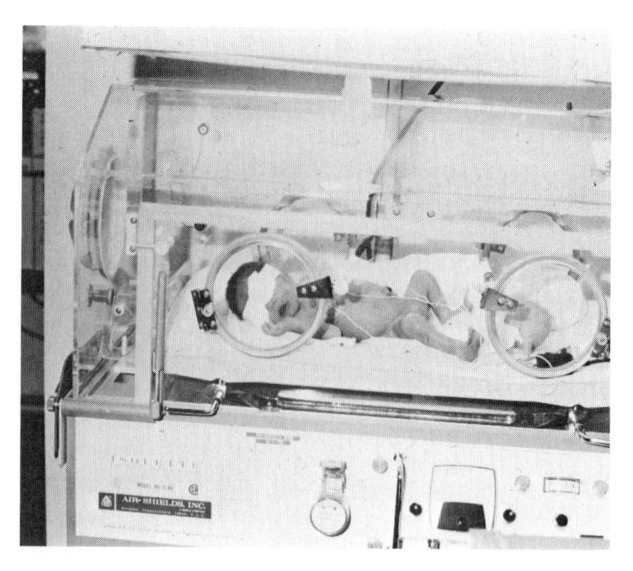

Figure 25–13. Infant receiving phototherapy. The phototherapy light is positioned over the Isolette. The infant is undressed to expose as much skin surface as possible, and bilateral patches must always be in place.

The neonate's temperature is monitored to prevent hypothermia or chilling. Stools and urine are evaluated for green color and amount. Loose green stools are often found with use of phototherapy. The neonate may require fluid replacement. Bronzing of the skin may occur, lasting two to four months with no sequelae if the neonate has a healthy liver. In addition to assessing the neonate's skin color for jaundice and bronzing, the nurse examines the skin for developing pressure areas. The neonate should be repositioned at least every two hours to permit the light to reach all skin surfaces, to prevent pressure areas, and to vary the stimulation to the infant.

The nurse keeps track of the number of hours each lamp is used so that each can be replaced before its effectiveness is lost.

Drug Therapy. Phenobarbital is capable of stimulating the liver's production of enzymes that increase conjugation of bilirubin and its excretion. This drug is effective if given to the mother prior to delivery; however, four to five days of treatment is needed to produce results postnatally. Infants who are already jaundiced or who are premature may not respond at all (Korones, 1976).

The nurse administers the medication as ordered and assesses its effectiveness in the treatment of hyperbilirubinemia. She must remain alert for signs and symptoms of negative reactions to the drug that is administered.

Other drugs have the capacity to increase conjugation of bilirubin and to keep bilirubin at levels lower than expected. These drugs are too risky to use for the prevention and treatment of neonatal jaundice.

Support of the Family

Many parents must face the mother's discharge while the neonate remains in the hospital for treatment of hyperbilirubinemia. The terms *jaundice, hyperbilirubinemia, exchange transfusion,* and *phototherapy* may sound frightening and threatening. Some parents may feel guilty that they have caused this situation to happen. On occasion, a multidisciplinary team (nurse, obstetrician, pediatrician, clergyman, genetic counselor, psychologist, or other) may collaborate in assisting the parents to cope with the situation. Under stress, parents may not be able to "hear" or understand the physician's first explanations. The nurse must expect that the parents will need explanations repeated and clarified and that they may need help voicing their questions and fears. Early eye and tactile contact with the neonate is encouraged and planned so that the nurse can be present while the parents visit the neonate. Parents are kept informed of their infant's condition and are encouraged to return to the hospital or to telephone at any time and to be involved in the care of their infant. (See the accompanying Nursing Care Plan for jaundice.)

NURSING CARE PLAN

Jaundice

Patient Data Base

History

Maternal

- Rh negative
- Presence of infection, such as syphilis, cytomegalovirus, rubella, toxoplasmosis
- Presence of familial blood dyscrasias (e.g., spherocytosis, G-6-PD deficiency)
- Medications: use of sulfonamides or salicylates interferes with conjugation or with serum albumin binding sites by competing for the sites
- Number and outcome of previous pregnancies
- Condition at birth and current health status of other children

Paternal

- Rh factor—negative or positive

Delivery

- Enlarged placenta (larger than 1/7 of neonate's weight)
- Delayed clamping of umbilical cord
- Traumatic delivery

Neonate

- Enclosed hemorrhage; hematoma; large bruises; intracranial bleeding
- Bacterial and/or viral infections can affect liver and thus decrease glucuronyl transferase activity
- Polycythemia (hematocrit of 60% or more)
- Biliary atresia

NURSING CARE PLAN Cont'd

Jaundice

Congenital hypothyroidism

Conditions that decrease available albumin binding sites:

1. Fetal or neonatal asphyxia decreases binding affinity of bilirubin to albumin
2. Chilling and hypoglycemia create free fatty acids to compete for binding sites
3. Prematures tend to have lower serum albumin levels and therefore less albumin to bind to

Physical examination

Generalized edema with pleural and pericardial effusion

Pallor or jaundice noted in first 24 to 36 hours

May have enlargement of spleen or liver

Changes in behavior (lethargy, irritability)

Dark, concentrated urine

Presence of hematomas or large bruises (assess for other signs of enclosed bleeding)

Assess vital signs

Laboratory evaluation

Coombs' test

Total bilirubin level:

Direct bilirubin greater than 3.7 mg requires exchange transfusion

Indirect bilirubin greater than 15-18 mg requires exchange transfusion

Total serum protein (provides measure of binding capacity)

CBC – assess anemia and polycythemia

Peripheral smear – evaluate red blood cells for immaturity or abnormality

CO_2 combining power – decrease is consistent with increased hemolysis

Blood glucose

Nursing Priorities

1. Observe signs of worsening conditions.
2. Monitor levels of bilirubin during therapy.
3. Provide adequate hydration.
4. Assess for signs of dehydration.
5. Provide tactile stimulation.
6. Provide parent education.

Problem	Nursing interventions and actions	Rationale
Prevention	Initiate feedings within 4 to 6 hr after delivery, if possible.	Early feeding in first 4 to 6 hr tends to discourage high bilirubin levels. Early feeding stimulates bowel activity and passage of bilirubin-containing meconium, thereby eliminating possibility of reabsorption of pigment from intestines.
	Keep infant warm.	Action necessary to prevent chill-induced acidosis, a condition that depletes serum albumin-binding sites.
	Administer phenobarbital per physician order.	Promotes hepatic clearance of bilirubin. Best results are obtained when given to mother before delivery and then administered to neonate for several days following birth.
	Identify risk factors.	Presence of risk factors necessitates more frequent assessment of neonate for development of jaundice and may include determining blood levels of bilirubin.

NURSING CARE PLAN Cont'd

Jaundice

Problem	Nursing interventions and actions	Rationale
Early identification of jaundice	Assess newborn for signs of jaundice.	Observation of jaundice may be initial sign of hyperbilirubinemia.
	1. Complete assessments in daylight, if possible.	Early detection is affected by nursery environment. Blue walls, artificial lights (with pink tint) may mask beginning of jaundice.
	2. Observe sclera.	Jaundice may first be noticed as a yellowing of the sclera.
	3. Observe skin color and assess by blanching.	Blanching the skin leaves a yellow color to the skin immediately after pressure is released.
	4. Check oral mucosa, posterior portion of hard palate, and conjunctival sacs for yellow pigmentation in dark-skinned neonates.	Underlying pigment of dark-skinned people may normally appear yellow.
Elevated level of bilirubin	Maintain treatment modalities.	Method of treatment depends on level of bilirubin, time of onset, and presence of other illness (disease states).
Bilirubin 5-9 mg/100 ml in first 24 hr or 10 to 14 mg/100 ml 24 to 48 hr after delivery	Phototherapy:	Photo-oxidation of bilirubin occurs in the skin with use of phototherapy. Photodecomposition products are largely water soluble, and can be excreted in stool and urine. Unconjugated bilirubin does not need to be bound to albumin for transport.
	1. Cover neonates eyes with eye patches while under phototherapy light.	Protects retina from damage due to high-intensity light.
	2. Remove neonate from under phototherapy light and remove eye patches during feedings.	Provides visual stimulation.
	3. Inspect eyes for conjunctivitis and corneal abrasions.	May be caused by irritation from eye patches.
	4. Cover only the diaper area.	Provides maximum exposure. Shielded areas become more jaundiced so maximum exposure is essential.
	5. Turn infant at regular intervals (e.g., every 2 hr).	Provides equal exposure of all skin areas and prevents pressure areas.
	6. Monitor neonate's skin and core temperature frequently until temperature is stable.	Hypothermia and hyperthermia are common complications of phototherapy.
	7. Provide extra fluid intake.	Assures adequate hydration.
	8. Closely assess infant's daily patterns to detect notable changes in food ingestion, bowel and urination patterns, sleeping and waking rhythms, irritability.	May indicate signs of worsening condition. Neonate may develop green, watery stools.
	9. Administer thorough perianal cleansing with each stool or change of perianal protective covering.	Frequent stooling increases risk of skin breakdown.
	10. Observe for bronzing of skin.	Uncommon complication. May last for 2 to 4 months.

NURSING CARE PLAN Cont'd

Jaundice

Problem	Nursing interventions and actions	Rationale
	11. Give 10% glucose feedings per physician order or protocol.	Increases peristalsis and excretion of bile before it can re-enter enterohepatic pathway.
	12. Record number of hours that lights have been used.	Lights may become ineffective after prolonged use.
	13. Observe signs of worsening condition (kernicterus): • hypotonia, lethargy, poor sucking reflex. • spasticity and opisthotonus. • fever. • gradual appearance of extra pyramidal signs. • impaired or absent hearing.	Deposition of bilirubin in brain leads to development of symptoms. NOTE: Treatment may be more aggressive in presence of neonatal complications such as asphyxia, respiratory distress, metabolic acidosis, hypothermia, low serum protein, signs of CNS deterioration (Avery, 1975).
Bilirubin level rising above 10 mg% in first 24 hr *or* >15 mg% after phototherapy treatment	Exchange transfusion (see Procedure 25-5):	
	1. Keep neonate NPO for 4 hr preceding exchange transfusion, or aspirate stomach contents.	Decreases chance of regurgitation and aspiration by neonate.
	2. Administer salt-poor albumin (1 gm/kg body weight) one hr before exchange transfusion.	Increases binding of bilirubin. Do not give to severely anemic or edemic neonate or to neonate with congestive heart failure, because of hazard of hypovolemia.
	3. Assess vital signs.	Provides a baseline.
	4. Position neonate in supine position and provide for warmth (see Figure 25-10).	Provides maximum visualization. Prevents chilling.
	5. Have resuscitation equipment available.	In case life support measures are necessary.
	6. Continuously monitor vital signs during exchange transfusion.	Provides data on status of neonate and response to treatment.
	7. Carefully check blood to be used for exchange.	Prevents error. Fresh O negative blood is usually used.
	8. Record time and amount of each withdrawal and addition of fresh blood.	Monitors progress.
	9. Inform physician when 100 ml of blood has been used.	Calcium gluconate is given IV after each 100 ml of blood, to decrease cardiac irritability.
	10. After the exchange, carefully monitor the following for 24 to 48 hr: • vital signs. • neurologic signs (lethargy, increased irritability, jitteriness, convulsion). • amount and color of urine. • presence of edema. • signs of necrotizing enterocolitis. • infection or hemorrhage at infusion site. • signs of increasing jaundice. • neurologic signs of kernicterus.	Provides information on status of neonate and identification of complications.
Dehydration	Assess dehydration: 1. Poor skin turgor. 2. Depressed fontanelles. 3. Sunken eyes.	Phototherapy treatment may cause liquid stools, which increases risk of dehydration. As bilirubin levels rise, neonate may become lethargic and more difficult to feed.

NURSING CARE PLAN Cont'd

Jaundice

Problem	Nursing interventions and actions	Rationale
	4. Decreased urine output. 5. Weight loss. 6. Changes in electrolytes.	
	Offer feedings every 3 to 4 hr.	
	Offer water between feedings.	Adequate hydration facilitates elimination and excretion of bilirubin.
	Administer IV fluids per physician order:	IV fluids may be used if neonate is dehydrated or in presence of other complications. IV may be started if exchange transfusion is anticipated.
	1. Monitor flow rate.	Prevents fluid overload.
	2. Assess insertion site for evidence of infection.	Identifies infection process.
Lack of tactile stimulation	Provide tactile stimulation during feeding and diaper changes.	Neonate has normal needs for tactile stimulation.
	Provide cuddling and eye contact during feedings. Talk to neonate frequently.	Provides comforting and decreased sensory deprivation.
	Encourage parents to come into nursery for feedings and to touch neonate.	Presence of equipment may discourage parents from interacting with neonate.
Inadequate parental information	Provide explanation of: 1. Infant's condition.	Parents may not understand what is happening or why.
	2. Treatment modalities.	Physician preference of treatment modalities may vary. Parents may not understand why their baby is not receiving a treatment that another baby with the same condition is receiving.
	3. Reasons that the mother may be asked to cease breast-feeding temporarily. 4. If breast-feeding is temporarily discontinued, assess mother's knowledge of pumping her breasts and provide information and support as needed.	Breast milk contains pregnanediol, which may suppress the conjugation process by inhibiting glucuronyl transferase. The serum bilirubin levels begin to fall within 48 hr after discontinuation of breast-feeding. Opinion of physicians varies regarding the need for discontinuing breast-feeding.
	5. Assist mother in reestablishment of breast-feeding.	Mother may need support and information to restart breast-feeding.

Nursing Care Evaluation

Kernicterus has been prevented.

Neonate has *no* or minimal residual damage.

Bilirubin levels are decreasing or normal.

Afebrile and vital signs are stable.

Adequate hydration and electrolyte balance has been achieved.

Tactile stimulation has been provided.

Parents understand the cause of the problem, the rationale for treatment, and subsequent care of the neonate.

If breast-feeding, the mother understands the reason for temporary discontinuation of breast-feeding, how to pump her breasts, and how to reinstate breast feedings.

NEONATAL ANEMIA

Neonatal anemia is often difficult to recognize by clinical evaluation alone. Normal hemoglobin in a neonate is about 17 gm/100 ml; infants with hemoglobin of less than 14 gm/100 ml are usually considered anemic. The most common causes of neonatal anemia are blood loss, hemolysis, and impaired red blood cell production.

Blood loss (hypovolemia) occurs in utero from placental bleeding (placenta previa or abruptio placentae). Postnatal blood loss may be fetomaternal, fetofetal, or the result of umbilical cord bleeding. Birth trauma to abdominal organs or the cranium may produce significant blood loss, and cerebral bleeding may occur due to hypoxia.

Excessive hemolysis of red cells is usually a result of blood group incompatibilities. Bacterial and nonbacterial infections and diseases are also associated with hemolytic anemias. The most common cause of impaired red cell production is a deficiency in G-6-PD (glucose-6-phosphate dehydrogenase). It is genetically transmitted, and anemia and jaundice are the presenting signs.

A condition known as "physiologic anemia" exists as a result of the normal gradual drop in hemoglobin for the first 6 to 12 weeks of life. Theoretically, the bone marrow stops production of red blood cells as a response to the elevated oxygenation of extrauterine respiration. When the hemoglobin becomes lower at about 6 to 12 weeks of age, the bone marrow begins to manufacture red blood cells again, and the anemia disappears spontaneously. Rarely does the hemoglobin level fall low enough to require a transfusion.

Clinically, anemic infants are very pale in the absence of other symptoms of shock and usually are found to have abnormally low red blood cell count. In acute blood loss, symptoms of shock may be present, such as pallor, low arterial blood pressure, and a decreasing hematocrit. The initial laboratory workup should include hemoglobin and hematocrit, reticulocyte count, examination of peripheral blood smear, direct Coombs' test of infant's blood, and examination of maternal blood smear for fetal erythrocytes.

Hematologic problems can be anticipated based on the obstetric history and clinical manifestations. The age at which anemia is first noted is also of diagnostic value. Management depends on severity and whether blood loss is acute or chronic. The infant should be placed on constant cardiac/respiratory monitoring. Mild or slow chronic anemia may be treated adequately with iron supplements alone or with iron-fortified formulas. Frequent determinations of hemoglobin, hematocrit, and bilirubin level (in hemolytic disease) are essential. In severe cases of anemia, transfusions are the treatment of choice.

The nurse must be aware of and promptly report any symptoms and should assist in obtaining blood specimens and taking care of specimen sites. Prophylactic measures carried out by the nurse include meticulous hand-washing and careful equipment cleaning to help prevent sepsis and subsequent hemolysis.

INFECTIONS

Sepsis Neonatorum

Neonates up to one month of age are particularly susceptible to infection, referred to as *sepsis neonatorum,* caused by organisms that do not cause significant disease in older children. Incidence of severe infection is 0.5–2 per 1000 live newborns.

One predisposing factor is prematurity. The general debilitation and underlying illness often associated with prematurity necessitates invasive procedures such as umbilical catheterization, intubation, resuscitation, ventilatory support, and monitoring. Even the full-term infant is susceptible because of his immature immunologic system, which lacks the complex factors involved in effective phagocytosis and the ability to effectively localize infection or to respond with a well-defined recognizable inflammatory response. Maternal antepartal infections such as rubella, toxoplasmosis, cytomegalic inclusion disease, and herpes may cause congenital infections and resulting disorders within the newborn. Intrapartal maternal infections such as amnionitis and those resulting from premature rupture of membranes and precipitous delivery are sources of neonatal infection. Passage through the birth canal and contact with colonization of the vaginal flora (β-hemolytic streptococci, herpes, listeria, and gonococci) exposes the infant to infection. With infection anywhere in the fetus or newborn, the adjacent tissues or organs are very easily penetrated, and the blood-brain barrier is ineffective. Septicemia is more common in males, except for those infections caused by group B β-hemolytic streptococcus.

The etiology of sepsis has changed in recent years. In the past, gram-positive organisms (that is, *Staphylococcus aureus* and A-streptococcus pneumococci) were the causative agents of significant neonatal illness. At present, gram-negative organisms (especially *Escherichia coli,* Aerobacter, Proteus, and *Klebsiella*) and the gram-positive organism B β-hemolytic streptococci are the most common causative agents. Pseudomonas is a common contaminant of fomites used for ventilatory support and oxygen therapy.

Clinical Manifestations and Diagnosis

Sepsis neonatorum is characterized by positive blood cultures and generalized clinical manifestations of illness, which are subtle and nonspecific and may be caused by other problems. Early detection of sepsis is extremely important. Symptoms are most often noticed by the nurse in her daily care of the neonate rather than during the sporadic contact of the physician. The most common symptoms are:

1. Usually a subtle behavioral change—infant "isn't doing well"; often lethargy, especially after first 24 hours, and hypotonia. Color changes may include pallor, duskiness, cyanosis, or a "shocky" appearance. Skin is cool and clammy.
2. Temperature instability, manifested by either hypothermia (recognized by a decrease in skin temperature) or hyperthermia (elevation of neonatal skin temperature) necessitating a corresponding increase or decrease in incubator temperature to maintain neutral thermal environment.
3. Poor feeding, evidenced by a decrease in total intake, abdominal distention, vomiting, poor sucking, lack of interest in feeding, and diarrhea.

Signs and symptoms may suggest central nervous system disease (jitteriness, tremors, seizure activity), respiratory system disease (tachypnea, labored respirations, apnea, cyanosis), hematologic disease (jaundice, petechial hemorrhages, hepatosplenomegaly), or gastrointestinal disease (diarrhea, vomiting, bile-stained aspirate, hepatomegaly). A differential diagnosis is necessary because of the similarity of symptoms to other more specific conditions.

Isolation of the causative agent is necessary to obtain the diagnosis of sepsis in a suspected case and to identify the drugs to which the pathogen is susceptible. The nurse must be prepared to assist in the aseptic collection of specimens for laboratory investigation. Before antibiotic therapy is begun, cultures are obtained (Gotoff and Behrman, 1970):

1. Blood culture is obtained from a peripheral, rather than umbilical, vessel, because catheters have yielded false positives resulting from contamination. Prepare the skin by cleansing with an antiseptic solution, such as one containing iodine; allow skin to dry and obtain the specimen with a sterile needle/syringe.
2. Spinal fluid culture is obtained following a spinal tap.
3. Urine culture is best obtained from a specimen obtained by a suprapubic bladder aspiration.
4. Skin cultures are obtained of any lesions or drainage from lesions or reddened areas.
5. Nasopharyngeal, rectal, or ear canal cultures may be obtained.

Other laboratory investigations include a complete blood count, chest x-ray examination, serology, and Gram's stains of cerebrospinal fluid, urine, skin exudate, and umbilicus. White blood count and differential may be helpful after 24 hours of age. A level of 30,000 WBC may be normal in the first 24 hours of life. Stomach aspirate should be sent for culture and smear if a gonococcal infection and amnionitis are suspected. Serum

IgM levels are elevated (normal level less than 20 mg/100 ml) in response to transplacental infections. Evidence of congenital infections may be seen on skull x-rays for cerebral calcifications (cytomegalovirus, toxoplasmosis), bone x-rays (syphilis, cytomegalovirus), and serum-specific IgM levels (rubella). Cytomegalovirus (CMV) infection is best diagnosed by urine cultures.

Nursing Management

Treatment

Because neonatal infection causes high mortality, therapy is often instituted before results of the septic workup are obtained. A combination of two broad-spectrum antibiotics in large doses is initiated until culture with sensitivities is received.

After the pathogen and its sensitivities are determined, appropriate specific antibiotic therapy is begun. Combinations of penicillin or ampicillin and kanamycin have been utilized in the past, but increasing kanamycin-resistant enterobacteria and penicillin-resistant staphylococcus necessitate increasing use of gentamycin. Duration of therapy varies from seven to ten days (Table 25-4).

In administration of antibiotics the nurse must be knowledgeable about: (a) the proper dose to be administered, based on the weight of the newborn; (b) the appropriate route of administration, as some antibiotics cannot be given intravenously; (c) admixture incompatibilities (some antibiotics are precipitated by intravenous solutions or by other antibiotics); and (d) side effects and toxicity.

In addition to antibiotic therapy, physiologic supportive care is essential in caring for a septic infant:

1. Observe for resolution of symptoms or development of other symptoms of sepsis.
2. Maintain neutral thermal environment with

Table 25-4. Neonatal Sepsis Antibiotic Therapy

Drug	Dose	Route	Schedule	Comments
Ampicillin	100-200 mg/kg/day	IM or IV	Every 12 hours*	Effective against gram-positive microorganisms and majority of *E. coli* strains
Gentamycin	3-7.5 mg/kg/day	IM or IV	Every 12 hours (preterm)* Every 8 hours (term)*	May be used instead of kanamycin, against penicillin-resistant staphylococci and *E. coli* strains and *Pseudomonas aeruginosa*
Kanamycin	15 mg/kg/day	IM	Every 8-12 hours	Initial sepsis therapy effective against almost all gram-negative organisms with exception of pseudomonas; not to be used for more than 12 days
Noficillin	50 mg/kg/day	IM or IV	Every 12 hours*	Effective against penicillin-resistant strains; nephrotoxic
Neomycin	50-100 mg/kg/day	Oral	Every 6 hours	Effective against enteropathic *E. coli*
Penicillin G (aqueous crystalline)	100,000 U/kg/day	IM or IV	Every 12 hours*	Initial sepsis therapy effective against most gram-positive microorganisms except resistant staphylococci; can cause heart block in infants

*Up to 7 days of age.

accurate regulation of humidity and oxygen administration.

3. Provide respiratory support—administer oxygen and observe and monitor respiratory effort.
4. Provide cardiovascular support—observe and monitor pulse and blood pressure; observe for hyperbilirubinemia, anemia, and hemorrhagic symptoms.
5. Provide adequate calories, because oral feedings may be discontinued due to increased mucus, abdominal distention, vomiting, and aspiration.
6. Provide fluids and electrolytes to maintain homeostasis.
7. Detect and treat metabolic disturbances, a common occurrence.
8. Observe for the development of hypoglycemia, acidosis, hyponatremia, and hypocalcemia.

Prevention

Protection of the newborn from infections starts prenatally and continues throughout pregnancy and through delivery into the world.

Prenatal prevention should include maternal screening for venereal disease and monitoring of rubella titers in mothers who are negative. Intrapartally, sterile technique is essential, smears from genital lesions are taken, placenta and amniotic fluid cultures are obtained if amnionitis is suspected and if genital herpes is present toward term, and delivery by cesarean section may be indicated. Local eye treatment with silver nitrate or an antibiotic ophthalmic ointment is given to all babies to prevent gonococcal damage.

In the nursery, environmental control and prevention of acquired infection is the responsibility of the neonatal nurse. Being the vanguard of infection control, the nurse must promote vigorous, strict hand-washing technique for all who enter the nursery, including nursing colleagues; physicians; laboratory, x-ray, and inhalation technicians; and parents. Scrupulous care of equipment—changing and cleaning of incubators at least every seven days, removal and sterilization of wet equipment every 24 hours, prevention of cross-utilization of linen and other equipment, periodic cleaning of sinkside equipment such as soap containers, and special care with the open radiant warmers (access without prior hand-washing is much easier than with the closed incubator)—will all prevent fomite contamination or contamination through improper hand-washing of debilitated, infection-prone newborns. An infected neonate can be effectively isolated in an incubator and receive close observation. Visitation of the nursery area by unnecessary personnel should be discouraged. Restriction of visiting parents has not been shown to have any effect on the rate of infection and may indeed be harmful for the baby's psychologic development. With instruction and supervision from the nurse, both parents should be allowed to handle the baby and participate in his care, even inside the incubators.

Syphilis

Because congenital syphilis is difficult to detect at birth, all infants of syphilitic mothers should be screened to determine the the necessity of treatment. Diagnostic serologic dilution tests are usually accurate between 3 and 6 months of age. The development and detection of the infant's own antibodies is essential for diagnosis.

By 3 months of age the congenitally infected infant exhibits the following signs:

1. Positive serology; elevated cord serum, immunoglobulin M (IgM).
2. Vesicular lesions over palms and soles.
3. Red rash around mouth and anus; copper-colored rash covering face, palms, and soles.
4. Hepatosplenomegaly.
5. Irritability.
6. Rhinitis (sniffles); fissures at mouth corners and on excoriated upper lip.
7. Pyrexia.
8. Painful extremities.
9. Bone lesions.
10. Generalized edema, particularly over joints.
11. Jaundice.
12. Small for gestational age (SGA) and failure to thrive (FTT).

The nursing management of these infants and their parents requires careful physical and psychologic care. Drug treatment of choice is penicillin. After proper treatment for 48 hours, the infant should not be contagious. Initially, nursing care includes use of isolation techniques. However, following treatment, general care may ensue. This would include basic assessment of axillary temperature every three to four hours; intake and output record; feedings; and infant's tolerances. The baby should be swaddled for comfort, and his hands should be covered to minimize trauma to his skin from scratching. Support to the parents is crucial. They need to be informed of the infant's prognosis as treatment continues and to be involved in care as much as possible. They need to understand how infection is transmitted. It is essential to avoid judging the parents, and encourage positive parental involvement.

Gonorrhea

Gonorrhea may be contracted by the fetus during vaginal delivery. Gonorrhea is usually manifested clinically as an eye infection, ophthalmia neonatorum. This is first diagnosed as a conjunctivitis that is indistinguishable from that caused by silver nitrate instillation. However, one clue is that chemical conjunctivitis disappears within 24 hours, whereas ophthalmia neonatorum becomes more readily apparent in the neonate on the third or fourth postnatal day. Other more severe clinical signs that develop are a purulent discharge and ulcerations of the cornea, which can be prevented if treatment is instituted promptly. In some cases, gonorrhea infection may be observed as temperature instability, poor feeding response, and/or hypotonia.

For neonates of all vaginal births, at delivery a 1% silver nitrate solution is instilled in the conjunctiva of the infant's eyes to prevent infection. It is imperative that delivery room nurses carefully instill the chemical and that they do not use normal saline to irrigate the eye following instillation. The normal saline precipitates the silver nitrate rapidly, making it ineffective. Therefore sterile water is used as an irrigant to decrease the chemical conjunctivitis caused by silver nitrate. Penicillin may also be administered topically and systemically, in lieu of silver nitrate. If allergy to penicillin is suspected, erythromycin, a tetracycline, or chloramphenicol may be substituted. If the infant's eyes are left untreated, partial or complete loss of vision may occur as a result of corneal ulceration. Some centers delay instillation of silver nitrate or any eye prophylactics until admission to the nursery in order to facilitate bonding in the delivery room; others postpone the instillation until after the neonate's first period of reactivity.

Herpesvirus Type 2

A wide variety of clinical manifestations of herpesvirus type 2 are noted in the neonate. Signs and symptoms are present at birth or by 3–4 weeks of age. The disseminated form is seen as a bleeding tendency, hepatitis with jaundice, hepatosplenomegaly, and neurologic abnormalities. About one-third of affected infants exhibit vesicular skin lesions in small clusters all over the body. The more localized form includes convulsions (focal or generalized), abnormal muscle tone, opisthotonus, a bulging fontanelle, and lethargy or coma and carries very high mortality rates. In the eyes, keratitis (cloudy corneas), conjunctivitis, and chorioretinitis are seen. Another form is asymptomatic at birth and can develop symptomatology up to 21 days after birth. Frequently the skin lesions are the only diagnostic finding.

In the absence of skin lesions, diagnosis is difficult, because the presenting clinical picture resembles septicemia (such as fever or subnormal temperature, respiratory congestion, dyspnea, cough, tachypnea, and tachycardia). It is therefore necessary to obtain cultures from the infant's lesions and throat and to identify the herpesvirus type 2 antibodies in the serum IgM fraction. Positive cultures are observable within 24 to 48 hours.

Therapy has consisted of treatment systemically with idoxuridine (IDU), which has been successful in some infants and of no avail in others (Korones, 1976). Other drug therapy includes cytosine arabinoside (ara-C) and adenine arabinoside (ara-A) (Amstey et al., 1976), all of which are immunosuppressive in nature. Careful handwashing and adequate infection-control methods are essential. Isolation measures should be instituted for all infants born to mothers known to have had third trimester infections.

Monilial Infection (Thrush)

Thrush (oral moniliasis) is caused by the fungus *Candida albicans*, contracted from a yeast-infected vagina during delivery. Clinically, it appears as white plaques distributed on the buccal mucosa, on the tongue, on the gums, inside the cheeks, and even on the lips. As it resembles milk curds, differentiation should be made by using a cotton-tipped applicator to gently attempt wiping away the patches. If the plaques are thrush, a raw bleeding area beneath them will be exposed. Involvement of the diaper area skin is seen as a bright red, well-demarcated eruption. On occasion, generalized moniliasis may be seen. Lesions are most frequently seen at about 5–7 days of age.

Care of the neonate infected with *Candida albicans* involves:

1. Maintaining cleanliness of hands, bedding, clothing, diapers, and feeding apparatus, because *Candida albicans* is present in the oral secretions and in the stools. Breast-feeding mothers should be instructed on treating their nipples with topical nystatin; otherwise a cycle of reinfection as well as sore nipples with breakdown of nipple tissue will occur.

2. Supporting physiologic well-being.

3. Administering drug therapy. Gential violet (1%–2%) is swabbed on oral mucosa, usually an hour after feeding once or twice a day; nystatin (Mycostatin) is instilled in the oral cavity with a medicine dropper. The mouth should be cleared of milk prior to instillation. It may also be swabbed over the oral mucosa. Topical nystatin is used for skin involvement.

4. Discussing with the parents that gential violet is a dye and will cause staining of the infant's mouth and possibly the infant's clothing if the saliva is gentian colored.

HEMORRHAGIC DISEASE

Several transient coagulation-mechanism deficiencies normally occur in the first several days of a newborn's life. Foremost among these is a slight decrease in the levels of prothrombin, resulting in a prolonged clotting time during the initial week of life. In order for the liver to form prothrombin (Factor II) and proconvertin (Factor VII) for blood coagulation, vitamin K is required. Vitamin K, a fat-soluble vitamin, may be obtained from food, but it is usually synthesized by bacteria in the colon, and consequently, a dietary source is unnecessary (Guyton, 1971).

Intestinal flora are practically nonexistent in the newborn, so he is unable to synthesize vitamin K. Although cow's milk contains more vitamins than breast milk, neither is a rich source. However, hemorrhagic disease of the newborn is more common in breast-fed babies. Bleeding due to vitamin K deficiency generally occurs on the second to third day of life, but it may occur earlier. Internal hemorrhage may occur. There may also be bleeding from the nose, umbilical cord, circumcision site, gastrointestinal tract, and scalp, as well as generalized ecchymosis.

This disorder may be completely prevented by the prophylactic use of an injection of vitamin K: 10 mg of Aquamephyton is given as part of the immediate care of the newborn following delivery. Larger doses are contraindicated, because they may result in the development of hyperbilirubinemia.

NECROTIZING ENTEROCOLITIS

With recent advances in the field of neonatology, severely ill infants who a decade ago would have succumbed are now surviving. With this increased survival, a group of infants are now being encountered with necrotizing enterocolitis. A previously unknown disease, necrotizing enterocolitis (NEC) occurs in the first weeks of life and may cause bowel perforation and ultimately death.

The occurrence of a "new" disease entity produces a flourish of theories as to the etiology. With NEC, the exact causation is not known, but some predisposing factors are associated with subsequent development of the disease.

An ischemic attack to the intestine may be precipitated by any condition in which systemic shock and hypoxia occur (Roback et al., 1974). Such conditions as fetal distress, neonatal shock and asphyxia, low Apgar score, respiratory distress syndrome, umbilical arterial catheters, infusion of hyperosmolar solution, and prematurity are associated with NEC. The diving reflex of the seal, in which blood is shunted to the heart and brain and away from the intestine and kidneys during prolonged dives, is thought to be analogous to the shunting of blood in asphyxial insults of the neonate.

Prolonged intestinal ischemia results in thrombosis in small intestinal vessels, infarction of affected bowels, and digestion of the mucosal lining of the intestine. Reestablishment of normal circulation enables restoration and regeneration of the damaged area if the damage is reversible (Touloukian et al., 1967).

The action of enteric bacteria on the damaged intestinal mucosa may serve to complicate the process, producing sepsis. Early feedings, advocated for promotion of adequate nutrition, provide excellent media for proliferation of intestinal bacteria. Gas formation and possible dissection of air into the portal system is a result of bacterial action upon the media provided by oral feedings. Some recent investigations have shown breast milk to be safer in feedings for the at-risk group. It is postulated that the antibodies present in breast colostrum act as a protector for the intestinal mucosa. Necrotic lesions are seen in any part of the intestine below the duodenum but are commonly seen in the lower ileum, the ascending and transverse colon, or both. The lesions are characterized by frequent mucosal ulcerations, pseudomembrane formation, and inflammation; radiologic examination reveals pneumatosis intestinalis and possible sequelae of perforation.

Clinical Manifestations and Diagnosis

The neonatal nurse, providing constant bedside care, is often the first person to observe the subtle signs and symptoms of early development of the disease. Recognition of the above-mentioned high-risk groups, careful observation for subtle, nonspecific symptoms, and prompt reporting of suspicions enable early, often life-saving treatment to begin. Onset usually occurs within the first two to three weeks of life. Systemic symptoms are those associated with sepsis—temperature instability (often hypothermia), respiratory changes (apnea, labored respirations), cardiovascular collapse, and behavioral changes such as lethargy or irritability. Gastrointestinal symptoms include abdominal distention and tenderness, feeding changes such as vomiting or increased gastric residual (bile-stained), poor feeding, abdominal wall cellulitis (development of an erythematous area on the abdominal wall), and blood in the stools (Hematest positive).

Clinical findings are corroborated by radiographic findings, which include (a) pneumatosis intestinalis—air in the bowel wall (extraluminal or intramural air bubble and strips); (b) adynamic ileus—a paralytic ileus with stasis; (c) bowel wall thickening and loops of unequal size, bubbly appearance of intestine; and (d) free air—pneumoperitoneum or free air in the portal vein (Touloukian et al., 1967).

Serial anteroposterior and lateral decubitus (or cross-table lateral abdominal) radiographic evaluation is recommended every four to six hours for detection of progression of the disease and determination of complications indicating surgical intervention (Master et al., 1974).

Complications

Complications or consequences of necrotizing enterocolitis include (a) surgical removal of the diseased intestine so that there is insufficient remaining small bowel to support life; (b) stenosis of the intestinal tract that develops secondary to NEC or surgery; (c) gastrointestinal dysfunction so that there is recurring intolerance to oral feedings, with vomiting, abdominal distention, water-loss diarrhea, and failure to gain weight; (d) parenteral hyperalimentation that predisposes to sepsis, thrombosis of major vessel, and metabolic complications such as hyperglycemia, glycosuria, acidosis, osmotic diuresis, dehydration, and hepatic damage; and (e) prolonged hospitalization with separation from parents and possible lack of appropriate developmental stimuli.

Interventions

Necrotizing enterocolitis is of increasing concern in the management of sick neonates. Survival of the infants depends on early recognition and treatment and meticulous nursing care.

Aggressive and early management may preclude the need for surgical intervention. Intensive nursing management consists of supportive therapy and constant observation of the neonate's condition (see the Nursing Care Plan on necrotizing enterocolitis). Gastric decompression, fluid and electrolyte replacement, correction of acidosis, correction of temperature instability, and parenteral antibiotics are common treatment techniques. Diffusion of volume expanders such as fresh frozen plasma may be necessary to correct existing hypotension and to improve peripheral perfusion, because large amounts of plasma protein are lost into the gut lumen and peritoneal cavity in the acute phase.

The nurse must be prepared to place a gastric tube for gastric decompression and drainage and must be prepared for possible instillation of oral

NURSING CARE PLAN

Necrotizing Enterocolitis

Patient Data Base

History

Prematurity

Gestational history: fetal distress, asphyxia, fetal acidosis

Neonatal history: low Apgar, hypovolemia, respiratory distress syndrome, utilization of umbilical catheters and/or infusion of hyperosmolar solution, bacterial infections; no clinical manifestations until about 1-2 weeks of age

Feeding patterns: changes, poor feeding, increased gastric residual

Physical examination

Hypothermia, apneic episodes, labored respirations, lethargy or irritability

Gastrointestinal signs: abdominal distention, shiny abdominal wall and tenderness, abdominal wall cellulitis, diarrheal stools

Vomiting (may be bile-stained)

Absence of bowel sounds

Laboratory evaluation

Hematest positive stools

Radiologic examination: pneumatosis intestinalis, adynamic ileus, thickening of bowel wall and bowel loops of unequal size, and pneumoperitoneum or free air in the portal vein

Nursing Priorities

1. Achieve early recognition by doing Hematests at least once per shift.
2. Determine and correct acid-base imbalances.
3. Provide support measures to maintain homeostasis; that is, maintain neutral thermal environment and provide adequate fluid and electrolytes.
4. Observe for progression of clinical manifestations indicating surgical intervention.
5. Preoperative management: maintain gastric decompression.
6. Provide for the emotional needs of the infant.
7. Provide parents with adequate explanation of treatment modalities and baby's condition plus anticipatory information about colostomy if surgery is pending.

Problem	Nursing interventions and actions	Rationale
Early recognition	Hematest stools at least every shift. Evaluate any changes in feeding patterns: 1. Poor feeding. 2. Bile-stained emesis. 3. Increase in gastric residual.	Increased gastric retention is caused by prolonged gastric emptying.

NURSING CARE PLAN Cont'd

Necrotizing Enterocolitis

Problem	Nursing interventions and actions	Rationale
	Auscultate bowel sounds. Measure abdominal girth every 4-6 hr if NEC is suspected.	
Ischemia of bowel	Discontinue oral feedings for 7-10 days.	Rests bowel.
	Insert gastric tube if not already being gavaged.	Provides for gastric decompression and drainage.
	Prevent trauma to abdomen: 1. Avoid diapers.	Diapers place pressure on lower abdomen and obstruct good observation of abdomen for any changes in condition.
	2. Pick up infant only when necessary.	Minimal handling prevents abdominal trauma.
	Observe for signs of perforation of bowel and peritonitis and increasing distention.	
	Take axillary temperature.	Rectal temperatures are contraindicated. Decreases trauma to rectal mucosa.
Acid-base imbalance	Administer parenteral fluid and electrolyte replacements as ordered. Observe vital signs. Monitor electrolytes.	Corrects acid-base imbalance.
Infection	Administer broad-spectrum parenteral antibiotic or oral antibiotic (through gastric tube). Obtain blood, urine, and stool cultures for sepsis workup.	Combats infectious process if present.
Shock	Observe for signs of shock (temperature instability, drop in blood pressure, apneic spells, bradycardia, listlessness).	
	Administer fresh frozen plasma per doctor's order.	Improves peripheral perfusion and corrects existing hypotension caused by shift of large amounts of plasma protein into gut lumen and peritoneal cavity.
	Administer dextran.	Dextran counters platelet adherence.
Lack of physical stimulation	Stroke hands and head. Talk to infant as often as possible, even in absence of tactile stimulation. Provide visual and auditory stimulation—mobiles, windup toys, music boxes, etc.	Meets emotional and sensory stimulation needs.

Nursing Care Evaluation

Stool Hematest is negative for three consecutive days.

Infant is afebrile and vital signs are stable.

Infant tolerates food and fluids.

Parents understand need for continual medical supervision.

Parent-infant bonding is appropriate.

antibiotics through the gastric tube and administration of parenteral fluids, calories, and antibiotics. Arterial oxygenation must be maintained. Constant observation of vital signs, oxygen concentration, development of increasing abdominal girth, and worsening clinical condition is the responsibility of the nurse.

Surgery is indicated at the development of intestinal perforation with pneumoperitoneum, intestinal infarction without perforation, progressive abdominal ascites and/or bowel wall thickening, and clinical deterioration. Even small or subtle changes may indicate rapid progression and worsening of the disease and the need for immediate surgical intervention.

Surgical intervention consists of removal of those areas of bowel that are necrotic or perforated. Intestinal areas of compromised circulation or questionable viability are usually preserved, in hopes of eventual recovery and regeneration. Primary anastomosis is not attempted because of the possibility of connecting areas of ischemic bowel. The infant returns with a gastrostomy in place to decompress the intestinal tract and an ostomy for drainage.

Meticulous nursing care is required in maintenance of skin integrity around the openings in these debilitated infants. Reestablishment of continuity of the intestines is done when the infant can tolerate oral feedings and when his general health is improved.

Recovery of the intestinal mucosa and return to proper small bowel functioning (in nutritional absorption) are delayed after enterocolitis (with or without surgical intervention). The small bowel mucosa must recover from the ischemia and regenerate to resume its function of absorption of nutrients. Meanwhile, parenteral hyperalimentation is utilized to maintain positive nitrogen balance, so that healing is promoted. After rest of the gastrointestinal tract, cautious feedings are begun, using elemental formulas (such as Vivonix) to promote easy absorption.

SUMMARY

The sick neonate—whether preterm, term, or postterm—must be managed within narrow physiologic parameters. These parameters (respiratory and thermal regulation) will maintain physiologic homeostasis and prevent introduction of iatrogenic stress to the already stressed infant. Maintenance of this physiologic environment must begin immediately, because lost ground is difficult or impossible to recover.

The nursing care of the neonate with special problems involves the understanding of normal physiology, the pathophysiology of the disease process, clinical manifestations, and supportive and corrective therapies. Only with this theoretical background can the nurse make appropriate observations concerning responses to therapy and development of complications. The neonate communicates his needs only by his behavior; the neonatal nurse, through objective observations and evaluations, interprets this behavior into meaningful information about the infant's condition.

SUGGESTED ACTIVITIES

1. Based on a prenatal record of a complicated pregnancy and labor and delivery, identify the potential risks to the neonate, appropriate nursing assessments, and necessary intervention.
2. In the classroom laboratory or a neonatal intensive care nursery, handle and determine the functioning of special equipment such as phototherapy units, open-bed radiant heaters, and incubators.
3. You are in the nursery and receive a telephone call from the delivery room nurse informing you that the delivery of a mother of 30 weeks' gestation is imminent. What preparation would you make for this infant?
4. While in the intensive care nursery, utilize the Silverman-Andersen scoring tool to assess the respiratory status of a premature infant with RDS and a premature infant in no distress. Compare your findings with your classmates' findings.
5. Locate the neonatal emergency drug box in your delivery room and intensive care nursery, identify the medicines, give the rationale for use of each, and describe the method of administration, drug range, and expected action.

REFERENCES

Amstey, M. S., et al. Jan. 1976. Herpesvirus infection in the newborn: its treatment by exchange transfusion and adenosine arabinoside. *Obstet. Gynecol.* 47(suppl.):33.

Avery, G. B. 1975. *Neonatology: pathophysiology and management of the newborn.* Philadelphia: J. B. Lippincott Co.

Behrman, R. E., ed. 1973. *Neonatology: diseases of the fetus and infant.* St. Louis: The C. V. Mosby Co.

Carson, B. S., et al. Nov. 1976. Combined obstetrical and pediatric approach to prevent meconium aspiration syndrome. *Am. J. Obstet. Gynecol.* 126:712.

Gluck, L., and Kulovich, M. May 1973. Fetal lung development. *Pediatr. Clin. N. Am.* 20:367.

Gotoff, S. P., and Behrman, R. D. 1970. Neonatal septicemia. *J. Pediatr.* 76:142.

Guyton, A. C. 1971. *Textbook of medical physiology.* 4th ed. Philadelphia: W. B. Saunders Co.

Jones, M. D. 1976. Equipment for neonatal resuscitation. Lecture at Perinatal Medicine Workshop, Snowmass, Colorado. University of Colorado School of Medicine.

Kempe, C. H., et al. 1978. *Current pediatric diagnosis and treatment.* Los Altos, Calif.: Lange Medical Publications.

Klaus, M. H., and Fanaroff, A. A. 1973. *Care of the high-risk neonate.* Philadelphia: W. B. Saunders Co.

Korones, S. B. 1976. *High-risk newborn infants: the basis for intensive nursing care.* 2nd ed. St. Louis: The C. V. Mosby Co.

Master, S., et al. Dec. 1973. Necrotizing enterocolitis. *Br. J. Radiol.* 46:1063.

Modanlou, H. D. 1976. Identification and resuscitation of the high-risk infant. Lecture on Critical Care of the Neonate. University of Colorado Medical Center.

Roback, S., et al. Aug. 1974. Necrotizing enterocolitis: an emerging entity in the regional infant intensive care facility. *Arch. Surg.* 109:314.

Saling, E. 1972. Technical and theoretical problems in electronic monitoring of the human fetal heart. *Internat. J. Gynecol. Obstet.* 10:211.

Silverman, W. A., and Andersen, D. H. 1956. A controlled clinical trial of effects of water mist on obstructive respiratory signs; death rate and necropsy findings among premature infants. *Pediatr.* 17:1.

Touloukian, R. J., et al. Oct. 1967. Surgical experience with necrotizing enterocolitis in the infant. *J. Pediatr. Surg.* 2:389.

ADDITIONAL READINGS

Abramson, H., ed. 1973. *Resuscitation of the newborn infant.* 3rd ed. St. Louis: The C. V. Mosby Co.

Affonso, D., and Harris, T. April 1976. CPAP: continuous positive airway pressure. *Am. J. Nurs.* 76:570.

Aladjem, S., ed. 1975. *Risks in the practice of modern obstetrics.* 2nd ed. St. Louis: The C. V. Mosby Co.

Aladjem, S., and Brown, A., eds. 1974. *Clinical perinatology.* St. Louis: The C. V. Mosby Co.

Bahr, J. E. Jan.–Feb. 1978. Herpesvirus: hominis type 2 in women and newborns. *MCN,* 3:16.

Bliss, V. J. Jan.–Feb. 1976. Nursing care for infants with neonatal necrotizing enterocolitis. *MCN.* 1:37.

Brazie, J. V., and Lubchenco, L. O. Oct. 1973. The newborn infant. In *Current pediatrics diagnosis and treatment.* 3rd ed. Los Altos, Calif.: Lange Medical Publications.

Brunner, L., and Suddarth, D., eds. 1974. *The Lippincott manual of nursing practice.* Philadelphia: J. B. Lippincott Co.

Gluck, L. May 1972. Surfactant. *Pediatr. Clin. N. Am.,* 19:325.

Goplerud, C., et al. 1973. The first Rh-isoimmunized pregnancy. *Am. J. Obstet. Gynecol.* 115:632.

Gregory, G. A. 1972. Respiratory care of newborn infants. *Pediatr. Clin. N. Am.* 19:311.

Hyperbilirubinemia and bacterial infection in the newborn. August 1975. *Arch. Dis. Child.,* 50:652.

Jensen, M., et al. 1977. *Maternity care: the nurse and the family.* St. Louis: The C. V. Mosby Co.

Massi, G., et al. 1974. Low dosage anti-immunoglobulin in the prevention of rhesus isoimmunization. *J. Obstet. Gynecol. Br. Commonw.* 81:87.

Meier, W. A. Sept.–Oct. 1977. Fetal respiratory development and adaptation to extrauterine life. *Perinatology/Neonatology.* 2:29.

Moncrieff, M. W., and Dunn, J. Feb. 1976. Phototherapy for hyperbilirubinemia in very low birthweight infants. *Arch. Dis. Child.* 51:124.

Nahmais, A. J., et al. Dec. 1972. Significance of herpes simplex virus infection during pregnancy. *Clin. Obstet. Gynecol.* 15:929.

Nalepka, C. D. Dec. 1975. The oxygen hood for newborn in respiratory distress. *AJN.* 75:85.

Pierog, S., and Nigam, S. Feb. 1976. Neonatal sepsis. *Pediatr. Ann.* 5:63.

Reid, W., and Shannon, M. March 31, 1973. Necrotizing enterocolitis: a medical approach to treatment. *Can. Med. Ass. J.* 108:573.

Reynolds, E. O. R., et al. 1975. Management of hyaline membrane disease. *Br. Med. Bull.* 31:1.

Richmond, J., and Mikety, V. 1975. Benign form of necrotizing enterocolitis. *Am. J. Radiol.* 123(2):301.

Roach, L. B. 1972. Skin changes in dark skin. *Nurs. '72.* 2:22.

Sinclair, J. C. 1970. Premature baby who "forgets to breathe." *N. Engl. J. Med.* 282:508.

Wilson, H. D., and Eichenwold, H. F. 1974. Sepsis neonatorum. *Pediatr. Clin. N. Am.* 21:571.

CHAPTER 26

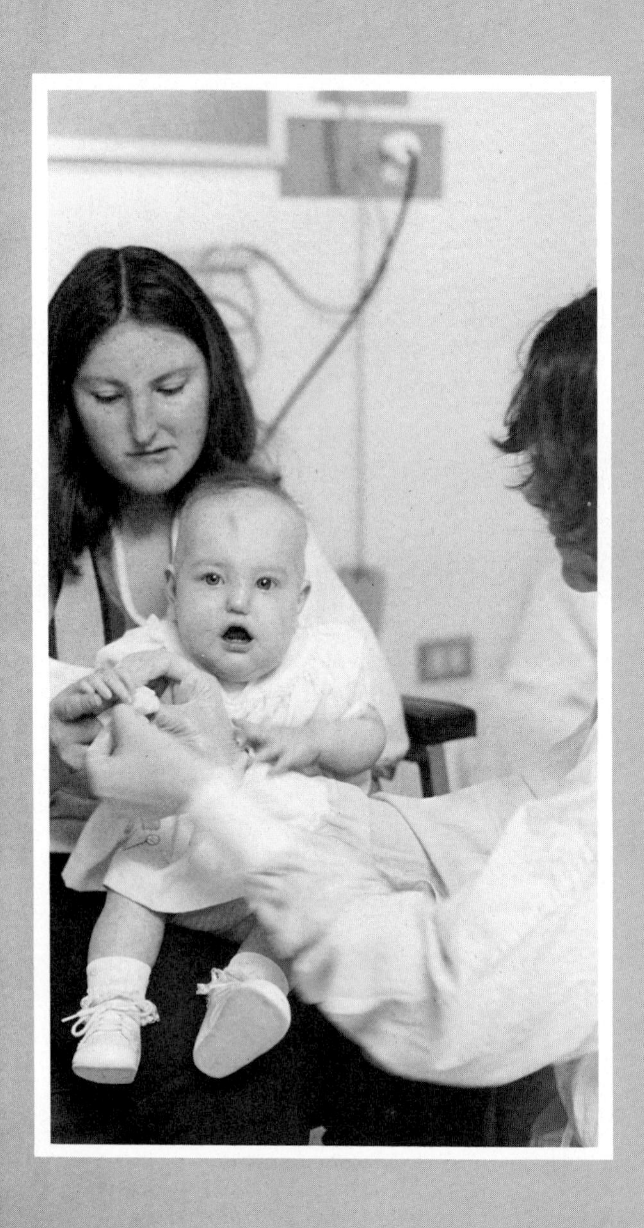

CONGENITAL ANOMALIES

OBJECTIVES

- Discuss the emotional impact on the family of the birth of a child with a defect.
- Identify methods a nurse may utilize to assist a family in dealing with the crisis produced by the birth of a defective child.
- Relate the pathophysiology of the Pierre Robin syndrome to the nursing care indicated for an infant with this disorder.
- Compare the nursing care of an infant with cleft lip to that of an infant with cleft palate.
- Identify the major types of esophageal atresia and tracheoesophageal fistula, and correlate the clinical manifestations with the anatomic malformations.
- Discuss the basic nursing care indicated for an infant with a gastrointestinal defect.
- Describe the clinical manifestations of a diaphragmatic hernia and explain why immediate surgical intervention is necessary.
- Discuss appropriate interventions in providing care to an infant born with an omphaloecele.
- Relate the pathophysiology of aganglionic megacolon to the clinical manifestations most commonly seen.
- Briefly describe the basic types of imperforate anus and the respective treatment and prognosis for each.
- Identify the prenatal and perinatal information and neonatal signs a nurse should assess in evaluating the status of an infant with an intestinal obstruction.
- Describe the nursing care indicated for an infant with exstrophy of the bladder.
- Discuss the physical assessment techniques utilized and the clinical manifestations of congenital dislocation of the hip.
- Discuss the immediate pre- and postsurgical (convalescent) nursing care of an infant with a meningocele or a meningomyelocele.
- Briefly describe the embryologic changes that occur in the development of the fetal heart.
- List the clinical manifestations of congenital heart disease commonly seen in infants.
- Discuss the pathophysiology of selected acyanotic and cyanotic heart defects.
- Discuss the nursing management of the infant with congestive heart failure.

INFANT WITH A DEFECT: CRISIS FOR THE FAMILY

The birth of a baby with a defect or disorder is a traumatic event with the potential for either total disruption or growth for the involved family. The fantasized fears of the mother become reality.

The need to grieve for the loss of the hoped-for perfect child is mandatory before the development of a positive relationship to the existing child can begin. Grief is expressed as shock and disbelief, denial of reality, anger toward self and others, guilt, blame, and concern for the future. Self-esteem and feelings of self-worth are jeopardized.

The period of waiting between suspected abnormality or dysfunction and the confirmation of the defect or disorder is a very anxious one for parents because it is difficult if not impossible to begin attachment to the baby if the baby's future is questionable. During the dilemma of the "not knowing period," parents need support and acknowledgment that this is a very anxious time and to be kept informed as to efforts to gather additional data and to maintain the infant's livelihood. Helfer and Kempe (1976) recommend that both parents be told about the defect at the same time, with the baby present. An honest discussion of the problem and anticipatory management at the earliest possible time by health professionals helps the parents (a) maintain trust in the physician and nurse, (b) appreciate the reality of the situation by dispelling fantasy and misconception, (c) begin the grieving process, and (d) mobilize internal and external support.

Nurses need to be aware that anger is a universal response and that it is best directed outward, because holding it in check requires great energy, which is diverted away from grieving and physical recovery from pregnancy and giving birth. Anger may be directed unjustifiably at the physician and/or nurse, at the food, at nursing care, or at hospital regulations and routines. Anger with the child is rarely demonstrated by parents, and can precipitate guilt feelings.

The heightened concern for self may erroneously be interpreted by health professionals as rejection of the baby. Both parents need time and understanding in order to deal with their own feelings before they can direct concern toward the infant. In a short span of time, the parent is confronted with the loss of the idealized child, the need to accept a child who deviates from normal, and a sense of personal failure. In addition, the new mother may be suffering from fatigue and sleep deprivation from her pregnancy and labor and from discomforts arising from cesarean section, episiotomy, inability to void, hemorrhoids, and afterpains. In the postpartum period concern for self and dependency are normal events.

In their very sensitive and vulnerable state, parents are acutely perceptive of others' responses and reactions (particularly nonverbal) to the child. Parents can be expected to identify with the responses of others. Therefore, it is imperative that medical and nursing staff be fully aware of their feelings and come to terms with those feelings so that they are comfortable and at ease with the child and the grieving family. Professional support and comfort fill the bank account from which parents can draw to nurture the child and themselves so that each can develop to full potential.

Nurses may feel uncomfortable, not knowing what to say or fearing confrontation with the intensity of their own and the parents' feelings. Each nurse must work out feelings with herself, her instructor, peers, clergy, parents, or significant others. It is helpful to have a stockpile of therapeutic questions and statements to initiate meaningful dialogue with parents. Opening statements can be as follows: "You must be wondering what could have caused this"; "Are you thinking you (or someone else) may have done something?"; "How can I help?"; "Go ahead and cry. It's worth crying about"; or "Are you wondering how you are going to manage?" Avoid statements such as "It could have been worse"; "It's God's will"; "You have other children"; "You are still young and can have more"; and "I understand how you feel." *This* child is important *now.*

Some nurses find relief for themselves or a means of escape from painful circumstances by overzealous and unrealistic reassurance that "everything will be all right" and by avoidance of the patient. Another means of self-defense used by many medical and nursing staff is the use of technical jargon and involvement in the technical aspects of the mother's care rather than taking time to talk about the situation. These approaches confuse the parents at a time when they need most to be understood and to understand.

Nurses show concern and support by planning time to spend with the parents, by being psychologically as well as physically present, by encouraging open discussion and grieving, by repetitious explanations (as necessary), by providing privacy as needed, and by encouraging contact with the baby. Identification and clarification of feelings and fears decreases distortions in perception, thinking, and feelings. Nurses invest the child with value in the eyes of the parents when they provide meticulous care to the baby, talk and coo (especially in the face-to-face position) while holding or providing care to the baby, refer to the baby by gender or name, and relate the baby's activities ("He took a whole ounce of formula"; "She burped so loud that . . ."; "He took hold of the blanket and just wouldn't let go"; "He voided all over the doctor"). Nurses should note the "normal" characteristics and capabilities of the baby as well as his needs.

Cues that the parents are ready to become involved with the child's care or planning for the future include their reference to the baby as "she" or "he" or by name and their questioning as to amount of feeding taken, appearance today, and the like.

Many physicians show parents "before" and "after" photographs of conditions requiring surgical intervention. Parents benefit from meeting other parents who have faced the same problem, such as at amputee centers or cleft palate groups. Specialists (plastic surgeons, neurosurgeons, orthopedists, oral surgeons, dentists, and rehabilitation therapists) can be reassuring and supportive of parents in their short- and long-term goals. However, these types of interventions must be carefully timed to the readiness of the parents and the family.

Mothers may be startled or feel guilty when they do not feel motherly toward their infant. One mother, looking at her child born with an ugly cleft lip and palate, said, "God help me. I can't stand looking at her. I wish she wasn't mine. What a horrid thing to say, but I can't . . . I just can't." She could not bring herself to hold or touch the child prior to cleft lip repair. She needed considerable assistance to talk of these feelings in a nonjudgmental and accepting atmosphere before she was able to hold the infant after surgery. She proceeded to learn to feed her daughter (whose cleft palate was not yet repaired) and become very "motherly" before the infant was discharged. Her husband, fortunately, facilitated the whole process by his continued love for and acceptance of his wife throughout the experience.

Occasionally a mother may become overprotective and overoptimistic shortly after the baby's birth. The nurse accepts her behavior but continues to remind the mother that it is okay and natural to feel disappointment, a sense of failure, helplessness, or anger. The overprotectiveness and overoptimism is a defense mechanism. To deny the negative feelings serves only to further entrench them, to delay their resolution, and to delay realistic planning.

Parental feelings toward the child are crucial. The child's feelings about his physical appearance and integrity and about his capabilities reflect those of his parents. Before confronting society at large, the child must have developed sufficient ego strength and social, intellectual, and physical skills. It is difficult for some parents to develop realistic expectations, to provide consistent discipline, and to expose the child to a healthy amount of frustration. The handicap or defect is a fact that necessitates some behavioral and goal changes, but modifications can prepare the child for constructive, self-actualizing, and satisfying pursuits as a responsible citizen in the community.

INFANT WITH FEEDING PROBLEMS

Congenitally produced feeding problems may result from the Pierre Robin syndrome, cleft lip and palate, or choanal atresia.

Pierre Robin Syndrome

Physiology and Pathophysiology

Hypoplasia of the mandible occurring prior to the 9th week of embryonic development results in a mouth too small to allow for normal development. Reduced mandibular size forces the tongue into the nasopharyngeal space, often preventing closure of the palate in the midline (cleft palate). In addition, micrognathia (small mandible) forces the tongue backward and upward (glossoptosis), thus partially or completely obstructing the airway. Respiratory distress, which can occur especially on inspiration, when the tongue is pulled down and back to lie against the epiglottis and posterior pharyngeal wall, and feeding problems are serious threats to the neonate's well-being.

Etiology of the Pierre Robin syndrome is not clearly understood. It may be transmitted by a dominant gene with variable expressivity, or it may be the result of polygenic or multifactorial inheritance.

Clinical Manifestations

Micrognathia (receding chin, small mandible), which gives the neonate a birdlike face, is apparent at birth. Cleft palate may be an associated defect. The neonate is usually of low birth weight. Respiratory distress is apparent at birth, accompanied by cyanosis and increased respiratory effort. An x-ray of the nasopharyngeal area demonstrates the narrowed airway.

Careful physical assessment may reveal other associated defects, especially affecting the cardiovascular system, central nervous system, ears, or extremities. Possible ocular defects include retinal detachment, microphthalmia, congenital glaucoma, and cataracts.

Differential Diagnosis

Treacher Collins syndrome (mandibulofacial dysostosis) differs from the Pierre Robin syndrome in that the mandible's overall shape is grossly deformed, it is often associated with other facial anomalies, and there is no basic improvement in facial appearance as mandibular growth proceeds.

Interventions

Neonates born with severe micrognathia and associated defects experience life-threatening respiratory difficulties. Intensive resuscitation measures must be instituted by the physician or nurse immediately, using endotracheal intubation, tracheotomy (in some cases), suction, and oxygen-air insufflation (see Chapter 25). Following these measures, the severely affected neonate is best treated in an intensive care unit.

Resuscitation efforts may need to occur in the presence of the neonate's parents, and explanations to support the parents during these efforts are important aspects of nursing care. Surgical suturing of the tongue to the lower lip to bring the tongue forward and away from the posterior pharynx and epiglottis may be necessary to alleviate and prevent recurring respiratory distress. The parents should be kept informed of the neonate's condition and the measures being taken in his care. They are encouraged to visit the nursery, touch their child, and participate in his care as much as possible.

Presence of the cleft palate necessitates special feeding techniques (see the Nursing Care Plan on cleft lip and palate). Occasionally the child may require feeding by gavage or gastrostomy tube, but he is weaned to oral feedings as soon as possible.

Prognosis

Prognosis depends on the degree of expression of this syndrome in the individual infant—on the severity of micrognathia and coexisting defects.

With adequate support of respirations and nutrition, most affected infants grow out of the condition by 3 to 4 months of age, at which time the mandible has grown sufficiently to allow the tongue to rest in the normal position. By the age of 4 to 6 years, the mandible, tongue, and air passageway are essentially normal. Distinctive characteristics, noted on x-ray, persist through adulthood, however.

If the infant has an associated cleft palate, ongoing treatment of cleft palate is necessary.

Cleft Lip and Palate

Several factors seem to be responsible for cleft lip and palate. Polygenic inheritance (combination of genes from different loci on different chromosomes), an occasional mutant gene, environmental factors (fetal viral infection, radiation, hypoxia), or interaction between genetic and environmental factors may be responsible for this malformation. Environmental factors, such as the teratogenic insult of drugs (corticosteroid or anticonvulsant drugs) during the latter part of the first trimester have also been implicated.

Differences have been noted in the incidence of cleft palate and cleft lip. The infant born with only a cleft palate generally has a lower birth weight, has a greater incidence of coexisting malformation (such as gastrointestinal tract defects), and tends to be female. Cleft lip, with or without a coexisting cleft palate, generally occurs more of-

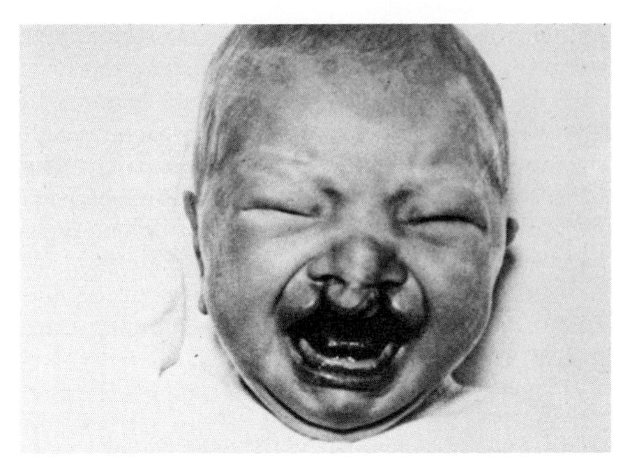

Figure 26–1. Bilateral cleft lip.

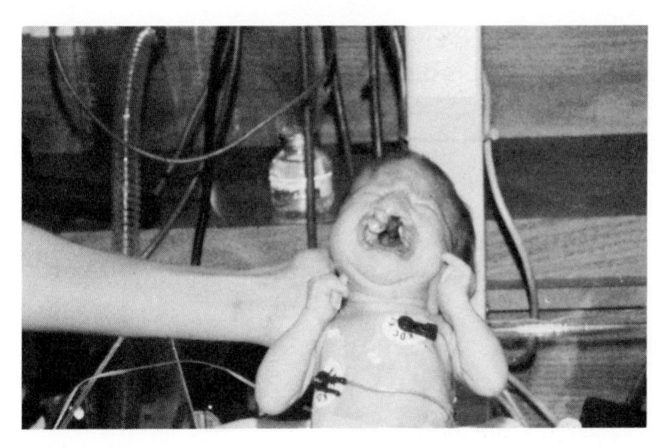

Figure 26–2. Cleft abnormality involving both hard and soft palate and unilateral cleft lip.

ten in the male. Parents should be referred for genetic counseling.

Physiology and Pathophysiology

Cleft lip occurs during the second month of embryonic development as a result of incomplete fusion of the nasomedial or intermaxillary process with the more laterally placed maxillary process. Because the fusion failure occurs during a period of rapid fetal growth, the structures of the face and mouth develop without the normal encircling restraints of the muscles of the lips. The characteristic depression or flattening of the infant's midfacial contour may result from the disruption of normal antagonistic forces across the midline and concomitant disturbance of growth of the facial segments involved. Facial clefts, even when not associated with cleft palate, may affect not only the lip but also the external nose, the nasal cartilages, the nasal septum, the alveolar process, and the alae (flesh flap forming the side of the nares) (Figure 26–1). The cleft is usually just beneath the center of one nostril. The more complete the cleft, the greater the incidence of missing, supernumerary, or malformed teeth in the line of the cleft. Failure of lip fusion by 35 days of gestation may impair the closure of the palatal shelves and may be a cause for cleft palate.

Palatal cleft refers to a fissure connecting the oral and nasal cavities. Cleft palate may involve the soft or soft and hard palate. The fissure is formed when embryonic fusion of the maxillary and premaxillary processes is incomplete. This abnormal development results in a complex syndrome initially involving any one or a combination of problems of respiration, feeding, or deglutition. Later consequences involve speech and hearing difficulties.

Clinical Manifestations

A cleft lip is readily visible at birth. The cleft palate may first be suspected when the neonate regurgitates formula through the nose. In the absence of a visible cleft, the palate is palpated for a possible submucous cleft that decreases the competence of the velopharyngeal valve. The fissure may involve only the uvula and soft palate or may extend forward to the nostril, involving the hard palate and the maxillary alveolar ridge. It also may occupy the midline posteriorly and as far forward as the alveolar process, where it causes deviation of the involved side, usually dividing the alveolar ridge between the upper lateral incisor tooth buds and the cuspid bud (Figure 26–2). The neonate may be of low birth weight. In addition, other malformations may be noted, especially of the craniofacial structures (see the discussion of the Pierre Robin syndrome, p. 845).

Interventions

The nursing and medical regimen focuses on repair of the lip, repair of the palate, speech development, and prevention of otitis media and dental abnormalities. The management of a cleft lip and palate is a team effort, with the nurse having an integral responsibility for fostering communications and coordinating all the various services for the parents and child.

Repair of Lip. The lip may be repaired during the first few days of life if the neonate's condition is good and weight is 2500 gm. Early labial repair for cosmetic effect has a positive influence on the developing parent-child relationship and permits the neonate to strengthen circumoral musculature. If possible, surgery is delayed until the infant weighs 10 lb and has a hemoglobin of 10 gm/100 ml, usually at about 3 months of age. The most common method of repair usually uses some modification of the Z-plasty, which produces a lip of sufficient depth without sacrificing the mucocutaneous line and with minimal scar formation.

Repair of Palate. The child is usually between 16 months and 2½ years of age. The aim of surgery is to obtain an air-tight closure of the palatal cleft and to preserve the mobility and length of the soft palate without disturbing tooth buds. Speech therapy is a valuable adjunct because the infant will develop deviant speech patterns if he begins to vocalize prior to closure of the palate. The child with a cleft palate is particularly vulnerable to middle ear infection and consequent dysfunction, because in addition to the normal horizontal placement of the eustachian tube in children, the child born with a cleft palate frequently has eustachian tube dysfunction.

Each neonate with a cleft palate is carefully examined for the existence of other malformations, especially those of the craniofacial structures.

The nurse works closely with the parents in determining the most successful approach to feeding the infant with a cleft lip or cleft palate. The difficulty they encounter may be a source of great frustration, so continued support and encouragement are essential. In addition, nursing efforts are directed to facilitating parent-infant bonding and acceptance of the defect. (See the Nursing Care Plan on cleft lip and palate.)

Choanal Atresia

Choanal atresia refers to the occlusion of the posterior nares, unilaterally or bilaterally, by either bone or membrane. Because infants are obligate nose breathers for at least the first few weeks of life, early symptoms include cyanosis even at rest, snorting respirations, and feeding difficulties, because the infant is unable to suck and breathe simultaneously. Failure to successfully pass a feeding tube through one or both of the infant's nares, coupled with the presence of the above symptoms, supports a diagnosis of choanal atresia.

Surgery is required to correct this disorder. Prior to surgery it may be necessary to tape a small airway in place in the infant's mouth to prevent respiratory distress. If necessary, feeding can be accomplished by nasogastric or orogastric tube until the child learns to eat and breathe at the same time.

INFANT WITH GASTROINTESTINAL DEFECT

Common congenital gastrointestinal defects include esophageal atresia and tracheoesophageal fistula, diaphragmatic hernia, omphalocele, aganglionic megacolon, imperforate anus, and intestinal obstruction.

Esophageal Atresia and Tracheoesophageal Fistula

The most common high gastrointestinal tract anomaly is atresia of the esophagus with tracheoesophageal fistula, occurring in approximately 1 in 3000 births.

Physiology and Pathophysiology

During embryonic development, the beginning cell structures of the esophagus dorsal wall may fail to grow and thereby fail to form a continuous hollow muscular tube connecting the pharynx to the stomach, forming instead a blind pouch *(atresia)*. In 87% of cases, the type III distal portion connects with the trachea (or a primary bronchus) near the bronchial bifurcation via an abnormal passageway known as a *fistula*. The tracheoesophageal fistula is caused by incomplete separation between the esophagus and trachea during

NURSING CARE PLAN

Cleft Lip and Palate

Patient Data Base

History

Pertinent prenatal and perinatal information, such as:

Genetic link or environmental factors (drugs, fetal viral infections, radiation, and hypoxia)

Complete physical assessment of neonate

Any significant respiratory difficulties at or soon after birth

Parents reactions to defect and initial information given to them

Physical examination

Cleft lip:
Obvious unilateral or bilateral visible defect, which may involve the external nares, nasal cartilages, nasal septum and the alveolar process

Characteristic depression or flattening of the infant's midfacial contour may be seen

Cleft palate:
Fissure connecting the oral and nasal cavity, which may involve the uvula and soft palate or may extend forward to the nostril involving the hard palate and maxillary alveolar ridge

Difficulty in sucking and feeding

May demonstrate expulsion of formula out through the nose

Nursing Priorities

1. Develop safe feeding practices and prevent complications.
2. Identify coexisting defects.
3. Encourage parents to participate in and cooperate in meeting short- and long-term rehabilitation goals.

Problem	Nursing interventions and actions	Rationale
Cleft lip		
Feeding preoperatively	Experiment with various nipples: Lamb's (longer-softer); asepto syringe (10 ml) with bulb and 1½ in. rubber tubing.	Select feeding technique best suited to infant. Choose simplest method to avoid further emphasis on child's difference to parents.
	Feed slowly.	Approximates normal stomach filling and prevents regurgitation.
	Burp frequently (after every ounce).	Prevents vomiting and discomfort from gas bubbles (infant has greater tendency to swallow air).
	Cleanse cleft with medicine dropper full of sterile water.	Prevents crusting to keep cleft in good condition for repair.
	Interact with infant as with any "normal" infant.	Assists in development of trust and serves as role model to mother and father.
Coexisting defects	Carefully assess, especially for defects of craniofacial tissues.	Assist physician to institute appropriate treatment; gather data for anticipatory guidance of parents.
Eliciting parental involvement and cooperation	Provide a role model in interacting with infant.	Parents internalize others' responses to their infant.
	Provide time for and encourage parents to grieve.	Grief must be resolved before parents can begin relating to this infant in positive manner and cooperate in child's rehabilitation.
	Teach parents method of feeding child prior to discharge if lip surgery is to be delayed.	Allows time for parents to gain self-confidence.
	Review with parents ways to decrease possibility of infection, especially upper respiratory infections. Encourage parents to have any upper respiratory infections treated by physician immediately.	Increases parents' self-confidence; specifies a definite course of action. Precaution against development of otitis media.

NURSING CARE PLAN Cont'd

Cleft Lip and Palate

Problem	Nursing interventions and actions	Rationale
Preoperative preparation	Assess for respiratory or gastrointestinal disorder and report to physician.	Avoid surgical/postsurgical complications.
	Feed infant by same method that will be used following surgery: asepto syringe with rubber catheter (a small gravy baster with 1½ in. rubber tube attached can be substituted).	Accustoms infant to changes. Avoids stress of sucking on suture line.
	Place catheter in side of mouth.	Avoids direct trauma to suture line.
	Drip formula onto surface of tongue.	Stimulates swallowing.
	Apply restraints:	Accustoms infant to restraints to decrease postsurgical distress:
	1. Elbow	1. Prevents trauma to suture line.
	2. Jacket	2. Necessary for child who is capable of turning over.
	In some instances, place infant in protective isolation.	Decreases possibility of cross-infection.
Postoperative recovery with cosmetic and functional repair of lip		
Adequate respiration	Observe for bleeding, airway obstruction (stridor, etc.) from edema or secretions.	Identifies possible complications following surgery that necessitate treatment.
	Place in croupette until respirations are normal.	Helps liquefy secretions and reduce edema.
	Lay infant in supine position; prop slightly under one side.	Facilitates drainage and respiration; prevents aspiration; protects suture line.
Adequate nutrition	Assess for hydration: adequacy of voiding; tenseness of fontanelle and appearance of eyeballs, skin turgor over abdomen and thighs, daily weight.	Aids calculation of daily fluid: type of fluid, rate of drip, total volume needed per day.
	Record intake and output.	
	Monitor IV hourly: type and amount of fluid infused, condition of infusion site.	Assures accuracy of flow to prevent fluid overload or inadequate fluid; prevents tissue trauma.
	Assess for adequate caloric intake; weigh daily; plot weight on chart.	Prevent inadequate intake to meet requirements of stress, surgical losses, repair and growth needs.
Feeding capabilities	When infant is fully aware, offer oral fluids as ordered; later, advance to clear fluid, then formula in 3–12 hr via method utilized prior to surgery.	Milk products increase mucus production and may cause crusting on suture line. Avoid solids, nipples, pacifiers to protect suture line.
	Assess response: Any chilling? Cyanosis? Abdominal distention? Type and amount of feeding? Was feeding retained? Swallowing and burping behavior? Fatigue? Activity?	Determines appropriate feeding method and appropriate time to advance feeding. Assists in identifying coexisting problems.
	Feed infant in cardiac chair or infant seat or hold upright, with head and chest tilted backward slightly; feed slowly.	Facilitates swallowing, burping, and retention of feeding and prevents aspiration or vomiting.
Intact suture line and even vermilion border	Treat suture line per physician/hospital preference: 1. Keep dressing moist with sterile saline at least every 2 hr. 2. Cleanse with gauze swab moistened with sterile saline or hydrogen peroxide. 3. Apply antibiotic ointment after feedings.	Prevents crusting with serosanguineous drainage, mucus, or feeding and prevents excessive scar formation.
	Continue use of restraints: elbow restraint pinned to shirt or mattress; jacket.	Prevent direct trauma to suture line.
	Remove restraints periodically. Remove one at a time for massage and exercise of muscles.	

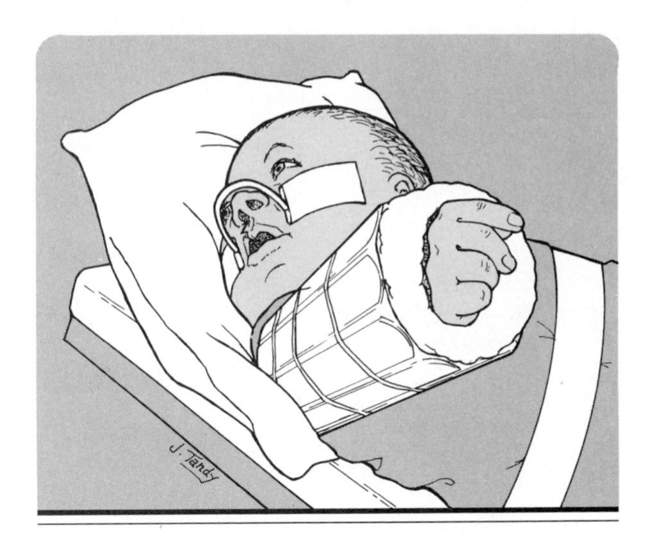

Figure 26–3. Cleft lip repair with Logan bar. Note the elbow restraints on the infant.

NURSING CARE PLAN Cont'd

Cleft Lip and Palate

Problem	Nursing interventions and actions	Rationale
	Check and replace adhesive tape securing the Logan bar (Figure 26–3), if used. If tape is loosened, remove, paint with tincture of benzoin, and apply new tape.	Maintains traction of Logan bar to prevent pull on suture line.
	Feed with rubber-tipped appliance placed into corner of mouth. Don't use nipple or pacifier.	Prevents direct trauma to suture line and discourages sucking.
	Prevent vomiting.	Prevents stress on line.
	Cuddle, hold, rock infant.	Prevents crying, which adds stress to suture line. Needs extra cuddling as he can't suck, which provides outlet for tension and anxiety.
Effects of immobility	Remove one restraint at a time, exercise limb, and reapply restraint.	Provides range of motion while maintaining protective restraints of unsupervised limbs. Provides kinesthetic and social stimulation.
	Check for reddened areas under restraints; keep all skin areas clean and dry.	Prevents skin breakdown.
	Turn from side to side; prop well.	Prevents skin breakdown and orthostatic pneumonia; immobilization protects suture line.
Infection	Administer antibiotics as prescribed by physician; carry out cleansing of suture line.	
Parent education	Supervise parents during feeding, restraining, exercising extremities, or whatever will be expected of them after infant's discharge home.	Instills self-confidence, feelings of self-worth and self esteem – provides avenue of learning about baby and developing positive relationship between parent and infant.
	Refer to community agencies as necessary, such as Homemaker's Service, Foster Home Care, and visiting nurse.	Frees mother to provide necessary care and stimulation or provides care for family that is unable to do so temporarily.
Cleft palate (prior to surgery)		
Adequate respirations	Place prone or in side-lying position.	Facilitates drainage.
	Suction gently, as needed.	Prevents aspiration or airway obstruction.

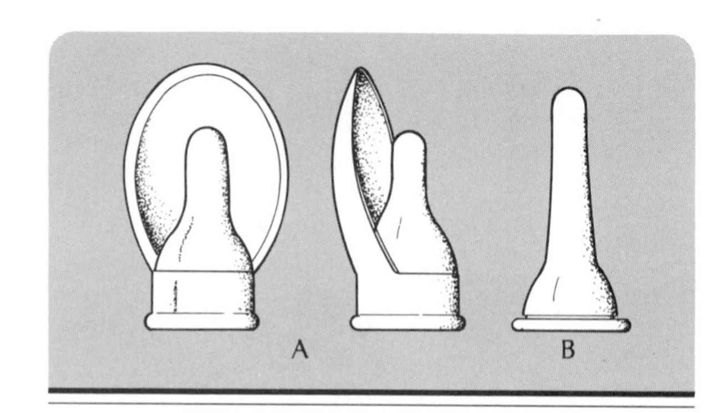

Figure 26–4. Cleft palate nipples. **A,** Side and front view of flanged nipple. **B,** Lamb's nipple.

NURSING CARE PLAN Cont'd

Cleft Lip and Palate

Problem	Nursing interventions and actions	Rationale
	Prevent upper respiratory infections and possible otitis media.	Prevents surgery delay or surgical complications since surgery isn't done until infant is about 16 months of age.
	Use appropriate feeding method (see section on cleft lip).	See section on cleft lip.
Adequate nutrition	Choose appropriate nipple: "winged", lamb's, nipple with flange cut to size, asepto syringe with bulb and 1½ in. rubber tip (Figure 26–4).	Deemphasizes child's "difference" to parents. Decreases possibility of formula entering nasal cavities, thus discouraging aspiration and respiratory distress.
	Be sure that nipples are soft and holes are slightly enlarged.	Assists feeding, because infant cannot create vacuum necessary for successful nursing.
	Support in upright position with head and chest tilted slightly backward.	Aids swallowing and discourages aspiration.
	Bubble frequently—after each ounce.	Aids removal of excessive air these infants tend to swallow; therefore, discourages vomiting and aspiration.
	Thicken formula per physician order.	Provides extra calories while utilizing gravity flow to prevent aspiration.
	Begin feeding with cup or from side of spoon.	Accustoms infant/toddler to postoperative situation.
	Irrigate mouth with water after feedings.	Prevents crusting.
	Plot pattern of weight gain.	Assesses adequacy of diet and readiness for surgery.

Nursing Care Evaluation

Infant suffers minimal emotional trauma from surgical interventions and hospitalizations.

Lip is repaired with improved appearance.

Otitis media is prevented or treated before hearing damage occurs.

Infant is feeding well and maintaining weight.

Parents develop positive relationship with the child, demonstrating positive parenting behaviors, and are able to meet own as well as child's needs.

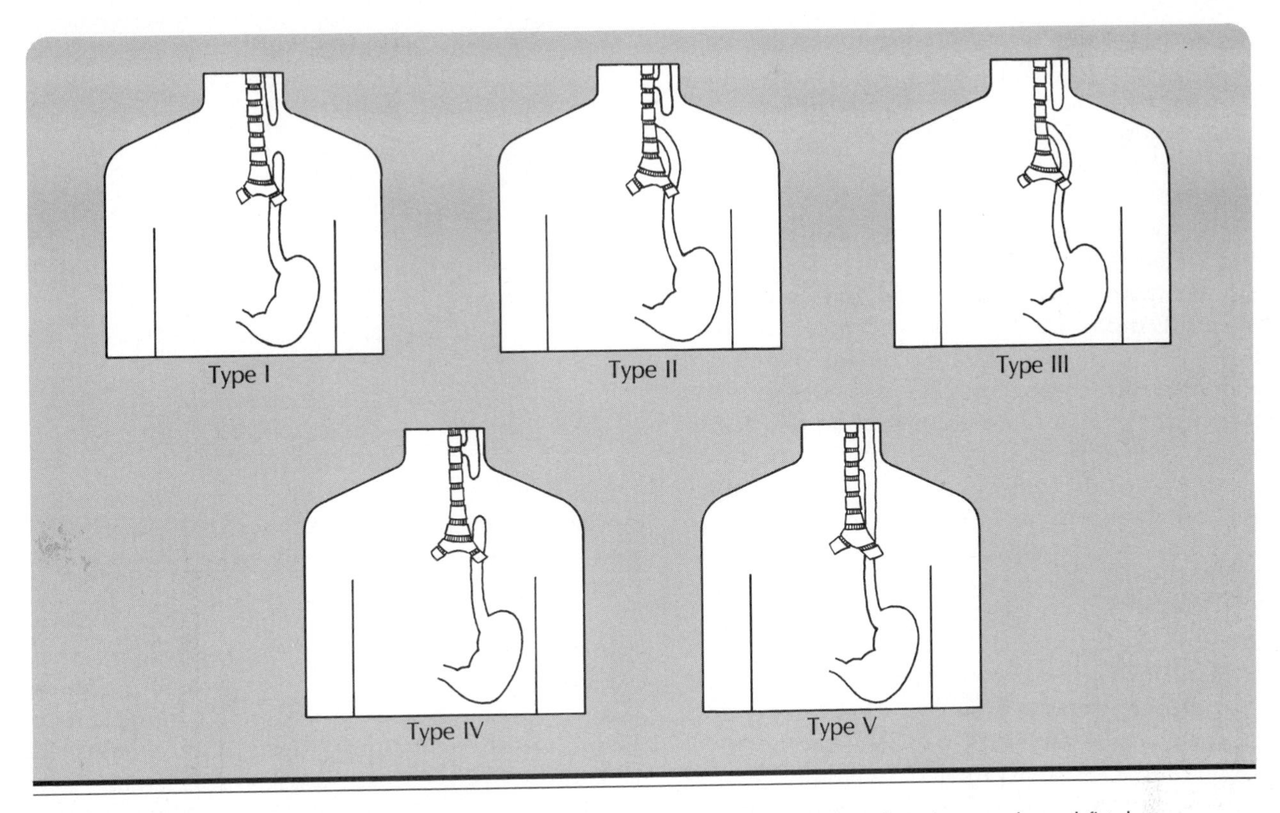

Figure 26–5. Five most frequently seen types of congenital esophageal atresia and tracheoesophageal fistula.

cleavage of the esophagotracheal groove or septum at 4 weeks' gestation.

Four other anatomic variations are less commonly seen. The upper and lower segments of the esophagus are atretic in 8% of cases (type I). The H-type of anomaly (type V, 4%) refers to a continuous esophagus that is connected by a fistulous tract to the trachea. In less than 2% of cases, the upper esophageal segment empties by a fistulous tract into the trachea, with some of these infants having the lower segment end in a blind pouch (type IV); in others it connects to the trachea (type II) (Figure 26-5). These infants may aspirate with the first feeding or develop pneumonia within a few days.

Clinical Manifestations

Maternal polyhydramnios is noted in about 40% of cases and is usually associated with the fetus who cannot swallow and excrete the amniotic fluid as the normal fetus does. From one-fourth to one-third of neonates with this anomaly are preterm (gestational age of 37 weeks or less). The neonate has excessive mucous secretions and drools almost constantly. Cyanotic episodes may occur secondary to aspiration of excessive mucus from the oropharynx. If the neonate is fed, there is immediate regurgitation, often through the nose as well as the mouth, after one or two swallows of fluid. The neonate gags, chokes, struggles, and turns cyanotic as the fluid enters the tracheobronchial tree. Abdominal distention begins to develop soon after birth if there is a tracheoesophageal fistula. Abdominal distention may occur, caused by air from the trachea via the fistula tract, or the neonate may pass abnormal amounts of flatus due to excess air being forced into the stomach. In contrast, the abdomen appears scaphoid (flat) if the distal segment of the esophagus does not connect to the trachea.

The neonate is examined for the presence of coexisting malformations, such as intestinal atresia, urologic disorders, and cardiovascular defects (patent ductus arteriosus, coarctation of the aorta).

Symptoms of aspiration pneumonia or chemical pneumonitis may occur with respiratory distress: tachypnea, flaring of nares, cyanotic episodes, retractions, rales, rhonchi, decreased breath sounds, unstable temperature (may be subnormal). Chemical pneumonitis results from regurgitation of gastric contents into the lungs in type

III. Gastric juices sear the lung tissue and may be fatal.

Diagnosis can be made by passing a well-lubricated soft No. 8 nasogastric catheter through the nose into the esophagus, where it will meet resistance.

X-ray examination reveals a radiopaque catheter coiled in the esophageal pouch, demonstrating the point of resistance and the end of the pouch. Fistulas are particularly difficult to diagnose as they are not constantly patent. Flat film of abdomen and chest shows the presence of air in the stomach and air in the upper blind pouch. Gas in the stomach and intestines indicates the presence of a fistula from the trachea to the esophageal segment into the stomach.

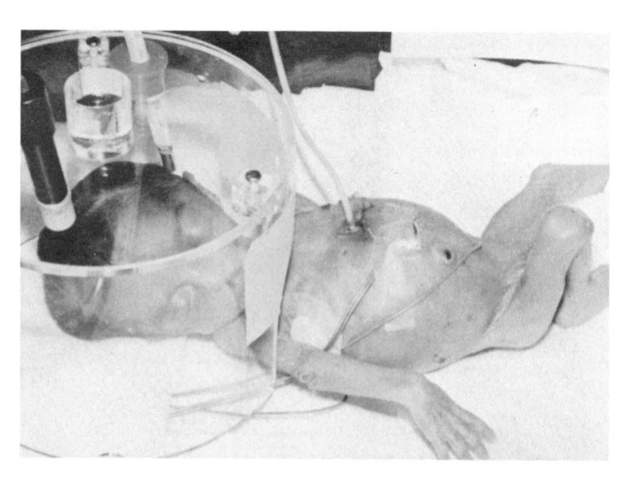

Figure 26–6. Infant with gastrostomy tube in place. Note that the tube is elevated. Oxygenation and temperature regulation are also monitored.

Interventions

Prompt surgical diversion or closure of the fistula is mandatory. Surgical correction of esophageal discontinuity is done in several stages, depending on the distance between the atresia and the lower segment as the child grows. When surgery must be postponed because of pneumonia, because of the absence of a lower esophageal portion, or because the distance between the lower and upper portions of the esophagus is too great, either (a) a double lumen nasogastric tube is inserted into the blind pouch and attached to continuous suction to prevent aspiration or (b) a cervical esophagostomy is performed and a gastrostomy is done for feeding purposes until a colon transplant or esophageal replacement can be accomplished (Figure 26-6). The cervical esophagostomy provides an outlet for secretions and allows "sham" feedings. Sham feedings allow the infant to be fed fluids and semisolids orally to provide for oral sucking needs and development of taste. (For nursing interventions, see the Nursing Care Plan on gastrointestinal defects.)

NURSING CARE PLAN

Gastrointestinal Defects

Patient Data Base

History

Pertinent information from the prenatal and perinatal record:

- Maternal history of polyhydramnios
- Choking, regurgitation immediately after 1 or 2 feedings and cyanotic episodes
- In H-type, recurrent aspiration pneumonia
- Failure to pass nasogastric tube and aspiration of mucus
- Current status of neonate—free from infections
- Parental reaction to situation

Physical examination

Esophageal atresia—excessive mucous secretions

Constant drooling

Scaphoid (flat) abdomen if distal esophageal segment does not connect to trachea

Symptoms of respiratory distress

With fistula type, same as above and abdominal distention that begins soon after birth

Laboratory evaluation

X-rays—visualization of radiopaque catheter coiled in esophageal pouch; if fistula is present, flat plate of abdomen and chest shows air in stomach and upper blind pouch

NURSING CARE PLAN Cont'd

Gastrointestinal Defects

Nursing Priorities

1. Support respiration by:
   - Preventing aspiration and aspiration pneumonia.
   - Preventing pneumonitis and entry of gastric juices into respiratory tree.
2. Maintain adequate nutrition.
3. Identify coexistent malformations.
4. Maintain infant in good physical condition for stress of surgery.
5. Prevent emotional trauma to infant.
6. Assist parents in coping with situation.
7. Prevent postoperative complications.
8. Foster parent-infant bonding.

Problem	Nursing Interventions and Actions	Rationale
Aspiration pneumonitis and reflux of gastric contents	Do not feed until assured of esophagus patency.	Decreases incidence of aspiration.
	Preoperatively:	
	Assess for presenting symptoms, i.e., excessive oral secretions and respiratory distress.	Identifies anomaly prior to respiratory problems.
	Quickly assess infant prior to putting baby to breast on delivery table.	
	Utilize sterile water for first feeding (if aspirated, does not create chemical pneumonitis).	
	Control saliva and mucus by suction with bulb syringe or oropharyngeal suction tube passed into pouch and attached to low intermittent suction per physician order.	Prevents aspiration pneumonia, which may be fatal.
	Place in warmed, humidified crib or isolette.	Liquefies mucus and facilitates its removal from trachea; protects from infection.
	Elevate head of bed 20° in semi-Fowler's position.	Prevents reflux flow of gastric juices through fistula into respiratory tree and resultant chemical pneumonitis.
	Postoperatively:	
	1. If chest tube is in place, keep tubing free of kinks and tension. Reposition or move infant carefully to avoid disrupting drainage system.	Promotes effective drainage of fluid from chest and facilitates lung inflation.
	Place clamp at head of crib; if tubing is dislodged, clamp it close to chest wall, stat.	Prevents pneumothorax.
	Measure and record amount and character of drainage.	Assists physician in assessing infant's progress and instituting appropriate measures.
	2. If gastrostomy tube has been inserted, keep open with injections of 2–4 ml of air and elevate (see Figure 26–6).	Promotes drainage.
	Do not suction or irrigate stomach.	Prevents direct trauma to stomach.
	3. Suction upper esophagus via nasal catheter as necessary.	Prevents direct trauma to incision sites.
	Replaced by physician daily.	Prevents infection and crusting.

NURSING CARE PLAN Cont'd

Gastrointestinal Defects

Problem	Nursing interventions and actions	Rationale
	4. Observe patency and maintain low intermittent suction.	
	5. Suction oropharynx with French (No. 8 or No. 10) soft rubber catheter. Watch for increasing edema.	Frequent suctioning may increase already-present surgical edema.
	6. Position head of bed at 30°; maintain position with rolled cloths or cloth sling or put infant in cardiac chair.	Promotes pooling of secretions at catheter tip if indwelling nasal catheter is in use.
	7. Reposition every 2 hr.	Prevents stasis pneumonia, skin breakdown.
	8. Keep in warmed, humidified crib or isolette.	Liquefies secretions and facilitates their removal.
	9. Assess vital signs and physical appearance: color, respiratory effort. Notify physician if respiratory distress persists despite suctioning.	Maintains ongoing record.
Adequate nutritional intake	Monitor parenteral fluids every hour pre- and postoperatively.	Prevents overhydration or underhydration.
	Assess for degree of hydration (see p. 749).	Prevents overhydration or underhydration.
	With gastrostomy tube in place, begin feedings when gastric juices move readily into duodenum.	Gastrointestinal motility must be established prior to feeding.
	Use syringe barrel, funnel, asepto to instill fluid.	Facilitates feeding process.
	Initially, introduce 5% dextrose water, slowly. Feed with warmed formula when dextrose water is tolerated and solution passes readily into duodenum.	Tests infant's tolerance or readiness for feeding.
	Gastrostomy feeding: Fill syringe barrel or funnel partially with fluid, attach to gastrostomy tube, then decompress tubing and slowly commence feeding via gravity, by raising level of feeding apparatus.	Decreases amount of air introduced into stomach, thus decreasing discomfort and regurgitation. Gravity flow decreases pressure on anastomosis.
	To discontinue feeding, compress gastrostomy tube as fluid level reaches tip of feeding apparatus. Fold tubing over itself and secure with clamp or rubber band in older children.	
	In infants, suspend gastrostomy tube; keep open to air.	With infant's small gastric capacity, open tubing prevents regurgitation of gastric contents up into esophagus and allows for fluctuation of feeding in tube until digested.
	Cleanse skin around gastrostomy tube and cervical esophagostomy and apply prescribed mild ointment i.e., aluminum paste or zinc oxide.	Prevents skin breakdown and infection.
	As stomach fills, give infant a pacifier.	Meets sucking needs and helps infant associate sucking with easing of hunger. Sucking also relaxes gastrointestinal musculature.
	Provide sham feedings via cervical esophagostomy.	Maintains sucking mechanism.
	Talk or sing to infant during feeding. Pick up infant for cuddling during and after feeding.	Helps infant associate pleasantness with feeding; facilitates normal gastrointestinal motility and avoids failure-to-thrive syndrome.
	Oral feedings: If continuity of esophagus has been achieved, begin feedings about 2 weeks postoperatively.	Assess infant's tolerance for feedings and readiness for removal of gastrostomy tube.
	Begin by offering 5% dextrose water and feed slowly. When water is well tolerated, advance to feeding with small amounts of formula by bottle.	Prevents possibility of coughing, choking, and regurgitation.
	Record intake and output; daily weight; plot pattern of weight gain.	Indicates adequacy of diet and method of feedings.
Possible coexisting malformation	Assess infant's anatomic appearance and physiologic functioning.	Enables physician to institute appropriate treatment; assesses readiness for surgery; provides more definitive anticipatory guidance to family.

NURSING CARE PLAN Cont'd
Gastrointestinal Defects

Problem	Nursing interventions and actions	Rationale
Emotional trauma to infant	Assign nurses for continuity of care.	Facilitates development of trust.
	Avoid loud talking, radios.	Facilitates rest; prevents overstimulation.
	Hold whenever possible; touch, stroke; carry infant around – pin gastrostomy asepto to clothing in infants. Respond to crying by stroking, talking, and cuddling.	Facilitates development of trust.
	Offer pacifier when child is being fed by gastrostomy. Feed while being held.	Assists infant to associate relief of hunger with sucking (he is getting nothing by mouth); strengthens muscles; exercises jaws; facilitates normal gastrointestinal functioning (e.g., stomach will not receive feeding if infant is upset). Associates feeding with comfort of being held.
	Encourage active parental participation in daily care of the infant.	Facilitates postive parent-infant relationship.
Parents' coping mechanisms	Keep parents informed: clarify and reinforce physician's explanations regarding malformation, surgical repair, pre- and postoperative care, and prognosis.	Knowledge is ego-strengthening.
	Encourage grieving for having child with defect.	Parents cannot begin positive relationship with this child until they grieve for the loss of desired perfect child.
	Involve parents in care of infant and in planning for future. Facilitate touch and eye contact.	Dispels feelings of impotence, increases self-esteem and self-worth. Potentiates incorporation of this child into family.
	Refer family to community agencies for financial assistance (defect necessitates long hospitalizations, specialized equipment and services).	Assists family with heavy financial burden.
	Refer to public health nurse to help keep parents motivated to return to physician or clinic at first signs of pulmonary infection or stricture of esophagus.	Maintains motivation and sense of hopefulness during lengthy treatment. Facilitates early identification and treatment to prevent serious complications.
Postoperative complications	Review with parents signs and symptoms of complications.	See discussion of preceding problems.

Nursing Care Evaluation

Neonate does not develop aspiration pneumonia or chemical pneumonitis.

Neonate's nutrition is adequate to maintain appropriate pattern of weight gain; dehydration is avoided.

Any coexisting malformations are identified and appropriate interventions are taken or planned.

Emotional trauma is minimized in infant.

Parents are able to cope with needs of not only affected infant but also themselves and rest of family.

Postsurgical complications do not occur.

Esophageal reconstruction is usually deferred until the infant is asymptomatic and between 6 months old to 2 years of age. The right or transverse portion of the colon is usually used to join the upper portion of the esophagus with the stomach.

The presence of an H-type fistula without esophageal atresia may not be identified during the first month of life. This rare lesion may be diagnosed after the infant suffers repeated bouts of coughing, choking, and aspiration pneumonia. At this time, surgical obliteration of the fistula is performed.

Complications of Surgery

Complications prior to surgical intervention result primarily from aspiration. The infant may have a brassy cough for six months to two years and upper respiratory infections such as recurrent pneumonitis, bronchopneumonia, and atelectasis. Postoperatively, the child may have difficulty swallowing due to edema or may have stenosis at the anastomosis site. Progressive dilatation of stricture by bougie (mercury-weighted dilators) is the usual treatment, but care must be taken as it can break the suture line if too tight. Ischemia causing total breakdown of the transplant is the most common postoperative complication.

Prognosis

Gestational age affects the survival rate. Approximately 50% of preterm infants and 90% of term infants survive.

Diaphragmatic Hernia

Diaphragmatic hernia occurs once in every 3000 live births, and the frequency of occurrence is equal in males and females.

Physiology and Pathophysiology

The neonate born with a diaphragmatic hernia requires immediate surgical intervention. Herniation of abdominal contents and malrotation into the thoracic cavity is possible, as the abdominal and thoracic cavity is one entity due to failure of the pleuroperitoneal folds (which comprise the diaphragm) to fuse completely by the 8th week of gestation. The diaphragm usually fuses anteriorly

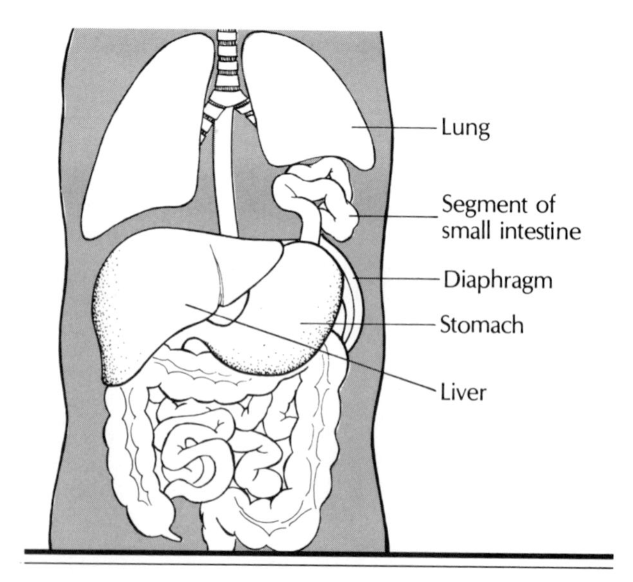

Figure 26–7. Diaphragmatic hernia. Note the compression of the lung by the intestine on the affected side.

to posterior. This abnormal connection between the thoracic and abdominal cavities is more common through the foramen of Bochdalek on the left side, as the liver blocks movement of the gut on the right (Figure 26–7). The size of the defect and the amount of abdominal viscera present in the thoracic cavity influence the success of surgical repair. In severe cases, the large amount of viscera in the thorax compresses lung space. The resultant pulmonary hypoplasia may be incompatible with life. The mediastinal structures are shifted to the side opposite the defect.

This otherwise normal-appearing neonate has difficulty initiating respirations. The affected side of the chest cannot expand. Absence of viscera in the abdomen gives the abdomen a scaphoid (flat) appearance. Neonates with severe herniation are hypoxic and rapidly develop respiratory and metabolic acidosis.

Clinical Manifestations

Breath sounds are absent on the left side. Respirations are gasping, with nasal flaring and chest retraction. Bowel sounds may soon be heard in the thoracic cavity (large barrel chest), and the abdomen appears scaphoid because of the presence of abdominal viscera in the chest. Respiratory and metabolic acidosis develop rapidly. The infant may vomit if fed. Heart sounds displaced to the right (diagnosis of dextrocardia), a chest full to auscultation, and spasmodic attacks of cyanosis and difficulty in feeding (resulting from dyspnea) are definitive signs of weakness. Cardiac action and respirations are further compromised as the bowel fills with gas. Signs of intestinal obstruction may also be seen due to associated malrotation of the intestines. Radiography reveals gas-filled bowels in the thoracic cavity and a displacement of the mediastinal structures to the side opposite the diaphragmatic defect. Lung collapse and hypoplasia due to early compression also provide differential diagnosis in cases of lung hematomas, paralysis of the diaphragm, eventuation of the diaphragm, and elevation in the diaphragmatic wall.

Interventions

The surgical procedure involves the removal of the bowels from the thoracic cavity and the closure of the diaphragmatic defect. The surgical approach is transthoracic when no intestinal obstruction is present and transabdominal when obstructive malrotation is present. If the defect is small, there is usually enough diaphragmatic tissue for closure; if not, a woven Teflon patch is used to close the defect.

Intestinal malrotation usually accompanies the hernia. This, too, must be repaired to prevent later duodenal obstruction. Because the abdominal cavity may be too small to hold all of the viscera, total closure may not be possible at this time. The peritoneum and muscle layers may be left open and the viscera covered with skin or Silastic plastic sheet, creating a ventral hernia. The compressed lung is not expanded during surgery because of the danger of a pneumothorax on the contralateral side. The compressed lung gradually expands in 7 to 14 days but may remain hypoplastic.

Nursing Management

A nursing history contains pertinent information from the prenatal and perinatal records; the summary of the neonate prior to surgery; the description of the type of defect (minimal or extensive abdominal malformations), preoperative presenting clinical picture, the postsurgical condition; and information on the chest tube, the type of abdominal closure, and the parental response to the neonate and the malformation.

Nursing priorities include maintaining adequate ventilation and nutrition, preventing postoperative complications (shock, bleeding, infection, pneumothorax), and assisting the parents to cope with the situation.

The nurse facilitates respirations by positioning the neonate in a high Fowler's position (infant seat may be used) in order to utilize gravity to keep abdominal organ pressure off the diaphragm. A chest tube is placed on the affected side, attached to a water seal on low suction, to relieve the surgical pneumothorax and to allow for gradual reexpansion of the lung on the affected side. Positive pressure ventilation may be used for several days postoperatively to relieve pneumothorax of the affected lung. The nurse is also responsible for maintaining chest tube function (see the discussion of esophageal atresia), placing the neonate in a warmed humidified environment, suctioning as necessary, placing the child on his affected side to facilitate unaffected lung expansion, and utilizing an appropriate feeding method. Gastric suction is continued immediately postoperatively to prevent abdominal distention and pressure on the diaphragmatic repair. Feeding may be accomplished initially by intravenous infusion and hyperalimentation, then by gavage on the second or third postoperative day to decrease air swallowing, then orally when tolerated without abdominal distention. Frequent burping is important.

The nurse assesses the neonate for adequacy of nutrition and hydration. A flexible feeding schedule is important in order to take advantage of the usually anorexic infant's increase in appetite and desire to eat. Care must be taken to decrease the swallowing of air, stomach compression, and predisposition to gagging and vomiting. Development of hiatal hernia is common. The parents may have difficulty coping with the situation because of the necessary rapidity of the surgery and the mechanical interventions, such as the respirator, needed to preserve their tiny infant's life.

Prognosis

Prognosis depends on the severity of the defect and the degree of pulmonary hypoplasia. Surgical intervention is successful in about 50% of the affected neonates. Mortality is highest in the first 24 hours after birth. For some children, the defect is asymptomatic during infancy and may be diagnosed years later, usually following recurrent episodes of respiratory infection (from compression of the lower lobe of the lung). These children have an excellent prognosis following surgery.

Omphalocele (Exomphalos)

Physiology and Pathophysiology

During embryologic development, midgut development occurs outside the abdomen. By the 10th week of gestation, the intestines reenter the abdominal cavity through the umbilical opening, and the anterior abdominal wall closes. Total or partial failure of the midgut to complete this migration results in omphalocele anomaly. The herniated intestines are covered with a fragile, transparent amniotic membrane that will degenerate within 12 hours after birth, becoming opaque, necrotic, and malodorous because of lack of blood supply. Large omphaloceles may contain the liver and spleen as well. The incidence is 1:10,000 births (Kempe et al., 1978).

About one-third of affected neonates demonstrate Beckwith's syndrome: high birth weight, rapid postnatal growth, macroglossia (hypertrophy of the tongue), facial nevus flammeus, and neonatal hypoglycemia. Coexistent malformations, such as cardiac anomalies, are common.

Clinical Manifestations

The presence of an omphalocele is obvious, with small intestine, colon, liver, and stomach (or any combination) in a sac or lying free if the sac is ruptured. Small omphaloceles may be confused with umbilical cysts or hematomas. Gastroschisis appears similar to omphalocele, as abdominal viscera protrude through an abdominal wall deficit; however, gastroschisis is located below and separate from the umbilicus and has no sac or covering. Chest x-rays are important in the diagnosis of cardiac malformations and the presence of atelectasis.

Interventions

Prior to surgery, the nurse protects the defect from infection, drying, and rupture by either sterile gauze moistened with warmed (body temperature) sterile saline or sterile petrolatum dressings and a firm (metal or plastic) shield. Sterile technique is essential. A nasogastric tube attached to low suction prevents distention of the lower bowel. Antibiotics are begun before surgery and are continued until the chance of infection has passed. Choice of corrective method depends on the general size and condition of the infant, on the presence of other abnormalities, on the size of the defect, and on the capacity of the sac.

Defects of 5 cm or less may be repaired in one procedure; larger defects require staged repairs. The viscera may not fit into the available abdominal space. Forcing the viscera into the abdominal cavity compresses the viscera, impairs venous return, and raises the diaphragm. When this occurs, within a matter of hours the infant develops respiratory distress and extreme fatigue and succumbs. Medium-sized defects are closed with skin flaps within 12 hours of birth until the peritoneal cavity has enlarged (approximately 6–12 months of age). Later a ventral umbilical herniorrhaphy is done as the final stage.

A nonsurgical treatment consists of painting the sac with 2% Mercurochrome surgical solution; Burow's solution may be used on large defects. The restrained neonate remains in an incubator until the sac thickens and toughens and a dry eschar forms. Several weeks later, after the eschar is sufficiently toughened and contracting and the mother has learned how to continue the application of the solution, the infant may be cared for at home. The defect closes, creating a ventral herniorrhaphy in a matter of weeks or months. However, complications may include late rupture of the sac and mercury poisoning.

Another method for correcting large defects or a ruptured sac is the creation of an articifical celom (sac) using a Silastic bag. The bag forms a pouch over the abdominal contents when it is sutured to the abdominal wall fascia. Then the bag is suspended from the top of the incubator by a flexible band. Every few days, pressure is exerted on the pouch, shortening it and forcing the organs back into the abdominal cavity and stretching the abdominal cavity to allow reentry and skin flap closure within 7–10 days.

Nursing activities include observing for respiratory distress that might result from pressure of abdominal organs on the diaphram, for fatigue, and for integrity of the operative site. The nurse also insures that the infant is properly positioned, clothed, and restrained in order to prevent trauma to the site. The nurse provides care of the surgical site according to physician's orders. In the nonsurgical corrective method, observations for mercury poisoning should be made; signs include edema, bright red spots on the skin other than areas being painted, lethargy, and seizures. Urinalysis is important, as mercury may be present in the urine before clinical signs appear. For care of intravenous feedings, assessing for adequate nutrition and hydration, and assisting parents, see the Nursing Care Plan for cleft lip and palate.

Prognosis

The prognosis depends on the presence and severity of the defect and the coexisting malformations: intestinal malrotation, abnormal obstructing bands across the duodenum, midgut volvulus, adhesions, intestinal atresia, congenital heart disease, cleft lip, and the like. About one-third of these infants suffer the hazards imposed by prematurity as well. The poorest surgical results and increased mortality are expected if the sac is more than 7 cm wide and contains the liver.

Aganglionic Megacolon

Physiology and Pathophysiology

Aganglionic megacolon is also known as Hirschsprung's disease, congenital megacolon, or aganglionosis. Parasympathetic nerve-ganglion cells are absent in the submucosa and muscles in the rectosigmoid colon. Without innervation, colonic peristalsis and passing of fecal material cannot occur in that segment. The intestine proximal to the aganglionic segment becomes grossly distended as fecal material accumulates. This motility disturbance results in intestinal obstruction, vomiting, constipation, fluid and electrolyte deficits, and hypoproteinemia. Aganglionosis is four times more common in males and is often associated with Down's syndrome or with a genetic predisposition.

Clinical Manifestations and Differential Diagnosis

Very mild cases may be undiagnosed for several years and may result in no symptoms except for persistent constipation, which is relieved by laxatives or enemas on occasion.

The neonate with this disorder may manifest the following symptoms: an absence of meconium, vomitus containing bile, constipation, and increasing abdominal distention and resultant respiratory distress (Figure 26–8). In older infants it is characterized by abdominal distention alternating diarrhea with obstinate constipation and large palpable fecal mass. If the condition is left untreated, the child becomes chronically ill, is malnourished, anemic, and lethargic, and may suffer respiratory embarrassment. A striking foul odor to his breath and stool is significant. The rectum may be tight or collapsed. Enterocolitis may develop. Complications of hyperthermia, neurogenic shock, and severe toxicity may be fatal if not treated immediately. Crisis is heralded by profuse vomiting, fever, and offensive diarrhea progressing to rapid dehydration and collapse of the empty rectum. On rectal digital exam, the rectum is tight and conical. Often there is expulsion of stool or gas after the exam.

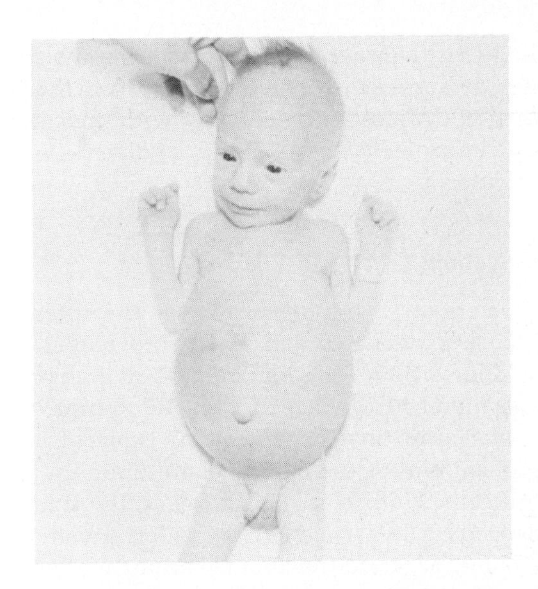

Figure 26–8. Infant with Hirshsprung's disease.

An anteroposterior radiography of the abdomen reveals a distended intestinal loop. An x-ray film of a barium enema shows a narrow rectum and sigmoid colon and a zone of conversion to the distended proximal colon. Usually the barium enema fails to be expelled. After abdominal decompression, a rectal biopsy is done to examine for absence of nerve-ganglion cells.

Histology shows an absence of parasympathetic ganglion cells of the intramural plexus in the narrowed segment. The physician must rule out meconium plug and ileus secondary to sepsis or volvulus. Diagnostic contrast enemas may be used to dislodge a meconium plug from the transverse or sigmoid colon, thus relieving this obstruction. Almost all neonates with meconium plug syndrome have no defect and remain well thereafter.

Interventions

An emergency colostomy relieves the intestinal obstruction, deflates and clears the bowel, and also allows time for improvement of nutritional and general health status until the optimal time for total correction. The colostomy is placed just at the distal end of the bowel where there are ganglion cells. Until corrective surgery, the infant is placed on a low residue diet and is given stool softeners; accurate intake and output records are kept, noting frequency and nature of stools. Just prior to corrective surgery, the bowel is emptied manually and with colonic irrigations of isotonic saline solutions. Drugs such as neomycin by mouth and by rectal instillation are given to reduce normal bowel flora. A nasogastric tube is inserted to decompress the stomach, and fluid and electrolyte replacements are carried out. Electrolyte imbalances are common as a result of vomiting and intestinal dysfunction. Final resection of the aganglionic segment and anastomosis of the proximal and distal portions are usually not done before 6 months of age and may be delayed for one year. Optimally the child is 12–18 months of age and weighs 20–25 lb (Jones, 1976).

The temporary colostomy is closed either during the total correction or usually one to two weeks later.

Nursing Management

The nurse plays an important role in the early diagnosis of this disorder. The nursing history contains pertinent information from the prenatal and perinatal records for familial history, the condition of the neonate from birth, and the onset of symptoms as previously described.

Nursing priorities prior to surgery include astute observations of symptoms (which assist in early diagnosis), maintenance of adequate nutrition and hydration, and assisting the parents to cope with the situation. These children tend to be finicky eaters. Frequent small feedings with consideration to likes and dislikes and developmental level should be offered, because they tend to eat slowly, have poor appetites, and become uncomfortable after eating, resulting in difficulties in establishing proper nutritional habits.

Following colostomy surgery, the nurse's priorities include the prevention of postoperative complications, maintenance of adequate nutrition and hydration, colostomy care, and preparation of the parents for the care of the colostomy and the infant until the corrective surgery is scheduled.

Colostomy care in the neonate requires conscientious care to prevent skin irritation and possible infection. Diapers and other clothing are changed frequently to keep the neonate clean, dry, and free from odor and to minimize skin breakdown with infection. The skin around the colostomy is cleansed with warm water, dried, then protected with a thin layer of aluminum paste, karaya gum, or Maalox. Periodic exposure to air is also beneficial. Drainage from the colostomy is assessed for amount, color, consistency, and the presence of mucus or blood. Fluid replacement is partially dependent on the amount of drainage. In the early period after the colostomy is constructed, the nurse observes the neonate for abdominal distention or obstruction. Obstruction may occur from peritonitis, which is manifested by increasing abdominal tenderness, hyperthermia, vomiting, or irritability.

The thought as well as the sight of a colostomy is very difficult for parents to accept. They require considerable support while they grieve over the situation, express their anger and frustration, and then, finally, learn to care for the infant and the colostomy. The parents notice each person's reaction to the colostomy and internalize these reactions. The nurse needs to plan time to be with the parents when they are visiting with the neonate to offer support and information. It is best if the parents have some idea what a colostomy will look like prior to surgery. The parents need to learn how to keep the child in a good nutritional state so that he will be ready for surgical repair later in infancy.

Postsurgical correction and the notation of feeding behaviors, pain upon elimination, and abdominal distention are important. Stools are tested for presence of bleeding and are measured to determine fluid and electrolyte losses. Initial replacement therapy based on the amount of stooling and electrolyte studies is instituted—intravenously at first until oral feedings are possible. Axillary temperature should be taken until rectal healing is complete. The infant may have nothing by mouth for long periods, so in order to meet his normal sucking needs a pacifier should be offered. Meticulous skin care around the perineal and anal regions is essential to prevent excoriations common with pull-through operations and postoperative diarrhea. When surgical correction is achieved, the primary focus is on the establishment of normal elimination. Patterns and amount of stooling should be assessed to determine the child's progression toward this goal.

Prognosis

Prognosis for normal bowel function and control depends on the length of the bowel segment that lacks the nerve-ganglia and on whether the rectum can be preserved.

Imperforate Anus

Physiology and Pathophysiology

Imperforate anus comprises a variety of lesions of the rectum and anus, ranging from a simple membrane at the anus to complex deformities. A brief review of embryonic development clarifies the development of this anomaly. In the normal embryonic process, a blind pouch within the abdomen moves downward to the perineum to meet another pouch invaginating upward from the anal area. The two pouches meet, fuse to form a continuous passageway, and the membrane that separates the rectum from the anus normally is absorbed during the 7th week of fetal life. Abnormality at any point in the pathway results in imperforate anus.

Imperforate anus is best classified according to the international classification of anorectal anomalies (Table 26–1). The "high" group are above the levator sling; the "intermediate" group are on the sling but not through it. The differentiation of these two supralevator groups is important in the operative decision. In the low group of imperforate anus anomalies (translevator group), the termination of the rectum is anterior to the external sphincter. In each group the bowel ends blindly or communicates by a fistula with the nearby viscera or the perineal skin. In all these deformities the internal anal sphincter is absent, but the external anal sphincter may be present in rudimentary form. Total sphincter absence does not necessarily produce fecal incontinence if the puborectalis is intact. Some slight staining may occur, because the external sphincter normally closes the anus.

The termination point of the descending bowel determines the success of surgical repair. A high anomaly that terminates above the puborectalis support of the levator ani musculature is more difficult to repair and is often associated with urologic and vertebral malformations, with increased mortality and morbidity. Surgical repair of a lower anomaly, which terminates after passing through the puborectalis sling, is anticipated to produce a better functional result.

Fistulous tracts originating in the intestinal pouch may terminate in the anal area or urinary tract in both sexes and in the vagina in females.

Imperforate anus is a common anomaly occurring in about 1 in 5000 births and is more common in males. In infants with high anomalies, 50% have associated neurologic defects that lessen the possibility of a well-functioning bowel after correction.

Clinical Manifestations

Several variations of the anatomic appearance of the perineum are possible. The anal opening may be absent with or without the presence of a sphincter musculature (Figure 26–9). The "wink" reflex may be absent. (A "wink" is elicited when one touches the normal sphincter muscle.) The anus may be abnormally placed. If only a thin membrane covers the anal opening, a black mass (meconium) may be seen behind the membrane. The examiner is unable to insert a lubricated thermometer (or tubing) into the anal opening. (Caution: If a rectal thermometer is used prior to the passage of meconium, the examiner must use extreme care so as not to traumatize or perforate an otherwise imperforate anus.)

The physiologic function is altered as well: No meconium is passed, and increasing abdominal distention is noted. Or meconium may be passed via an ectopic opening from the vagina or urethra. Meconium in the urine of males indicates a fistula to the urinary tract.

Diagnosis is based on examinations to determine the anatomic level of the anomaly, the location of the fistula and its ectopic opening, and the presence of coexisting malformations. An Invertogram roentgenogram (Wagenstein-Rice method), of the neonate tilted upside down, to determine the level of intestinal pouch is not always accurate, because it takes time (at least 18–24 hours) for air to reach the apex of the blind pouch. Lumbosacral vertebral malformations may be visualized on x-ray, especially sacral agenesis, which affects neural pathways. A micturating cystourethrogram (MCU) identifies urologic malformations and rectourinary communication that may accompany this defect.

Interventions

If only a simple membrane is covering the anus, it is excised or treated with a cruciate incision followed by dilatation of the anus at periodic intervals to keep the opening the size of the little finger, thereby preventing stricture and scar formation.

Table 26-1. International Classification of Anorectal Anomalies*

Male	Female
Supralevator anomalies	
A. High anomalies	
1. Anorectal agenesis	1. Anorectal agenesis
(a) Without fistula	(a) Without fistula
Anorectal agenesis (no fistula)	Anorectal agenesis (no fistula)
(b) With fistula	(b) With fistula
(i) Rectovesical	(i) Rectovesical
(ii) Rectourethral	(ii) Rectocloacal
	(iii) Rectovaginal (mid and high)
2. Rectal atresia	2. Rectal atresia
B. Intermediate anomalies	
1. Anal agenesis	1. Anal agenesis
(a) Without fistula	(a) Without fistula
Anal agenesis (no fistula)	Anal agenesis (no fistula)
(b) With fistula	(b) With fistula
Rectobulbar	(i) Rectovaginal (low)
	(ii) Rectovestibular
2. Anorectal stenosis	2. Anorectal stenosis
Translevator low anomalies	
1. At normal anal site	1. At normal anal site
(i) Covered anus—complete†	(i) Covered anus—complete†
(ii) Anal stenosis‡	(ii) Anal stenosis‡
2. At perineal site	2. At perineal site
(i) Anterior perineal anus	(i) Anterior perineal anus
(ii) Anocutaneous fistula (covered anus—incomplete)	(ii) Anocutaneous fistula (covered anus—incomplete)
	3. At vulvar site
	(i) Vulvar anus
	(ii) Anovulvar fistula
	(iii) Anovestibular fistula

*From Smith, E. D. 1976. Anorectal anomalies. In *Clinical paediatric surgery: diagnosis and management.* 2nd ed. Ed. P. G. Jones. Oxford: Blackwell Scientific Publications, p. 87.

†Includes imperforate anal membrane.

‡Includes anal membrane stenosis.

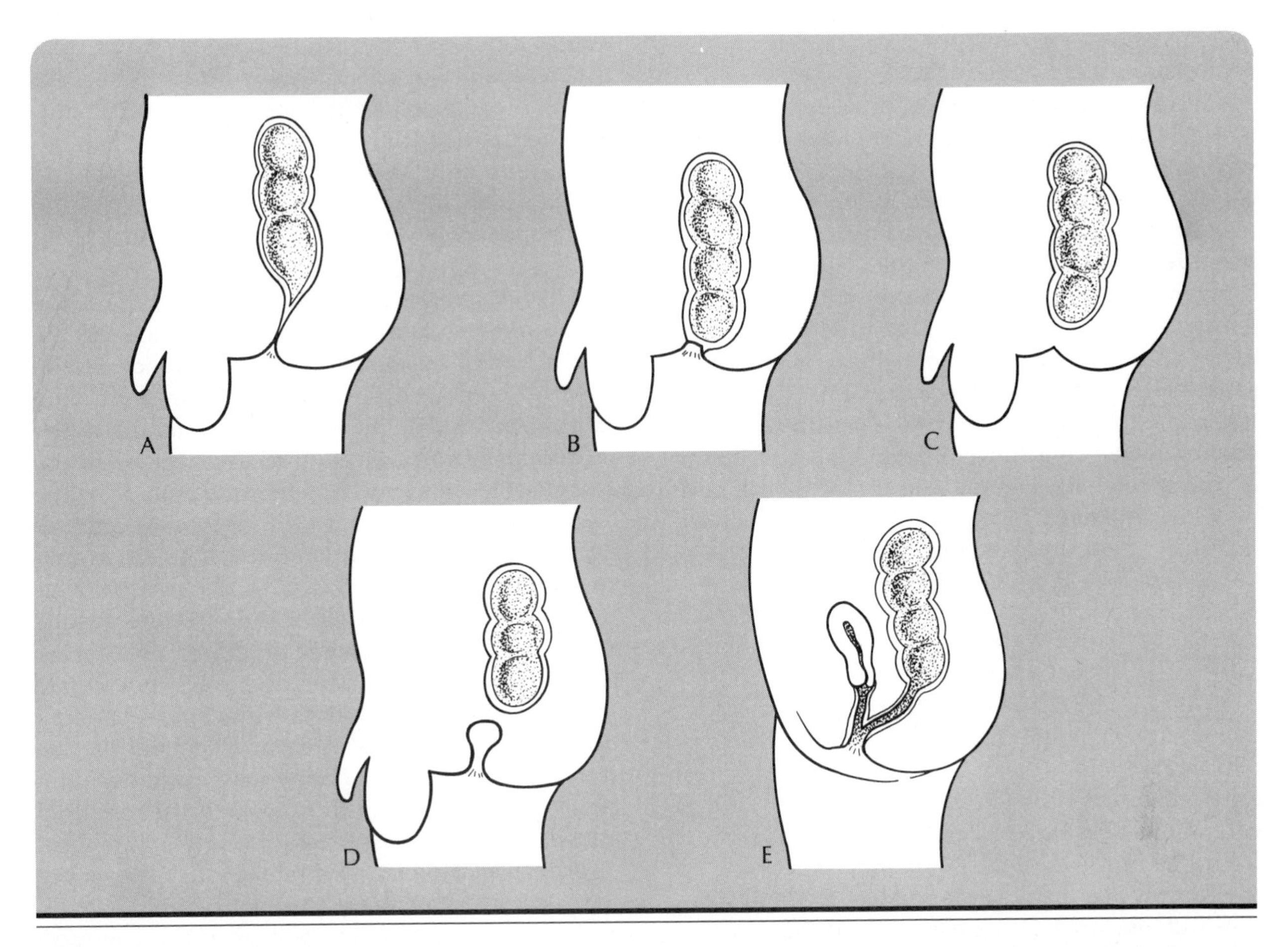

Figure 26–9. Variations in imperforate anus and anal rectal stenosis. **A,** Congenital stenosis of the anus. **B,** Anal opening covered by thin membrane. **C,** Anal agenesis. **D,** Rectal atresia. **E,** Rectal vaginal fistula.

Low anomalies (short length of rectal agenesis—less than 1.5 cm from perineal skin) are corrected to make a continuous passageway by means of either a perineal approach "cutback" procedure or anoplasty followed by anal dilatation at periodic intervals initiated as soon as initial healing occurs.

High anomalies (those in which the blind pouch is farther than 1.5 cm away from the perineal skin) are treated in at least two stages: sigmoid colostomy above the fistulous tract to protect the urinary system from fecal contamination and corrective surgery (to make a continuous passageway) at about 9–12 months of age. Usually a sacro-abdomenoperineal rectoplasty is done, which exposes and delineates the puborectalis sling, then via the abdominal route the rectum is mobilized, the fistula is divided, and the bowel is brought down within the puborectalis sling to the perineum. For intermediate anomalies a sacroperineal rectoplasty is done.

Nursing Management

A complete nursing history based on careful observation of the neonate's anatomic appearance and physiologic functioning assists in the identification and early treatment of this congenital anomaly. Notation is made of the parental reactions to the situation and the infant. Regardless of the surgical treatments, parents need assistance in coping with the birth of a child with a defect. Parents need to be encouraged to see and touch the infant early and often. Postoperative care is directed toward colostomy and pull-through care (discussed in the section on aganglionic megacolon, p. 862). Immediately postoperatively, diapers are not used, and immediate cleansing of the anal area after each stool is very important. The infant should be positioned and turned from side to side but never allowed to lie with his legs pulled up under him, as this puts pressure on the suture area. Anal dilatations may cause emotional trauma because of the preoccupation with the anal area and its by-products.

Depending on the surgical procedure, parents may need to be taught to perform anal dilatation with catheters or the little finger or to perform colostomy care (see the section on aganglionic megacolon, p. 862). Parents need to be advised that even if continuity of the bowel is achieved, some infants with high anomalies will have problems with fecal continence throughout life, which can lead to problems in school and with interpersonal relationships. Toilet training is a difficult milestone to achieve; it may take months or years or may never be achieved, producing a stressful situation for both parents and child. In the case of a low anomaly, toilet training is achieved by learning to use the puborectalis muscle.

Complications

Anal strictures readily develop after anoplasty or rectoplasty, and anal dilatation is required at regular intervals for at least three months. Strictures can lead to constipation and colonic inertia, development of a large hypertrophied and dilated rectum, and incontinence. Ischemic sloughing of the rectum may result from inadequate mobilization and tension. Fistulas may recur if their initial closure was inadequate. Urinary complications and perineal or pararectal abscess may develop.

Prognosis

Prognosis depends on the severity of the anomaly and on the presence of associated malformations.

Intestinal Obstruction

Physiology and Pathophysiology

Intestinal atresia and stenosis may result from intrauterine interferences of blood supply to the embryonic bowel or from failure to reestablish the lumen during fetal bowel development. The atresia may take the form of a septum in the lumen of the intestines, complete atresia of varying lengths, or separated multiple blind pouches. Most of these malformations occur distal to the opening of the bile and pancreatic ducts (duodenum), so that vomitus is bile-stained. The annular pancreas may constrict the duodenum. If the stricture is incomplete, symptoms may not occur during the first month of life. This anomaly is often coincident with Down's syndrome. Duodenal and ileal atresias are most common. Atresias are not common between the duodenum and the lower ileum.

Meconium ileus refers to an obstruction of the intestine by thick, inspissated meconium. In the neonate with cystic fibrosis, a deficiency of the pancreatic enzyme trypsin causes the meconium in utero to become puttylike and to adhere to the intestinal mucosa. Meconium ileus may become complicated by rupture of the intestine proximal to the obstruction, spillage of meconium into the peritoneum, and consequent development of meconium peritonitis.

Volvulus, the twisting of the intestine, results from abnormal embryonic development. Either the colon (ileocecal structure) does not rotate properly as the intestines enter the abdomen through the umbilical area and remains in the right upper quadrant, or the mesentery does not attach properly during the 10th week of gestation, allowing the bowel to twist upon itself. Remnants of normal peritoneal attachments of the cecum to the right abdominal wall in embryonic development may exist, extending from the cecum and ascending colon across the descending duodenum, further causing obstruction. In addition to intestinal obstruction, a severe complication of volvulus is infarction and necrosis. Volvulus is possible any time during the first few years of life but is most common in early infancy.

Meconium plug syndrome results from an accumulation of meconium in the rectum. The meconium becomes inspissated and firm, thus obstructing the lower bowel. All the symptoms of intestinal obstruction are seen.

Clinical Manifestations

Neonates with intestinal obstruction usually fail to pass any meconium, and prenatal polyhydramnios is present. Increasing abdominal distention is noted. If the distention progresses, the neonate's respiratory rate increases. Vomiting may be bilious (green) or fecal. Volvulus may be palpable. Without surgical intervention, the neonate loses weight, becomes dehydrated, and develops hypoproteinemia, hypokalemia, hyponatremia, metabolic acidosis, and shock.

Differential Diagnosis

With intestinal atresia, barium-contrast x-rays show the characteristic "double bubble," indicating a large amount of barium in the stomach and a smaller amount in the duodenum only.

Ileal atresia and meconium ileus may be difficult to differentiate. Symptoms of both include abdominal distention and fecal-contaminated vomitus and absence of stooling if the condition is not diagnosed and treated soon enough. X-rays show larger fluid-air levels in ileal atresia, as opposed to tiny air bubbles in viscid meconium in meconium ileus. Meconium ileus is suspected if there is a familial history of cystic fibrosis (mucoviscidosis). Volvulus is differentiated from high intestinal atresia by use of upper gastrointestinal films and barium enema. Meconium plug syndrome x-rays show distended gaseous loops, usually without fluid levels.

Interventions

Management of intestinal atresia or stricture of the duodenum from an annular pancreas is surgical resection of the affected intestinal segment with end-to-end anastomosis or duodenal bypass procedure (duodenoduodenostomy or duodenojejunostomy) for duodenal atresia. Treatment for jejunal or ileal atresia is excision of atretic and distended portions followed by end-to-end anastomosis (jejunojejunostomy or ileostomy). The pancreas is not incised, because this procedure is often followed by pancreatitis or fistula formation.

Management of volvulus is surgical (Ladd procedure) to relieve the twisting, to divide any constricting bands, to reduce the volvulus, and to reattach the bowel if necessary.

Management of meconium ileus is surgical, with removal of inspissated meconium after irrigations of acetylcysteine, an aproteolytic enzyme solution. The infant is assessed for cystic fibrosis, and management focuses on preventing complications of that disease if it is diagnosed.

Diagnostic tests for intestinal obstruction may relieve the meconium plug. The examiner's finger or the barium enema may force the expulsion of the meconium and pent-up gas. If the obstruction is not relieved, normal saline enemas (plain water enema should never be used, because it could lead to water intoxication), followed by an instillation of 5 ml of acetylcysteine solution, usually stimulate the expulsion of the meconium obstruction. Neonates with meconium plug syndrome are otherwise normal. To verify the accuracy of the diagnosis, neonates are observed for a time (days or months) to rule out Hirschsprung's disease, hypothyroidism, or cystic fibrosis.

Nursing Management

A complete nursing history with a record of day-by-day observation is invaluable in identifying symptomatology that can lead to an early definitive diagnosis and appropriate intervention.

In addition to recognizing symptomatology described in the preceding pages, the nurse needs to know how to pass an orogastric tube for aspiration; how to assess vomitus, stooling, and stools; and how to evaluate for abdominal distention.

Assessment of Vomiting and Vomitus. Note the following concerning vomiting:

1. Time in relation to the beginning or completion of the feeding.
2. Type:
   a. Regurgitation, or "spitting up," is usually a nonforceful "spilling out" of fluid unaccompanied by abdominal contractions. Overfeeding or inadequate bubbling is the probable cause.
   b. Nonprojectile vomiting is that which is mildly ejected and is often accompanied by abdominal contractions.
   c. Projectile vomiting is a forceful ejection of vomitus up to a distance of 5 feet. Pyloric stenosis or brain injury may be the underlying cause.

Identify the nature of the vomitus as follows:

1. Unchanged formula: formula that is unchanged by gastric juices and that usually occurs shortly after the feeding is started. Esophageal atresia is suspected.
2. Curdled milk: formula has been modified by gastric juices.
3. Greenish color: bile (turns green on exposure to air) in vomitus. Although this may be nonpathologic in nature, intestinal obstruction below the duodenum is probable.
4. Fecal contamination: obstruction of the lower gastrointestinal tract is suspected.

5. Bloody: one nonpathological cause is swallowing of blood during birthing. Pathologic causes include a bleeding ulcer.

Assessment of Stooling and Stools. Note the following:

1. Passage or lack of passage of meconium. One or two small stools can be passed even in the presence of obstruction.
2. Appearance of meconium:
   a. Light-colored (acholic) due to absence of bile in intestine.
   b. Inspissated (firm, thick) usually because of lack of the pancreatic enzyme trypsin.
3. Appearance of stool:
   a. Bloody. If unaccompanied by pain, may be due to a Meckel's diverticulum or a rectal polyp.
   b. Bloody diarrhea—may be due to ulcerative colitis.
   c. Presence of mucus.
4. Pain. (Infant draws legs up to abdomen, paroxysmal bouts of crying, demonstrates facial grimaces and clenches fists.)
5. Constipation. If severe, it is accompanied by lower abdominal pain and tenderness, and the child may display anxiety and apprehension. Constipation may be due to Hirschsprung's disease.

Evaluation of Abdominal Distention. Determine the location of the distention:

1. Abdominal distention. Visible waves of peristalsis seen passing from left to right across the epigastrium and distention high in the abdomen indicate that the obstruction is at the level of the duodenum.
2. Marked generalized abdominal distention is commonly associated with lower intestinal tract obstruction.
3. Distention may be accompanied by respiratory distress as the diaphragm is forced upward.

Nursing priorities include identifying symptoms of intestinal obstruction prior to onset of complications (respiratory distress, fluid and electrolyte imbalance, damage to intestinal tract or other signs of toxicity), preventing postoperative complications (or the early treatment of complications to prevent untoward sequelae), and assisting the parents to cope with the situation.

INFANT WITH GENITOURINARY DEFECT

Exstrophy of the Bladder

Failure of the anterior abdominal wall and symphysis pubis to unite results in the exposure of the posterior and lateral walls of the bladder and trigone. This anomaly of unknown etiology may be accompanied by other defects of the intestinal tract and genital system. The folds of deep-red exposed bladder mucosa are sensitive when touched and are susceptible to ulceration. Urine seeps directly out over the skin, causing excoriation.

The exposed bladder mucosa with continual seepage of urine is evident at birth. Frequently associated malformations include undescended testes, inguinal hernia, vaginal agenesis, epispadias, short penis, and cleft labia (in females). When older, the child demonstrates a waddling or unsteady gait.

The objectives of treatment are continuing adequate renal function, preventing infections, and cosmetic reconstruction as needed to improve the child's appearance and meet physiologic needs. Cosmetic reconstruction is particularly important for the male child with abnormalities of the penis. Early treatment consists of collecting urine and protecting the bladder mucosa from the seeping urine with a prosthesis applied to the surrounding skin. Several weeks or months later, surgery is performed. Minor defects may be corrected completely, and the patient will void normally. Major defects may require complete removal of the bladder tissue, transplantation of ureters into the colon, and plastic repair of the abdominal wall. Bladder reconstruction has been limited in its success, and treatment of choice is urinary diversion. Urinary diversion, such as ureterosigmoidostomy with antireflux urethral anastomosis is usually performed at 15–18 months of age. If chronic urethral reflux symptoms are present, this procedure frees the child from an external appliance. Complications are hydroureters, hydronephrosis, and pyelonephritis. Surgery or braces may be needed for the pelvic deformity.

Nursing priorities include protecting the exposed bladder wall and skin surrounding it from infection, as well as the respiratory and gastrointestinal tracts; preventing emotional trauma to the infant; preventing postoperative complications; and assisting the parents to cope with the situation. Convalescent priorities include control of urination and the development of an acceptable gait.

Several nursing actions help to prevent infection and direct trauma to the bladder mucosa. These include propping the neonate on his side, covering the defect per physician's orders (sterile petrolatum gauze or a firm covering), changing diapers frequently, cleansing the surrounding area with each diaper change, and periodically exposing the area to the air. The surrounding skin may be protected by a thin layer of aluminum paste, karaya gum, or Maalox.

Should a urine specimen be needed, the infant can be held over a sterile basin to collect the drops of urine.

Because surgery is scheduled weeks or months later, the parents are taught to care for the defect. Parents are encouraged to hold, cuddle, and assist in their infant's care as soon after birth as they possibly can. The nurse encourages the parents to grieve for the birth of a child with a defect and provides physical and verbal support while the parents view and work with the defect.

INFANT WITH DISTURBANCE OF LOCOMOTION

Many skeletal anomalies are apparent in the neonatal period, although others are not identified until months later, usually when the child begins to walk. Early recognition and treatment is necessary for successful correction.

Two of the most common skeletal malformations apparent in the neonatal period are clubfoot and congenital dysplasia of the hip. Other disturbances of locomotion are caused by spina bifida and phocomelia.

Talipes Equinovarus (Clubfoot)

Physiology and Pathophysiology

Talipes equinovarus (clubfoot) is the most serious and most common deformity of the foot. The fixed postural deformity typically is in a position of inversion (varus) and adduction of the heel and forefoot (the bottom of the foot faces the midline), marked plantar flexion (equinus) at the ankle, and shortening of the Achilles tendon (Figure 26–10,*A*). Passive correction is impossible because of the tightness of the affected structures. Genetic and environmental factors (intrauterine position) are implicated. This condition occurs in 1 of every 1000 births (Ferguson, 1975). Recurrence in a family with one affected child is from 1 in 35 to 1 in 10. Males are affected about twice as often as females. Unilateral clubfoot is slightly more common than bilateral.

About 5% of the cases of clubfoot are classified as talipes calcaneovalgus. The typical position is with the foot dorsiflexed (the heel turns outward and the anterior part of the foot is elevated on the outer border) and deviating laterally.

Clinical Manifestations

The infant has an obvious fixed deformity of the foot, as described above. Calf size and degree of internal or external torsion of the tibia should be noted. In true fixed clubfoot, the calf on the affected side is smaller or atrophied; the foot lies in external torsion in relation to the knee; and the peroneal muscles, stimulated by stroking the lateral side of the foot, demonstrate weakness and an inability to evert the foot. The Achilles tendon is always shortened, and the tibial tendons are contracted in proportion to the severity. When the infant cries, the deformity is exaggerated, whereas a positional mobile "deformity" corrects itself when the child is crying or can be passively

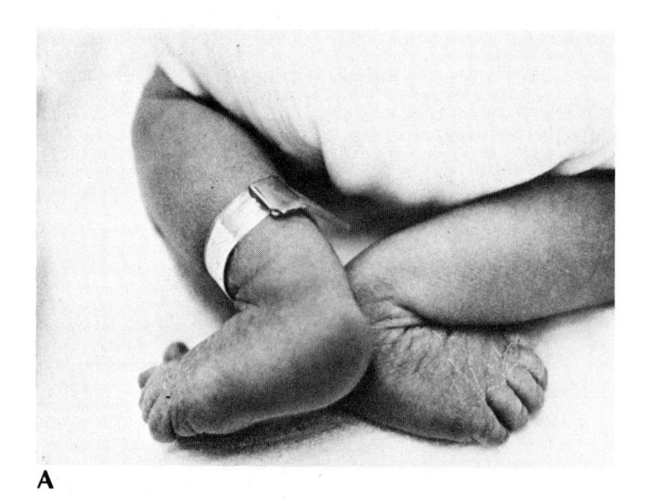

A

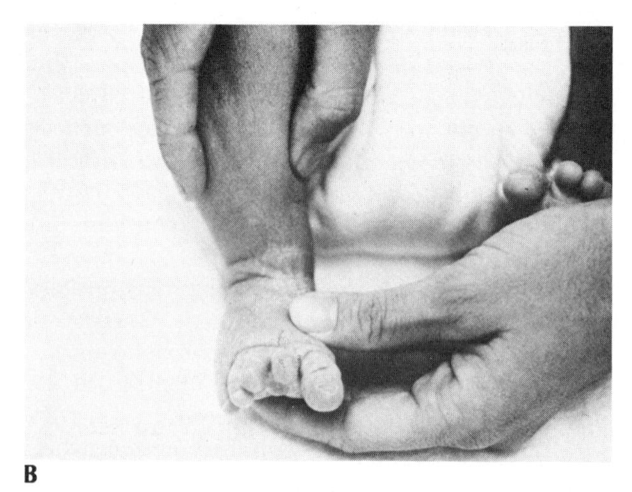

B

Figure 26–10. **A,** Bilateral talipes equinovarus seen with infant in supine position. **B,** To determine the presence of clubfoot, the nurse moves the foot to the midline. Resistance indicates true clubfoot.

manipulated into correct position (Figure 26–10,*B*). The child must be examined for possible coexisting malformations, such as hip dysplasia, spina bifida, and meningomyelocele. Clubfoot associated with meningomyelocele is particularly resistent to correction because of the lack of nerve supply.

Interventions

Intervention is aimed at correcting all elements of the deformity and at maintaining correction throughout the early growth years.

Plaster casts are applied in the neonatal period during the nursery stay, when the ligaments are still relaxed from maternal hormones. Depending on the severity of the deformity and physician preference, conservative methods are employed:

1. The Kite method of wedge casting is a gradual corrective measure that systematically, by means of plaster casts and wedges, deals with the different aspects of the deformity.

2. Manipulation and casting is the most common technique, using a series of corrective casts applied after forcible manipulation. Frequent changes of casts are required. The best results are achieved with weekly change.

3. Denis Browne splints are used for infants under 1 year of age. The appliance is made of two foot plates attached to a crossbar. Feet are attached to the splint either by strapping with adhesive tape or by slipping the foot into a shoe already attached to the plates. After the child starts to walk, he is given special shoes with an elevated outer edge, thereby forcing him to walk in a more correct position. Night splints are continued for a year or longer. Denis Browne splints may be used in conjunction with other conservative methods, such as correction by casting; the splint is used to maintain correction. Lower leg braces with special shoes may be used when the child is walking.

Because clubfoot has a tendency to recur even following appropriate treatment, the affected child must be watched throughout childhood. Occasionally surgery may be required. Usual treatment involves lengthening of the Achilles tendon or Achilles tendon transfer, release of the medial ligaments, and ankle joint capsulotomy. Surgery on the bone (osteotomies) may be required for maximum correction in some patients. Families can be referred to community agencies for financial support and to public health departments for continued moral support and supervision.

Nursing care of the child with talipes equinovarus is directed toward promoting parental acceptance of the child and the deformity and toward education of the parents regarding their infant's needs for care. Care of an infant in a cast or splint is discussed, and symptoms of complications are reviewed. It is essential for a successful outcome that the parents recognize the long-term nature of the treatment program and be willing to cooperate fully.

Prognosis

Repair is usually very good with proper treatment at an early age. The condition may recur later during childhood and will again require treatment. Exercises may be required for many years.

Dysplasia of the Hip

Physiology and Pathophysiology

Congenital dislocation of the hip in the neonatal period refers to a potential rather than a true dislocation. The term implies that the head of the femur is out of the acetabulum at birth, but this is not always true, and there are varying degrees of dysplasia of the hip joint.

Dysplasia refers to an inadequate formation of the acetabulum. The acetabulum and femoral head are potentially normal but remain in the fetal cartilaginous state with delay of ossification. The hip capsule, which ordinarily holds the femoral head in the acetabulum, is stretched, and the acetabulum is shallow and rimmed with cartilage instead of being deep and completely ossified. As a result of the capsule failure to hold the femoral head in the acetabulum, some degree of displacement occurs, and there is an increased upward slant of the acetabulum roof and anteversion of the head and neck of the femur.

This potentially crippling deformity is a result of an interaction between genetic influences and environmental factors such as insufficient femoral head pressure in the acetabulum during fetal life, position of the fetus in utero, or hormonal influence. It is seen four to seven times as often in females as in males (the female pelvis appears more affected by the maternal hormones, which relax maternal pelvic ligaments), involves the left hip three times more often than the right, occurs more frequently in breech presentations, and is twice as common unilaterally as bilaterally. Relaxation of the joint capsule and ligaments in response to maternal hormones initially abets the dislocation. Early recognition and treatment is important so that the cartilaginous structures are not malformed through muscle pull pressures and early weight bearing.

The depth of the acetabulum determines the degree of dislocation, and an infant can progress from the stage of dysplasia to subluxation to luxation or complete dislocation. *Subluxation* refers to a partial or incomplete dislocation (that is, the femoral head rides on the lateral third edge of the acetabulum, with partial displacement from the acetabulum and some degree of anteversion of the head of the femur). Subluxation is more common than dislocation but, if untreated, may result in complete dislocation. Early signs are limited abduction of the hip in a flexed position or a click sign while the hip is being abducted. The mother may note an inability to abduct the hip during diaper changes.

Luxation is present when the femoral head is completely dislocated above the acetabular rim. Anteversion of the femur is usually quite marked. It can occur during intrauterine life or can follow an untreated subluxation some time after birth. In either case, it demands early recognition, while it is possible to reduce the dislocation easily and to begin correction of the defect. Without treatment, the stretched capsule and ligaments become more rigid, the head of the femur may press a socket in the ileum above the acetabulum, and the hip abductor muscles may shorten. This development results in painful and basically untreatable crippling deformity in adulthood.

The incidence of dysplasia varies in different parts of the world. The highest incidence is among the Lapps and certain American Indian tribes, who swaddle babies for the first year of life. The next highest incidence (3 in 1000) is in Italy, France, and Japan. An incidence of 1 in 1000 exists in England and Sweden. Dysplasia is rarely seen among blacks.

Clinical Manifestations

Upon examination, it is noted that folds on the dorsal gluteal and popliteal surfaces are asymmetrical and appear higher on the affected side. There is limited abduction of the leg at the hip on the affected side (under 60°). The greater trochanter on the affected side is prominent and elevated, and the perineum on the affected side is broadened (Figure 26–11). Marked bilateral broadening is seen if both hips are dislocated. Later, after the child has begun to bear weight, marked prominence of the greater trochanter and flattening of the buttock on the affected side can be seen. With a characteristic limp, the child lurches or sways to the affected side. The child may demonstrate lumbar lordosis and protuberant abdomen. In unilateral dislocation, there is marked shortening of the affected leg, possible

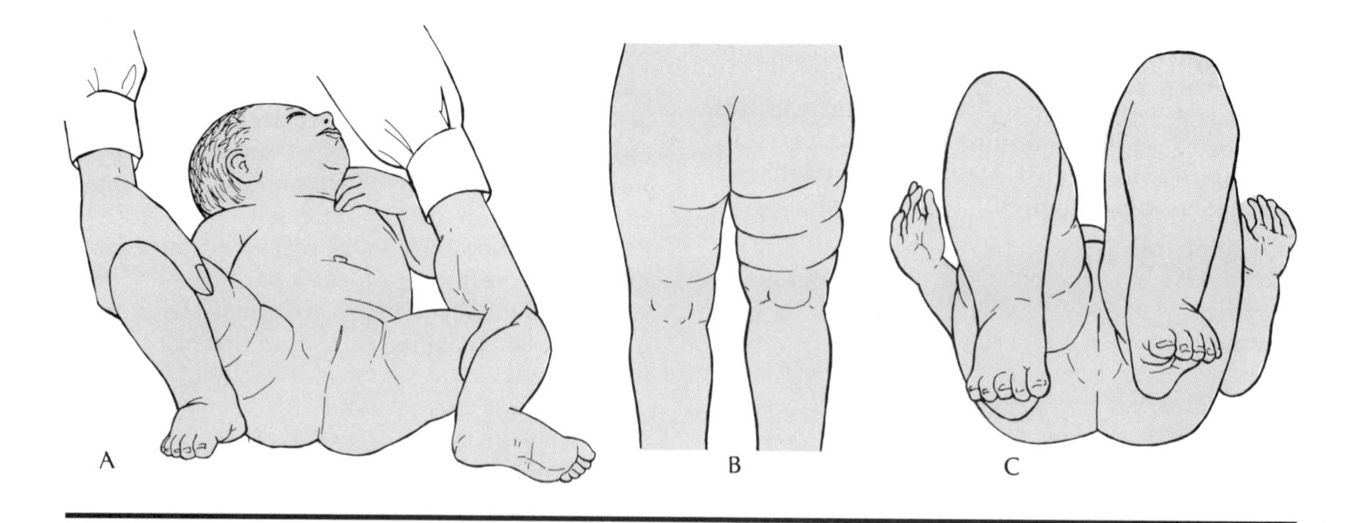

Figure 26–11. Early signs of congenital dislocation of the right hip. **A,** Limitation of abduction. **B,** Asymmetry of skin folds and prominence of trochanter. **C,** Shortening of femur. (Courtesy Ross Laboratories, Columbus, Ohio.)

functional scoliosis, and abduction and flexion contractures of the involved hip. The examiner may be unable to feel the femoral pulse over the head of the femur.

Several maneuvers assist in a definitive diagnosis:

1. *Ortolani's maneuver.* With the infant supine on a firm surface, flex hips to 90° and abduct fully; bend knees. As the hip is reduced during abduction, an audible click is produced by the head of the femur as it enters the acetabulum. Then, with forefinger on the greater trochanter and thumb on the lesser trochanter, adduct hip to elicit a palpable click. This maneuver is not always suitable in the neonatal period, because movement of the head of the femur out of the socket may be smooth and quiet or a luxated hip may not reduce and therefore not produce a click. It is best used to detect an already-dislocated hip.

2. *Barlow's maneuver.* This is a modification of the Ortolani maneuver but is more suitable for the neonatal period and detects a potentially dislocated hip. With the infant supine on a firm surface, flex hips to 90° and flex the knee completely. With the forefingers on the greater trochanters, apply pressure posteriorly with thumbs on the lesser trochanters. The head of the femur will slip out of an unstable hip and slip back when thumb pressure is stopped.

3. *Galeazzi's sign.* With the infant supine, flex hips at right angles. Lowering of the knee length (due to apparent shortening of the thigh when the head of the femur is out of the socket) is a positive sign.

X-ray studies of the pelvis and hips are of little value in the neonatal period but may be diagnostic after 4 to 5 months of age.

Differential Diagnosis

The limited abduction characteristic of hip dysplasia is also seen in cases of voluntary resistance, spina bifida due to weak hip abductors and adduction contracture, hip joint infection, Still's disease, rickets, cerebral palsy with spastic paralysis (which causes a stretch reflex in the abductors that limits reduction), and polio. Developmental coxa vara with deformity of the femoral neck presents a clinical picture similar to congenital dysplasia but is unusual before the age of 4.

Interventions

Early recognition and treatment is imperative to the successful correction of the abnormality. The longer the condition goes unrecognized, the more severe the anomaly becomes, the more difficult the treatment, and the less favorable the prognosis. The regimen depends on the age of the child and the severity of the dysplasia. The goal is prevention of dislocation and promotion of normal hip joint formation by maintaining the femoral head within the acetabulum.

Medical management of the neonate consists of manipulating then maintaining the hips in abduction. A stable position of hip flexion, abduction, and external rotation is achieved by the use of appliances such as a Frejka pillow, orthopedic abduction splint, or numerous diapers. For about 75% of infants, the hip will revert to normal in a few weeks, but the splints should be continuously used for approximately two to three months and then used only at night. The Frejka pillow splint is applied over diapers and is reapplied with each diaper change. The infant's mother or caretaker must be careful to maintain the desired position. Even with the splint, the emotional needs must be remembered—the child needs to be picked up and cuddled and allowed to sit in a high chair as any baby would.

Some physicians (Ferguson, 1975) have noted an increased incidence of avascular necrosis in conservative closed reduction via abductor splints without preuse of traction and prefer a surgical medial adductor approach and hip spica casting in children under 2 years of age. A very unstable hip may necessitate reduction by manipulation under anesthesia and a hip spica cast for about a month until the capsule tightens and the femoral head pressure stimulates the development of an adequate acetabulum. Immobilization may be as long as six to nine months, depending on hip joint development as seen on x-rays.

If treatment is begun after the first few months, traction, followed by open reduction and a hip spica cast, is used.

As with talipes equinovarus, nursing responsibilities focus on early detection, facilitation of parent-infant bonding, and parent education regarding the treatment plan.

Prognosis

With early and adequate treatment, an adequate hip can be achieved. When treatment is delayed for several months or even years, crippling can be anticipated, despite surgical intervention.

Spina Bifida: Failure of Closure of the Neural Axis

Physiology and Pathophysiology

Malformations in the closure of the spinal canal are termed *spina bifida.* Defects range from a small slit in the vertebras to the absence of several spinous processes and laminae as a result of failure of the neural tube to close at around the fourth month of gestation (Figure 26–12). Three of the most common defects are spina bifida occulta, meningocele, and meningomyelocele.

Spina bifida occulta, nonclosure of the posterior arches of the spine, is found at lumbar 5 in about 30% of the normal population and is of no consequence. This defect becomes of clinical significance when its presence is associated with underlying abnormalities that may be suspected by the presence of a dimple, a tuft of hair, a hemangioma, or a lipoma in the lumbosacral area.

Meningocele is a cystic outpouching of the meninges through the spina bifida without associated abnormalities of the spinal cord and nerve roots.

Meningomyelocele is a cystic herniation of meninges that also contains spinal cord and nerve roots. There is a neurologic deficit below the level of this lesion. The lower the level (lumbar 5 to sacral 1), the greater the probability of functional ambulation, although braces may be required.

Meningomyelocele and meningocele usually communicate with the subarachnoid space and therefore contain cerebrospinal fluid. The pressure of the fluid enlarges the cystic sac and may cause it to rupture. This direct access to cerebrospinal fluid may predispose to meningitis.

The Arnold-Chiari lesion is frequently associated with spinal malformation such as meningomyelocele. It occurs in varying degrees of abnormality, the most serious of which is the downward displacement of the tonsils of cerebellum through the foramen magnum and the downward displacement and folding over of the medulla oblongata and fourth ventricle onto the cervical spinal cord, causing a noncommunicating type of hydrocephalus. Etiology is unknown, but it is *not* due to traction on the cord, as was first assumed. Symptoms may be absent in early life or may be expressed in the neonatal period as lower cranial nerve palsies or vocal cord paralysis. Surgical repair of the meningomyelocele may result

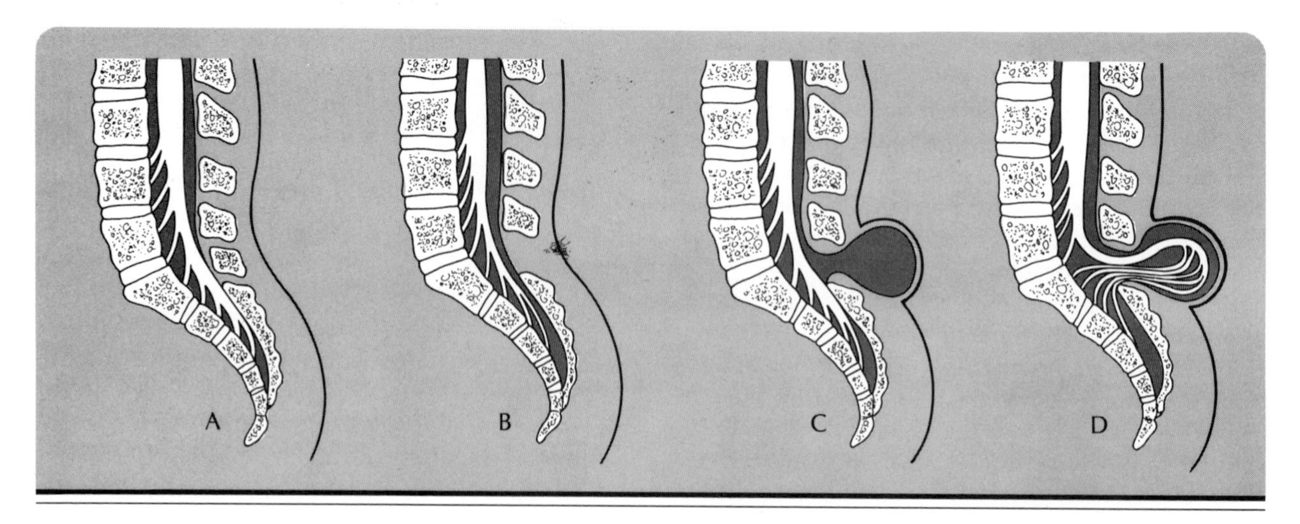

Figure 26–12. Midsagittal view of spinal column with various degrees of neural defect. **A,** Normal. **B,** Spina bifida occulta. Note posterior vertebral arches have not fused. There is no herniation of cord or meninges. **C,** Meningocele. Meninges protrude through the spina bifida forming a saclike cyst visible on the infant's back. **D,** Meningomyelocele. Meninges, elements of the cord with its nerves, and spinal fluid protrude through the spina bifida. This defect resembles a meningocele externally.

in symptoms by compressing the medulla and tonsils into the foramen magnum, unless ventricular drainage is also established.

Between 1 and 3 live births per 1000 present with this lesion (spina bifida). It is more common in females but tends to be more severe in males. Spina bifida is seen more frequently in the firstborn and beyond the sixth pregnancy. It occurs with greater frequency in white populations.

Clinical Manifestations

Spina bifida occulta is asymptomatic in most cases. If the defect is associated with underlying abnormalities, the area is identifiable by the presence of a dimple, tuft of hair, hemangioma, or lipoma. Occasionally spina bifida is diagnosed in early childhood by disorders of sphincter control or muscular weakness in the lower extremities.

Meningocele is seen as a cystic outpouching in the midline over the spine. The skin may be defective as well, so that the sac is covered with a transparent fragile membrane containing the meninges. Because spinal cord or nerve roots are not involved, muscles are usually not affected. The sac may enlarge from the pressure of cerebrospinal fluid and rupture if the defect is not surgically treated. Hydrocephalus may be coincident or may occur after surgical repair of the sac. *Hydrocephalus* refers to the abnormal increase of cerebrospinal fluid in the cranial vault. It may result from obstruction of flow, faulty reabsorption, or increased production. Symptoms include enlargement of the head, "sunset" eyes, weakness, irritability, brain atrophy and retardation, and convulsions.

Meningomyelocele is also seen as a cystic outpouching in the midline, usually over the lumbosacral spine. Because this sac contains spinal cord and nerve roots, several associated neurologic problems are apparent. The degree of dysfunction depends on the level of the lesion. Lesions of lumbar 3–5 and sacral 1–3 sympathetic may result in musculoskeletal malformation and dysfunction (deformed feet, immobile joints of the lower extremities, flaccid paralysis of the lower extremities); proprioceptive dysfunction and absence of sensation to the level of the lesion; or autonomic nervous system dysfunction (inability to sweat, dry and cool skin, and so on). Lesions at lumbar 1 and below may result in loss of bowel and bladder control (constant seepage of urine); stasis of urine in the malfunctioning bladder with recurrent infections and possible eventual upper urinary tract and kidney damage; incontinence or retention of feces; or obstruction of cerebrospinal fluid (CSF) flow, causing hydrocephalus. Arnold-Chiari malformation may be associated with the hydrocephaly.

Surgical exposure and exploration of the lesion reveals the existence and extent of the underlying abnormality. Electromyographs identify the extent and degree of muscular denervation. Careful sensory and motor testing during early infancy predicts with a high degree of reliability the prognosis and effects of therapy.

Interventions

There is usually no therapy for spina bifida occulta unless neurologic abnormalities appear and progress.

Meningocele is surgically corrected, usually in a fairly simple procedure within 24 hours after birth to prevent meningitis if the sac ruptures. Following surgery, the infant usually shows no neurologic deficit. However, the infant must be observed for the development of hydrocephaly.

Surgical correction of meningomyelocele is complex and difficult and often requires several procedures. Surgery is performed within 24 hours after birth to prevent continuing deterioration of nerves and to prevent infection if the sac should rupture. Coexisting abnormalities (hydrocephalus, clubfoot) must also be repaired. In addition to closure of the defect after reinserting nerve tissue, several other surgeries may be needed. These include: (a) shunting (and repetitive shunting if a high meningomyelocele exists) for hydrocephalus in 60%–75% of cases (Figure 26–13); (b) an ileal loop for urologic complications in 90% of cases; and (c) possible transplanting of muscles and tendons and casting along with braces for the orthopedic defects. Frequently, the skin above the repaired defect breaks down, necessitating further treatment and perhaps therapy for meningitis as well. About 30% of live-born infants survive past the first two years of life. The family is referred for psychological support and social services.

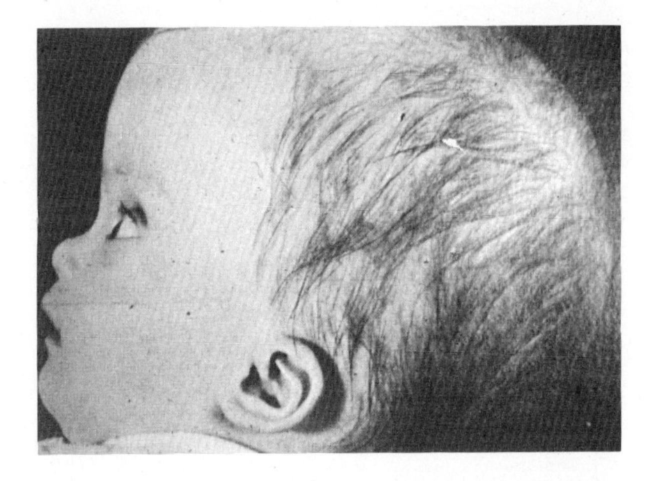

Figure 26–13. Hydrocephaly. Note enlarged occiput area and lateral view of the sunset eyes.

A plan of care for the years succeeding the early surgical repair of the herniated sac focuses on emotional development, education, control of urinary and orthopedic complications, and physical therapy.

Preoperative nursing intervention is directed to protection of the sac, careful assessment of the infant's status and functioning, and parental support. Postoperative intervention includes careful monitoring of vital functions, observation for the development of hydrocephalus and other complications, and supportive care measures. In addition, it is vital to assist the parents in dealing with the long-term implications of this disorder and their child's rehabilitation needs. (See the Nursing Care Plan on meningocele/meningomyelocele.)

NURSING CARE PLAN

Meningocele/Meningomyelocele

Patient Data Base

History

Course of pregnancy and birth

Neonate's condition at birth and apparent malformations noted at birth

Assessment of infant's anatomic appearance and physiologic functioning as described under clinical picture

Parental reactions and any teaching accomplished with parents

NURSING CARE PLAN Cont'd

Meningocele/Meningomyelocele

Physical examination

Round bulging sac on infant's back.

No response or varying response to sensation below the level of the sac.

Spontaneous movement below defect is absent or minimal.

May have constant dribbling of urine.

Incontinence or retention of stool; anal opening may be flaccid.

May develop hydrocephalus.

Nursing Priorities

1. Assess each neonate's anatomic and physiologic functioning to assist in identification of lesions.
2. Protect herniated meningeal sac from drying and rupture.
3. Protect infant with meningomyelocele from trauma to body below lesion.
4. Assess for hydrocephalus.
5. Protect infant from psychologic trauma.
6. Assist parents in coping with situation.

Problem	Nursing interventions and actions	Rationale
Protection of sac from drying, rupture, and infection	Position neonate on abdomen or prop on side very carefully; restrain if necessary. (Some hospitals use Bradford frame.)	Avoids pressure and direct trauma.
	Avoid touching sac with diaper, if one is used.	Avoids pressure and direct trauma.
	Scrupulously cleanse and dry buttocks and genitals frequently. Use meningocele apron. Position apron below the defect.	Avoids contamination of sac from constantly dripping urine and feces and therefore decreases possibility of infection (meningitis).
	If ordered, cover defect with plastic, sterile dressing, sterile petrolatum gauze, or doughnut-shaped appliance with gauze covering (some physicians order Varidase dripped onto sac).	Prevents urine/fecal contamination. Keeps sac moist; prevents drying and cracking.
	Observe sac for oozing of fluid or pus.	Indicates rupture or infection.
	Provide passive exercises to joints in lower extremities as ordered by physician.	Prevents deformity.
Development of hydrocephalus	Measure along suboccipital bregmatic line on admission to nursery.	Provides baseline measurement of neonatal head. This may be inaccurate during the first 24 hr due to molding.
	Measure chest circumference at nipple line.	Chest normally equals or is slightly smaller than head circumference.
	Check fontanelle with infant in upright position for bulging and separation of suture lines.	Tenseness indicates possible increase in intracranial pressure.
	Assess for change in behavior, irritability.	May indicate increased intracranial pressure.
Prevention of trauma to infant's body below lesion	Evaluate urological function—note constant or intermittent dripping.	
	Does urine have good stream?	
	If constant dripping exists, use Credé method of emptying bladder. That is, press gently but firmly starting at umbilical area, downward and under symphysis pubis toward anus, every 2 hr during day and at least once per night.	Prevents stasis, which can lead to infection and damage to renal system.
	Teach parents this method of evaluating anal sphincter functioning. Is there a dimple? Does it constrict to the touch—"wink"?	Determines degree of innervation to area and degree of possible incontinence.
	Support parts of body with rubber pads or cloth	Prevents pressure areas.

NURSING CARE PLAN Cont'd

Meningocele/Meningomyelocele

Problem	Nursing interventions and actions	Rationale
	rolls. Change position from abdomen to side every 2 hr. Provide passive exercises to joints in lower extremities as ordered by physician.	Prevents pressure areas and hypostatic pneumonia. Prevents deformity.
Postoperative period Development of hydrocephalus	Assess frequently vital signs, color, tension of fontanelle, neurologic status, behavior (high-pitched cry, irritability or lethargy, vomiting); measure head circumference once per day.	Facilitates early diagnosis and treatment of postoperative complications. Indicates increased intracranial pressure.
	Raise foot of infant's bed for first few hours.	Lessens pressure of spinal fluid at site of defect and maintains pressure of cerebrospinal fluid in brain.
	Change position from abdomen to side frequently.	Prevents hypostatic pneumonia.
	Assess for and report abdominal distention and symptoms of respiratory distress.	Paralytic ileus and distention of bladder follow spinal cord surgery and embarrass respiration by upward pressure on diaphragm.
Protection of surgical site from trauma and infection	Position on abdomen or prop on side.	Prevents pressure and direct trauma.
	Observe for signs of local infection: redness, warmth.	Early treatment may prevent breakdown of skin repair.
	Provide scrupulous skin care as previously described under preoperative care.	Prevents contamination of operative site and prevents excoriation and infection of surrounding skin areas.
Prevention of trauma to other parts of body		See discussion of preoperative care.
Prevention of emotional trauma to neonate	In addition to content under preoperative care: 1. Hang colorful mobile or place toy where neonate can view it. 2. Put musical toy in crib. 3. Talk or sing to infant while providing care.	Provides visual and auditory stimulation.
	4. Respond to crying by attending infant, stroking, holding, talking, or feeding.	Facilitates development of parent-infant bonding.
Parents' ability to cope with situation	In addition to content discussed previously: 1. Refer to community agencies: community public health, birth defect clinics with a multidisciplinary staff, physical and occupational therapy, parent groups who share the same problem.	Assists with financial, emotional, and rehabilitation burden.
	2. If parents are considering admitting infant to special care facility or placing for adoption, encourage expression of feelings about this. Refer to social service. Do not pass judgment on parents.	After parents are presented with all possible alternatives other than surgical care of defect, final decision must be parents'. Support parents' right to make own decision.
	3. Reinforce, clarify physician's explanations of repair and prognosis.	Under stress, people have difficulty hearing what is said. Repetition is also needed as people work to incorporate information and its meaning for them.
	4. Encourage parents to participate in infant's care; teach in small doses; stand close by as parent attempts infant's care. Praise where appropriate.	Facilitates development of more positive relationship to child. Provides opportunity to see where infant is normal. Builds feelings of self-worth and self-esteem, and helps parents be less overwhelmed.
	5. Prepare parents for future therapy. Teach them how to check anterior fontanelle and head circumference and when to report findings.	Assists parents by encouraging "worry work" and planning for rest of family as well as for affected child. Assures early identification of hydrocephalus.

NURSING CARE PLAN Cont'd

Meningocele/Meningomyelocele

Nursing Care Evaluation

All lesions are identified and appropriate treatment is instituted.

Prior to surgery, herniated sac does not rupture and does not become infected.

Child's bowel and bladder function is maintained without complications and acceptable degree of ambulation is achieved.

Hydrocephalus is diagnosed and treated immediately if it develops.

Parents are able to come to acceptable decision regarding infant's placement outside home or acceptance within home; parents learn to provide physical and emotional care for infant; needs of all family members are met and each has opportunity to develop to full potential.

With other members of the health team, the nurse teaches parents how to provide physical care. Parents learn safe methods of holding, turning, positioning, and giving passive exercise. Techniques of feeding do not differ significantly for this infant, except that it is more difficult to burp him. Care of elimination is more complex. Parents are taught Credé's method of emptying the bladder or care of an ileostomy or indwelling catheter, if one is present. Glycerin suppositories or enemas may be needed to prevent impaction of feces. Parents are assisted in putting the child on a regular routine for bowel emptying as soon as possible. The nurse can be instrumental in developing a bowel and bladder program with the mother of the child with a meningomyelocele.

Phocomelia

Pathophysiology and Clinical Manifestations

Phocomelia ("seal limbs") is an abnormality of one or more extremities. Phocomelia caused by the drug thalidomide is characterized by deformity or absence of an intermediate part or by deformity of the distal part. Even one dose of thalidomide (100 mg) taken during the period of limb formation (days 28 to 42) can cause the deformity.

Parents are especially concerned about the etiologic cause of the deformity. A complete family history is taken, events of the pregnancy are investigated, and genetic causes are explored.

The etiology of sporadic incidence of stunting or amputation of limbs is unknown. However, since the 1960s, when thalidomide was implicated in the limb deformities of thousands of infants (especially in Germany), the United States Food and Drug Administration has tightened regulations governing approval of drugs.

Interventions

The medical regimen is concerned with making the differential diagnosis, identifying any coexisting malformations, and coordinating the rehabilitation plan.

Nursing Management

Pertinent information from the prenatal and perinatal records is noted in the nursing history. The results of investigating the cause of the deformity, the proposed treatment plan, and the teaching accomplished with parents are necessary components of the history and are also vital so that a firm data base is established for the long-term care plan.

The nursing priority is to assist the parents in coping with the situation. Although the child usually has no other malformation, he requires special care.

Rehabilitative problems are complex and require a multidisciplinary approach. Prostheses are fitted early and require frequent changes as the child grows. Parents need assistance in the use of prostheses and in training the child to use them in all daily activities. Child amputee centers throughout the United States provide such assistance.

The family is taught about the child's developmental needs and how to improvise to help him meet these needs. For instance, children without this anomaly experience kinesthetic satisfaction from kicking their feet and waving and reaching with their arms. Such movements, plus the satisfaction of the hand-to-mouth movement for self-gratification and exploring the environment, are not possible for the child with phocomelia. Pillows propped under the chest when he is prone on a flat surface assist him to look around and perhaps to touch things with his hands. A positive body image and self-concept are the result of internalizing the reflection of positive feelings toward him from significant others. The family needs assistance in coping with their feelings and the situation before they can develop positive attitudes. The family will continue to require information and other assistance for many years.

CONGENITAL HEART DEFECTS

Although the incidence of congenital heart defects is less than 1% of all births, they account for 50% of deaths caused by all types of congenital defects in the first year of life. Because accurate diagnosis and surgical treatment are now available, many such deaths can be prevented. Thus it is crucial for the nurse to have comprehensive knowledge of congenital heart disease in order to detect deviations from normal and to initiate nursing interventions.

Normal Anatomy and Physiology of the Heart

Embryology

Early formation of the cardiovascular system is necessary, because the human ovum lacks sufficient yolk to provide nutrients for the rapidly growing embryo. On about the 15th to 18th day, a small cluster of cells, called the cardiogenic plate, can be identified. The cardiogenic plate is located at the cephalic end of the embryo in front of the tissue that will become the head. A small U-shaped cavity rapidly encircles the cardiogenic plate. The outer layer of this evolving structure will become the pericardium, the inner layer will develop into the myocardium and epicardium, and the remaining cells will migrate to form the endocardium. The head of the embryo grows forward as the pericardial cavity swings under, so that the early heart tissue becomes part of the developing thorax. Within the pericardial cavity, cells arrange themselves in long side-by-side strands. These strands develop into two thin-walled vessels that fuse together and form a single vessel that functions as a simple tubular heart. The tubular heart attaches itself to the pericardium at the cephalic and caudal ends. The cephalic end is the arterial end and will later divide to form the pulmonary artery and aorta. The caudal portion is the venous end, from which will emerge the superior and inferior venae cavae as well as the pulmonary veins. By the end of the third week, this tubular heart has rhythmic contractions, forcing blood through primitive vessels in the developing embryo (Toronto, 1972).

The tubular heart grows much more rapidly than the pericardial chamber within which it finds itself. In order to accommodate, it first folds into a simple U-shaped bend and then into a spiral S shape. As the tubular heart folds and doubles on itself, the venous end swings up toward the arterial end, and slight constrictions appear, dividing it into the primitive atrium and the primitive ventricle. As the heart continues to grow, complex rotation of the chambers occurs, until the ventricle becomes situated below the atrium. At this time, the embryo is 6 weeks old and one-half inch long, and its heart shows the general shape and markings that it will carry permanently (Toronto, 1972).

From the 5th to the 7th week, partitions are formed, and a four-chambered heart is developed. First, masses of endocardial tissue, called *endocar-*

dial cushions, grow together from the dorsal and ventral portions of the atrioventricular groove, forming the tricuspid and mitral valves and separating the atria from the ventricles. At the same time, a septum develops from the interventricular groove and grows toward the base of the heart, separating the right and left ventricles, but this septum is not completely developed until the 8th week.

The ventricular septum is derived from three components: membranous, muscular, and bulbar. *Membranous septum,* originating from the endocardial cushions, grows downward to meet the muscular septum. The upper part of the membranous septum divides the left ventricle from the right atrium as the tricuspid valve and the mitral valve develop. *Muscular septum* originates as an upward projection from the primitive ventricle floor and grows toward the endocardial cushion tissue. *Bulbar septum*—the most cephalad ventricular septum component—separates the outflow tracts of the ventricles (the infundibulum of the right ventricle and the vestibule of the left) (King, 1975). The proximal part of this septum consists of the proximal part of the bulbospinal septum. Distal partition divides the arterial end of the primitive tube, making two vessels out of one. One vessel becomes the aorta, which is connected to the left ventricle. The other vessel is the pulmonary artery and is connected to the right ventricle (Rushmer, 1976).

A crescentic ridge appears on the dorsocephalic part of the atrium, forming a septum that rapidly grows toward the ventricle. Before it reaches the ventricle and closes completely, a new opening develops higher up in the septum. A second thin septum grows down and extends like a curtain over the aperture. This structure is called the *foramen ovale,* a unidirectional valve permitting blood to flow only from the right atrium into the left (Toronto, 1972).

The venous end of the primitive tube divides and separates, forming veins that empty into the atrium. These veins migrate and arrange themselves so that the superior vena cava, the inferior vena cava, and the coronary sinus empty into the right atrium and the pulmonary veins empty into the left atrium.

Circulation

The lungs of the fetus do not function in utero; therefore, it is necessary to have a special circulatory system that will bypass the blood supply to the lungs. See p. 147 for a discussion of fetal circulation. At the time of birth, marked changes occur in the cardiovascular system. See p. 780 for a discussion of circulatory changes that normally occur at birth.

Heart Rate

The normal heart rate for an infant is 100–130 beats per minute while asleep and 140–160 while awake and may go as high as 200 while crying. Apical pulse rates should be obtained by auscultation for one full minute, preferably when the infant is asleep. The child's pulse rate steadily decreases until adolescence, when the pulse rate is approximately 60–75 beats per minute.

Heart Murmurs

Murmurs are usually produced by turbulent blood flow. Murmurs may be heard when blood flows across an abnormal valve or across a stenosed valve, when there is an atrial septal or ventricular septal defect, or when there is increased flow across a normal valve. About 50%–60% of normal children have what are called innocent or functional murmurs. In young children, a low-pitched, musical murmur heard just to the right of the apex of the heart is fairly common. There appears to be no structural or underlying reason for these murmurs. Functional murmurs are always short in duration and midsystolic, never diastolic.

Occasionally significant murmurs will be heard, including the murmur of a patent ductus arteriosus, the murmur of aortic or pulmonic stenosis, or the murmur of a small ventricular septal defect.

Overview of Congenital Heart Defects

Congenital cardiac malformations are the result of failure of the gene-directed developmental phenomenon to time each move at exactly the right moment for everything to fall accurately into place. Factors that might influence this phenomenon can be classified as environmental or genetic. Viruses such as rubella and Coxsackie B that affect the mother during pregnancy have been implicated. Thalidomide and, more recently, some of the anticonvulsants have been shown to cause congenital malformations of the heart. Infants born with chromosomal abnormalities have an increased incidence of cardiovascular anomalies. About 40% of Down's syndrome babies have cardiac malformations. Trisomy E and trisomy D individuals also show frequent heart lesions. Increased incidence and increased risk of recurrence of specific defects occur in families. At the present time, 10% of cardiovascular malformations can be attributed to genetic factors, 5% to chromosomal abnormalities, 10% to environmental factors, and 75% to unknown causes (Doyle and Rutbowski, 1970).

General signs and symptoms in infants are as follows: dyspnea, difficulty in feeding, stridor or choking spells, pulse rate over 200, recurrent respiratory infections, failure to gain weight, heart murmurs, cyanosis, cerebral vascular accidents, and anoxic attacks.

The three most common ways in which infants with congenital cardiac abnormalities first manifest their problem are in cyanosis, with a detectable heart murmur, or in congestive heart failure, a frequent sequela.

It is customary to divide congenital malformations of the heart into *acyanotic*—those that do not present with cyanosis—and *cyanotic*—those that do present with cyanosis. Normally, if an opening is present between the right and left sides of the heart, blood will flow from the area of greater pressure (left side) to the area of lesser pressure (right side). This process is referred to as a left-to-right shunt and does not produce cyanosis. If pressure in the right side of the heart, due to obstruction of normal flow, exceeds that in the left side, unoxygenated blood will flow from the right side to the left side of the heart and out into the system, producing a right-to-left shunt and resulting in cyanosis. If the opening is large, there may be a bidirectional shunt with mixing of blood in both sides of the heart, also producing cyanosis.

Acyanotic Lesions

Acyanotic congenital defects include patent ductus arteriosus, atrial septal defects, ventricular septal defects, endocardial cushion defects, coarctation of the aorta, and aortic stenosis.

Patent Ductus Arteriosus

Patent ductus arteriosus is an abnormal persistence of the fetal connection between the aorta and the pulmonary artery (Figure 26-14). Increased incidence is noted in females, in certain families, after maternal rubella during the first trimester of pregnancy, in infants born at high altitudes, and especially in premature infants. Respiratory distress syndrome with hypoxemia can cause persistent patency of the ductus arteriosus because of lowered oxygen saturation of blood shunted through the ductus and decreased pressure in the lungs (Ziai et al., 1975).

The hemodynamics consist of a left-to-right shunting of oxygenated blood from the high-pressure system of the aorta to the lower-pressure system of the pulmonary artery. The blood is recirculated through the lungs, with eventual overloading of the left ventricle due to increased output and work load in an effort to maintain systemic circulation.

The child with this problem is usually asymptomatic except for some impairment in growth. He tends to be small, short in stature, and slender and tends to have frequent upper respiratory infections. The condition is often discovered on careful auscultation. At the upper left sternal border, just beneath the left clavicle, the typical continuous murmur can be heard. It is called a machinery-type murmur and is heard throughout both systole and diastole. The child may also show a great difference between systolic and diastolic blood pressures. This wide pulse pressure is due to a low diastolic pressure, because the shunting of blood reduces peripheral resistance.

X-ray findings are often normal when shunting is of a small amount. X-rays of hearts with larger shunts show left ventricular and left atrial enlargement, a dilated ascending aorta, a prominent pulmonary artery, and increased pulmonary vascularity with the increased blood flow to the lungs. A cardiac catheterization is not necessary for diagnosis but may be performed to rule out associated defects.

Treatment is surgical ligation of the ductus arteriosus. This is major surgery and involves opening the chest but does not require the use of a heart-lung machine. Surgery is usually done some time after 1 year of age unless the infant develops complications earlier.

Atrial Septal Defects

An *atrial septal defect* is an abnormal opening in the atrial septum. It is more common in females and occurs frequently in Down's syndrome infants. Atrial septal defects are of three types. The major type of defect is within the area of the foramen ovale. Patency is caused by a short valve, a perforated valve, or an enlarged opening at the valve site. A defect high in the atrial septum, called ostium secundum, is less common and results from failure of the septum to develop completely. It can exist as one large or several small openings. The third type, called ostium primum, is caused by failure of the correct fusion of the atrial septum, the ventricular septum, and the endocardial cushions (see Figure 26–14). It is uncommon and more complicated, usually involving the mitral and tricuspid valves (Polansky, 1970).

There is a left-to-right shunt with recirculation of oxygenated blood through the lungs, which produces abnormally high pulmonary blood flow. Eventually there will be right heart failure due to sustained overload. Atrial septal defects are often not detected in early infancy, because the murmur of a minimal left-to-right shunting of blood is scarcely detectable. As pressure differences become greater, the shunt becomes larger and a systolic murmur becomes audible over the second left intercostal space. With very large shunts, a diastolic rumbling murmur is present at the lower left sternal border.

The child with a small atrial septal defect may be asymptomatic. If the defect is large, he may have frequent respiratory infections, failure to

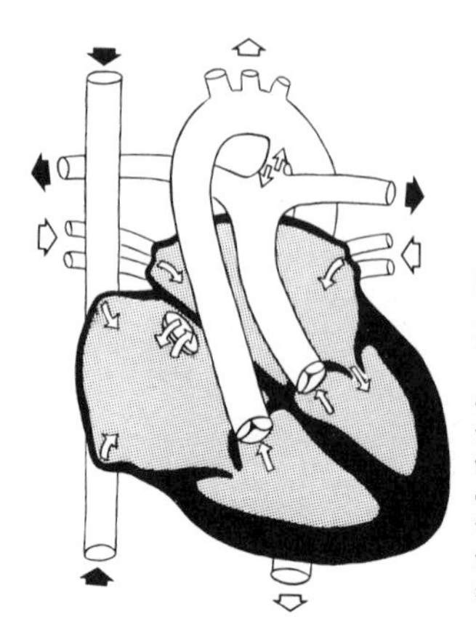

Complete Transposition of Great Vessels

This anomaly is an embryologic defect caused by a straight division of the bulbar trunk without normal spiraling. As a result, the aorta originates from the right ventricle, and the pulmonary artery from the left ventricle. An abnormal communication between the two circulations must be present to sustain life.

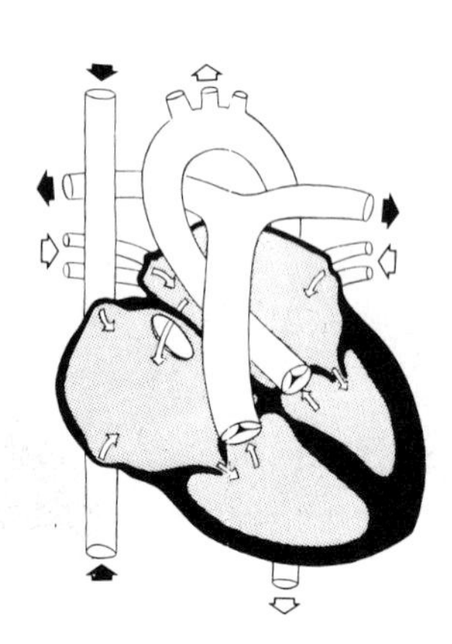

Atrial Septal Defects

An atrial septal defect is an abnormal opening between the right and left atria. Basically, three types of abnormalities result from incorrect development of the atrial septum. An incompetent foramen ovale is the most common defect. The high ostium secundum defect results from abnormal development of the septum secundum. Improper development of the septum primum produces a basal opening known as an ostium primum defect, frequently involving the atrio-ventricular valves. In general, left to right shunting of blood occurs in all atrial septal defects.

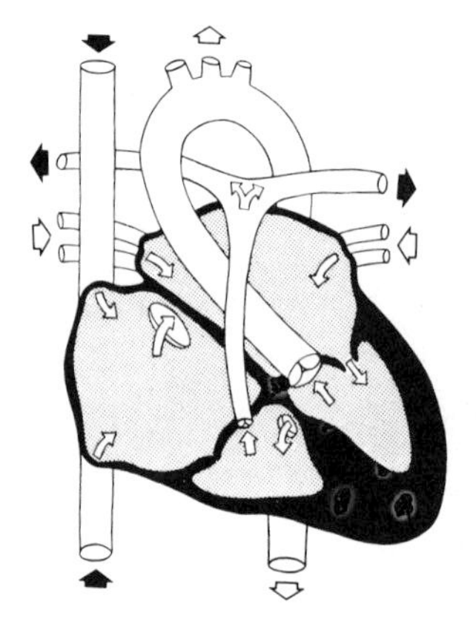

Tricuspid Atresia

Tricuspid valvular atresia is characterized by a small right ventricle, large left ventricle and usually a diminished pulmonary circulation. Blood from the right atrium passes through an atrial septal defect into the left atrium, mixes with oxygenated blood returning from the lungs, flows into the left ventricle and is propelled into the systemic circulation. The lungs may receive blood through one of three routes: 1) a small ventricular septal defect 2) patent ductus arteriosus 3) bronchial vessels.

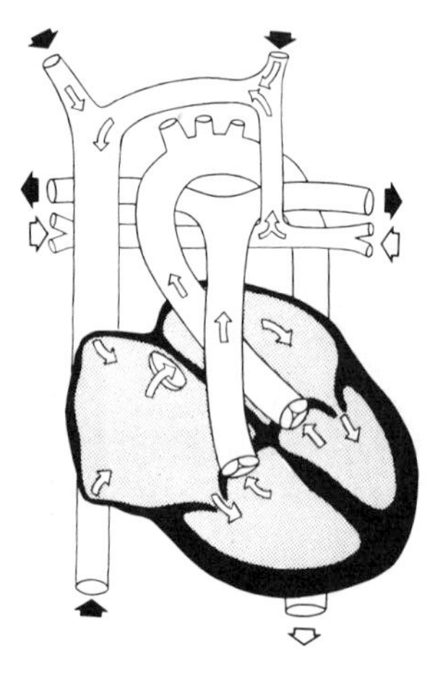

Anomalous Venous Return

Oxygenated blood returning from the lungs is carried abnormally to the right heart by one or more pulmonary veins emptying directly, or indirectly through venous channels, into the right atrium. Partial anomalous return of the pulmonary veins to the right atrium functions the same as an atrial septal defect. In complete anomalous return of the pulmonary veins, an interatrial communication is necessary for survival.

Figure 26–14. Congenital heart abnormalities. (From Congenital heart abnormalities. Clinical Education Aid No. 7. Ross Laboratories, Columbus, Ohio.)

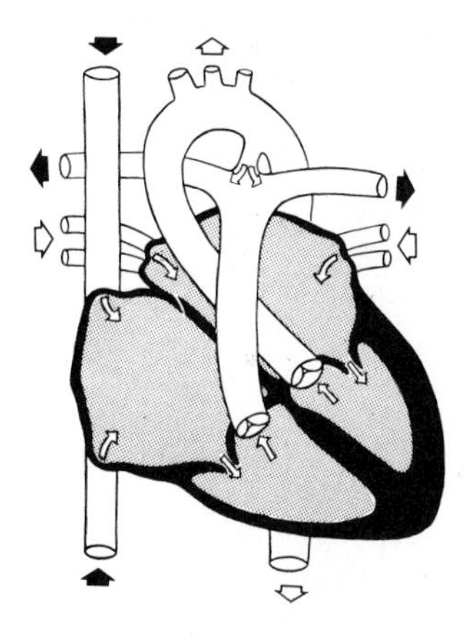

Patent Ductus Arteriosus

The patent ductus arteriosus is a vascular connection that, during fetal life, short circuits the pulmonary vascular bed and directs blood from the pulmonary artery to the aorta. Functional closure of the ductus normally occurs soon after birth. If the ductus remains patent after birth, the direction of blood flow in the ductus is reversed by the higher pressure in the aorta.

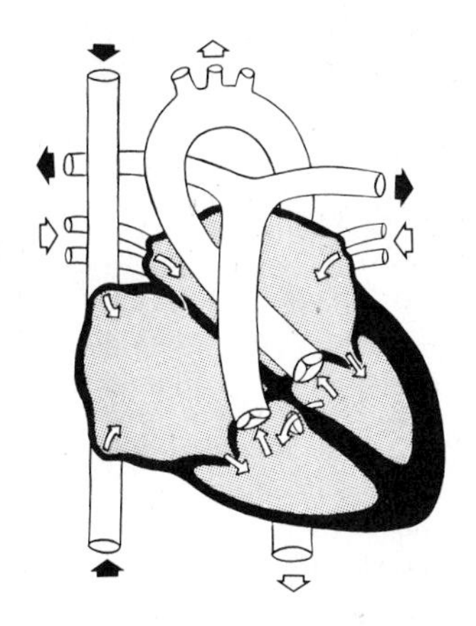

Ventricular Septal Defects

A ventricular septal defect is an abnormal opening between the right and left ventricle. Ventricular septal defects vary in size and may occur in either the membranous or muscular portion of the ventricular septum. Due to higher pressure in the left ventricle, a shunting of blood from the left to right ventricle occurs during systole. If pulmonary vascular resistance produces pulmonary hypertension, the shunt of blood is then reversed from the right to the left ventricle, with cyanosis resulting.

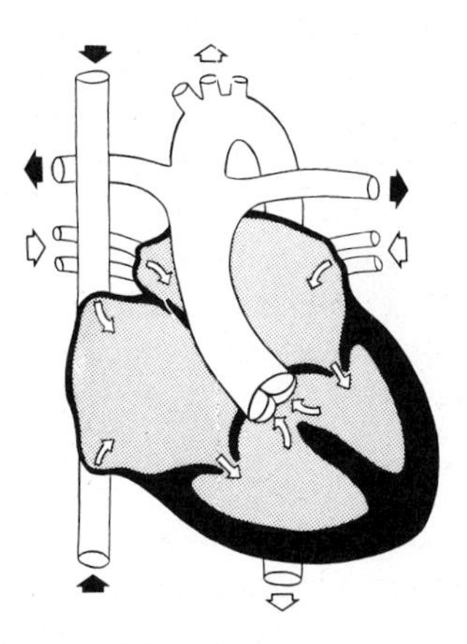

Truncus Arteriosus

Truncus arteriosus is a retention of the embryologic bulbar trunk. It results from the failure of normal septation and division of this trunk into an aorta and pulmonary artery. This single arterial trunk overrides the ventricles and receives blood from them through a ventricular septal defect. The entire pulmonary and systemic circulation is supplied from this common arterial trunk.

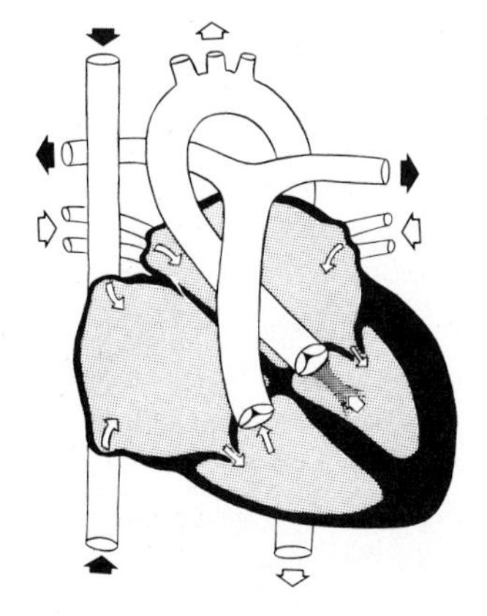

Subaortic Stenosis

In many instances, the stenosis is valvular with thickening and fusion of the cusps. Subaortic stenosis is caused by a fibrous ring below the aortic valve in the outflow tract of the left ventricle. At times, both valvular and subaortic stenosis exist in combination. The obstruction presents an increased work load for the normal output of the left ventricular blood and results in left ventricular enlargement.

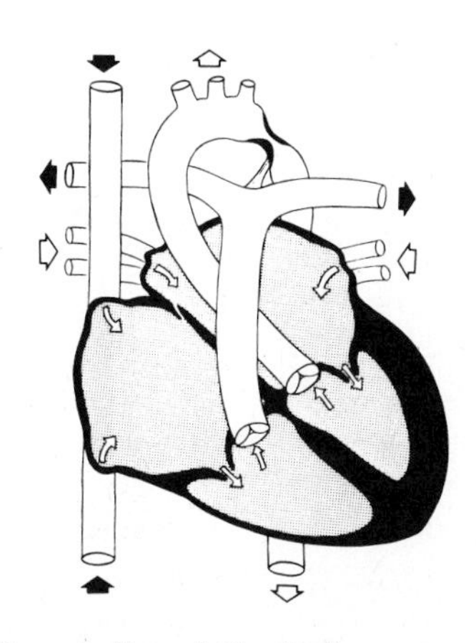

Coarctation of the Aorta

Coarctation of the aorta is characterized by a narrowed aortic lumen. It exists as a preductal or postductal obstruction, depending on the position of the obstruction in relation to the ductus arteriosus. Coarctations exist with great variation in anatomical features. The lesion produces an obstruction to the flow of blood through the aorta causing an increased left ventricular pressure and work load.

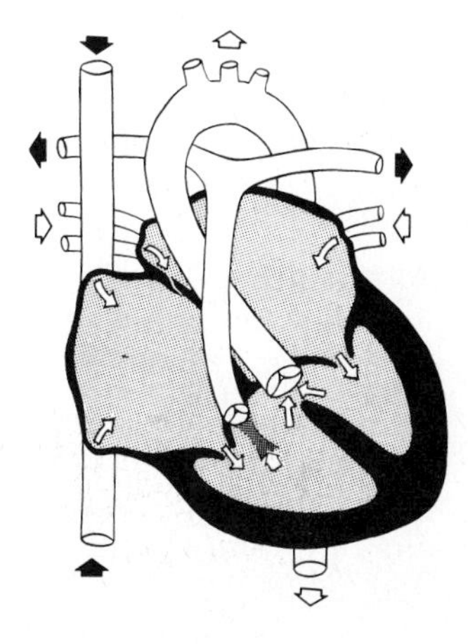

Tetralogy of Fallot

Tetralogy of Fallot is characterized by the combination of four defects: 1) pulmonary stenosis 2) ventricular septal defect 3) overriding aorta 4) hypertrophy of right ventricle. It is the most common defect causing cyanosis in patients surviving beyond two years of age. The severity of symptoms depends on the degree of pulmonary stenosis, the size of the ventricular septal defect, and the degree to which the aorta overrides the septal defect.

thrive, poor exercise tolerance, a thin build due to abnormally high pulmonary blood flow and poor tissue perfusion, and episodes of congestive heart failure.

Prevention of infection and aggressive treatment with antibiotics when infections develop is essential. Open-heart surgery with the help of the heart-lung machine is required to repair atrial septal defect.

Ventricular Septal Defects

A *ventricular septal defect* is an abnormal opening in the ventricular septum (see Figure 26–14). It is the most common congenital cardiovascular anomaly and occurs more frequently in males than in females. The abnormal opening is usually located in the membranous portion of the septum but occasionally occurs in the muscular portion of the ventricular septum. The smallest defects are called maladie de Roger. They are associated with a minor left-to-right shunting of blood through the opening in the ventricular septum. The pressure in the right ventricle is not markedly increased and stays within normal range. At birth, pressures in the right and left ventricles are almost equal, so very little shunting occurs for the first few weeks of life.

These infants are asymptomatic, but by the end of the first month of life, a loud, blowing systolic murmur can be heard in the third and fourth left interspace. X-ray usually shows the heart to be of normal size and shape and without increased pulmonary blood flow. Cardiac catheterization is not usually done, as no treatment is required for these infants. Spontaneous closure occurs in 50% of children with ventricular septal defects.

In large membranous defects, the left-to-right shunting of blood is greater and does result in increased right ventricular pressure and right ventricular hypertrophy. There is a middiastolic murmur heard best at the left lower sternal border. Congestive heart failure may develop between 6 weeks and 2 months of age. Children exhibit rapid respirations, growth failure, and feeding difficulties. Chest x-ray shows cardiac enlargement and increased pulmonary blood flow. Electrocardiogram demonstrates left ventricular hypertrophy and, if the defect is very large, may show combined ventricular hypertrophy.

Medications such as Lanoxin and diuretics are used to control the congestive heart failure, and

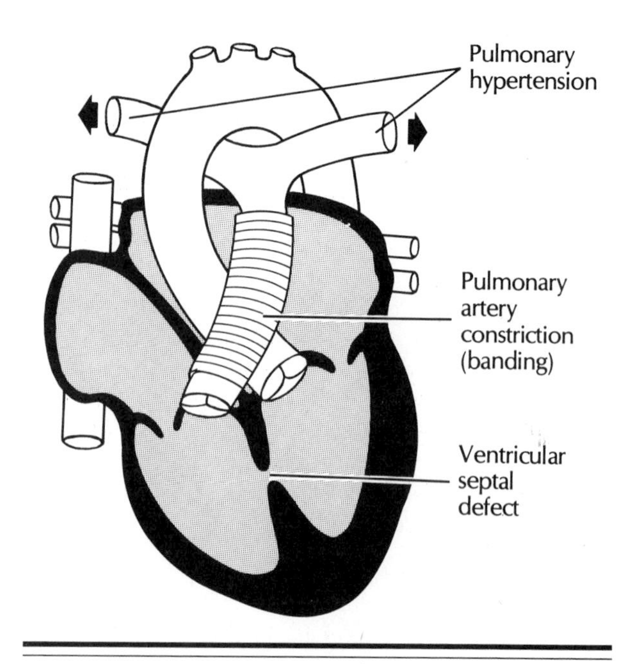

Figure 26–15. Pulmonary banding for ventricular septal defect to decrease blood flow through the pulmonary artery.

the infant is usually followed for a period of time, because even large ventricular defects may close spontaneously. Cardiac catheterization reveals higher oxygen saturation in the right ventricle than in the right atrium. Pressures in the right ventricle and pulmonary artery are frequently increased.

When pressures in the right ventricle and pulmonary artery begin to approach the same pressure as the systemic pressure of the left ventricle, pulmonary hypertension due to pulmonary arterial changes is occurring and surgical intervention is necessary. Surgery may also be performed when cardiac catheterization demonstrates that the pulmonary blood flow is twice the systemic blood flow. In the past, a palliative procedure called a *pulmonary artery banding* was done during the first year of life (Figure 26–15). A constricting Teflon band was placed around the pulmonary artery to reduce blood volume to the lungs. When the child was older, the band was released, his pulmonary artery was reconstructed, and his ventricular septal defect was closed with a Dacron patch. At the present time, an initial correction of the defect with a Dacron patch is being done more frequently because of the increased success of the surgery with fewer long-term complications.

Endocardial Cushion Defects

There are four embryologic centers of growth, called *endocardial cushions* (pods of embryonic endothelium-covered connective tissue that bulge into the embryonic atrioventricular canal), that develop into the mitral valve, the tricuspid valve, a portion of the atrial septum, and a portion of the ventricular septum. When development of these growth centers is not complete, a group of cardiac lesions called *endocardial cushion defects* occurs. Endocardial cushion defects are common in Down's syndrome babies. The defect may involve the atrial septum, the ventricular septum, or both septa. The mitral valve does not completely close due to a cleft in one section of the valve, and sometimes the tricuspid valve also has a cleft with incomplete closure. These infants have left-to-right shunting of blood at the site of the defect and also leakage of blood from ventricle to atrium through the defective valves.

When there is a large ventricular defect, it is usually accompanied by pulmonary hypertension, and many of these children are very ill. About 50% of them die from congestive heart failure and pneumonia during the first year of life. An apical diastolic murmur accompanies the left-to-right shunt. If a mitral defect is present, a systolic murmur is also heard, and the pulmonary hypertension causes a loud second heart sound. On chest x-ray, the heart size is enlarged, varying with the severity of the condition. Increased pulmonary blood flow is demonstrated by extra markings in the lungs. Cardiac catheterization is performed to study the location and severity of the defects. Open-heart surgery reduces the left-to-right shunting of blood and repairs the valvular defects. Usually repair is not completely successful, and most children have continuing cardiac problems (Polansky, 1970).

Coarctation of the Aorta

Coarctation of the aorta is a congenital narrowing of a segment of the aorta (see Figure 26-14). The coarctation may involve either a short or long section of the aorta and can occur anywhere but is most often located in the aortic arch near the ductus arteriosus. Difficulties occur in infants and children who also have a patent ductus arteriosus or a ventricular septal defect, because of increased left-to-right shunting of blood through these defects.

Important physical findings may be detected by an astute nurse during the newborn assessment. Absent or diminished femoral pulsation should alert the nurse to listen for a late systolic heart murmur, heard best in the left interscapular region, and decreased systolic blood pressure in the lower extremities when compared with blood pressure in the upper extremities, due to increased blood volume in upper extremities and diminished blood volume in major arteries of the lower extremities. Obstruction of blood flow through the aorta causes an increased left ventricular pressure and work load. Collateral vessels arise, chiefly from the branches of the subclavian artery, and bypass the constricted aorta to supply circulation to the lower extremities. The chest x-ray shows an enlarged heart, with most of the increased size due to enlargement of the left ventricle. The indented area of the narrow segment of the aorta can usually be identified. Some infants and children remain generally asymptomatic, but others present in severe congestive heart failure at about 7-12 days of age.

If the coarctation is not complicated by other cardiac lesions, these infants usually respond well to medical management, and surgical correction is delayed until the child is beyond 6 years of age. Management includes monitoring left ventricular hypertrophy, observing for signs of early heart failure, and monitoring growth and development to maintain within normal parameters.

If the coarctation is accompanied by a patent ductus arteriosus or a ventricular septal defect, the response to medical management is generally poor and surgery is required. The coarctation is resected, and with short defects, the ends of the aorta are anastomosed. With longer defects, a prosthetic graft of Dacron may be inserted to bridge the gap in the aorta after resection. The patent ductus arteriosus is tied off, and a Teflon band may be placed around the pulmonary artery if pulmonary blood flow is excessive. The mortality rate is very low when surgery is done on older children to correct coarctation of the aorta, but it is high when the operation must be performed as an emergency measure for heart failure in infancy (Ziai et al., 1975).

Aortic Stenosis

Aortic stenosis may be divided into four types: first, and most common, is a defective valve with limited ability to open; second is subvalvular, a result of obstruction beneath the valve caused by hypertrophy of ventricular muscle; third is also subvalvular and involves membranous ridges of obstructive tissue beneath the valve; and fourth is supravalvular and consists of a coarctation immediately above an otherwise normal aortic valve (see Figure 26–14). Any type of aortic stenosis presents as an obstruction that causes an increased work load on the left ventricle and results in left ventricular hypertrophy. A systolic murmur heard in the second right interspace is usually associated with a palpable thrill.

Children with mild to moderate aortic stenosis may have few symptoms. Fainting spells may occur when children are under stress, due to increased heart rate and decreased cardiac output, and sudden death associated with excessive physical exertion is a possibility. Chest x-ray may reveal a normal heart or may show some enlargement of the left ventricle.

In severe cases, open-heart surgery is utilized either to remove the obstructive tissue or to replace the aortic valve in order to alleviate the obstruction (Ziai et al., 1975).

Cyanotic Lesions

Cyanosis in congenital heart diseases results from shunting unoxygenated venous blood into the systemic arterial circuit. *Cyanosis* is defined as blue discoloration of the skin, nail beds, and mucous membranes resulting from the presence of approximately 5 gm/100 ml of reduced hemoglobin in the blood. Cyanosis depends on the total hemoglobin as well as on the arterial oxygen saturation. In profound anemia, cyanosis may not be seen because of insufficient amounts of reduced hemoglobin. In contrast, in an infant with polycythemia there may be peripheral cyanosis due to an increased amount of reduced hemoglobin, even though the degree of arterial unsaturation is minimal. Generally, cyanosis is associated with anoxia or a low arterial partial pressure of oxygen.

The nurse must differentiate between central and peripheral cyanosis. *Central cyanosis* is manifested as follows: The tongue and mucous membranes of the mouth are blue, and the blood leaving the heart contains an excess of reduced hemoglobin; arterial oxygen saturation is low; arteriovenous oxygen difference is normal; extremities are warm; and cardiac output is normal. Central cyanosis is produced by the admixture of unsaturated venous blood into the systemic circulation, resulting from a large right-to-left intracardiac shunt or intrapulmonic shunt. In *peripheral cyanosis*, only the extremities are blue, and the central blood contains sufficient oxygenated hemoglobin. Peripheral cyanosis results from profound oxygen unsaturation of capillary blood and is seen in cases of marked vasoconstriction or advanced cardiac failure associated with low cardiac output. It is most commonly seen when cardiac output is reduced by an obstructive lesion such as mitral stenosis, pulmonic stenosis, or low-output congestive heart failure.

The usual causes of central cyanosis in the neonate are pulmonary disorders, heart defects, hematologic abnormalities, and central nervous system disorders. In central nervous system disorders the newborn infant is usually full term, with a history of the mother having had a difficult labor or delivery. Often some visible signs of trauma to the neonate can be seen. The infant's respirations are slow, shallow, and irregular. Administration of 100% oxygen may improve cyanosis, especially if ventilation is also increased. With hematologic abnormalities, the only differentiating factor is the laboratory analysis of the circulating hemoglobin.

The leading pulmonary disorder is respiratory distress syndrome. Neonates with RDS are born prematurely and show obvious signs of respiratory difficulties. At least at the onset of respiratory distress, placing the infant in 100% oxygen improves the cyanosis, and ventilatory assistance causes marked improvement. In contrast, infants with cyanotic heart disease are usually full term and frequently have rapid respirations with intense cyanosis but without the other signs of respiratory distress. Their cyanosis does not improve significantly with administration of 100% oxygen (Harris, 1976).

Tetralogy of Fallot

Tetralogy of Fallot is thought to be the most common congenital cardiovascular defect causing cyanosis in children (see Figure 26–14). It is identified by its classical combination of four defects: pulmonary stenosis, ventricular septal defect, aorta overriding both ventricles, and hypertrophy of the right ventricle. Pulmonary stenosis may be caused by either a defective pulmonary valve or obstruction in the infundibular area of the right ventricle directly below the pulmonary valve. This obstruction decreases the outflow of blood through the pulmonary circulation and increases the work load and pressure of the right ventricle. When the pressure in the right ventricle becomes greater than the pressure in the left ventricle, a right-to-left shunting of unoxygenated blood into oxygenated blood through the ventricular septal defect occurs, and cyanosis develops. The overriding aorta is situated over the high ventricular septal defect, and much of the shunted unoxygenated blood flows directly into it and further increases cyanosis.

Infants may be cyanotic at birth or may develop cyanosis during the first months of life. The child with this disorder is small, his growth rate is very slow due to poor nutrition caused by decreased circulation, and he has difficulty with feeding. The circulating blood volume tends to pool in the extremities, causing clubbing of the fingers and toes. The body responds to the low oxygen saturation of the blood and attempts to compensate by increased secretion of erythropoietin, which accelerates red blood cell production. The resulting polycythemia causes increased viscosity of the blood and puts the child at risk for cerebral thrombosis. Low hemoglobin is also a constant threat, because poor nutrition and rapid red blood cell production easily deplete the infant's iron stores. A normal or low hemoglobin level may contribute to increased hypoxia and dyspnea. Anoxic spells, the result of suddenly decreased cardiac output, are usually precipitated by exertion or emotional stress. The crying infant exhibits increased cyanosis and then suddenly becomes limp and unresponsive due to decreased circulation and oxygen to the brain. Placing the infant in a knee-chest position often alleviates the anoxia somewhat. If the defect is severe, right ventricular hypertrophy may be extensive enough to cause protrusion of the left chest. A harsh systolic murmur can be heard along the left sternal border.

X-ray examination reveals a heart of small or normal size with a boot-shaped appearance, caused by the small pulmonary artery. There are also diminished markings in the lung fields due to decreased pulmonary blood flow and a prominent or enlarged aorta.

The goal of medical management is to prevent dehydration and intercurrent infections and to alleviate paroxysmal dyspneic attacks. Indications for surgical intervention are severe anoxic attacks and severe dyspnea on exertion, which prevents the child from leading a normal life. The current surgical approach is for complete correction through open-heart surgery with use of the heart-lung machine. Obstructive infundibular tissue is removed from the right ventricle below the pulmonary artery, or the stenotic pulmonary valve is incised, whichever is necessary to increase pulmonary circulation. A Dacron patch is used to close the ventricular septal defect and extend the left ventricle to the right of the overriding aorta, thereby removing the right-to-left shunting of unoxygenated blood.

Palliative surgery may be done when the child is too ill or too small to tolerate total correction. The goal of such surgical intervention is to increase blood flow to the lungs and to decrease the degree of cyanosis. The procedure that has been used for the longest period of time is the Blalock-Taussig operation, in which the subclavian artery is anastomosed to the pulmonary artery. An artificial patent ductus arteriosus is constructed to shunt blood into the pulmonary circulation for reoxygenation. In the Potts-Smith-Gibson operation, the aorta is joined to the pulmonary artery by a side-by-side anastomosis to create this shunt (Figure 26–16). A direct anastomosis of the aorta and the pulmonary artery is also done in the Waterston-Cooley procedure but at a different site. The Potts-Smith-Gibson operation creates a shunt in the descending aorta, and the Waterston-Cooley operation uses the ascending aorta. When the child is older, or when his condition is more stable, the shunt is removed and a total correction is done, using open-heart surgery.

Pulmonary Stenosis

Pulmonary stenosis may exist alone or in combination with other cardiovascular defects. When pulmonary stenosis exists alone, the symptoms and physical findings vary from asymptomatic to dyspnea, easy tiring, cyanosis, and heart failure. There is usually a loud ejection systolic murmur, heard best at the upper left sternal border.

In mild cases, the chest x-ray is normal. With severe problems, it may show right ventricular hypertrophy and right atrial hypertrophy, with decreased pulmonary blood flow. A child with mild to moderate pulmonary stenosis often requires no specific treatment except for careful well-child care. More extensive stenosis requires surgical correction with the use of the heart-lung machine.

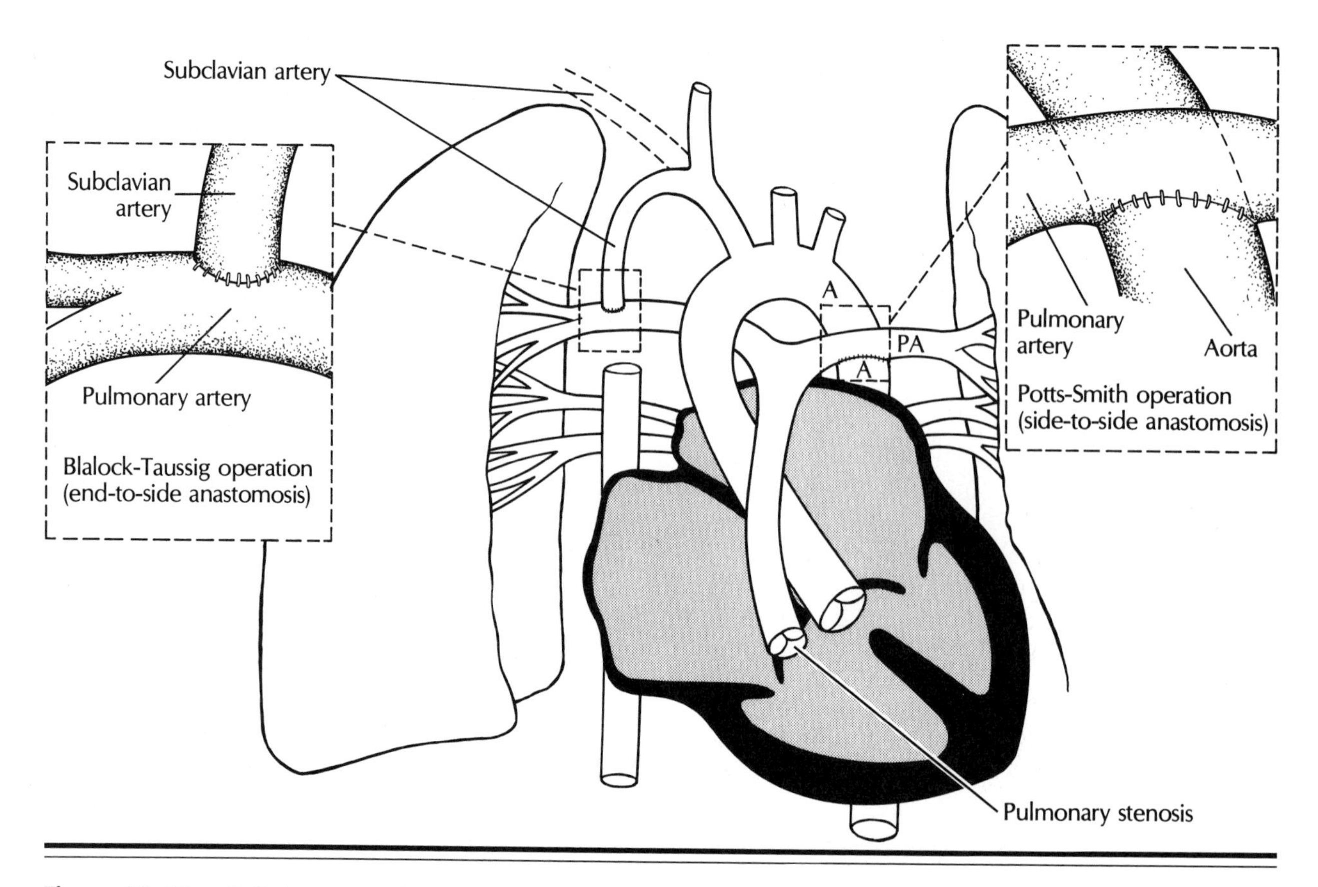

Figure 26–16. Palliative surgery for tetralogy of Fallot.

Transposition of the Great Vessels

In transposition of the great vessels, the aorta arises from the right ventricle and the pulmonary artery from the left ventricle. Unoxygenated venous blood from the body returns to the right side of the heart and is pumped through the aorta out to the body tissues without reoxygenation. Oxygenated blood from the lungs returns through the pulmonary veins to the left side of the heart and is pumped through the pulmonary artery back to the lungs again. The neonate cannot live unless a communication between the two circulations is present. The ductus arteriosus is usually patent during the first few days after birth and creates some mixing of blood from the two separate circulations through shunting (see Figure 26–14). If closure of the ductus begins to occur, the infant quickly enters a critical state with the threat of death from heart failure or hypoxia.

Some medical centers are using intravenous infusions of prostaglandins to inhibit or prevent closure of the ductus arteriosus. Some prostaglandins have vasoconstrictive properties, and others function as vasodilators. E-type prostaglandins appear to be able to cause vasodilatation, especially of the ductus arteriosus in the newborn (Olley et al., 1976). Another possible communication between the two circulations is the shunting of blood through a patent foramen ovale or an atrial septal defect. A ventricular septal defect is a commonly associated defect that creates a communication between the two separate circulations. Pulmonary stenosis may also be an associated defect.

Because the infant never has adequate oxygen saturation of his systemic circulation, he is always cyanotic. Heart failure may occur due to overwork or when pulmonary stenosis is not present because of congestion due to increased pulmonary blood flow. Transposition of the great vessels occurs more frequently in males than in females and in infants of diabetic mothers. The affected infant is usually large. Transposition of the great vessels is thought to be more common than tetralogy of Fallot, but because many infants with this defect

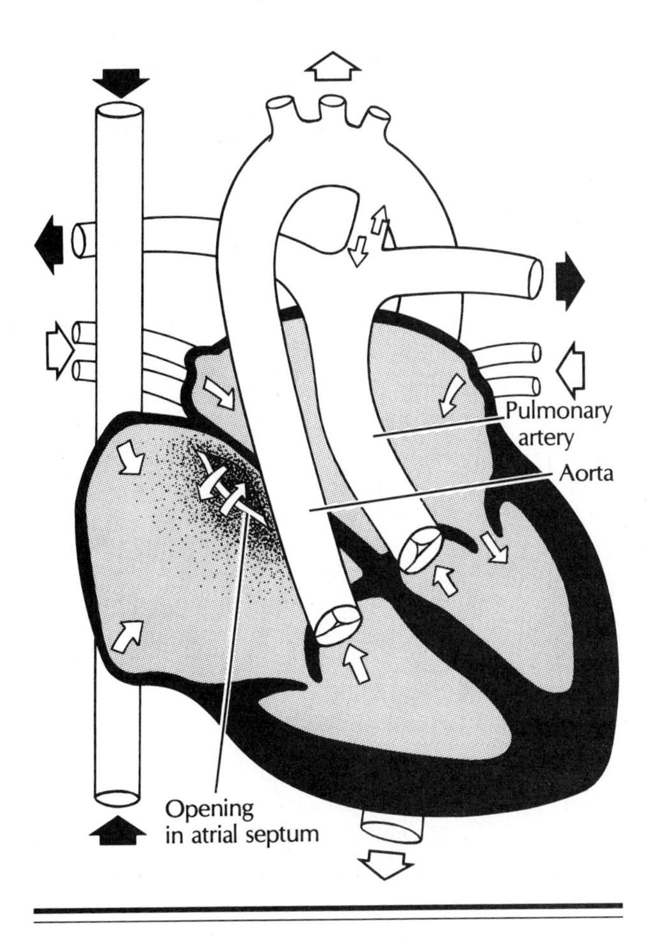

Figure 26–17. Palliative surgery for transposition of great vessels is accomplished by enlarging or creating an atrial septal defect.

die early, more children over 2 years of age are seen with tetralogy of Fallot. Recent management is greatly increasing survival during the first year of life for infants with transposition of the great vessels, so these statistics may soon change.

Cyanosis is present at birth or occurs within three days. Murmurs are present in relation to the blood flow through the various shunts—patent ductus arteriosus, ventricular septal defect, or atrial septal defect—and when present, the murmur of pulmonary stenosis can be heard. Although large at birth, these infants have rapid respirations, tire easily, feed poorly, and fail to grow and develop at a normal rate. The deep cyanosis causes polycythemia and early clubbing of fingers and toes due to decreased oxygen to tissues of the kidney, which stimulates the production of erythropoietin, which in turn increases red blood cell production by the bone marrow. The infant has anoxic paroxysmal dyspneic attacks with loss of consciousness.

The chest x-ray shows cardiac enlargement and the classic configuration, described as an "egg on its side." When pulmonary stenosis is not present, the x-ray also shows evidence of increased pulmonary blood flow. An electrocardiogram demonstrates right ventricular hypertrophy, which is considered normal for the newborn infant. A cardiac catheterization displays an increased right ventricular pressure and identifies the various defects.

If the mixing of blood does not appear to be adequate for the infant to survive, a Rashkind balloon atrial septostomy can be performed with the cardiac catheterization (Figure 26–17). A balloon-tipped catheter is passed from the right atrium through the foramen ovale into the left atrium. The balloon is inflated with radiopaque material and then forcefully withdrawn into the right atrium. This tear in the atrial septal tissue allows a bidirectional blood flow. It usually causes an immediate increase in arterial oxygen saturation and a decrease in left atrial pressure. If the balloon septostomy is not successful, a Blalock-Hanlen operation—the surgical creation of an atrial septal defect—might be done. Open-heart surgery is done, and the tissue dividing the two atria is excised.

In some infants with large ventricular septal defects and without pulmonary stenosis, increased pulmonary blood flow may require a pulmonary banding surgical procedure. At the present time, a complete repair of the total defect with open-heart surgery, Mustard's operation, is being done early, even at less than 1 year of age. In this procedure, the remaining part of the atrial septum is excised, and a baffle of pericardium is sutured in place in a manner that directs the oxygenated pulmonary venous return into the right ventricle and aorta, whereas the systemic venous circulation enters the left ventricle and pulmonary artery. Other anomalies—such as patent ductus, pulmonary stenosis, or ventricular septal defect—are also repaired at the same time. Selection of the proper time for the total repair varies with the child's particular defect and clinical progress and with the experience of the cardiologic and surgical teams.

Truncus Arteriosus

Truncus arteriosus occurs when the arterial end of the primitive tube fails to partition itself into two vessels, the pulmonary artery and the aorta. The truncus arteriosus, a large single vessel, situates itself in the middle of the ventricles over a large ventricular septal defect (see Figure 26-14). It receives blood from both ventricles, and the entire pulmonary and systemic circulation is supplied through this large single vessel. Pulmonary arteries do develop at various sites along the truncus arteriosus. Mixing of oxygenated and unoxygenated blood causes cyanosis. Pulmonary hypertension and decreased pulmonary blood flow increase cyanosis. If pulmonary blood flow is high, the infant will have difficulty with congestive heart failure and respiratory infections.

The child with truncus arteriosus has polycythemia and dyspnea, tires easily, feeds poorly, and shows failure to thrive. A loud pansystolic murmur is heard at the lower left sternal border. X-ray studies show an enlarged heart with a large single vessel arising from its center. An electrocardiogram demonstrates right, left, or combined ventricular hypertrophy. Cardiac catheterization reveals ventricular shunting of blood, with similar pressures in both ventricles and the truncus. At the present time, a highly successful surgical procedure is not available for this defect. Many children die in infancy; some survive longer with careful management.

Atresia of Tricuspid Valve

Defects of the tricuspid valve are not common. *Atresia of the tricuspid valve* is characterized by an imperforate underdeveloped valve, an atrial septal defect, a small right ventricle with diminished pulmonary circulation, and a large left ventricle (see Figure 26-14). There is a right-to-left shunting of blood through the atrial septal defect, with unoxygenated blood from the right atrium mixing with oxygenated blood in the left atrium. The child shows considerable cyanosis and marked left ventricular overload, because the right ventricle is receiving very little blood. Another communication with shunting must be present so that the lungs can receive blood. The most common is either a ventricular septal defect with left-to-right shunting due to increased pressure in the left ventricle or a patent ductus arteriosus with blood shunting from the aorta to the pulmonary artery.

This child shows the usual clinical manifestations of cyanotic heart disease—growth retardation, clubbing of fingers and toes, paroxysmal dyspneic attacks, polycythemia, and squatting. A harsh systolic murmur can be heard along the left sternal border. Chest x-ray reveals decreased pulmonary vascularity, a small right ventricle, and a small pulmonary artery. The electrocardiogram shows left ventricular hypertrophy. During cardiac catheterization, the right ventricle cannot be entered and the right atrial pressure is elevated.

Surgery at the present time is palliative. A Potts-Smith-Gibson or Blalock-Hanlen procedure may be done to increase pulmonary blood flow by an anastomosis to the pulmonary artery. One of the procedures to enlarge the atrial septal defect may be performed. An anastomosis of the superior vena cava to the right pulmonary artery has also been used to increase pulmonary blood flow. Surgery usually has to be done during the first year of life to prevent death. The results are only partially successful, and the child continues to manifest the problems of cyanotic heart disease.

Anomalous Venous Return of the Pulmonary Veins

Anomalous return of the pulmonary veins may be either complete or partial. In complete anomalous return all of the pulmonary and systemic veins empty into the right atrium. An atrial septal defect must be present for blood to reach the left side of the heart. In partial anomalous return, some of the pulmonary blood flow returns to the left atrium, and the rest is emptied into the right atrium. Part of the increased blood volume in the right atrium is shunted through an atrial septal defect into the left atrium, resulting in a mixture of unoxygenated and oxygenated blood being pumped into the system circulation.

The infant presents with cyanosis, fatigue, dyspnea, tachycardia, and frequent respiratory infections. He may develop right-sided heart failure due to the increased pulmonary blood flow. Chest x-ray reveals cardiac enlargement and a large pulmonary artery with increased pulmonary circulation. The electrocardiogram shows right ventricular hypertrophy. Cardiac catheterization is done to identify all existing defects and to assess their severity. Oxygen saturation of the blood in the right atrium is higher than normal, and the pressure in the right atrium is increased.

Complete anomalous return of pulmonary veins requires surgical correction at an early age. The heart-lung machine is used to perform an open-heart procedure in which the anomalous veins are detached from the right atrium and transplanted to the left atrium, and the atrial septal defect is repaired. Partial anomalous venous return may or may not be severe enough to require surgical correction.

Hypoplastic Left Heart Syndrome

In hypoplastic left heart syndrome, the left ventricle is nonfunctional; there may be hypoplasia of the aorta, mitral atresia or stenosis, or aortic valve atresia. The right ventricle is large, dilated, and hypertrophied in an attempt to maintain the entire heart action. The infant may appear normal at birth, but within a few hours to days he develops cyanosis and congestive heart failure. There is a nonspecific soft systolic murmur heard best just left of the sternum. Palpation of extremities reveals diminished pulses. Chest x-ray shows cardiac enlargement with increased or normal pulmonary blood flow. The electrocardiogram demonstrates right ventricular hypertrophy. There is no effective treatment for hypoplastic left heart syndrome, and these infants rarely live longer than two weeks.

Congestive Heart Failure

Hospitalization for congestive heart failure is one of the most common situations requiring nursing care for infants with congenital heart defects. Infants and children with left-to-right shunts and many with obstructive lesions may first present with congestive heart failure. It occurs with greatest frequency during the first year of life but can occur at any age, prior to surgery or as a postsurgical complication.

Physiology and Pathophysiology

The simplest definition of heart failure is the inability of the heart to pump blood in accordance with body needs. When the *right ventricle* fails, output through the pulmonary artery is diminished, and residual blood volume in the right ventricle and right atrium is increased. Pressure rises in the right ventricle, the right atrium, and the venous circulation. Right-sided failure occurs most often in children with tricuspid valve anomalies, pulmonary stenosis, or large atrial septal defects. Because of the systemic venous hypertension, these children have hepatomegaly (venous engorgement of the liver) and edema due to venous pressure exceeding plasma protein pressure, with resulting loss of fluid from capillaries into surrounding tissue. Also impaired is the removal of interstitial fluid by the lymphatics.

When the *left ventricle* fails, output through the aorta is diminished, and residual blood volume in the left side of the heart is increased. Decreased renal perfusion results in retention of sodium and water. Pressure increases in the left ventricle, left atrium, and the pulmonary veins, with subsequent pulmonary venous congestion. Left-sided failure occurs most frequently in infants and children with hypoplastic left heart syndrome, coarctation of the aorta, or aortic stenosis. These infants have tachypnea and dyspnea, often accompanied by rales; bloody, frothy sputum; wheezing; and cyanosis.

Left- and right-sided failure often appear concomitantly in infants and children. They can occur as a component of transposition of the great vessels, ventricular septal defect, total anomalous venous return of the pulmonary veins, and patent ductus arteriosus. The heart dilates and enlarges in an effort to accommodate the increased residual blood volume. The dilatation at first increases the force of the heart's contraction. When this mechanism reaches its maximum, the heart's next compensatory effort is to increase its rate (tachycardia) (Goldring, 1971).

Clinical Manifestations

The alert nurse might first notice easy fatigability, which the infant frequently demonstrates as an inability to feed well, requiring many rests before finishing even one or two ounces of formula. Fatigue at feeding might be accompanied by perspiration, with beads of moisture appearing on the upper lip and forehead. Failure to gain weight may also be seen, because of this poor feeding pattern and perhaps also because of poor absorption of nutrients and the frequent respiratory infections occurring commonly in these small, weak infants. Chronic hacking cough, if present, is caused by pulmonary venous pressure creating congested bronchial mucosa. The presence or development of an increase in respiratory rate reflects the increased pulmonary blood flow. Excess venous blood flow to the lungs can result not only in tachypnea but also in difficult respirations, with retraction of the chest, wheezing, and coughing. Congestion of blood flow in the liver can result in hepatomegaly, which is easily palpated in the abdomen of the small infant. Tachycardia of more than 160 beats per minute and cardiac enlargement are invariably present.

Pulsus alternans is detected by slowly releasing the sphygmomanometer until every second atrial beat is heard as pressure drops another 5–10 mm—the number of sounds doubles suddenly and becomes equal to the apex beat. The gallop rhythm so commonly used as a sign of failure in adults is not so significant in infants and young children, because a third heart sound can frequently be heard in children with no cardiac abnormality. Edema is a late manifestation and usually does not occur in infants. If it does occur, generally periorbital edema occurs first, followed by edema of the face. The skin generally appears very pale and moist. Peripheral pulses are decreased, and if heart failure is severe, peripheral vasoconstriction can occur, resulting in low blood pressure, low urine output, acidosis, and shock.

Interventions

Care of infants with congestive heart failure has four major goals: to reduce the energy requirements of the body, to increase cardiac efficiency, to increase oxygenation of the blood, and to reduce retention of fluids in the tissues. Bed rest, often with the use of morphine for sedation, is required. Morphine is thought to allay anxiety and to decrease peripheral and pulmonary vascular resistance, which results in decreased tachypnea. The appropriate dosage for infants and children is 0.1 to 0.2 mg per kg of body weight, given no more often than every four to six hours during distress. Infants and children in congestive heart failure are more comfortable in a semi-Fowler's position.

Cardiac efficiency is increased by medical management. Digitalization will be ordered by the physician. Digoxin (Lanoxin) is given either by mouth or intravenously. It also has a diuretic effect due to increased kidney perfusion. Digoxin is fast-acting (10–30 minutes), has a short half-life of one and a half days, and is excreted mainly by the kidneys.

When the infant or child has dyspnea or cyanosis, oxygen must be given by an oxygen hood, tent, mask, cannula, or oxygen prongs. Mist is often ordered given with oxygen to infants, making the use of an oxygen hood or tent necessary. Oxygen administration should always be accompanied by humidity, and the air should be warmed to decrease the drying effects of cold, dry oxygen. Vital signs are carefully monitored for evidence of tachycardia, tachypnea, expiratory grunting, and retractions.

During cardiac failure, the blood supply to the kidneys is reduced, and the diminished perfusion of the glomeruli and tubules results in increased sodium and water retention. Renin is also released, which promotes aldosterone secretion and causes more sodium retention by the kidneys. Diuretics are given to block the reabsorption of sodium in the kidneys. Furosemide (Lasix) is the one most often used at the present time. The usual dose is 1 mg per kg of body weight, and it may be given either orally or intravenously. The onset of diuresis varies from about five minutes when given intravenously to about two hours when given orally.

The most common problem occurring with the use of furosemide is hypokalemia. Potassium levels should be monitored and a potassium supplement given to the child as needed. When furosemide is taken orally by children, gastrointestinal irritation may also occur (Graef and Cone, 1974). If congestive heart failure occurs over a long period of time, sodium restriction may be necessary. Infants may be placed on low-sodium formulas, such as SMA S-26, Lonalac milk powder, or Similac PM 60/40. The infant's weight should be monitored about every eight hours, and a careful record of his fluid intake and urine output should be kept.

Preparation of the parents for home care should begin early in the infant's hospitalization. Information provided should include medication administration, techniques of isolating the infant from others with infection, availability of community resources, and public health referrals. It is also essential to provide a nonjudgmental atmosphere in which the parents can express their concerns and voice their anger.

DEVELOPMENTAL CONSEQUENCES OF CONGENITAL ANOMALIES

The infant who is born prematurely, is ill, or has a malformation or disorder is at risk in his emotional and intellectual, as well as physical, development. The risk is directly proportional to the seriousness of the problem and the length of treatment. Resolution of a meconium plug syndrome during the expected hospital stay, allowing the infant to be discharged with his mother, is not expected to alter the child's developmental course. However, the physical appearance, immediate and repeated surgeries, and complex rehabilitation problems of exstrophy of the bladder or meningomyelocele precludes a normal developmental course.

Medical, surgical, and technical advances in recent years have been responsible for salvaging increasing numbers of premature and ill neonates. The necessary physical separation of family and child and the tremendous emotional and financial burden have adversely affected the parent-child relationship. A considerable percentage of these children have been rescued only to be emotionally or physically battered by the parents. The most recent trend in many hospitals is to involve the parents with the neonate early, repeatedly, and over protracted periods of time. Early and continued involvement may only mean opportunities to look at the baby or to stroke his skin. Later, when the mother's and baby's conditions warrant it, the mother participates in her baby's care (to the extent she is willing) and in planning for the future. This type of involvement facilitates early bonding, attachment, and emotional investment. The parents need a sense of personal success, self-worth, self-esteem, and confidence from knowledge that they can cope with the situation. This atmosphere aids the child as well—he may escape from battering and may instead be assisted toward self-actualization.

Mothers of babies who are gravely ill are unable to chance an emotional investment in their child. These mothers need assistance in perceiving the cues and hearing the words that indicate the child is going to survive. They need time and support to establish a positive relationship with the child. A mother who is unable to develop maternal feelings may reject the child or overcompensate because of underlying guilt feelings; in either case an unproductive relationship may develop. The child may then be further handicapped by inability to relate well to others and by seeing the world as unsatisfying and painful.

The parents must have a clear picture of the reality of the handicap and the types of developmental hurdles ahead. Unexpected behaviors and responses from the child due to his defect or disorder can be upsetting and frightening. For example, parents find it difficult to cope with the child's lack of motor or social responsiveness and tend to interpret them as a form of rejection. The parents may in return respond with rejection, and an unfortunate cycle is begun.

It is difficult for many to discipline a handicapped child, to say no to him, to expect the same behaviors of him as are expected of "normal" children. The child who is given free rein can feel unworthy as well as be unable to develop more mature behavior patterns. Every child requires some exposure to delayed gratification, separation, and frustration in order to develop mastery over his feelings aroused by such situations. If the child is aware of limit-setting for his siblings, he feels unwanted, insecure, and unworthy of parental love and concern if he is denied the same limits to his behavior. He may be prompted to provocativeness and to testing limits to the point of irritation and possible rejection by those around him.

The demands of care of the child and disputes regarding his management or behavior stress family relationships. One or more members of the family may scapegoat the child. Another may become his champion to the exclusion of others. One or the other spouse may feel pushed aside or lacking in attention and thus may leave the family unit. Parents or siblings may feel that their own needs (schooling, material goods, freedom of movement) are being set aside while all assets (financial and other) go to support the one child's needs.

The child who has been overprotected has little chance to develop the intrapersonal and interpersonal skills needed to achieve in social situations, in school, and at work. Each child must have the opportunity to experience and explore the environment, to learn about it, to learn how to use it, and to learn how to cope with it. Deficient motor skills in particular can hamper exploration and mobility. Unless the child is motivated to explore and experience, the concept of the self and one's world is limited.

The parents and the child must confront daily an outside society that values normality. If the parents cannot develop a positive attitude toward the child, the child may see himself as not good—perhaps even as responsible for the predicament.

Fortunately, many children have parents who can accept them and help them cope with their "differentness." These children can explore and grow personally without unusual amounts of frustration and anxiety.

The entire multidisciplinary team may need to pool their resources and expertise to help parents of children born with defects or disorders so that both parents and children can thrive.

SUMMARY

Early assessment and appropriate intervention to prevent possible complications are essential in the nursing management of the infant with a congenital anomaly. It is incumbent upon the neonatal nurse to be knowledgeable about possible congenital anomalies and to utilize assessment skills to identify and then initiate appropriate interventions.

The nurse should be skilled in preoperative management so that valuable time is not lost and unnecessary complications do not occur. It is imperative that the nurse understand the emotional process associated with the birth of an infant with a congenital problem, as she is a key person in the establishment of the parent-infant relationship in this crucial early attachment period.

SUGGESTED ACTIVITIES

1. With two other classmates, role play a situation in which you, as a nurse, attempt to assist the parents of a defective infant to express their feelings.
2. Tour your local crippled children's facility to observe the services available.
3. Select one infant (inpatient or outpatient) with a congenital anomaly and do a case study based on his development, needs, and care.

REFERENCES

Doyle, E., and Rutbowski, M. 1970. Etiology of congenital heart disease. In *Cardiovascular clinics,* vol. II, no. 1, ed. A. N. Brest. Philadelphia: F. A. Davis Co.

Ferguson, A. 1975. *Orthopedic surgery in infancy and childhood.* 4th ed. Baltimore: The Williams & Wilkins Co.

Goldring, D., et al. 1971. The critically ill child: care of the infant in cardiac failure. *Pediatrics.* 47(6):1056.

Graef, J. W., and Cone, T. E. 1974. *Manual of pediatric therapeutics.* Boston: Little, Brown & Co.

Harris, H. 1976. Cardiorespiratory problems in the newborn. *Postgrad. Med. J.* 60(7):92.

Helfer, R. E., and Kempe, C. H. 1976. *Child abuse and neglect: the family and the community.* Cambridge: Ballinger Publishing Co.

Jones, P. G. 1976. *Clinical paediatric surgery: diagnosis and management.* 2nd ed. Oxford: Blackwell Scientific Publications.

Kempe, C. H., et al. 1978. *Current pediatric diagnosis and treatment.* Los Altos, Calif.: Lange Medical Publications.

King, O. M. 1975. *Care of the cardiac surgical patient.* St. Louis: The C. V. Mosby Co.

Olley, P. M., et al. 1976. E-type prostaglandins: new emergency therapy for certain cyanotic congenital heart malformations. *Circulation.* 53:728.

Polansky, B. J. 1970. Congenital heart disease. In *Medicine,* ed. C. S. Keefer and R. W. Wilkins. Boston: Little, Brown & Co.

Rushmer, R. F. 1976. *Cardiovascular dynamics.* Philadelphia: W. B. Saunders Co.

Smith, E. D. 1976. Anorectal anomalies. In *Clinical paediatric surgery: diagnosis and management.* 2nd ed., ed. P. G. Jones. Oxford: Blackwell Scientific Publications.

Toronto, A. F. 1972. *Structure and function of the heart.* Salt Lake City: Zion's Book Co.

Ziai, M., et al. 1975. *Pediatrics.* 2nd ed. Boston: Little, Brown & Co.

ADDITIONAL READINGS

Adler, J., and Brown, G. E. 1977. Patient assessment: abnormalities of the heartbeat. *Am. J. Nurs.* 77(4):647.

Aladjem, S., and Brown, A., eds. 1974. *Clinical perinatology.* St. Louis: The C. V. Mosby Co.

Altshulter, A. 1971. Complete transposition of the great arteries. *Am. J. Nurs.* 71:96.

Applebaum, A., et al. 1976. Surgical treatment of truncus arteriosus, with emphasis on infants and small children. *J. Thorac. Cardiovasc. Surg.* 71(3):436.

Ashcraft, K. W., and Tyson, K. R. 1975. For earlier correction of great-artery transposition. *RN.* 38(10):108.

Behrendt, D. M., et al. 1975. The Blalock-Hanlen procedure: a new look at an old operation. *Ann. Thorac. Surg.* 29(4):424.

Behrman, R., ed. 1973. *Neonatology: disease of the fetus and infant.* St. Louis: The C. V. Mosby Co.

Blackstone, E. H., et al. 1976. Optimal age and results in repair of large ventricular septal defects. *J. Thorac. Cardiovasc. Surg.* 72(5):661.

Bland, J. W., Jr., et al. 1976. Anesthetic technic using profound hypothermia for correction of congenital heart defects in infants and small children. *South. Med. J.* 69(7):831.

Breckenridge, I. M., et al. 1973. Correction of total anomalous pulmonary venous drainage in infancy. *J. Thorac. Cardiovasc. Surg.* 66(3):447.

Brest, A. N. ed. 1970. *Cardiovascular clinics.* Philadelphia: F. A. Davis Co.

Brown, M. S., and Alexander, M. M. 1974. Physical examination. II. Examining the heart. *Nursing.* 4(12):41.

Brunner, L., and Suddarth, D., eds. 1974. *The Lippincott manual of nursing practice.* Philadelphia: J. B. Lippincott Co.

Burr, B. D., et al. 1974. Clinical conference: cardiac surgery for congenital heart disease in a multiproblem family. *J. Fam. Practitioners.* 1(1):64.

Christensen, A. Jan.–Feb. 1977. Coping with the crisis of premature birth—one couple's story. *MCN.* 2:24.

Clarke, D. R., et al. 1976. Patent ductus arteriosus ligation and respiratory distress syndrome in premature infants. *Ann. Thorac. Surg.* 22(2):138.

Clarkson, P. M., and Orgill, A. A. 1974. Continuous murmurs in infants of low birth weight. *J. Pediatr.* 84(2):208.

Coats, K. 1975. Non-invasive cardiac diagnostic procedures. *Am. J. Nurs.* 75(11):1980.

Devine, A., and Goodchild, L. 1974. Total anomalous pulmonary venous connection. *NAT News.* 11(2):10.

Everson, S. 1977. Sibling counseling. *Am. J. Nurs.* 77(4):644.

Finley, K. H., et al. 1974. Intellectual functioning of children with tetralogy of Fallot: influence of open heart surgery and earlier palliative operations. *J. Pediatr.* 85(3):318.

Floyd, C. July–Aug. 1977. A defective child is born: a study of newborns with spina bifida and hydrocephalus. *J. Obstet. Gynecol. Nurs.* 6(4):56.

Foster, S. B. 1974. Pump failure. *Am. J. Nurs.* 74(10):1830.

Freed, M. D., and Bernhard, W. F. 1975. Prosthetic valve replacement in children. *Progr. Cardiovasc. Diseases.* 17(6):475.

Friedman, B. 1974. Skilled nursing during the postoperative period. *Nurs. '74.* 4:37.

Gerbode, F. 1976. A simple test to identify coarctation of the aorta. *Ann. Surg.* 184(4):615.

Gersony, W. M. 1973. Persistence of the fetal circulation: a commentary. *J. Pediatr.* 82(6):1103.

Gillon, J. E. 1973. Behavior of newborns with cardiac distress. *Am. J. Nurs.* 73(2):254.

Gray, R. V. 1974. Grief. *Nurs. '74.* 4:25.

Griepp, E., et al. 1975. Is pulmonary artery banding for ventricular septal defects obsolete? *Circulation.* 50(2):14.

Gruenwald, M. 1976. *Nursing care of the child having open-heart surgery.* Salt Lake City: University of Utah.

Gundermuth, S. 1975. Mothers' reports of early experiences of infants with congenital heart disease. *MCN.* 4:155.

Guntheroth, W. G. 1976. Neonatal and pediatric cardiovascular crises. *Emergency Med.* 8:39.

Hardgrove, C., and Warrick, L. 1974. How shall we tell the children? *Am. J. Nurs.* 74:448.

Harris, H. 1976. Cardiorespiratory problems in the newborn. *Postgrad. Med. J.* 60(7):92.

Hilt, N. April 1976. Care of the child in a hip spica cast. *RN.* 39:27.

Hogarth, W. 1975. Cardiopulmonary bypass in infants under two years. *Nurs. Times.* 71(24):921.

Howarth, E. 1973. Transposition of the great vessels. *Nurs. Times.* 69(36):1147.

Hurd, J. July–Aug. 1975. Assessing maternal attachment: first step toward the prevention of child abuse. *J. Obstet. Gynecol. Neonatal Nurs.* 4:25.

Hurst, J., and Loque, R. B. 1974. *The heart.* 3rd ed. New York: McGraw-Hill Book Co.

Hurwitz, R. A., and Girod, D. A. 1976. Percutaneous balloon atrial septostomy in infants with transposition of the great arteries. *Am. Heart J.* 91(5):618.

Isler, C. 1970. Open heart surgery: pre and post op nursing care. Part 2. *RN.* 33:44.

Jackson, P. L. 1974. Chronic grief. *Am. J. Nurs.* 74(7):1288.

Jensen, M., et al. 1977. *Maternity care: the nurse and the family.* St. Louis: The C. V. Mosby Co.

Kaye, H. H., and Tynan, M. 1974. Balloon atrial septostomy via the umbilical vein. *Brit. Heart J.* 36(10):1040.

Laks, H.; Marco, J. D.; and Willman, V. L. 1975. The Blalock-Taussig shunt in the first six months of life. *J. Thorac. Cardiovasc. Surg.* 70(4):687.

Lam, C. R. 1976. A safe technique for closure of the recurrent patent ductus arteriosus. *J. Thorac. Cardiovasc. Surg.* 72(2):232.

Lavoie, D. Oct. 1973. Spina bifida and immediate concerns—long term goals. *Nurs. '73.* 3(10):43.

Laycock, D. 1972. Waterston's operation for Fallot's tetralogy. *Nurs. Times.* 68(21):632.

Leifer, G. 1972. *Principles and techniques in pediatric nursing.* 2nd ed. Philadelphia: W. B. Saunders Co.

Linde, L. M., et al. 1966. Attitudinal factors in congenital heart disease. *Pediatrics.* 38:92.

Long, M., et al. 1974. Cardiopulmonary bypass. *Am. J. Nurs.* 74(5):860.

Lu, O. July–Aug. 1977. Orthopedic management of a child with a spinal cord disorder. *Pediatr. Nurs.* 3:37.

Mair, D. D., et al. 1974. Selection of patients with truncus arteriosus for surgical correction: anatomic and hemodynamic considerations. *Circulation.* 49(1):144.

Miller, J. E., et al. 1976. Atrial septal defect: review of ten year experience. *J. Med. Ass. Georgia.* 65(1):27.

Miller, R. 1974. Children and their hearts. *Postgrad. Med. J.* 55(3):121.

Moller, J. H., and Anderson, R. C. 1971. Cyanosis. *Hosp. Med.* 7:105.

Nadas, A. S., and Fyler, D. C. 1972. *Pediatric cardiology.* 3rd ed. Philadelphia: W. B. Saunders Co.

Neches, W. H., et al. 1973. Balloon atrial septostomy in congenital heart disease in infancy. *Am. J. Dis. Child.* 125(3):371.

Nora, J. J., and Morriss, J. H. 1973. Clinical clues to congenital heart disease in infants. *Medical Times.* 101(11):53.

O'Grady, R. 1971. Feeding behavior in infants. *Am. J. Nurs.* 71(4):736.

Pediatric care viewed by a mother. 1975. *Nurs. Times.* 71(44):4.

Pierce, W. S., and Waldhausen, J. A. 1972. Surgical approaches in congenital heart disease. *Pediatr. Clin. N. Am.* 19(2):333.

Posey, R. A. 1974. Creative nursing care of babies with heart disease. *Nursing.* 4(10):40.

Raffensperger, J. G. 1970. *The acute abdomen in infancy and childhood.* Philadelphia: J. B. Lippincott Co.

Rao, P. O. 1973. The femoral route for cardiac catheterization of infants and children. *Chest.* 63(2):239.

Reif, K. 1972. A heart makes you live. *Am. J. Nurs.* 72:1085.

Richardson, J. P., and Clarke, C. P. 1976. Tetralogy of Fallot: risk factors associated with complete repair. *Brit. Heart J.* 38(9):926.

Roberts, F. B. 1972. The child with heart disease. *Am. J. Nurs.* 72:1080.

Robinson, S. J. 1970. Diagnosis of congenital heart disease: clues from the history and physical examination. *Cardiovasc. Clin.* 2(1):77.

Rosenthal, A. 1975. The patient with congenital heart disease after surgical repair: an overview. *Prog. Cardiovasc. Dis.* 17(6):401.

Rosenthal, A., and Castanedo, A. 1975. Growth and development after cardiovascular surgery in infants and children. *Progr. Cardiovasc. Dis.* 18(1):27.

Ross Laboratories. 1975. Congenital heart abnormalities. *Ross Laboratories Clinical Education Aid.* Number 7. Teaching Reference. Columbus, Ohio.

Sade, R. M., and Castanedo, A. 1976. Recent advances in cardiac surgery in the young infant. *Surgical Clin. N. Am.* 56:451.

Schwartz, J. L., and Schwartz, L. H., eds. 1977. *Vulnerable infants: a psychosocial dilemma.* New York: McGraw-Hill Book Co.

Shirkey, H., ed. 1972. *Pediatric therapy.* 4th ed. St. Louis: The C. V. Mosby Co.

Slade, C., et al. March–April 1977. Working with parents of high-risk newborns. *J. Obstet. Gynecol. Neonatal Nurs.* 6:21.

Tatooles, C. J. 1975. Palliative cardiac surgery in the infant. *Surgical Clin. N. Am.* 55(1):89.

Taylor, J. R., et al. 1976. Proceedings: repair of ventricular septal defects in infancy. *Brit. Heart J.* 38(5):535.

Tooley, W. J., and Stanger, P. 1972. The blue baby—circulation or ventilation or both? *N. Engl. J. Med.* 287(19):983.

Truccone, N. J., et al. 1976. Cardiac output in infants and children after open heart surgery. *J. Thorac. Cardiovasc. Surg.* 71(3):410.

Vaughan, V. C. and McKay, R. J. *Nelson's textbook of pediatrics.* 9th ed. Philadelphia: W. B. Saunders Co.

Waechter, E. H. 1970. The birth of an exceptional child. *Nurs. Forum.* 9:202.

Waechter, E. H. 1970. Developmental correlates of physical disability. *Nurs. Forum.* 9:90.

Waechter, E., and Blake, F. 1976. *Nursing care of children.* 9th ed. Philadelphia: J. B. Lippincott Co.

Walker, D. R. 1976. Surgical treatment of truncus arteriosus. *Nurs. Times.* 72(2):49.

Whaley, L. 1974. *Understanding inherited disorders.* St. Louis: The C. V. Mosby Co.

Winward, R. 1974. Nursing care study: closure of ventricular septal defect. *Nurs. Mirror.* 139(7):74.

Young, R. Jan.–Feb. 1977. Chronic sorrow: parents' response to the birth of a child with a defect. *MCN.* 2:38.

UNIT VI

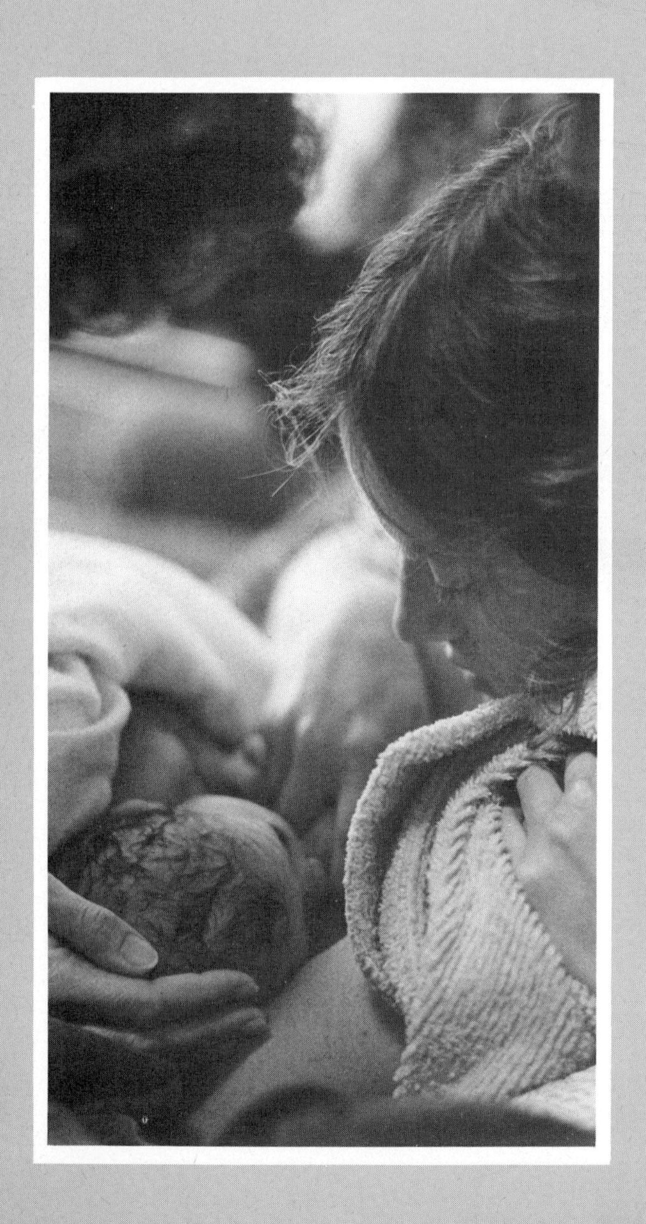

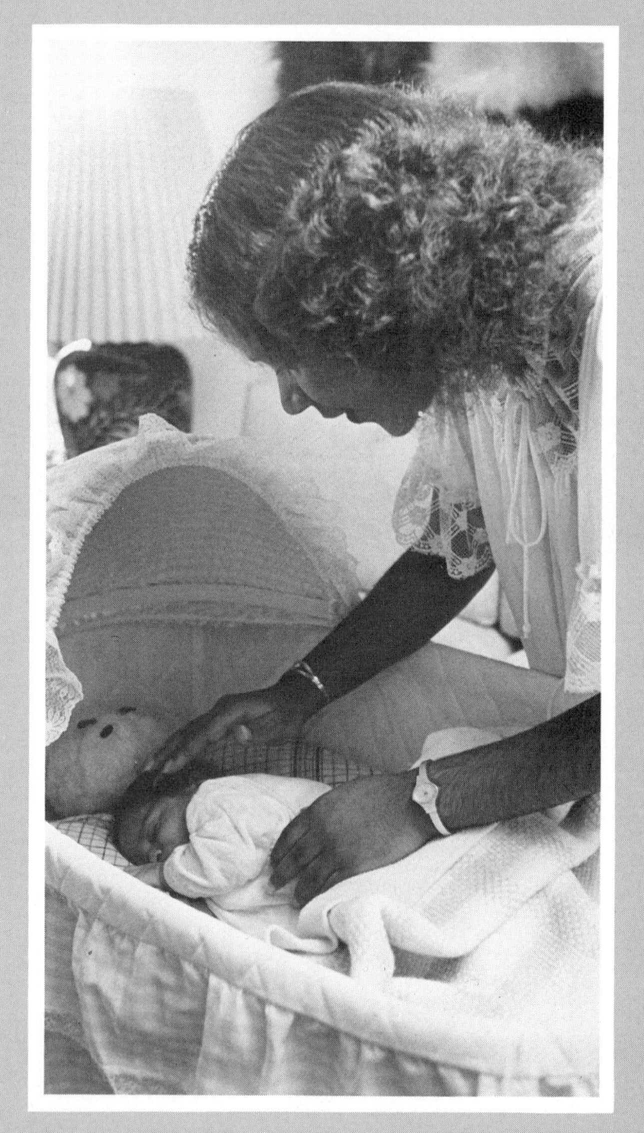

THE PUERPERIUM

CHAPTER 27

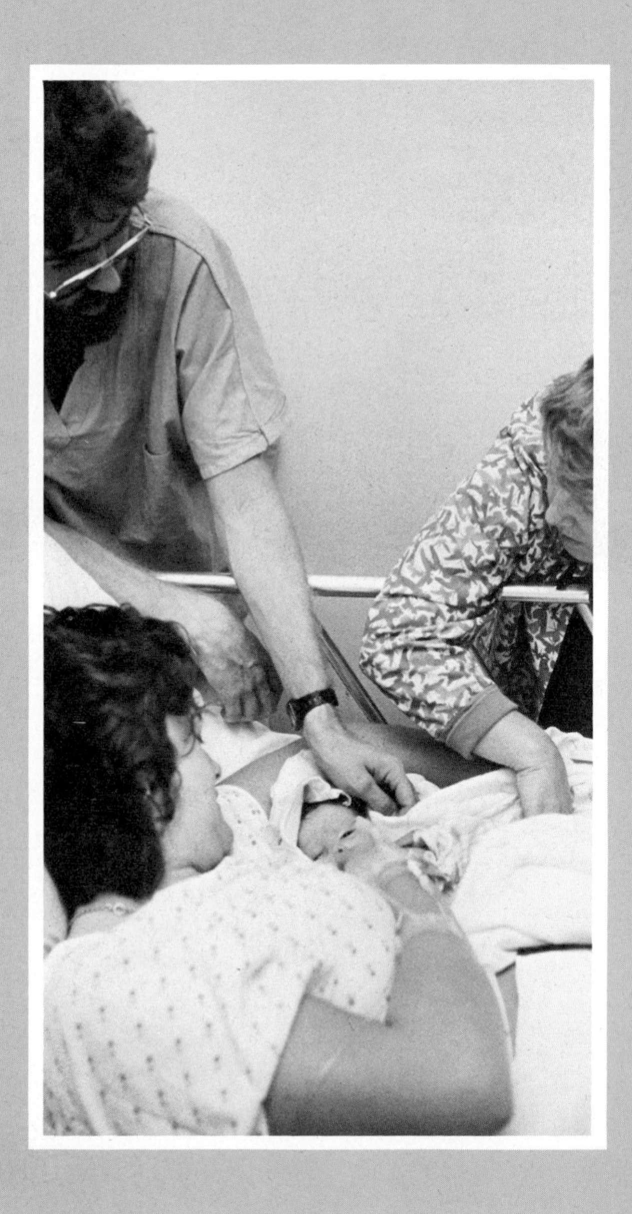

THE POSTPARTAL FAMILY: ASSESSMENT, NEEDS, AND CARE

OBJECTIVES

- Identify the systemic adaptations and physiologic changes of the postpartal period.
- Describe the normal psychologic changes of the postpartal family.
- Discuss assessment and nursing management of the postpartal family.
- Delineate the nursing responsibilities for patient education about various feeding methods.
- Discuss the concept of the fourth trimester as it relates to the provision of nursing care for the postpartal family.

The *puerperium* may be described as that period of time during which the body adjusts, both physically and psychologically, to the process of childbearing. By definition, it begins immediately after delivery and proceeds for approximately six weeks or until the body has completed its adjustment and has returned to a near prepregnant state. Some have referred to the puerperium as "the fourth trimester," and whereas the time span does not necessarily cover three months, this terminology demonstrates the idea of continuity.

Postpartum does not occur as an isolated period and is significantly influenced by the processes that have preceded it. During pregnancy the body adjusted gradually to the physical changes, but now it is forced to respond more rapidly. The method of delivery and circumstances associated with the delivery alter the speed with which the body reacts. Changes in body image and assumption of new roles often influence the outcome and ultimate adaptation to childbearing. Nursing interventions during postpartum must take into account a history of the total process and reactions of all family members in order to effect a healthy adjustment.

Certain premises form the basis for the provision of effective nursing care during the puerperium:

1. The best postpartal care is that provided with a family-centered focus and with minimal disruption of the family unit. This approach consolidates the family's resources and enhances an early and smooth adjustment to the newborn by all family members.

2. Establishing a normative base for the physiologic as well as psychologic adaptations required during the postpartal period allows for early recognition of alterations and subsequent early intervention. Communicating this knowledge to the family facilitates their adjustment.

3. Emphasis in providing care is focused on assessment of the individual's needs and consideration of factors that could influence the outcome or nursing requirements. Nursing interventions are then planned to accomplish specific goals. It should be remembered that needs overlap, as does nursing intervention, so that one need should not be seen as being isolated from other needs.

PUERPERAL PHYSICAL ADAPTATIONS

Comprehensive nursing assessment is first based on a sound understanding of the normal anatomic and physiologic processes of the puerperium.

Reproductive Organs

Involution of Uterus

Immediately following the expulsion of the placenta, the uterus contracts firmly to the size of a large grapefruit, reducing uterine size by over one-half. The fundus can be located by observation and palpation approximately halfway between the symphysis pubis and the umbilicus and is situated in the midline (Figure 27-1). The walls of the contracted uterus are in close proximity and measure approximately 4 cm × 5 cm each. In contrast to the dusky color of the congested pregnant uterus, the puerperal uterus appears more ischemic due to the compression of the uterine vessels by the myometrium. Within 12 hours after delivery the fundus of the uterus rises to one finger breadth (1.0 cm) above the umbilicus. If the uterus is higher than one finger breadth or is deviated from the midline and is boggy, the most probable cause of its displacement is a distended urinary bladder. Because the uterine ligaments are still stretched, the uterus can easily be moved by the full bladder. The uterus should be evaluated immediately after emptying the bladder and the change in height and position recorded. On each succeeding postpartum day the fundus should descend into the pelvis approximately one finger breadth. If the mother is breast-feeding, the involution of the uterus is facilitated by the release of oxytocin from the posterior pituitary as a response to suckling, and the uterus may descend more rapidly into the pelvis.

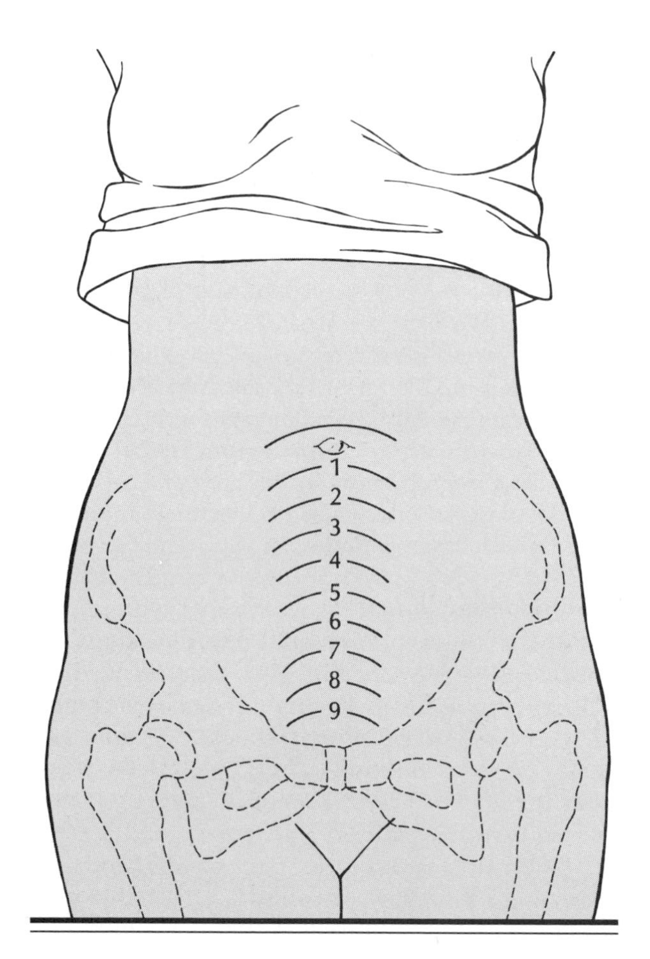

Figure 27–1. Involution of the uterus. The height of the fundus decreases about one finger breadth (approximately 1 cm) each day.

Following delivery the uterus remains about the same size for two days and then begins to atrophy so rapidly that within two weeks postpartum, the fundus becomes a pelvic organ and is no longer palpable abdominally (Pritchard and MacDonald, 1976). Barring complications such as infection or retained secundines, the uterus approximates the nonpregnant size by five to six weeks. Changes in the weight of the uterus are equally dramatic. Although it weighs 1000–1200 gm at term, the uterus decreases to 500 gm at one week, 300 gm at two weeks, and 100 gm after the third week (Pritchard and MacDonald, 1976). This reduction in weight is not due to a decreased number of muscle cells but occurs because the individual cells become thinner. With the dramatic decrease in the levels of circulatory estrogen and progesterone following placental separation, the uterine cells atrophy, and hyperplasia of pregnancy begins to reverse. Proteolytic enzymes are released, and macrophages migrate to the uterus to promote autolysis (self-digestion). Protein material in the uterine wall is broken down and absorbed. Thus the process is basically one of cell size reduction rather than a radical decrease in cell number. The term "involution" is used to describe the rapid reduction in size and the return of the uterus to a normal condition similar to its nulliparous state.

Following separation of the placenta, the decidua of the uterus is irregular, jagged, and varied in thickness. The spongy layer of the decidua is cast off as lochia, and the basal layer of the decidua remains in the uterus to become differentiated into two layers within the first 48–72 hours after delivery. The outermost layer becomes necrotic and is sloughed off in the lochia. The layer closest to the myometrium contains the fundi of the uterine endometrial glands, and these glands lay the foundation for the new endometrium. Except at the placental site, the endometrium is formed by the proliferation of the fundi of the endometrial glands and of the stroma from the interglandular connective tissue (Pritchard and MacDonald, 1976). This process is completed in approximately three weeks.

Involution of the placental site follows a similar process and is generally thought to take six weeks for completion. Following separation, the placental site contracts to an area about 8–9 cm in diameter that appears raised and irregular. Bleeding from the larger uterine vessels is controlled by compression of the retracted uterine muscle fibers. The placental site consists of multiple thrombosed vascular sinusoids that are treated by the body as any other vascular clot. Some of these vessels are eventually obliterated and replaced by new vessels with smaller lumens (Greenhill and Friedman, 1974).

Rather than forming a fibrous sac in the decidua, the placental site heals by a process of exfoliation. This process consists of the undermining of the site by the growth of the endometrial tissue both from the margins of the site and from the fundi of the endometrial glands left in the basal layer of the site. The infarcted superficial tissue then becomes necrotic and is sloughed off.

Exfoliation is one of the most important aspects of involution in an otherwise unremarkable postpartum course for two reasons:

1. If the healing of the placental site were to

leave a fibrous scar, the area available for future implantation would be limited, as would the number of possible pregnancies.

2. Failure of the placental site to undergo normal involution may result in late puerperal (delayed postpartum) hemorrhage or subinvolution, which is characterized by persistent lochia, failure of the uterus to decrease in size progressively, lack of uterine tone, and painless fresh bleeding.

Some of the factors that retard uterine involution are prolonged labor, anesthesia or excessive analgesia, difficult delivery, grandmultiparity, a full bladder, and incomplete expulsion of the products of conception. Some factors that enhance involution include an uncomplicated labor and delivery, complete expulsion of the products of conception, breast-feeding, and early ambulation. In some regions an oxytocic agent is given to aid involution. However, research has demonstrated no appreciable difference in the involutional process except for an increase in the amount of pain experienced by the women receiving oxytocins (Pritchard and MacDonald, 1976).

It is necessary to determine not only location but also consistency of the uterus, for it is the state of uterine contraction that controls bleeding, preventing hemorrhage. The uterus should be palpated at frequent intervals: every 15 minutes during the fourth stage of labor, every 30 minutes for the next two to three hours, then every eight hours to maintain firm consistency and to evaluate the rate of involution of the uterus. Care should be taken not to overmassage, which tires the muscle, resulting in atony. The patient may be instructed and encouraged to gently massage the uterus at intervals to enhance uterine contraction.

The vaginally delivered patient presents little difficulty for palpation of the uterus, but modifications are required for patients delivered by cesarean section. Often with abdominal dressings it becomes difficult to determine the position of the fundus. Firmness and position may be determined by gently palpating on each side of the incision. With the cesarean section patient it is essential to observe the amount of lochia to assess for relaxation of the uterus.

If oxytocic drugs are given following delivery, caution should be exercised. Although side effects are uncommon when the drugs are correctly administered, they include hypertension, bradycardia, dyspnea, headache, nausea and vomiting, dizziness, cramps, and chest pain. With prolonged use, water intoxication may also occur. Once the medications are discontinued, the patient should be monitored closely for relaxation of the uterus.

Lochia

One of the most unique capabilities of the uterus is the ability to rid itself of the debris remaining after delivery. This discharge is termed lochia and is classified according to its appearance and contents. *Lochia rubra* takes its name from the dark red color of the discharge. It occurs for the first two to three days and contains epithelial cells, erythrocytes, leukocytes, shreds of the decidua, and occasionally fetal meconium, lanugo, and vernix caseosa. Lochia should not contain large clots; if it does, the cause should be discovered without delay. *Lochia serosa* follows from approximately the third until the tenth day. It is characterized by a pinkish color and serosanguineous consistency. It is composed of serous exudate (hence the name), shreds of degenerating decidua, erythrocytes, leukocytes, cervical mucus, and numerous microorganisms.

Gradually the blood cell component decreases, and a creamy or yellowish discharge persists for an additional week or two. This final discharge is termed *lochia alba* and is composed primarily of leukocytes; large, irregular round or spindle-shaped mononucleated decidual cells; both flat and cylindrical epithelial cells; fat; cervical mucus; cholesterol crystals; and bacteria. When the lochia stops, the cervix is considered closed, and chances of infection ascending from the vagina to the uterus decrease.

Lochia, similar to menstrual discharge, has a musty, stale odor that is not offensive. Microorganisms are always present in the vaginal lochia, and by the second day following delivery the uterus is contaminated with the vaginal bacteria. Researchers speculate that infection does not develop because the organisms involved are relatively nonvirulent. In addition, by the time the bacteria reach the raw, exposed surface of the uterus the process of granulation has begun, forming a protective barrier (Greenhill and Friedman, 1974). Any foul smell to the lochia or used peri-pad suggests infection and the need for prompt assessment.

The amount of lochia varies from woman to woman, but the average is 251–277 gm during the first five to six postpartal days (Pritchard and MacDonald, 1976). A gradual reduction in volume occurs until the average daily amount ranges between 2–5 gm. Discharge is heavier in the morning than at night, but whether this difference is real or apparent is unclear. A logical explanation would be that the recumbent position at night would tend to cause pooling of the lochia in the vagina and uterus, and this accumulation would subsequently be discharged when the upright position is achieved. The amount of lochia may also be increased by exertion or breast-feeding.

Evaluation of lochia is necessary not only to determine the presence of hemorrhage but also to assess uterine involution. The type, amount, and consistency of lochia determine the state of healing of the placental site, and a progressive change from bright red to pink to white/clear discharge should be observed. Persistent discharge of lochia rubra or a return to lochia rubra indicates subinvolution or late postpartal hemorrhage (see Chapter 29).

Caution should be exercised in the evaluation of bleeding immediately after delivery. The continuous seepage of blood is more consistent with cervical or vaginal lacerations and may be effectively diagnosed when the bleeding is evaluated in conjunction with the consistency of the uterus.

Until recently, it was fairly common to administer an oxytocic agent such as 0.2 mg methylergonovine maleate (Methergine) orally every four hours for the first 24–72 hours postpartum as a prophylactic measure against postpartal hemorrhage. It was also believed to facilitate involution. Currently routine use of oxytocic agents is no longer being practiced. Oxytocic agents may be ordered for patients who are at risk for involution problems, such as those with prolonged labor, intrapartal hemorrhage, or overdistention of the uterus during pregnancy.

Cervical Changes

Following delivery the cervix is spongy, bruised, flabby, and formless. The external os has a markedly irregular outline suggestive of multiple small lacerations. The os closes slowly, and by the end of the first week only a fingertip opening remains.

The shape of the external os is permanently changed following the first childbearing. The characteristic dimplelike os of the nullipara changes to the lateral slit (fishmouth) os of the multipara. If there has been a significant cervical laceration or several lacerations, the cervix may appear lopsided.

Vaginal Changes

Careful inspection of the vagina following delivery demonstrates that the vagina appears edematous and bruised. Small superficial lacerations may be evident, and the rugae have been obliterated. The hymen has been lacerated in several places. The apparent bruising of the vagina is due to pelvic congestion, and resolution takes place rapidly following the birth. The torn edges of the hymen do not reanastomose but rather stay separate and heal along the torn edges. These small tags of hymen are the carunculae myrtiformes and indicate a previous vaginal birth.

Vaginal rugae begin to return by three weeks, which facilitates the gradual return to realistic but not nulliparous dimensions. Tightening of the vaginal orifice may require perineal tightening exercises, which may begin soon after delivery and should be incorporated into the exercise regimen. The labia majora and labia minora are more flabby in the woman who has borne a child than in the nullipara.

Perineal Changes

During the second stage of labor the pelvic floor muscles are thinned and stretched by the pressure of the advancing fetal head. The pressure is greater in primigravidas and in women with large babies. In the United States, it is common medical practice to incise the perineum by performing an episiotomy. The overstretching and trauma of birth may cause weakening of the perineal muscles. This condition predisposes to rectocele and cystocele, common sequelae of childbirth, especially if the woman has borne more than one child. In some regions of the country physicians and nurse-midwives are delivering the parturient in a sidelying or sitting position. It is thought that either of these positions is better physiologically, decreases the stress and stretching of the perineum during delivery, and decreases the need for performing an episiotomy.

During the early postpartal period the soft tissue in and around the perineum may become edematous with some bruising. The edges of the episiotomy appear to be approximated within the first 24 hours and should not have any ecchymoses, as these will delay healing.

Recurrence of Ovulation and Menstruation

It has been generally thought that menstruation reoccurs in non-breast-feeding women within 6–8 weeks following delivery. However, it has been demonstrated that about 25% of non-breast-feeding women resume menstruation in 6 weeks. 61% resume menstruation by the end of the 12th week, and 77% within 24 weeks following delivery. At 12 weeks following delivery about 33% of lactating primiparas are menstruating (Greenhill and Friedman, 1974). These periods may be ovulatory or anovulatory. In the lactating, amenorrheic, anovulatory woman there is evidence that there are normal amounts of gonadotropin in the urine, but the ovaries are temporarily not affected by this stimulus for reasons as yet not known (Pritchard and MacDonald, 1976).

Abdomen

The peritoneum, if it were visible during the puerperium, would appear to drape the lower part of the uterus in uneven folds. These folds usually disappear during the first several days. Likewise, the uterine ligaments (notably the round and broad ligaments) are stretched, but they require a much longer time to recover. The abdominal wall itself has also been stretched and will appear loose and somewhat flabby for a time. Within two to three months, with exercise, abdominal muscle tone improved greatly. In the grandmultipara, in the woman in which overdistention of the abdomen has occurred, or in the woman with poor muscle tone before pregnancy, the abdomen may fail to regain good tone and may remain somewhat flabby. Diastasis recti abdominis is a separation of the recti muscle, which may occur with pregnancy, especially in women with poor abdominal muscle tone. Diastasis recti abdominis and poor muscle tone respond well to abdominal exercises. Improvement is also dependent on the physical condition of the mother, the total number of pregnancies, and the type and amount of physical exercise. Exercise may begin immediately after a vaginal delivery and within a few weeks following a cesarean section.

The striae (stretch marks), which occurred as a result of stretching and rupture of the elastic fibers of the skin, are red to purple at delivery. These gradually fade and after a time appear as silver or white streaks.

Lactation

During pregnancy increased levels of estrogen stimulate breast duct proliferation and development, and elevated progesterone levels promote the development of breast lobules and alveoli in preparation for lactation.

Colostrum, a premilk substance, may be expressed from the breasts by the sixth or seventh month of pregnancy. It is a yellowish fluid containing more protein, vitamin A, and inorganic salts than breast milk but less fat and carbohydrates. It also contains colostrum corpuscles, formed by the fatty degeneration of large masses of secreting cells. High levels of immunoglobulins are present in colostrum, but their ability to provide immunity for the infant is questionable because of poor intestinal absorption.

The initiation of lactation requires the interplay of a variety of hormones. During pregnancy the high levels of circulating estrogen and progesterone exert an inhibitory effect upon prolactin secretion. Delivery results in a rapid drop in estrogen and progesterone with a concomitant increase in the secretion of prolactin by the anterior pituitary. This hormone promotes milk production by stimulating the alveolar cells of the breasts. When the infant sucks on the mother's nipple, oxytocin is released from the posterior pituitary. This hormone increases the contractility of the myoepithelial cells lining the walls of the mammary ducts, and a flow of milk results. This "letdown" reflex may be initiated by tactile stimulation or suckling but may also be triggered by psychic factors such as the sound of an infant's cry. Mothers have described the letdown reflex as a prickling or tingling sensation during which they feel the milk coming down. It is not unusual for the breasts to leak some milk prior to feeding or when the baby cries as a result of the ejection (letdown) reflex.

Emotional problems, fatigue, pain, or worry may inhibit the letdown reflex. To prevent this the feeding environment should be restful and private, pain relief measures to promote maternal comfort should be employed, and emotional support should be provided. After lactation is established, suckling is the most important factor in the maintenance of milk production. "The afferent stimuli from the nipple reach the hypothalmus and initiate a complex response mediated by dopamine which results in suppression of prolactin-inhibiting factor, a substance ordinarily present to inhibit the release of prolactin. The net result is a temporary increase in prolactin secretion which stimulates the milk-producing epithelium of the alveoli" (Danforth, 1977, p. 710).

After several weeks of nursing the production of prolactin diminishes somewhat and subsequent maintenance of milk production is not as clearly understood. It has been suggested that the mother's response to her infant's presence or cry may play a role in continued milk production as well as in milk release (Danforth, 1977).

Milk production is decreased with repeated inhibition of the letdown reflex. Failure to empty the breasts frequently and completely also decreases production, because as milk accumulates and is not withdrawn, the buildup of pressure in the alveoli suppresses secretion. The administration of androgens and estrogens also inhibits lactation. With frequent nursing (every 2–3 hours) milk production may be reestablished even in the woman who received drugs to suppress lactation.

It requires two to four days following delivery for milk to replace colostrum in the breasts of a nursing mother, although multigravidas may begin producing milk as early as 24 hours after delivery. Because the law of supply and demand influences milk production, mothers who feed early and more frequently may experience earlier milk production (Nichols, 1978).

Gastrointestinal System

Hunger following delivery is common, and the mother may enjoy a light diet. Frequently the mother is quite thirsty and will begin drinking large amounts of fluid as soon as she is permitted to do so. She may continue to drink large amounts of water to replace water lost in labor, in the urine, and through perspiration (Greenhill and Friedman, 1974).

The bowel tends to be sluggish after delivery, due to decreased hormonal levels, decreased muscle tone in the intestine, and decreased intra-abdominal pressure. Other contributing factors are less often cited for constipation during the puerperium. One is the questionable routine of administering a labor room "admission" enema; another is the fasting (sometimes up to 24 hours) that laboring women are subjected to. Both may result in decreased transit time in the bowel. Finally, the pain from an elective episiotomy (especially a mediolateral), any lacerations, and hemorrhoids encourages women to delay elimination for fear of increasing their pain or in the belief that their stitches will be torn by the strong bearing-down pressure. In refusing or delaying the bowel movement, the patient may cause increased constipation and more pain when elimination finally occurs.

Bowel elimination may become a problem after the patient resumes a diet, because the woman has probably received a cleansing enema as a part of the admission procedure in labor and has not received solid foods while in labor. Fluids and solid food should be delayed for one to two days for the cesarean patient, until peristalsis is resumed. It may take a few days for the bowel to regain tone. Stool softeners may be ordered to increase bulk and moisture in the fecal material and to facilitate more comfortable and complete evacuation. Constipation should be avoided to prevent pressure on sutures that increases discomfort. Encouraging ambulation, forcing fluids, and providing fresh fruits and roughage in the diet enhance bowel elimination and assist the patient in reestablishing her normal bowel pattern.

Urinary Tract

Edema, hyperemia of the bladder, and submucous extravasation of blood are frequent occurrences following labor and birth. These conditions—combined with an increased capacity for and a decreased sensitivity to fluid pressure, swelling and bruising of the tissues around the urethra, decreased sensation of bladder filling, and inability to void in the recumbent position—put the puerperal woman at risk for overdistention, incomplete emptying, and buildup of residual urine.

Women who have been subjected to conductive anesthesia have inhibited neural functioning of the bladder and are more susceptible to bladder complications. Urinary output increases during the early postpartal period (first 12–24 hours) due to puerperal diuresis. The kidneys must eliminate an estimated 2000–3000 ml of extracellular fluid associated with a normal pregnancy. With eclampsia and preclampsia, hypertension, and diabetes, an even greater fluid retention is experienced, and postpartum diuresis is accordingly increased.

Bladder elimination presents an immediate problem. If stasis exists, there is an increased chance of a urinary tract infection because of bacteriuria and the presence of dilated ureters and renal pelves, which persist for about 4 weeks after delivery (Pritchard and MacDonald, 1976). A full bladder may also increase the tendency of relaxation of the uterus by displacing the uterus and interfering with its contractility, leading to hemorrhage.

The postpartal patient should be encouraged to void every four to six hours. A careful monitoring of intake and output should be maintained until the patient demonstrates complete emptying of the bladder with each voiding. The nurse may employ techniques to facilitate voiding, such as perineal care with warm water to promote relaxation of the perineum. If catheterization is required, the technique must be gentle, and when the catheter is removed, accurate measuring of the amount of urine is essential until voiding is no longer a problem. The surgical postpartal patient may have a catheter inserted prophylactically. The same considerations should be made in evaluating emptying once the catheter is removed.

Hematuria, resulting from bladder trauma, is not unusual following delivery. If hematuria occurs in the second or third postpartal week, there may be a bladder infection. Acetone may be present in the urine of diabetics or of patients with prolonged labor and dehydration. Proteinuria occurs in about 40% of women following labor and may persist for about three days (Greenhill and Friedman, 1974). Proteinuria may be associated with an infectious process (cystitis, pyelitis) and should be further evaluated. A urine specimen contaminated with lochia may be the cause of proteinuria, so any specimen should be obtained as a midstream or a catheterized specimen. The preeclamptic patient may demonstrate proteinuria for a week or more following delivery.

In the absence of infection, the dilated ureters and renal pelvis will return to prepregnant size by the end of the fourth week.

Vital Signs

During the postpartal period, with the exception of the first 24 hours, the patient should be afebrile and normotensive. A temperature of 100.4F (38C) may occur following delivery as a result of the exertion and dehydration of labor. Infection must be considered in the patient with a temperature of 100.4F or above on any two of the first ten postpartal days sequentially, excluding the first 24 hours, if the temperature is taken at least four times per day.

Blood pressure readings should remain stable following delivery. A decrease may indicate physiologic readjustment to decreased intrapelvic pressure, or it may be related to uterine hemorrhage. Blood pressure elevations, especially when accompanied by headache, suggest preeclampsia, and the patient should be evaluated further.

Puerperal bradycardia with rates of 50–70 beats per minute commonly occurs during the first six to ten days of the postpartal period. It may be related to decreased cardiac strain, the decreased vascular bed following delivery, contraction of the uterus, and increased stroke volume. Tachycardia occurs less frequently and is related to increased blood loss or difficult, prolonged labor and delivery.

Blood Values

The blood values should return to the prepregnant state about one week postpartum. However, pregnancy-associated activation of coagulation factors may continue for variable amounts of time. This condition, in conjunction with trauma, immobility, or sepsis, predisposes the patient to development of thromboembolism. Plasma fibrinogen is maintained at pregnancy levels for a week, accounting for the higher sedimentation rate observed in the early postpartum period.

Other hemodynamic changes include leukocytosis with elevated white blood counts (WBC) of 15,000– 20,000, primarily due to an increased number of granulocytes. Eosinophils are rarely found, and lymphocytes may be reduced.

Blood loss averages 300–400 ml with a vaginal delivery and 700–1000 ml with cesarean section. Because rapid red blood cell destruction does not occur following delivery, the decrease in numbers occurs gradually according to their life span. Hemoglobin and erythrocyte values vary during the early puerperium, but they should approximate or exceed prelabor values within two to six weeks as normal concentrations are reached. As extracellular fluid is excreted, hemoconcentration occurs, with a concomitant rise in hematocrit. A drop in values indicates an abnormal blood loss. A convenient rule of thumb: A 4-point drop in hematocrit equals 1 pint of blood loss.

Weight Loss

An initial weight loss of 10–12 lb occurs as a result of the delivery of infant, placenta, and amniotic fluid. Puerperal diuresis accounts for the loss of an additional 5 lb during the early puerperium. By the sixth to eighth week following delivery, the patient has returned to approximately her prepregnant weight if the patient has gained the average 24–28 pounds.

Postpartal Chill

Frequently the mother experiences a shaking chill immediately following delivery, which is related to a nervous response or to vasomotor changes. If not followed by fever, it is clinically innocuous but uncomfortable to the patient. Many hospitals cover the patient with warmed bath blankets to alleviate the chill. The mother may also find a warm beverage helpful. Later in the puerperium, chills and fever indicate infection and require further evaluation.

Postpartal Diaphoresis

The elimination of excess fluid and waste products via the skin during the puerperium produces greatly increased perspiration. Diaphoretic episodes frequently occur at night, and the patient may awaken drenched with perspiration. The practice of covering the mattress with a protective plastic pad also contributes to the patient's discomfort. This perspiration is not significant clinically, but the mother should be protected from chilling. The plastic pad should be covered with both a pad and a sheet to decrease skin contact, and the bed linens and patient gown should be changed if diaphoresis occurs. Patient comfort is also enhanced with a daily shower.

Afterpains

Afterpains more commonly occur in multiparas than primiparas and are caused by intermittent uterine contractions. Although the uterus of the primipara usually remains consistently contracted, the lost tone of the multipara results in alternate contraction and relaxation. This phenomenon also occurs if the uterus has been markedly distended, as with multiple pregnancies or polyhydramnios, or if clots or placental fragments were retained. These afterpains may cause the mother severe discomfort for two to three days following delivery. The administration of oxytocic agents stimulates uterine contraction and increases the discomfort of the afterpains. Because oxytocin is released when the infant suckles, breast-feeding also increases the severity of the afterpains. The nursing mother may find it helpful to take a mild analgesic approximately one hour before feeding her infant. An analgesic is also helpful at bedtime if the afterpains interfere with the mother's rest.

POSTPARTAL NURSING MANAGEMENT

Comprehensive care is based on a thorough assessment, with identification of individual needs or potential problems.

Physical Assessment

Several principles should be remembered in preparing for and completing the assessment of the postpartal patient. First, as in any assessment, select the time that will provide the most accurate data. Palpating the fundus when the patient has a full bladder will not result in a true indication of involution, and assessing the condition of the episiotomy following a sitz bath may produce data that would indicate complications. Second, an explanation of the purpose of regular assessment should be given the patient. Third, the patient should be as relaxed as possible, and the procedures should be accomplished as gently and smoothly as possible to avoid unnecessary discomfort. Examining the patient who is experiencing afterpains only intensifies her pain, increases tension of muscles, and possibly necessitates medicinal relief. Finally, the data obtained during the assessment should be recorded and reported as clearly as possible.

A sample assessment form (Figure 27–2) has been included to assist the student nurse in organizing and charting the postpartal physical assessment. Staff nurses may want to devise a similar format as part of the patient's hospital chart in order to assure continuity and quality of care.

POSTPARTAL PHYSICAL ASSESSMENT

Student			Date
Patient	Postpartum Day	Breast Feeding	Bottle

VISUAL INSPECTION:

BREAST	RIGHT	LEFT
Size	small average large	small average large
(Bra cup size)	A B C or D	A B C or D
Shape	bell pendulous other (describe)	bell pendulous other (describe)
Tension	soft firm hard nodular caked	soft firm hard nodular caked
Skin	taut with striae no striae	taut with striae no striae
Color	same as color of body reddened	same as color of body reddened
Other (describe)		
AREOLA	**RIGHT**	**LEFT**
Size	small (size of quarter) average (size of half dollar) large (size of silver dollar)	small (size of quarter) average (size of half dollar) large (size of silver dollar)
Tension	soft engorged	soft engorged
NIPPLE	**RIGHT**	**LEFT**
	erect inverted caked flat clean	erect inverted caked flat clean
Tissue integrity	color even with protusions of mammary glands reddened, cracks/fissures, bleeding	color even with protusions of mammary glands reddened, cracks/fissures, bleeding
COLOSTRUM	**RIGHT**	**LEFT**
Amount	Nothing with expression with gentle expression lactating freely	Nothing with expression with gentle expression lactating freely
Color	bluish white cream dark yellow mixed	bluish white cream dark yellow mixed

MOTHER'S REPORT:

BREAST	RIGHT	LEFT
General feeling	tingling sensation of fullness backache painful	tingling sensation of fullness backache painful
NIPPLE	**RIGHT**	**LEFT**
Soreness	none since last nursing none during nursing none as baby goes to breast	none since last nursing none during nursing none as baby goes to breast

BREAST SUPPORT (Bra)

☐ Proper support includes shoulder straps not cutting; nonelastic straps; nipples elevated with breasts supported; no wrinkles in bra cup

☐ Poor support includes cutting into shoulders; constriction of thoracic cavity; nipples not elevated; breast overlapping bra cup; breast support depends on straps

Figure 27–2. Postpartal physical assessment.

1. DIASTASIS Rectus abdominis
   a. Length (cm) ______
   b. Width (cm) ______
2. FUNDUS
   a. Height in finger breadths in relationship to umbilicus ______
   b. Position ______
   c. Tenderness ______
      (1) with touch ______
      (2) constant ______
3. LOCHIA
   a. Amount ______
   b. Color ______
   c. Consistency ______
   d. Odor ______
4. PERINEUM
   a. Intact ______
   b. Episiotomy ______
      (1) type ______
      (2) healing ______
         (a) REEDA scale ______
   c. Hygiene ______
5. CVA TENDERNESS ______
6. HOMANS' SIGN ______
   a. Superficial varicosities ______
7. BOWEL AND BLADDER HABITS ______
8. SLEEP PATTERNS ______
9. MENTAL OUTLOOK ______
10. NUTRITIONAL INTAKE ______
11. ADJUSTMENT TO INFANT ______
12. EVALUATION ______

Nurses' notes would then concentrate on aspects of care: physical, such as the progression of involution and the establishment of lactation; maternal-infant bonding; parenting behaviors; and teaching activities and return demonstrations.

While the nurse is performing the physical assessment, she should also be teaching the patient. Assessing the breast provides an optimal time to discuss milk formation, the letdown reflex, and breast self-examination. Mothers are very receptive to instruction on postpartal abdominal tightening exercises when the nurse assesses the patient's fundal height and diastasis. The assessment also provides an excellent time to teach the body's physical and anatomical changes postpartally as well as danger signs to report.

Breasts

Beginning with the breasts, the nurse should first assess the fit and support provided by the bra. A properly fitting bra provides support to heavy breasts, thereby promoting maternal comfort. It also helps maintain the shape of the breasts by limiting undue stretching of connective tissue and ligaments. If the mother is breast-feeding, the straps of the bra should be cloth, not elastic, and they should be easily adjustable. The back should be wide and should have at least three rows of hooks to adjust for fit. Underwires are not necessary unless the breast is large (C cup or larger). Traditional nursing bras have a fixed inner cup and a separate half cup or flap that can be unhooked to allow for breast-feeding while continuing the support of the breast. Some companies have designed the nursing flap to open and close with a plastic snap rather than the traditional loop and hook. Some mothers find the snap much easier and quicker to operate.

Although one brand should not be recommended, several brands of bras can be purchased by the hospital and made available as demonstrators so the mother can compare the benefits of one bra against another before investing in a brand and finding out that she would have preferred another had she known about it. Some women prefer a standard bra that hooks in front, and if the breast is not heavy this is acceptable. It is wise for mothers to purchase a nursing bra with a cup one to two sizes too large. The breast increases in size with milk production, and a bra that fits well during pregnancy will be too tight during lactation.

Once the bra has been assessed, it should be removed so that the breasts may be examined. First, the nurse should note the size and shape of the breasts and any abnormalities, reddened areas, or engorgement. One breast is usually slightly larger than the other, which is most noticeable by observing the placement of the nipples. Next, the nurse should palpate the breasts lightly, checking for heat, edema, engorgement, and caking (swelling of the lobules due to a blockage of the duct), which usually begins in the upper outer quadrant. The mother should be asked whether she has any tenderness or pain, and if so, that area should be examined carefully. The nipples should be checked for fissures, cracks, soreness, and erectility. This check is done by placing the thumb and first finger on each side of the nipple and gently pulling the nipple out from the breast. When released, the nipple and areola should show some signs of erectility. The procedure may need to be performed several times before results are produced. Finally, an evaluation of milk production is achieved by manually expressing a small quantity of milk from the ducts behind the areola. To do this, the nurse should place the thumb and first finger at the edge of the areola, press slightly back toward the breast, and then gently squeeze the areola. Small beads of colostrum or milk will appear on the nipple. Colostrum can be distinguished from milk by its color and consistency; it appears ivory colored to dark yellow and has a creamy appearance. Milk, on the other hand, has a whitish to bluish white color and may look thin and watery. The nurse should wipe the nipples with a dry tissue.

The nursing mother needs to be reminded to keep the nipples supple, with the use of lanolin-based creams, and to keep them well cleansed, avoiding a buildup of secretions that could irritate the nipples. Perfumed lotions and creams should not be used because they can cause excessive drying of the tissues. Exposing the nipples to air is a technique that promotes healing and toughens them so that suckling by the infant is less irritating and painful.

The nonnursing mother should be assessed for evidence of breast discomfort. Medications such as Tace or Diatate are given to dry up the milk, but tenderness may still occur. The mother may alleviate this by wearing a well-fitting bra and by the judicious use of analgesics. Ice packs may also be used as needed. Heat and massage

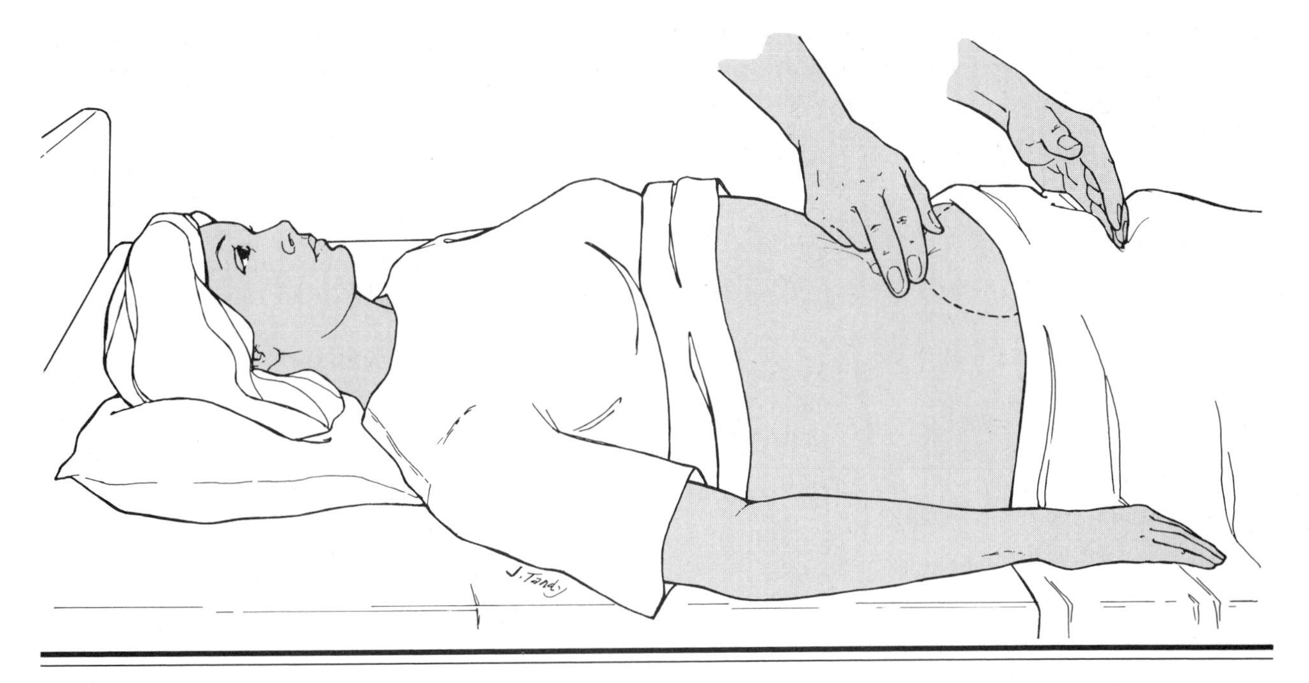

Figure 27–3. Measurement of descent of the fundus. The fundus is located two finger breadths below the umbilicus.

stimulate milk production and should be avoided. The mother may be encouraged to let the shower water flow over her back rather than her breasts.

Abdomen and Fundus

Prior to examination of the abdomen, the patient should void. This practice assures that a full bladder is not causing any uterine atony; if atony is present, other causes need to be investigated. The nurse should determine the relationship of the fundus to the umbilicus. Because of the relaxation of the abominal wall, the uterus is usually clearly outlined, except in the most obese of patients. The nurse should gently place one hand on the lower segment of the uterus to provide support and then place the first finger of her other hand on top of the fundus and should measure in finger breadths the relationship to the umbilicus. If the fundus is more than one finger breadth in either direction, she should place additional fingers on the abdomen (Figure 27–3). Fundal height is recorded in finger breadths: that is, "2 FB ↓ U; 1 FB ↑ U." Once fundal height has been assessed, the nurse should check whether the uterus is deviated from the midline and should then assess the tone of the uterus. Usually the nurse has already ascertained uterine tone when first palpating the fundus. If not, the fingers of the examining hand are placed gently on the fundus.

A well-contracted uterus feels as firm as the uterus does during a strong labor contraction. If handled gently, the uterus should not be tender. Excessive pain during postpartal examination should alert the nurse to possible genital tract infection. If the uterus is not firm, the nurse should gently massage the fundus with the fingertips of the examining hand, then assess the results. If the uterus becomes firm, the chart should read "Uterus: boggy → firm c̄ light massage." A good habit for the nurse to develop during the postpartal examination is to have the patient lie on her back with head comfortably elevated and legs relaxed. Then the nurse can release the peri-pad to observe the results of uterine massage based on the amount of expelled blood.

The boggy uterus that does not contract with light, gentle massage may need more vigorous massage. Be sure to assess the amount and character of any expelled blood obtained while massaging the fundus. The nursing care involved with a patient who has postpartal uterine atony is to:

1. Reevaluate for full bladder; if the bladder is full, have the patient void.
2. Question the patient on her bleeding history since delivery or last examination.
3. Put the baby to the mother's breast to stimulate oxytocin production.

4. Reassess the fundus; if the fundus is still boggy, alert the certified nurse-midwife or physician.

In the majority of patients the uterus will be firm; however, it is important to keep in mind the complications that cause postpartal uterine atony and the effect on the patient of a postpartal hemorrhage. The alert nurse will observe, assess, plan, and implement a care plan quickly.

Following the uterine assessment and prior to assessing the lochia, the nurse should examine the diastasis recti. In the event of diastasis of the rectus muscle, part of the abdominal wall has no muscular support but is formed by only skin, subcutaneous fat, attenuated fascia, and peritoneum (Pritchard and MacDonald, 1976). The separation in the rectus muscle is evaluated according to its length and width. The student nurse should use a tape measure that measures in centimeters; the skilled practitioner can accurately estimate the distance visually. (A disposable paper tape measure like the one used in the nursery for measuring babies is preferred.) The separation is palpated first just below the umbilicus, and the width is ascertained. Then the separation is palpated for length toward the symphysis pubis and toward the xiphoid process. If palpation is difficult due to abdominal relaxation, the patient is asked to lift her head unassisted by the nurse. This action contracts the rectus muscles and more clearly defines their edges.

Methods of charting these results vary from institution to institution. Some prefer recording the diastasis measured from the umbilicus down and then from the umbilicus up:

Diastasis: U ↓ 4 cm by 1 cm
U ↑ 2 cm by 1 cm

Others prefer recording the entire length:

Diastasis: 6 cm by 1 cm

Either method is acceptable.

Lochia

The next aspect to be evaluated is the lochia, which is assessed for character, amount, odor, and the presence of clotting. During the first one to three days the lochia should be dark red, similar in appearance to menstrual flow. Clotting is abnormal, and the cause should immediately be investigated. After two to three days, the lochia appears more pinkish or serous. As it is unusual to observe a patient during the full involutional period, the loss of all color in the lochia of the hospitalized patient should be suspected.

Lochia should never exceed a moderate amount, such as four to eight peri-pads daily, with an average of six. The patient should be questioned about the length of time the current pad has been in use, whether the amount is normal, and whether any clots were passed prior to this examination, such as during voiding. If heavy bleeding is reported but not seen, put a clean peri-pad on the patient and check the pad in one hour. If the patient needs to void before the hour is up, ask her to save the pad for your inspection. Usually the flow is moderate, but the patient, who is used to menstrual flow, may consider it heavy. If clots are reported but not seen, ask the patient to save all pads with clots or not to flush the toilet if clots were expelled during urination. Clots and heavy bleeding may be caused by uterine atony or retained placental fragments and require further assessment. Because of the manipulation of the uterine cavity during cesarean section, women with such surgery have less lochia after the first 24 hours than mothers who deliver vaginally. Often they need wear no pad. Therefore, amounts of lochia that would be normal in vaginally delivered women are suspect in women who have undergone cesarean section.

The odor of the lochia is nonoffensive and never foul. If odor is present, so is an infection.

The amount of lochia is charted first, followed by character. For example:

- Lochia: moderate amount rubra
- Lochia: small rubra/serosa
- Lochia: scant/serosa

Perineum

The perineum is observed with the patient lying in a Sims position, with the top leg positioned over the bottom leg. Either side is acceptable. The buttock is lifted to expose the perineum and anus (Figure 27–4). If the perineum has not been incised, it is charted as "Perineum: intact." If an episiotomy was performed or a laceration necessitated suturing, the wound is assessed. Davidson (1974) has developed a method of evaluating the episiotomy by identifying five components that indicate the state of healing. The REEDA method allows for a systematic evaluation of the episiot-

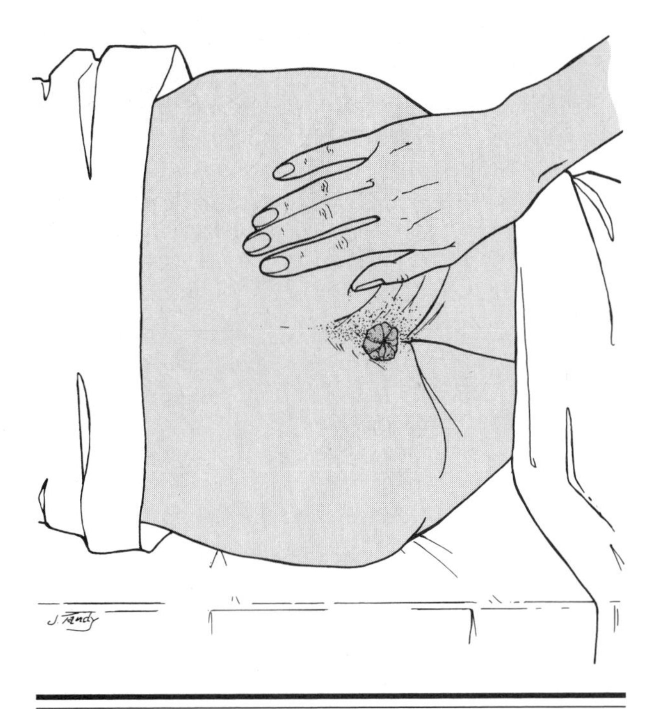

Figure 27–4. Intact perineum with hemorrhoids. Note how the examiner's hand raises the upper buttocks to fully expose the anal area.

omy for Redness, Edema, Ecchymosis, Discharge, and Approximation (see Table 29–1). For example, the incision should be approximated and nontender and may have some edema from the time it is repaired to 12 to 24 hours later. After 24 hours some edema may still be present, but the skin edges should be "glued" together so that gentle pressure does not separate them. Gentle palpation should elicit minimal tenderness, and there should be no hardened areas suggesting infection. These observations provide good evidence that the episiotomy/laceration is healing normally. Ecchymosis interferes with normal healing, as does infection.

The nurse should next assess the state of any hemorrhoids present around the anus for size, number, and pain or tenderness. Some examples of charting for this portion of the postpartal assessment:

- Perineum: intact, no hemorrhoids.
- Perineum: episiotomy—skin edges approximated, slight edema; two medium-sized nontender hemorrhoids.
- Perineum: laceration—nontender, nonedematous, healing well; three large, swollen, painful hemorrhoids.

In the patient delivered by cesarean section, the abdominal incision should be observed for any indications of infection. Foul odors associated with drainage from an abdominal or perineal incision indicate infection. Further observation of the incision for separation should also be made.

Thrombophlebitis

The incidence of thrombophlebitis is 1 in 2000 in pregnancy but rises 5 to 10 fold in the postpartal period (Barber and Graber, 1974). Mothers who are at increased risk in the postpartal period are those with dehydration, a traumatic delivery, postpartal hemorrhage, sepsis, and delivery by cesarean section and those who have received synthetic estrogens to suppress lactation (Barber and Graber, 1974).

If thrombophlebitis occurs, the most likely site will be in the patient's legs. To evaluate the patient, her legs should be stretched out straight and should be relaxed. The foot is then grasped and sharply dorsiflexed. No discomfort or pain should be present. If pain is elicited, the nurse-midwife or physician is notified that the patient has a positive Homans' sign. The pain is caused by inflammation of the vessel. The legs are also evaluated for edema. This may be done by comparing both legs, since usually only one leg is involved. Any areas of redness, tenderness, and increased skin temperature should also be noted. Early ambulation is an important aspect in the prevention of thrombophlebitis. Most women are able to be up shortly after delivery. The cesarean section patient requires passive range of motion exercises until she is ambulating more freely.

Vital Signs

Alterations in vital signs may be an indication of complications such as hemorrhage or infection. There may be a slight alteration in blood pressure as the blood volume peaks immediately after delivery, but this should not present significant problems for the patient. Conversely, there may be a drop in blood pressure as a result of blood loss.

The pulse rate during the immediate postpartal period may be low but presents no cause for alarm. Rates of 56 beats/min are not unusual as the body attempts to adapt to the decreased pressures intraabdominally as well as to the reduction of the vascular bed with the contraction of the uterus. Pulse rates return to prepregnant norms very quickly unless complications arise.

Temperature elevations may be a sign of infection but must be carefully evaluated. The normal process of wound healing, as well as dehydration and breast engorgement, may also increase body temperature. Temperature elevation from normal processes should last for only a few days and should not be associated with other clinical manifestations of infection.

There is an increased maternal risk for infections with the rise in invasive techniques for diagnosing and treating high-risk pregnancies, such as amniocentesis and fetal blood sampling. Gram-negative pathogens are becoming more prominent as causative agents for infection. They are not as familiar as gram-positive organisms, nor do they respond so effectively to the commonly used antibiotics. It is interesting to note that "less than 50 percent of patients who require systemic antibiotics for postpartal infection satisfied the temperature criteria for standard morbidity" in studies reported by Ledger (1974). It becomes essential to evaluate temperature elevations in light of other symptomatology as well as in a careful review of history to identify factors such as premature rupture of membranes or prolonged labor, which might increase the incidence of infections in the genital tract.

The remainder of the physiologic assessment usually consists of the patient's subjective complaints and answers to questions on sleep, mood, elimination, appetite, and comfort.

Psychologic Assessment

Adequate assessment of the mother's psychologic adjustment is an integral part of postpartal evaluation. This assessment focuses on the mother's general attitude, feelings of competence, available support systems, and caregiving skills. It also evaluates her fatigue level, sense of satisfaction, and ability to successfully accomplish her developmental tasks. See p. 922 for further discussion of emotional status of the postpartal patient.

Problem cues might include excessive fatigue, marked depression, excessive preoccupation with physical status and/or discomfort, evidence of low self-esteem, lack of support systems, marital problems, inability to care for or nurture the child, and current family crises (such as illness, unemployment, and so on). These characteristics frequently indicate a potential for maladaptive parenting, which may lead to child abuse or neglect (physical, emotional, intellectual) and cannot be ignored. Utilization of public health nurse referrals or other available community resources may provide greatly needed assistance and may alleviate potentially dangerous situations.

Interventions

The physical and psychologic assessment are used as a basis for identifying normal progress and evaluating problem areas. The plan of care is based on the following objectives:

1. Provision of comfort and relief of pain.
2. Promotion of rest and graded activity.
3. Promotion of psychologic well-being.
4. Education of parents.
5. Promotion of successful infant feeding.
6. Promotion of family wellness.
7. Promotion of parent-infant bonding and attachment.

Provision of Comfort and Relief of Pain

Pain may be present to varying degrees in the postpartal patient and may be of multiple origin. The perineum is often edematous after delivery. An episiotomy presents an additional source of pain. There may be lacerations or extensions that further traumatize the perineum and that may create sufficient pain to impede ambulation, elimination, or maintaining a comfortable position. Greater pain is manifested in patients with a mediolateral episiotomy, because muscles have been severed. Observations should be made for the development of hematomas, which account for pain and are also a source of blood loss not evident as overt bleeding. Patients may be taught to tighten their buttocks prior to sitting to avoid direct trauma to the perineum. Lateral positions may also be useful during the most painful period. Perineal care is given to promote comfort, to enhance healing, and to provide cleansing. Sitz baths are particularly useful with the severely traumatized perineum, as moist heat not only increases circulation to promote healing but also relaxes the tissue to promote comfort and decrease edema. Dry heat in the form of heat lamps may be used. The perineum should be cleansed prior to the use of the heat lamp to prevent drying of secretions on the perineum. Local heat applications (warm moist pads) are also soothing when hemorrhoids are present. Local anesthetics may be applied in different forms as well as astringents to decrease pain sensations and reduce swelling. Perineal care should be encouraged after each elimination to provide cleansing of the perineum and subsequently to promote comfort. Most agencies provide "peri-bottles," which the patients fills with warm water that is squirted over the perineum following elimination. The patient should be instructed to cleanse from front to back to prevent contamination of the vulva from the anal area. When toilet tissue is used the patient will be more comfortable if she uses a blotting motion. The patient should also be instructed to apply the perineal pad from front to back so as to prevent contamination from the anal area.

Afterpains are commonly experienced postpartum, particularly in the multiparous patient and the one who is breast-feeding. These cramplike contractions of the uterus are more severe during the first few days and may interfere with the establishment of an early positive mother-child relationship. If nursing personnel are able to anticipate needs and to administer medications before the pain is excessive, greater comfort will be provided to the patient. A breast-feeding mother may experience increased discomfort with breast-feeding due to the release of oxytocin and its subsequent effect of increasing uterine contractions. If she is experiencing afterpains an hour before feeding, administration of an analgesic will promote comfort during the feeding and enhance the mother-infant interaction.

Some mothers experience hemorrhoidal pain following delivery. Relief measures include the use of sitz baths two to three times per day; ointments, rectal suppositories, or witch hazel pads applied directly to the anal area may also provide comfort. The mother should be encouraged to maintain an adequate fluid intake, and stool softeners or laxatives should be administered to insure greater comfort with bowel movements. The hemorrhoids usually disappear a few weeks after delivery if the mother did not have them prior to this pregnancy.

Nurses should be alert to both nonverbal as well as verbal manifestations of pain and should intervene with appropriate measures. The physical response to pain may be influenced by the patient's possible lack of acceptance of the pregnancy and new baby, or other situational crises, which trigger psychologic crises that will ultimately affect the family's adjustment. The first alternative to pain relief may not necessarily be medication; frequently, changing positions or encouraging the patient to ventilate her feelings in an atmosphere of acceptance may be sufficient to promote relaxation. Drugs should be available if other measures fail. (See the Nursing Care Plan on the postpartal period.)

NURSING CARE PLAN

Postpartal Period

Patient Data Base

History

1. Delivery information
   a. Gravida, para
   b. Date and time of delivery
   c. Anesthesia and analgesia
   d. Course of labor and delivery
2. Support people available (such as father)
3. Parenting information or beliefs
4. Condition of infant

Physical examination

Uterus – firm and in the midline

Cervix – healing as evidenced by lochia

Perineum – note presence of episiotomy or lacerations and evaluate for healing

Rectum – may have hemorrhoids

Abdomen – muscles stretched, may have striae on skin

Breast – soft, nipple erect, no reddening of tissues, colostrum with gentle expression, no nipple soreness, utilization of proper supporting bra

Pulse – may be slowed to 56 beats/min

NURSING CARE PLAN Cont'd
Postpartal Period

Blood pressure – minimal fluctuation from admission

Temperature – may rise to 38C (100.4F) during first 24 hours postpartum

Weight – may have loss of 10 lb

Laboratory evaluation

Second day

Hemoglobin – not more than 2 mg less than admission

Hematocrit – drop less than 3% from admission

Urine – presence of red blood cells is considered normal; no glucose; specific gravity 1.020; no bacteria

Nursing Priorities

1. Restore body to approximately nonpregnant state with minimal complications.
2. Establish successful infant feeding patterns, whether breast-fed or bottle-fed.
3. Develop a healthy family-child relationship with total integration of the newly born into family unit.
4. Provide patient education, including all aspects of self-care, infant care, maternal-child bonding, integration of newborn into family, and continued medical supervision for mother and child.

Problem	Nursing interventions and actions	Rationale
Delayed involution	Observe, record, and report involution process, including: 1. Evaluation of fundus daily for height, position, and consistency. 2. Observation of lochia for color, amount, odor.	Involution is monitored to evaluate process of healing in female reproductive system following delivery of fetus.
Perineal trauma	Promote healing of perineum by: 1. Assessing episiotomy for REEDA. 2. Local application of heat. 3. Teaching proper perineal care. 4. Monitoring vital signs. Pulse may be as low as 56/min (normal); blood pressure should have minimal fluctuation; temperature may rise to 38C (100.4F) in first 24 hr but should not be elevated after that. Continued temperature elevation may represent presence of infection.	Perineum is traumatized during birth from stretching by baby's head, cutting during episiotomy, or tearing during delivery. Application of heat promotes healing through increase of circulation. Perineal area should always be cleaned from front to back or from clean to dirty area. Vital sign variations alert professional staff to possible presence of complications.
Pain	Complete physical assessment will identify factors/conditions that may cause pain. Implement specific comfort measures, including: 1. Episiotomy: a. Sitz bath. b. Perineal light. c. Spray such as Dermaplast. 2. Hemorrhoids: a. Sitz bath. b. Tucks or ointment. c. Stool softeners to prevent constipation.	Pain may be present in varying degrees and may be multiple in origin. Pain is increased by exhaustion, and by emotional factors such as acceptance of pregnancy and of new baby. Pain may interfere with establishment of early mother-child relationship.
	3. Afterpains: a. Administer analgesics. b. May administer analgesics to nursing mothers 1 hr before feeding to facilitate mother's comfort.	Infant suckling at breast stimulates release of oxytocin, which in turn stimulates uterine contractions resulting in afterpains.

NURSING CARE PLAN Cont'd

Postpartal Period

Problem	Nursing interventions and actions	Rationale
	4. Cesarean section: a. Ambulation. b. Position changes. c. Analgesics. 5. Breast engorgement (breast-feeding mother): a. Increase frequency of feedings. b. Warm compresses. c. Manual expression of milk. d. Supportive brassiere. e. Ointments and exposure to air for cracked nipples. 6. Breast engorgement (non-breast-feeding mothers): a. Medication to suppress lactation (such as Diatate, Tace). b. Supportive brassiere. c. Avoid stimulation of breast. d. Cool compresses. e. Do not express milk manually. f. Keep fluid intake minimal for 24-48 hr after engorgement.	Cesarean-section patients may have additional pain due to interference of greater number of nerve endings. Also, manipulation of abdominal contents and anesthesia lead to decreased intestinal motility. Exaggeration of normal venous and lymphatic secretions produces distended, full, firm breasts. Breast engorgement in non-breast-feeding mothers inhibits letdown reflex.
Difficulty in elimination	Encourage voiding every 6-8 hr. Monitor intake and output until complete bladder emptying is established. Create positive attitude that enhances relaxation of patient through: 1. Teaching. 2. Assisting patient to bathroom if possible. 3. Pouring warm water over perineum. 4. Leaving faucet running (sound of running water is suggestive). Evaluate bladder for distention. Encourage increased intake of fluids. Catheterize if absolutely necessary. Assist patient in establishing normal bowel pattern by: 1. Encouraging ambulation and fluids. 2. Providing fresh fruit and roughage in diet. 3. Administering stool softeners as indicated. 4. Administering enema if necessary.	Close proximity of urethra to birth canal results in increased trauma during delivery. Pressure of larger uterus before delivery causes changes in position and capacity of bladder. Medications given at delivery cause decreased sensation of bladder filling. Development of diuresis postpartally causes bladder to fill more quickly. Stasis leads to increased risk of urinary tract infection. Full bladder increases tendency of uterus to relax by displacing uterus and interfering with its contractility, which leads to hemorrhage. Bowel is sluggish due to decreased peristalsis. Rectal soreness, episiotomy, extensions, and hemorrhoids create difficulty with bowel elimination. Patient may anticipate painful elimination and tense up. Cleansing enema during labor and omission of solid foods may add to elimination problem. Constipation increases pressure on sutures and increases discomfort.
Fatigability	Evaluate individual rest needs. Encourage rest by organizing activities to avoid frequent interruptions. Provide rest periods prior to feeding times. If mother is rooming-in, encourage mother to rest while her baby sleeps, which is an activity she may continue at home. Initiate activities gradually with frequent rest periods. Patient may become overzealous in an exercise regimen if she is concerned about her protruding abdomen.	Physical exertion during labor may leave patient exhausted. Level of physical fatigue often influences many adjustments and functions of new mother. For example, milk flow may be reduced, increasing problems with establishing breast-feeding. Energy is required in order to make psychologic adjustments to new baby and to assume new roles. Adjustments to unknown and unexpected are most smoothly accomplished when adequate rest is obtained.

NURSING CARE PLAN Cont'd

Postpartal Period

Problem	Nursing interventions and actions	Rationale
	Have patient do the following several times a day for 5 min at a time: 1. Perineal tightening. 2. Head raising and placing chin on chest. 3. Pelvic rocking to strengthen muscles in lower back and abdomen. 4. Leg raises. 5. Defer sit-ups for approximately 2 weeks. Teach patient to reevaluate her activity and to make necessary alterations if she has an increase in lochia or pain.	
Infection	Observe, record, and report signs and symptoms of infection, including: 1. Fever. 2. Foul-smelling lochia. 3. Separation, edema, discharge, poor healing of episiotomy. 4. Urinary urgency, frequency, pain. 5. Abnormal pain in abdomen, legs, etc. Implement treatments as prescribed. Document effectiveness of care.	See discussion of specific infections in Chapter 29.
Assimilation of new roles and tasks	Assess learning needs of patient/family and readiness to learn. Utilize demonstration and allow opportunity for return demonstration. Suggested areas of teaching: infant feeding, burping, diapering, bathing, safety; mother's hygiene needs, care of breasts, activity, exercises, parenting skills, nutrition. Support mother as she takes on mothering role; time teaching to her ability to accept new information.	All postpartal patients have teaching needs (some for new information, some for review or reordering). During teaching, emphasize principles rather than encouraging mimicking of demonstrated techniques.

Nursing Care Evaluation

Infection is absent in episiotomy (incision) site.

Infant feeding techniques are established.

Mother can care for herself and implement postpartal exercises.

Mother-infant and father-infant bonding process is established.

Parents understand infant care techniques and can demonstrate knowledge of infant care, feeding, bathing, safety, cord care, circumcision care, and continued medical supervision (including immunization schedule).

The patient who has delivered by cesarean section may experience additional pain caused by the interference of greater nerve endings. Because of the manipulation of abdominal contents, this patient experiences the discomfort of flatus, which may be relieved with ambulation. Discomfort may also be caused by immobility, because the patient who has been in stirrups for any length of time may experience muscular aches from such extreme positioning. It is not unusual for women to complain of joint pains and muscular pain in both arms and legs, depending on the effort they exerted during the second stage of labor.

Breast engorgement may be a source of severe pain for the postpartal patient. Around the time their milk initially comes in, many mothers complain of feelings of engorgement. Their breasts are hard, painful, and warm and may appear taut and shiny. Contrary to popular belief, this is caused by venous congestion, not by excessive milk retention. Because the breast is quite hard, nursing may be difficult for the infant and painful for the mother. Manual expression of milk or the use of a breast pump to initiate the flow may be helpful, as is the judicious use of analgesics. Warmth is often quite soothing, and the mother who has problems with engorgement may find a warm shower very comforting. In order to prevent excessive stimulation, it is advisable to avoid having the spray beat directly on the nipples and breasts. Warm, moist cloths may also be used for relief. Additional relief measures include the use of ice packs between feedings, with hot packs applied 20 minutes prior to a feeding. The engorgement is generally relieved within 12 to 24 hours.

Personal hygiene actions during the postpartal period are essential in promoting comfort. Because diaphoresis is an expected occurrence as the body attempts to dispose of the extra fluids retained during pregnancy, a daily shower is very refreshing for the patient. The patient may become dizzy when she first sits up and should be closely supervised during her initial shower. Patients who have remained NPO (having nothing by mouth) for any length of time require mouth care. Assisting the patient with these basic needs makes her more comfortable. During the puerperium the patient is frequently thirsty as she recovers from delivery and experiences postpartal diuresis. The patient should have a filled pitcher of cold water within reach and should be offered milk and fruit juice frequently.

Early ambulation should be encouraged postpartally. Studies have demonstrated the benefit of activity not only in promoting psychologic wellbeing but also in reducing the incidence of complications such as constipation and thrombus formation. Assistance may be required immediately postpartum, with alterations in equilibrium from fatigue or drugs being common.

Promotion of Rest and Graded Activity

The physical exertion experienced during labor and delivery leaves the patient exhausted and in need of rest. The patient who has participated in the delivery process may be euphoric and full of psychic energy immediately after delivery, ready to relive the experience of birth repeatedly with whoever will listen. Essential nursing activities must be done frequently in order to adequately assess the patient's condition; however, they may create an environment of constant activity, making rest a luxury and not a routine in most maternity units. Rather than being totally frustrated by these circumstances, the nurse must be astute in evaluating individual needs, always with the goal of providing opportunities for rest during hospitalization. If rest is achieved while in the hospital, there is a greater likelihood that the patient will arrange such opportunities at home, adjusting her schedule to meet this important need. For the excited, euphoric patient, the nurse may allow a period for airing of feelings, then insist on a period of rest.

Physical fatigue often influences many other adjustments and functions with the new mother, such as reduction of milk flow, thereby increasing problems with establishing breast-feeding. Energy is required in order to make the psychologic adjustments to a new baby and to assume new roles. Many women are not able to anticipate their behavior and are often surprised at their response to the birth process. Adjustments to the unknown and unexpected are most smoothly accomplished when adequate rest is obtained.

The nurse may encourage rest by organizing her activities to avoid frequent interruptions for the patient. Rest times should be provided prior to encounters with the baby if rooming-in is not utilized. If it is, the mother should be encouraged to rest as the baby sleeps, which is an activity she may continue at home.

Activities should be initiated gradually, with frequent periods of rest. Many of the activities will be initiated in the form of postpartal exercises to improve muscle tone. Often women are so concerned with their protruding abdomen that they become overzealous in an exercise regimen. The patient should be encouraged to begin with simple exercises while in the hospital and to repeat them several times a day for approximately five-minute intervals. These exercises include perineal tightening, head raising, placing the chin on the chest, and pelvic rocking to strengthen muscles in the low back and abdomen. Leg raises may be initiated next, with sit-ups delayed for approximately two weeks. With the appearance of increased lochia or pain, the patient should be encouraged to reevaluate her activity and to make necessary alterations.

Promotion of Maternal Psychologic Well-being

The birth of a child, with the changes in role and the increased responsibilities it produces, is a time of emotional stress for the new mother. This stress is increased because tremendous physiologic changes are transpiring as her body adjusts to a nonpregnant state. During the early postpartal days the mother is emotional, labile. Mood swings are common, and she may become tearful at the slightest provocation.

During the early postpartal days, the mother may repeatedly discuss her experiences of labor and delivery. This review seems necessary to assist the mother in integrating her experiences in order to adjust to her new role. If, in her opinion, she did not cope well with labor and delivery, she may have feelings of inadequacy to work through. Reassurance from the nurse that she did well is frequently very helpful. However, this reassurance is effective only if the nurse has established a warm, supportive relationship with the mother. In addition, the mother must adjust to the loss of her fantasized child in order to deal effectively with the child she has borne. This may be more difficult if the infant is not of the desired sex or if he exhibits birth defects. Follow-up visits from the nurse who assisted her in labor and delivery provide additional opportunities for the mother to relive her experiences and to come to terms with them.

Two major stages of emotional adjustment occur in the puerperium. These stages represent a reversal of the inward focusing that characterized labor. During that time the mother's energies focused increasingly inward as she drew on her personal strength to cope with the stress of labor. In the postpartal period, the focus turns outward from herself to her child, husband, other family members, and then to those in the immediate environment. Slowly she resumes her normal role and functions and also accepts the new ones resulting from the birth of her child.

Rubin (1961) describes the first period of adjustment as the *taking-in phase.* This period, lasting two to three days, is marked by maternal passivity and dependence. The mother follows suggestions, is hesitant about making decisions, and is still somewhat preoccupied with her own needs. Food and sleep are a major focus for her. Mealtime is eagerly awaited and food-related dicussions are common with the mothers. During this phase the new mother is talkative but passive.

The *taking-hold phase* begins on about the second or third day following delivery. The mother has had time to relive her experiences, to adjust to her new life, to rest, and to recover from childbirth. Now she is ready to resume control of her life. Initially this phase involves control of her bodily functions. She is concerned about bowel and bladder elimination. If she is breast-feeding, she may be concerned about the quality of her milk and her ability to successfully nurse her child. She requires constant reassurance that she is performing well. This desire to succeed is also apparent in concerns about her ability to be a "good" mother. If the baby is sleepy during a feeding or spits up, the mother may view this occurrence as a personal failure. The nurse who is extremely proficient in handling the child reinforces these feelings of inadequacy, which can be exhausting and demoralizing for the mother. Skillful intervention by the nurse, with constant reassurance that she is a successful mother, is vital. During this time the mother is most receptive to teaching, and tactful instruction and demonstration assist her in mothering effectively. The nurse must carefully avoid "taking over" the infant. By functioning as an adviser and allowing the mother to perform the actual care, the nurse demonstrates her confidence in the mother's skill and ability, which in turn increases the mother's self-confidence about her effectiveness as a parent.

The "postpartum blues" are a transient period of depression occurring during the puerperium. It may be manifested by anorexia, tearfulness, difficulty in sleeping, and a "letdown" feeling. This depression frequently occurs during hospitalization, although it may occur at home, too. Ego adjustment and hormonal changes are both thought to be causal factors, although fatigue, discomfort, stimulation overload, or stimulation deprivation may also play a part. The mother requires reassurance that these feelings are normal and an explanation as to why they occur. A therapeutic environment that permits the mother to cry without feelings of guilt is vital. Her privacy should be protected. The nurse should also indicate her interest if the mother feels a need to talk. In rare instances initial depression leads to a pathologic condition known as postpartum psychosis (see Chapter 29).

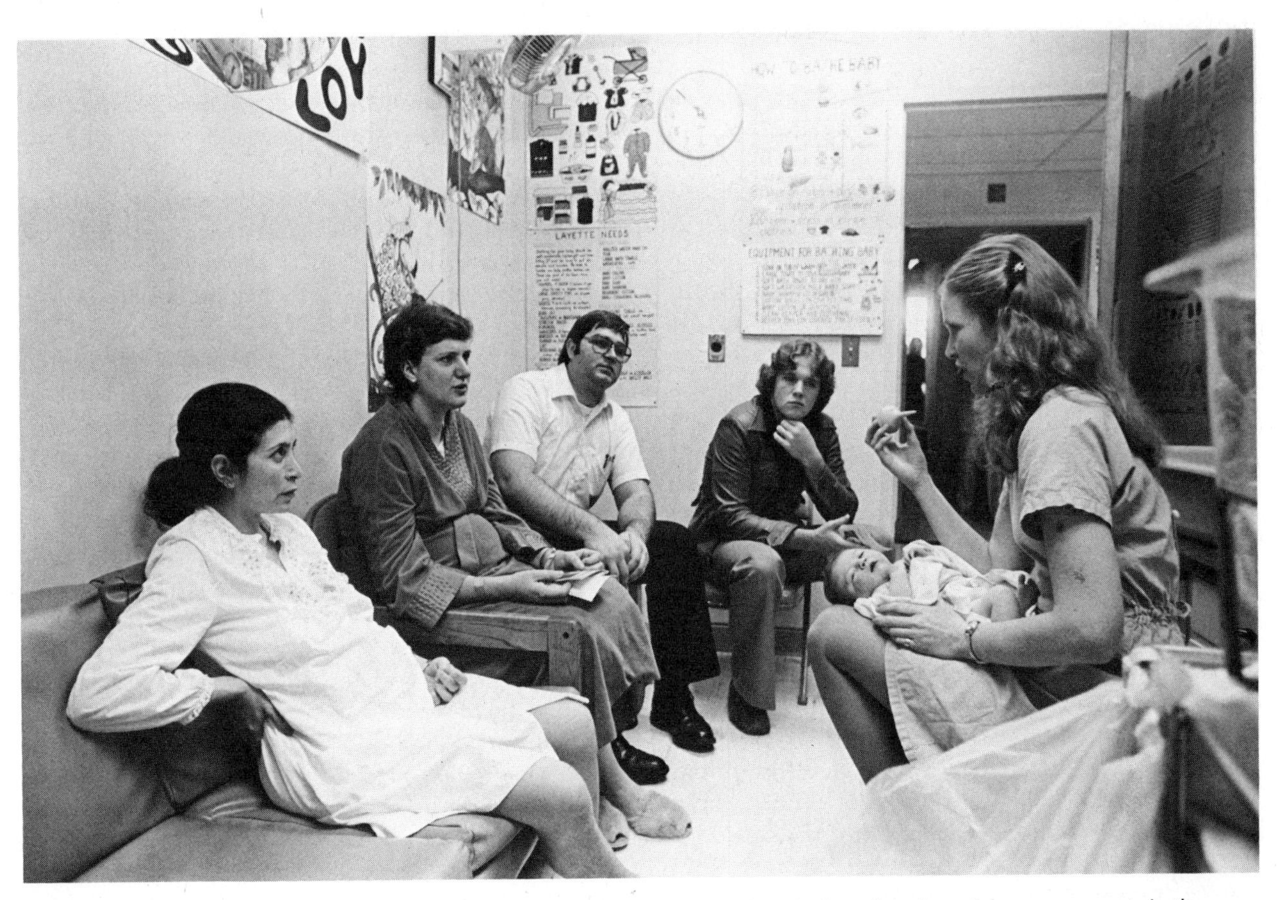

Figure 27–5. One of the most important postpartal nursing responsibilities is the education of the new parents in the care of their baby.

Education of Parents

All postpartal patients have education needs, whether they are primiparas who are unfamiliar with physiologic changes, feeding techniques, and infant care or are multiparas who need reinforcement of previous knowledge or suggestions about how to deal with sibling rivalry (Figure 27–5).

Techniques for teaching an adult learner and for assessing the new mother's stage of restoration must be taken into consideration. Both factors influence the individual's response to teaching and her retention of knowledge. The nurse should tailor her techniques to the family members who are present for the sessions. The nurse's primary responsibilities with younger children are to answer questions and to describe characteristics of the newborn that influence handling and basic needs fulfillment.

Emphasizing principles rather than encouraging mimicking of demonstrated techniques is most useful. The nurse may utilize demonstration as a form of transmitting information, but she should provide for return demonstrations to evaluate understanding of the instructions. It is often better to have the individual complete the task or procedure, such as infant bathing, while the nurse offers suggestions or reinforces principles, including supporting the infant's head, cleansing the genitals from front to back, bathing from clean to dirty areas with warm water, and preventing exposure of the infant that will reduce body temperature. This way, the nurse does not impose her methods on the couple and allows for their individual approach. The nurse should remember to praise the couple's effort, reminding them that they and the baby will learn together and that techniques may vary as long as principles of care are carried through.

Rubin (1961) has provided useful information in identifying maternal behavior during the phases of restoration. This information must also be considered when initiating teaching with the new mother. During the taking-in phase, the patient is concerned with body functions, is attempting to incorporate the experience of birth, and is more oriented to instructions in self-care. If the nurse proceeds with instructions on infant bathing, diapering, and cord or circumcision care during this time, they will only have to be repeated when the mother reaches the taking-hold phase and assumes more responsibility for her own care as well as care of the baby. Repetition may be required, but by assessing the stage of restoration and integrating this information into the teaching plan, the nurse better utilizes the time she has with the parents.

Various types of media may be effectively utilized with the new family, with the content geared to the educational levels of family members. Whatever methods are employed, the nurse should provide for follow-up to continuously evaluate areas needing clarification or additional information.

In preparation for discharge, the nurse may provide anticipatory guidance in helping the family cope with the realities of a new baby. The imposition on individuals' time and the added responsibilities that require strength and energy and that may alter the perceived role for the individual need to be anticipated. If the family is aware of the possible behaviors and their origin, they are better able to cope and are less likely to evaluate expected occurrences as abnormal. Consultation also provides an opportunity to develop sensitivities to new modes of communication, which are often required among family members.

Promotion of Successful Infant Feeding

Although the selection of the method for feeding should have been determined during pregnancy for optimal preparation, some attempt should be made during the postpartal period to assess reaction of the family to the particular method chosen. Observations made during the first feeding encounter may give useful data regarding feelings. If the father is not present, or if the mother experienced a difficult labor or a delivery by cesarean section, the situation must be carefully evaluated. The inability to select between breast- and bottle-feeding, or the "I think I'll try . . ." response, may provide more reliable information as to the mother's true feelings regarding the method selected. The nurse's primary responsibility is to support the decision and to assist the family to achieve a positive result, regardless of the feeding method utilized. No woman should be made to feel inadequate or superior because of her choice in infant feeding. There are advantages and disadvantages to breast- and bottle-feeding, but positive bonds in parent-child relationships may be developed with either method.

The nurse should determine what preparations for feeding have been made during the pregnancy. With this information, she may adapt her teaching methods to incorporate or to reinforce the unapplied knowledge during the initial feeding experiences. Teaching tapes and parent classes may be useful in meeting this goal. Any new instructions or techniques should be given with consideration for physicians' directions to parents and should be coordinated so that the family is not confused by conflicting information.

Parenting is a learned behavior, not one acquired instinctively. As an expression of personality, the response of the infant to caring is important. Early behavior of the infant may be internalized as rejection, which may alter the progress of parent-child relationships. A parent may interpret the sleepy baby's refusal to suck or inability to retain formula as evidence of his or her incompetence as a parent. Likewise, the breast-feeding mother may deduce that the baby does not like her if he fails to take her nipple readily. Conversely, infants pick up messages from the muscular tension of those holding them. Therefore, the early feeding periods should be learning experiences for the family, and the nurse should be present to provide information or to give positive feedback and reassurance as the techniques for parenting are developed.

Immediately prior to the feeding, the mother should be made as comfortable as possible. Preparations may include voiding, washing her hands, assuming a position of comfort, or arranging the environment so that privacy is maintained while assistance is readily available. The breast-feeding mother is encouraged to experiment with different positions to find the best position for her and the baby, whether it is lying on her side or sitting upright. The cesarean section mother may need support so that the baby does not rest on her abdomen for long periods of time. Providing for comfort contributes to the success of the feeding.

Depending on the infant's level of hunger, the parents may want to use the time prior to the feeding to get acquainted with the baby. For the sleepy baby, this period of playful activity may increase his alertness so that, when the feeding is initiated, the baby is ready and eagerly sucks. It may allow the active baby an opportunity to calm down so that he can find and grasp the nipple effectively. Following the feeding, when the baby is satisfied and asleep, parents may explore the characteristics unique to their baby. Hospital routines must be flexible enough to allow this time for the family. Rooming-in offers spontaneous, frequent encounters for the family and provides opportunities to practice skills of handling, thereby increasing confidence in care after discharge. It may also allow for demand rather than scheduled feeding times, which should be encouraged.

Bottle-feeding

For the bottle-feeder, it is necessary to remember several important principles:

1. Bottles should always be held, not propped. Positional otitis media may develop when the infant is fed horizontally, because milk and nasal mucus may occlude the eustachian tube. Holding the baby provides a rest for the feeder, social and close physical contact for the baby, and an opportunity for parent-child interaction and bonding. Once feeding is initiated, the child should be held close to provide physical closeness and to facilitate eye contact (Figure 27–6).

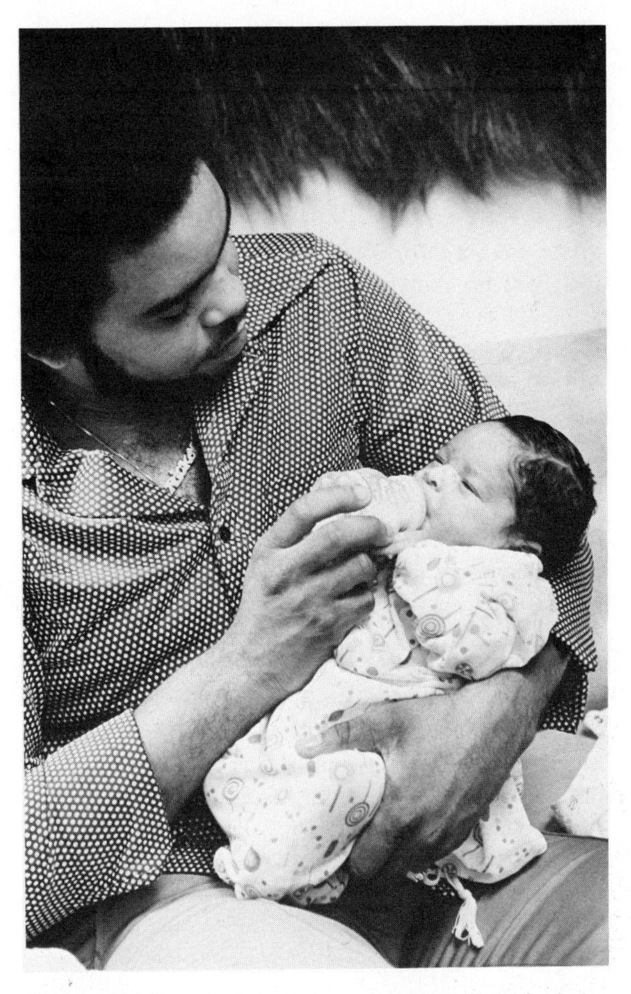

Figure 27–6. An infant is supported comfortably during bottle-feeding.

2. The nipple should have a hole big enough to allow milk to flow in drops when the bottle is inverted. Too large an opening may cause overfeeding or regurgitation because of too-fast feeding. If feeding is too fast, the nipple should be changed and the infant should be helped to eat more slowly by stopping the feeding frequently for burping and cuddling.

3. The nipple should be pointed directly into the mouth, not toward the palate or tongue, and should be on top of the tongue. This position creates greater suction and a more controlled flow of milk. The nipple should be full of liquid at all times to avoid ingestion of extra amounts of air, which decreases the amount of feeding and increases discomfort.

4. The infant should be burped at intervals, preferably at the middle and end of the feeding. Burping is done by holding the infant upright and by gently massaging or patting his back. Too-frequent burping confuses the baby as he attempts to learn to coordinate sucking, swallowing, and breathing simultaneously.

5. A fat baby is not necessarily a healthy one. Avoid overfeeding or feeding the baby every time he cries. The infant should be encouraged but not forced to feed and should be allowed to set his pace once feedings are established. Research suggests that mothers tend to set artificial goals—"The baby must take all five ounces"—and tend to

work with the child until he meets those goals, even though he may not be hungry. Overfeeding results in infant obesity. During early feedings, however, the infant may need simple tactile stimulation—such as gently rubbing feet and hands, adjusting clothing, and loosening coverings to expose him to room air—in order to maintain adequate sucking for a sufficient time to complete a full feeding.

Formula preparation and sterilization techniques are always important to discuss with families. Professional personnel frequently spend time describing detailed procedures that are time-consuming, that are not followed at home, and that are not necessary because of the milk processing required by law. However, cleanliness remains an essential component. Bottles may be effectively prepared in dishwashers (nipples may be weakened by the temperature of dishwashers and therefore should be washed thoroughly by hand with soap and water and rinsed well). Tap water, if from an uncontaminated source, may be used for mixing powdered formulas, which are less expensive than the concentrated or ready-to-use prepared formulas. Whole or evaporated milk may be diluted with water and sweetened with a sugar source such as corn syrup, depending on the age of the infant and his caloric requirements. If the water source is questionable, the terminal heat method of sterilization or single-bottle method of preparation should be used. If more than one bottle is prepared at a time, they should be stored in the refrigerator and warmed slightly before feeding.

Breast-feeding

The baby who is breast-feeding should be put to breast as soon as possible, depending on the situation of birth and on the amount of drugs required. Some infants are not interested so soon, but for those who are, breast-feeding affords a soothing experience and has considerable physiologic and psychologic benefit for the mother. Colostrum, available since the fourth month of pregnancy, has sufficient nutrients (as well as providing immunoglobulins) to satisfy the infant until milk is established in two to four days. Establishment of lactation depends on the strength of the infant's suck and the frequency of nursing. The principles involved in breast-feeding are (a) to provide adequate nutrition (b) to establish an adequate milk supply, and (c) to prevent trauma to the nipples. All instructions are aimed toward these goals.

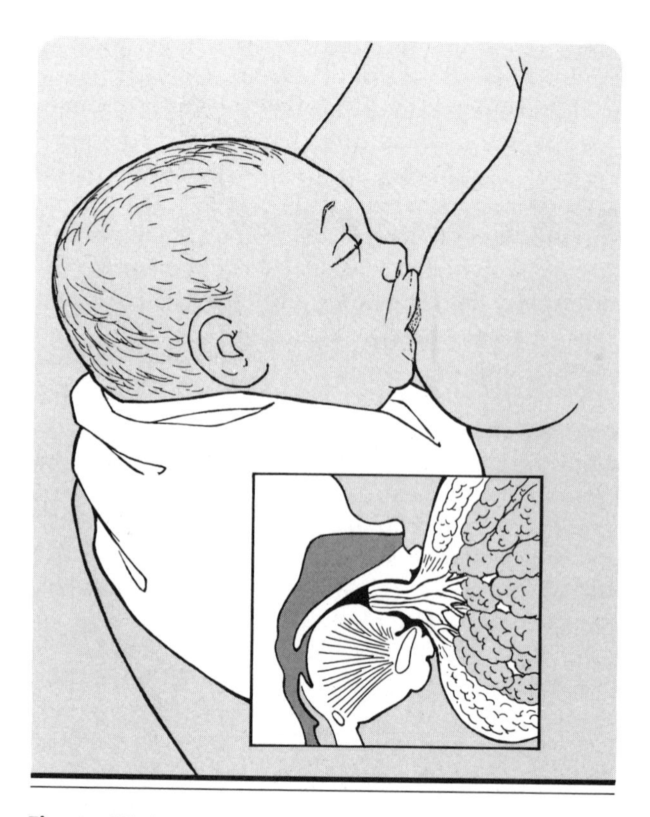

Figure 27–7. To nurse effectively, it is important that the infant's mouth covers the majority of the areola to compress the ducts below. (Courtesy Ross Laboratories, Columbus, Ohio.)

Positioning of the baby at the breast is a critical factor. The entire body of the infant should be turned toward the mother's breast, with his mouth adjacent to the nipple. The mother should not have to lift her shoulder or breast to direct the nipple into the infant's mouth. The nipple should be directed straight into the mouth, not toward the palate or tongue, and as much of the areola as possible should be included so that, as the baby sucks, his jaws compress the ducts that are directly beneath the areola (Figure 27–7). To do this the mother places her index finger above the nipple and her middle finger below. She then compresses the areolar area and guides the nipple into the infant's mouth. Through the rooting reflex, the infant can locate the nipple. Avoid stimulation of both cheeks, which only confuses the hungry infant.

If the mother does not have a prominent or everted nipple, she may try rolling the nipple between her thumb and forefinger or stretching the nipple by pressing in and outward around the nipple prior to the feeding. Nurses should avoid the temptation to substitute a nipple shield to correct nipple positions. The shield tends to confuse the baby, as artificial nipples are softer and easier to feed from, and the baby may refuse the human nipple when it is reoffered. Following feedings, the nipples should be assessed for trauma so that corrections may be made in position and technique for the next feeding.

The mother will find that the beginning of the feeding, when the baby has his most active sucking reflex, is the most uncomfortable, but this situation should subside when the nipples become tougher and more resilient. The length of time at the breast also has a significant influence on trauma and degree of comfort. Initially it is less traumatic for the mother to nurse more frequently than for long periods at one time. Often the mother is reluctant to terminate the feeding if the infant is sucking well, but if she allows the infant to suck as long as he wants to, by the time her milk is established she will be too uncomfortable to tolerate the initial sucking of the infant. Nipple soreness may also be decreased by encouraging the mother to rotate positions when feeding the infant. Because the area of greatest stress to the nipple is in line with the baby's chin and nose, the alternating use of the cradle hold, football hold, and maternal-sidelying position rotates the focus of greatest stress and promotes more complete breast emptying (Dutton, 1979).

Breasts should be alternated at each feeding, beginning with five minutes on each side and progressing to seven to ten minutes by the third or fourth day and ultimately to ten minutes on each side. A convenient way for the mother to remember which breast to use is to fasten a small safety pin to the bra cup on that side. The infant will empty the breasts during this time, and any additional time may meet an oral need for the baby but may also cause increased breast trauma. Once feedings are established, length of nursing time on the second breast may be extended to meet this oral need, because the sucking reflex will not be so strong once the infant is partially satisfied with nourishment from the first breast. While the infant is nursing, the mother should press the breast away from the infant's nares to prevent obstruction of his nasal passageway, thus allowing him to breathe (Figure 27–8).

The mother should be instructed in techniques for breaking suction prior to removing the infant from the breast. By inserting a finger into the infant's mouth beside the nipple, she can break the suction, and the nipple may be removed without trauma. Burping between feedings on each breast and at the end of the feeding continues to be necessary. If the infant has been crying, it is also advisable to burp him prior to beginning feeding.

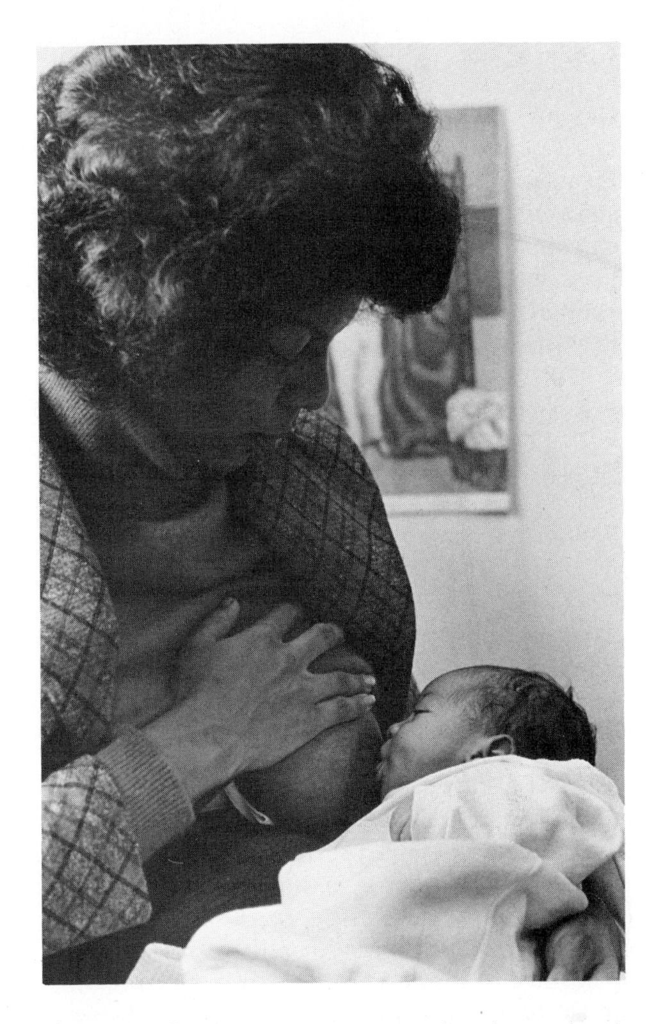

Figure 27–8. Breast-feeding. Note that the mother is holding her breast away from the baby's nostrils so that breathing is not obstructed.

Initially more milk is produced than is required by the infant (see Chapter 23). Later the amount of milk will be produced to meet his nutritional need, manifested through sucking. Milk may tend to leak until supply meets demand, and the mother should expect this, utilizing breast pads in her bra to absorb the secretions. She should be cautioned to remove wet pads frequently to avoid irritation to the nipples or the possibility of infection. The mother may also be taught to apply direct pressure to the breast with her hand or forearm. This will often stop the leaking.

The use of supplementary feedings for the breast-feeding infant may weaken or confuse the sucking reflex and may interfere with successful outcome. Often parents are concerned because they have no visual assurance regarding the amount consumed. If the infant appears to gain weight and has six or more wet diapers a day, he is receiving adequate amounts of milk. Activity levels and intervals between feedings may also indicate how satisfied the infant is. Parents should know that, because breast milk is more easily digested than formulas, the breast-fed infant becomes hungry sooner. Thus the frequency of breast feedings may be greater, particularly after discharge, when fatigue or excitement may decrease milk supply temporarily. Increasing the frequency of feedings alleviates problems during these periods. The parents may also expect the infant to demand more frequent nursing during periods when growth spurts are expected, such as ten days to two weeks, five to six weeks, and three months. There is a lag in nursing due to increased activity and interest in surroundings at four to six months, seven months, and nine months to a year (Slattery, 1977).

The mother may be taught to manually express her milk and to freeze it for bottle-feeding if she will be absent for a scheduled feeding. Breast milk should be frozen in plastic bottles because if glass bottles are used the antibodies will adhere to the sides of the bottle and their benefits will be lost. Manual expression is also advisable if the mother must go several hours without feeding, to relieve maternal discomfort and to maintain the milk supply, which decreases unless the breasts are emptied regularly (Figure 27-9).

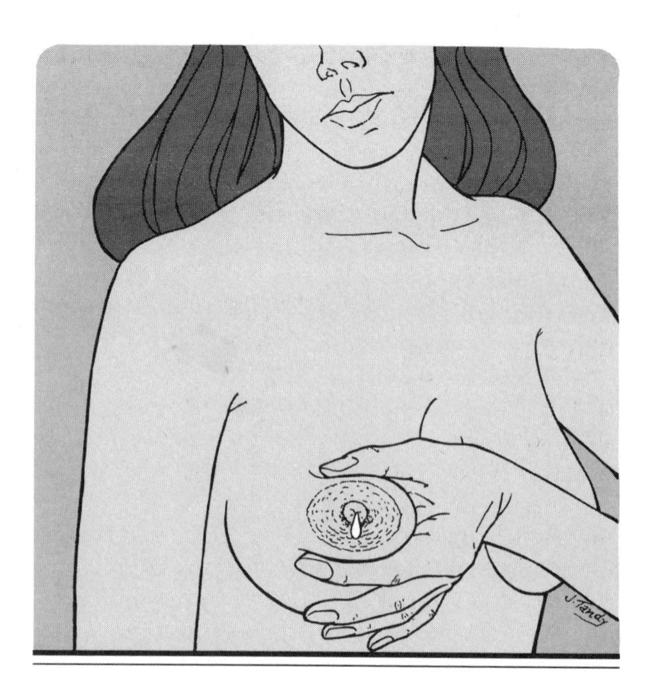

Figure 27-9. Manual expression of milk.

Numerous medications, when administered to the mother, are secreted in the milk. These include salicylates, bromides, antibiotics, most alkaloids, some cathartics, alcohol, and the majority of addicting drugs (Pritchard and MacDonald, 1976). The mother should receive information about this and should also be instructed to inform her physician that she is nursing, should she require medical treatment at a later time.

Numerous resources in the form of pamphlets and organized La Leche League activities are available to parents to assist with the establishment of successful breast-feeding. The mother needs the support of all family members, her pediatrician, her obstetrician, and nursing personnel, because it is often the attitudes reflected by these people that ultimately lead the mother to success or failure.

Promotion of Family Wellness

The promotion of family health encompasses several areas of concern, including a satisfactory maternity experience, the need for follow-up and continued medical supervision for the mother and infant with checkups every six weeks, infant immunizations, and birth control (see Appendix for schedule of infant immunizations). Regular health assessment of individual family members is important to maintain health and to prevent problems. Assessment of physiologic restoration should be a vital part of postpartal follow-up care. The new or expanding family may also have needs for information about adjustment of siblings, resuming sexual relations, and family planning.

Rooming-in

The trend to truly family-centered maternity care must, of necessity, be continued in the postpartal period. The tendency to separate the infant from his parents is being displaced by a flexible concept—rooming-in—that provides increased opportunities for parent-child interaction.

In rooming-in, the infant shares his mother's unit, and they are cared for together. Rooming-in provides continuous opportunities for the mother to begin to know her child, to bond with him, and to learn how to effectively care for him. The infant's crib is placed near the mother's bed, where she can easily see her child. The crib should be a self-contained unit well stocked with items that the mother might require in providing care, including diapers, shirts, blankets, crib sheets, cotton balls, A & D ointment, and a comb or hairbrush. A bulb syringe should be readily accessible in the crib for suctioning the mouth or nares, and the mother should be familiar with its use.

Mothers are frequently extremely tired following delivery, so the responsibility for providing total infant care could be overwhelming. The rooming-in policy must be flexible enough to permit the mother to return the baby to the nursery if she finds it necessary because of fatigue or physical discomfort. The woman with children at home may require additional rest, and a modified form of rooming-in may best meet her needs. The babies may return to the central nursery at night, allowing their mothers more time for uninterrupted rest if they desire.

Rooming-in is very conducive to a self-demand feeding schedule. The lactating mother may find it especially beneficial to be able to nurse her child every two to three hours if necessary. This type of schedule meets the infant's needs, promotes milk production, and helps prevent the nipple soreness caused by the ever-vigorous suck of the very hungry infant.

Fathers are also able to participate in the care of their infants with a rooming-in arrangement. They are asked to scrub their hands and usually wear a cover gown over their street clothes. Caps or masks are not required. Opportunities to hold and care for the child promote paternal self-confidence and foster paternal bonding. With rooming-in, father, mother, and infant have the opportunity to begin functioning as a family unit.

Reactions of Siblings

Although the parents have prepared their child for the presence of a new brother or sister, the actual arrival of the infant necessitates some adjustments. If small children are waiting at home, it is helpful if the father carries the baby inside. This practice keeps the mother's arms free to hug and touch her older children. She thereby reaffirms her love for them before introducing them to their new sibling. Many mothers have found that bringing a doll home with them for the older child is helpful. The child cares for the doll alongside his mother or father, thereby identifying with the parent. This identification helps decrease anger and the need to regress for attention. If the child is "too old" for receiving a doll, or if he is a boy to whom parents do not wish to give a doll, the child can be allowed to work alongside the parents in caring for the newborn. With constant supervision, the child may be permitted to hold the baby and to hold the bottle during feeding. In one instance, when the mother was breast-feeding, her 2½-year-old son sat next to her with his T-shirt pushed up and a doll to his breast. (Some parents may be distressed to observe this normal behavior.) The older child learns acceptable behavior toward the newborn, feels a sense of accomplishment, and learns tenderness and caring—qualities appropriate for both males and females. The nurse and parents can come up with numerous ways unique to their own environment and life-styles to show the older child or children that they too are valued, important, and have their own places in the family.

It is inevitable that an older child will at one time or another try to hurt the baby (or will hurt the baby unintentionally, not knowing his own strength or the effect of hitting). Parents are guided to respond by saying things like "I won't let you hurt (the baby) just as I won't let someone else hurt you."

The remaining umbilical cord or the unhealed stump may provoke anxiety in the older child. Parents are encouraged to point out what its function was, that it will fall off soon, and that it will look somewhat like the umbilical stump they too have.

The child, especially one of the opposite sex from the newborn, will raise queries about the appearance of the genitals as compared to his own. A simple explanation, such as "That's what little girls (boys) look like," is often sufficient.

Sexual Relations Between Parents

Nursing intervention in the postpartal period considers the parent as a sexual person as well. An unprepared mother who experiences a sexual response (feels "turned-on") by her baby's suckling at the breast may feel abnormal or guilty. Interdiction against sexual intercourse until the sixth week postpartum is scientifically unfounded and psychologically undesirable. Episiotomies should be healed and the lochial flow abating by the end of the third week. The woman's partner can test for vaginal tenderness by inserting one clean finger (lubricated with a water-based compound such as K-Y jelly) into the vaginal orifice. If no tenderness is experienced, two fingers may be inserted. If this illicits no tenderness, the vaginal vault is almost certainly healed. Because the vaginal vault is "dry" (hormone-poor) as yet, some form of lubrication (K-Y jelly or contraceptive foam) may be necessary during intercourse.

To avoid pregnancy, it is best for the male to use a condom with a spermaticide and for the female to use contraceptive foam. Many couples believe that breast-feeding provides contraceptive protection. *Breast-feeding has no contraceptive value.* There may occasionally be some dyspareunia for the first time or two. Without knowledge about this dyspareunia, couples are apt to be reluctant to repeat the sexual experience, and they may enter a disruptive communication cycle.

Breast-feeding couples need to be forewarned that, during orgasm, milk may spout from the nipples due to the release of oxytocin with sexual excitement and/or orgasm. Some couples find this pleasurable; other couples choose to have the woman wear a bra during sex.

Many couples have been frustrated during lovemaking by the baby's crying ("There's nothing like his crying to turn a guy off"). Some men as well as women are repulsed by the woman's changed body—the stretch marks, flabby abdominal skin, or breast changes. Maternal sleep deprivation may interfere with a mutually satisfying sexual relationship during this period. Couples may also be frustrated if there are changes in the woman's physiologic response to sexual stimulation. These changes are due to hormonal changes and may persist for about three months.

Anticipatory guidance during the prenatal and postnatal period can forewarn the couple of these eventualities and of their temporary nature. Anticipatory guidance is enhanced if the couple can discuss their feelings and reactions as they are experienced. Postpartal discussion groups reassure and support couples.

THE FOURTH TRIMESTER

The disparity between the quality and consistency of care provided to a woman during the intrapartal period and during the initial weeks of the postpartal period has received increased recognition by both consumers and health care providers. The term "fourth trimester" is frequently used to define this period.

During the postpartal period, the mother must accomplish certain physical and developmental tasks, including restoring physical condition, developing competence and skill in caring for and meeting the needs of her dependent infant, establishing a relationship with her new child, and adapting to altered life-styles and family structure resulting from the addition of a new member (Gruis, 1977).

Although physical restoration is fairly predictable, the new mother may have an inadequate or incorrect understanding of what to expect during the weeks following delivery. Concern over the restoration of her figure is often high, especially if she has retained some weight or had not expected a soft abdomen, stretch marks, or changes in her breasts. If her husband seems disappointed in her appearance, the problem may be compounded and the new mother may secretly fear that the physical changes in her body are permanent.

Continued physical discomfort frequently represents an unexpected element, too. Breast enlargement and nipple tenderness may produce discouragement for the breast-feeding mother, and episiotomy and hemorrhoidal pain may interfere with elimination and sexual relations and may promote fatigue. Fatigue is perhaps the most pervasive yet underestimated problem during the initial weeks.

Increased social mobility has decreased the availability of family support systems to assist a new family in adjusting. If the husband is unable to provide assistance and if there are other small children in the family, obtaining adequate rest becomes especially difficult. The constant, consistent needs of the new child for care also contribute to the problem as mother and child attempt to establish a mutually acceptable routine.

Developing competence and skill in caring for an infant may be especially anxiety-provoking for a new mother. Nurses and other health care providers have attempted to alleviate this anxiety by offering classes in child care both prenatally and in the postpartum unit. However, the psychologic changes occurring during the immediate postpartal period, coupled with the excitement and anxiety of parenthood, may serve as blocks to complete learning. Then, too, small unanticipated concerns may become monumental to a mother home alone attempting to cope. Her feelings of awkwardness or inadequacy may cause her to perceive herself as a failure. If she has family or friends nearby, she will generally ask for their assistance and advice, but many new mothers do not have adequate support systems and thus experience increased feelings of isolation.

The maternal-infant attachment process begins during pregnancy, intensifies in the period following delivery, and continues into the postpartal period. As the mother-child relationship develops, it is vital that the mother understand both normal growth and development and her child's distinct patterns of behavior, crying, eating, and sleeping. She should also be aware of the interaction capacity, behavioral response, and mood or temperment of the infant.

The woman's developmental task of adapting to the new family member involves developing a realistic acceptance of changed roles, retaining a sense of autonomy while developing a sense of "family," establishing and maintaining healthful routines, sharing parenting responsibilities, and maintaining a satisfactory personal relationship with her husband (Duvall, 1971). Efforts to achieve these tasks frequently produce stress, even if the child was planned. It is difficult to be adequately prepared for the changes a child brings, and a certain degree of grief for the lost life-style is to be expected. Sibling problems must be anticipated and dealt with as other children also seek to adjust to the new family member (Gruis, 1977).

Nursing Management

Nurses have been in the forefront of health providers in attempting to rectify the deficiencies in care currently existing during the postpartal period. Many obstetricians and nurse practitioners now routinely see all postpartal patients one to two weeks following delivery in addition to the routine six-week checkup. This extra visit provides an opportunity for physical assessment as well as assessment of the mother's psychologic and informational needs.

Two- and Six-Week Examinations

The routine physical assessment, which may rapidly be made, focuses on the woman's general appearance, breasts, reproductive tract, bladder and bowel elimination, and any specific problems or complaints. (See the accompanying Postpartal Physical Assessment Guide.) In addition, conversation is used to determine nutrition patterns, fatigue level, family adjustment, and psychologic status of the mother (see the accompanying Psychologic Assessment Guide). Any problems with child care are explored, and referral to a pediatric nurse practitioner or pediatrician is made if needed. Available community resources, including a Public Health Department follow-up, are mentioned when appropriate.

Discussion of family planning is appropriate at this time, and information regarding birth control methods is provided.

The couple may wish to resume a method that they used before the pregnancy or may require information regarding alternative birth control methods (see Chapter 7). Contraceptive methods are reinstated at various times following delivery. Vaginal foams, jellies, spermaticides, and condoms may be used as soon as sexual activity resumes. A diaphragm needs to be refitted after delivery due to possible change in the size of the vaginal vault; this is usually done at the postpartal check-up. An IUD may be inserted 3 to 6 weeks after delivery with no resultant increased risk of perforation of the uterus, expulsion of the device, or pregnancy (Pritchard and MacDonald, 1976). Birth control pills may be restarted at 3 weeks postpartum as long as there are no contraindications, and there is no increase in morbidity rates (Pritchard and MacDonald, 1976).

In ideal situations a family approach involving husband and infant (and possibly other siblings) would permit a total evaluation and provide an opportunity for all family members to ask questions and express concerns. In addition, disturbed family patterns might be more readily diagnosed so that therapy could be instituted to prevent future problems of neglect or abuse.

POSTPARTAL PHYSICAL ASSESSMENT GUIDE: TWO WEEKS AND SIX WEEKS AFTER DELIVERY

Assess	Normal findings	Deviations and possible causes*	Nursing interventions[†]
Vital signs			
Blood pressure	Return to normal prepregnant level	Elevated blood pressure (anxiety, essential hypertension, renal disease)	Review history, evaluate normal baseline. Refer to physician if necessary.
Pulse	60-90 beats/min (or prepregnant normal rate)	Increased pulse rate (excitement, anxiety, cardiac disorders)	Count pulse for full minute, note irregularities. Marked tachycardia or beat irregularities require additional assessment and possible physican referral.
Respirations	16-24/min	Marked tachypnea or abnormal patterns (respiratory disorders)	Evaluate for respiratory disease. Refer to physician if necessary.
Temperature	36.2C-37.6C (98F-99.6F)	Increased temperature (infection)	Assess for signs and symptoms of infection or disease state.
Weight	2 weeks: probable weight loss of 14-20+ lb	Little or no weight loss (fluid retention, subinvolution, poor dietary habits)	Evaluate dietary habits and nutritional state. Review blood pressure to evaluate fluid retention or blood losses.
	6 weeks: returning to normal prepregnant weight	Retained weight (poor dietary habits)	Determine amount of daily exercise. Refer to dietician if necessary for dietary counseling.
		Extreme weight loss (excessive dieting)	Discuss appropriate diets; refer to dietician if necessary.
Breasts			
Nonnursing	2 weeks: may have mild tenderness; small amount of milk may be expressed; breasts returning to prepregnant size	Some engorgement (incomplete suppression of lactation)	Engorgement usually seen only when no medication has been given to suppress lactation. Advise patient to wear a supportive well-fitted bra, avoid hot showers, etc. (see p. 912).
	6 weeks: soft, with no tenderness; return to prepregnant size	Redness, marked tenderness (mastitis) Palpable mass (tumor)	Evaluate for signs and symptoms of mastitis (rare in nonnursing mothers).
Nursing	Full, with prominent nipples; lactation established	Cracked, fissured nipples (feeding problems) Rednesss, marked tenderness; may even be abscess formation (mastitis)	Counsel about nipple care (see p. 912). Evaluate patient condition, evidence of fever. Refer to physician for initiation of antibiotic therapy.

*Possible causes of deviations are placed in parentheses.
[†]Nursing interventions are directed primarily toward identified deviations.

POSTPARTAL PHYSICAL ASSESSMENT GUIDE Cont'd

Assess	Normal findings	Deviations and possible causes*	Nursing interventions†
		Palpable mass (full milk duct, tumor)	Opinion varies as to value of breast examination for nursing mothers. Some feel a nursing mother should examine her breasts monthly, after feeding, when breasts are empty. If palpable mass is felt, refer to physician for further evaluation. For breast inflammation instruct the mother to: 1. Keep breast empty by frequent feeding. 2. Rest when possible. 3. Take aspirin for pain. 4. Force fluids. If symptoms persist for more than 24 hours, instruct her to call her physician.
Abdominal musculature	2 weeks: improved firmness, although "bread dough" consistency is not unusual, especially in multipara Striae pink and obvious	Marked disastasis recti (relaxation of muscles)	Evaluate exercise level. Provide information on appropriate exercise program.
	C-section incision healing	Drainage, redness, tenderness, pain, edema (infection)	Evaluate for infection. Refer to physician if necessary.
	6 weeks: muscle tone continues to improve; striae may be beginning to fade, they may not achieve a silvery appearance for several more weeks Linea nigra fading		
Elimination pattern			
Urinary tract	Return to prepregnant urinary elimination routine	Urinary incontinence, especially when lifting, coughing, laughing, etc. (urethral trauma)	Assess for cystocele. Instruct in appropriate muscle tightening exercises; refer to physician.
		Pain or burning when voiding, urgency and/or frequency, pus or WBC in urine, pathogenic organisms in culture (urinary tract infection)	Evaluate for urinary tract infection. Obtain clean catch urine. Refer to physician for treatment if indicated.

*Possible causes of deviations are placed in parentheses.
†Nursing interventions are directed primarily toward identified deviations.

POSTPARTAL PHYSICAL ASSESSMENT GUIDE Cont'd

Assess	Normal findings	Deviations and possible causes*	Nursing interventions†
	Routine urinalysis within normal limits (proteinurea disappeared)	Sugar or ketone in urine—may be some lactose present in urine of breast-feeding mothers (diabetes)	Evaluate diet. Assess for signs and symptoms of diabetes. Refer to physician.
Bowel habits	2 weeks: may still be some discomfort with defecation, especially if patient had severe hemorrhoids or 3° extension	Severe constipation or pain when defecating (trauma or hemorrhoids)	Discuss dietary patterns; encourage fluid, adequate roughage. Continue use of stool softener if necessary to prevent pain associated with straining. Continue sitz baths, periods of rest for severe hemorrhoids. Assess healing of episiotomy and/or lacerations. Severe constipation may require administration of laxatives, stool softeners, and an enema.
	6 weeks: return to normal prepregnancy bowel elimination	Marked constipation	See above.
		Fecal incontinence or constipation (rectocele)	Assess for evidence of rectocele. Instruct in muscle tightening exercises. Refer to physician.
Reproductive tract			
Lochia	2 weeks: lochia alba, scant amounts, fleshy odor	Foul odor, excessive in amounts (infection) Return to lochia rubra or persistence of lochia rubra or serosa	Assess for evidence of infection and/or subinvolution; culture lochia. Refer to physician.
	6 weeks: no lochia, or return to normal menstruation pattern	See above	See above.
Pelvic examination	2 weeks: uterus no longer palpable abdominally; external os closed; uterine muscles still somewhat lax and uterus may be displaced; introitus of vagina still lacking tone—gapes when intraabdominal pressure is increased by coughing or straining	External cervical os open, uterus not decreasing appropriately (subinvolution, infection) Evidence of redness, tenderness, poor tissue approximation in episiotomy and/or laceration (wound infection)	Assess for evidence of subinvolution and/or infection. Refer to physician if indicated.

*Possible causes of deviations are placed in parentheses.
†Nursing interventions are directed primarily toward identified deviations.

POSTPARTAL PHYSICAL ASSESSMENT GUIDE Cont'd

Assess	Normal findings	Deviations and possible causes*	Nursing interventions†
	Episiotomy and/or lacerations healing; no signs of infection		
	6 weeks: almost returned to prepregnant size with almost completely restored muscle tone Cervix completely closed with only transverse slit apparent	Continued flow of lochia, some opening of cervical os, failure to decrease appropriately in size (subinvolution)	Assess for evidence of subinvolution and/or infection. Refer to physician for further evaluation and for dilatation and curettage if necessary.
	Good return of muscle tone to pelvic floor	Marked relaxation of pelvic floor muscles (uterine prolapse)	Assess for evidence of uterine prolapse. Discuss appropriate perineal exercises. Refer to physician if indicated.
Papanicolaou test	Normal cells on Pap smear (class 1 or 2)	Abnormal cells, classes 3, 4, or 5 (cancer of cervix)	Refer to physician for further evaluation and treatment.
Hemoglobin and hematocrit level	6 weeks: Hgb 12 gm/100 ml Hct 37% ± 5%	Hgb $<$ 12 gm/100 ml Hct 32% (anemia)	Assess nutritional status, begin (or continue) supplemental iron. For marked anemia (Hgb 9 gm/100 ml) additional assessment and/or physician referral may be necessary.

*Possible causes of deviations are placed in parentheses.
†Nursing interventions are directed primarily toward identified deviations.

PSYCHOLOGIC ASSESSMENT GUIDE

Assess	Normal findings	Deviations and possible causes*	Nursing interventions†
Attachment	Evidence of bonding process demonstrated by soothing, cuddling and talking to infant, appropriate feeding techniques, eye-to-eye contact, calling infant by name	Failure to bond demonstrated by lack of behaviors associated with bonding process, calling infant by nickname that promotes ridicule, inadequate infant weight gain, infant is dirty, hygienic measures are not being maintained, severe	Provide counseling. Refer to public health nurse for continued home visit.

*Possible causes of deviations are placed in parentheses.
†Nursing interventions are primarily directed toward identified deviations.

PSYCHOLOGIC ASSESSMENT GUIDE Cont'd

Assess	Normal findings	Deviations and possible causes*	Nursing interventions†
		diaper rash, failure to obtain adequate supplies to provide infant care (malattachment)	
Adjustment to parental role	Parents are coping with new roles in terms of division of labor, financial status, communication, readjustment of sexual relations, and adjusting to new daily tasks	Inability to adjust to new roles (immaturity, inadequate education and preparation, ineffective communication patterns, inadequate support, current family crisis)	Provide counseling. Refer to parent groups.
Education	Mother understands self-care measures	Inadequate knowledge of self-care (inadequate education)	Provide education and counseling.
	Parents are knowledgeable regarding infant care	Inadequate knowledge of infant care (inadequate education)	
	Siblings are adjusting to new baby	Excessive sibling rivalry	
	Parents have chosen method of contraception		

*Possible causes of deviations are placed in parentheses.
†Nursing interventions are primarily directed toward identified deviations.

Telephone Follow-up

Another approach to improving care during the fourth trimester is the telephone follow-up, usually initiated by nurses from the postpartal unit of the agency where the mother delivered. The initial contact is made during the first week following discharge. If the call is delayed beyond this time, the family may have already adopted unsatisfactory methods of dealing with problems. For instance, a new nursing mother discouraged by sore nipples may elect to give up breast-feeding because she is not aware of measures she could employ to improve her comfort.

The nurse has five major functions to accomplish when telephoning:

1. Initiating contact with the family during the especially stressful first week. Frequently the family recognizes that problems exist, but they are unaware of where to seek help or are reluctant to do so.

2. Assessing the mother and family in order to evaluate their status.

3. Providing follow-up as indicated, utilizing all available resources.

4. Reinforcing existing knowledge and provides additional health teaching as indicated.

5. Communicating the results of her assessment, intervention, and evaluation to appropriate agencies and/or health care providers (Donaldson, 1977).

The hospital identification numbers for both mother and baby are saved and utilized as a reference when phoning. Most agencies also utilize an assessment form (Figure 27–10) to provide for consistency and information in the event that additional follow-up is indicated.

Although the focus of concern in a follow-up

TELEPHONE POSTPARTAL FOLLOW-UP RECORD

Patient name ______________________ Date DC ____________ Date TC ____________

OB ______________________ Ped ______________________

Help at home ______________________ Other supports ______________________

NURSING ASSESSMENT

Maternal physical

☐ Feels generally well ("I'm__________________")
☐ Fatigue ("Do you have help in the home?")
☐ Perineum
☐ No or minor discomfort
☐ Complaints of suture discomfort
☐ Scant, appropriate flow
☐ Moderate flow, clots
☐ Other abnormal flow ______________

Breasts
☐ Lactating: ☐ Soft ☐ Engorgement
☐ Sore nipples ☐ Cracked nipples
☐ Nonlactating: ☐ Soft ☐ Leaking ☐ Pain

Elimination
☐ Complaints of constipation
☐ Urination sufficient
☐ Frequency, burning, on medication ______________

Nutrition
☐ Good appetite ☐ Poor appetite ☐ PNV

C-section
☐ Suture line clean, dry
☐ Discharge ______________
☐ Pain at incision site

Miscellaneous
☐ Headache ☐ Backache ☐ Other ______________
☐ Postpartal follow-up appointment made or reminded

Caregiving skills and family adjustment

☐ Growing competence and confidence
☐ Generally comfortable in caregiver role, relaxed, seems confident
☐ Seems overwhelmed ☐ Many questions
☐ Lack of interest ☐ Anxious
☐ Father active as caregiver ☐ Supporting as father
☐ Nonsupportive
☐ Baby up for adoption
☐ Siblings ______________
☐ Adjusting well ☐ Not adjusting well

Baby

☐ Breast-feeding every 3-4 hours with little or no additional bottle-feeding required following breast feeding
☐ Formula ______________ ☐ No problems
☐ Feeding problems ______________
☐ "The baby is ______________ "
☐ Cord on ☐ Off ☐ Circumcision healing
☐ Discharge cord ☐ Discharge circumcision
☐ Alert when awake ☐ Active ☐ Responsive
Consolability: ☐ Easily consoled
☐ Fussy ☐ Irritable
☐ SGA ☐ Preterm ☐ LGA

☐ Jaundiced ☐ Had phototherapy
☐ Special problems ______________

INTERVENTIONS

☐ Reinforce appropriate activity limits
☐ Reevaluate priorities ______________
☐ Increase rest ☐ Decrease activity
☐ Utilize available resources
☐ Tucks ☐ Sitz baths as per obstetrician
☐ Report excessive flow to obstetrician

☐ Binding, icing, engorgement instruction
☐ Demand/supply reviewed
☐ Air ☐ Nipples ☐ Expose to light
☐ Masse cream
☐ Limit nursing time to________ minutes per side
☐ Pc glucose water or form ☐ Shield
☐ As per pediatrician ☐ Massage
☐ Hot packs ☐ Shower

☐ Increase fluid intake
☐ Fruits
☐ Roughage intake
☐ Laxative as per obstetrician
☐ Opportunity

☐ Healing needs discussed ☐ Basic Four
☐ Sexuality discussed
☐ Postpartal exercise discussed
☐ Family planning teaching
☐ Postpartal transitions and stresses discussed
☐ Self-nurturing options explored

☐ Reassurance
☐ Answer questions

☐ Advise about infant's needs, rhythms, nurturing

☐ Explore expectations and needs of sibling adaptation
☐ Infectious disease in home — advised about control, hygiene, ventilation, TLC
☐ Cord care reviewed
☐ Circumcision care reviewed

☐ Report to pediatrician ☐ Nurse ☐ Patient
____
☐ Report to obstetrician ☐ Nurse ☐ Patient
____

Recommendations

☐ Discontinue follow-up
☐ Refer to obstetrician
☐ Refer to pediatrician
☐ Refer to Public Health for follow-up
☐ Repeat telephone call ______________

Figure 27–10. Telephone postpartal follow-up record. (Modified from Hoag Memorial Hospital Presbyterian, Newport Beach, Calif.)

call may vary, concern is frequently directed toward specific aspects of infant care (Sumner and Tritsch, 1977). However, a written evaluation of a group of mothers by Gruis (1977) found that the group's major worry was the return of their figures to normal. Because of this variation in concerns, the nurse must be prepared to discuss physical hygiene problems or worries, basic infant care, sibling difficulties, maternal attachment, paternal engrossment, and the status of the family as a whole. The goal of the follow-up is to promote confidence and independence while serving as a source of assistance and a guide to other resources when necessary (Donaldson, 1977).

The data obtained during the follow-up call should be preserved and incorporated into the maternal record, which is useful in providing information to the physician or community agencies and may be a helpful reference during subsequent births.

SUMMARY

The puerperium begins with the delivery of a newborn and extends through the next six weeks. During this period numerous changes are occurring within the mother's body. The involutional process involves changes in the majority of the body systems as they return to the prepregnant state. The addition of a new family member necessitates a reordering and restructuring of the family unit. These changes may produce a time of stress for the new family. There are many new tasks to be learned and new adjustments to be made.

Through an understanding of expected changes and assessment of numerous physical and psychologic factors, the nurse can intervene more appropriately and assist the new family as they take on the parenting role. In these modern times of increased mobility and lack of family members in close proximity, the new family looks to the nurse as a resource person who can assist them in learning their new tasks.

SUGGESTED ACTIVITIES

1. Identify, through patient assessment, the physiologic changes in the mother on delivery day and on the first and second postpartal days.
2. Provide a baby bath demonstration and return demonstration to a new mother and father.
3. Develop a postpartal patient education program with appropriate resources.
4. Conduct three telephone follow-up calls and determine appropriate nursing interventions.
5. Prepare a home care handout for maternal-infant needs, and discuss its application with three mothers.
6. In a small group, discuss methods to facilitate sibling adjustment in the postpartal family.

REFERENCES

Barber, H. R., and Graber, E. A. 1974. *Surgical disease in pregnancy.* Philadelphia: W. B. Saunders Co.

Danforth, D. N. 1977. *Obstetrics and gynecology.* 3rd ed. Hagerstown, Md: Harper & Row Publishers, Inc.

Davidson, N. Summer 1974. REEDA: evaluating postpartum healing. *J. Nurse-Midwifery.* 9(2):6.

Donaldson, N. E. July 1977. Follow-up at home. *Am. J. Nurs.* 77(7):1176.

Dutton, M. A. May–June 1979. A breastfeeding protocol. *J. Obstet. Gynecol. Neonatal Nurs.* 8(3):151.

Duvall, E. 1971. *Family development.* Philadelphia: J. B. Lippincott Co.

Greenhill, J. P., and Friedman, E. A. 1974. *Biological principles and modern practice of obstetrics.* Philadelphia: W. B. Saunders Co.

Gruis, M. May–June 1977. Beyond maternity: postpartum concerns of mothers. *Am. J. Maternal-Child Nurs.* 2(3):182.

Ledger, W. J. March–April 1974. The new face of puerperal sepsis. *J. Obstet. Gynecol. Neonatal Nurs.* 3(2):26.

Nichols, M. March–April 1978. Effective help for the nursing mother. *J. Obstet. Gynecol. Neonatal Nurs.* 7(2):22.

Pritchard, J. A., and MacDonald, P. C. 1976. *In Williams obstetrics.* 15th ed. New York: Appleton-Century-Crofts.

Rubin, R. Nov. 1961. Basic maternal behavior. *Nurs. Outlook.* 9:683.

Slattery, J. S. March–April 1977. Nutrition for the normal healthy infant. *Am. J. Maternal-Child Nurs.* 2(2):105.

Sumner, G., and Tritsch, J. May–June 1977. Postnatal parental concerns: the first six weeks of life. *J. Obstet. Gynecol. Neonatal Nurs.* 6(3):27.

ADDITIONAL READINGS

Cahill, A. S. Jan.–Feb. 1975. Dual purpose tool for assessing maternal needs and nursing care. *J. Obstet. Gynecol. Neonatal Nurs.* 4(1):28.

Campbell, S., and Smith, J. July 1977. Postpartum assessment guide. *Am. J. Nurs.* 77(7):1179.

Carlson, S. E. Sept.–Oct. 1976. The irreality of postpartum observations on the subjective experience. *J. Obstet. Gynecol. Neonatal Nurs.* 5(5):28.

Clark, A. L., and Affonso, D. D. March–April 1976. Mother-child relations—infant behavior and maternal attachment: two sides to the coin. *Am. J. Maternal-Child Nurs.* 1(2):94.

Clausen, J. P. 1972. Efficient postpartum checks. *Nurs. '72.* 2:24.

Countryman, B. A. Sept.–Oct. 1973. Breast care in the early puerperium. *J. Obstet. Gynecol. Neonatal Nurs.* 2(5):36.

Crummette, B. D. Summer 1975. Transitions into motherhood. *Am. J. Maternal-Child Nurs.* 4(2):65.

Danforth, D. N., ed. 1977. *Obstetrics and gynecology.* New York: Harper & Row Publishers, Inc.

Derthick, N. Fall 1974. Sexuality in pregnancy and the puerperium. *Birth Family J.* 1(4):5.

Edwards, M. Winter 1973–1974. The crises of fourth trimester. *Birth Family J.* 1(1):19.

Erickson, M. P. March–April 1978. Trends in assessing the newborn and his parents. *Am. J. Maternal-Child Nurs.* 3(2):99.

Haight, J. Sept.–Oct. 1977. Steadying parents as they go—by phone. *Am. J. Maternal-Child Nurs.* 2(5):311.

Johnson, N. W. Jan.–Feb. 1976. Breast-feeding at one hour of age. *Am. J. Maternal-Child Nurs.* 1(1):12.

Kilker, R., and Wilkerson, B. May 1973. Eight point postpartal assessment. *Nurs. '73.* 3:56.

Kyndely, K. Jan.–Feb. 1978. The sexuality of women in pregnancy and postpartum: a review. *J. Obstet. Gynecol. Neonatal Nurs.* 7(1):28.

Ludington-Hoe, S. M. 1977. Postpartum: development of maternicity. *Am. J. Nurs.* 77(7):1171.

Miller, D. L., and Baird, S. F. March–April 1978. Helping parents to be parents—a special center. *Am. J. Maternal-Child Nurs.* 3(2):117.

Nichols, M. G. March–April 1978. Effective help for the nursing mother. *J. Obstet. Gynecol. Neonatal Nurs.* 7(2):22.

Rubin, R. 1961. Puerperal change. *Nurs. Outlook.* 9:753.

Rubin, R. Nov. 1963. Maternal touch. *Nurs. Outlook.* 11:828.

Rubin, R. Oct. 1975. Maternity nursing stops too soon. *Am. J. Nurs.* 75(10):1680.

Scahill, M. C. March–April 1975. Helping the mother solve problems with feeding her infant. *J. Obstet. Gynecol. Neonatal Nurs.* 4(2):51.

Schmidt, J. May–June 1978. Using a teaching guide for better postpartum and infant care. *J. Obstet. Gynecol. Neonatal Nurs.* 7(3):23.

Schroeder, M. A. May–June 1977. Is the immediate postpartum period crucial to the mother-child relationship? A pilot study comparing primiparas with rooming-in and those in a maternity ward. *J. Obstet. Gynecol. Neonatal Nurs.* 6(3):37.

Swenden, L. A., et al. March–April 1978. Role supplementation for new parents—a role mastery plan. *Am. J. Maternal-Child Nurs.* 3(2):84.

Tanner, L. M. 1971. Assessing needs of new mothers in the postpartum unit. In *Current concepts in clinical nursing,* vol. 3, eds. M. Duffy et al. St. Louis: The C. V. Mosby Co.

Williams, J. K. July 1977. Learning needs of new parents. *Am. J. Nurs.* 77(7):1173.

CHAPTER 28

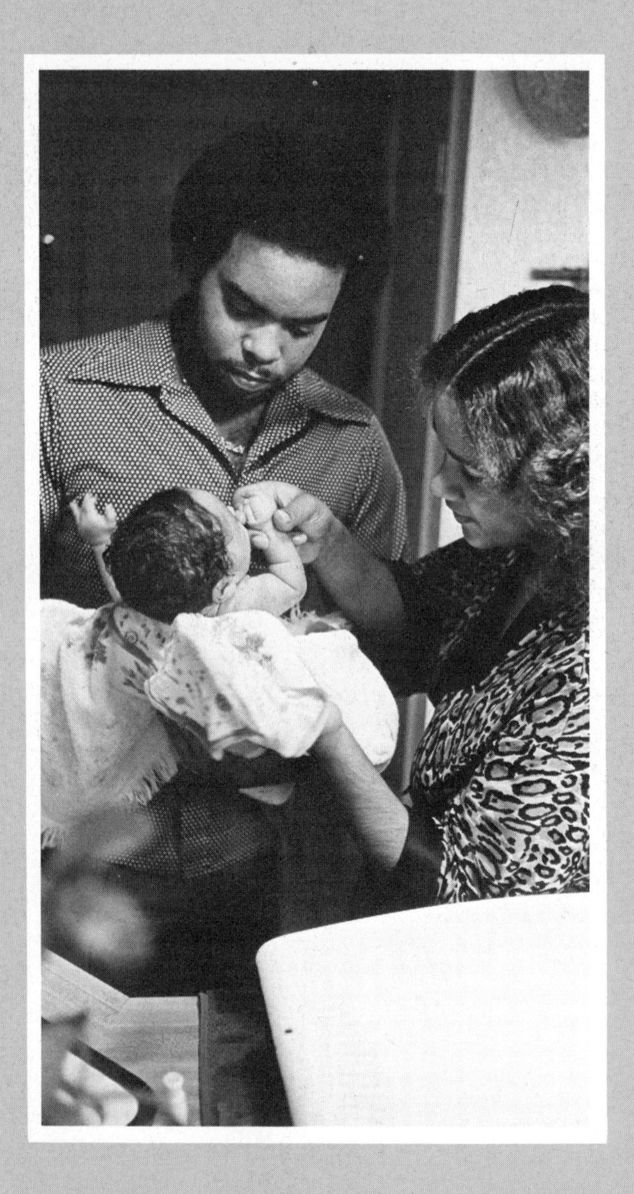

ATTACHMENT

OBJECTIVES

- Describe the attachment process, including the phases of maternal-infant interaction.
- List methods the nurse can use to facilitate a positive attachment process.
- Compare the factors influencing the first maternal-infant interaction.
- Explain the types of questions used for evaluating the maternal-infant relationship.
- Contrast the factors affecting family member interactions with the infant.

When a baby is born, two unique individuals who have been biologically united for nine months—mother and child—now and for the first time have a potential for direct interpersonal interaction. What will that interaction be like? What feelings will come into the mother's awareness and be expressed—or remain unexpressed? What continuities in maternal feelings will carry over from the time before the pair was separated by birth? What do they portend for the quality of the future relationship? What will be the baby's contribution to that relationship? These are not easy questions to answer. Yet nurses are being challenged to predict such outcomes in order to plan for individual and family interventions and community programs. What kinds of information can be helpful in making realistic assessments of the various phases of the maternity cycle? What are the appropriate interventions?

WHAT THE MOTHER BRINGS TO THE FIRST INTERACTION

It is often important in developing an understanding of a mother-infant dyad to become aware of certain aspects of the mother's life history that may have significance for the relationship between the two. Each mother brings to the first meeting with her infant a broad range of life experiences—pleasant, unpleasant, neutral, or mixed.

Life History

The mother brings the total of her years of experience as a participating family member in her family of origin. The number of years can vary considerably, but she has been an infant, a child, an adolescent, and probably a young adult within a particular family setting. Although the experiential content of those years, in pattern and meaning, is unique to each mother, certain aspects of the family can be viewed as potentially important to the present interaction:

1. The mother was born into a specific ordinal position in her family, which in part determined the nature of some life experiences. For example, she could have been first-born, last-born, middle child, only child, or only girl. Each position could have influenced the quality of parenting she received, limited her opportunities for practice with young babies, or shaped her feelings for a baby of similar position. For example, if the mother has sought out and experienced encounters with infants and young children, she is more likely to be aware of their abilities and therefore have realistic expectations of her own baby. Early interest in young children has been found to be predictive of postpartum maternal adaptation (Shereshefsky and Yarrow, 1973).

2. Her family could be described as relatively stable or unstable in terms of geographical location, employment, persons available, and physical and mental health of its members. Instability in any of these areas adds situational stresses to the developmental stresses of a growing child. Poverty, poor housing, fears of unemployment, geographical mobility, and undernutrition are all environmental factors that can affect a mother's ability to relate well to her infant or child.

3. Her family utilized communication patterns that were relatively effective or ineffective in meeting the emotional and educational needs of individual family members or in maintaining the healthy functioning of the family system.

4. Significant persons in the family who were responsible for her nurturance had a greater or lesser capacity to express interpersonal tenderness and warmth through caring for another human being.

The constellation and characteristics of the mother's family provide the model on which she is most likely to base her mothering practices. The exact nature of the past family experiences, only suggested above, helped fashion the blueprint for family development and childrearing that the new mother carries within her. Part of the design is in conscious awareness; part lies hidden from view, waiting to be provoked in unpredictable ways by situations that arise in the course of mother-infant interaction.

Personality

The mother brings to the first interaction with her infant the self she has become. Her genetic potential has shaped and been shaped by family and other experiences over time. She has developed into an extremely complex and unique personality with a number of characteristics of importance in her relationship with her infant:

1. The level of basic trust this mother has been able to develop in reaction to her life experiences. Does she view the world as a generally friendly or hostile place? Does she consider humans to be fundamentally good or evil? The feelings accompanying her views can influence her motivation for childbearing and her philosophy of childrearing, both of which are reflected in direct interactions.

A mother with adequate levels of basic trust can accept her baby as an individual with unique and changing needs that should be gratified as much as possible. If she cannot trust that her baby is capable of expressing his needs and will not make unnecessary demands, she is put in the position of deciding whether to respond to his fussing or crying each time it occurs. Such a decision-making burden can delay maternal responses and can also result in inconsistencies in mothering behavior. In addition, a prevailing mistrust of others can result in unwillingness to reach out for emotional and informational support and in an inability to benefit from support when it is received (Kennedy, 1969).

2. Level of self-esteem. How much does she value herself as a person, as a woman, as a wife and potential mother? Does she feel relatively competent or generally ineffective in coping with tasks, transitions, and adjustments?

3. Capacity for enjoying oneself. Is the mother able to find pleasure in everyday activities and in human relationships?

4. Interest in and adequacy of knowledge about childbearing and childrearing. A mother's beliefs about the course of pregnancy, the capacities of infants, and the nature of maternal emotions can set up expectations for both self and infant that may influence her behavior at first contact with the infant and in later interactions.

5. Her prevailing mood, or usual feeling tone. Is the woman predominantly content, angry, depressed, or anxious? Does she tend to express or withhold her feelings, positive or negative? Is her expression appropriate and authentic, devious, oblique, or nonverbal? Is she sensitive to her own feelings and those of others? These capacities will help determine her ability to understand and accept her own needs and to obtain support in meeting them.

In an extensive study of essentially normal middle-class families, Shereshefsky and Yarrow (1973) reported that two personality factors—ego strength and nurturance—were predictive of maternal adjustment during pregnancy and in the postpartum period. *Ego strength* was described as a woman's overall level of maturity and emotional adaptation and included, among other qualities, her self-acceptance and ability to provide for her own enjoyment. *Nurturance* was a woman's ability and willingness to respond to others in a giving way. The authors concluded that a woman's "adaptation to pregnancy and maternity tends to be consistent with her characteristic patterns of response and her adaptive behavior in general." Another recent study indicates that personality qualities (self-confidence, self-image, and others) observable in early pregnancy can be predictive of overall pregnancy adjustment and adaptation to motherhood (Leifer, 1977).

Sexual-Reproductive Experience

Each mother brings to her first meeting with her newborn a mixture of past experiences related to the reproductive function. Some of the experiences are indirect or vicarious. Stories related by relatives, friends, acquaintances, and strangers have become a part of her store of information. More often than not, it is the unpleasant or fearful experiences that are remembered, exaggerated, misinterpreted, and transmitted, creating or confirming fears and negative expectations.

A mother's direct experiences with sexuality can influence her view of herself as a mother-to-be and her expectations of her baby. If she experienced menstruation negatively—as a painful condition, a sickness, or a vulnerable state—or if she considers her genital expression of sexuality as less than adequate or normal, she might also question the outcome of her procreative efforts. A period of infertility can also reduce maternal self-confidence. A prior reproductive loss through spontaneous abortion, premature delivery, stillbirth, or sudden infant death syndrome can diminish a mother's ability or willingness to develop an emotional tie to the next baby. Having previously delivered a genetically defective, developmentally disabled, or physically ill infant can have a similar effect.

Present Pregnancy

Each mother brings to her first visual contact with her infant her reactions to that particular pregnancy, from conception through birth. The pregnancy evolved and developed in an emotional climate. The conception was planned or unplanned, the baby was wanted or unwanted—for any number of reasons. The course of the pregnancy was predominantly either pleasant and worry-free or filled with discomfort and anxieties. The mother felt encouraged and supported in her nine months, or she experienced disapproval and felt isolated. Ongoing life events essentially unrelated to her pregnant condition may have enhanced her pregnancy or depleted the energy reserves and coping ability so necessary to pregnancy adjustments (Kennedy, 1969). The stresses of pregnancy, in combination with low adaptive potential, can influence the pregnancy's vulnerability to a variety of complications (Nuckolls et al., 1972).

Most important, perhaps, is the fact that each mother, by the time of expected delivery, has developed an emotional orientation of some kind toward the fetus, based on a tactile-kinesthetic awareness combined with her fantasy images and perceptions. It has been suggested that there are several patterns of developing maternal feeling observable during the course of pregnancy (Leifer, 1977). One type of mother feels an emotional closeness to the fetus very early in the pregnancy. This feeling becomes deeper at quickening and grows in intensity through the second and third trimester. By the time of labor, this mother feels a close relationship and interaction between herself and the fetus. A different type of mother feels no attachment early in pregnancy, develops positive feelings shortly after feeling fetal movement, and has a well-established maternal bond by the end of pregnancy. In a third pattern, the mother experiences little or no positive feeling even by the end of the third trimester. Fetal movement is viewed as an intrusion and is reacted to with irritation. In this case the emotional orientation toward the expected infant is essentially negative.

Leifer (1977) found that women who did not plan to become pregnant or who conceived for reasons of status or security were frequently among those who had minimal feelings of closeness to the fetus throughout the pregnancy. Those who felt well adjusted in their marriage and emotionally ready to have a baby were able to develop strong affectionate feelings and to interact with the fetus, demonstrating a positive orientation toward the baby even before the birth.

In summary, it appears that a woman's total life history, up to the time of birth, can be predictive of the nature of her adaptation to motherhood. However, a large part of her postpartal adjustment relates to the new arrival in the family, who until the moment of birth is essentially an unknown factor in the equation.

WHAT THE NEWBORN BRINGS TO THE FIRST INTERACTION

When there are two partners in an interpersonal interaction, each contributes in some way to the process. In years past, the infant's influence on the beginning mother-infant relationship was treated as nonexistent or minimal. More recently, research on the capacities of the newborn and very young infant has shown that he is indeed an active partner in the exchange and takes part in shaping his own human environment from the moment of birth. He does this by virtue of who he is and what he does—his appearance and behavior.

Appearance

At the moment of birth certain information about the baby's external appearance is available to the mother. Each characteristic may have a special meaning for the mother as it relates to her hopes, fears, and expectations. The relatively obvious things are usually noted first: sex, size, shape, color, and presence or absence of abnormality or injury.

Behaviors

The baby has, and may demonstrate at birth, certain functional behaviors, such as crying, sucking, eliminating, looking, listening, and startling. These behaviors do not occur in a random fashion. The normal newborn comes into the world programmed to respond positively to the expected maternal stimuli. For example, in the very first days of life, the infant has been shown to selectively attend to the human face, to prefer the human voice over other sounds, and to become quiet and alert when picked up and held over the shoulder (Korner and Thoman, 1970; Goren et al., 1975).

In addition to having behaviors in common with other infants, each newborn, like his mother, is already a unique combination of genetic potential and life experience. His life experience is shorter and more limited in scope, of course, but it can have a powerful effect on his observable behavior.

This simplified overview of significant background factors in the initial meeting of mother and infant points up the fact that the exact feelings, reactions, and interactional responses of each mother at the culmination of each delivery defy prediction. The past history and present personality of each mother combine with the characteristics and behavior of her infant to influence the quality and direction of the maternal-infant relationship. Two unique individuals are blending into an equally unique interactional system that changes with time and as the actors change and grow.

Precise prediction seems impractical, but is it feasible to develop some guidelines of normality for evaluating maternal-newborn interaction? What behaviors should alert us to watch for the disordered relationship? What behaviors should allows us to feel comfortable about the future direction?

THE SETTING

We cannot possibly consider setting up behavioral norms for mother and infant at first contact unless we can first describe the variables of physical context, human environment, and condition of the interactors.

Physical Environment

No drama takes place without a stage. In the case of the first dialogue between infant and mother, the prerequisite delivery may have occurred in one of a variety of places. The most frequent setting by far is a maternity unit of a hospital. The physical surroundings are, in all probability, relatively strange to the woman as she moves from the admitting area to the labor room, delivery room, recovery area, and thence to her room in the postpartal unit. She sees and comes in contact with "sickness and operation" furniture, materials, and routines. Noise levels are usually high, and many sounds are of uncertain origin and meaning for the mother. Food is usually withheld until after delivery. The strain and concomitant psychic stress of frequent accommodations to the physical environment can interfere with the progress of labor and delivery and with the comfort of mother-infant interaction.

An increasing number of women are deciding to give birth in their homes. This setting differs from the conventional hospital in that the physical environment is stable and familiar. In most instances of home birth, the mother-to-be has taken the major responsibility for selecting, furnishing, and equipping the birth environment.

Consumer and professional efforts to increase the comfort of hospital births while decreasing the risks inherent in home birth have produced an intermediate type of setting—hospital-independent birth centers or hospital birthing rooms. These facilities are more homelike in appearance and do not require moves from one module to another during the progression from labor through early recovery.

Human Environment

It appears to be a human characteristic to carry out the acts of labor and giving birth in a social setting. Very few women express the wish to be alone during parturition; most respond with distress to the idea of abandonment at such a time. Hospitals, now and in the past, have generally provided for fairly constant nursing supervision of women in active labor, in the course of delivery, and in the early hours after birth. Usually, however, there is a different caretaker present in each phase of the childbearing activities. Each nurse is relating to an unknown patient at each step, and each patient is relating to a series of unknown nurses. The nurse may systematically receive pertinent information about the patient, but the patient typically gets no help in orienting herself to interaction with each new nurse—and each has different advice, expectations, attitudes, and relating skills.

A number of hospitals have changed routines to permit the father or another significant person to be present at her labor and delivery. This practice increases the possibility that a woman will have the support of one trusted person for the whole childbirth experience. The quality of support available from professionals or laypersons varies considerably according to their clinical and psychosocial skills. There are indications that a woman's perceptions of her physical care and emotional support and her reactions to the nonhuman elements of the environment can influence her mothering responses.

Condition of the Interactors

When the postbirth conditions are optimal, mother and infant are ready to relate effectively to each other and to benefit from the interaction. The mother is emotionally high and alert, primed for maternal responsiveness by her hormonal state. The infant is in a quiet, alert state, capable of attending to his mother's face and voice. However, several commonly occurring conditions act to diminish or divert the physical and psychologic energies available to the mother for relating with her infant. Fatigue, pain, cold, hunger, and thirst are discomforts frequently reported by mothers after delivery. Not uncommonly, the postpartal mother experiences a spell of uncontrollable shaking of the legs. In the typical labor, the mother has received medication for relaxation and pain relief and is encumbered in her movements by intravenous tubing.

Certain conditions in the infant indicate lowered potential for human interaction. In addition to the physiologic adaptations immediately necessary to extrauterine existence, physical maturity, nutritional adequacy, neurologic intactness, bodily discomfort, extremes of temperature, and levels of analgesic and anesthetic agents have all been related to the infant's behavioral responses in the first hours of life—and later. Prophylactic eye treatments interfere with the infant's ability to keep his eyes open and focused on the mother's face. Generally speaking, any situation, condition, or stimulus that detracts from the energy either partner can direct toward attending to the other diminishes the probability of optimal interaction between the two.

MOTHER-INFANT INTERACTIONS

Introductory Bonding

Observers of very early mother-infant interactions in hospital settings have presented evidence that a fairly regular pattern of maternal behaviors is exhibited at first contact with the normal newborn (Rubin, 1963; Klaus et al., 1970). In a progression of touching activities, the mother proceeds from fingertip exploration of the baby's extremities toward palmar contact with the larger body areas and finally to enfolding the infant with the whole hand and arms. The time taken to accomplish these steps varies from minutes to days, depending, it appears, on the timing of the first contact, the clothing barriers present, and the physical condition of the baby. Maternal excitement and elation tend to increase during the time of the initial meeting. The mother also increases the proportion of time spent in the *en face* position. She arranges herself or the infant so that direct face-to-face and eye-to-eye contact is facilitated. There is an intense interest in having the baby's eyes open. When the eyes are open, the mother characteristically greets the infant and talks to him in high-pitched tones.

Clinical observations indicate that behaviors differ somewhat in nonconventional delivery situations. Home birth and LeBoyer deliveries seem to speed up and otherwise modify the behaviors described. Often after a home birth the mother turns almost immediately to pick up and hold the baby and to rub its cheek with her fingertip. The baby is often offered the breast before the placenta is expelled. In a delivery patterned after the LeBoyer method, the mother, and sometimes the father, is encouraged to gently massage the infant's whole body while waiting for the placenta to be delivered.

In most instances the mother relies heavily on her senses of sight, touch, and hearing in getting to know what her baby is really like. She tends also to respond verbally to any sounds emitted by the baby, such as cries, coughs, sneezes, and grunts. The sense of smell may also be involved, although this possibility has not been adequately studied as yet.

In addition to acting upon and interacting with the baby, the mother is undergoing her own emotional reactions to the whole happening and, more specifically, to the baby as she perceives him. Sometimes direct comments and nonverbal cues clearly reflect the felt emotions; sometimes the mother reports only later on her feelings at the time. The frequency of the "I can't believe" reaction leads to the speculation that human gains as well as losses might initially be responded to with a degree of shock, disbelief, and denial. A feeling of emotional distance from the newborn is quite common: "I felt he was a stranger." On the other hand, feelings of connectedness between the baby and the rest of the famiy can be expressed in positive or negative terms: "She's got your cute nose, Daddy" or "Oh, God, no! He looks just like the first one, and he was an impossible baby." A mother's facial expressions or the frequency and content of her questions may demonstrate concerns about the infant's general condition or normality, especially if her pregnancy was complicated or if a previously delivered baby was not normal.

Some of the more common emotional reactions to the infant at birth have been noted briefly. There is, of course, a wide range of possible maternal feelings seen at delivery—positive, negative, and mixed. There are also differences in the intensity of feeling and in the mode of expression. For example, intense pleasure may be shown in smiles or in tears. In general, extremely negative feelings are predictive of later problems in the mother-infant relationship.

During the initial mother-infant interaction the baby, too, is continuously communicating. Although he behaves without conscious intent to convey interpersonal messages or to influence the behavior of others, elements of his appearance and behavior are perceived by the mother as if they represented intentionality and interpersonal dialogue, and they do influence her responses. The baby's size says to the mother, "You nourished me well—you did a good job." Individual features say, "I am a part of you, or of my father. I belong with you." Even the time of birth can be read as a message: "I'm cooperative—or uncooperative." The intensity, timing, configuration, and other elements of the newborn's observable activity, however reflexive, are regularly responded to as a very personal communication from the baby to his mother.

What are the characteristic behaviors of a newborn? Unless care is taken to effect a gentle birth, a number of noxious stimuli impinge on the senses of the newly born infant. He is probably suctioned, held by the feet with his head down, exposed to bright lights and cool air, and in some way cleaned. He usually responds by crying. In fact, he is typically stimulated to cry to reassure his caretakers that he is well and normal. When he no longer needs to concentrate most of his energy in physical and physiologic response to the immediate crisis of birth, he is able to lie quietly with eyes open, looking about, moving limbs occasionally, making sucking motions, possibly attempting to get hand to mouth. Placed in appropriate proximity to his mother, he appears to focus briefly on her face and to attend to her voice repeatedly in the first moments. When mother is talking and he is attending, he is likely to move parts of his body—arms, legs, fingers, eyelids—in an exact synchrony with his mother's minute voice changes (Condon and Sander, 1974). This synchrony between rhythms of speech and body movements of an infant can clearly be seen only with stop-frame analysis of films, but the mother probably has, at some level, an awareness of its occurrence.

The introductory mother-infant interaction proceeds on the basis of identified, mutually elicited behaviors, occurring simultaneously and in multiplicity between the partners. The significant

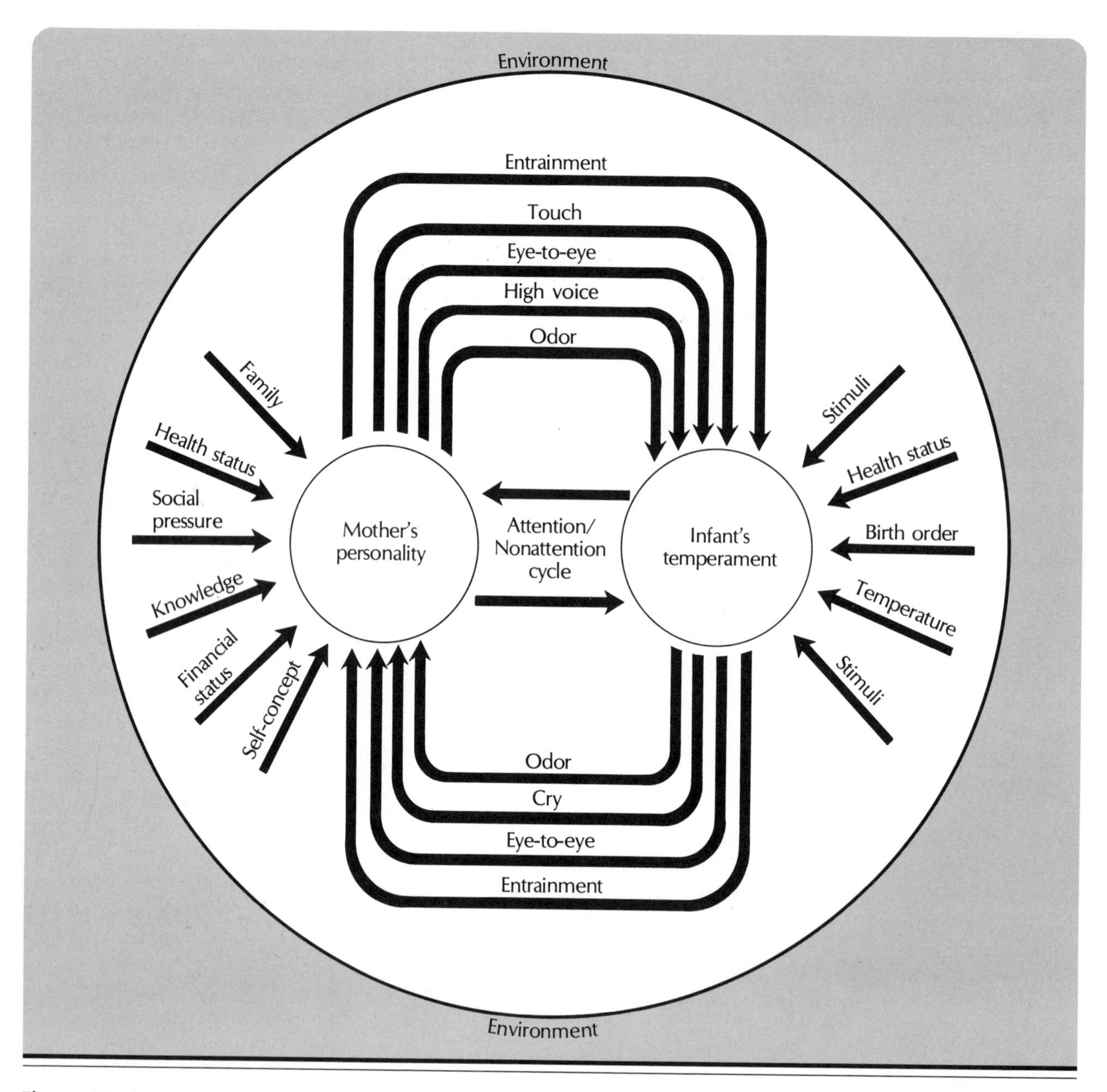

Figure 28–1. Reciprocity system.

behavioral cues that shape the dyadic interaction at the first and subsequent contacts are illustrated in Figure 28–1.

Another kind of mutuality of experience may bring the mother into emotional closeness with her infant. If the birthing has been essentially normal and the partners are not prevented from immediate contact, they share in common the experiences of surviving a traumatic event, being brought to a state of alertness, gathering information about the other through direct interaction, and, if time permits, subsiding into a sleep of recovery. Both have demonstrated to each other the heightened capacity for interaction that has been observed during the first hours after birth.

Much evidence has accumulated to show that facilitation of this apparent readiness to relate to each other results in an increased maternal responsiveness to the infant's needs that endures over time (Lozoff et al., 1977). In a number of related studies, some groups of mothers were given earlier and/or more extended contact with their newborn than was the routine for control groups of similar mothers and then were observed in later interactions with their infants. Mothers allowed earlier contact and/or increased in-hospital contact smiled more at their infants, showed more face-to-face behavior, and were quicker to use soothing and comforting behaviors when their infants exhibited distress. They appeared to enjoy subsequent contact with their infants more than the control group of mothers did. Differences between the groups were observable two years later. Klaus et al. (1970) and others have concluded that there is a period of increased maternal sensitivity in the early minutes and hours after birth, during which mother-infant contact is likely to enhance the development of the emotional bond between the mother and her infant and to influence the nature and direction of the relationship in the early years. The term *bonding* might well be reserved for application to the time of the attraction peak immediately after birth, when first contact occurs.

Acquaintance Phase

During the introductory contact after birth, the mother gathers a certain amount of information about her baby. This learning about the partner is the first step in any interpersonal acquaintance. As described in relation to adults (Newcomb, 1961), the acquaintance process includes the following components: the acquisition of knowledge about the other, assessment of the other's attitude, and either reinforcement or change in existing states of orientation toward the other. From the remarks, questions, and activities of a new mother in the earliest postpartal days, it is apparent that she is applying herself to the task of getting acquainted with her baby. She wants to know what kind of baby she is taking into her family system and what the baby's reaction to her is. She is also consciously involved in clarifying the nature of her own developing feelings toward the baby. In part she is becoming acquainted with herself as the mother of this particular infant.

There is some indication that the degree to which a mother develops feelings of affectionate closeness or attachment to the fetus before birth is generally predictive of the course of maternal feelings toward the baby immediately after birth and in the acquaintance phase (Leifer, 1977). Minimal closeness before birth seems to lead to less enjoyment of the baby, less responsiveness to his needs, and less empathy when the infant is in distress. Women who feel an intense attachment and interaction before birth appear to pick up the relationship at that level after delivery and to develop increased feelings of closeness in the acquaintance phase. They eagerly respond to the infant's needs and are gratified by the infant's apparent well-being. In addition, they are likely to be more successful at initiating and maintaining breast-feeding than are minimally attached mothers. Liking the baby at the start apparently contributes to the woman's understanding of her infant as an individual with unique needs and adds to her willingness to respond to those needs. The positive orientation at the beginning of contact probably also influences the woman toward a positive perception of her infant's attitude toward her as a mother. It helps her believe that her baby appreciates her.

Just as in the bonding phase, the infant plays an important part in determining the outcome of the acquaintance phase of the mother-infant relationship. He can either assist or confound the mother as she attempts to learn his embryonic personality, his characteristic abilities and behaviors. If he is relatively well organized in his responses to the usual caretaking stimuli and is regular in his biologic rhythms, he tends to be easy to understand. If he gives clear behavioral cues about his needs, his responses to mothering will be predictable. Such predictability makes a mother feel effective and competent—a pleasant feeling. If the baby responds to motherly ministrations with a predominantly positive mood rather than with irritability, and if he has relatively long periods of being quietly awake and attentive, he is pleasant to be near and to interact with. Other behaviors that make a baby more attractive to his caretakers are smiling, grasping a finger, nursing eagerly, cuddling, and being easy to console.

At the same time that he is unknowingly facilitating or providing obstacles to the mother's acquaintance with him, the infant is also becoming acquainted. Thrust unexpectedly into a strange environment, he is gathering what information he can about his new world. He is attending to sights, sounds, tastes, and smells. He is experiencing different tactile and kinesthetic sensations. Within a few days after birth, he shows signs of recognizing recurrent situations and responding to changes in routine. To the extent that the world is his mother, it can be said that he is actively acquainting himself with her.

The peak of the acquaintance phase appears to occur simultaneously with one of the phases of maternal puerperal restoration described by Rubin (1961). In the "taking-in" phase, which lasts for two or three days, the mother has a need to replenish her physical and emotional resources. Her inclination is to take in food, praise, information, sleep, and nurturance, in a rather undiscriminating and passive way. She seems impelled to review and to integrate every detail of her labor and delivery. So much happened in such a short time that it was difficult to take it all in while it was happening.

When the taking-in phase of rest and recuperation draws to a close and the acquaintance phase is well under way, the "taking-hold" phase of active maternal involvement with self and infant begins. The mother acts to regain control of her bodily functioning, to initiate mothering tasks, and to reintegrate herself with her family in the new role of mother with baby.

Phase of Mutual Regulation

In the performance of the necessary tasks of infant care, such as feeding, bathing, and comforting, the new mother develops an awareness, on some level, that there is a degree of discrepancy between her wishes and needs and her baby's needs and desires. This awareness ushers in a phase of mutual regulation of behaviors. The degree of control to be exerted by each partner in the interpersonal adjustment is an issue in the early postpartal weeks. Maternal goals related to the resolution of this issue of control, are, of course variable, both among different mothers and within the same mother at different times. In some mother-infant pairs, the maternal goal is primarily to change the infant to meet the mother's needs. In other pairs it is quite apparent that the mother's intent is primarily to interpret correctly and to gratify completely all of her infant's needs. Either of those approaches is likely to result in relational disturbances, the degree of distress and tension depending to a large extent on the infant's reactions to the maternal behaviors used to reach the goal. For example, the mother who wishes to adjust her baby rather than adjust to him will have a smoother postpartal course if she is blessed with a highly adaptive baby who is positive in mood. The mother who is bent on meeting every need of her child at the same moment it arises will meet with failure very quickly if she has produced an infant who is unpredictable, is irregular in daily rhythms, and presents behavioral cues that are difficult to interpret. This kind of infant can easily take on the role of "spoiled" baby in a family.

The ideal solution to the control issue would be somewhere between the two extremes. A mother who realizes that she is a person with her own needs will be less vulnerable to the buildup of anger, frustration, anxiety, and guilt. In all but the most ideal situations, each partner must undergo disappointments, and each must at some time subordinate his or her own needs to the needs of the other. The most important consideration is that each should obtain a good measure of enjoyment from the ongoing interactions.

Generally speaking, it would seem that enjoyment is enhanced during the early months if the infant is sufficiently organized to clearly indicate his needs and if the mother's personality allows her to let him lead the interaction. Mutual maternal-infant regulation is never instantaneous; it is a process that continues to some degree throughout infancy and childhood. Fortunately, there appears to be a tendency toward improved organization of behavior in the newborn period and an increasing ability to nurture in the mother during the same time.

It is during the mutual adjustment phase that negative maternal feelings are likely to surface or intensify. Because "everyone knows that mothers love their babies," these negative feelings often go unexpressed and are allowed to build up. If they are expressed, the response of friends, relatives, or health care personnel is often to deny the feeling to the mother: "You don't mean that"; "You can't feel that way"; "Your baby is not ugly, she is beautiful." Some negative feelings are normal in the first few days following delivery, and the nurse should be supportive when the mother vocalizes these feelings.

In the adjustment phase a mother may become ready to learn more about infants in general and about her infant in particular (Adams, 1963). The mothering problems to be addressed have already arisen and become clarified. Information is needed to develop effective solutions. If valid information is available, the solutions will be more appropriate and more lasting than those based on inadequate data.

When mutual regulation arrives at the point where both partners have achieved a predominance of enjoyment in each other's company, it is usually obvious to an observer that things are going well in the relationship. It may be said that reciprocity has been achieved. A high degree of reciprocity is characteristic of successful mutual regulation.

Reciprocity

The mother-infant interaction process can be visualized as a system. This system is concerned with the mother-infant unit, the interactions between them, and the environment within which they operate. The interpersonal interaction is a reciprocal process that relies on cues from each member to instigate and maintain it. As in any dynamic interpersonal system, certain reactions are expected and anticipated, but individual behavioral input may vary, thus producing variations in the system's functioning.

Reciprocity within a mother-infant system may be described as an interactional cycle that occurs simultaneously between the mother and the infant (Brazelton et al., 1974). It involves mutual cuing behaviors, expectancy, rhythmicity, and synchrony. There are intimations of reciprocity in the early hours of life. The mother and her infant are like two actors who respond to each other's cues. During several weeks of interactive continuity, they establish a pattern of behavior in which they mesh with each other. When this meshing or synchrony is attained, the couple perform a reciprocal dance of cyclical attention and nonattention. Brazelton and his colleagues have studied this reciprocal process in the laboratory and have carefully analyzed the component parts. He has described five phases of the cycle: (a) initiation, (b) orientation, (c) acceleration, (d) deceleration, and (e) turning away. The first two phases establish the partner's expectations regarding the interaction. Both mother and infant utilize clusters of behaviors as the interaction develops. Feedback between partners enables them to modulate their behaviors. Sensitivity and adjustment by the mother allows the infant to maintain his homeostatic state and to develop an expanding attention cycle. The infant may begin to develop recognizable patterning of behavior by about 2 weeks of age, and it is often well established by 6 weeks.

If the observer is aware of what to look for, the segments of an interactional cycle can be described as they are observed. The following is a hypothetical example of an interactional period, as it is likely to appear when things are going well:

Initiation: The infant is being held on the mother's knee, facing her. He looks toward her with a relaxed expression and makes slow movements with his arms and hands.

Orientation: As the infant makes eye contact with his mother, his eyes brighten and become alert, and he turns his whole body toward her, extending arms and legs in her direction. He reaches toward the mother.

State of attention: The mother smiles and talks to the infant, and he responds by smiling, moving his arms and legs in pedaling motions, cooing, and making other sounds. The eyes alternately become alert and dull as he responds to the smiles and words of his mother. The limbs move rhythmically, and if watched carefully, the ebb and flow of movement can be seen to keep time with the mother's voice. There is a constant slow smooth reaching and circular movement occurring as the tension within the infant's body rises and falls. The infant assumes the look of expectancy.

Acceleration: The infant continues to move, to wave his hands and feet about, and to increase his smiling activity. His eyes are bright and alert. He strains toward his mother in the intensity of the interaction, all the time watching her and cuing to her smile. For the most part, the body movement is smooth, but there may be occasional jerkiness.

Peak of excitement: As the infant becomes wholly involved in the interaction, his movements may become jerky and intense. He brings his hand to his mouth and tries to insert his thumb while still smiling and cooing. The other hand clutches his thigh and he leans forward to his mother as she continues to smile at him. As he endeavors to reach forward, his back arches and his body tends to twist toward one side.

Deceleration: The excitement begins to pass off as the infant's movements slow. There is a gradual decrease in body movement, the bright look dims, the eyes become dull, and the lids appear to droop. The smiles fade, and vocalization decreases. Suddenly the infant yawns and begins to suck his thumb as he leans away from his mother. His hands drop to his lap with the fingers widespread, and he appears to be relaxing.

Withdrawal or turning away: The infant's activity slows down almost completely. He slumps against his mother's hands with his body half turned away from her. His eyes are dull and focused in the direction of an object to the side. There is a faint smile on his face. The mother stops smiling and talking to the infant. She just sits holding him quietly, waiting for his next cue. The mother briefly raises her head and glances beyond the infant. This prompts a reaction in the infant. He looks toward his mother, smiles briefly, and looks away again, then turns back to the mother, ready to resume another period of interaction.

The responsibility for monitoring cues and for sensitively initiating or maintaining the interaction rests primarily with the mother. The infant uses the nonattention time to recover from the tension of interaction, to organize his behavior, and to process what he has taken in during the attentive periods.

The development of reciprocity between a mother and her infant is evidence of the bond or attachment that has formed between them. It enables the mother to let go of the infant as she knew him during pregnancy. A new relationship now develops with an individual who has his own unique character and who evokes a response entirely different from the fantasy response of pregnancy. When reciprocity is synchronous, the interaction between mother and infant is mutually gratifying and is sought and initiated by both partners. Pleasure and delight develop in each other's company, and there is mutual development of love and growth.

Not all mothers fall in love with their infant instantaneously. Reciprocity may take weeks to develop, and it requires sensitive stimuli from both actors. As the infant becomes more organized in his behavior and as his senses develop, he is able to give positive feedback to his mother. He transmits the appearance of listening, he follows voice and movements, and he responds with intentionality to her as an individual whom he recognizes and seeks to communicate with.

In cases where either the mother or the infant is sick and the initial acquaintance is delayed, there is likely to be a concomitant delay in the development of reciprocity. In some cases the lag may be so detrimental to the process that reciprocity never develops.

Overstimulation or inappropriate stimulation by the mother may interfere with the synchrony of the interaction. In the resultant dyssynchrony, the mother may be in the attention phase of the reciprocal process when the infant is in the nonattention phase. This dyssynchrony can lead to frustration on the part of either partner or both and may lead to a disharmonious relationship as both become established in their interactional patterns. In extreme instances mother and infant may cease to communicate with each other.

Infants vary in their strategies for dealing with an overload of stimulation. Four types of reaction have been described in infants responding to unpleasant and inappropriately timed stimuli (Brazelton et al., 1974): active physical withdrawal, rejection, decreased sensitivity, and communication of distress. An infant can move away form the source of stimulation, can push the stimulus away from him, can lapse into drowsiness or sleep, or can fuss and cry. Some of these strategies, if they become characteristic of an infant's behavior, are easier to live with than others; they interact with a mother's expectations and her personality.

It is quite possible that the nurse will have the opportunity to observe reciprocity developing between a mother and her infant in the early weeks of life. If she recognizes the appearance of dyssynchrony, she may be able to initiate intervention before the dyssynchronous behaviors become firmly established.

The ultimate goals of nursing care in the maternity cycle are the continuation of life and the enhancement of the quality of that life in terms of physical and mental health. There is reason to believe that a state of mutual attachment or an enduring emotional bond between a parent (or parent surrogate) and an infant is essential to the infant's optimum health. It appears also that a new mother's feelings of closeness or attachment to her infant have a positive effect on her own continued personal growth. The same is probably true of a new father. Therefore, the facilitation of parent-infant attachment is a significant goal to pursue. But what is attachment, and how is it most effectively established and maintained between members of a beginning family?

NATURE OF ATTACHMENT

"To him who in the love of nature holds communion with her visible forms she speaks a various language." Those lines, written by the poet William Cullen Bryant, could have been written to describe parent-infant attachment. The naked, thumbnail-sized newborn kangaroo demonstrates its attachment to its mother by climbing upward virtually unaided from the birth opening into the pouch and by physically attaching mouth to nipple in such a way that the force required to separate the two would rupture tissue before breaking the bond. In the case of an ibex, the dynamics are quite different. The young is born so nimble and quick that he goes off up the rocky terrain by leaps and bounds and his mother must follow him in the first hours to establish a bond of closeness.

Mothers and infants throughout the natural world emit and receive communications by certain sensory modalities—the varied languages of smell, taste, touch, sight, and sound. A hen turkey will kill her own young if she does not hear the cheeping sounds that are characteristic of newly hatched turkeys. A mother deer will abandon a fawn that has been handled by a human, who thus alters its olfactory signal. A graylag goose tends to attach to the first object it sights after leaving the egg.

What is the language of human attachment? How can the concept of attachment apply to so many different patterns of behavior? Those who have studied attachment in the past 40 years have approached the topic with different goals, out of varying professional backgrounds, and from opposite directions. Among the purposes of the research on attachment have been to describe it, to operationally define it, to relate it to outcomes in cognitive and social development, to support or refute psychologic theories, and to determine public child care policy. The background disciplines of researchers and clinicians interested in attachment include psychoanalysis, psychiatry, psychology, pediatrics, obstetrics, social work, teaching, child development, ethnology, and nursing.

The two major directions of attachment that are investigated are from mother to infant and from infant to mother. The early literature on attachment related primarily to the infant's tie to its mother, which was understood to occur in the second half of the first year of life, when the infant was capable of recognizing the mother. This literature was derived in part from experience with maternally deprived infants. More recently, and motivated in part by disorders and failures in mothering, researchers have investigated the attachment of mothers to infants. The importance of fathers and siblings as attachers and attachees is in the early stages of exploration.

Just this brief glimpse at the past history of the concept of attachment makes it easy to understand why the language of attachment research is indeed a various one. Definitions of the term, when found, vary in specificity and generality.

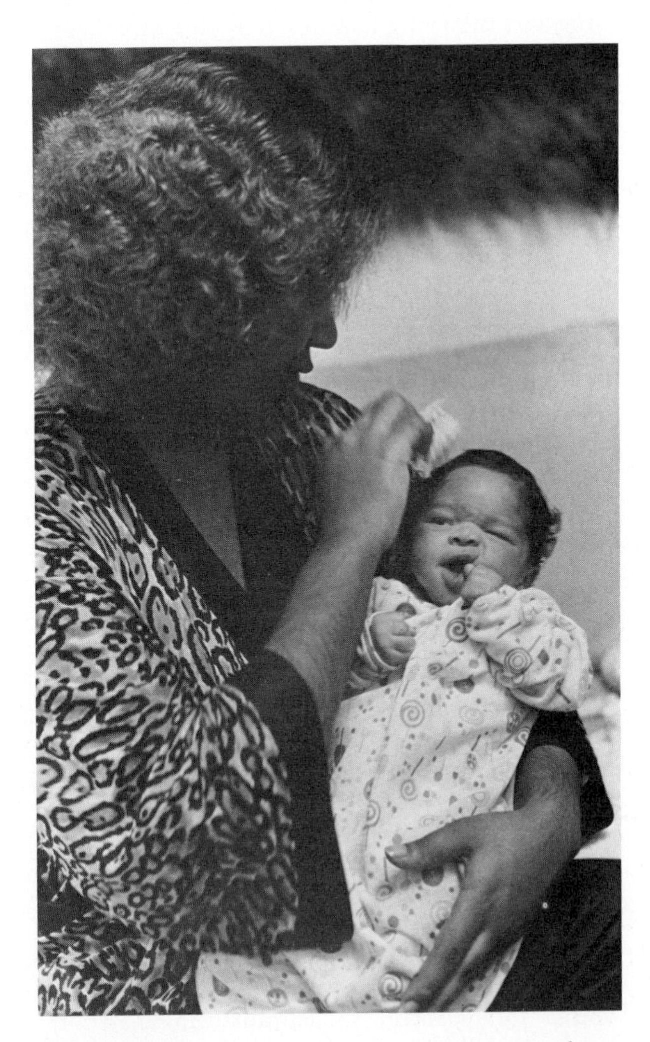

Figure 28–2. The way in which the mother performs her caretaking tasks is a good indication of her maternicity.

Behaviors said to indicate attachment vary. Terms such as *bond, affectional tie,* and *affiliation* are often treated interchangeably and are used as synonyms for attachment without themselves being defined.

Whichever definition or description of attachment is accepted, everyone involved in the investigation or facilitation of healthy parent-infant interaction is in agreement that the chances for optimum growth and development of both parents and infants increase as the quality of attachment is enhanced. Because the facilitation of parent-to-infant attachment has become an accepted goal in maternal-child health nursing, an important first step toward that goal is the achievement of a clear understanding of the nature of attachment. Following is a proposed definition of parent-to-infant attachment designed to help nurses who are in direct contact with members of beginning and enlarging families. It is a tentative working definition, presented for consideration, which takes the form of an ideal outcome to be pursued.

Attachment is an attraction to and inclination to nurture one's infant that is consistently acted upon, intelligently and sensitively, with predominately positive feeling. This definition implies a cycle of feelings that lead to mothering activities, which are in turn accompanied or followed by feelings. Ludington-Hoe (1977) has termed the physical caretaking tasks "mothering" and the emotional aspects "maternicity." She suggests *maternicity* as a nursing diagnostic term for the emotional component of the maternal role. It includes qualities that enable the mother to feel warmth, affection, attachment, protectiveness, and devotion to the child. The physical tasks of the mother's role can be observed and evaluated when the nurse is with the interacting pair. Maternicity is not as easily noted and assessed, as it can be expressed in a variety of ways at different times in the maternity cycle. However, many of the activities that provide clues to the quality of maternal bonding also provide useful guides to the degree of maternicity the mother has developed (Figure 28–2).

FATHER-INFANT INTERACTIONS

In the past 25 years, the typical perinatal experience of an expectant father has changed considerably. Many maternity nurses can remember a time when fathers-to-be kissed their wives goodby at the admitting room door and went home to await the obstetrician's phone call announcing the new arrival. Often the father and mother were not reunited for several hours after the birth, as the mother was recovering from anesthesia. The infant was usually viewed through the nursery window, and the father was not permitted to touch or hold him until all three were reunited on the day of hospital discharge. Under present, more humanized hospital practices, increasing numbers of fathers have the opportunity to become directly involved in the life of their infant from the moment of birth.

Traditionally, the father has been seen as the primary source of support for his wife. He contributed to the growth and development of his young infant indirectly by nurturing and supporting his wife through the pregnancy and the early postpartal weeks. As women became interested in a different kind of childbearing experience and began to attend classes to prepare themselves for more participation in the birth process, they came to value husbands, and the hospital staff, as an additional support during labor. But for years after the father was permitted to coach his wife in labor, he was still left behind at the delivery room door to await a doctor's report of the birth and a brief reunion with mother and baby as they left the delivery room. Gradually couples became less willing to be separated from each other during any part of the childbearing experience, and they became more vocal about expressing their wishes. At the same time, health care workers became more cognizant of the emotional and educational needs of the whole family and more willing to permit paternal participation during the entire hospital stay.

Out of commitment to a family-centered approach to maternity care, there developed an interest in understanding the experiences and feelings of the new father. The formerly ignored and little understood father became the willing subject of a number of research endeavors. Some of these indicate that a father experiences feelings

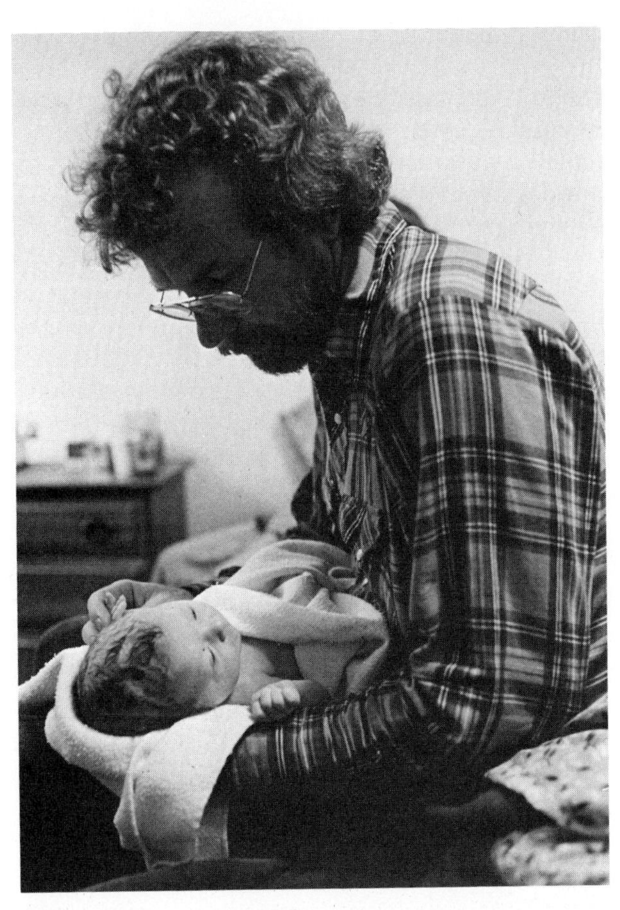

Figure 28–3. The bond between father and infant develops.

toward his newly born infant that are quite similar to the mother's feelings of attachment. In the past the significance of any psychologic response called fatherliness has been minimized. It was implied that, because the man did not have deep physiologic roots of fatherliness, his feelings were somehow of less importance than the mother's and were weaker and longer in developing. There is increasing evidence that a father does have a strong attraction to his newborn and highly positive emotional reactions to first contact. The first hours after delivery appear to be significant in the development of the father-infant bond as well as the mother-infant bond.

Greenberg and Morris (1974) have noted the reactions of first-time fathers to early contact with their infants. They used the term *engrossment* to label characteristic aspects of the impact of the newborn on the father—his sense of absorption, preoccupation, and interest in the infant. From this engrossment, the attachment bond between the father and his infant develops. As a result of their study of new fathers, the authors have described the characteristics of engrossment commonly found among fathers in the early postpartal days.

In general, the father is strongly attracted to his newborn and enjoys looking at him. He sees the baby as a unique individual with personal features and qualities that distinguish him from other newborns. The baby's face is particularly attractive and beautiful. Many fathers see their babies as perfect. The body contact involved in holding the newborn, touching the skin, and feeling the limb movements is extremely pleasurable and is sought out (Figure 28–3). The emotional reaction to first sight of the infant and later contacts is very positive. Greenberg and Morris (1974) found that nearly all the fathers studied felt elated and gave indication of increased self-esteem.

These heightened feelings and perceptions of new fathers can be compared to those present in an infatuation. The degree of involvement in the love affair with his baby can draw a man's time and energy away from the ongoing husband-wife relationship. The husband who has been encouraged to support his wife in her new mothering role may feel some guilt about preoccupation with the baby, and the wife may feel ignored or excluded from a significant relationship. It seems likely that couples who shared experiences, relationships, and material things before the birth will be better able to share their baby's attention after the birth and to share the responsibilities of parenting, too.

When he is pulled as if by a magnet into contact with his infant, the new father initiates direct interaction, and the infant responds and initiates behaviors. As with the mother-infant interaction, the infant contributes his part. He cries and moves, indicating his aliveness and well-being. His spontaneous and reflexive movements and grimaces are interpreted by the father as personal dialogue with him, and the father responds by voice and touch. From the beginning, the father's interactive behaviors are different from the mother's, and these differences are perceptible to the infant. A father's odor, voice pitch, appearance, and touch qualities are all different from a mother's. In a face-to-face "play situation," a mother tends to use her hands to enfold and enclose her baby's body and limbs, gently modulating and smoothing out motions, whereas the father punctuates his conversation with finger pokes and more exaggerated changes in facial expression, which act to increase the baby's excitement level. Observers have noted differences in a baby's responses to interaction with mother or father as early as two weeks after birth.

Mothers, too, appear to notice a difference. Often in the early weeks, when asked if they play with the baby, mothers say, "No, but my husband does." It seems as if one function of the father-infant interaction is to further acquaint the mother with her baby's range of possible behaviors in the context of a shared relationship.

In families where the husband-wife relationship has not developed adequate stability, evidence of the baby's increased excitement and entrancement when interacting with the father can be interpreted by the mother in ways that are dangerous to the family system. For example, feelings of competition, resentment, or incompetence can arise and become detrimental to all family members.

Goals for family-centered nursing care during pregnancy should include an assessment of the couple's ability to share the experience of pregnancy through various forms of communication. Often each partner has important feelings, hopes, fantasies, and fears that have not been communicated to the other. They often unknowingly share the same concerns, which neither speaks of for fear of worrying the other. By stimulating open discussion about matters relating to the pregnancy, a nurse can help develop patterns of communication and sharing for continued use in family living.

It might be helpful if, during the pregnancy, nurses explain the potential for engrossment of the father after birth. If both parents are aware that each has needs at this time, they may be better able to support each other's growing relationship to this added family member. Many fathers in the Greenberg and Morris study were surprised and amazed at the extent of their feelings toward the newborn. The unexpectedness of the feelings seemed to increase the father's preoccupation with his relationship to the infant. Further study is needed to describe the ways in which couples successfully cope with their own feelings and needs while continuing to support each other in the childbearing experience. In order to make nursing goals appropriate and intervention effective, more knowledge is also needed about the long-term effects of different levels of direct paternal involvement on the quality of the father-child relationship and other family relationships.

SIBLINGS AND OTHERS

Little is known about the components of bonding between the new baby and his siblings. Most parents endeavor to prepare their children for the advent of a new baby. The type and extent of the preparation may depend on the age of the children and the type of relationships that exist in the home. If the new baby is seen as nonthreatening to the relationships the children have with their parents, there will probably be minimal disruption, and the new baby will be accepted without serious problems (Figure 28-4).

The conventional view of the bonding or attachment process has been that the infant was capable of forming only one bond at a time and that this bond should be to the mother. Bowlby (1958) called this tie *monotropy.* More recent work with infants has shown that they are capable of maintaining a number of attachments. These attachments may include siblings, grandparents, aunts, and uncles. Some infants were found to be capable of forming attachments with five or more people simultaneously without loss of quality. The social setting and personalities of the individuals would appear to be significant factors in permitting the development of multiple attachments.

EVALUATION AND INTERVENTIONS IN MOTHER-INFANT RELATIONSHIPS

Nurses come into professional contact with women and their families at any point in the maternity cycle. The nurse may be operating as a representative of an agency—such as a public health office, hospital, doctor's office, child protection center, or a childbirth education group—

face-to-face contact, and eye contact? Is she actively reaching out or only passively receiving? Does she hold the infant on her left side? Is attraction increasing or decreasing? If the mother does not exhibit increasing attraction, why not? Do the reasons lie primarily within her, in the baby, or in the environment?

It is not enough to report a deficiency. Appropriate intervention is called for, and it requires an understanding of precipitating influences. Such knowledge guides the nurse in selecting measures to increase attraction.

2. Is the mother inclined to nurture her infant? Is she progressing through the stages of taking in, taking hold, and letting go in her interactions with her infant? Has she selected a rooming-in arrangement if it is available?

3. Does she act consistently? Is she developing a consistent and predictable approach to the care of her infant? Does she tend to respond to the same situation in the same way from day to day? If not, is the source of unpredictability within her or her infant?

4. Is her mothering intelligently carried out? Does she seek information and evaluate it objectively? Does she develop solutions based on adequate knowledge of valid data? How did she prepare herself for the parenting role? Does she evaluate the effectiveness of her maternal care and make appropriate adjustment?

5. Is she sensitively responsive to the infant's needs as they arise? How quickly does she interpret infant behavior and react to cues? How much of this ability and willingness to respond is related to the baby's nature and how much to her own?

6. Is she experiencing pleasure in the interaction with her infant? What times are most and least enjoyable? What interferes with the enjoyment?

When these questions are addressed and the facts have been assembled by the nurse, the feelings she experienced and her background of knowledge should combine to answer three more questions: Is there a problem in attachment? What is the problem? What is its source? Each nurse can then devise a creative approach to the problem as it presents itself in the context of a unique developing mother-infant relationship.

It is necessary for nurses to creatively design on-the-spot measures for each situation, for two reasons. First, each situation is unique and extremely complex. Second, there are few intervention designs that have proven effective for general application to clinical practice in maternal-infant care. Longitudinal studies of families from early pregnancy through six months or a year after birth are needed. Patterns of nursing intervention need to be explicated in detail and carefully evaluated as to results obtained in varying situations of personality descriptions, past histories, pregnancy outcomes, infant temperaments, family environments, and medical settings. Health delivery systems that allow for continuity of nursing care by one nurse or by a few effectively communicating nurses are in a position to facilitate nursing research that could eventually lead to increased efficiency in the use of health care resources in the area of maternal-infant interaction.

SUMMARY

A mother's feelings for and her behavior toward her newborn are determined by multiple factors. Past experiences, personality, pregnancy experiences, human environment, and physical setting combine to shape a mother's potential for nurturant interaction with her baby. The father is important both in his contribution to the emotional climate within which the fetus and infant is nurtured by the mother and as a nurturing and interacting figure in his own right. The infant is born with interactive capacities, which continue to develop through appropriate adult social stimulation. Generally speaking, when the lives and relationships of the procreating pair are going well, they are likely to continue in a positive direction through the course of pregnancy and adjustment to the new family member. When emotional resources and social skills are lacking in a couple and when they are generally discontent, a pregnancy and postpartal adjustment period will tend to be negatively perceived, and positive feeling for the baby will be diminished or delayed.

It would be nice if there were simple nursing measures to change negative maternal feelings to positive, but such is not the case. Instead, the nurse, who ideally has achieved emotional maturity and a measure of psychosocial skills, is challenged to understand each mother-infant pair within its unique context. Such a level of patient and family knowledge is made possible only through the development of a nurse-patient relationship of mutual trust, which is facilitated by continuity of interpersonal contact. In the absence of opportunity for an ongoing relationship, continuous communication of data relevant to the developing mother-infant relationship is essential to effective maternal support. Helping to initiate and maintain a healthy attachment in all its many aspects is a primary preventive goal of importance to family life. Improvement of disordered relationships is another priority goal. Nurses can support these goals through direct patient care, through initiating changes in health care delivery systems, and through research for evaluation of nursing interventions.

SUGGESTED ACTIVITIES

1. Observe, without intervening, three mother-infant interactions. Identify the maternal-infant interaction phase, and determine whether positive attachment is occurring.
2. Observe three father-infant interactions, and describe differences from mother-infant interactions.
3. Make a collection of pictures illustrating mother-infant, father-infant, and sibling-infant interactions.

REFERENCES

Adams, M. 1963. Early concerns of primigravida mothers regarding infant care activities. *Nurs. Res.* 12:72.

Bowlby, J. 1958. The nature of the child's tie to his mother. *Internat. J. Psychoanal.* 39:350.

Brazelton, T. B., et al. 1974. The origins of reciprocity: the early mother-infant interaction. In *The effect of the infant on its caregiver,* eds. M. Lewis and L. A. Rosenblum. New York: John Wiley & Sons, Inc.

Condon, W. S., and Sander, L. W. June 1974. Synchrony demonstrated between movements of the neonate and adult speech. *Child Dev.* 45:456.

Goren, C. C., et al. 1975. Visual following and pattern discrimination of face-like stimuli by newborn infants. *Pediatrics.* 56:544.

Greenberg, M., and Morris, N. 1974. Engrossment: the newborn's impact upon the father. *Am. J. Orthopsychiatry.* 44:520.

Kennedy, J. C. 1969. *The little stranger: mother-infant acquaintance in the first two weeks.* Unpublished doctoral dissertation, Boston University.

Klaus, M. H., et al. 1970. Human maternal behavior at first contact with her young. *Pediatrics.* 46:187.

Korner, A. F., and Thoman, E. B. 1970. Visual alertness in neonates as evoked by maternal care. *J. Exploratory Child Psych.* 10:67.

Leifer, M. 1977. Psychological changes accompanying pregnancy and motherhood. *Genet. Psychol. Monographs.* 95:55.

Lozoff, B., et al. 1977. The Mother-newborn relationship: limits of adaptability. *J. Pediatr.* 91:1.

Ludington-Hoe, S. L. 1977. Postpartum: development of maternicity. *Am. J. Nurs.* 77:1171.

Newcomb, T. M. 1961. *The acquaintance process.* New York: Holt, Rinehart & Winston, Inc.

Nuckolls, K. B., et al. 1972. Psychological assets, life crisis and the prognosis of pregnancy. *Am. J. Epidemiology.* 95:431.

Rubin, R. 1961. Puerperal change. *Nurs. Outlook.* 9:753.

Rubin, R. 1963. Maternal touch. *Nurs. Outlook.* 11:828.

Shereshefsky, P. M., and Yarrow, L. J. 1973. *Psychological aspects of a first pregnancy and postnatal adaptation.* New York: Raven.

ADDITIONAL READINGS

Bromwich, R. M. 1976. Focus of maternal behavior in infant intervention. *Am. J. Orthopsychiatry.* 40:439.

Broussard, E. R., and Hartner, M. S. 1970. Maternal perception of the neonate as related to development. *Child Psychiatry Hum. Develop.* 1:16.

Rubin, R. 1977. Bonding-in in the postpartum period. *Maternal-Child Nurs. J.* 6:67.

Sander, L. W., et al. 1972. Continuous 24-hour interactional monitoring in infants reared in two caretaking environments. *Psychosomatic Med.* 34:270.

CHAPTER 29

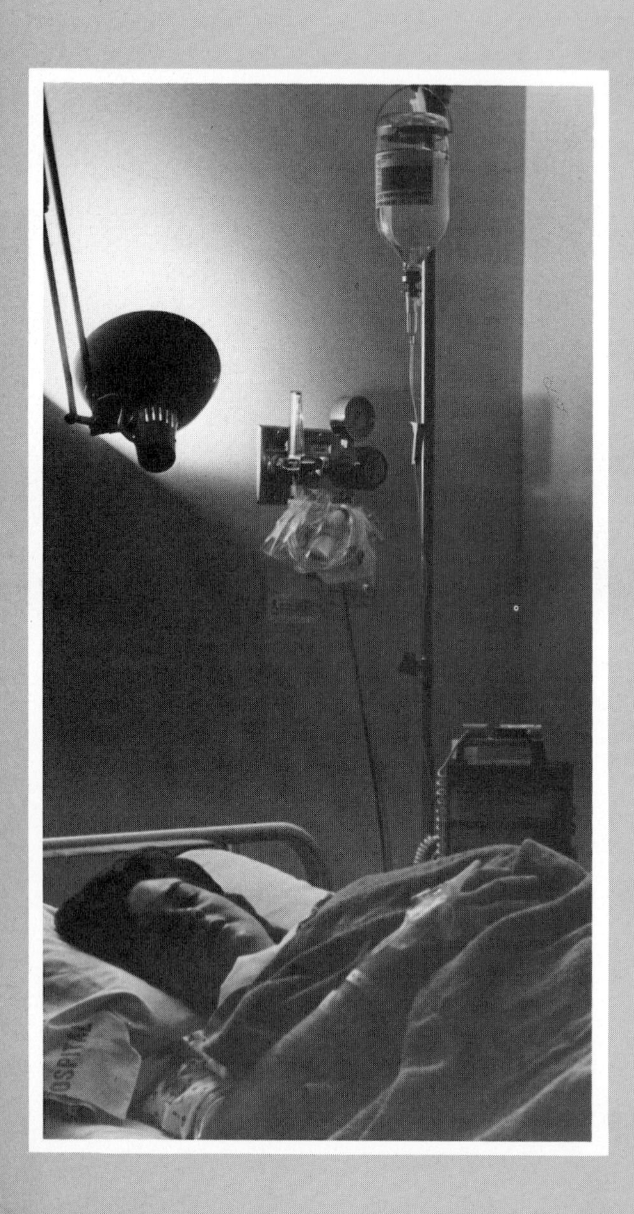

COMPLICATIONS OF THE PUERPERIUM

OBJECTIVES

- Discuss the causative factors, pathophysiology, and nursing interventions of puerperal infections.
- Identify the three complications of the puerperium that account for one-half of the maternal mortality in the United States.
- List the causes and nursing interventions of hemorrhage during the fourth stage of labor.
- Define subinvolution.
- Discuss causative factors, pathophysiology, and nursing interventions for thromboembolic disease of the puerperium.
- Describe puerperal cystitis and its implications for maternal nursing care.
- Differentiate disorders of the breast and complications of lactation.
- List the types of complications that can affect the maternal-infant attachment process.
- Identify the possible precipitating factors associated with puerperal psychiatric disorders.

The puerperium is classically that segment of the maternity cycle that begins with the delivery of the infant and ends when the involutionary process is complete, approximately six weeks later. In few if any other normal physiologic conditions is there such a rapid series of catabolic events. The normal involutionary process, establishment and maintenance of lactation, and the nursing care involved have been covered elsewhere (Chapter 27). This chapter deals with the broad area of complications during the puerperium and the nursing intervention and care that is appropriate. Physiologic complications to be considered include puerperal infection, subinvolution, hemorrhage, hematomas, disorders of the breast and complications of lactation, urinary tract and renal system disorders, and thromboembolic disease. Psychosocial and developmental complications include postpartum depression and puerperal psychosis and disorders of the mother-infant bonding process.

PUERPERAL INFECTIONS

Puerperal infection is an infection of the genital tract associated with parturition and generally encompasses the time from delivery to ten days postpartum. The infection most common is metritis/endometritis and is limited to the uterine cavity. However, it can spread by way of the lymphatics and blood vessels to become a progressive disease resulting in peritonitis or pelvic cellulitis. The patient's prognosis is directly related to the stage of the disease at the time of diagnosis, the invading organism, and the patient's state of health and her ability to resist the disease state.

Because infection accounts for a large percentage of postpartum morbidity, it is useful to remember the definition of puerperal morbidity published by the Joint Committee on Maternal Welfare (Pritchard and MacDonald, 1976):

> Temperature of 100.4°F (38.0°C) or higher, the temperature to occur on any two of the first ten portpartum days, exclusive of the first 24 hours, and to be taken by mouth by a standard technique at least four times a day.

Historical Perspective

Prior to the modern use of bacteriologic culturing and antibiotic therapy, childbearing women stood a considerable risk of developing infections that were often fatal. References to puerperal sepsis and childbed fever are rife even in popular literature today. Hippocrates described a fatal puerperal infection in 460 BC in his Third Book of the Epidemics. He hypothesized that the infection was caused by suppression of the lochia and that the lochia was possibly carried to the mother's head, where it acted as a toxin. The physicians Galen (a Greek) and Avicenna (an Arab) supported the belief that infection was caused by retention of lochia, and Willis published a thesis on *febris puerperarum* in the 1600s.

The modern term *puerperal fever* is generally attributed to Strother (1716). Leake (1772) was the first physician to suggest that this infection was contagious, and Hamilton stated this positively in 1781. In 1773, White recommended a semirecumbent position for postpartal women to facilitate the drainage of the stagnant lochia, and he also demanded meticulous cleanliness, improved ventilation of the lying-in room, and strict isolation of infected patients. Jordon described the epidemic properties of puerperal infection in 1795. As discussed in Chapter 1, the American physican Oliver Wendell Holmes (1843), in a paper on *The Contagiousness of Puerperal Fever,* clearly showed that the epidemic nature could be traced to the lack of precautions by doctors and nurses in the lying-in wards. Semmelweiss in 1847 began his classical investigation of puerperal morbidity in the Vienna Lying-In Hospital (described in Chapter 1). He related the high mortality in the hospital to a wound infection caused by infectious material on the physician's hands being introduced into the woman at the time of vaginal examination. Following his investigation, Semmelweiss insisted that all personnel disinfect their hands by washing them in chlorine water before examining the laboring woman. Unfortunately, his contributions were generally ignored by the physicians of his time, and it was left to Pasteur and the development of microbiology and to Lister and the use of aseptic technique to bring about a reduction in puerperal morbidity and mortality.

Epidemics of puerperal infection have been reported in the literature in modern times, but they are fortunately rare.

Causative Factors

Antibiotic therapy alone has not caused the decrease in morbidity and mortality that we see today. Aseptic technique, fewer traumatic operative deliveries, a better understanding of labor dystocia, improved surgical intervention, plus a population that is generally at less risk from malnutrition and chronic debilitative disease have also contributed to this reduction.

The vagina and cervix of approximately 70% of all healthy pregnant women contain pathogenic bacteria that alone or in combination are sufficiently virulent to cause extensive infections. Why the organisms do not cause infection during pregnancy is not altogether clear; however, recent studies indicate that more than the presence of a pathogen in the woman's genital tract is necessary for infection to begin. The uterus is essentially a sterile cavity prior to rupture of the fetal membranes, and the placental site, episiotomy, lacerations, abrasions, and any operative incision are all potential portals for bacterial entrance and growth. Hematomas are easily infected and enhance the possibility of sepsis. Tissue that has been compromised through trauma is less able to marshal the necessary forces to combat infection.

Gorbach and Bartlett in 1974 demonstrated that anaerobic bacteria as well as the aerobic bacteria commonly found in the bowel are capable of causing, indeed are likely to cause, puerperal infection. The bacteria reported in this study include the following:

- *Anaerobic bacteria:* peptostreptococcus, peptococcus, *Bacteroides fragilis, Clostridium perfringens,* clostridium (other)
- *Aerobic bacteria: Escherichia coli,* klebsiella, enterobacteriaceae, *Proteus mirabilis,* pseudomonas, hemolytic streptococcus groups A and B, hemolytic streptococcus group D, *Staphylococcus aureus, Neisseria gonorrhoeae*

Pathophysiology

Endometritis

Following delivery of the placenta, the placental site provides an excellent culture medium for bacterial growth. The site (in the contracted uterus) is a 4 cm round, dark red, elevated area with a nodular surface composed of numerous veins, many of which become occluded due to clot formation. The remaining portion of the decidua is also susceptible to pathogenic bacteria because of its thinness (approximately 2 mm) and its hypervascularity. The cervix may also present a bacterial breeding ground because of the multiple small lacerations attending normal labor and spontaneous delivery.

The pathogens deposited at the cervix during vaginal examination and those already present invade the decidua and eventually involve the entire mucosa. If the infection is confined to the surface of the mucosa, this area will become necrotic and be sloughed off within three to five days. In this instance the discharge is scant (or profuse), bloody, and foul-smelling.

Pelvic Cellulitis and Peritonitis

If the infection spreads by way of the lymphatic system, peritonitis or pelvic cellulitis (parametritis) may result. Pelvic abscess may form in the case of puerperal peritonitis and most commonly is found in the uterine ligaments, Douglas' cul-de-sac, and the subdiaphragmatic space. Pelvic cellulitis or infection of the pelvic connective tissue may be a secondary result of pelvic vein thrombophlebitis. This condition occurs when the clot becomes infected and the wall of the vein breaks down from necrosis, spilling the infection into the connective tissues of the pelvis. Another mechanism for spread of pelvic cellulitis is cervical laceration that has extended into the connective tissue of the broad ligament. This laceration then serves as a direct pathway that allows the pathogens already in the cervix to spread into the pelvis.

As the course of pelvic cellulitis advances, a mass of exudate develops along the base of the broad ligament that may push the uterus toward the opposite wall (if the infection is unilateral), where it will become fixed. If the exudate spreads into the rectocervical septum, a firm mass develops behind the cervix instead. The abscess that results should be drained or resolved through appropriate antibiotic therapy to avoid rupture of the abscess into the peritoneal cavity and development of a possibly fatal peritonitis.

There has been a concern in recent years that the increased use of internal fetal monitoring, especially when followed by cesarean birth, would proportionally increase puerperal morbidity. Wiechetek et al. (1974) reported no statistical differences between monitored and unmonitored groups, regardless of the method of delivery (that is, vaginal deliveries versus cesarean), whereas Hagen (1975) found that patients monitored internally prior to cesarean section did have a higher morbidity than a similar group with internal monitors whose labors were the same length but who delivered vaginally. Because sufficient data are not yet available to disprove the need for vigilance on the nurse's part, it is safe to assume that any patient who has been monitored, especially one who was delivered by cesarean, should be monitored closely for signs and symptoms of infection during the puerperal period.

Localized Infections

A less severe complication of the puerperium is the localized infection of the episiotomy or of lacerations to the perineum, vagina, or vulva. Wound infection of the abdominal incision site following cesarean section is also not infrequent. The skin edges become reddened, edematous, firm, and tender. The skin edges then separate, and purulent material, sometimes mixed with sanguineous liquid, drains from the wound.

Interventions and Nursing Care

Management of an infectious process begins with assessment of presenting signs and symptoms. The first 24–48 hours of the infectious process may be accompanied by a temperature of no more than 38.3–38.9C (101–102F) and a white blood count that remains in the normal range. As the infection progresses, the patient has a sustained temperature elevation and such other symptoms as pain, tenderness, and malaise. Diagnosis of the infection site is accomplished by a complete physical examination, blood work, and urinalysis.

Cultures of urine and any body discharges assist in diagnosing and identifying the causative organism. Specific treatment regimens are determined by the infection site and by the causative organism.

The Nursing Care Plan on puerperal infection presents the nursing management for the more common types of infections. General and specific aspects of nursing care are identified for the major patient problems.

NURSING CARE PLAN
Puerperal Infection

Patient Data Base

History

1. Predisposing health factors include:
   a. Malnutrition
   b. Anemia
   c. Debilitated condition
2. Predisposing factors associated with labor and delivery include:
   a. Prolonged labor
   b. Hemorrhage
   c. Premature and/or prolonged rupture
   d. Soft tissue trauma
   e. Invasive techniques

Physical examination

1. Localized episiotomy infections may present the following signs and symptoms:
   a. Complaints of unusual degree of discomfort
   b. Reddened edematous lesion
   c. May have associated purulent drainage
   d. Failure of skin edges to approximate
   e. Fever (generally below 101F)
2. Endometritis
   a. Mild case may be asymptomatic or characterized only by low-grade fever, anorexia, and malaise

NURSING CARE PLAN Cont'd
Puerperal Infection

b. More severe cases may demonstrate
   (1) Fever of 101-103F+
   (2) Anorexia, extreme lethargy
   (3) Chills
   (4) Rapid pulse
   (5) Lower abdominal pain
   (6) Lochia – appearance varies depending on causative organism: may appear normal, be profuse, bloody, and foul-smelling, may be scant and serosanguineous to brownish and foul-smelling
   (7) Severe afterpains

3. Pelvic cellulitis (endoparametritis)
   a. Signs and symptoms of severe infection (see discussion of endometritis, above)
   b. Severe abdominal pain, usually lateral to the uterus on one or both sides and apparent with both abdominal palpation and pelvic examination
4. Puerperal peritonitis
   a. Above symptoms plus severe abdominal pain
   b. Abdominal rigidity, guarding, rebound tenderness
   c. Vomiting and diarrhea may occur
   d. If paralytic ileus develops, marked bowel distention will be evident

Laboratory evaluation

1. Elevated white blood count (WBC), although it may be within normal puerperal limits (10,000-15,000/mm^3) initially
2. Culture of intrauterine material reveals causative organism
3. Urine culture should be normal but is done to rule out an asymptomatic urinary tract infection

Nursing Priorities

1. Promote healing of perineum, uterus, and pelvic area without exposure to infectious agents.
2. Assess signs and symptoms of impending infections with prompt interventions.
3. Explain through a patient-education program the signs and symptoms, course of condition, treatment methods, self-care to enhance cleanliness and promote healing of tissue, and home care routine for postpartal infections.

Problem	Nursing interventions and actions	Rationale
Wound infection	Promote normal wound healing by utilizing: 1. Sitz baths 2-3 times daily for 10-15 min. 2. Peri-light 2-3 times daily for 10-15 min. 3. Peri-care following elimination. 4. Frequent changing of peri-pads. 5. Early ambulation. 6. Diet high in protein and vitamin C. 7. Fluid intake to 2000 ml/day.	Warm water is cleansing, promotes healing through increased vascular flow to affected area, and is soothing to patient. Peri-care promotes removal of urine and fecal contaminants from perineum.
	Evaluate degree of healing by applying REEDA Scale (Table 29-1).	REEDA Scale provides consistent, objective tool for evaluation of wound healing.
	Observe, record, and report signs and symptoms of wound infection, including: 1. Redness. 2. Edema. 3. Excessive pain. 4. Inadequate approximation of wound edges. 5. Purulent drainage.	

Table 29–1. REEDA Scale Utilized to Evaluate Healing*

Points	Redness	Edema	Ecchymosis	Discharge	Approximation
0	None	None	None	None	Closed
1	Within 0.25 cm of incision bilaterally	Perineal, less than 1 cm from incision	Within 0.25 cm bilaterally or 0.5 cm unilaterally	Serum	Skin separation 3 mm or less
2	Within 0.5 cm of incision bilaterally	Perineal and/or vulvar, between 1 to 2 cm from incision	Between 0.25 to 1 cm bilaterally or between 0.5 to 2 cm unilaterally	Serosanguineous	Skin and subcutaneous fat separation
3	Beyond 0.5 cm of incision bilaterally	Perineal and/or vulvar, greater than 2 cm from incision	Greater than 1 cm bilaterally or 2 cm unilaterally	Bloody purulent	Skin, subcutaneous fat, and fascial layer separation
Score:	_______	_______	_______	_______	_______
					Total _______

*From Davidson, N. 1974. REEDA: Evaluating postpartum healing. *J. Nurse-Midwifery.* 19:7.

NURSING CARE PLAN Cont'd

Puerperal Infection

Problem	Nursing interventions and actions	Rationale
	6. Fever, anorexia, malaise.	
	Obtain culture from wound site and administer antibiotics, per physician order.	Antibiotic therapy based on knowledge of causative organism is treatment of choice for localized infection.
	Increase wound drainage by: 1. Assisting physician in opening wound for drainage, when indicated. 2. Anticipating packing of a cavity greater than 2–3 cm with iodoform gauze.	Abscesses may develop when infected material accumulates in closed body cavity. Iodoform packing maintains patency of opening so drainage can continue.
	Assess pain level and administer analgesics per physician orders if pain is not relieved through nursing measures.	
	Prevent spread of infection through: 1. Careful hand-washing techniques by staff, patient, and visitors. 2. Special disposal of infected materials such as disposable bed chux, peri-pads, and contaminated linen.	
	Promote and maintain mother-infant interaction by: 1. Encouraging mother to continue feeding her infant. 2. Reassuring mother that infant is not likely to become infected by her localized infection.	Success at feeding infant generally enhances the patient's outlook, encourages mother-infant interaction, and prevents patient from dwelling on herself to exclusion of infant. Breast-feeding is not affected by localized infection and should be encouraged. Some institutions still insist on separation of the mother and infant if an infection is present. The mother must be instructed in pumping her breasts (if

NURSING CARE PLAN Cont'd

Puerperal Infection

Problem	Nursing interventions and actions	Rationale
		breast-feeding) and will need support during this separation.
Metritis/endometritis	Care of the patient is essentially the same as for wound infections, including antibiotics, analgesics, and careful cleansing techniques.	
	Newborn: Assess breast-feeding infant's mouth for signs of thrush, which is a common side effect of antibiotics ingested by infant in mother's milk. Treatment should be initiated but breast-feeding need not be stopped.	Thrush, a monilial infection caused by *Candida albicans,* often occurs when normal oral flora are destroyed by antibiotic therapy.
Pelvic cellulitis	Observe, record, and report signs and symptoms of severe infection, including: 1. Fever spiking to 103-104F. 2. Elevated white blood count. 3. Chills. 4. Extreme lethargy. 5. Lower abdominal pain, especially lateral to uterus. 6. Nausea and vomiting.	Infection produces characteristic signs and symptoms.
	Administer IV fluids and antibiotics as ordered.	IV fluids maintain proper hydration of patient.
	Assist physician in pelvic examination for detection of abscess. Be prepared for surgical incision and drainage if necessary. In cases where all management fails, removal of infected uterus, tubes, and ovaries may be necessary.	
	Promote patient comfort by providing: 1. Adequate periods of rest. 2. Emotional support. 3. Judicious use of antibiotics. 4. Maintenance of cleanliness and warmth.	
Peritonitis	Observe, record, and report signs and symptoms of severe infection, such as nausea, vomiting, and abdominal rigidity.	Paralytic ileus is frequently associated with peritonitis.
	Maintain continuous nasogastric suction per physician order.	Continuous nasogastric suction is used to decompress bowel when paralytic ileus complicates clinical course.
	Administer IV fluids and antibiotics as ordered. Monitor intake and output, urine specific gravity, vital signs, and level of hydration.	Vigorous fluid and electrolyte therapy is necessary not only because of vomiting and diarrhea, but also because both fluid and electrolytes become sequestered in lumen and wall of bowel.
	Provide narcotic analgesics for alleviation of severe pain, per physician order.	
	Transfer patient to intensive care or provide critical care services by skilled registered nurse.	Patient with peritonitis is in critical condition, and quality of nursing care this patient receives will weigh the balance between recovery and demise.
	Provide emotional support, including: 1. Anticipate maternal depression. 2. Provide opportunities for mother to see, touch, and hold infant when possible, taking proper precautions to protect infant. 3. Assist breast-feeding mothers to pump breasts in order to maintain milk production. 4. Encourage husband/family/support persons to become involved with patient's care and with infant.	Critically ill patient may become very depressed not only from disease process but also because her anticipated postpartal course is now denied to her, and she may interpret this as a failure of her ability to mother her infant.

NURSING CARE PLAN Cont'd
Puerperal Infection

Nursing Care Evaluation

Purulent drainage, odor, edema, elevated temperature, and wounds are controlled or relieved.

Wound is healing.

Patient is ambulating.

Patient understands condition, treatment regimen, prevention of spread of infection, infant care, and necessity of continued medical supervision.

Discharge Planning

The mother with a puerperal infection needs assistance when she is discharged from the hospital. If the family cannot provide this home assistance, a referral to the community homemakers' service is needed. The community health/visiting nurse service can also be contacted as soon as the patient is diagnosed so that the nurse can meet with the patient for a family and home assessment and development of a home care plan. The community health nurse is aware of the community resources available to assist the patient, and planning with the patient/family before discharge will assure continuity of care after discharge.

The family needs instruction in the care of a newborn, including feeding, bathing, cord care, immunizations, and significant observations that should be reported. A well-baby appointment should be scheduled. Breast-feeding mothers should be instructed to inspect the baby's mouth for signs of thrush and to report the finding to their physician.

The mother should be instructed regarding activity, rest, medications, diet, and signs and symptoms of complications, and she should be scheduled for a return medical examination.

PUERPERAL HEMATOMAS AND HEMORRHAGE

Hemorrhage, hypertension, and infection together account for one-half of the maternal mortality in the United States. This portion of the chapter deals with puerperal hematomas and hemorrhage.

Hematomas

Hematomas are usually the result of injury to a blood vessel without noticeable trauma to the superficial tissue. Hematomas occur following spontaneous as well as forceps deliveries.

Because of the dorsal recumbent position following delivery, the most frequently observed hematomas are of the external genitals, particularly of the vagina and vulva. The soft tissue in the area offers no resistance, and hematomas containing 250–500 ml of blood develop rapidly. The patient complains of severe pain, usually from her "stitches" or "down there," or of severe rectal pressure. On examination, the large hematoma appears as a unilateral bulging mass at the introitus or encompassing the labia majora. The bleeding may not be as apparent as described above, so the observant nurse checks for unilateral bluish or reddish discoloration of skin of the perineum and buttocks. The area feels firm and is painful to the touch. The nurse should estimate the size of the hematoma carefully with the first assessment, in order to better estimate the potential blood loss.

Hematomas can also occur in the upper portion of the vagina and bleed into the broad ligament or lateral walls of the vagina. Pain is the most common symptom, and careful investigation by the physician through manual examination is needed to confirm the diagnosis.

Large hematomas generally require surgical intervention to evacuate the clot and to achieve hemostasis. General anesthesia is usually required, and if the hematoma is not accessible vaginally, a laparotomy must be performed.

Continuous assessment of the vaginal bleeding is required following surgery. If the hematoma was of the vulva or perineum, the nurse should check for recurrence. It should be standard procedure for the nurse giving report to the new shift to assist the next shift in examining the patient so that baseline data can be obtained. The nurse assuming responsibility for the oncoming shift should record her findings immediately and state that the patient was examined by both nurses together.

Hemorrhages

Puerperal hemorrhage is classically divided into early and late postpartal hemorrhage. Early postpartal hemorrhage is generally due to uterine atony or lacerations of the genital tract and is dealt with before the patient leaves the delivery room.

After the first hour postpartum, most hemorrhage is due to retained cotyledons, retained fetal membranes, or subnormal or abnormal involution of the placental site. The fundus easily demonstrates the progress of involution by its relationship to the patient's umbilicus. Generally, the fundus should be well contracted, in the midline, firm, and below the umbilicus immediately following delivery. Gradually it expands to a one-finger breadth above the umbilicus on the first postpartal day. On each succeeding day the fundus should recede toward the pelvis another finger breadth; that is, on the second postpartal day the fundus is 1–2 finger breadths below the umbilicus, and so on. Breast-feeding encourages the involution process and is an additional benefit to the mother for nursing her baby. Subinvolution occurs when the uterus fails to follow this normal pattern of involution but remains enlarged (see Chapter 27).

Failure of the lochia to progress from rubra to serosa to alba, or a return to rubra after the first several days postpartum, is another symptom of subinvolution.

Careful observation and documentation of vaginal bleeding (often by way of pad count or weighing of the peri-pad) is important if medical intervention is to be elicited. A boggy uterus that does not stay contracted without constant massage is atonic, whereas a uterus that does not involute appropriately needs to be investigated for possible retained placental tissue and infection. The most commonly employed intervention is a continuous infusion of fluids and oxytocin. If the patient is normotensive, intramuscular injections of methylergonovine or ergonovine may be employed, followed by orally administered ergonovine. (Typical dosage is ergonovine 0.2 mg every 4 hours × 6 doses.) If this treatment is not effective or if a placental fragment is retained for several days, curettage is usually indicated, together with the administration of antibiotics to prevent puerperal infection.

THROMBOEMBOLIC DISEASE

Although thromboembolic disease is not limited to the puerperium, it does occur at that time and may have grave sequelae.

Superficial thrombophlebitis is limited to the superficial saphenous veins, whereas deep thrombophlebitis generally involves most of the deep venous system from the foot up to (and including) the iliofemoral area. The major risk from thrombophlebitis at this or any time is, of course, the development of pulmonary emboli.

Causative Factors

A balance exists in the blood between the coagulation system, which assists in clot formation, and the fibrinolytic system, which breaks down clots

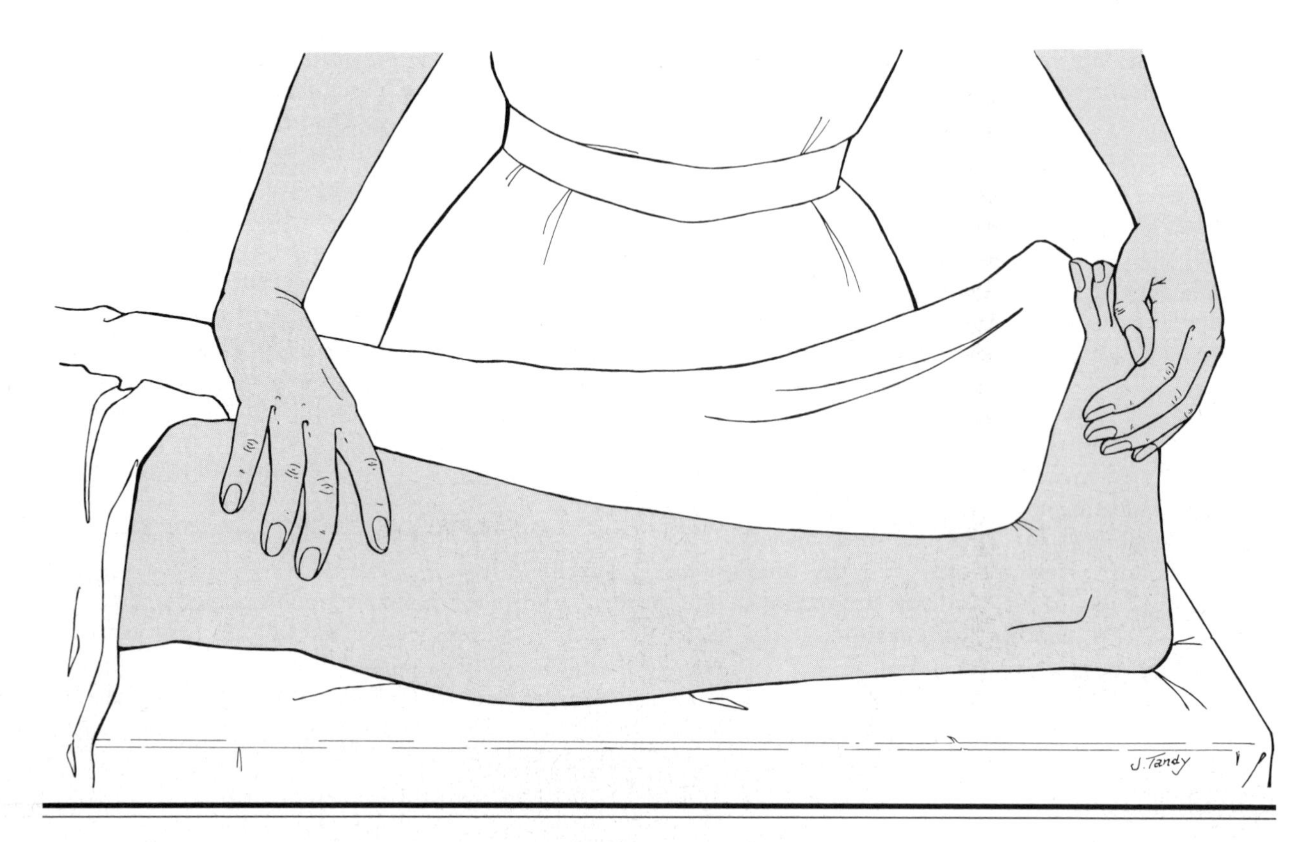

Figure 29–1. Homans' sign. While holding the patient's knee flat, the nurse dorsiflexes the patient's foot. Pain in the patient's foot or leg is indicative of a positive Homans' sign.

already formed. During a normal pregnancy, this balance shifts in favor of clot formation. Shortly after delivery the balance returns, but it swings again in favor of clot formation during the puerperium. The danger of thrombosis is highest in the puerperium, when both blood fibrinogen content and platelet count increase and when those platelets present become more sticky (Cooper, 1976).

Slowing of the blood flow in the legs is another factor, and prolonged inactivity (as from bedrest following cesarean section) facilitates clot formation (Turnbull et al., 1971).

The suppression of lactation with estrogen may add a tenfold risk of thrombus formation (Daniel, 1969; Cooper, 1976).

Additional risk factors include maternal age (over 30), especially in combination with high parity, operative delivery, obesity, previous thrombophlebitis/thromboembolic disease, and possibly familial tendency (Tindall, 1968; Turnbull et al., 1971).

Thrombophlebitis is often the result of the spread of infection along the venous pathways and is generally unilateral. The veins most frequently involved are the ovarian veins (probably because of their proximity to the infected placental site). When the infection spreads via the left ovarian vein, it may reach the left renal vein and involve the kidney, as in a renal abscess. If the infection spreads via the right ovarian vein, the inferior vena cava may become involved. In certain cases the common iliac veins are also involved if the uterine rather than the ovarian veins provide the pathway for spread of the infection. The presence of a clot in the vein may stop the spread of the disease by providing a barrier to the bacteria; however, the clot itself can also support bacterial growth, and the surrounding vein wall will become necrotic.

The classic picture of lower extremity puerperal thrombophlebitis is one of sudden onset of pain, tenderness and turgidity of the calf, redness and increased skin temperature, positive Homans' sign, and edema of the calf or thigh (Figure 29–1). Because of reflex arterial spasm, the affected leg may also appear pale and cool, with decreased peripheral pulses. Unfortunately, many cases present few if any of these classic signs and symptoms. According to Cooper (1976), only 20% of cases have a positive Homans' sign. Pelvic thrombosis is especially elusive unless it has become so extensive as to prevent venous return. In this case, the nurse may note pain and tenderness over the groin area.

Pulmonary Emboli

A sudden onset of dyspnea accompanied by sweating, pallor, cyanosis, confusion, systemic hypotension, and increased jugular pressure may indicate the possibility of pulmonary emboli. Chest pain that mimics cardiac ischemia, coupled with the patient's verbalized fear of imminent death and complaint of pressure of the bowel and rectum, should alert the nurse to the extensive size of the embolus. A gallop (heart) rhythm may be present even if respiratory inspiration is normal, although smaller emboli may present with only transient syncope, tightness of the chest, or unexplained pyrexia.

Even x-ray and ECG changes and laboratory data are not always reliable. If a case of pulmonary embolism is suspected, prompt treatment should begin even in the absence of collaborative data.

Interventions and Nursing Care

For nursing management of thrombophlebitis and pulmonary embolism, see the accompanying Nursing Care Plan.

NURSING CARE PLAN

Thrombophlebitis and Pulmonary Embolism

Patient Data Base

History

1. Predisposing factors include:
   a. Obesity
   b. Prolonged labor with associated pressure of the fetal head on the pelvic veins
   c. Preeclampsia-eclampsia
   d. Heart disease
   e. Hypercoagulability of the early puerperium
   f. Anemia
   g. Hemorrhage
2. Initiating factors may include:
   a. Trauma to deep leg veins due to faulty positioning for delivery
   b. Operative delivery, including cesarean section
   c. Abortion
   d. Postpartal pelvic cellulitis

Physical examination

1. Superficial thrombophlebitis
   a. Tenderness along the involved vein
   b. Areas of palpable thrombosis
   c. Warmth in the involved area
2. Deep vein thrombosis
   a. Positive Homans' sign (pain occurs when foot is dorsiflexed while leg is extended)
   b. Calf tenderness and pain
   c. Fever
   d. Edema in affected extremity

NURSING CARE PLAN Cont'd

Thrombophlebitis and Pulmonary Embolism

Laboratory evaluation

1. Thrombophlebitis
   a. Doppler ultrasonography demonstrates increased circumference of affected extremity
   b. Venography confirms diagnosis
2. Pulmonary embolism
   a. Electrocardiogram may reveal indications of right-sided heart strain
   b. Lung scan or pulmonary angiography may reveal evidence of pulmonary embolism but may not be definitive
   c. SGOT and LDH may be elevated

Nursing Priorities

1. Prevent circulatory stasis through correct positioning in delivery stirrups, early ambulation, avoiding crossing legs, leg exercise, and applications of support stockings.
2. Maintain maternal-infant interrelations.
3. Instruct through patient education program about cause of condition, treatment regimen, medications, infant care, necessity of continued medical supervision, and means to avoid circulatory stasis.
4. Promote mental health through patient's expressions of fears, acceptance of change in body image, and alternatives to infant care when activities are restricted.

Problem	Nursing interventions and actions	Rationale
Thrombophlebitis	Initiate and maintain actions to prevent development of thrombophlebitis, including: 1. Careful positioning of patient in stirrups for delivery. 2. Early active ambulation. 3. Use of support stockings following operative deliveries. 4. Instruction as to necessity for doing leg exercises regularly when confined to bed.	Prolonged pressure, resulting in venous stasis and trauma to the vein wall, is contributing factor to development of thrombophlebitis. Movement and support encourage venous return and decrease tendency to venous stasis.
	Observe, record, and report signs and symptoms of thrombophlebitis (refer to section on physical examination).	
	Maintain bed rest and warm, moist soaks as ordered. Administer analgesics for relief of pain per physician order.	Bedrest is ordered to decrease possibility that portion of clot will dislodge and result in pulmonary embolism. Warmth promotes blood flow to affected area.
	Administer intravenous heparin as ordered, by continuous intravenous drip, heparin lock, or subcutaneously, including: 1. Monitor IV or heparin lock site for signs of infiltration. 2. Obtain Lee White clotting times per physician order and review prior to administering heparin. 3. Observe for signs of anticoagulant overdose with resultant bleeding, including: a. Hematuria. b. Epistaxis. c. Ecchymosis. d. Bleeding gums.	Heparin does not dissolve clot but is administered to prevent further clotting. It is safe for breast-feeding mothers because heparin is not excreted in mother's milk.
	4. Provide protamine sulfate, per physician order, to combat bleeding problems related to heparin overdosage.	Protamine sulfate is heparin antagonist, given intravenously, which is almost immediately effective in counteracting bleeding complications caused by heparin overdose.

NURSING CARE PLAN Cont'd

Thrombophlebitis and Pulmonary Embolism

Problem	Nursing interventions and actions	Rationale
	5. Initiate progressive ambulation following the acute phase. Provide properly fitting elastic stockings prior to ambulation.	Elastic stockings or "Teds" help prevent pooling of venous blood in lower extremities.
Pulmonary embolism	Observe, record, and report signs and symptoms of pulmonary embolism, including: 1. Sudden onset of severe chest pain, often located substernally. 2. Apprehension and sense of impending catastrophe. 3. Cough (may be accompanied by hemoptysis). 4. Tachycardia. 5. Fever. 6. Hypotension. 7. Diaphoresis, pallor, weakness. 8. Shortness of breath. 9. Neck vein engorgement. 10. Friction rub and evidence of atelectasis upon auscultation.	Signs and symptoms may occur suddenly and require immediate emergency treatment. Prognosis is related to size and location of embolism.
	Initiate or support emergency treatment and additional treatment, including: 1. Combat hypoxia: a. Administer oxygen. b. Assist physician with tracheal intubation if necessary. 2. Monitor vital signs, ECG. 3. Administer medications as ordered: a. Sedative. b. Digitalis. 4. Prepare patient for embolectomy if ordered. 5. Additional treatment involves anticoagulants, bed rest, and analgesics and is similar to treatment for thrombophlebitis.	Sedation is used to control pain and anxiety. Digitalis is administered to improve myocardial function.
Prevention of maternal/infant deprivation	Maintain mother-infant attachment when mother is on bed rest by: 1. Providing frequent contacts for mother and infant; modified rooming-in possible if crib placed tangent to mother's bed or if Baby Bonding Crib is used.	Evidence indicates that first few days of life may be crucial to development of maternal-infant bonds, and separation during this period should be avoided.
	2. Encouraging continuation of breast-feeding or breasts may be pumped for acutely ill patients.	Flow of milk is contingent on emptying of breast, either by placing infant to breast or pumping milk from breast. Many institutions utilize milk pumped from mother's breasts for feeding infant.

Nursing Care Evaluation

Presenting signs and symptoms are relieved or controlled.

Patient is stabilized on anticoagulant medication.

No inflammatory process is evident.

Patient is ambulatory without pain.

Patient applies elastic stocking.

Patient knows to avoid constrictive clothing; to avoid placing legs in dependent positions; purposes of medications, including dosage, untoward effects of anticoagulant medications, frequency, symptoms to report to physician; and necessity of continued medical supervision.

Maternal-infant bonding is established.

PUERPERAL CYSTITIS

The puerperal woman is a likely candidate for development of cystitis. Diuresis is a normal physiologic function during the immediate postpartal period. The body uses this mechanism to begin to eliminate the extra fluid volume that was accumulated during pregnancy. The bladder has a normal increase in capacity following delivery and is less sensitive to fluid retention than during pregnancy or in the nonpregnant state.

Stretching or trauma to the base of the bladder occurs to some degree in any vaginal delivery, and in rare instances the resulting edema of the trigone is great enough to obstruct the urethra and to cause acute retention. Obstruction by large hematomas is not unknown and should be investigated when other causes of acute urinary retention have been ruled out.

Modern obstetric practice has also contributed to the increased risk of puerperal cystitis. Routine administration of intravenous fluids increases the circulating fluid volume that must be filtered out and eliminated following delivery. General anesthesia temporarily inhibits the normal neural control of the bladder and facilities rapid filling and overdistention. However, except in the case of emergency and cesarean sections, general anesthesia is rarely seen in enlightened obstetrics today. Conductive anesthesia, popular among some obstetricians, inhibits the normal functioning of the bladder to an even greater extent.

Overdistention of the bladder also leads to increased bleeding during the puerperium. As described earlier, the bladder fills the pelvic cavity and possibly the lower abdominal cavity, preventing the uterus from contracting sufficiently.

Emptying the bladder is vital. Women who are not sufficiently recovered from the effect of anesthesia cannot void spontaneously, and catheterization is necessary.

Retention of residual urine, bacteria introduced at the time of catheterization, and a bladder traumatized by delivery combine to provide an excellent environment for the promotion of cystitis.

Overdistention

The overdistended bladder appears as a large mass, reaching sometimes to the umbilicus and displacing the uterine fundus upward. There is increased vaginal bleeding, and the patient may complain of cramping.

Overdistention, if discovered in the recovery room, is often managed by draining the bladder with a straight catheter as a onetime measure. If the overdistention is recurrent or is diagnosed later in the postpartal period, an indwelling catheter is generally ordered for 24 hours. When the catheter is discontinued, normal bladder functioning is evaluated by one of the two following measures. First, the patient who is able to void within 4 hours is catheterized for residual urine. If the residual is greater than 100 ml, the catheter is left in for another 24 hours. Second, if the patient is unable to void within 4 hours, the bladder is catheterized, and if the amount measured is greater than 200 ml, the catheter is retained for an additional 24 hours. If the amount is less than 200 ml, the catheter is removed and the patient is given another 4-hour trial. In the case of a patient who is required to void within 4 hours following removal of an indwelling catheter, it is important to encourage fluid intake.

Diligent monitoring of the bladder during the recovery period and preventive health measures greatly reduce the number of women who need to be treated for overdistention of the bladder. Encouraging the mother to void spontaneously and assisting her to use the toilet or the bedpan (if possible) if she has received conductive anesthesia prevent the largest percentage of overdistention. If catheterization becomes necessary, a Foley catheter should always be used, and meticulous aseptic technique should be employed.

As previously mentioned, the vagina and vulva are traumatized to some degree by vaginal delivery, and edema is common. If forceps have been used (a frequent adjunct to conductive anesthesia), the trauma is greater, and edema, especially of the vestibule, is marked. This edema may obscure the urinary meatus, and the nurse needs to be extremely careful in cleansing the vulva and inserting the catheter. It is imperative to discard a catheter that has inadvertently been introduced into the vagina and thus contaminated. (Catheterization, an uncomfortable procedure at any time, is generally painful during the puerperium due to the trauma and edema of the tissue. Therefore, the nurse should be especially careful, considerate, and gentle not only in inserting the catheter but also in handling and cleansing the perineal area.)

If the amount of urine siphoned from the bladder reaches 900–1000 ml, the catheter should be clamped, the Foley bag inflated, and the catheter attached firmly to the patient's leg. The physician should be notified, and the procedure, including the patient's vital signs before and after the procedure and her responses, should carefully be charted. After one hour, the Foley may be unclamped and placed on straight drainage. By following this technique, the bladder is protected, and rapid intraabdominal decompression is avoided. When the indwelling catheter is removed, a urine sample is automatically sent to the laboratory, and usually the tip of the catheter is removed and sent for culture also. If catheterization for residual urine is to be performed, a Foley should again be used in anticipation of having to leave the catheter in place. Failure to use a Foley catheter might necessitate an additional catheterization and increase the risk of cystitis.

Clinical Manifestations

The initial symptoms of cystitis may include frequency, urgency, dysuria, and nocturia. Costal vertebral angle (CVA) tenderness may also be present.

Interventions and Nursing Care

When cystitis is suspected in the puerperium, a catheterized urine specimen is obtained for microscopic examination, culture, and sensitivity. Antibiotic therapy is begun, and a urinary tract antispasmodic or analgesic agent may also be ordered.

In all probability, the nurse will be the first to suspect puerperal cystitis. Careful examination and questioning of the patient at each shift elicits the required information on normal bladder functioning and augments or reinforces the prenatal teaching the patient received on normal body functioning, self-help, and preventive health care maintenance.

When suspect symptomatology is discovered, the physician should be notified immediately so that prompt treatment can be instituted. Prompt treatment, it is hoped, will prevent the infection from spreading to the upper urinary tract. Once cystitis has been diagnosed, the nurse needs to encourage fluids to help flush the urinary tract and to encourage active ambulation to assist in mobilizing the remaining extra fluid volume of pregnancy. Active involvement with the new baby decreases the mother's concentration on her problem while strengthening the maternal-infant bond. As previously mentioned, breast-feeding of the infant need not be curtailed, although the choice of antibiotic agents may need to be reconsidered.

DISORDERS OF THE BREAST AND COMPLICATIONS OF LACTATION

The physiology of lactation and the maternal-infant benefits derived from breast-feeding have been discussed elsewhere (see Chapter 27). This section discusses engorgement, mastitis, nipple disorders, breast abscess, and suppression of lactation.

Engorgement and Suppression of Lactation

Separation of the placenta triggers the release of prolactin from the anterior pituitary, resulting in the initiation of lactation (see p. 906). Stagnation of fluids in the lymphatic and venous systems may become so marked as to cause the breast to enlarge and to become hard, painful, and engorged. This fullness is not related to the overdistention of the milk ducts that may later be present during weaning. It has been reported that early and frequent breast-feeding all but eliminates engorgement as a complication of normal lactation (Pryor, 1973; Rees, 1976).

With the increase in the number of women who breast-feed their babies, suppression of lactation is becoming less common. Historically, suppression of lactation has been accomplished by mechanical means, that is, breast binders and ice bags to inhibit vascular filling. Drug suppression with estrogens (stilbestrol) was highly favored in the 1940s and 1950s. Hodge (1967) reports a 12% failure rate of women who lactated despite estrogen treatment, as opposed to a 65% failure rate for mechanical suppression. Unfortunately, estrogen administered during the puerperium has been reported to provide up to a tenfold risk of development of thromboembolism (Daniel et al., 1967) and thus is no longer recommended. Current use of a long-acting steroid/testosterone combination given at the time of delivery has shown itself to be effective; however, Markin and Wolst (1960) reported a complication rate of 20%–40%. These complications include delayed engorgement with pain and increased lochia. Because these complications occur following hospital discharge of the patient, some maternity nurses have remained uninformed about this important area of anticipatory guidance.

Interventions and Nursing Care

Nonnursing Mothers

Currently, Deladumone or Diatate-DS combined with oral analgesics is the most common lactation suppressant utilized clinically. Mothers who are not nursing should avoid pumping the breasts, because this activity stimulates milk production and delays the "drying-up." Many folk remedies are still found in ethnic cultures both to stimulate milk production and to assist drying up of the breast. (A common folk remedy for engorgement and for assisting drying up is for the mother to express her milk into a silver cup and to throw the milk onto the bare ground. This procedure is supposed to demonstrate that the milk is not needed, and the absorption into the soil symbolizes the reabsorption that will take place in the mother's breasts.)

In addition to analgesics and ice packs, use of a good supporting brassiere that covers the entire breast should be encouraged day and night. A nursing pad can be inserted into the bra to collect any leaking milk, but care should be taken to change the pads frequently to avoid maceration of the nipples.

Breast-feeding Mothers

Mothers who have been encouraged to breast-feed and who have been given appropriate support by the nursing staff rarely have engorgement. The cure for engorgement is then, of course, one of prevention. If the breasts become tender and feel full to the touch, the mother should be encouraged to nurse her baby more often. This practice will not only stimulate milk production but will also increase circulation in the breast and help move the fluid that may lead to engorgement. When engorgement is seen in lactating mothers, it can usually be credited to poor nursing care, separation of mother from baby, non-family-centered maternity services, uninformed or unsympathetic medical care, and restrictive feeding schedules.

When suckling is limited to 2–4 minutes and not gradually lengthened to 7–10 minutes, letdown does not completely occur, and colostrum or milk is retained within the breast. The resultant back pressure interferes with blood circulation to the breast. Impeded circulation in turn affects hormonal control of milk secretion and letdown. As a result, engorgement occurs, and a vicious cycle is initiated (Rees, 1976).

If engorgement should occur, the mother should be assisted to express some milk from her breast, either manually or with a nontraumatic pump, such as the Lapoca manual breast pump. Expression of milk decreases the tension in the lactiferous sinuses and provides the infant a better chance to begin nursing. Frequent nursing (every 1½–2 hours), even during the night, soon alleviates the problem. Mild analgesics should be administered, because engorgement is very painful. Minimal amounts of the medication may be transferred to the infant through the milk, but this amount does not appear to have any deleterious effect on the infant. Many mothers find relief from engorgement by standing under a warm shower while performing breast massage. This combination helps mobilize stagnant fluids and makes expression of milk and nursing easier.

Sore, Cracked, Fissured, or Abnormal Nipples

Successful breast-feeding is most easily accomplished when the nipples have been properly prepared during pregnancy. Nipples that are soft and supple adapt more easily to the stretching and pulling exerted by the nursing infant's mouth, whereas the dry, sensitive nipple becomes painful during lactation and is more prone to fissuring (Rees, 1976) (Figure 29–2).

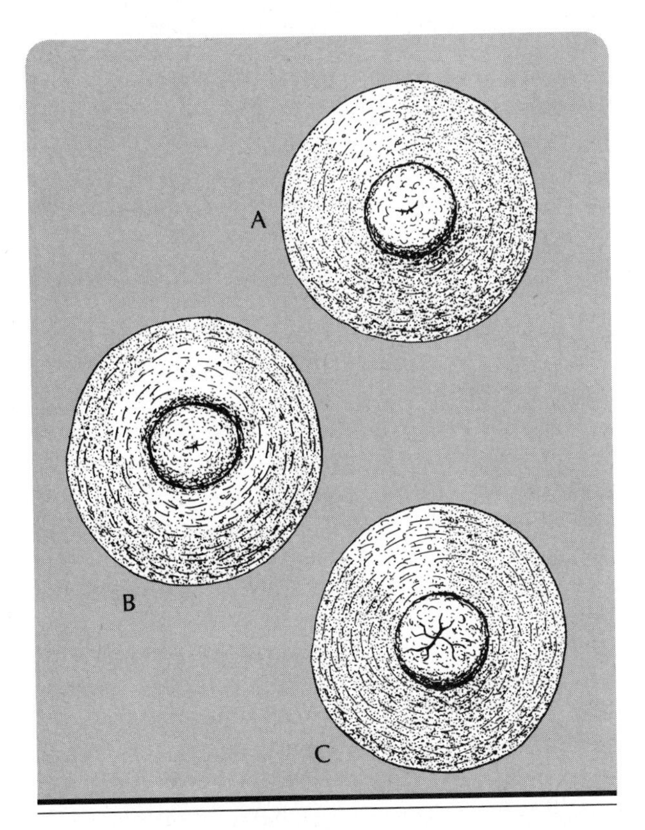

Figure 29–2. **A,** Normal nipple. **B,** Inverted nipple. **C,** Fissured nipple. (From *The mammary glands and breast-feeding.* Clinical Education Aid No. 10. Ross Laboratories, Columbus, Ohio.)

Nurses should advise mothers to avoid astringents and soaps because of their drying effect. Breasts should be washed in warm water only, and perfumed creams or ointments should be avoided. Lanolin-based bland creams, such as Massé cream, are often used to relieve sore nipples. The chapstick normally used on the lips may be very effective in the prevention or treatment of sore or cracked nipples. Exposing the breasts to air between feedings and for 10–15 minutes after each feeding or the use of a heat lamp may also be helpful. More frequent breast-feeding is also advocated, based on the theory that engorgement can be decreased and overly vigorous sucking can be avoided. Oral thrush infection of the infant can also cause very sore nipples for the mother. In addition to treating the infant, the mother should be treated by applying Mycolog cream to the nipples.

Inverted nipples should be corrected prior to the onset of lactation, if possible (see Figure 29–2). The truly inverted nipple rarely appears inverted or flat until stimulated. When stimulated, the nipple appears to retract into the breast rather than to become erect. Hoffman (1953) recommended exercises to loosen the adhesions at the base of the nipple that are responsible for the inversion, then use of Woolwich Shields or Netsy Swedish Milk Cups to apply gentle pressure at the edge of the areola; such practices gradually increase the nipple's protractility. For the majority of women, inverted or flat nipples are a variation of normal that can be corrected (Otte, 1975).

Mastitis and Breast Abscess

A distinction needs to be made between true mastitis and the localized inflammation of the breast resulting from a blocked milk duct. The latter is usually a benign condition that responds readily to breast massage and frequent nursing. The former is a bacteria-caused infection that necessitates vigorous intervention if the disease is to be controlled.

Pathophysiology

Mastitis is generally caused by *Staphylococcus aureus;* however, bacteroides can also be cultured from the abscess that forms around the areolae (Pearson, 1967). The source of the invading organism is usually the nose and mouth of the infant. The organism is then deposited on the mother's nipple and areola. If there are lesions or fissures of the nipples, the organism then ascends into the lactational system. Stasis of the milk provides a medium for growth of the organism.

Mastitis epidemics have occurred in lying-in wards and nurseries. Usually an infant becomes colonized first, and the infection spreads from infant to infant. Poor hand-washing technique by nursery personnel is generally the culprit.

Clinical Manifestations

Blocked milk ducts often present as a hard, warm, reddened, and tender area, usually in the upper outer quadrant of the breast (Figure 29–3). This area (the alveola) appears to be a hard, fixed, irregularly shaped mass that feels like cauliflower under the skin. True mastitis or suppurative mastitis may appear as marked engorgement, pain, chills, fever, and tachycardia. In untreated cases, singular or multiple abscesses may form.

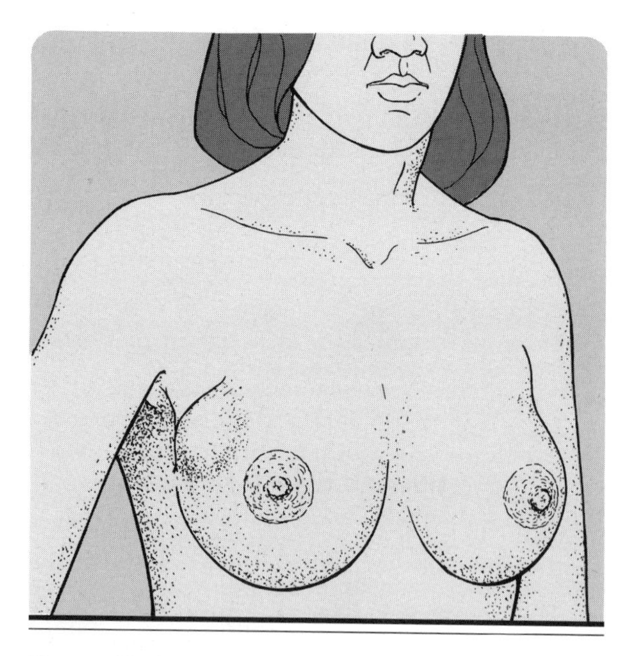

Figure 29–3. Mastitis. Erythema and swelling are present in the upper outer quadrant of the breast. Axillary lymph nodes are enlarged and tender.

Interventions and Nursing Care

True mastitis needs to be treated with appropriate antibiotics, analgesics, and local application of heat. A sample of the mother's milk is sent for culture and sensitivity. If abscesses form, they must be incised and drained, usually under general anesthesia.

Meticulous hand-washing by all personnel is obviously the primary measure in preventing epidemic nursery infections and subsequent maternal mastitis. Periodic nasal cultures of all nursery personnel identify bacteria carriers, who can then be treated. Prompt attention to mothers who have blocked milk ducts eliminates the stagnant milk as a growth medium for bacteria. Frequent breast-feeding of the infant, as previously mentioned, usually prevents mastitis.

If a mother finds that one area of the breast feels distended (caked), several simple methods will help. First, she can rotate the position of the baby for nursing so that the baby's gums compress different sinuses each time. Second, if the affected breast has not been emptied at a particular feeding, manual expression or a nontraumatic breast pump can be employed to assure that the breast is emptied. Third, as the infant is nursing, the mother should massage the caked area, starting from the point farthest away from the nipple and gently stroking down toward the nipple. (Be sure that the mother doesn't accidentally break the infant's suction.) This technique manually stimulates emptying the alveola.

Opinion varies as to whether breast-feeding should be discontinued in the presence of mastitis. Those advocating cessation of breast-feeding suggest that a vicious cycle of reinfection may develop as the baby ingests infected milk, becomes reinfected, and in turn reinfects his mother.

Those favoring continuation of breast-feeding raise several points in support of their beliefs. First, if the milk contains bacteria, it also contains the antibiotic that the mother is taking. Second, if the baby is the initial carrier of the infection, he should also be under treatment. And third, sudden cessation of lactation will certainly cause caking and severe engorgement, which may be much more painful than continuing to breast-feed. Breast-feeding adds an additional benefit in that it stimulates circulation and moves bacteria-containing milk out of the breast, instead of leaving the affected milk to stagnate in the breast.

Should the condition lead to formation of abscesses, the nurse needs to prepare the patient for surgical intervention. If multiple abscesses are present, the patient may have multiple incisions. A sterile packing is generally placed in each incised abscess to provide drainage. Because the breast is then covered with a sterile surgical dressing, access to the breast will temporarily be inhibited and breast-feeding will become impossible. Once the dressings, drains, and packing have been removed and the incisions are healing well, careful breast-feeding may resume, closely supervised by the experienced nurse.

COMPLICATIONS OF MATERNAL-INFANT ATTACHMENT

Klaus and Kennell (1976), Kempe and Helfer (1972), and Brazelton (1963) have demonstrated the needs of mothers and babies to establish bonds of affection and love. These bonds are in rudimentary form during pregnancy; labor develops the bonds further, and it is not until several weeks or months following delivery that the bonding process is complete. The literature gives many guidelines to assist the maternity/pediatric nurse in evaluating the bonding process. (The normal process is discussed in Chapter 28, and the complications that arise when the baby is premature or ill are discussed in Chapters 24 and 26.)

The mother who has a high-risk labor and delivery or who has complications in the immediate postpartal period has an increased risk of having difficulties in attachment. She is more likely to have had medications, analgesia, or anesthesia during the intrapartal period, which may influence early interaction with her newborn infant. In the immediate postpartal period she may be more likely to receive medications or analgesics or have problems that limit her energy. Complications involving the mother or infant may necessitate separation during the critical early stages of attachment. Although these are only a few of the factors that may be present, they may be significant if they interfere with the bonding or attachment process.

Unfortunately, there are insufficient data available in the assessment of the bonding process when the mother is ill. It would be an oversimplification to state that the effects of bonding when the mother is sick are essentially the same as the effects of early separation, because the psychologic effect of illness has not been considered. The mother may have to work through her own ambivalence about the illness and the infant's role as the possible cause of the illness. Mothers may express this anxiety in many ways. Three expressions that nurses frequently encounter are: (a) clearly blaming the infant (pregnancy) for the illness; (b) blaming herself and the infant, especially when the pregnancy was unplanned or unwanted; and (c) blaming the infant and infant's father, as if a conspiracy existed to cause the illness.

Assessment of attachment behaviors has become increasingly important in light of current theories that correlate malattachment with an increased incidence of parenting problems, failure to thrive, and child neglect or abuse. When assessing attachment behaviors, the nurse should be careful not to generalize or give too much importance to any one factor. Adaptive behavior may vary from one situation to the next. Cultural factors such as decreased eye contact should also be considered. All cultures may not recognize or value the same behaviors that we in the Western culture value.

Assessment of the mother-infant (or father-infant) interaction should be made on various occasions to avoid attaching too much significance to one behavior on a given occasion. Books are available that provide comprehensive material and guidelines for identifying maladaptive behaviors. Some behaviors that may indicate a maladaptive attachment process include refusal by the mother to see her infant, failure to progress from fingertip to palm when holding or exploring the infant, making no attempt to establish eye-to-eye contact, inability to choose a name, or choosing a name that is so unusual or different that it brings ridicule (such as "Jim Beam," "Spirits," "Tornado").

The observed behaviors should be recorded objectively to validate the nursing assessment. An example of objective recording is: "At 9 AM mother fed her infant while holding him across her knees. She did not place her hands on the infant. During a 20 minute continuous observation the mother did not establish eye contact and did not talk to the infant. Mother refers to her infant as 'it' when talking with the nursing staff." Subjective documentation of the same situation would be: "Mother fed baby at 9 AM. Mother does not appear to like her baby." Subjective documentation includes the observer's values or biases and is not as beneficial as objective data.

When maladaptive behaviors are identified, there are various interventions that can be used. A team approach involving all three nursing shifts is advised. Any positive behaviors are communicated so that each staff member can continue to offer support and stimulate further development of such strengths.

Hospital practices should be examined for factors that may inhibit or exaggerate the maladaptive behaviors. Hospital practices such as strict adherence to four-hour feedings, discouraging the mother from unwrapping and looking at her infant, or prolonged separation may create a problem for some mothers.

The mother needs a supportive, understanding person she can interact with as she works through her feelings about the infant. At times, in the presence of severe emotional disorders, a referral to a psychologist or psychiatrist may be necessary. Referral to community agencies such as the Public Health Department is advised so that follow-up care can be established. The referral should be accompanied by a summary of the hospital course, the identified strengths and maladaptive behaviors, the educational process that was accomplished in the hospital, and the mother's response. Personal or telephone contact may be maintained after dismissal so that the mother can continue to have contact with a supportive person with whom she is already acquainted. The mother should be encouraged to call the postpartal unit or newborn nursery if she has questions.

PUERPERAL PSYCHIATRIC DISORDERS

Since Hippocrates first misdiagnosed puerperal infection for puerperal psychosis in 460 BC, health care providers have continued to believe that there is a psychologic, physiologic, endocrine, or metabolic rationale that makes women susceptible to "mental breakdown" following childbirth. Even today, the literature continues to hypothesize a multitude of reasons to account for "the phenomenon" of puerperal psychosis.

Many different types of psychiatric problems may be encountered in the puerperium and only rarely is the disorder serious. Approximately 70%–80% of women experience a transient depression during the first week, which is most common on the third postpartal day (Danforth, 1977). This transient depression is usually accompanied by tearfulness and is a self-limiting, brief episode.

Occasionally, the psychiatric problem is more serious and may be accompanied by lack of tearfulness, apathy, and lack of interest in the newborn. Danforth (1977) reports that in former years problems occurred primarily in women who had minimal contact with the baby in the hospital, had minimal education in child care or minimal first-hand knowledge of baby care (which increased feelings of inadequacy), or who functioned in a more dependent role in which they were not involved in the decision-making process. Nilsson et al. (1971) related puerperal psychosis to insufficient gender role development in the mother. Kaplan and Blackman (1969) found that the husband's cruelty, ineffectuality, or neglect greatly influenced the severity of the psychosis. Other contributing causes include use of general anesthesia; social class and ethnic origin; illegitimacy of offspring; planned versus unplanned pregnancy; breast-feeding; narcissism; perineal soreness; preexisting personality patterns; and pituitary and thyroid insufficiency.

The conclusion, if any can be reached from these diverse theories, is probably stated best by Brown and Shereshefsky (1972), who observed that "childbirth, if it plays any etiological role at all, functions as a nonspecific stress." Melchior (1975) concurs and encourages nurses to be prepared to do crisis intervention and to refer any mother who demonstrates coping dysfunction or decompensation.

The psychiatric disorders of the puerperium range from "postpartum blues" to full-blown psychoses, although the latter are rare and generally occur in patients with a history of emotional problems. In these cases, the stress associated with pregnancy, delivery, and motherhood functions as a precipitating factor rather than a causative agent.

Psychiatric Interventions

The type of interaction between the mother and newborn may be one of the first clues of a puerperal psychiatric disorder. A mother who has difficulty in interacting or in holding or feeding her infant may be demonstrating that she is not accepting the newborn. The nurse is able to observe the mother over a longer period of time and is available to talk with her at intervals throughout the day. When the mother is discharged, a referral may be made to the Public Health Department to provide follow-up. The public health nurse can be a resource person for the mother.

SUMMARY

The normal puerperium is a dynamic period during which major physiologic changes must take place in order for the body to return to its nonpregnant state. When the nurse is keenly aware of these normal physiologic changes, she can then quickly assess whether deviations occur in the involutional process. These deviations place additional stress on the body, creating a risk situation for the mother that necessitates immediate intervention and evaluation. In addition to the dynamic physiologic changes of the partpartal period, there are new psychologic needs to be met as the mother and family adapt to the challenge of their new roles and responsibilities as parents and as an expanded family.

SUGGESTED ACTIVITIES

1. Develop a written nursing care plan for a patient with a puerperal infection.
2. Complete a home visit with a community health/visiting nurse for a mother with a puerperal complication. Describe the resolution of the complication and assess the patient's involution progress.
3. Weigh several peri-pads to determine the amount of vaginal bleeding and to identify how they compare to the normal amount of vaginal bleeding.
4. Mrs. Lee complains of a sudden onset of dyspnea accompanied by sweating, pallor, cyanosis, confusion, systemic hypotension, and increased jugular pressure. Identify the complication and critical nursing management for Mrs. Lee's care.
5. Assess in several patients: involution, breast changes, bladder changes, episiotomy healing. Identify any deviations from the normal.

REFERENCES

Brazelton, T. B. 1963. The early mother-infant adjustment. *Pediatrics.* 32:931.

Brown, W. A., and Shereshefsky, P. May 1972. Seven women: a prospective study of postpartum psychiatric disorders. *Psychiatry.* 35:139.

Cooper, K. March 11, 1976. Thrombosis and embolism in obstetrics. *Nurs. Mirror.* 142:65.

Danforth, D. N., ed. 1977. *Obstetrics and gynecology.* Hagerstown, Md.: Harper & Row Publishers, Inc.

Daniel, D. G. Nov. 1969. Estrogen and puerperal thromboembolism. *Am. Heart J.* 78:720.

Daniel, D. G., et al. Aug. 5, 1967. Puerperal thromboembolism and suppression of lactation. *Lancet.* 2:287.

Hagen, D. Sept. 1975. Maternal febrile morbidity associated with fetal monitoring and cesarean section. *Obstet. Gynecol.* 46:260.

Hodge, C. Aug. 5, 1967. Suppression of lactation by stilbestrol. *Lancet.* 2:286.

Hoffman, J. B. Aug. 1953. A suggested treatment for inverted nipples. *Am. J. Obstet. Gynecol.* 66:346.

Gorbach, S. L., and Bartlett, J. G. May 23, 1974. Anaerobic infections, part I. *N. Eng. J. Med.* 290:1177.

Kaplan, E. H., and Blackman, L. H. 1969. The husband's role in psychiatric illness associated with childbearing. *Psychiatr. Quarterly.* 43:396.

Kempe, C. H., and Helfer, R. E. 1972. *Helping the battered child and his family.* Philadelphia: J. B. Lippincott Co.

Klaus, M. H., and Kennell, J. H. 1976. *Maternal-infant bonding: the impact of early separation or loss on family development.* St. Louis: The C. V. Mosby Co.

Markin, K. E., and Wolst, M.D. 1960. A comparative controlled study of hormones used in the prevention of postpartum breast engorgement and lactation. *Am. J. Obstet. Gynecol.* 80:128.

Melchior, July 1975. Is the postpartum period a time of crisis for some mothers? *Can. Nurs.* 71:30.

Nilsson, A., et al. 1971. Parental relations and identification in women with special regard to para-natal emotional adjustment. *Acta Psychiatr. Scand.* 47:57.

Otte, M. J. March 1975. Correcting inverted nipples. *Am. J. Nurs.* 75:454.

Pearson, H. E. Oct. 1967. Bacteroides in areolar breast abscesses. *Surg. Gynecol. Obstet.* 125:800.

Pritchard, J. A., and MacDonald, P. C. 1976. *Williams obstetrics.* 15th ed. New York: Appleton-Century-Crofts.

Pryor, K. 1973. *Nursing your baby.* Rev. ed. New York: Harper & Row Publishers, Inc.

Rees, D. April-June 1976. Sore nipples are a pain. *Keeping Abreast J.* 1:125.

Tindall, V. R. Dec. 1968. Factors influencing puerperal thromboembolism. *J. Obstet. Gynecol. Brit. Comm.* 75:1324.

Turnbull, A. C., et al. June 1971. Antenatal and postnatal thromboembolism. *Practitioner.* 206:727.

Wiechetek, W. J., et al. May 15, 1974. Puerperal morbidity and internal fetal monitoring. *Am. J. Obstet. Gynecol.* 119:230.

ADDITIONAL READINGS

Antle, K. 1975. Psychologic involvement in pregnancy by expectant fathers. *J. Gynecol. Nurs.* 4(4):40.

Applebaum, R. M. 1969. *Abreast of the times.* Miami: Applebaum.

Applebaum, R. M. 1970. The modern management of successful breast feeding. *Pediatr. Clin. N. Am.* 17:203.

Applebaum, R. M. 1974. Breastfeeding and care of the breasts. In Davis' *Gynecology and obstetrics,* vol. 1, no. 32. Hagerstown, Md.: Harper & Row Publishers, Inc.

Avery, J. L., ed. 1976. Good news of "innies": up front facts about inverted nipples. *Keeping Abreast J.* 1(1):46.

Babson, S. G., and Benson, R. C. 1971. *Management of high risk pregnancy and intensive care of the neonate.* 2nd ed. St. Louis: The C. V. Mosby Co.

Barnes, J. 1975. The aftermath of childbirth; physical aspects. *Proceed. Royal Soc. Med.* 68:223.

Brazelton, T. B. 1969. *Infants and mothers.* New York: Delacorte Press.

Brazelton, T. B. 1974. *Toddler and parents.* New York: Delacorte Press.

Brazelton, T. B. 1976. *Doctor and child.* New York: Delacorte Press.

Butts, H. F. May 1968. Psychodynamic and endocrine factors in postpartum psychoses. *J. Nat. Med. Assoc.* 60(3):224.

Butts, H. F. March 1969. Postpartum psychiatric problems. *J. Nat. Med. Assoc.* 61(2):136.

Clausen, J. P., et al. 1977. *Maternity nursing today.* 2nd ed. New York: McGraw-Hill Book Co.

Cohen, R. Dec. 1971. Breast-feeding without pregnancy. *Pediatr.* 48:996.

Coulton, D. Jan. 1966. Prenatal and postpartum uses of hypnosis. *Am. J. Clin. Hypnosis.* 8(3):192.

Division of Maternal and Perinatal Studies, Department of Health, New South Wales. March 1972. Thromboembolic phenomena in the puerperium: a retrospective survey. *Med. J. Australia.* 1:628.

Garibaldi, R. A., et al. 1974. Bacteriuria during indwelling urethral catheterization. *N. Engl. J. Med.* 291:215.

Helfer, R. E., and Kempe, C. H. 1976. *Child abuse and neglect: the family and the community.* Cambridge, Mass.: Bollinger.

Hurd, J. 1975. Assessing maternal attachment: first step toward the prevention of child abuse. *J. Gynecol. Nurs.* 4:25.

Kennell, J. H., et al. 1974. Maternal behavior one year after early and extended postpartum contact. *Develop. Med. Child Neurology.* 16:172.

Klaus, M., and Kennell, J. 1972. Maternal attachment: importance of the first postpartum days. *N. Engl. J. Med.* 286:460.

Klaus, M., and Kennell, J. 1973. Care of the mother. In *Care of the high risk neonate.* Philadelphia: W. B. Saunders Co.

Klaus, M., et al. 1970. Human maternal behavior at the first contact with her young. *Pediatr.* 46:187.

Koshiishi, T., et al. 1971. A double blind study of the effects of kimotab on engorgement of the breast. *Acta Obstet. Gynaec. Jap.* 18:222.

La Leche League International. 1956. *The womanly art of breast feeding.* Franklin Park, Ill.: The League.

Moir, D. D., and Davidson, S. 1972. Postpartum complications of forceps delivery performed under epidural and pudendal nerve block. *Br. J. Anesthesia.* 44:1197.

Nau, J. Jan.–March 1976. When baby has surgery. *Keeping Abreast J.* 1(1):38.

Newton, M., and Newton, N. 1970. The normal course and management of lactation. *Child and Family.* 9(2):102.

Nilsson, A., et al. 1967. Postpartum mental disorder in an unselected sample: The importance of the unplanned pregnancy. *J. Psychosomatic Res.* 10:341.

Raphael, D. 1973. *The tender gift: breastfeeding.* Englewood Cliffs, N.J.: Prentice-Hall, Inc.

Rising, S. S. 1974. The fourth stage of labor—family integration. *Am. J. Nurs.* 74(5):870.

Robson, K. 1967. The role of eye-to-eye contact in maternal-infant attachment. *J. Child Psych. Psychiatry.* 8:13.

Rosenwald, G. C., and Stonehill, M. W. March–April 1972. Early and late postpartum illnesses. *Psychosomatic Med.* 34(2):129.

Rothenburg, R. 1975. *The complete book of breast care.* New York: Crown Publishers.

Rubin, R. Nov. 1961. Basic maternal behavior. *Nurs. Outlook.* 9:683.

Rubin, R. Nov. 1963. Maternal touch. *Nurs. Outlook.* 11:828.

Seward, E. M. March 1972. Preventing postpartum psychosis. *Am. J. Nurs.* 72(3):520.

Stevens, B. C. Dec. 1971. Psychoses associated with childbirth: a demographic survey since the development of community care. *Soc. Science Med.* 5:527.

Wiedenbach, E. 1964. *Clinical nursing: a helping art.* New York: Springer Verlag New York, Inc.

Wiedenbach, E. 1967. *Family centered maternity nursing.* New York: Putnam.

CHAPTER 30

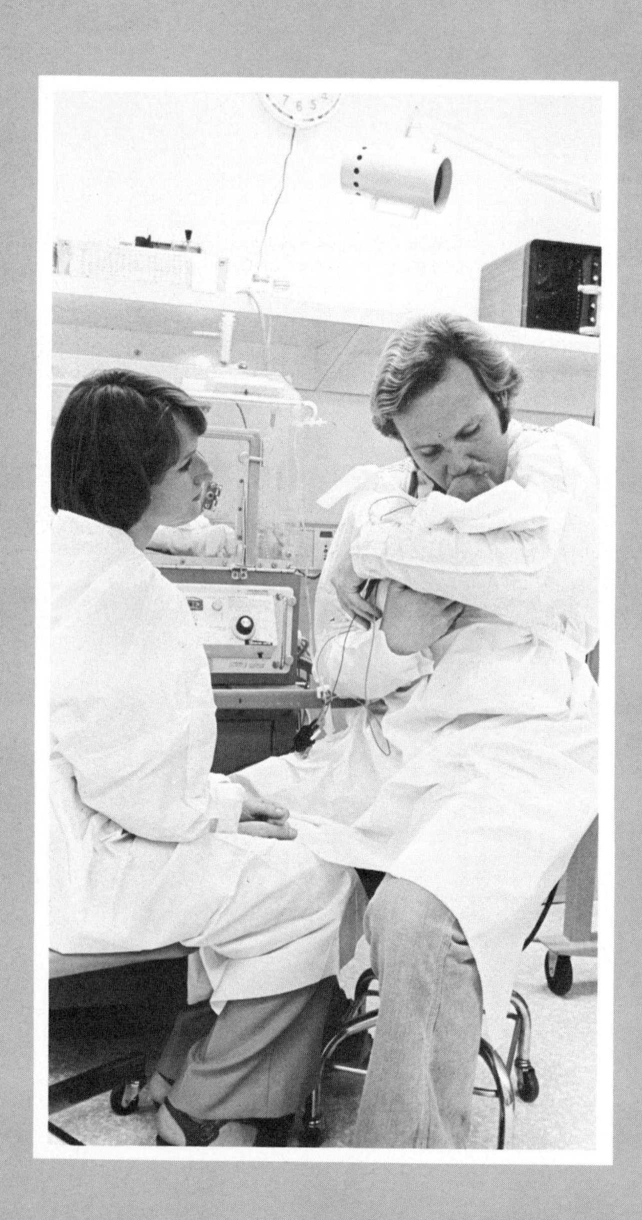

FAMILIES IN CRISIS AND THE ROLE OF THE NURSE

OBJECTIVES

- Define the term *family crisis.*
- List the types of crises that may occur within a family.
- Compare the process of crisis intervention to the nursing process.
- Describe crisis intervention as applied to maternity nursing.

The postpartal period is a stressful time for the family. The new mother and father must adjust to their new roles and responsibilities. Siblings must accept the entrance of the newest family member. Life-style changes are necessary, and daily activities are disrupted. The lives of family members, especially the parents, often revolve around the needs of the new baby.

Many families find that their coping resources are tapped beyond their limit during this postpartal period because of overwhelming stress arising from various problems. The nurse who follows postpartal families can identify those families suffering from a crisis. The members of these families may be behaving in obviously maladaptive ways, or the nurse may pick up subtle clues indicating the presence of a problem.

The nurse may be required to apply crisis intervention techniques when caring for postpartal families who are not functioning optimally. This chapter describes some of the crises requiring nursing intervention during the postpartal period.

FAMILIES AND CRISIS

When one or more members of a family cannot successfully cope with stress, a crisis may occur. A *crisis* is defined as any situation that cannot be coped with adequately by the usual living patterns of the family. Two types of crises are generally recognized: maturational crisis and situational crisis. Maturational crises are those rated to the normal processes of growth and development. A maturational crisis generally evolves more slowly, is characterized by feelings of disequilibrium, and requires the individual to make character changes. Adolescence is seen as a common maturational crisis (Aguilera and Messick, 1974). A situational crisis is seen by Lindemann (1956) as an event in the life of an individual that generates intense emotional strain and stress and that requires successful adaptation in order to master the situation. Common situational crises include bereavement, birth of a defective child, and loss of employment.

The breakdown in coping mechanisms associated with a crisis can result from internal or external pressures. Families with fewer resources may be expected to have more trouble coping with a crisis. Families typically feel the effects of particular pressures at certain stages of the family life cycle (see Chapter 3) more than at other times. For example, economic pressures are generally greatest in the first and last years of a marriage. In the middle years, after the children have left home, a couple usually has a higher income and fewer expenses.

Increased social pressures take their toll on families. Political and economic factors, influences by the media, governmental policies, and various other environmental variables affect family structure. Some people decry the degeneration of the institution of the family; others believe that social development has made certain changes in the family necessary. Various life-styles have made divorce and family dissolution more prevalent. In the event of a crisis, unless the individual members have values that support the integrity of the family, the crisis often becomes the stimulus for family breakdown.

Examples of family crises are as follows:

1. Loss within family
   a. Hospitalization
   b. Loss of child
   c. Loss of spouse
   d. Loss of parents
   e. Separation (work, military service, etc.)
2. Loss of standing in community
   a. Disgrace (drug addiction, spouse or child abuse, delinquency, alcoholism)
   b. Marital infidelity
   c. Nonsupport or poverty
   d. Progressive dissention
3. Addition of new members
   a. Pregnancy and birth
   b. Adoption
   c. Relative moves in
   d. Reunion after separation
   e. Remarriage

4. Other crises
   a. Divorce
   b. Annulment
   c. Desertion by spouse
   d. Illegitimate birth
   e. Imprisonment
   f. Institutionalization
   g. Runaway child
   h. Suicide of member
   i. Homicide
   j. Birth of deformed or premature child

The postpartal family must deal with several of these events simultaneously. For example, the birth of a healthy child and the stress of adjusting to the new member can precipitate disruption within a family. If other factors are present, such as economic problems, the family may not have the coping mechanisms to deal with the crisis adaptively. Without adequate adjustment, these crises can prevent a family from adequately performing the task of nurturing its members.

A significant feature of the family in crisis is the phenomenon of *scapegoating*. An individual within the family becomes the focus of the underlying disturbance and carries most of the blame for the disturbance by "acting out" in certain unacceptable ways. If the family is dealt with as a unit, it can be seen that the family member who is acting out does so in the context of disturbed social relations within the family group. In other words, the individual is not the only one in need of treatment—the entire family needs to be treated. An individual acts in the context of his environment and in response to those around him. For example, the woman who suffers from severe postpartal depression may be responding to a situation in which she is receiving no help from other family members or in which her spouse demands the same kind of attention that he received before the baby arrived.

Conflict about an issue may gradually erode a family if ineffective means of coping with conflict are utilized. The individual who attempts to escape the situation by desertion, divorce, or separation, who submits to domination, or who uses physical force is contributing to his or her family's crisis state (Duvall, 1975).

How a family crisis is met depends on the personalities involved, on the family structure, and on previously existing problems. It is also determined by the family's previous experience with crises and patterns of problem solving. Responses may range from defeatism and self-pity to acceptance to belief in the situation as a challenge. Situations that cause a crisis may differ from family to family. Family adjustment depends on family philosophy and outlook, family policies and practices, and personal resources of family members.

Factors that aid in the weathering of a crisis include adaptability, a value system in which family closeness is of greater importance than material gain, sharing of tasks by husband and wife, accurate perception of problems, the attitude that an individual's emotional problems are a family concern, problem-solving skills of the wife, and personal adjustment of husband and wife (Hill et al., 1953). Constructive coping mechanisms during a family crisis include such measures as open communication of feelings and wishes among family members, empathy, competency in role-playing and role reversal, negotiation until the family members are satisfied, mental health maintenance for the family as a whole, consultation with competent resource persons, and consolidation of the family's goals (Duvall and Hill, 1960).

It is important to recognize that a crisis cannot continue forever. The high anxiety level existing in a crisis state moves the individual to some action to end the crisis, and the outcome of a crisis is significantly influenced by the amount of support the family or individual receives. Several outcomes are possible for the family or individual:

1. The family can return to its precrisis state. This may be the result of effective problem solving. Growth has not necessarily taken place; the family has simply returned to its previous level of functioning.

2. The family may grow from the crisis experience. For example, marriage may be strengthened as a result of a difficult situation that the partners overcame together. A couple may become better parents because of a crisis with their child.

3. The intolerable tension of a crisis may be reduced by neurotic behavior such as resorting to alcoholism or drug dependency. Possibly one or both of the partners in a marriage may desire dissolution of the relationship, thus seeking to end

the tension of a crisis. Desertion or breakdown of a family member's mental health may occur.

The purpose of crisis intervention is to recognize the potential negative outcomes for each family and to prevent their occurrence. The utilization of crisis intervention by skilled professionals can lessen the effects of crises and can assist the family in returning to a state of equilibrium.

CRISIS INTERVENTION

Crisis intervention is a form of psychotherapy. The main differences between crisis intervention and traditional psychoanalysis or psychotherapy are in the amount of time involved, the focus of the therapy, and the role of the therapist (Aguilera and Messick, 1974). Psychoanalysis may continue for a number of years before the goal of restructuring the personality is attained. The psychoanalyst is passive and nondirective. Traditional psychotherapy focuses on removing specific symptoms and preventing the development of neurosis or psychosis. The psychotherapist is more active than the psychoanalyst, but he or she still assumes an indirect role or that of a participating observer. There are up to twenty sessions in brief psychotherapy.

Crisis intervention, on the other hand, focuses on the immediate crisis. It is not necessary to know the history or the personalities of the people in crisis. The therapist's role is direct, active, and participating. Getz et al. (1974) describe the qualities necessary for crisis intervention counseling:

1. Empathy, or perception of the patient's feelings.
2. Warmth, or a communication of acceptance and an effort to understand.

Table 30–1. Major Differences Among Psychoanalysis, Psychotherapy, and Crisis Intervention Methodology*

Dimension	Psychoanalysis	Psychotherapy	Crisis intervention
Goals of therapy	Restructuring the personality	Removal of specific symptoms	Resolution of immediate crisis
Focus of treatment	1. Genetic past	1. Genetic past as it relates to present situation	1. Genetic present
	2. Freeing the unconscious	2. Repression of unconscious and restraining of drives	2. Restoration to level of functioning prior to crisis
Usual activity of therapist	1. Exploratory 2. Passive observer 3. Nondirective	1. Suppressive 2. Participant observer 3. Indirect	1. Suppressive 2. Active participant 3. Direct
Indications	Neurotic personality patterns	Acutely disruptive emotional pain and severely disruptive circumstances	Sudden loss of ability to cope with a life situation
Average length of treatment	Indefinite	From one to twenty sessions	From one to six sessions

*From Aguilera, D., and Messick, J. 1978. *Crisis intervention.* 3rd ed. St. Louis: The C. V. Mosby Co.

3. Genuineness, which leads to a trusting relationship.

The techniques of crisis intervention are relatively simple and do not require extensive training. Time is limited; usually one to four sessions are all that are needed, because a crisis lasts no longer than four to six weeks. A crisis may be prolonged past six weeks depending on the events that precipitated it. Some families have chronic crisis due to a long-term illness or disability. (Table 30–1 outlines the main differences in therapy.)

The primary goals of crisis intervention (Getz et al., 1974) are (a) to help the patient deal with the crisis and to regain his or her equilibrium, that is, to return to the precrisis state; and (b) to enable the person to grow from the experience, to gain more self-awareness, and to improve coping skills.

The specific problem-solving steps involved in the technique of crisis intervention as outlined by Aguilera and Messick (1974) are similar to the steps in the nursing process: (a) assessment, (b) planning of therapeutic intervention, (c) intervention, and (d) evaluation.

Assessment

The first step in the assessment is to clearly define the situation before any action is taken and to identify the crisis-precipitating event. The patient's perception of the event is examined. What does the event mean to the patient? Is the perception distorted or realistic? Assessment is then made of the person's support systems (family, friends, and religious beliefs). The individual's coping skills are evaluated. How does this person usually handle tension, depression, or anxiety? Questions from the counselor may help the patient remember methods he or she has used successfully in the past. At this point, the counselor may determine that the person needs more extensive therapy. For example, the person may seem suicidal, may be in danger of hurting others, or may be out of touch with reality.

Planning the Therapeutic Intervention

Further data must be collected at this point. How much has the crisis disrupted the individual's life? How does the family feel about the problem? Tentative approaches are proposed to the individual and examined for their usefulness.

Intervention

Planned intervention may include one technique or a combination of several. A direct approach may help the patient gain an intellectual understanding of the crisis. This approach includes interpretation and confrontation and must be used carefully to avoid further raising the patient's anxiety. Allowing the person to express his or her feelings freely stimulates the person to explore these feelings. The counselor should be very attentive and relaxed. Other resources (such as therapy groups) may be included when necessary; a knowledge of community resources is valuable. Assertiveness training sessions may benefit the patient by increasing self-esteem. When a trusting relationship has been established, reassurance based on truth and concrete evidence can be a powerful tool to alleviate anxiety and to give moral support. Feedback is important for increasing the person's confidence in the progress being made and thus hastening it.

Experience helps the counselor to become familiar with several other methods of intervention. For example, *modeling* might be helpful. Modeling is introducing the behavior of others as examples through role-playing or by having the patient talk with someone who has mastered a similar crisis.

A counselor might try *self-disclosure*—sharing one's own experiences with the patient. This method is effective in stimulating a person in crisis to talk about the problem. The counselor must be careful that he or she does not add to the patient's problem. The patient is not there to resolve the counselor's crises.

Any positive coping mechanisms that can be added to the patient's repertoire will help this individual handle future stressful situations more easily. The counselor can teach the patient relaxation techniques as an effective means of dealing with anxiety. One that nurses have found to be helpful is an adaptation of the relaxation and breathing techniques used by women in labor.

Evaluation

Evaluation is an ongoing process throughout planning and intervention. Various approaches are tried and then discarded or modified depending on their success. As the crisis is resolved, attention is turned to anticipatory planning. The adaptive coping mechanisms that the patient has used successfully are reinforced. Discussion can include ways in which the present experience may help in coping with future problems.

THE NURSE AS CRISIS INTERVENTION COUNSELOR

To help an individual or family in crisis, a counselor needs to learn the scope of the crisis as perceived by the individual or family members and its consequent impact on the entire family. Because nursing has traditionally emphasized family-centered care, the nurse can be an effective crisis counselor.

According to Caplan (1961), nurses have another advantage in the role of crisis counselor. They are especially close to their patients in many ways:

1. *Close in space.* The nurse is physically close in the home, in the hospital, and at the bedside.
2. *Close in time (contact time).* The nurse is often present throughout a crisis, as during labor and delivery.
3. *Psychologic closeness.* The nurse becomes involved with the family members, forms trusting relationships, and gives emotional support.
4. *Sociologic closeness.* Communications between the nurse and family members can be open. Patients feel free to ask questions.

Other functions the nurse can easily perform include *case-finding.* The nurse is able to observe family interaction and interpersonal relationships and thus can recognize and identify crisis situations. The nurse can also motivate patients to seek help because of their unique, trusting relationship.

The nurse is in a good position to explain a patient's situation to other team members or support personnel and to interpret their recommendations to the patient. The nurse can serve as the primary coordinator of the crisis intervention program for the family. Her teaching skills are useful for crisis resolution in maternity nursing.

FAMILIES AT RISK

Many human experiences are predictable, such as progress through developmental stages and addition of family members. With precautionary measures, one can avoid some crises. Role changes occur when a person leaves school, attains employment, marries, becomes a parent, and eventually retires. When a person cannot or does not prepare for these events, crisis may result. For example, with adequate family planning a newly married couple need not start a family immediately but can determine the optimal time when they are economically and emotionally secure.

Unpredictable life events also occur within families, including death of a significant other, serious physical illness, natural disasters resulting in personal or financial loss, stillbirth, and birth of an infant with congenital anomalies. These, too, may result in crisis if normal coping mechanisms are not adequate.

Through the process of assessment, nurses and other health care professionals are responsible for identifying families at risk. Assessment should discover crisis states in families and identify whether a particular family or individual is in crisis.

After determination that the family is, in fact, in a crisis or precrisis state, the information obtained from careful assessment becomes the basis for the plan for crisis intervention. Hoff (1978) suggests that the following key questions be answered before formulating a plan for help:

1. To what extent has the crisis disrupted the family's normal life pattern?

2. Are there any family members not able to go to school or to hold a job?
3. Can family members handle the responsibilities involved in the activities of daily living—for example, eating or personal hygiene?
4. Has the crisis situation disrupted the lives of others?
5. Is a family member suicidal, homicidal, or both?
6. Does the family or a family member seem to be on the brink of despair?
7. Has the high level of tension distorted one or more individual's perception of reality?
8. Is the family's usual support system present, absent, or exhausted?
9. What are the resources of the nurse or agency in relation to the family's assessed needs?*

Essential data are identified from the answers to these and related questions. These data are used for the intervention plan. Following are key features of an effective intervention plan (Hoff, 1978):

1. The plan is problem oriented, with a focus on the immediate concrete problem.
2. The plan considers the family's functional level and dependency needs.
3. The plan is appropriate to the family's culture and life-style.
4. The plan is inclusive of all family members and their social milieu.
5. The plan is practical, has a specified time frame, and is concrete.
6. The plan is dynamic and renegotiable.
7. The plan includes an arrangement for follow-up contact.

Active involvement of the family in the plan for crisis resolution is essential for the success of the intervention plan.

Many of the crises affecting families postpartally require an intervention plan directed toward loss and grief. The family that suffers loss of an infant or that faces the task of caring for a deformed or seriously ill child is a family at risk for serious disruption.

LOSS AND GRIEF

Loss is a state of being deprived or being without something one has had. Some losses are natural and predictable, whereas others are unpredictable. Losses can be sudden or gradual, traumatic or nontraumatic.

The most serious loss is the loss of a loved one by death. Loss can also be through divorce or separation. Serious illness can cause partial loss because of disability.

One can also lose an aspect of "self," which is how we feel about ourselves, our ideas, our worth, and our capacities. Loss of health, loss of body parts, loss of pride, and loss of independence are all examples of loss of self.

Object loss refers to the loss of an object that has special value and emotional meaning to a person.

Losses are experienced throughout life. For example, there are numerous developmental losses. A mother feels a tremendous loss (of a part of herself) when giving birth and later feels a loss whenever her baby is separated from the breast. Such losses produce strong emotional responses. Other losses are hardly noticeable, but they still evoke responses. How a person responds or adapts to the resultant change contributes to the development of that person's personality.

Grief is an emotional state, a reaction to loss. Studies have shown that the grief reaction is similar whether the loss is of a loved one, a body part, or a body function (Schoenberg et al., 1970).

Grief has been studied by Freud, Deutsch, and many others in the past, but it was Lindemann's classic report, "Symptomatology and Management of Acute Grief" (1944), that brought the medical, psychologic, and sociologic implications of separation, grief, and bereavement to the attention of medical and social scientists. Lindemann

*Modified from Hoff, L. A. 1978. *People in crisis: understanding and helping.* Menlo Park, Calif.: Addison-Wesley Publishing Co., p. 53.

observed that *acute grief* is a definite syndrome and described five features he considered to be characteristic of this syndrome:

1. Somatic distress characterized by sighing respiration, a complaint of lack of strength and of exhaustion, digestive symptoms, and lack of appetite.
2. An intense preoccupation with the image of the deceased and feelings of unreality.
3. Strong feelings of guilt, self-accusation, and feelings of negligence in relation to the deceased.
4. A disturbing loss of warmth in relationship to other people, feelings of irritability, and anger.
5. A disorganized pattern of conduct, such as restlessness.

Grief work is the inner process of working through or managing the bereavement (Schoenberg et al., 1974). The first stage of this process is disbelief, which is similar to the denial stage of dying (Kübler-Ross, 1969). It is common for people to say, "No, no . . . it can't be!" The second stage is a questioning one. The person who suffers the loss looks for reasons why the death occurred, asking "What happened?" and "How?" This search for reasons is an attempt to make the event believable. Questioning is usually followed by anger (stage 3). Anger is often expressed as, "Why did this happen?" Anger at God may be expressed. The fourth stage is anger combined with desperation. The person seems resigned, dismayed, and in despair. This stage is the first indication of acceptance, which is necessary before the final stage can be reached—resolution.

The duration of grief is variable, and it can last up to six months or a year, but the acute stage should be over in one or two months. Brief upsurges of these feelings will occur in later months, especially when the bereaved person is faced with reminders of the loss. The best indicator of the resolution of grief is a gradual return to the preloss level of functioning. New interests and relationships are formed. According to Engel (1964), the clearest indication that grieving has successfully been completed is the ability to realistically and completely remember both the pleasures and disappointments of the lost relationship.

Grief work can be helped or hindered by a person's emotional status and by the ability of family members or significant others to allow the person to express grief. If the person does not successfully complete the grief work, he or she may have prolonged or distorted grief reactions.

For example, delayed grief may occur if affected persons are maintaining the morale of others and therefore are repressing their own reactions. Or they may be attempting to respond to our culture's expectation of controlled behavior.

Chronic grief is a response that represents a denial of the reality of the loss. There can be no resolution if there is no acceptance. One manifestation of chronic grief is retaining the lost loved one's belongings as they were during his or her lifetime.

Anticipatory grief reactions are seen when there is a threat of death or separation (Lindemann, 1944). Because the dynamics of anticipatory grief have much in common with those of acute grief, one might expect that working through anticipatory grief would diminish the acute grief when the loss finally does occur. This may be the case with some, but many people cannot work through feelings of denial. These feelings are supported by the hope that accompanies anticipatory grief. Kübler-Ross (1969) has noticed this with the dying patient. However, hope must be gone before acceptance of death can be complete. (This is especially true with parents of very ill children.)

There are often ambivalent feelings about the dying loved one that relatives find difficult to accept or to recognize. The difference in the impact of ambivalence on the anticipatory grief of family members is that the target of the ambivalent feelings is not only still alive but also particularly vulnerable (Schoenberg et al., 1974). The ambivalence may be interpreted as a death wish—which is too unacceptable to admit—and so these feelings are repressed.

The stable family, with healthy coping mechanisms and strong support both from within the family structure and from friends and other ties, can weather the crises of life. However, the high-risk family may need the help and support that crisis intervention can give.

CRISIS INTERVENTION DURING IMMEDIATE POSTPARTAL PERIOD

The postpartal period is a time of disequilibrium and of emotional changes. It is also a period of increased susceptibility to situational crises because of changes in roles of family members and because of the many economic and social pressures that are encountered (Caplan, 1961). Although the stable family can usually cope and even grow in strength, family members need help to handle certain highly stressful events that can occur during the maternity cycle. These include fetal death and birth of a low-birth-weight infant or of a defective child.

Loss of Newborn

The loss of a newborn evokes intense mourning reactions whether the baby lives one hour, lives several days, or is stillborn; whether the baby is a nonviable 500 gm fetus or a 4000 gm healthy child; and whether the baby is planned or not. Until recently, it was not realized that both parents show the same grief reactions (Klaus and Fanaroff, 1973). The father may have more difficulty expressing his grief because, while supporting and comforting his wife, he may be suppressing his own feelings and thus delaying his grief work. He may have not worked through ambivalent feelings of guilt. Thus, denial mechanisms may be persistent, with the anger being directed outward—perhaps at his wife. Disturbance in communication between husband and wife could lead to serious disturbances within the family, as a recent study shows (Cullberg, 1972). One or two years after perinatal death, one-third of the mothers have had emotional problems.

If the father is not included in the grief work and if his needs are not recognized, he may feel alienated from his wife at a time when she needs him the most. This alienation increases his feelings of helplessness, and he may withdraw.

Nursing Intervention

A major goal of the nurse should be to facilitate and to encourage communication between parents who have experienced the loss of a newborn (see the accompanying Nursing Care Plan on stillbirth). The nurse should encourage them not to hold back their feelings—to cry if they feel like it. Unless they are told what reactions to expect, their feelings may worry them and further interfere with their relationship. Once denial is overcome and the questioning phase starts, the nurse can clarify the reality of situations in which mothers blame themselves for the death. It is usual for the woman to review the pregnancy over and over. The nurse should allow her to express her feelings of anger, which may be directed toward the physician, the staff, or God. The mother's feelings may be turned inward. The nurse should watch for feelings of shame and guilt, which are destructive to the mother's self-esteem and can delay her grief work. The nurse must be as positive as possible but should avoid such meaningless phrases as "Don't worry" or "Everything will be fine." Especially important is avoiding comments on future pregnancies ("You are young, you can have other babies"). Such remarks negate this baby. Remember, good crisis intervention concentrates on the immediate problem.

A diagnosis of intrauterine death before or during labor is extremely stressful for parents and staff. Shock and disbelief plus the physical discomfort of labor produce overwhelming stresses. Denial is maintained by most mothers up to the moment of delivery, often combined with anger, bargaining, and depression, as described by Kübler-Ross (1969). Allowing the woman to express her feelings facilitates her working through her acute grief in a healthy manner when the death is confirmed at delivery.

Never leave the mother alone in labor. For optimum emotional support, continuity of care (one caregiver) should extend through the labor and delivery and into the immediate postpartal period.

Nurses may be shocked at their own feelings of anger and despair and therefore find it extremely difficult to work effectively with grieving parents. Nurses who recognize that they, too, are going through the grief process must not suppress these feelings, so that they can move through the phases quickly. Nurses who suppress or deny their reactions tend to remove themselves from the situation, to increase their physical and psychologic distance from patients, and thus to reduce their effectiveness. Each nurse must assess her reactions: How are you expressing your anger? Are you venting your anger on your peers or your family? With your patient, are you nonjudgmental, helpful, and approachable?

NURSING CARE PLAN

Stillbirth

Patient Data Base

History

1. Prenatal history
   a. Uneventful? High-risk?
   b. Fetal death before labor? During labor? Totally unexpected?
2. Family history
   a. Interactions, communications – are they mutually supportive? Blaming?
   b. Grief response – are normal reactions manifested?

Nursing Priorities

1. Facilitate the normal grief process.

Problem	Nursing interventions and actions	Rationale
Communications between parents	Encourage them to express feelings, to cry. Provide support.	Disturbance in communication can delay resolution of grief and cause possible long-range disturbances within family.
Father's needs	Include father in intervention.	Both parents have same grief responses. Each needs support of the other.
Acceptance of reality of the situation	Listen. Correct any misconceptions, answer questions.	Misconceptions reinforce guilt feelings and lower self-esteem.
	Make it possible for parents to see infant. Explain the reasons for the infant's death, if known. Prepare them fully for the experience.	Acceptance is facilitated and resolution will follow more smoothly.

Nursing Care Evaluation

There is evidence that normal grief work is in process.

Disbelief phase has been worked through, followed by questioning and anger. Feelings have been expressed freely, and acceptance has begun.

Because crisis lasts 4-6 weeks, resolution will not be evident in the hospital. Further support may be needed to help parents cope, because acute grief can be recurrent. Referral can be made to community mental health agency, to appropriate parent groups, or to visiting community health nurse.

A month or six weeks after the stillbirth, parents are regaining their equilibrium, to precrisis level. Their coping skills have been strengthened, and family relationships are even closer than before.

Without resolution, guilt feelings and lack of communication between parents may not only lead to abnormal grief reactions (delayed or chronic grief) but may lead to disorganization of family unit.

Recent research indicates that most mothers want to see and touch their dead babies (Seitz and Warrick, 1974; Kowalski and Osborn, 1977). It is felt that this practice facilitates grief work, because acceptance and then resolution follow more smoothly. The nurse who has been caring for the mother and has established a trusting and therapeutic relationship with the parents is able to pick up feelings and concerns that parents may have about seeing the baby. If parents wish to see the child and are denied their wish, they may imagine something far worse than the reality. If parents do not want to see their child, the nurse should support their decision. If the parents are prepared by descriptions of what they will see and by explanations of what happened when there is evidence of trauma to the fetus, the experience is less stressful. Point out all normal and positive aspects of the child. Mothers who have seen their dead babies (even those who are macerated or deformed) have stated that the reality was not so bad as they had imagined. For the mother unable to face the task, some benefit may be realized from answering her questions concerning the delivery and the child.

Premature Birth

The delivery of a premature baby is an acute crisis situation for a family. Acute grief reactions are evident, as there is the loss of the perfect full-term baby they have fantasized. Also, the premature birth has interrupted the attachment process, denying the mother the last few weeks of pregnancy that seem to prepare her psychologically for the stress of birth. Attachment at this time is fragile, and interruption of the process by separation can affect the future mother-child relationship. Many studies on the crisis of prematurity focus on this aspect. A healthy mother-infant relationship depends upon a successful resolution of the crisis.

Kaplan and Mason (1960) have identified four psychologic tasks that must be mastered for successful resolution. The first task, at time of delivery, prepares the mother for possible loss of the child. It is anticipatory grief, involving a withdrawal from the attachment process. She can still hope for the child's survival but is prepared for its death. The second task is to face the reality of the loss. The anticipatory grief and depression the mother exhibits are normal responses and show that she is mastering these tasks. When the baby's survival is certain, the third task is undertaken—the resumption of the attachment process. Her outlook is then one of hope and anticipation. The fourth task is understanding and learning the special needs of the premature infant in preparation for assuming responsibilities of care.

Table 30-2 illustrates the maternal emotional and situational differences between term and premature births. The factors listed may be commonly found in mothers but are by no means universal. These factors may be influenced or altered by the mother's past experiences, her personality, the specifics of her situation, and the amount of education and support she may receive concerning her situation. The following case study contains many of the factors identified in the table.

Case Study*

Eric was born 8 weeks premature to Mrs. V. He weighed approximately 1790 gm at birth and subsequently reduced to 1680 gm. He remained in the neonatal intensive care unit for over five weeks, had abdominal surgery for pyloric stenosis, and nearly died from surgical complications.

This was Mrs. V's third pregnancy. Her first son was stillborn. Her second son was born after a high-risk pregnancy, a fetus-threatening virus, and two months of strict maternal bed rest.

Mrs. V's labor and delivery occurred before she was psychologically ready and her child physically ready for birth. Because she perceived a malfunctioning of her reproductive system, her self-esteem was lowered. She was very anxious and showed limited confidence in her ability to give birth with a good outcome. At a time that should have been filled with happiness and joy because personal expectations were being met, Mrs. V perceived yet another reproductive failure and exhibited unhappiness, grief, and disappointment about not meeting her expectations.

During the delivery, Mrs. V was allowed to be only a passive participant. She told the health care team to do whatever was necessary to save her baby. An air of emergency filled the delivery room as additional staff rushed to assist with and to make decisions about the birth process. Immediately after delivery, her infant was rushed to the neonatal intensive care unit. Mrs. V was not given an opportunity to see or to hold him.

Postpartal stress is extremely great for Mrs. V because she is anxious about her ill infant's health. He appears small and unattractive when she compares him to full-term babies. She expresses concern about her ability to care for her son. She fears emotional attachment to her infant, because of his uncertain health. The memories of her previous stillbirth surface, which increases the stress. Mrs. V watches the nurses and physi-

*Modified from material prepared by Lauri Lowen, Chairman of Parents of Prematures, Seattle, Washington.

Table 30–2. Comparison of Maternal Emotional and Situational Factors in Term and Premature Births*

Factors	Term birth	Premature birth
Emotional factors at time of birth	More likely to be regarded as rewarding experience	May be regarded as less than rewarding experience; frustration and a sense of missing something
	More likely to have good self-image regarding body functioning	May have poor self-image regarding imperfectly functioning body
	Pleasurable experience	Anxiety-producing experience
	Confident in ability to give birth with good outcome	Not confident in ability to give birth with good outcome
	Little fear of danger to baby	Great fear of danger to baby
	Great sense of achievement; pride in success	Little sense of achievement; no pride in failure; guilt
	Emotionally prepared for outcome as planned and expected	Shocked; emotionally unprepared for outcome, which is different from plans and expectations
	Previous pregnancy and birth experience likely to have been considered favorable	Previous pregnancy and birth experience probably considered unfavorable if previous reproductive failure occurred
	Happiness and joy	Unhappiness and grief
	Meets expectations	Disappointment; does not meet expectations
Situational factors at time of birth	Able to choose option of active role in birth	Possibly forced to play passive role by circumstances
	More in control of situation; more opportunity for voluntary decisions	Less in control of situation; decisions often made for her
	More opportunity to be independent	Dependent
	Nonemergency atmosphere	Emergency and crisis atmosphere
Postpartal emotional factors	Pleased at appearance of baby	Shocked at appearance of baby
	Identifies with other mothers in her chosen role	Does not identify with other mothers; did not choose this strange role; does not know exactly what her role is
	Loss of fantasized child; replaced by different but probably equally acceptable child	Loss of fantasized child; replaced by less acceptable sick or imperfect child
	Usually under less than severe stress	Under severe stress
	Happy with successful completion of pregnancy	Regrets unsuccessful completion of pregnancy; feels "empty"
	Less anxious about baby's health than mother of premature	Very anxious about baby's health

*Copyright © 1980, Lauri Lowen, Chairman of Parents of Prematures, Seattle, Washington.

Table 30–2. Cont'd

Factors	Term birth	Premature birth
	Sees baby as better than average; feels proud	Sees baby as better than average premature baby but not as good as average term baby; may feel envious
	Confident in ability to care for child	Not confident in ability to care for child
	Naturally inclined and eager to increase attachment to child	Naturally inclined to increase attachment to child, but may be hindered by question of baby's survival
	Attachment process free of many obstacles	Attachment process more difficult, with more obstacles
	Realistic expectations	May have unrealistic expectations; less able to anticipate outcome
	Baby seems to be parents' possession	Baby seems to be hospital's possession
Postpartal situational factors	Baby is responsive to mother	Baby is less responsive to mother
	Major caregiver; role as major caregiver begins early; caregiving requires moderate energy and effort	Not major caregiver; role as major caregiver begins late; caregiving requires more energy and effort
	Recognition by others of identity as mother	Less recognition by others of identity as mother
	Gives pregnancy up in exchange for possessing baby	Gives pregnancy up but cannot possess baby
	Many opportunities for contact with baby	Fewer opportunities for contact with baby
	Information about parents' situation readily available	Information about parents' situation not readily available
	Family unit can be together	Family unit may be divided due to hospitalization of baby

cians as they touch, feed, diaper, and care for her son. She feels that it should be she who takes care of her infant but that instead her son "belongs" to the hospital staff.

Mrs. V leaves the hospital carrying not her child but flowers. Her role as a new mother is not recognized by others because she does not have a baby in her arms. Although she has few opportunities to have contact with the baby, she participates by bringing her breast milk for Eric and by breast-feeding him when his condition allows. She expends much time and energy traveling to the hospital and telephoning to ask about Eric's condition.

When Eric is discharged from the hospital, Eric's responsiveness to Mrs. V increases as he matures. Mrs. V begins to receive more recognition as a new mother.

Nursing intervention in Mrs. V's case requires identification of the immediate crisis situation, appropriate action directed toward each problem contributing to the crisis, and evaluation of the effectiveness of the intervention.

Nursing Intervention

Nursing intervention should be family-centered, focusing on helping the parents cope with the crisis. The nurse should assess their relationship. Are they able to share their feelings? The nurse should share their concerns and encourage them to express their feelings. What is their perception of the sequence of events? The nurse should clarify and correct any misconceptions, explaining as soon as possible the status and condition of the baby and arranging for them to see and to touch their child. Few parents take the initiative, because persons in crisis feel helpless. Without aid and encouragement, many hours might pass, further delaying optimum resolution of the crisis.

The nurse should accompany the parents to the intensive care nursery, preparing them ahead of time as much as possible for what they will see. Not only should the baby's appearance and condition be described but also the equipment and procedures. The nurse should encourage questions and anticipate as many as possible. Experience makes one aware of which aspects of care alarm the parents the most. The parents should be made to feel welcome so that they feel free to return whenever they wish. As soon as feasible (and depending on the infant's condition), the parents should be included in the child's care (Figure 30–1). Being a part of the team increases the mother's self-esteem and helps her feel less futile by doing something useful and positive. It is especially important to include the parents in planning for the baby's care at home.

The evaluation of this intervention should be ongoing. For example, the nurse should be careful not to give the mother a caretaking task too difficult for her. Failure reinforces her feelings of inadequacy. Further evaluation after the infant has gone home is useful in determining whether the crisis has been resolved satisfactorily. The parents are usually given the intensive care nurse's telephone number to call for support and advice. It is suggested here that the staff follow up this family with visits or telephone calls at intervals for several weeks to assess and evaluate the baby's (and parents') progress.

Caplan et al. (1965) identified indicators for healthy and unhealthy outcomes in parent-child relationships and in parenting skills. The best indicator, they found, was the frequency of the parents' visits to the child in the nursery. Why are some parents hesitant to visit their baby? One reason might be the staff's pessimism about the baby's chance of survival (Klaus and Fanaroff, 1973). While the bonds of affection are still forming, they can be damaged by such pessimism. If the mother abandons hope, anticipatory grief becomes acute grief and can move rapidly toward resolution, which in reality is detachment. If the baby lives, attachment will be a difficult task.

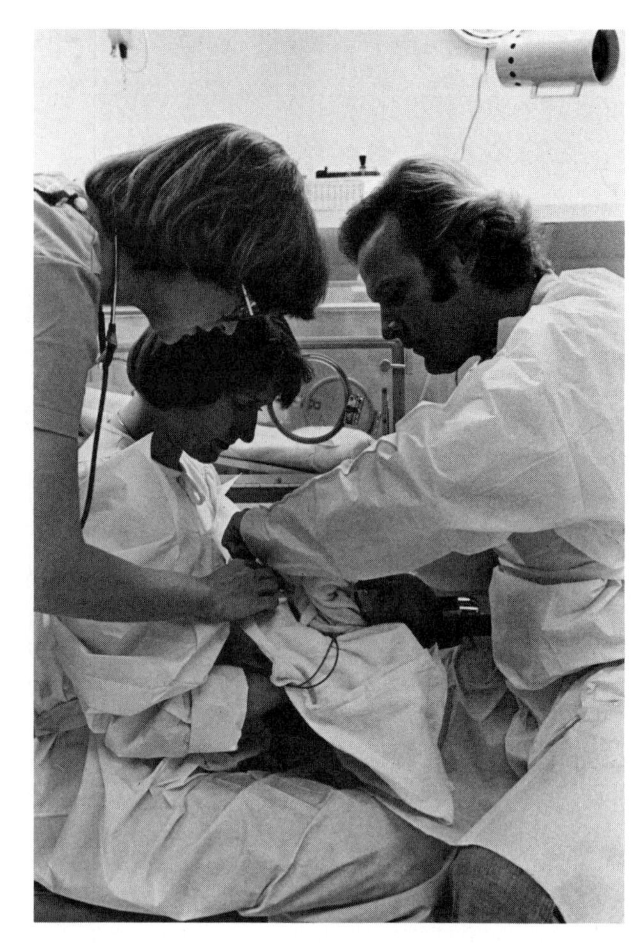

Figure 30–1. The parents of this premature infant are learning how to take care of their child.

Another parental behavior signaling future problems is the inability to accept help that has been offered (DuBois, 1975). Some parents are unwilling or unable to share their fears with each other and with other family members and friends. They need these support systems and should be encouraged to express their feelings.

It is healthy for the future parent-child relationship if the new parent seeks information about the baby's condition, prognosis, and treatment. The emotionally healthy mother is aware of ambivalent and negative feelings and is willing to express them. It is unhealthy for the future relationship if the parents do not seek information, cannot express feelings, and show no anxiety.

It is important to identify possible poor-outcome parents and to help them avoid negative patterns of behavior through prompt, active intervention. Intervention is a possibility, because persons in crisis usually have an increased desire to be helped and are more susceptible to influence

(Caplan et al., 1965). Identification and assistance to these parents could reduce the incidence of mothering disorders. Consequences of mothering disorders range from minor abnormalities, such as persistent overconcern, to the most severe—the battered child syndrome. Klaus and Kennell (1970) believe that the whole range of problems may be due in part to maternal-infant separation during the early newborn period. Statistics show that 21%–41% of battered children were premature. Green and Solnit (1964), in their report on the vulnerable child syndrome (children who are expected by their parents to die prematurely and who develop severe emotional disturbances), observed that 44% of these infants were separated from their parents in the first weeks of life because of prematurity or severe illness.

Many of the interesting psychologic aspects of prematurity are undergoing research. For example, a recent study suggests that stress may be a factor in the cause of prematurity (Schwartz and Schwartz, 1977). Mothers of premature infants were compared to mothers of full-term infants. Results showed that mothers of premature infants showed significantly higher numbers of life changes preceding and during pregnancy.

Obviously, prematurity is a psychologic as well as a medical problem. High-risk mothers can be identified, and early crisis intervention may be useful in reducing the levels of stress and perhaps the incidence of prematurity.

Defective Newborn

The crisis created by the birth of a defective infant is devastating. Not only is there the loss of the expected normal child, but both parents feel a severe loss of self-esteem and self-confidence. The grief reactions become prolonged and recurrent because as long as the child lives there can be no resolution of grief. Guilt and ambivalent feelings are overwhelming. As time elapses, the unresolved grief becomes less intense. The term chronic sorrow has been used to describe the long-term effect (Young, 1977). Although there is no resolution, acceptance of the reality of the disability can be reached with either maladaptive or adaptive outcomes.

With *maladaptive responses,* acceptance can be precarious. Persistent denial can make it almost impossible to care for the infant. Or overwhelmed by guilt, the mother may spend all her time with the affected child, ignoring her other children. Social life is often restricted because of the time involved in care. Marriages, under a tremendous strain, often break down.

Olshansky (1962) has described a grief reaction in parents of defective or mentally retarded children that he terms "chronic sorrow." The parents begin this process with the birth of the child and the grieving or sorrow continues throughout the lifespin as they face subsequent developmental milestones that their child is unable to meet. For the first few months their child may not be very different from other children, but as their child reaches the age when the "normal child" would be walking and talking, toilet-training, going to school, or learning to drive a car, their sorrow is reinforced. The process continues until they are elderly and concerned with what will happen to their child when they die.

The needs of siblings should not be overlooked. They have been looking forward to the new baby, and so they, too, suffer a degree of loss. The siblings have grief work to do, and they are frightened and confused by their ambivalent feelings. Younger children may react with hostility and older ones with shame. Both reactions make them feel guilty. Parents, preoccupied with working through their own feelings, cannot give the other children the attention and support they need. Sometimes another child becomes the focus of family tension. Anxiety thus directed can take the form of finding fault or of overconcern. It is a form of denial; the parents cannot face the real worry—the congenital anomaly of the new child. The observant nurse could, after assessing the situation, see that another family member or friend step in and give the needed support to the siblings of the afflicted baby.

With the *adaptive response,* the parents accept the reality and learn to cope with the crisis. They attempt to face the consequences of the child's defect, and they take part in his or her care. Support systems (family and friends) are mobilized. There are many ups and downs, with parents alternating between maladaptive and adaptive responses. The goal of nursing intervention (and crisis intervention) is to enhance adaptation. Emotional support, acceptance of often intense reactions, and explanations as indicated help families toward acceptance of the child and his defect. As with the premature infant, the rationale for early contact with the baby is the establishment of a positive parent-child relationship. The nurse should help the parents assess their strengths and coping

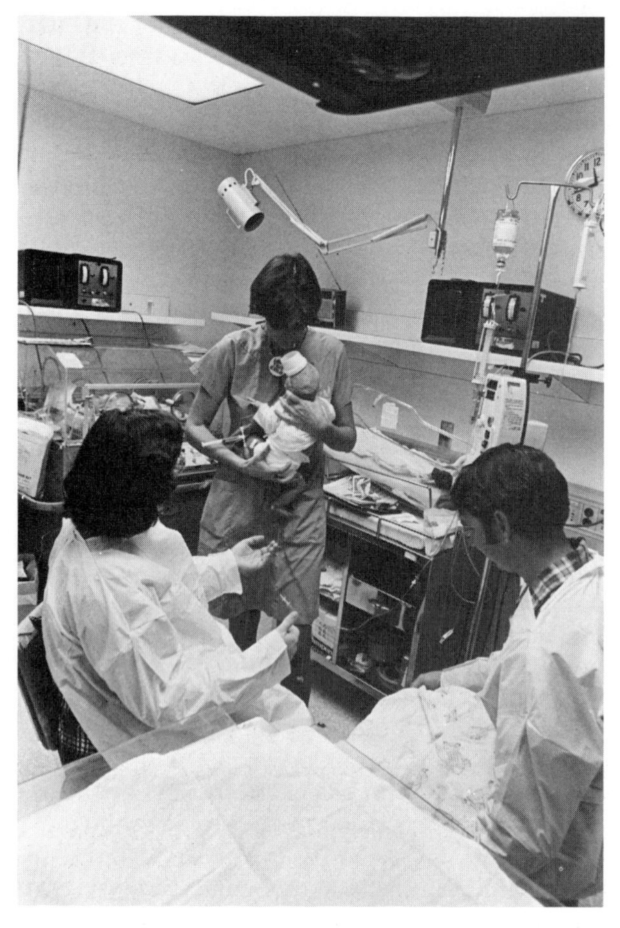

Figure 30–2. It is essential that the nurse recognize the emotional needs of parents of children with defects or complications.

skills. Their perception of the problem is often distorted by strong guilt feelings. Correcting these perceptions helps relieve some of the self-blame and helps them move toward acceptance. Referral to agencies for financial assistance or referral to parent groups increases the range and depth of support for the family. Again, knowledge of community resources is important. If genetic counseling is indicated, the nurse should prepare the family with thorough explanations and support to reduce possible stress and should make sure they understand the counseling.

A multidisciplinary approach is needed to adequately care for the affected child and his family, including perhaps a social worker, a family counselor, medical specialists, and various agencies. This approach can be overwhelming for the family; if continuity of care is not maintained, they may feel fragmented and confused. The nurse can often interpret the many facets of care.

Parents have expressed deep appreciation of the nurse who cares, listens, and shares their feelings and concerns (Figure 30–2). As one mother of an infant born with an encephalocele said, "Someone came to my bed and identified herself as a nurse from pediatrics. She asked me if I would like to *hold* my baby. I couldn't believe it! Someone finally cared about the here and now for me and my child. This nurse seemed to realize my strong need to hold the child I had carried nine months" (Donnelly, 1974).

Many families do adapt, accept the child as he is, and find fulfillment in caring for him. For these families, even a crisis as profound as the birth of a defective child can be a strengthening experience for the individual and for the family unit.

CRISIS INTERVENTION DURING POSTPARTAL FOLLOW-UP

In this section, we consider child abuse, malattachment, and single-parent families. Child abuse is a tragedy, and when it is discovered, action should be taken immediately to ensure the safety of the children and to resolve the emotional problem of the parents. Single-parenthood is a situation that carries the risk of potential crisis. Economic and social factors may place intense stress on the single parent, and the problems of the parent ultimately affect his or her children.

Nurses often deal with families suffering from other kinds of crises (for example, alcoholism, drug dependency, poverty, and other serious problems that can contribute to the malfunctioning of a family). An in-depth discussion of all these problems is beyond the scope of this text. However, during the postpartal follow-up evaluation, the nurse should be attuned to all clues indicating a family in crisis.

Child Abuse

Child abuse refers to the physical, emotional, verbal, or sexual harming of a child, either by the child's parents or by older siblings. Child abuse arises in part from the cultural sanctioning of physical disciplining of children by their parents. Among the many serious effects of child abuse are physical handicaps, a poor self-image, inability to love others, antisocial or violent behavior in later life, and death (Hoff, 1978).

The parents of an abused child are rarely malevolent and hateful. In fact, child abuse is an emotional crisis for the parents as well as for the child. In some cases the abused child is one whose behaviors provoke the parent to violent action. The parent feels shaken by hurting the child, is riddled by guilt, is in many cases fearful for the child's life, worries about being prosecuted for the act, and is afraid of future uncontrolled outbursts of anger toward the child.

It is important for the nurse to understand the emotional needs of abusive or neglectful parents in order to provide the proper intervention. Such parents tend to be emotionally immature, unhappily married, unsure of themselves as parents, unrealistic in their expectations for their children, themselves survivors of a deprived or abused childhood, and victims of frequent life crises.

Nursing Intervention

In order to help abused children and their parents, the nurse must first be aware of the signs of child abuse. Hoff (1978) lists the following indications of child abuse in a family:

1. Repeated injury of a child with unconcern on the part of the parents or with unlikely explanations.
2. Aggressive behavior by the child, which is really a cry for help.
3. Generally neglected appearance of the child.
4. A "supercritical" attitude on the part of the parents.

Once the nurse has identified a family in need of help, crisis intervention should begin by encouraging the parents to express their feelings about the situation. Of particular value is actively involving the parents in planning the medical care for the child so that they feel that they are doing something positive and perhaps "making up" for the harm.

The nurse should explain to the parents the function of the child welfare authorities, pointing out that such people are there to help the parents carry out their responsibilities. The nurse can also help by referring the parents to such self-help groups as Parents Anonymous and Parents in Crisis. Such groups can help parents to express their feelings and to realize that there are others who have experienced similar situations. Additional counseling from appropriate sources can help the parents to deal with possible underlying emotional problems that contributed to their child abuse behavior.

Attachment Problems

During the past 15 years a body of evidence has grown that clearly demonstrates that the most common element in the lives of parents who neglect or abuse their children is a "lack of empathic mothering" in their own lives (Steele and Pollack, 1968). This phrase describes inadequate responses of the caretaker to the infant, frequently beginning in the perinatal period and related to poorly developed maternal-infant attachment or insufficient bonding (Helfer and Kempe, 1976). Because of this finding attention has been given to the promotion of adequate parent-infant bonding in order to prevent malattachment and its related sequelae. Factors that may retard the formation of maternal-infant attachment include "an abnormal pregnancy, an abnormal labor or delivery, neonatal separation, other separation in the first six months, illnesses in the infant during the first year of life, and illnesses in the mother during the first year of life" (Helfer and Kempe, 1976, p. 29).

In the prenatal period, warning signs that may indicate lack of acceptance of the pregnancy and a potential for malattachment include: negative maternal self-perception, excessive mood swings or emotional withdrawal, failure to respond to quickening, excessive maternal preoccupation with appearance, numerous physical complaints, and failure to prepare for the infant during the last trimester (Helfer and Kempe, 1976).

At delivery, signs of maladaptive responses may include lack of interest in seeing the baby; withdrawal, sadness, or disappointment; negative comments such as "She's such an ugly thing"; or expressions of marked disappointment when told of the baby's sex. When shown the infant, the mother may avoid looking at it or may regard it without expression. She may decline to hold it, or if she does hold it she may not touch or stroke the infant's face or extremities. The mother may also avoid asking questions or talking to the infant and may suddenly decide she doesn't really want to breast-feed (Johnson, 1979).

During the early postpartal period, evidence of maladaptive mothering may include limited handling of or smiling at the infant, lack of preparation or questions about his needs and care, and failure to snuggle the newborn to her neck and face. The mother may also describe her infant negatively or use animal characteristics hostilely in referring to the infant: "He looks just like a withered old monkey to me!"

The father, too, may exhibit signs of malattachment to his infant. Examples of maladaptive paternal behaviors include inattentiveness and indifference toward the child, rough, unrelaxed handling, and tense, rigid posture. The father may also choose inappropriate types of play and exhibit no protective behavior toward his child (Johnson, 1979).

Interventions to promote healthy parent-infant attachment should begin during the prenatal period. The health history should include questions that provide the caregivers with some initial understanding of the parents' attitudes, fears, and knowledge. Questions such as "Do you have family or close relatives nearby?" "How often do you see them?" and "Are there things that have happened in the past that make you worry about the baby or being pregnant?" may provide invaluable information.

As the pregnancy progresses, further information may be elicited and teaching instituted. During the third trimester the caregivers should begin looking for evidence that the parents have started to prepare for the infant. Has the mother made arrangements for the care of other infants, if any, while she is hospitalized? Have the parents chosen names or prepared a room or area for the baby? Lack of preparation suggests continued rejection of the pregnancy.

A tour of the maternity unit is often helpful in decreasing fear of the unknown and fostering confidence in the parents so that they will be able to cope.

It is essential that whenever possible mother, father, and newborn have a period of time alone to begin getting acquainted. The baby should be undressed so that the parents can explore him thoroughly, and the mother may nurse if she so desires. To facilitate eye contact, eye prophylaxis may be delayed until after this parent-infant meeting (Helfer and Kempe, 1976).

During the postpartal period, continued family interaction should be encouraged by a supportive staff, liberal visiting policies, and educational offerings for both father and mother. Staff should be trained in assessment techniques and alert for evidence of malattachment, so that appropriate interventions may be initiated. If necessary, referrals to the community health nurse or social services may provide the ongoing assistance needed. Telephone "hotlines" may provide a useful resource for a frustrated parent, as may classes or parents' groups during the early weeks following delivery.

Single-Parent Families

In the United States in 1975, 12.1 million children (17%) under 18 years of age lived with one parent—1.9 million with their fathers and 10.2 million with their mothers. Single-parent homes most commonly develop as a result of divorce, desertion, or death of a spouse. Such parents are faced with problems related to maintaining their own positive self-concept in the face of depression, guilt, and lowered self-esteem. They must decide how to answer questions the children raise about family disruption and must avoid the urge to become a "superparent" in the wake of guilt associated with the effects of loss on the children.

Single-parent homes also occur when the child's parents are unmarried and the child lives with either his mother or father. The stigma of illegitimacy is decreasing, and children raised in these situations are less apt to be labeled negatively because of it. Positive acceptance of the single woman parent is readily available in the Chicano and black communities. Many single women rear their children with the support of their extended families.

Single-parent homes may also occur as a result of adoption. This phenomenon, although still relatively rare, is increasing. For instance, the Los Angeles County Department of Adoptions reported that from 1965 to March 1975 they placed 265 children (1.3% of all their placements) with single parents; 251 of these parents were women, and 14 were men. Single parenthood as a result of adoption requires an individual to consider the meaning not only of adoption but also of being single and a parent.

In the book *The Single-Parent Experience,* Klein (1973) lists four implications that single "expectant" parents male or female, ought to consider prior to accepting the single-parent role:

1. What will being a single parent mean with respect to family, employment, and social relations?
2. What are the social implications for the child raised by a parent in a particular state, region, and neighborhood?
3. What child care facilities are available?
4. What are the options available with respect to sexual identity formation of the child?

Hazards to successful childrearing do exist for single-parent families. It is extremely important that, as children pass through certain developmental stages, they be provided with opportunities to relate to individuals of the same and the opposite sex to learn sex roles. In a single-parent family these opportunities may not be readily available, and provision for substitute experiences must be made. A relative or close friend may assist the single parent in providing the needed experiences. An additional drawback in a single-parent family is the lack of opportunities for the child to observe parental husband-wife interactions. Furthermore, the parent in a single-parent situation is usually employed outside the home. Thus, the parent must handle the demands of job and family alone. With adequate support from the extended family, from friends and groups such as Parents Without Partners, single parents can successfully raise healthy, mature children. This task requires careful recognition of potential problems, evaluation of the needs of both child and parent, realistic planning and provision for day-to-day living, and use of available support and assistance when necessary.

Nursing Intervention

The nurse will be able to counsel the single parent more effectively if she has an understanding of the stresses and demands of parenting a child. A single parent is more likely to have minimal support.

The nurse can begin by assessing the parent's educational needs and then providing information as needed. Counseling may include investigation into the availability of child care facilities and referral to single parent support groups within the community. Support groups offer opportunities for socialization, sharing of problems, and opportunities to expose the child to a group setting in which there are members of the opposite sex, which may facilitate sexual identity formation.

SUMMARY

The nurse is often in a position of first contact with families in the grip of a crisis brought about by health care problems. The death of a child, the birth of a deformed infant, and the arrival of a premature child are various types of crises that may be seen in obstetric nursing. Successful coping on the part of the maternity patient and her family can be facilitated by the health care professional skilled in crisis intervention. Even though the nurse may be unsure of her skills in crisis intervention, she may still be the person in the position to make a referral for a family in crisis. The recognition of the stresses that contribute to a crisis and the insight to make a referrral to a skilled crisis intervention counselor can constitute positive nursing care for a grieving family or couple.

Recognition of the dynamics of loss and grieving are important for the nurse practitioner; she may therefore better aid her patients who experience these life situations. It is a realistic part of nursing care to assess the emotional turmoil in a patient and plan intervention to aid the patient in returning to a harmonious level of functioning.

SUGGESTED ACTIVITIES

1. Identify obstetric-related crises and propose appropriate crisis intervention for each situation.
2. Develop a plan of crisis intervention that could be used with a family in a crisis during the postpartal period.
3. Observe an obstetric patient who has just experienced loss. Identify the patient's stage of grief and suggest interventions to facilitate the grief process.
4. In a small group, discuss maternity nursing situations that may result in a malfunctioning of the family unit.

REFERENCES

Aguilera, D. C., and Messick, J. M. 1974. *Crisis intervention: theory and methodology.* 2nd ed. St. Louis: The C. V. Mosby Co.

Caplan, G. 1961. *An approach to community mental health.* New York: Grune & Stratton, Inc.

Caplan, G., et al. 1965. Four studies of crisis in parents of prematures. *Community Mental Health J.* 1:149.

Cullberg, J. 1972. In *Psychosomatic medicine in obstetrics and gynaecology.* 3rd International Congress, Basel. New York: S. Karger.

Donnelly, E. 1974. The real of her. *J. Obstet. Gynecol. Neonatal Nurs.* 3:48.

DuBois, D. R. 1975. Indications of an unhealthy relationship between parents and premature infants. *J. Obstet. Gynecol. Neonatal Nurs.* 4:21.

Duvall, E. M. 1975. *Marriage and family development.* 5th ed. Philadelphia: J. B. Lippincott Co.

Duvall, E., and Hill, R. 1960. *Being married.* New York: Association Press.

Engel, G. 1964. Grief and grieving. *Am. J. Nurs.* 64:93.

Getz, W., et al. 1974. *Fundamentals of crisis counseling.* Lexington, Mass.: D. C. Heath.

Green, M., and Solnit, A. J. 1964. Reactions to the threatened loss of a child: the vulnerable child syndrome. *Pediatrics.* 34:58.

Helfer, R. E., and Kempe, C. H. 1976. *Child abuse and neglect.* Cambridge, Mass.: Ballinger Publishing Co.

Hill, R., et al. 1953. *Eddysville's families.* Chapel Hill: University of North Carolina.

Hoff, L. A. 1978. *People in crisis: understanding and helping.* Menlo Park, Calif.: Addison-Wesley Publishing Co.

Johnson, S. H. 1979. *High risk parenting: nursing assessment and strategies for the family at risk.* Philadelphia: J. B. Lippincott Co.

Kaplan, D., and Mason, E. 1960. Maternal reactions to premature birth viewed as an acute emotional disorder. *Am. J. Orthopsychiatry.* 30:539.

Klaus, M. H., and Fanaroff, A. A. 1973. *Care of the high-risk neonate.* Philadelphia: W. B. Saunders Co.

Klaus, M. H., and Kennell, J. H. 1970. Mothers separated from their newborns. *Pediatr. Clin. N. Am.* 17:1015.

Klein, C. 1973. *The single-parent experience.* New York: Walker and Co.

Kowalski, K., and Osborn, M. R. Jan.-Feb. 1977. Helping mothers of stillborn infants to grieve. *Am. J. Maternal-Child Nurs.* 2:29.

Kübler-Ross, E. 1969. *On death and dying.* New York: The Macmillan Co.

Lindemann, E. 1944. Symptomatology and management of acute grief. *Am. J. Psychiatry.* 101:141.

Lindemann, E. 1956. The meaning of crisis in individual and family. *Teachers Coll. Rec.* 57:310.

Olshansky, S. 1962. Chronic sorrow: a response to having a mentally defective child. *Soc. Casework.* 43:190.

Schoenberg, B., et al. 1970. *Loss and grief: psychological management in medical practice.* New York: Columbia University Press.

Schoenberg, B., et al. 1974. *Anticipatory grief.* New York: Columbia University Press.

Schwartz, J. L., and Schwartz, L. H., eds. 1977. *Vulnerable infants.* New York: McGraw-Hill Book Co.

Seitz, P. M., and Warrick, L. H., Nov. 1974. Perinatal death: the grieving mother. *Am. J. Nurs.* 74(11):2028.

Steele, B., and Pollock, C. 1968. A psychiatric study of parents who abuse infants and small children. *The Battered Child,* eds. R. Helfer and C. H. Kempe. Chicago: University of Chicago Press.

Young, R. K. 1977. Chronic sorrow: patient's response to the birth of a child with a defect. *Am. J. Maternal-Child Nurs.* 2:38.

ADDITIONAL READINGS

Burgess, E. W. 1968. The family as a unit of interacting personalities. In *Family roles and interactions: an anthology,* ed. J. Heiss. Chicago: Rand McNally & Company.

Burgess, E. W. 1971. *The family: from traditional to companionship.* New York: Van Nostrand Reinhold Company.

Duvall, E. 1971. *Family development.* 2nd ed. Philadelphia: J. B. Lippincott Co.

Holmes, T., and Rahe, R. 1967. The social readjustment rating scale. *J. Psychosom. Res.* 11:213.

Kantor, D., and Lehr, W. 1975. *Inside the family.* San Francisco: Jossey-Bass, Inc., Publishers.

Mercer, R. T. 1977. *Nursing care for parents at risk.* Thorofare, N.J.: Charles B. Slack, Inc.

Novak, E. R., et al. 1971. *Textbook of gynecology.* 8th ed. Baltimore: The Williams & Wilkins Co.

Patterson, G. R. 1977. *Families: applications of social learning to family life.* Champaign, Ill.: Research Press.

Putt, A. M. *General systems theory applied to nursing.* Boston: Little, Brown & Co.

APPENDICES

- That the family is viewed as a whole unit within which each member is an individual enjoying recognition and entitled to consideration;
- That childbearing and childrearing are unique and important functions of the family;
- That childbearing is an experience that is appropriate and beneficial for the family to share as a unit;
- That childbearing is a developmental opportunity and/or a situational crisis, during which the family members benefit from the supporting solidarity of the family unit.

To this end, the family-centered philosophy and delivery of maternal and newborn care is important in assisting families to cope with the childbearing experience and to achieve their own goals within the concept of a high level of wellness, and within the context of the cultural atmosphere of their choosing.

The implementation of family-centered care includes recognition that the provision of maternity/newborn care requires a team effort of the woman and her family, health care providers, and the community. The composition of the team may vary from setting to setting and include obstetricians, pediatricians, family physicians, certified nurse-midwives, nurse practitioners, and other nurses. While physicians are responsible for providing direction for medical management, other team members share appropriately in managing the health care of the family, and each team member must be individually accountable for the performance of his/her facet of care. The team concept includes the cooperative interrelationships of hospitals, health care providers, and the community in an organized system of care so as to provide for the total spectrum of maternity/newborn care within a particular geographic region.[1]

As programs are planned, it is the joint responsibility of all health professionals and their organizations involved with maternity/newborn care, through their assumptions and with input from the community, to establish guidelines for family-centered maternal and newborn care and to assure that such care will be made available to the community regardless of economic status. It is the joint concern and responsibility of the professional organizations to commit themselves to the delivery of maternal and newborn health care in settings where maximum physical safety and psychological well-being for mother and child can be assured. With these requirements met, the hospital setting provides the maximum opportunity for physical safety and for psychological well-being. The development of a family-centered philosophy and implementation of the full range of this family-centered care within innovative and safe hospital settings provides the community/family with the optimum services they desire, request and need.

In view of these insights and convictions, it is recommended that each hospital obstetric, pediatric, and family practice department choosing this approach designate a joint committee on family-centered maternity/newborn care encompassing all recognized and previously stated available team members, including the community. The mission of this committee would be to develop, implement, and regularly evaluate a positive and comprehensive plan for family-centered maternity/newborn care in that hospital.

In addition, it is recommended that all of this be accomplished in the context of joint support for:

- The published standards as presented by The American College of Obstetricians and Gynecologists, The American College of Nurse-Midwives, The Nurses Association of The American College of Obstetricians and Gynecologists, The American Academy of Pediatrics, and the American Nurses' Association.[2–7]
- The implementation of the recommendations for the regional planning of maternal and perinatal health services, as appropriate for each region.[1]
- The availability of a family-centered maternity/newborn service at all levels of maternity care within the regional perinatal network.

Potential Components of Family-Centered Maternity/Newborn Care

No specific or detailed plan for implementation of family-centered maternity/newborn care is uniformly applicable, although general guidance as to the potential components of such care is commonly sought. The following description is intended to help those who seek such guidance and is not meant to be uniformly recommended for all maternity/newborn hospital units. The attitudes and needs of the community and the providers vary from geographic area to geographic area, and economic constraints may substantially modify the utilization of each component. The detailed implementation in each hospital unit should be left to that hospital's multidisciplinary committee established to deal with such development. In addition to the maternal/newborn health care team, community and hospital administrative input should be assured. In this manner, each hospital unit can best balance community needs within economic reality.

The major change in maternity/newborn units needed in order to make family-centered care work is attitudinal. Nevertheless, a description of the potential physical and functional components of family-centered care is useful. It remains for each hospital unit to implement those components judged feasible for that unit.

I. *Preparation of families:* The unit should provide preparation for childbirth classes taught by appropriately prepared health professionals. Whenever possible, physicians and hospital maternity nurses should participate in such programs so as to maximize cohesion of the team providing education and care. All class approaches should include a bibliography of reading materials. The objectives of these classes are as follows:

   A. To increase the community's awareness of their responsibility toward ensuring a healthy outcome for mother and child.

   B. To serve as opportunities for the community and providers to match expectations and achieve mutual goals from the childbirth experience.

   C. To serve to assist the community to be eligible for participation in the full family-centered program.

   D. To include a tour of the hospital's maternity and newborn units. The tour should be offered as an integral part of the preparation for childbirth programs and be available to the community by appointment. The public should be informed of a mechanism for emergency communication with the maternity/newborn unit.

II. *Preparation of hospital staff:* A continuing education program should be conducted on an ongoing basis to educate *all levels* of hospital personnel who either directly or indirectly come in contact with the family-centered program. This education program may include:

   - Content of local preparation for childbirth classes.
   - Current trends in childbirth practices.
   - Alternative childbirth practices: safe and unsafe, as they are being practiced.
   - Needs of childbearing families to share the total experience.
   - Ways to support those families experiencing less than optimal outcome of pregnancy.
   - Explanation of term "family" so that it in-

6. American Nurses' Association. *Standards of Maternal-Child Health Nursing Practice,* 1973.
7. (a). The American College of Obstetricians and Gynecologists, the American College of Nurse-Midwives, and The Nurses Association of The American College of Obstetricians and Gynecologists. *Joint Statement on Maternity Care.* 1971.
(b). The American College of Obstetricians and Gynecologists, the American College of Nurse-Midwives, and The Nurses Association of The American College of Obstetricians and Gynecologists. *Supplement to Joint Statement on Maternity Care.* 1975.

APPENDIX B UNITED NATIONS DECLARATION OF THE RIGHTS OF THE CHILD

Preamble

Whereas the peoples of the United Nations have, in the Charter, reaffirmed their faith in fundamental human rights, and in the dignity and worth of the human person, and have determined to promote social progress and better standards of life in larger freedom,

Whereas the United Nations has, in the Universal Declaration of Human Rights, proclaimed that everyone is entitled to all the rights and freedoms set forth therein, without distinction of any kind, such as race, color, sex, language, religion, political or other opinion, national or social origin, property, birth or other status,

Whereas the child, by reason of his physical and mental immaturity, needs special safeguards and care, including appropriate legal protection, before as well as after birth,

Whereas the need for such special safeguards has been stated in the Geneva Declaration of the Rights of the Child of 1924, and recognized in the Universal Declaration of Human Rights and in the statutes of specialized agencies and international organizations concerned with the welfare of children,

Whereas mankind owes to the child the best it has to give

NOW THEREFORE
THE GENERAL ASSEMBLY
PROCLAIMS

This Declaration of the Rights of the Child to the end that he may have a happy childhood and enjoy for his own good and for the good of society the rights and freedoms herein set forth, and calls upon parents, upon men and women as individuals and upon voluntary organizations, local authorities and national governments to recognize these rights and strive for their observance by legislative and other measures progressively taken in accordance with the following principles:

PRINCIPLE 1

The child shall enjoy all the rights set forth in this Declaration. All children, without any exception whatsoever, shall be entitled to these rights, without distinction or discrimination on account of race, color, sex, language, religion, political or other opinion, national or social origin, property, birth or other status, whether of himself or of his family.

PRINCIPLE 2

The child shall enjoy special protection, and shall be given opportunities and facilities, by law and by other means, to enable him to develop physically, mentally, morally, spiritually and socially in a healthy and normal manner and in conditions of freedom and dignity. In the enactment of laws for this purpose the best interests of the child shall be the paramount consideration.

PRINCIPLE 3

The child shall be entitled from his birth to a name and a nationality.

PRINCIPLE 4

The child shall enjoy the benefits of social security. He shall be entitled to grow and develop in health; to this end special care and protection shall be provided both to him and to his mother, including adequate pre-natal and post-natal care. The child shall have the right to adequate nutrition, housing, recreation and medical services.

PRINCIPLE 5

The child who is physically, mentally or socially handicapped shall be given the special treatment, education and care required by his particular condition.

PRINCIPLE 6

The child, for the full and harmonious development of his personality, needs love and understanding. He shall, wherever possible, grow up in the care and under the responsibility of his parents, and in any case in an atmosphere of affection and of moral and material security; a child of tender years shall not, save in exceptional circumstances, be separated from his mother. Society and the public authorities shall have the duty to extend particular care to children without a family and to those without adequate means of support. Payment of state and other assistance toward the maintenance of children of large families is desirable.

PRINCIPLE 7

The child is entitled to receive education, which shall be free and compulsory, at least in the elementary stages. He shall be given an education which will promote his general culture, and enable him on a basis of equal opportunity to develop his abilities, his individual judgment, and his sense of moral and social responsibility, and to become a useful member of society.

The best interest of the child shall be the guiding principle of those responsible for his education and guidance; that responsibility lies in the first place with his parents.

The child shall have full opportunity for play and recreation, which shall be directed to the same purposes as education; society and the public authorities shall endeavor to promote the enjoyment of this right.

PRINCIPLE 8

The child shall in all circumstances be among the first to receive protection and relief.

PRINCIPLE 9

The child shall be protected against all forms of neglect, cruelty and exploitation. He shall not be the subject of traffic, in any form.

The child shall not be admitted to employment before an appropriate minimum age; he shall in no case be caused or permitted to engage in any occupation or employment which would prejudice his health or education, or interfere with his physical, mental or moral development.

PRINCIPLE 10

The child shall be protected from practices which may foster racial, religious and any other form of discrimination. He shall be brought up in a spirit of understanding, tolerance, friendship among peoples, peace and universal brotherhood and in full consciousness that his energy and talents should be devoted to the service of his fellow men.

APPENDIX C NEONATAL INTENSIVE CARE—SUPPLEMENT TO OBSTETRIC, GYNECOLOGIC, AND NEONATAL NURSING FUNCTIONS AND STANDARDS (1974)*

Allied personnel in such areas as respiratory therapy, radiology, laboratory, social services, and the chaplaincy must be able to adapt their skills to the needs of the ill newborn and his parents. The neonatal intensive care unit needs 24-hour a day coverage by these allied departments.

Clerical and ancillary personnel and services should also be available to the unit for optimal functioning of the professional staff.

When medical and nursing students or other special students are in the neonatal intensive care unit for clinical experience, their roles and responsibilities must be clearly defined in writing as part of the unit's protocols. Nursing students should not be included in the nurse-infant ratios.

Job descriptions must be written for all cate-

*Reprinted with permission from Neonatal Intensive Care—Supplement to Obstetric, Gynecologic, and Neonatal Nursing Functions and Standards; published by The Nurses Association of the American College of Obstetricians and Gynecologists.

gories of personnel and used as a basis for appraising employees' performance. These descriptions must be reviewed and updated at least once a year.

A structured orientation program for each new staff member is essential. Completion of the program must be documented in the employee's permanent record.

Continuing education is essential to neonatal intensive care nursing, and is the responsibility of the individual nurse. Participation by nurses in medical rounds and conferences in the unit is important for optimal team care of the ill newborn. A pertinent reference library in the unit, provision by the institution of continuous and ongoing in-service educational programs, and participation in workshops are necessary for continuing preparation of staff. Participation in formal academic programs is desirable.

Facilities and Equipment

The design of the unit must be in keeping with the philosophy and standard of care and must provide for parental visiting and education, diagnostic and treatment services, infection control, staff and storage needs, and safety requirements. Various aspects of each of these categories must be considered, including:

1. Parental visiting and education
   a. Viewing windows
   b. Conference rooms
2. Diagnostic and treatment services
   a. Respiratory therapy
   b. Radiology
   c. Laboratory
3. Infection control
   a. Housekeeping
   b. Clean and dirty utilities
   c. Separation of patient areas from staff work areas
4. Staff and storage needs
   a. Staff lounges with locker and toilet facilities
   b. On-call staff facilities
   c. Office space
   d. Equipment storage areas
   e. Supply storage areas
5. Safety requirements
   a. Oxygen and compressed air
   b. Vacuum valves
   c. Electrical outlets

A system for preventive maintenance of all equipment and surveillance for electrical hazard must be established and enforced. Electrical fuse boxes, oxygen and other gas supplies, and vacuum valves must be clearly and specifically marked to avoid confusion in emergency situations. Each nurse must be able to operate all equipment and to recognize malfunctions and hazards.

Listed below are categories of basic equipment needed for neonatal intensive care. This list is not intended to be all-inclusive.

1. Monitoring devices
   a. Respiratory
   b. Cardiac
   c. Electrocardiograph
   d. Blood pressure: internal and external transducers
   e. Temperature
   f. Oxygen analyzers
   g. Infusion controllers and pumps with lower limits of 0.1 cc
2. Beds
   a. Incubators with servocontrol
   b. Overhead radiant warmer with treatment surface
   c. Transport incubator with independent life-support mechanisms
3. Treatment equipment
   a. Ventilators with tubing support frames
   b. Continuous positive airway pressure
   c. Oxygen administration
      - Hoods
      - Masks
      - Positive pressure bags, capable of delivering 100 per cent oxygen
      - Heated nebulizers
      - Portable cylinders
   d. Phototherapy lights
   e. Closed chest drainage systems
   f. Heat shields
   g. Sterile trays and instruments

h. Nasogastric tubes with radiopaque markers
i. Umbilical catheters with radiopaque markers
j. Blood analyzers

4. Resuscitation and emergency equipment. This equipment should be kept ready and easily available in a movable cart or box.
   a. Laryngoscopes, extra bulbs, blades, batteries
   b. Suction catheters
   c. Endotracheal tubes, adaptors
   d. Forceps for insertion of endotracheal tubes
   e. Positive pressure bags, capable of delivering 100 per cent oxygen
   f. Sterile trays and instruments
   g. Medications
5. Scales
   a. Sling model
   b. Metric table model
6. Examination
   a. Stethoscope at each bedside
   b. Special cardiac stethoscope
   c. Otoscope
   d. Ophthalmoscope
   e. Transluminator
   f. X-ray viewing box
7. Stimuli to foster normal growth and development and infant-caretaker interaction
   a. Visual; e.g., brightly colored objects/toys, with and without patterns; these may be stationary or mobile
   b. Auditory; e.g., rhythmical sounds produced by mechanical devices or human voice, e.g., rattles, bells, other objects/toys
   c. Tactile; e.g., objects/toys of various textures and shapes
   d. Thermal; e.g., objects/toys that do not insult normal temperature
   e. Vestibular; e.g., changes in horizontal and/or vertical positions

Basic facilities and equipment for the newborn nursery are discussed in the American Academy of Pediatrics manual, *Standards and Recommendations for Hospital Care of Newborn Infants,* The American College of Obstetricians and Gynecologists manual, *Standards for Obstetric-Gynecologic Services* and the NAACOG manual, *Obstetric, Gynecologic and Neonatal Nursing Functions and Standards* and in state and local health regulations.

Policies and Procedures

Departmental policies and procedures should be established by representatives from the administrative, medical, and nursing staff and reviewed annually. Nursing policies, procedures, and protocols should be evaluated on a regular basis and revised as needed.

All policies must be clearly written and specific, including exceptions and delegations of authority. Procedures should be written in clearly understandable terms, explaining the equipment needed, the steps in the procedure, and who performs each step.

Policies and procedures for a normal newborn nursery (see NAACOG manual, pages 34–36) are the basis for the intensive care unit. The following are additional areas to be covered:

1. Allied departments. Policies must describe areas of cooperation.
2. Identification of newborn.
3. Informed consents. Policies must specify which procedures and treatments require consent, and who secures the consent.
4. Admission and discharge. Policies must prescribe criteria for admission to and discharge from each clinical component of the nursery, must specify who makes the decision for admission and discharge, and must establish routine procedures to be performed.
5. Consultations. Policies for inter- and intrainstitutional consultations must be established.
6. Referrals. Policies must specify who may initiate referrals and the procedure to be followed.
7. Visitors.
8. Emergency plans. Policies must provide for internal and external disasters and for failure of life-support systems.
9. Release of information to news media. Policies must define the kind of information that may be released, who obtains the consent for release, and who may release the information.
10. Research. Policies must note government and

other regulations to which research projects must conform.

Special Nursing Functions

The specially prepared nurse in a neonatal intensive care unit may perform certain functions that were previously reserved for physicians. The nurse's role may vary from one unit to another, but in any given unit it must always remain within the limits set by that unit's written protocols. The specific functions of the individual nurse will be determined by the requirements of the state's nursing practice act with documented evidence of preparation in conjoint agreements among medical and nursing directors of the nursery and the individual nurses. Listed below are examples of functions of the specially prepared nurse. The list is not intended to be all-inclusive.

1. Procedures
   a. Care of hyperalimentation infusions, including filter and dressing changes
   b. Endotracheal intubation
   c. Reinsertion of tracheotomy tubes
   d. Peripheral venipuncture for intravenous fluids
   e. Peripheral arterial puncture for blood gases
   f. Care and emergency reinsertion of chest tubes
   g. Intravenous push medications and blood
   h. Electrocardiography
   i. Urethral catheterization
   j. Needle and syringe aspiration of pleural cavity to rule out pneumothorax
2. Patient Assessment
   a. Evaluation of laboratory, x-ray, monitoring data
   b. Awareness of variations or deviations
   c. Evaluation of infant-caretaker interaction
3. Initiation and/or maintenance of diagnostic and treatment regimens (based on department protocols).
   a. Oxygenation, continuous positive airway pressure
   b. Mechanical and clinical monitoring
   c. Nutrition: intravenous, oral, gavage, hyperalimentation
   d. Standardized laboratory and x-ray procedures
4. Assessment of family needs
   a. Physical
   b. Psychological
   c. Social
   d. Economic
   e. Spiritual

Parent Education

For the parents of a critically ill newborn child, education is of the utmost importance. Rapport with the parents should be established as soon as possible, and the parents should be encouraged to come to the unit to see their infant and talk with members of staff. The unit should keep open visiting hours to make parental visits easier.

Conferences in a quiet atmosphere will help the nurse meet the parents' needs for information and emotional support, and will help them accept the nurse as caretaker of their child. Questions should be encouraged and should be answered accurately and with sensitivity to the parents' need and readiness for information.

Awareness of the normal grief response and other characteristic psychological responses of parents of the critically ill newborn is essential. Parents must be permitted to air their feelings. Active listening is one of the most effective tools in initiating and maintaining communication with parents. Each member of the team should also be aware of his or her own feelings and behavior and how they may affect relationships with parents.

If the critically ill infant must be transferred to a distant hospital where he will be separated from his parents, the nurses and physicians in both hospitals must try to keep the parents informed of the infant's condition.

The continuation of family-staff interactions after the discharge or death of the infant should be encouraged. Followup care after discharge is essential to the infant's continued well-being, and its importance should be impressed on the family.

Documentation of all parental visiting and education is essential.

Discharge Planning, Referrals, and Followup

Discharge planning should begin at the time of admission. It should be based on the expected outcome, the needs of the family, and the resources available to them.

Each unit must maintain a file of current information on local, state, and national organizations that provide financial and other resources for ill newborns and their families. Methods for putting families in touch with these helping organizations must be developed by the unit's administrative, medical, and nursing staffs in cooperation with community agencies.

The need for appointments for supervision and maintenance of health care of the infant after discharge must be impressed on the parents. They should be encouraged to continue using the resources of the hospital and other agencies as long as they need to.

Documentation of Nursing Care

Assessment, planning, implementation, and evaluation of nursing care, parent education, discharge planning, and referrals must be documented in the nursing care plan and in the patient's permanent record. Requests for nursing consultations and any resulting recommendations must also be documented in the permanent record.

The use of bedside flow sheets is recommended. Each flow sheet must be designed by and for the health team, and should include treatments and procedures specific to the level of care. Data not reflected on the flow sheet must be recorded in the nurse's notes.

Quality of care must be assessed at regular intervals through use of prospective and retrospective audits. Use of space, personnel, equipment, records, and funds should also be reviewed at regular intervals.

Neonatal Transport

Each state and regional area may have different transport needs, but the basic standards of care are similar for all.

Essential requirements include:

1. Physicians available for consultation 24 hours a day
2. Surface and/or air transport service available 24 hours a day with specially prepared neonatal personnel, life-support equipment, and supplies.

Personnel

The preferred protocol would call for a minimum number of persons specially prepared to maintain life en route and initiate emergency life support procedures. The minimum staff should be a physician or a specially qualified registered nurse, and a respiratory therapist. In situations where the number of specially qualified personnel is limited and patient care requirements are high, an on-call team may be the best method for facilitating transport.

In some cases the referring hospital may need to transport the neonate to the regional center without a specially prepared team. In these situations, transport may be performed in accord with local protocol and the level of care required.

Equipment

The level of care delivered during transport should approximate the care delivered in the intensive care unit. Equipment and supplies for resuscitation and life support are essential. Listed below are categories of basic equipment needed. The list is not intended to be all-inclusive.

1. Monitoring devices
   a. Stethoscope
   b. Portable cardiac monitor
   c. Temperature
   d. Portable blood pressure doppler
   e. Oxygen analyzers
2. Beds
   a. Transport incubator with independent power source
3. Treatment equipment
   a. Oxygen hood with heated nebulizer and thermometer
   b. Portable oxygen supply
   c. Portable compressed air supply
   d. Nasogastric tubes
   e. Umbilical catheters
   f. Ventilators/continuous positive airway pressure
4. Resuscitation and emergency equipment
   a. Portable suction machine
   b. Suction catheters, bulb syringe and mucous traps

c. Positive pressure bags, capable of delivering 100 per cent oxygen
d. Face masks of various sizes
e. Endotracheal tubes, adaptors
f. Forceps for insertion of endotracheal tubes
g. Emergency kit with syringes, needles, drugs, and miscellaneous supplies

5. Items transported with the infant must include:
   a. A copy of the mother's chart, with antepartum, labor and delivery history
   b. A copy of the infant's chart, with electrocardiogram tracings and x-ray films, if any were made
   c. Maternal blood sample
   d. Cord blood sample
   e. Informed consents for transport, hospital care, surgical procedures

Policies and Procedures

The designated regional center has the responsibility for establishing specific transport policies and procedures and disseminating them to the referring hospitals. The policies and procedures should include:

1. Protocols for initiation, consultation, and transport
2. Protocol for admission
3. Personnel and their responsibilities
   a. Number and preparation
   b. Maintenance of infant prior to transport
   c. Stabilization prior to transport
   d. Provision for contact with family members
   e. Provision for contact of infant with family prior to transport
   f. Emergency and continuing care
   g. Securing written authorization for transport and care
4. Records, x-ray and blood specimens that must accompany the infant
5. Arrangements for surface and/or air transportation
6. Protocols for using military transport assistance where applicable
7. Return of newborn to referring hospital after critical period
8. Media announcements and interviews at both referring and receiving hospitals
9. Written agreements concerning authority during transport with commercial surface and/or air carriers

Documentation

Informed consent forms for transport, medical and nursing care must be obtained before transport takes place, and must become part of the permanent record at the receiving hospital. All care given at the referring hospital and during transport must be documented and become part of the patient's permanent record.

Parent Education

Contact between the infant and family and between transport team and the family must be established prior to transport. Before transport, the family must also be given written instructions on keeping in touch with the infant and the receiving hospital.

APPENDIX D TECHNOLOGY IN MATERNAL-NEWBORN CARE

The purpose of this appendix is to familiarize students with some of the equipment used in obstetrics. The devices shown here are made by various manufacturers. Our selection is not meant to promote any one product.

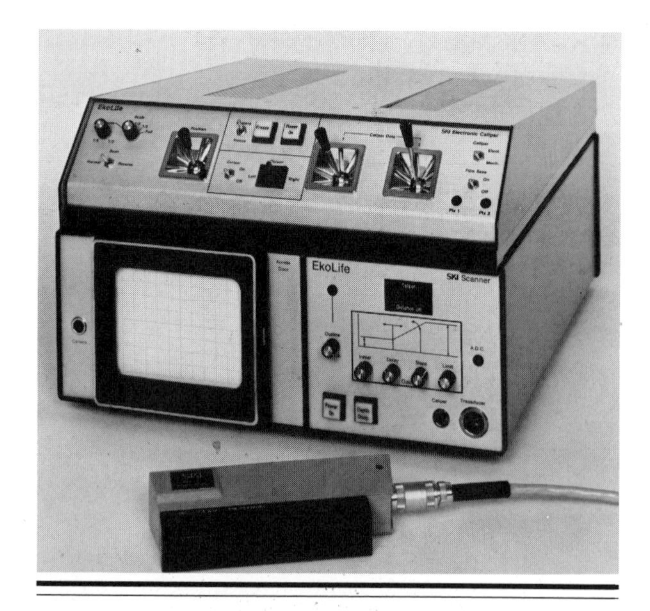

Figure D–1. The EkoLife real-time scanner is used to obtain and record images of the fetus in utero. M-mode tracings of fetal breathing and limb activity are recorded, and biparietal diameters and crown-rump measurements can be determined and displayed. (Courtesy SmithKline Instruments, Inc., Sunnyvale, Calif.)

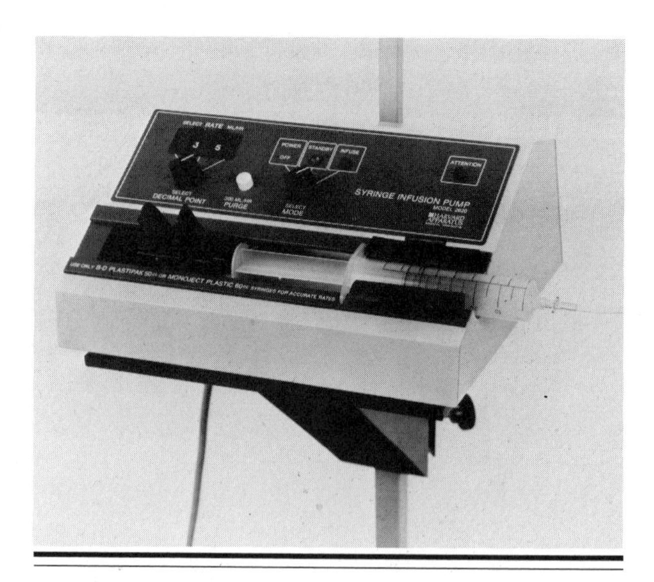

Figure D–2. The Harvard Syringe Infusion Pump continuously monitors and administers intravenous infusions. Obstetric applications include administration of oxytocin for labor induction and administration of medication to maternity patients and newborns requiring critical care. The Harvard Pump also has nonobstetric uses, such as dialysis and chemotherapy. (Courtesy Harvard Apparatus, an Ealing Company, So. Natick, Mass.)

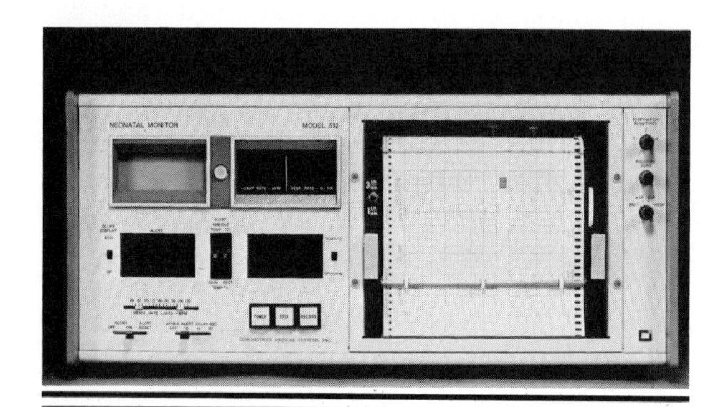

Figure D–3. The Neonatal Monitor measures, displays, and records vital signs during the neonatal period, including arterial and central venous blood pressures, heart rate variability, and skin, core, and ambient temperatures. This device may be ordered with delivery room capability and used to measure and record fetal heart rate variability and uterine activity. (Courtesy Corometrics Medical Systems, Inc., Wallingford, Conn.)

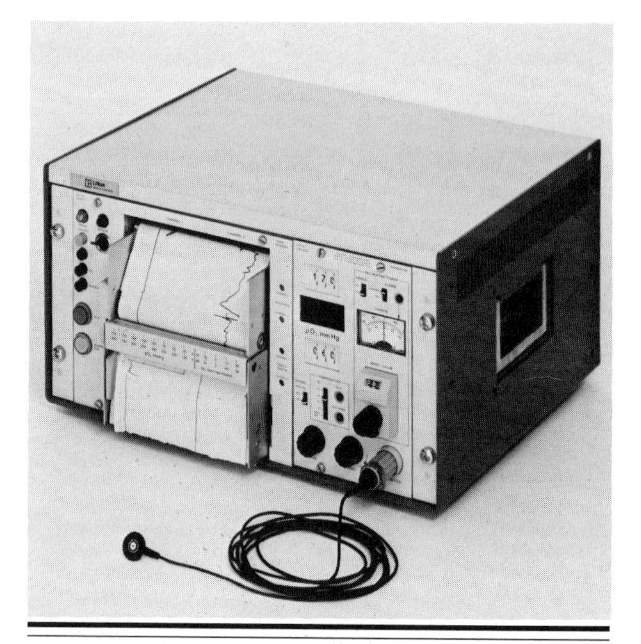

Figure D–4. The Oxymonitor is used to monitor Po_2 levels in the newborn transcutaneously. This device can detect hypoxemia and hyperoxemia. (Courtesy Litton Medical Electronics, Elk Grove, Ill.)

APPENDIX E EVALUATION OF FETAL WEIGHT AND MATURITY BY ULTRASONIC MEASUREMENT OF BIPARIETAL DIAMETER*

Biparietal Diameter (cm)	Grams	Weight Pounds	Ounces	Weeks of Gestation
1.0	NA	NA		9
1.1	NA	NA		9
1.2	NA	NA		9.5
1.3	NA	NA		10.0
1.4	NA	NA		10.0
1.5	NA	NA		10.5
1.6	NA	NA		11.0
1.7	NA	NA		11.0
1.8	NA	NA		11.5
1.9	NA	NA		12.0
2.0	NA	NA		12.0
2.1	NA	NA		12.5
2.2	NA	NA		13.0
2.3	NA	NA		13.0
2.4	NA	NA		13.5
2.5	NA	NA		14.0
2.6	NA	NA		14.0
2.7	NA	NA		14.5
2.8	NA	NA		15.0
2.9	NA	NA		15.0
3.0	NA	NA		15.5
3.1	NA	NA		16.0
3.2	NA	NA		16.0
3.3	NA	NA		16.5
3.4	NA	NA		17.0
3.5	NA	NA		17.0
3.6	NA	NA		17.5
3.7	NA	NA		18.0
3.8	NA	NA		18.0
3.9	NA	NA		18.5
4.0	NA	NA		19.0
4.1	NA	NA		19.0
4.2	NA	NA		19.5
4.3	NA	NA		20.0
4.4	NA	NA		20.0
4.5	NA	NA		20.5
4.6	NA	NA		21.0
4.7	NA	NA		21.0
4.8	NA	NA		21.5
4.9	NA	NA		22.0
5.0	NA	NA		22.0
5.1	NA	NA		22.5
5.2	42.6		2	23.0
5.3	119.9		5	23.0
5.4	197.1		6	23.5
5.5	274.3		10	24.0
5.6	351.5		13	24.0
5.7	428.7		14	24.5
5.8	514.9	1	2	25.0
5.9	583.2	1	5	25.0
6.0	660.4	1	8	25.5
6.1	737.6	1	10	26.0
6.2	814.8	1	13	26.0
6.3	892.1	2		26.5
6.4	969.3	2	2	27.0
6.5	1046.5	2	5	27.0
6.6	1123.7	2	8	27.5
6.7	1200.9	2	10	28.0
6.8	1278.2	2	13	28.0
6.9	1355.4	3		28.5
7.0	1432.6	3	3	29.0
7.1	1509.8	3	5	29.0
7.2	1587.0	3	8	29.5
7.3	1664.3	3	11	29.5
7.4	1741.5	3	14	30.0
7.5	1818.7	4		30.5
7.6	1895.9	4	3	30.8
7.7	1973.1	4	5	31.0
7.8	2050.4	4	8	31.7
7.9	2127.6	4	11	32.0
8.0	2204.8	4	14	32.7
8.1	2282.0	5		33.0
8.2	2359.2	5	3	33.6
8.3	2436.5	5	6	34.0
8.4	2513.7	5	8	34.6
8.5	2590.9	5	11	35.0
8.6	2668.1	5	14	35.5
8.7	2745.3	6		36.0
8.8	2822.6	6	3	36.5
8.9	2899.8	6	6	37.0
9.0	2977.0	6	8	37.4
9.1	3054.2	6	11	38.0
9.2	3131.4	6	14	38.4
9.3	3208.7	7	2	39.0
9.4	3285.9	7	3	39.0
9.5	3363.1	7	6	39.8
9.6	3440.3	7	10	40.0
9.7	3517.5	7	11	40.8
9.8	3594.8	7	14	41.0
9.9	3672.0	8	2	41.7
10.0	3749.2	8	3	NA
10.1	3826.5	8	6	NA
10.2	3903.6	8	10	NA
10.3	3980.9	8	13	NA
10.4	4058.1	8	14	NA
10.5	4135.3	9	2	NA
10.6	4212.5	9	5	NA

*Data from Hellman and Kobayashi.

APPENDIX F CERVICAL DILATATION ASSESSMENT AID

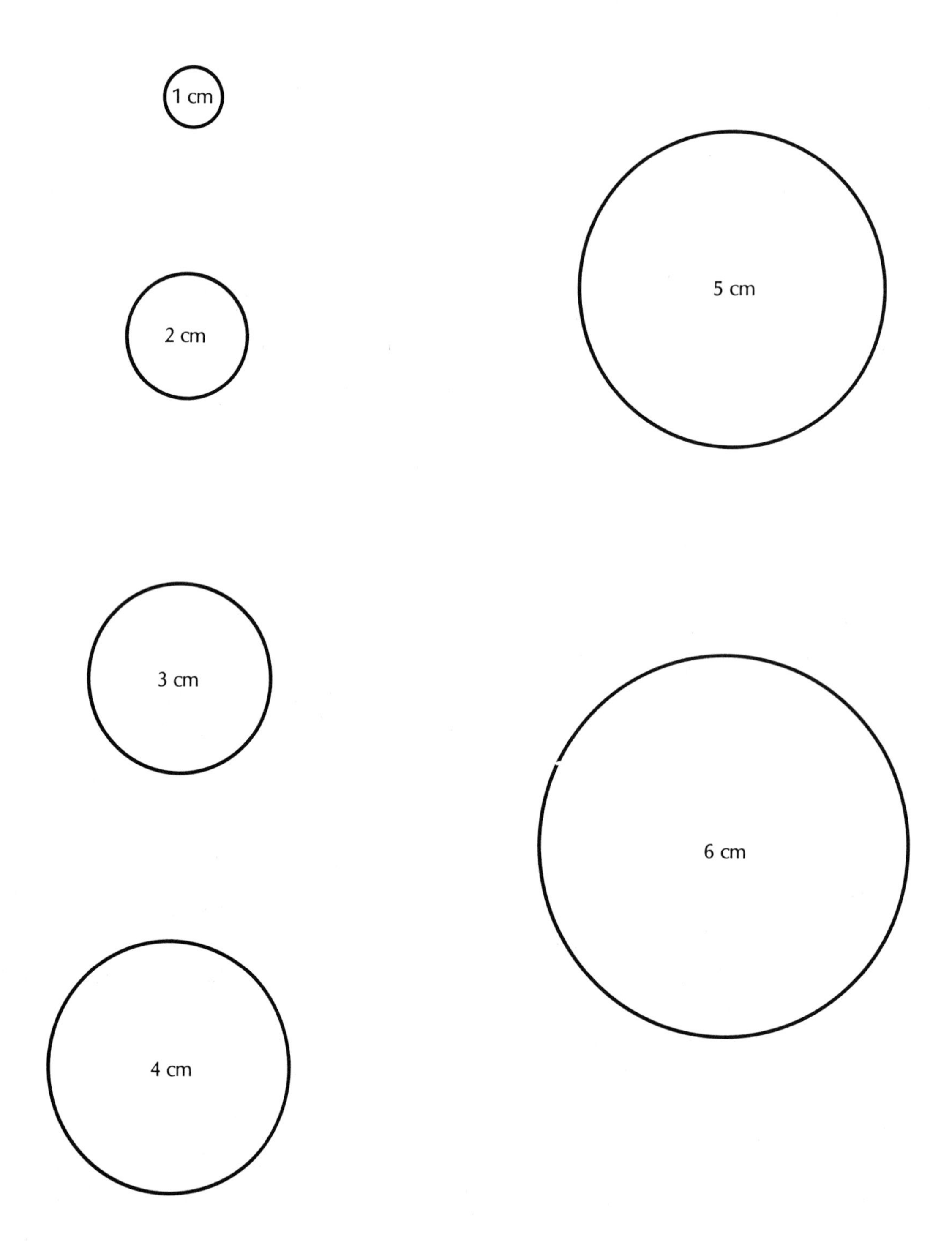

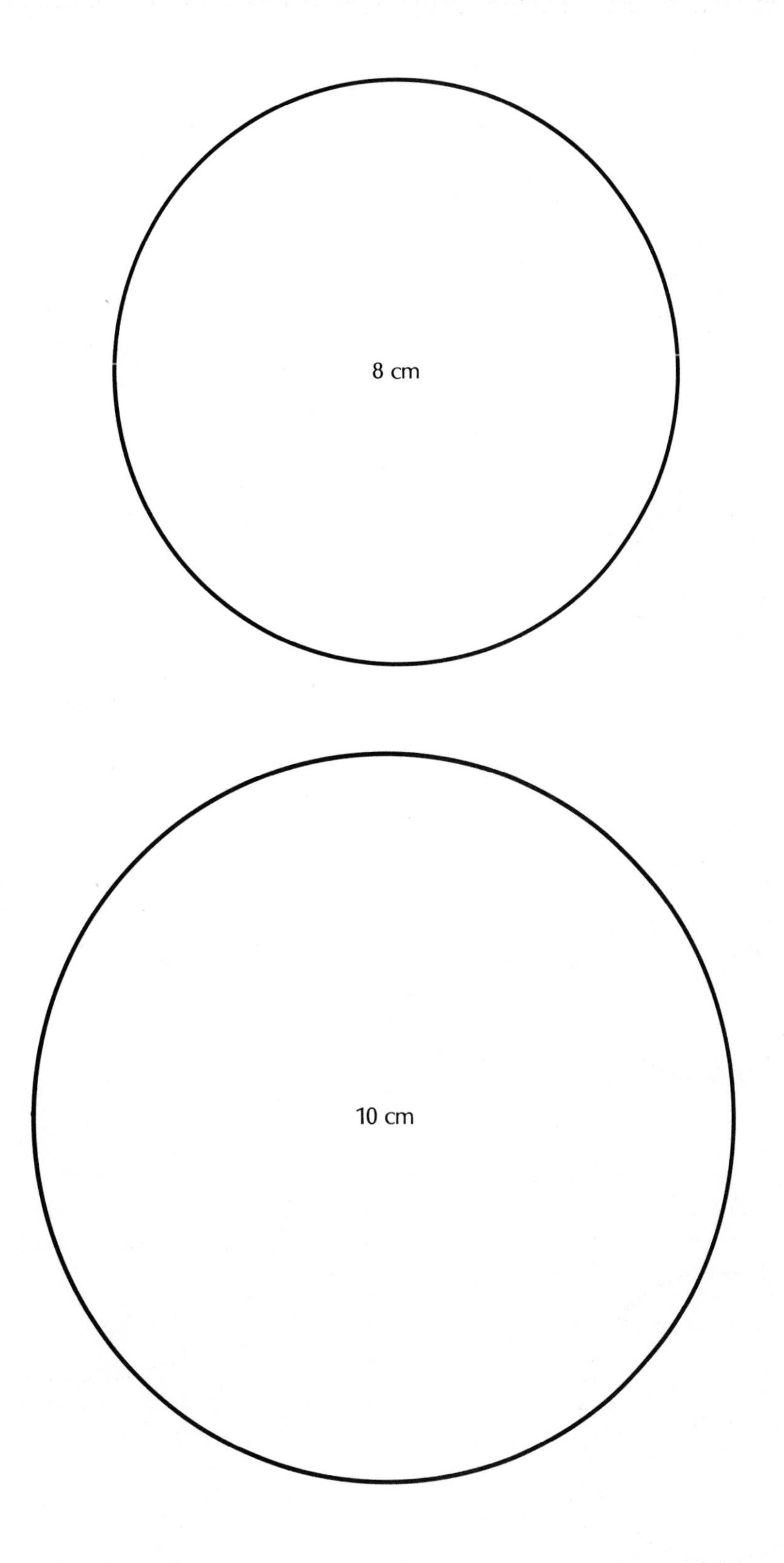
8 cm
10 cm

APPENDIX G PHYSICAL GROWTH NATIONAL CENTER FOR HEALTH STATISTICS PERCENTILES

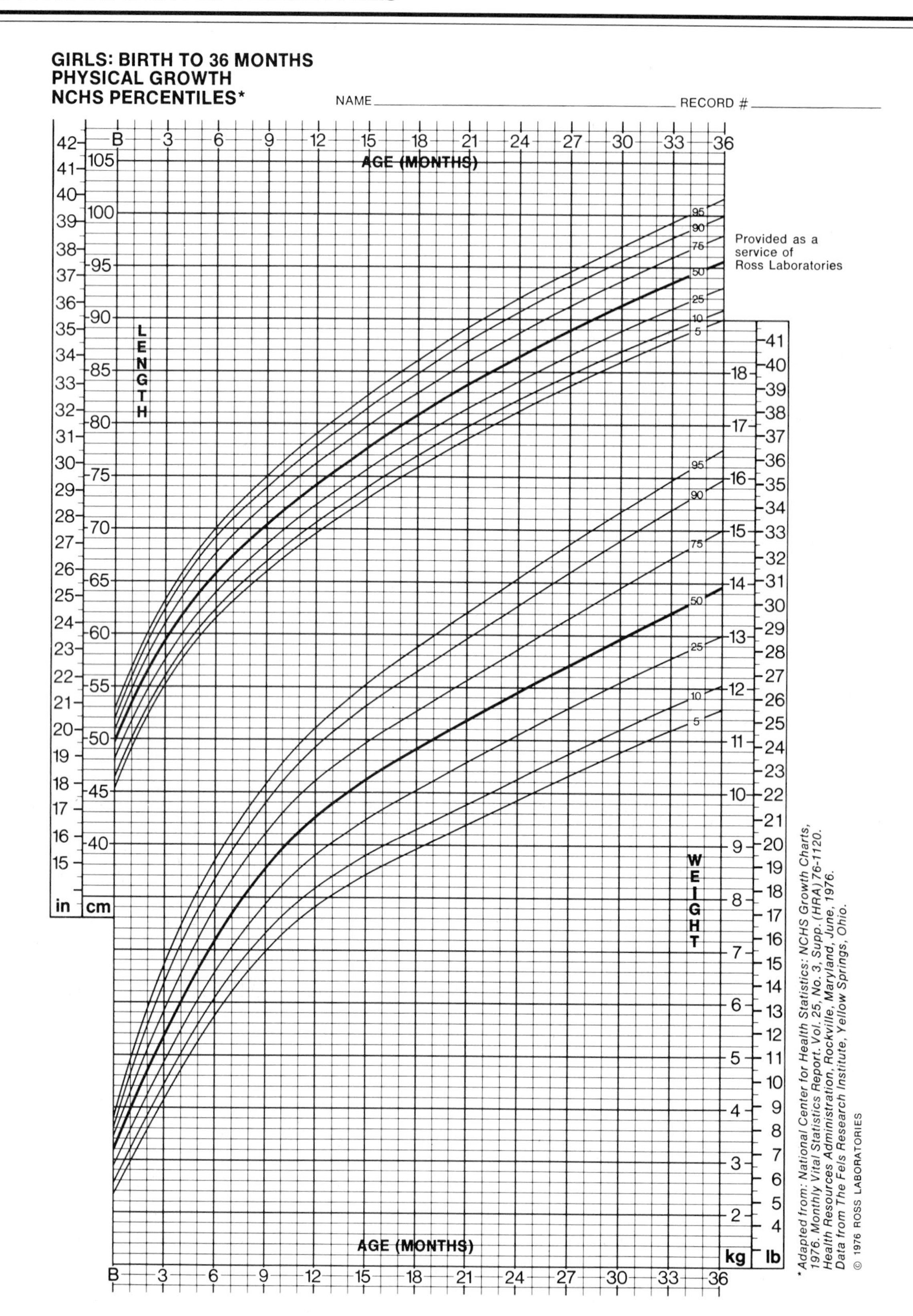

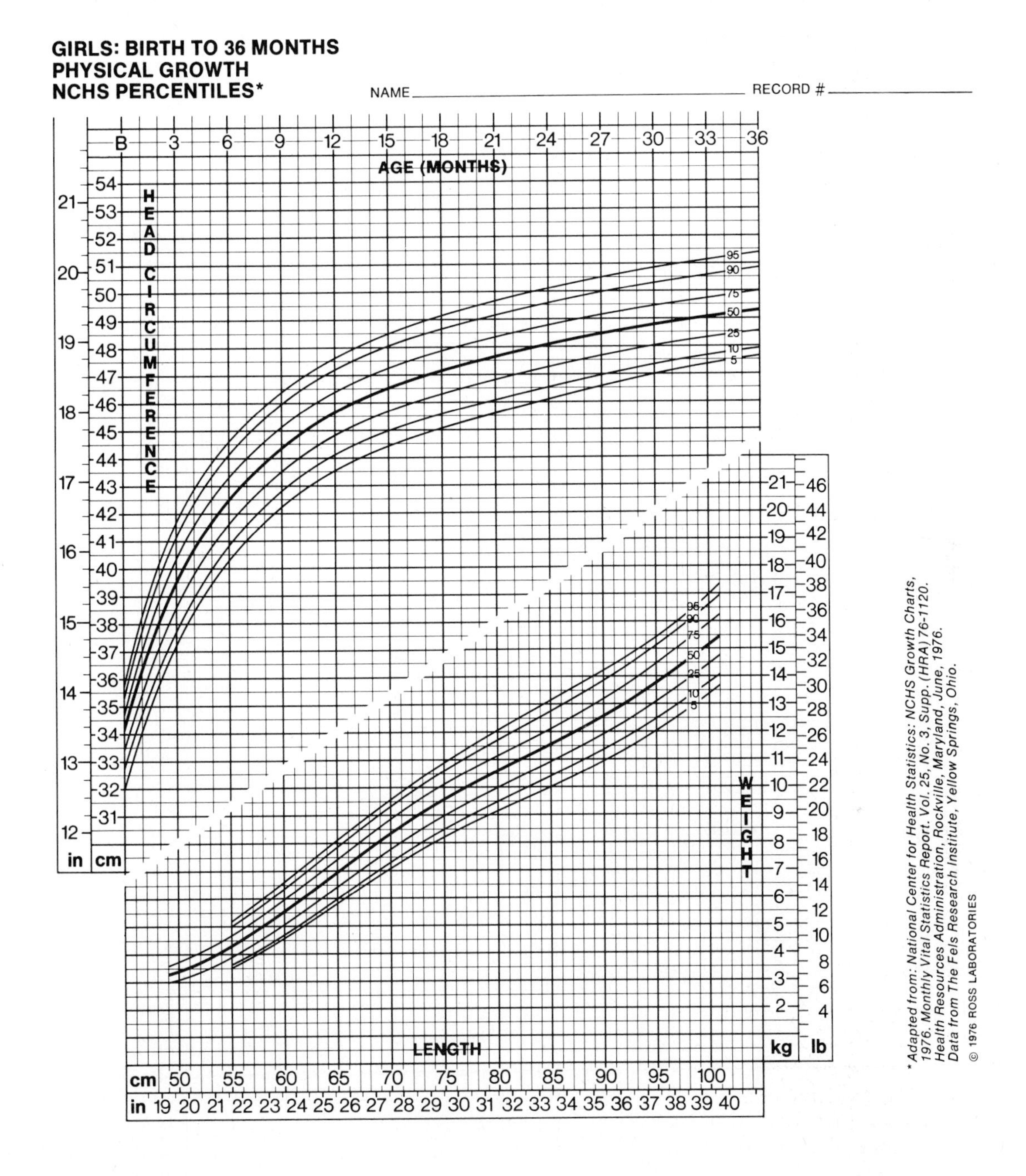

DATE	AGE	LENGTH	WEIGHT	HEAD C.
	BIRTH			

DATE	AGE	LENGTH	WEIGHT	HEAD C.

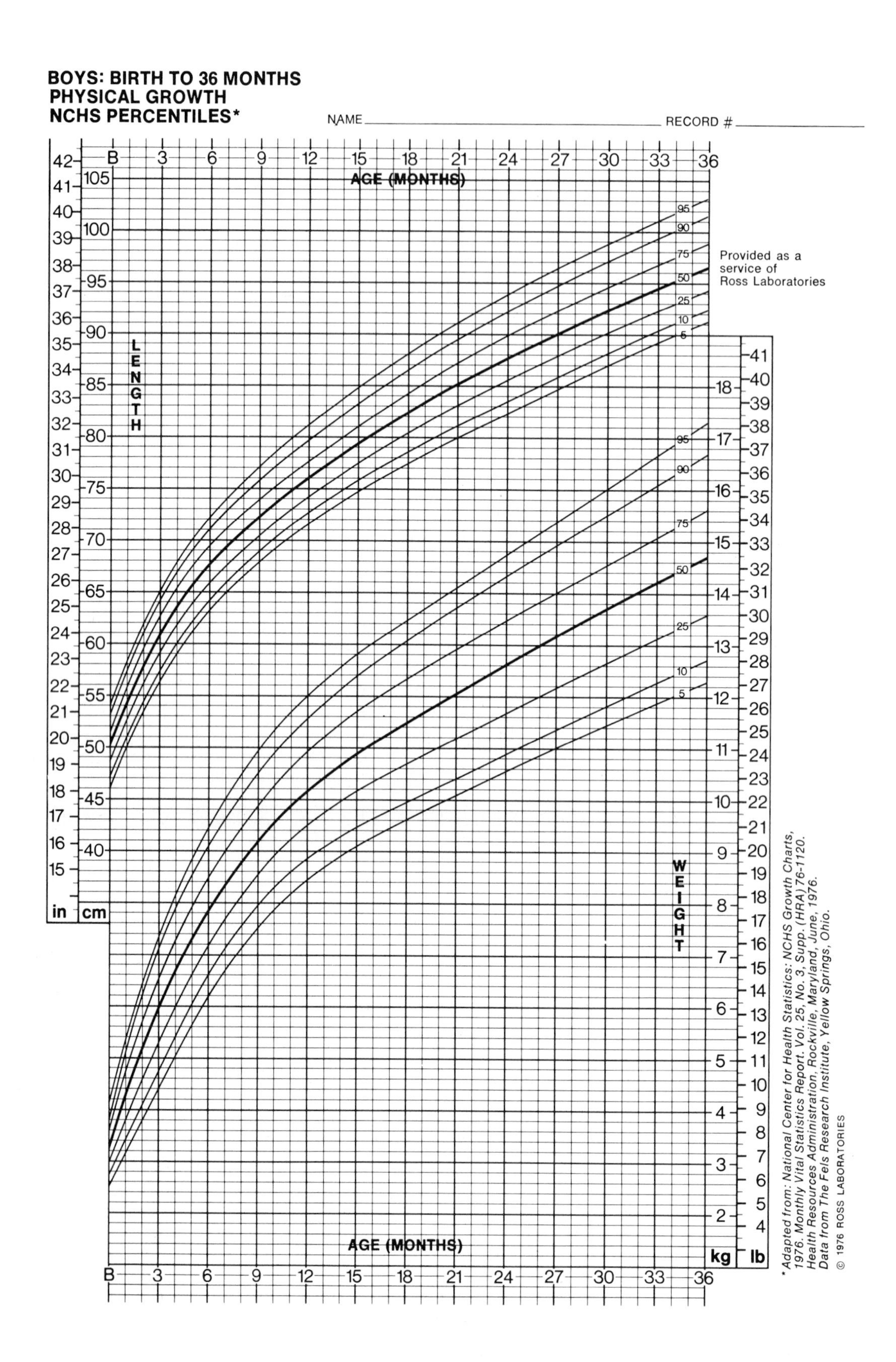
BOYS: BIRTH TO 36 MONTHS
PHYSICAL GROWTH
NCHS PERCENTILES*
NAME
RECORD #
AGE (MONTHS)
LENGTH
WEIGHT
in
cm
kg
lb
Provided as a service of Ross Laboratories
* Adapted from: National Center for Health Statistics: NCHS Growth Charts, 1976. Monthly Vital Statistics Report. Vol. 25, No. 3, Supp. (HRA) 76-1120. Health Resources Administration, Rockville, Maryland, June, 1976. Data from The Fels Research Institute, Yellow Springs, Ohio.
© 1976 ROSS LABORATORIES

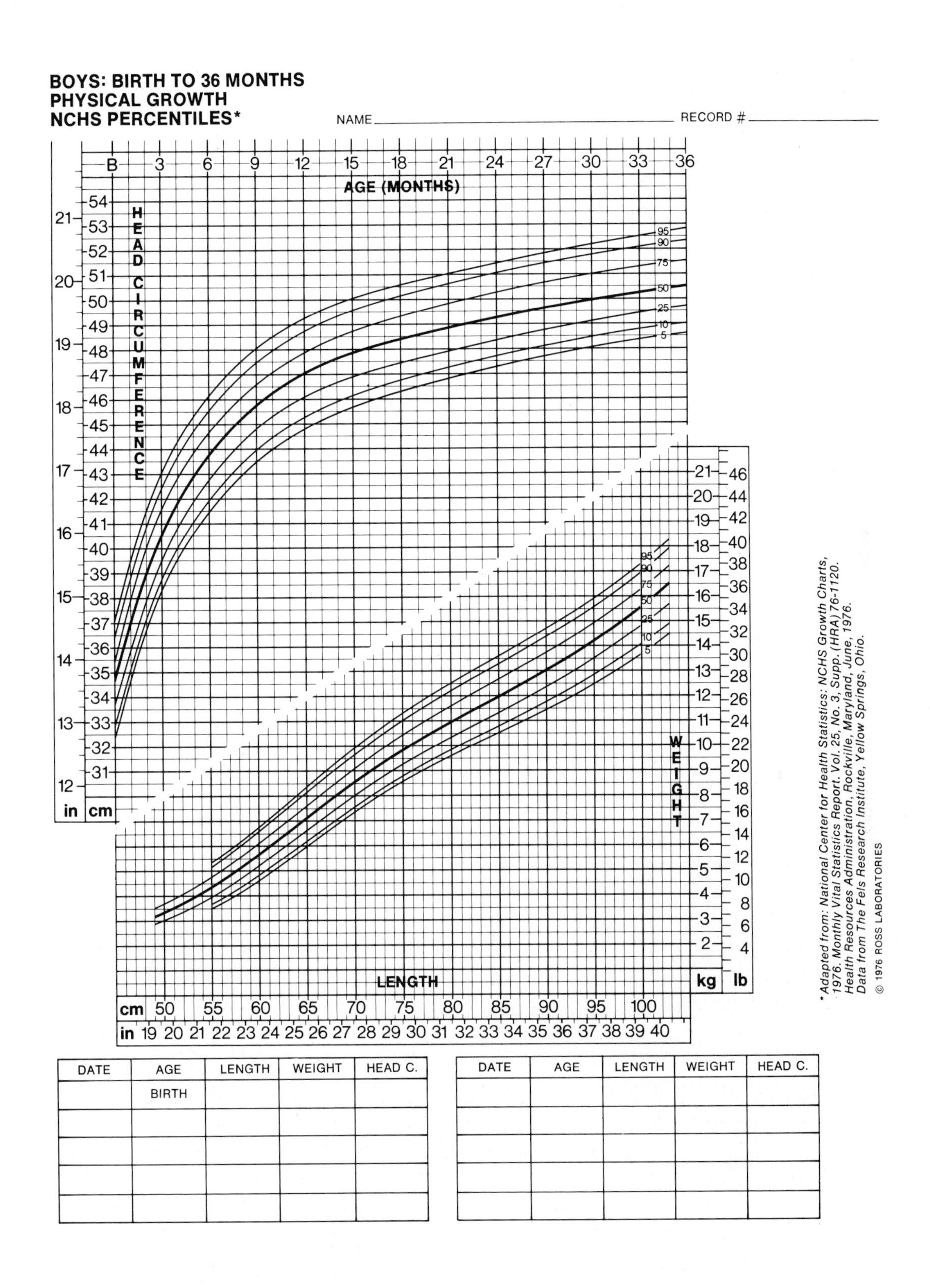

DATE	AGE	LENGTH	WEIGHT	HEAD C.
	BIRTH			

DATE	AGE	LENGTH	WEIGHT	HEAD C.

APPENDIX H IMMUNIZATION SCHEDULES

Recommended Schedule for Active Immunization of Normal Infants and Children*

Age	Immunization
2 months	DTP, TOPV[†]
4 months	DTP, TOPV
6 months	DTP, TOPV
12 months	Tuberculin test
15 months	Measles, mumps, rubella
18 months	DTP, TOPV
4-6 years	DTP, TOPV
14-16 years	Td[‡] (repeat every 10 years)

*Modified from the *Report of the Committee on Infectious Diseases.* 1977. Evanston, Ill.: American Academy of Pediatrics.

[†]DTP—diphtheria and tetanus toxoids combined with pertussis vaccine.
TOPV—Trivalent oral poliovirus vaccine.

[‡]Td—combined tetanus and diphtheria toxoids.

Recommended Schedules for Children Not Immunized During Infancy*

Under 6 years of age	
First visit	DTP, TOPV, tuberculin test
Interval after first visit	
1 month	Measles, mumps, rubella
2 months	DTP, TOPV
4 months	DTP, TOPV
10-16 months later or preschool	DTP, TOPV
6 years of age and older	
First visit	Td, TOPV, tuberculin test
Interval after first visit	
1 month	Measles, mumps, rubella
2 months	Td, TOPV
8-14 months	Td, TOPV
Age 14-16 years	Td (repeat every 10 years)

APPENDIX I CONVERSIONS AND EQUIVALENTS

Temperature Conversion

(Fahrenheit temperature − 32) × 5/9 = Celsius temperature
(Celsius temperature × 9/5) + 32 = Fahrenheit temperature

Selected Conversions to Metric Measures

Known value	Multiply by	To find
inches	2.54	centimeters
ounces	28	grams
pounds	454	grams
pounds	0.45	kilograms

Selected Conversions from Metric Measures

Known value	Multiply by	To find
centimeters	0.4	inches
grams	0.035	ounces
grams	0.0022	pounds
kilograms	2.2	pounds

Conversion of Pounds and Ounces to Grams

POUNDS	OUNCES 0	1	2	3	4	5	6	7	8	9	10	11	12	13	14	OUNCES 15
0	–	28	57	85	113	142	170	198	227	255	283	312	340	369	397	425
1	454	482	510	539	567	595	624	652	680	709	737	765	794	822	850	879
2	907	936	964	992	1021	1049	1077	1106	1134	1162	1191	1219	1247	1276	1304	1332
3	1361	1389	1417	1446	1474	1503	1531	1559	1588	1616	1644	1673	1701	1729	1758	1786
4	1814	1843	1871	1899	1928	1956	1984	2013	2041	2070	2098	2126	2155	2183	2211	2240
5	2268	2296	2325	2353	2381	2410	2438	2466	2495	2523	2551	2580	2608	2637	2665	2693
6	2722	2750	2778	2807	2835	2863	2892	2920	2948	2977	3005	3033	3062	3090	3118	3147
7	3175	3203	3232	3260	3289	3317	3345	3374	3402	3430	3459	3487	3515	3544	3572	3600
8	3629	3657	3685	3714	3742	3770	3799	3827	3856	3884	3912	3941	3969	3997	4026	4054
9	4082	4111	4139	4167	4196	4224	4252	4281	4309	4337	4366	4394	4423	4451	4479	4508
10	4536	4564	4593	4621	4649	4678	4706	4734	4763	4791	4819	4848	4876	4904	4933	4961
11	4990	5018	5046	5075	5103	5131	5160	5188	5216	5245	5273	5301	5330	5358	5386	5415
12	5443	5471	5500	5528	5557	5585	5613	5642	5670	5698	5727	5755	5783	5812	5840	5868
13	5897	5925	5953	5982	6010	6038	6067	6095	6123	6152	6180	6209	6237	6265	6294	6322
14	6350	6379	6407	6435	6464	6492	6520	6549	6577	6605	6634	6662	6690	6719	6747	6776
15	6804	6832	6860	6889	6917	6945	6973	7002	7030	7059	7087	7115	7144	7172	7201	7228
16	7257	7286	7313	7342	7371	7399	7427	7456	7484	7512	7541	7569	7597	7626	7654	7682
17	7711	7739	7768	7796	7824	7853	7881	7909	7938	7966	7994	8023	8051	8079	8108	8136
18	8165	8192	8221	8249	8278	8306	8335	8363	8391	8420	8448	8476	8504	8533	8561	8590
19	8618	8646	8675	8703	8731	8760	8788	8816	8845	8873	8902	8930	8958	8987	9015	9043
20	9072	9100	9128	9157	9185	9213	9242	9270	9298	9327	9355	9383	9412	9440	9469	9497
21	9525	9554	9582	9610	9639	9667	9695	9724	9752	9780	9809	9837	9865	9894	9922	9950
22	9979	10007	10036	10064	10092	10120	10149	10177	10206	10234	10262	10291	10319	10347	10376	10404

Approximate Weight Equivalents: Metric and Apothecaries' Systems

Metric	Apothecaries'	Metric	Apothecaries'
0.1 mg	1/600 grain	4 mg	1/15 grain
1.12 mg	1/500 grain	5 mg	1/12 grain
0.15 mg	1/400 grain	6 mg	1/10 grain
0.2 mg	1/300 grain	8 mg	1/8 grain
0.25 mg	1/250 grain	10 mg	1/6 grain
0.3 mg	1/200 grain	12 mg	1/5 grain
0.4 mg	1/150 grain	15 mg	1/4 grain
0.5 mg	1/120 grain	20 mg	1/3 grain
0.6 mg	1/100 grain	25 mg	3/8 grain
0.8 mg	1/80 grain	30 mg	1/2 grain
1 mg	1/60 grain	40 mg	2/3 grain
1.2 mg	1/50 grain	50 mg	3/4 grain
1.5 mg	1/40 grain	60 mg	1 grain
2 mg	1/30 grain	100 mg (0.1 gm)	11/2 grains
3 mg	1/20 grain	150 mg (0.15 gm)	21/2 grains

Metric	Apothecaries'	Metric	Apothecaries'
200 mg (0.2 gm)	3 grains	7.5 gm	120 grains (2 drams)
300 mg (0.3 gm)	5 grains	10 gm	2½ drams
400 mg (0.4 gm)	6 grains	30 gm	1 ounce (8 drams)
500 mg (0.5 gm)	7 1/2 grains	500 gm	1.1 pounds
600 mg (0.6 gm)	10 grains	1000 gm	2.2 pounds (1 kilogram)
1 gram	15 grains		
1.5 gm	22 grains		
2 gm	30 grains		
3 gm	45 grains		
4 gm	60 grains (1 dram)		
5 gm	75 grains		
6 gm	90 grains		

Approximate Volume Equivalents: Metric, Apothecaries', and Household Systems

Metric	Apothecaries'	Household
0.06 ml	1 minim	1 drop (g+)
0.3 ml	5 minims	
0.6 ml	10 minims	
1 ml	15 minims	15 drops
2 ml	30 minims	
3 ml	45 minims	
4 ml	60 minims (1 fluid dram)	60 drops (1 tsp)
8 ml	2 fl. drams	2 teaspoons
15 ml	4 fl. drams	4 tsp. (1 tbsp)
30 ml	8 fl. drams (1 fl. ounce)	2 tablespoons
60 ml	2 fl. ounces	
90 ml	3 fl. ounces	
200 ml	6 fl. ounces	1 teacup
250 ml	8 fl. ounces	1 large glass
500 ml	16 fl. ounces (1 pint)	1 pint
750 ml	1½ pints	
1000 ml (1 liter)	2 pints (1 quart)	1 quart
4000 ml	4 quarts	1 gallon

GLOSSARY

abdominal belonging or pertaining to the abdomen, its functions and disorders.

abdominal delivery see *cesarean section.*

abdominal gestation pregnancy within the abdominal cavity but outside the uterus.

abdominal hysterectomy surgical removal of the uterus through an incision in the abdominal wall.

abduct to draw away from the median plane of the body or one of its parts.

abortion loss of pregnancy before the baby is viable outside the uterus; miscarriage.

abruptio placentae premature separation, partially or totally, of a normally implanted placenta.

abstinence refraining voluntarily, especially from indulgence in food, alcoholic beverages, or sexual intercourse.

acceleration periodic increase in the baseline fetal heart rate.

acini cells secretory cells in the human breast that create milk from nutrients in the bloodstream.

acme peak or highest point; time of greatest intensity (of a uterine contraction).

acrocyanosis cyanosis of the extremities.

acromion projection of the spine of the scapula, which forms the point of the shoulder.

adduct to draw toward the main axis of the body.

adenomyoma tumor that affects the glandular and smooth muscle tissue, such as the muscles of the uterus.

adnexa adjoining or accessory parts of a structure, such as the uterine adnexa: the ovaries and fallopian tubes.

adolescence period of human development initiated by puberty and ending with the attainment of young adulthood.

afibrinogenemia absence of or decrease in fibrinogen in the blood plasma, so that the blood does not coagulate. This condition may be acquired or congenital, and it may result from such obstetric complications as abruptio placentae and retention of a dead fetus.

afterbirth placenta and membranes expelled after the birth or delivery of the child, during the third stage of labor; also called *secundines.*

afterpains cramplike pains due to contractions of the uterus that occur after childbirth. They are more common in multiparas, tend to be most severe during nursing, and last two to three days.

agalactia absence or failure of the secretion of breast milk.

alae nasi nostrils.

albinism a congenital absence of normal skin pigmentation.

albuminuria readily detectable amounts of albumin in the urine.

allantois tubular diverticulum of the posterior

part of the embryo's yolk sac that passes into the body stalk. The allantoic blood vessels develop into the umbilical vein and paired umbilical arteries.

allele one of a series of alternate genes at the same locus; one form of a gene.

alopecia natural or abnormal loss of hair. May be partial or complete, local or generalized.

alveolus a saclike cavity.

ambient surrounding; that which is around us.

amblyopia reduced vision that is not caused by visible changes in the eye or by refractive error.

amelia absence of a limb.

amenorrhea suppression or absence of menstruation.

amnesia loss of memory.

amniocentesis removal of amniotic fluid by insertion of a needle into the amniotic sac. Amniotic fluid is used for assessment of fetal health or fetal maturity and for providing information to aid in decisions about therapeutic abortion.

amniography x-ray examination of the amniotic sac following the injection of radiopaque dye into the amniotic fluid.

amnion the inner of the two membranes that form the sac containing the fetus and the amniotic fluid.

amnionitis infection of the amniotic fluid.

amniotic relating or pertaining to the amnion.

amniotic fluid the liquid surrounding the fetus in utero. It absorbs shocks, permits fetal movements, and prevents heat loss.

amniotic sac the bag or sac formed by the amnion and containing the fetus.

anaerobic catabolism the breakdown of organized substances into simple compounds in the absence of free oxygen, with the release of energy.

analgesic drug that relieves pain and does not cause unconsciousness.

androgen substance producing male characteristics, such as the male hormone testosterone.

android pelvis male-type pelvis.

anencephaly congenital deformity in which the cerebrum, cerebellum, and flat bones of the skull are absent.

anesthesia partial or complete loss of sensation with or without loss of consciousness.

anomaly a malformation; an organ or structure that is abnormal in position, structure, or form.

anovular menstrual period cyclic uterine bleeding that is not preceded by ovulation.

anoxia deficiency of oxygen.

antenatal before birth.

antepartal before the onset of labor.

anterior pertaining to the front.

anterior fontanelle diamond-shaped area between the two frontal and two parietal bones just above the newborn's forehead.

anteroposterior repair surgical reconstruction of the upper and lower walls of the vagina to correct relaxed tissue.

anthropoid pelvis pelvis in which the anteroposterior diameter is equal to or greater than the transverse diameter.

antibody a specific protein substance developed by the body in response to specific antigens in order to restrict or destroy them.

antigen a substance formed within the body or introduced into it that induces the formation of antibodies.

antitoxin an antibody that is capable of neutralizing a specific toxin and that is produced by the body in response to the presence of the toxin.

Apert syndrome an autosomal dominant disorder characterized by mental deficiency, irregular craniosynostosis, high full forehead and flat occiput, flat facies, hypertelorism, narrow palate, and syndactyly.

apnea a condition that occurs when respirations cease for more than 25 seconds, with generalized cyanosis.

areola pigmented ring surrounding the nipple of the breast.

Arnold-Chiari malformation a condition in which the inferior poles of the cerebellar hemispheres and the medulla protrude and may herniate through the foramen magnum. This is one of the causes of hydrocephaly and is usually accompanied by spina bifida or meningomyelocele.

articulation connection of bones in the skeleton; joint. Classified as (1) immovable, (2) slightly movable, and (3) freely movable.

artificial insemination introduction of viable semen into the vagina by artificial means for the purpose of impregnation.

Aschheim-Zondek test a test for pregnancy in which the woman's urine is injected into a mouse subcutaneously. After five days, the animal is killed and its ovaries examined. Enlarged ovaries and maturing follicles indicate pregnancy.

asphyxia a condition caused by a decreased amount of oxygen or an excess amount of carbon dioxide in the body.

aspiration syndrome a condition that occurs with fetal hypoxia: the anal sphincter relaxes and meconium is expelled; reflex gasping movements draw meconium and other particulate matter in the amniotic fluid into the bronchial tree, thereby obstructing air flow after birth.

asynclitism an oblique presentation of the fetal head; the pelvic planes and those of the fetal head are not parallel.

atelectasis a condition in which the lungs of a fetus remain unexpanded at birth; it involves alveolar collapse. May be partial or complete.

atony lack of normal muscle tone.

atresia congenital absence or pathologic closure of a normal anatomic opening. See also *biliary atresia; choanal atresia.*

attitude an assumed body posture; behavior toward a group, person, or thing based on a conscious or unconscious view.

auscultation process of listening for sounds produced within the body in order to detect abnormal conditions.

autosome a chromosome that is not a sex chromosome.

axis a line, real or imaginary, that a part revolves around or that runs through the center of the body.

azoospermic absence of spermatozoa in the semen.

bag of waters the membrane containing the amniotic fluid and the fetus.

balanced translocation rearrangement of chromosomal material in which a piece of one chromosome is broken off and joined to another chromosome. An individual with a balanced translocation has the normal amount of genetic material but it is arranged abnormally, making the individual at risk for producing offspring with chromosomal abnormalities.

ballottement a technique of palpation to detect or examine a floating object in the body. In obstetrics, the fetus, when pushed, floats away and then returns to touch the examiner's fingers.

Bandl's ring a thickened ridge of uterine musculature between the upper and lower segments that occurs following a mechanically obstructed labor, with the lower segment thinning abnormally.

Barr body deeply staining chromatin mass located against the inner surface of the cell nucleus. Found only in normal females; also called *sex chromatin.*

Bartholin's glands two small mucous glands situated on each side of the vaginal orifice that secrete small amounts of mucus during coitus.

battledore placenta placenta in which the umbilical cord is inserted on the periphery rather than centrally.

Beckwith syndrome syndrome of unknown etiology characterized by macroglossia, omphalocele, macrosomia, ear creases, neonatal polycythemia, diastasis recti, and cryptorchidism.

Beau's lines white lines across the fingernails. May appear spontaneously or during acute illness.

Bell's palsy distortion of the face caused by a lesion of the facial nerve, resulting in peripheral facial paralysis.

bicornuate uterus anomalous uterus resulting from incomplete union of the müllerian ducts. May be double or single with two horns.

biliary atresia absence of the bile duct.

bilirubin orange or yellowish pigment in bile; a breakdown product of hemoglobin that is carried by the blood to the liver, where it is chemically changed and excreted in the bile or is conjugated and excreted in the stools.

bimanual performed with both hands.

bimanual palpation examination of the pelvic organs by placing one hand on the abdomen and one or two fingers of the other hand into the vagina.

biopsy excision of a small piece of tissue for microscopic examination and diagnosis.

birth rate number of live births per 1000 population.

birth stool a small wooden chair that a woman may sit on during labor and delivery.

blastoderm germinal membrane of the ovum.

bleeding diathesis predisposition to abnormal blood clotting.

born out of asepsis (BOA) a birth that takes place without the use of sterile technique.

brachial palsy partial or complete paralysis of portions of the arm. Results from trauma to the brachial plexus during a difficult delivery.

bradycardia slow heart rate.

Braxton Hicks sign intermittent contractions of the uterus that are painless and that may occur every 10 to 20 minutes. They occur more frequently toward the end of pregnancy and are sometimes mistaken for true labor pains.

Braxton Hicks version a maneuver designed to turn the fetus from an undesirable position to a more desirable one in order to facilitate delivery.

breast milk jaundice yellowing of the infant's skin caused by pregnandiol in the mother's milk. Pregnandiol inhibits glucuronyl transferase, the enzyme necessary for the conjugation of bilirubin.

breech presentation a delivery in which the buttocks and/or feet are presented instead of the head. Occurs in approximately 3% of all deliveries.

bregma juncture of the coronal and sagittal sutures of the skull; the area of the anterior fontanelle of the fetus; the brow.

brim the edge of the superior strait of the true pelvis; the inlet.

brown fat fat deposits in neonates that provide greater heat-generating activity than ordinary fat. Found around the kidneys, adrenals, and neck, between the scapulas, and behind the sternum.

Brudzinski's sign in the presence of meningitis, bending the patient's neck produces flexion of the patient's lower extremities.

café-au-lait spots light brown (coffee with cream) marks that appear on the body. The presence of more than six such spots may be accompanied by a neurologic disorder.

caked breasts accumulation of milk in the secreting ducts of the breast after delivery; see also *engorgement*.

calcaneus the heel bone, which articulates with the cuboid bone anteriorly and with the astragalus bone above.

calcemia increased amount of serum calcium.

Candida albicans a fungus causing infections such as moniliasis and thrush.

caput the head; the occiput of the fetal head, which appears at the vaginal introitus prior to delivery of the head.

caput succedaneum swelling or edema occurring in or under the fetal scalp during labor.

carotinemia (pseudojaundice) yellowing of the skin caused by carotene in the blood.

carrier (1) an individual possessing an abnormal gene or chromosome who manifests no outward signs but who can pass the abnormality on to offspring. (2) A person who harbors a specific pathogenic organism in the absence of identifiable disease and is capable of spreading the disease to others.

catamenia menses.

catarrhal symptoms symptoms associated with inflammation of the mucous membranes, causing redness and mucoid drainage.

caudal anesthesia regional anesthesia used in childbirth in which the anesthetic agent is injected into the caudal area of the spinal canal through the sacral hiatus, affecting the caudal nerve roots and thereby providing anesthesia to the cervix, vagina, and perineum.

caul membranes or portions of the amnion covering the fetal head during delivery.

cautery method of destroying tissue by the use of heat, electricity, chemicals, or freezing.

centimeter unit of measurement used to describe cervical dilatation. Used interchangeably with "fingers" (one "finger" equals 2 cm).

cephalhematoma subcutaneous swelling containing blood; found on the head of a baby several days after delivery. Usually disappears within a few weeks to two months.

cephalic pertaining to the head.

cephalic presentation delivery in which the fetal head is presenting against the cervix.

cephalopelvic disproportion (CPD) a condition in which the infant's head is of a shape, size, or position that it cannot pass through the mother's pelvis.

cerebral palsy nonprogressive form of brain damage appearing up to the third year of life and resulting in motor dysfunction.

certified nurse-midwife see *midwife.*

cervical amputation surgical removal of the neck of the uterus.

cervical cauterization destruction of the superficial tissue of the cervix by heat, electric current, or freezing.

cervical conization excision of a cone-shaped section of tissue from the endocervix.

cervical erosion chronic irritation or infection that causes an alteration in the epithelium of the cervix.

cervical esophagostomy surgical formation of an opening from the esophagus to the neck region.

cervical os the small opening of the cervix that dilates during the first stage of labor. See also *external os; internal os.*

cervical polyp a small tumor or a stem or pedicle attached to the inside of the cervix.

cervical stenosis narrowing of the canal between the body of the uterus and the cervical os.

cervicitis infection of the cervix.

cervix the "neck" between the external os and the body of the uterus. The lower end of the cervix extends into the vagina.

cesarean hysterectomy surgical removal of the uterus immediately after cesarean delivery.

cesarean section delivery of the fetus by means of an incision into the abdominal wall and the uterus; also called *abdominal delivery.*

Chadwick's sign violet bluish color of the vaginal mucous membrane caused by increased vascularity; visible from about the fourth week of pregnancy.

chalazion a small hard tumor that develops on the eyelids; formed by distention of the meibomian gland with secretion.

change of life see *climacteric.*

childbed fever see *puerperal sepsis.*

chloasma brownish pigmentation over the bridge of the nose and the cheeks during pregnancy and in some women who are taking oral contraceptives. Also called *mask of pregnancy.*

choanal atresia complete obstruction of the posterior nares by membranous or bony tissue.

chorioamnionitis an inflammation of the amniotic membranes stimulated by organisms in the amniotic fluid, which then becomes infiltrated with polymorphonuclear leukocytes.

chorioepithelioma carcinoma of the chorion, with rapid malignant proliferation of the epithelium of the chorionic villi.

chorion the fetal membrane closest to the intrauterine wall; it gives rise to the placenta and continues as the outer membrane surrounding the amnion.

chorionic villi threadlike projections growing in tufts on the external chorionic surface that project into the maternal uterine sinuses; they help form the placenta and secrete human chorionic gonadotropin.

chromatids the two longitudinal halves of each chromosome.

chromosomes the threadlike structures within the nucleus of a cell that carry the genes.

cilia hairlike processes that project from epithelial cells and that serve to propel mucus, pus, and dust particles.

circumcision surgical excision of the prepuce (foreskin) of the penis.

circumoral cyanosis bluish appearance around the mouth.

circumvallate placenta a placenta with a thick white fibrous ring around the edge.

cleavage rapid mitotic division of the zygote; cells produced are called blastomeres.

cleft palate incomplete closure of the roof of the mouth, producing a passageway between the mouth and nasal cavity. May be unilateral or bilateral, complete or incomplete.

climacteric period marking the cessation of

menstruation and the end of a woman's reproductive abilities; the body undergoes significant physiologic and psychologic changes. Also called *change of life* or *menopause*.

clitoris female organ homologous to the male penis; a small oval body of erectile tissue situated at the anterior junction of the vulva.

clubfoot see *talipes equinovarus*.

coccyx a small bone at the base of the spinal column.

colostrum secretion from the breast before the onset of true lactation; contains mainly serum and white blood corpuscles. It has a high protein content, provides some immune properties, and cleanses the baby's intestinal tract of mucus and meconium.

colpectomy surgical excision of the vagina.

colporrhaphy suturing of the vagina.

colpotomy incision into the wall of the vagina.

complementary feeding additional feeding given to the infant if he is still hungry after breast-feeding.

complete dilatation occurs when the cervix is sufficiently dilated for the baby to pass through; usually 10 cm or five "fingers."

conception union of male sperm and female ovum; fertilization.

conceptional age the number of complete weeks since the moment of conception. Because the moment of conception is almost impossible to determine, conceptional age is estimated at two weeks less than gestational age.

condyloma wartlike growth of the skin, usually seen on the external genitals or anus. There are two types, a pointed variety and a broad, flat form usually found with syphilis.

congenital present at birth.

conjoined twins twins attached to each other, either at one small part of the body or in varying degrees up to complete sharing of the body with two heads. One twin may be small and underdeveloped, attached to the other twin parasitically.

conjugate important diameter of the pelvis, measured from the center of the promontory of the sacrum to the back of the symphysis pubis. The diagonal conjugate is measured and the true conjugate estimated.

conjunctivitis inflammation of the mucous membrane lining the eyelids.

consanguinity blood relationship by descent from a common ancestor.

consultand individual seeking counseling.

contraception the prevention of conception or impregnation.

contraction tightening and shortening of the uterine muscles during labor, causing effacement and dilatation of the cervix; contributes to the downward and outward descent of the fetus.

Coombs' test a test for antiglobulins in the red cells. The indirect test determines the presence of Rh-positive antibodies in maternal blood; the direct test determines the presence of maternal Rh-positive antibodies in fetal cord blood.

copulation sexual intercourse; coitus.

Cornelia DeLange syndrome characterized by micromelia, a down-turning upper lip, shortness of stature, mental retardation, microbrachycephaly, bushy eyebrows, long curly eyelashes, high-arched palate, micrognathia, hirsutism, simian crease. Etiology unknown.

corona radiata a ring of elongated cells surrounding the zona pellucida.

corpus luteum a small yellow body that develops within a ruptured ovarian follicle; it secretes progesterone in the second half of the menstrual cycle and atrophies about three days before the beginning of menstrual flow. If pregnancy occurs, it continues to produce progesterone until the placenta takes over this function.

cotyledon one of the rounded portions into which the placenta's uterine surface is divided, consisting of a mass of villi, fetal vessels, and an intervillous space.

couvade in some cultures, the male's observance of certain rituals and taboos to signify the transition to fatherhood.

Couvelaire uterus purplish discoloration and boardlike rigidity of the uterus caused by accumulation of blood in the interstitial myometrium of the uterus from premature separation and subsequent hemorrhage of the placenta.

CPD see *cephalopelvic disproportion*.

cradle cap an oily, yellowish crust that may appear on the newborn's scalp and that is caused by excessive secretion of the sebaceous glands in the scalp; also called *seborrhea dermatus.*

craniosynostosis premature closure of cranial sutures.

Credé's method an obsolete method of expelling the placenta by downward manual pressure on the uterus through the abdominal wall.

Credé's prophylaxis instillation of 1% silver nitrate solution into the conjunctiva of the newborn infant to prevent ophthalmia neonatorum.

crepitus (1) sound produced when pressure is applied to tissues containing abnormal amounts of air; (2) grating sound heard when broken bone ends are moved; (3) noise of gas being expelled from intestines.

cretinism condition caused by congenital lack of thyroid gland secretion; characteristics include arrested physical and mental development.

cri-du-chat chromosomal disorder characterized by microcephaly, downward slant of palpebral fissures, catlike cry, low birth weight, mental deficiency, hypotonia, and simian crease. Caused by partial deletion of the short arm of chromosome number 5.

crisis any naturally occurring turning point, such as courtship, marriage, pregnancy, parenthood, death.

Crouzon's syndrome an autosomal dominant disorder of variable expression characterized by premature craniosynostosis, maxillary hypoplasia, and shallow orbits.

crowning appearance of the presenting part of the baby at the vaginal orifice.

cul-de-sac of Douglas retrouterine pouch formed by an extension of the peritoneal cavity that lies between the rectum and the posterior wall of the uterus.

culture the ideas, customs, traditions, arts, and so on of a particular group of people.

curettage removal of the contents of the uterus by scraping of the endometrial lining with a curette. Done to obtain specimens for diagnostic purposes or following an abortion.

cutis marmorata purplish discoloration of skin on exposure to cold. A transient vasomotor response occurring primarily over the extremities of the infant; occasionally seen in an infant in respiratory distress.

cyesis pregnancy.

cystocele hernia of the bladder. Injury to the vesicovaginal fascia during delivery may allow herniation of the bladder into the vagina.

cytogenetics branch of genetics dealing with the study of chromosomes and associated gene behavior.

deceleration periodic decrease in the baseline fetal heart rate.

decidua endometrium or mucous membrane lining of the uterus in pregnancy that is shed after giving birth.

decidua basalis the part of the decidua that unites with the chorion to form the placenta. It is shed in lochial discharge after delivery.

decidua capsularis the part of the decidua surrounding the chorionic sac.

decidua vera nonplacental decidua lining the uterus.

decrement decrease or stage of decline, as of a contraction.

deletion in genetics, the loss of a chromosomal segment.

delivery expulsion of the baby with placenta and membranes from the mother at birth.

democratic family a family in which there is a high degree of equality and mutuality.

deoxyribonucleic acid (DNA) intracellular complex protein carrying genetic information; consists of two purines (adenine and guanine) and two pyrimidines (thymine and cystosine).

dermatoglyphics study of the surface markings and skin ridge patterns on fingers, toes, palms of hands, and soles of feet; useful in identification and in genetic studies.

desquamation shedding of the epithelial cells of the epidermis.

diagonal conjugate distance from the lower posterior border of the symphysis pubis to the sacral promontory; may be obtained by manual measurement.

diaphragmatic hernia failure of the diaphragm

to fuse, resulting in protrusion of the abdominal contents through the diaphragm into the thoracic cavity. May be congenital or traumatic.

diastasis recti abdominis separation of the recti abdominis muscles along the median line. In women, seen with repeated childbirths or multiple gestation. In the newborn, usually caused by incomplete development.

diathesis hereditary predisposition to some abnormality or disease. See also *bleeding diathesis.*

dilatation of the cervix expansion of the external os from an opening a few millimeters in size to an opening large enough to allow the passage of a baby.

dilatation and curettage (D and C) stretching of the cervical canal to permit passage of a curette, which is used to scrape the endometrium to empty the uterine contents or to obtain tissue for examination.

dilatational phase of labor phase in which active cervical dilatation takes place.

diploid containing a set of maternal and a set of paternal chromosomes. In humans the diploid number of chromosomes is 46.

discordance discrepancy in size (or other indicators) between twins.

disparate twins twins that are different from one another, as in weight or appearance; most likely fraternal twins.

dizygotic twins fetuses that develop from two fertilized ova; also called *fraternal twins.*

Döderlein bacillus gram-positive bacterium found in normal vaginal secretions.

dominant gene a gene that is expressed in the heterozygous state. In a dominant disorder the mutant gene overshadows the normal gene.

Down's syndrome an abnormality resulting from the presence of an extra chromosome number 21 (trisomy 21); characteristics include mental retardation and altered physical appearance. Formerly called mongolism or mongoloid idiocy.

dry labor lay term referring to labor in which amniotic fluid has already escaped. In reality, there is no such thing as a "dry labor."

ductus arteriosus a communication channel between the main pulmonary artery and the aorta of the fetus. It is obliterated after birth by a rising PO_2 and changes in intravascular pressure in the presence of normal pulmonary functioning. It normally becomes a ligament after birth but sometimes remains patent (patent ductus arteriosus), a treatable condition.

ductus venosus a fetal blood vessel that carries oxygenated blood between the umbilical vein and the inferior vena cava, bypassing the liver; it becomes a ligament after birth.

Duncan's mechanism occurs when the maternal surface of the placenta presents upon delivery rather than the shiny fetal surface.

dyscrasia incompatible mixture, such as fetal and maternal blood incompatibility.

dysfunctional uterine bleeding abnormal bleeding from the uterus for reasons that are not readily established.

dysmenorrhea painful or difficult menstruation; may be primary or secondary.

dyspareunia painful sexual intercourse.

dyspnea difficult or labored breathing.

dystocia difficult labor due to mechanical factors produced by the fetus or the maternal pelvis, or due to inadequate uterine or other muscular activity.

ecchymosis bleeding into tissue caused by direct trauma, serious infection, or bleeding diathesis.

eclampsia a major complication of pregnancy of unknown cause. It occurs more often in the primigravida and is accompanied by elevated blood pressure, albuminuria, oliguria, tonic and clonic convulsions, and coma. May occur during pregnancy (usually after the 20th week of gestation) or within 48 hours after delivery.

ectoderm outer layer of cells in the developing embryo that give rise to the skin, nails, and hair.

ectopic in an abnormal position.

ectopic pregnancy implantation of the fertilized ovum outside the uterine cavity; common sites are the abdomen, fallopian tubes, and ovaries; also called *oocyesis.*

EDC estimated date of confinement.

effacement thinning and shortening of the cervix that occurs late in pregnancy or during labor.

effleurage gentle stroking used in massage.

ejaculation ejection of the seminal fluids from the penis.

Ellis-Van Creveld syndrome autosomal recessive syndrome characterized by small stature with disproportionally short extremities, polydactyly of fingers and/or toes, hypoplastic nails, and short upper lip. One half the patients also have a cardiac defect.

embolus undissolved matter present in a blood vessel brought there by the blood or lymph current; may be solid, liquid, or gaseous.

embryo the early stage of development of the young of any organism. In humans, the period from about two weeks' to eight weeks' gestation, which is characterized by cellular differentiation and predominantly hyperplastic growth.

empathy objective awareness of and insight into the emotions, feelings, and behavior of another person and their meaning and significance.

en face an assumed position in which one person looks at another and maintains his or her face in the same vertical plane as that of the other.

enanthem eruption of the mucous membrane, such as Koplik's spots.

endocervical pertaining to the interior of the canal of the cervix of the uterus.

endocrine glands glands that secrete special substances (hormones) that regulate body functions.

endoderm the inner layer of cells in the developing embryo that give rise to internal organs such as the intestines.

endometriosis ectopic endometrium located outside the uterus in the pelvic cavity. Symptoms may include pelvic pain or pressure, dysmenorrhea, dyspareunia, abnormal bleeding from the uterus or rectum, and sterility.

endometrium the mucous membrane that lines the inner surface of the uterus.

engagement the entrance of the fetal presenting part into the superior pelvic strait and the beginning of the descent through the pelvic canal.

engorgement vascular congestion or distention. In obstetrics, the swelling of breast tissue brought about by an increase in blood and lymph supply to the breast, preceding true lactation.

enuresis involuntary urination; may be complete or partial, diurnal or nocturnal, depending upon pathologic or functional causes.

enzygotic developed from one fertilized ovum.

epicanthus a fold of skin that extends from the top of the nose to the median end of the eyebrow, covering the inner canthus.

episiotomy incision of the perineum to facilitate delivery and to avoid laceration of the perineum.

epispadias congenital opening of the urethra on the dorsum of the penis, or opening by separation of the labia minora and a fissure of the clitoris (rare).

Epstein's pearls small, white blebs found along the gum margins and at the junction of the soft and hard palates; commonly seen in the newborn as a normal manifestation.

Erb's palsy paralysis of the arm and chest wall as a result of a birth injury to the brachial plexus or a subsequent injury to the 5th and 6th cervical nerves.

ergot a drug that stimulates the smooth muscles of blood vessels and the uterus, causing vasoconstriction and uterine contractions. Obtained from *Claviceps purpurea*, a fungus.

erythema toxicum innocuous pink papular rash of unknown cause with superimposed vesicles that appears within 24 to 48 hours after birth and resolves spontaneously with a few days.

erythroblastosis fetalis hemolytic disease of the newborn characterized by anemia, jaundice, enlargement of the liver and spleen, and generalized edema. Caused by isoimmunization due to Rh incompatibility or ABO incompatibility.

escutcheon pattern of distribution of pubic hair.

esophageal atresia a malformation in which the esophagus ends in a blind pouch or narrows into a thin cord, failing to form a passage to the stomach.

estrangement in obstetrics, a condition that occurs when the mother is diverted from establishing a normal relationship with her baby because of separation caused by illness or prematurity.

estriol metabolic product of estrone and estradiol found in the urine of pregnant women.

estrogen the hormones estradiol and estrone, produced by the ovary.

estrus cyclic period of sexual activity in female mammals.

eugenics the science that deals with the improvement of the human race through control of genetic factors.

euthenics the science that deals with the improvement of the human race through control of environmental factors.

exanthem any eruption of the skin; frequently accompanies infectious diseases.

exchange transfusion the replacement of 70%–80% of circulating blood by withdrawing the recipient's blood and injecting a donor's blood in equal amounts, for the purpose of preventing the accumulation of bilirubin or other byproducts of hemolysis in the blood.

exostosis benign cartilage-covered bony growth on the surface of a bone, often caused by chronic irritation.

exotoxin a toxin produced by microorganisms and excreted into the surrounding medium.

expiratory grunt a sign of respiratory distress indicative of the baby's attempt to hold air in the alveoli for better gaseous exchange.

expressivity the extent to which a gene is expressed in an individual.

expulsive contractions labor contractions that are effective in contracting the uterine muscle; characteristic of the second stage of labor.

exstrophy of the bladder exposure and eversion of the posterior and lateral walls of the bladder and trigone because of failure of the anterior wall and symphysis pubis to unite.

external os the opening between the cervix and the vagina.

extraperitoneal occurring or located outside the peritoneal cavity.

extrauterine occurring outside the uterus.

extrauterine pregnancy ectopic pregnancy in which the fertilized ovum implants outside the uterus.

facies pertaining to the appearance or expression of the face; certain congenital syndromes typically present with a specific facial appearance.

failure to thrive (FTT) term used to describe the infant or child whose growth and development pattern falls below the norms for his age.

fallopian tubes tubes that extend from the lateral angle of the uterus and terminate near the ovary; they serve as a passageway for the ovum from the ovary to the uterus and for the spermatozoa from the uterus toward the ovary. Also called *oviducts* and *uterine tubes.*

false labor contractions of the uterus, regular or irregular, that may be strong enough to be interpreted as true labor but that do not dilate the cervix.

familial the presence of a trait or disorder in more than one member of a family; not necessarily inherited.

family a group of people united by marriage, blood, or adoption, residing in the same household, maintaining a common culture, and interacting with each other on the basis of their roles within the group. See also *democratic family; nuclear family; traditional family.*

fecundation impregnation; fertilization.

fertility ability to reproduce.

fertility rate number of births per 1000 women age 15 to 44 in a given population per year.

fertilization impregnation of an ovum by a spermatozoon.

fetal pertaining or relating to the fetus.

fetal alcohol syndrome (FAS) syndrome caused by maternal alcohol ingestion and characterized by microcephaly, intrauterine growth retardation, short palpebral fissures, and maxillary hypoplasia.

fetal alveoli terminal pulmonary sacs that in fetal life are filled with fluid that is a transudate of fetal plasma.

fetal death death of the developing fetus after 20 weeks' gestation. Also called *fetal demise.*

fetal distress evidence that the fetus is in jeopardy, such as a change in fetal activity or heart rate.

fetal heart rate the number of times the fetal

heart beats per minute; normal range is 120–160 beats per minute.

fetal heart tones (FHTs) the fetus' heartbeat as heard through the mother's abdominal wall.

fetal lie relationship of the long axis of the fetus to the long axis of the mother.

fetotoxic destructive or poisonous to the fetus.

fetus the child in utero from about the seventh to ninth week of gestation until birth.

FHTs see *fetal heart tones.*

fibroid fibrous, encapsulated connective tissue tumor, especially of the uterus.

fimbria any structure resembling a fringe; the fringelike extremity of the fallopian tubes.

first stage of labor period of time extending from the onset of regular contractions to the complete dilatation of the cervix.

fissure an open crack or groove in tissue.

fistula an abnormal tubelike passage that forms between two normal cavities or to a free surface; may be congenital or caused by trauma, abscesses, or inflammatory processes.

flaccid flabby, relaxed; absent or defective muscle tone.

flaring of nostrils widening of nostrils during inspiration in the presence of air hunger; a sign of respiratory distress.

flexion in obstetrics, a situation that occurs when resistance to the descent of the baby down the birth canal causes its head to flex, or bend, the chin approaching the chest, thus reducing the diameter of the presenting part.

follicle a small secretory cavity or sac.

follicle-stimulating hormone (FSH) hormone produced by the anterior pituitary during the first half of the menstrual cycle, stimulating development of the graafian follicle.

fontanelle in the fetus, an unossified space or soft spot consisting of a strong band of connective tissue lying between the cranial bones of the skull.

footling a breech presentation in which one or both feet present.

foramen ovale septal opening between the atria of the fetal heart. Normally, the opening closes shortly after birth; if it remains open, it can be surgically repaired.

forceps obstetric instruments occasionally used to aid in delivery.

Fordyce spots yellowish white papules on the oral mucosa; may be present at birth.

foreskin loose skin covering the end of the penis or clitoris; prepuce.

fornix a body with a vaultlike or arched shape.

fornix of the vagina the anterior and posterior spaces into which the upper vagina is divided; formed by the protrusion of the cervix into the vagina.

fossa shallow depression or furrow.

fourchette transverse fold of mucous membranes at the posterior angle of the vagina that connects the posterior ends of the labia minora.

fraternal twins see *dizygotic twins.*

fremitus vibratory tremors felt through the chest wall by palpation.

frenulum thin ridge of tissue extending from the floor of the mouth to the inferior surface of the tongue along its midline.

Friedman graph a method of describing and recording labor progress.

Friedman's test modification of the Aschheim-Zondek pregnancy test in which the woman's urine is injected into a mature, unmated female rabbit. After two days, the rabbit's ovaries are examined; the presence of fresh corpora lutea or hemorrhagic corpora constitutes a positive test.

FSH see *follicle-stimulating hormone.*

fundus the upper portion of the uterus between the fallopian tubes.

funic souffle hissing sound synchronous with the fetal heartbeat and considered to be produced in the umbilical cord.

funis a cordlike structure, such as the umbilical cord.

furuncle a boil.

galactagogue an agent that causes the flow of milk to increase.

galactorrhea excessive secretion of milk.

gamete a mature germ cell; an egg or sperm.

gargoylism a hereditary condition, associated with Hurler's syndrome, characterized by deformed limbs and hands and grotesque facies, with thickening of the lips, nostrils, and ears.

gastroschisis congenital herniation of the bowel or other abdominal viscera through an extraumbilical defect in the abdominal wall with no external covering membrane.

gastrula the stage in early embryonic development that follows the blastula.

gavage feeding by means of a tube passed into the stomach.

gene smallest unit of inheritance; genes are located on the chromosomes.

generative involved in reproduction of the species.

genetic compound a situation in which an individual has two different mutant alleles at a given locus.

genetic heterogeneity a situation that occurs when a trait or disease can be caused by gene pairs located at different loci but presenting a similar clinical picture.

genetics the science that deals with the genetic transmission of characteristics from parents to offspring.

genocopy a mutant gene that produces a phenotype indistinguishable from that produced by a different mutant gene.

genotype the genetic composition of an individual.

gestation period of intrauterine development from conception through birth; pregnancy.

gestational age the number of complete weeks in fetal development, calculated from the first day of the last normal menstrual cycle.

glycosuria presence of glucose in the urine.

gonad sex gland; the ovaries in the female and the testes in the male.

gonadotropin a hormone that stimulates the sex glands.

Goodell's sign softening of the cervix that occurs during the second month of pregnancy.

graafian follicle the ovarian cyst containing the ripe ovum; it secretes estrogens.

gravid pregnant.

gravida a pregnant woman.

gynecoid pelvis typical female pelvis in which the inlet is round instead of oval.

gynecology study of the diseases of the female, especially of the genital, urinary, and rectal organs and the breasts.

habitus physical appearance indicating a tendency or predisposition to disease or abnormal conditions.

haploid half the diploid number of chromosomes. In humans, there are 23 chromosomes, the haploid number, in each germ cell.

harlequin fetus a newborn with skin that resembles a thick horny armor; the skin is divided into areas by deep red fissures. These infants die within a few days.

harlequin sign a rare color change that occurs between the longitudinal halves of the newborn's body, such that the dependent half is noticeably pinker than the superior half when the newborn is placed on one side; of no pathologic significance.

HCG see *human chorionic gonadotropin.*

Hegar's sign a softening of the lower uterine segment found upon palpation in the second or third month of pregnancy.

hematoma a swelling or collection of blood in the tissues; a bruise or blood tumor.

hemianopsias blindness for half the field of vision in one or both eyes.

hemizygous having only one allele for a given trait instead of a pair.

hemoconcentration increase in the number of red blood cells resulting from a decrease in plasma volume or from increased erythropoiesis.

hemorrhagic disease of newborn hemorrhaging during the first few days of life caused by inadequate supply of prothrombin or by a delay in the production of vitamin K.

hemorrhoids varicose veins of the rectum; may be external or internal.

hereditary able to be passed from one generation to the next through the gametes of the parents.

heterozygous a genotypic situation in which two different alleles occur at a given locus on a pair of homologous chromosomes.

high risk having an increased possibility of suffering harm, damage, loss, or death.

hirsutism excessive growth of hair or growth of hair in unusual places.

Homans' sign pain in the calf when the foot is passively dorsiflexed; an early sign of phlebothrombosis of the deep veins of the calf.

homiothermic warm-blooded.

homologous similar in origin or structure but not necessarily in function.

homologous chromosomes a matched pair of chromosomes.

homozygous a genotypic situation in which two similar genes occur at a given locus on homologous chromosomes.

hordeolum inflammation of a sebaceous gland of the eyelid.

hormone a substance produced in an organ or gland and conveyed by the blood to another part of the body in order to exert an effect.

human chorionic gonadotropin (HCG) a hormone produced by the chorionic villi and found in the urine of pregnant women; also called *prolan.*

Hurler's syndrome lipochondrodystrophy.

hyaline membrane disease respiratory disease of the newborn infant characterized by interference with ventilation at the alveolar level, thought to be caused by the presence of fibrinoid deposits lining the alveolar ducts. Also called *respiratory distress syndrome (RDS).*

hydatidiform mole degenerative process in chorionic villi, giving rise to multiple cysts and rapid growth of the uterus with hemorrhage.

hydramnios an excess of amniotic fluid, leading to overdistention of the uterus. Frequently seen in diabetic pregnant women even if there is not coexisting fetal anomaly. Also called *polyhydramnios.*

hydrocele accumulation of serous fluid in a saclike cavity, especially in the sac that surrounds the testicle, causing the scrotum to swell.

hydrocephalus increased accumulation of cerebrospinal fluid within the ventricles of the brain, resulting from interference with normal circulation and absorption of the fluid and especially from destruction of the foramens of Magendie and Lushka; caused by congenital anomalies, infection, injury, or brain tumors.

hydrops fetalis see *erythroblastosis fetalis.*

hymen membranous fold that normally partially covers the entrance to the vagina.

hymenal tag normally occurring redundant hymenal tissue that protrudes from the floor of the vagina and that disappears spontaneously a few weeks after birth.

hyperbilirubinemia excessive amount of bilirubin in the blood; indicative of hemolytic processes due to blood incompatibility, intrauterine infection, septicemia, neonatal renal infection, and other disorders.

hypercapnia an increased amount of carbon dioxide in the blood; acts as a respiratory depressant.

hypercholesterolemia excessive amount of cholesterol in the blood.

hyperemesis gravidarum excessive vomiting during pregnancy, leading to dehydration and starvation.

hyperlipidemia excessive amount of fat in the blood.

hypermagnesemia excessive amount of magnesium in the blood.

hyperplasia excessive increase of normal cells in the normal tissue arrangement of an organ.

hypersomnia excessive need for sleep.

hypertelorism abnormal width between two paired organs.

hypertrophy increase or enlargement in size of existing cells; usually applies to any increase in size as a result of functional activity.

hypofibrinogenemia lowered levels of fibrinogen in the blood.

hypogalactic pertaining to deficient secretion of milk.

hypogastric arteries branches of the right and left iliac arterties that carry deoxygenated blood from the fetus through the umbilical cord (where they are known as umbilical arteries) to the placenta.

hypoglycemia abnormally low level of sugar in the blood.

hypomagnesemia abnormally low amount of magnesium in the blood.

hypospadias abnormal congenital positioning

of the male urethra on the undersurface of the penis or a urethral opening into the vagina.

hypotensive drugs drugs that lower blood pressure.

hypovolemic shock a condition in which the patient exhibits lowered blood pressure and increased pulse rate; caused by a decrease in the volume of circulating blood in the body.

hypoxemia insufficient oxygenation of the blood, resulting in metabolic acidosis.

hypoxia insufficient availability of oxygen to meet body tissue metabolic needs.

hysterectomy surgical removal of the uterus. See also *abdominal hysterectomy; panhysterectomy; subtotal hysterectomy; total hysterectomy.*

hysterotomy surgical incision into the uterus.

icterus neonatorum jaundice in the newborn.

ideopathic respiratory distress syndrome see *hyaline membrane disease.*

iliopectineal line bony ridge on the inner surface of the ilium and pubis, dividing the true and false pelvis.

immature baby considerably underdeveloped newborn weighing less than 1134 gm (2½ lb) at birth.

imperforate anus congenital closure of the anal opening, usually by a membranous septum; may be associated with a fistulous tract.

impetigo a skin disease caused by streptococci or staphylococci and characterized by pustules.

implantation embedding of the fertilized ovum in the uterine mucosa six or seven days after fertilization; also called *nidation.*

impotence inability of the male to perform sexual intercourse.

impregnate to make pregnant or to fertilize.

inanition condition of malnutrition caused by lack of sufficient food; may be due to lack of food supply or to malabsorption.

inborn error of metabolism a hereditary deficiency of a specific enzyme needed for normal metabolism of specific chemicals.

incompetent cervix a mechanical defect in the cervix making it unable to remain closed throughout pregnancy; produces dilatation and effacement leading to abortion, usually during the second trimester or early third trimester.

increment increase or addition; to build up, as of a contraction.

incubation (1) care of a premature infant in an incubator; (2) the development of an impregnated ovum; (3) interval between exposure to an infection and the appearance of first symptoms.

incubator apparatus used for premature infants in which the temperature can be regulated.

index case the closest affected relative to the consultand; also known as the proband or propositus/proposita.

induction the process of causing or initiating labor by use of medication or surgical rupture of membranes.

inertia inactivity or sluggishness; absence of weakness of uterine contractions during labor.

infant child under 1 year of age.

infant death rate number of deaths of infants under 1 year of age per 1000 live births in a given population per year.

infantile uterus failure of the uterus to attain adult characteristics.

infertility diminished ability to conceive.

infiltration process of substance being passed into or being deposited within a tissue, such as a local anesthetic drug.

inlet passage leading to a cavity.

inlet of the pelvis upper opening into the pelvic cavity.

innominate bone the hip bone, ilium, ischium, and pubis.

internal os an inside mouth or opening; the opening between the cervix and the uterus.

intervillous spaces irregular spaces in the maternal portion of the placenta that are filled with maternal blood, serving as sites of maternal-fetal gas, nutrient, and waste exchange.

intrathecal within the subarachnoid space.

intrauterine device (IUD) small metal or plastic form that is placed in the uterus to prevent implantation of a fertilized ovum.

intrauterine growth retardation (IUGR) fetal undergrowth due to any etiology, such as intrauterine infection, deficient nutrient supply, or congenital malformation.

introitus opening or entrance into a cavity or canal, such as the vagina.

intromission insertion or placing of one part into another, such as insertion of the penis into the vagina.

in utero within or inside the uterus.

inversion of the uterus condition in which the fundus of the uterus protrudes through the cervix and sometimes through the vaginal introitus; may occur immediately postpartum as a result of too vigorous placental expression while the placenta is still fixed in the uterus.

involution rolling or turning inward; the reduction in size of the uterus following delivery.

ischium lower portion of the hip bone.

ischogalactic causing suppression of breast milk.

IUD see *intrauterine device.*

IUGR see *intrauterine growth retardation.*

jaundice yellow pigmentation of body tissues caused by the presence of bile pigments. See also *pathologic jaundice; physiologic jaundice.*

Kahn test test used for diagnosing syphilis.

kalemia the level of potassium in the blood.

karyotype the set of chromosomes arranged in a standard order.

kernicterus an ecephalopathy caused by deposition of unconjugated bilirubin in brain cells; may result in impaired brain function or death.

Kernig's sign nuchal rigidity; stiffness of the neck.

Klinefelter's syndrome a chromosomal abnormality caused by the presence of an extra X chromosome in the male; characteristics include tall stature, sparse pubic and facial hair, gynecomastia, small firm testes, and absence of spermatogenesis.

labia external folds of skin on either side of the vulva.

labia majora the larger outer folds of skin on either side of the vulva.

labia minora the smaller inner folds of skin on either side of the vulva.

labor the process by which the fetus is expelled from the maternal uterus; also called childbirth, confinement, or parturition.

laceration in obstetrics, a tear in the perineum, vagina, or cervix as a result of stretching of the tissues during childbirth.

lactation process of producing and supplying breast milk.

lactiferous ducts tiny tubes within the breast that conduct milk from the acini cells to the nipple.

lactogenic hormone hormone produced by the anterior pituitary to promote growth of breast tissue and to stimulate the production of milk.

lactosuria excretion of lactose in the urine during late pregnancy and lactation.

lambdoidal suture line forming the base of the triangular posterior fontanelle, separating the occipital bone from the two parietal bones.

lanugo fine, downy hair found on all body parts of the fetus after 20 weeks' gestation, with the exception of the palms of the hands and the soles of the feet.

large for gestational age (LGA) excessive growth of a fetus in relation to the gestational time period.

lay midwife a person who gives care during the prenatal, labor and delivery, and postpartal periods. Education varies from apprenticeship to self-teaching to short-term programs. Skills may be passed from one midwife to another.

Leopold's maneuvers series of four maneuvers designed to provide a systematic approach whereby the examiner may determine fetal presentation and position.

letdown reflex pattern of stimulation, hormone release, and resulting muscle contraction that forces milk into the lactiferous ducts, making it available to the baby; milk ejection reflex.

LGA see *large for gestational age.*

leukorrhea mucous discharge from the vagina or cervical canal that may be normal or pathologic, as in the presence of infection.

LH see *luteinizing hormone.*

lie relationship of the long axis of the fetus and

the long axis of the mother; also called *presentation.*

ligation suturing or tying shut, as in the suturing closed of the fallopian tubes to prevent pregnancy *(tubal ligation).*

lightening moving of the fetus and uterus downward into the pelvic cavity; engagement.

linea nigra line of darker pigmentation extending from the pubis to the umbilicus noted in some women during the later months of pregnancy.

linkage occurs when genes for different traits are located near one another on the same chromosome.

lithotomy position position in which the patient lies on her back with thighs drawn up toward her chest and with her knees flexed and abducted.

lochia discharge of blood, mucus, and tissue from the uterus that may last for several weeks after the birth of a baby.

lochia alba white vaginal discharge that follows lochia serosa and that lasts from about the 10th to 21st day following delivery.

lochia rubra red, blood-tinged vaginal discharge that occurs following delivery and lasts 2 to 4 days.

lochia serosa pink, serous, and blood-tinged vaginal discharge that follows lochia rubra and lasts until the 7th to 10th day after delivery.

locus the position that a gene occupies on a chromosome.

L/S ratio the ratio of the phospholipids lecithin and sphingomyelin produced by the fetal lungs; useful in assessing fetal lung maturity.

LTH see *luteotropin.*

lunar month a 28-day cycle corresponding to the phases of the moon. A normal pregnancy lasts ten lunar months.

lung compliance degree of distensibility of the lung's elastic tissues.

lutein cells yellow ovarian cells involved in the formation of the corpus luteum.

luteinizing hormone (LH) anterior pituitary hormone responsible for stimulating ovulation and for development of the corpus luteum.

luteotropin (LTH) lactogenic hormone; prolactin.

lysis of adhesions surgical procedure to release organs tied together by bands of tissue.

lysozyme enzyme with antiseptic properties found in blood cells, saliva, sweat, tears, and breast milk.

maceration wasting away, degeneration, or breaking down of fetal skin, as seen with postterm infants or a fetus retained in the uterus after its death.

macroglossia hypertrophy of the tongue, as in infants with Down's syndrome, or a tongue too large for present oral cavity development, as seen in some premature neonates.

macrosomia condition seen in some neonates of large body size and high birth weight, as those born of prediabetic and diabetic mothers.

macule a flat, discolored skin lesion smaller than 1 cm.

magnesemia level of magnesium in the blood.

mammary glands compound glandular elements of the breast that in the female secrete milk to nourish the infant.

Marfan's syndrome an inherited disorder characterized by abnormally long, thin extremities, spidery fingers and toes, defects of the spine and chest, and congenital heart disease.

mask of pregnancy see *chloasma.*

mastalgia breast pain or tenderness.

mastectomy surgical removal of the breast.

mastitis inflammation of the breast.

maternal mortality number of deaths from any cause during the pregnancy cycle per 100,000 live births.

maturation in reproduction, the process of cell division that reduces the number of chromosomes in the sperm and ova to one half the number carried in the somatic cells of the species.

meatus external opening for a passageway to an internal organ, such as the urethral meatus.

mechanism process by which results are obtained, as in labor and delivery of a fetus.

meconium dark green or black material present

in the large intestine of a full-term infant; the first stools passed by the newborn.

meconium-stained fluid amniotic fluid that contains meconium because fetal distress has caused increased intestinal activity and relaxing of the fetus's anal sphincter.

meiosis the process of cell division that occurs in the maturation of sperm and ova that decreases their number of chromosomes by one half.

membrane thin, pliable layer of tissue that covers an organ or that divides structures, as in the amnion and chorion surrounding the fetus.

menarche beginning of menstrual and reproductive function in the female.

meningomyelocele a defect in the spinal column with resulting protrusion of the spinal cord and membranes.

menopause see *climacteric.*

menorrhagia excessive or profuse menstrual flow.

menstrual cycle cyclic buildup of the uterine lining, ovulation, and sloughing of the lining occurring approximately every 28 days in nonpregnant females.

menstruation (menses) shedding of the uterine lining at the end of the menstrual cycle, resulting in a bloody discharge from the vagina.

mentum the chin.

mesoderm the intermediate layer of germ cells in the embryo that give rise to connective tissue, bone marrow, muscles, blood, lymphoid tissue, and epithelial tissue.

metrorrhagia abnormal uterine bleeding occurring at irregular intervals.

microcephalic having an abnormally small head in relation to total body size.

micrognathia abnormally small lower jaw.

midwife see *lay midwife; nurse-midwife*

migration in obstetrics, movement of the ovum from the ovary down the fallopian tube to the uterus.

milia tiny white papules appearing on the face of a neonate as a result of unopened sebaceous glands; they disappear spontaneously within a few weeks.

milk-leg phlebitis and thrombosis of the femoral vein, resulting in venous obstruction and edema of the affected leg.

miscarriage see *spontaneous abortion.*

mitochrondria slender filament or granular component of cytoplasm in which oxidative reactions occur that provide the cell with energy.

mitosis process of cell division whereby both daughter cells have the same number and pattern of chromosomes as the original cell.

molding shaping of the fetal head by overlapping of the cranial bones to facilitate movement through the birth canal during labor.

Mongolian spot dark flat pigmentation of the lower back and buttocks noted at birth in some infants; usually disappears by the time the child reaches school age.

Mongolism see *Down's syndrome.*

moniliasis yeastlike fungus infection caused by *Candida albicans.*

monosomy the presence of only a single chromosome of a homologous pair.

monozygotic twins two fetuses that develop from a single divided fertilized ovum; identical twins.

Montgomery's glands small nodules located around the nipples that enlarge during pregnancy and lactation.

mons veneris fleshy tissue over the symphysis pubis of the female from which hair develops at puberty.

morbidity incidence of diseased persons in relation to a specific population.

morning sickness nausea and vomiting occurring during the first trimester of pregnancy; may occur at any time during the day.

Moro reflex flexion of the newborn infant's thighs and knees accompanied by fingers that fan then clench as the arms are simultaneously thrown out and then brought together as though embracing something. This reflex can be elicited by startling the newborn with a sudden noise or movement; also called the *startle reflex.*

mortality incidence of deaths in relation to a specific population.

morula developmental stage of the fertilized ovum in which there is a solid mass of cells.

mosaic an individual who has two or more cell lines different from each other in chromosome number or morphology; generally some cells are normal while others contain chromosomal aberrations.

mottling discoloration of the skin in irregular areas; may be seen with chilling, poor perfusion, or hypoxia.

mucous membrane mucus-secreting tissue layer lining cavities and canals of the body.

mucous plug a collection of thick mucus that blocks the cervical canal during pregnancy; also called *operculum.*

mucus thick, viscid fluid.

multigravida female who has been pregnant more than once.

multipara female who has had more than one pregnancy in which the fetuses were viable.

multiple pregnancy more than one fetus in the uterus at the same time.

mutagen an environmental agent, either physical, chemical, or biologic, capable of inducing mutation.

mutation change or alteration in gene or chromosome structure that may be transmitted to offspring.

myometrium uterine muscular structure.

nadir the lowest point.

Nägele's rule a method of determining the estimated date of confinement (EDC): after obtaining the first day of the last menstrual period, one subtracts three months and adds 7 days.

natal relating to birth.

natural childbirth prepared childbirth, in which the couple attends a prenatal education program and learns exercises and breathing patterns that are used during labor and childbirth.

navel area of the abdomen where the umbilical cord emerged from the fetus; the *umbilicus.*

neonatal mortality rate number of deaths of infants in the first 28 days per 1000 live births.

neonate infant from birth through the first 28 days of life.

neurofibromatosis syndrome autosomal dominant syndrome characterized by café-au-lait spots, freckling in the axilla, and subcutaneous dyplastic tumors that may appear along the nerves or in the meninges or eye.

nevus mole, blemish, or mark.

nevus cavernosus a blemish or mark that may be well circumscribed and elevated or with poorly defined borders and that is composed of large venous channels; the overlying skin has a red-blue discoloration. The nevus enlarges when the infant cries or strains.

nevus flammeus large port-wine stain.

nevus vasculosus "strawberry mark"; raised, clearly delineated, dark red, rough-surfaced birth mark commonly found in the head region.

nidation see *implantation.*

nondisjunction failure of separation of paired chromosomes during cell division.

nuclear family family group consisting of one or more adults and one or more children.

nulligravida female who has never been pregnant.

nullipara female who has not delivered a viable fetus.

nurse-midwife a certified nurse-midwife (CNM) is an R.N. who has received special training and education in the care of the family during childbearing and the prenatal, labor and delivery, and postpartal periods. After a period of formal education, the nurse-midwife takes a certification test to become a CNM.

nystagmus involuntary rhythmic oscillation of the eyeball in any direction.

obstetrics the branch of medicine concerned with the care of women during pregnancy, childbirth, and the postpartal period.

occiput posterior part of the skull.

OCT see *oxytocin challenge test.*

ocular hypertelorism abnormal width between the eyes.

oligohydramnios deficiency or absence of amniotic fluid, which may indicate a fetal urinary tract defect.

oliguria decrease in urine secretion by the kidney (100–400 ml/24 hours).

omphalic concerning the umbilicus.

omphalitis infection of the umbilicus.

omphalocele congenital herniation or protrusion of the abdominal contents into the base of the umbilicus.

oocyesis see *ectopic pregnancy.*

oophorectomy surgical removal of the ovary.

operculum see *mucous plug.*

ophthalmia neonatorum purulent infection of the eyes or conjunctiva of the newborn, usually caused by gonococci.

opisthotonis backward flexion of the head and feet due to tetanic spasm.

orifice normal outlet of a body cavity.

Ortolani's maneuver a manual procedure performed to rule out the possibility of congenital hip dysplasia.

os opening, mouth. See also *cervical os.*

ossification conversion into bone.

osteogenesis imperfecta a dominant inherited disease characterized by blue sclerae and hypoplasia of osteoid tissue and collagen, which results in bone fractures with slight trauma.

outlet dystocia inadequate pelvic size, causing the fetal head to be pushed backward toward the coccyx, making extension of the head difficult.

ovary female sex gland in which the ova are formed and in which estrogen and progesterone are produced. Normally there are two ovaries, located in the lower abdomen on each side of the uterus.

oviducts see *fallopian tubes.*

ovulation normal process of discharging a mature ovum from an ovary approximately 14 days prior to the onset of menses.

ovum female reproductive cell; egg.

oxygen toxicity excessive levels of oxygen therapy that result in pathologic changes in tissue.

oxytocics drugs that accelerate childbirth and lessen postnatal hemorrhage by stimulating uterine contractions.

oxytocin hormone normally produced by the posterior pituitary, responsible for stimulation of uterine contractions and the release of milk into the lactiferous ducts.

oxytocin challenge test (OCT) test designed to evaluate the circulatory-respiratory status of the fetoplacental unit to determine the ability of the fetus to withstand the stress of labor. While externally monitoring uterine contractions and FHR, oxytocin is administered to stimulate contractions. The FHR pattern is then assessed for evidence of a late deceleration pattern. The test is negative when there are three contractions in a ten-minute period without late deceleration.

palpation use of fingers or hands to manually determine the characteristics of tissues or organs; see also *bimanual palpation.*

palsy loss of or decreased ability to initiate or control muscle movement; paralysis.

panhysterectomy removal of the entire uterus, the ovaries, and the fallopian tubes.

Papanicolaou (Pap) smear procedure to detect the presence of cancer of the uterus by microscopic examination of cells gently scraped from the cervix.

papule a small, raised, sharply circumscribed lesion less than 1 cm in size that may be colored or flesh tone.

para a woman who has borne offspring who reached the age of viability.

parabiotic syndrome anomaly occurring in a small percentage of identical twins, in which one twin is anemic and the second suffers polycythemia as a result of a fetofetal blood transfer via placental vascular anastomoses.

parametritis inflammation of the parametrial layer of the uterus.

parametrium layer of muscle and connective tissue extending between the broad ligaments and surrounding the uterus.

parity the condition of having borne offspring who had attained the age of viability.

parturient pertaining to the act of childbirth.

parturition the process of giving birth.

pathologic jaundice jaundice that occurs within 24 hours of birth, secondary to an abnormal condition such as ABO–Rh incompatibility.

patulous open widely or spread apart.

pedigree a graphic picture using symbols representing an individual's family tree.

pelvic pertaining to the pelvis.

pelvic axis imaginary curved line that passes through the centers of all the anteroposterior diameters of the pelvis.

pelvic phase of labor the deceleration phase, in which active descent occurs.

pelvimeter instrument for the measurement of the diameters and capacities of the pelvis.

pelvis the lower portion of the trunk of the body bounded by the hip bones, coccyx, and sacrum.

pemphigus neonatorum impetigo bullosa.

penis the male organ of copulation or reproduction.

perforation of the uterus a hole made in the uterus.

perinatal mortality both neonatal and fetal deaths per 1000 live births.

perinatal period the time frame extending from the 28th week past conception to the 28th day past birth.

perinatologist a physician specializing in fetal and neonatal care.

perineal body wedge-shaped mass of fibromuscular tissue found between the lower part of the vagina and the anal canal.

perineorrhaphy suturing of the perineum, usually performed following a laceration.

perineotomy a surgical incision through the perineum.

perineum the area of tissue between the anus and scrotum in the male or between the anus and vagina in the female.

periodic breathing sporadic episodes of apnea, not associated with cyanosis, which last for about 10 seconds and commonly occur in premature infants.

peritoneum a serous membrane that lines the abdominopelvic walls.

pessary a device inserted into the body to support an organ or structure, such as a pessary inserted into the vagina to support the uterus in place.

petechia pinpoint, raised, round, purplish red spot caused by minute capillary hemorrhage.

phenocopy an environmentally induced phenotype mimicking one usually produced by a specific genotype.

phenotype the whole physical, biochemical, and physiologic make-up of an individual as determined both genetically and environmentally.

phenylalanine a naturally occurring amino acid essential for optimal growth and nitrogen balance in humans.

phenylketonuria (PKU) a recessive hereditary metabolic error that causes the buildup of phenylalanine, leading to mental retardation, brain damage, light pigmentation, and other characteristics. Can be treated with a low-phenylalanine diet.

phimosis abnormal tightness of the foreskin so that it cannot be retracted over the glans; analogous to tightening of the clitoral hood.

phlebitis inflammation of a vein.

phlebothrombosis presence of a clot within a vein without associated symptoms of vein inflammation.

phlegmasia alba dolens postpartal ileofemoral-thrombosis (milk-leg).

phocomelia absence of or incomplete formation and development of arms, forearms, thighs, and legs. Hands and feet are present but may be abnormally developed.

phototherapy the treatment of disease by exposure to light.

physiologic pertaining to normal or expected functioning of a body or organ.

physiologic jaundice a harmless condition caused by the normal reduction of red blood cells, occurring 48 or more hours after birth, peaking at the fifth to seventh day, and disappearing between the seventh to tenth day.

Pierre-Robin syndrome syndrome characterized by mandibular hypoplasia that occurs prior to the ninth week of embryologic development. The mandibular hypoplasia results in micrognathia, glossoptosis, and possibly a cleft in the soft palate. The infant's mandible generally shows normal growth catch-up by 12–24 months of age.

pigeon chest chest deformity in which the sternum is prominent. Transverse diameters may be shortened.

pilonidal cyst a hair-containing cavity in the sacrococcygeal area.

pinna the part of the ear that lies outside the skull.

PKU see *phenylketonuria.*

placenta specialized disk-shaped organ that connects the fetus to the uterine wall for gas and nutrient exchange; also called *afterbirth.*

placenta accreta partial or complete absence of the decidua basalis and abnormal adherence of the placenta to the uterine wall.

placenta previa abnormal implantation of the placenta in the lower uterine segment. Clasification of type is based on proximity to the cervical os: *total*—completely covers the os; *partial*—covers a portion of the os; *marginal*—in close proximity to the os.

placental pertaining to the placenta.

placental dystocia difficulty in the delivery of the placenta.

placental dysfunction placental insufficiency; the placenta fails to meet fetal requirements.

placental souffle soft blowing sounds produced by blood coursing through the placenta; has the same rate as the maternal pulse.

platypelloid pelvis an unusually wide pelvis, having a flattened oval transverse shape and a shortened anteroposterior diameter.

plethora a reddened florid complexion, usually caused by an excessive amount of blood in the area.

pneumomediastinum accidental or diagnostically introduced air or gas into the mediastinal area, which could lead to pneumothorax, pneumopericardium, or pneumoperitoneum.

pneumothorax air within the chest cavity between the lung tissue and chest wall, creating a positive pressure space instead of negative pressure.

podalic version a technique designed to produce a change in fetal position or polarity in order to convert an abnormal presentation to a breech presentation.

polycythemia an abnormal increase in the number of total red blood cells in the body's circulation.

polydactyly a developmental anomaly characterized by more than five digits on the hands or feet.

polygenic determined by the action of more than one gene.

polyhydramnios see *hydramnios.*

polymorphous pertaining to lesions in various stages of change.

polyuria passage of excessive amounts of urine within a given time period.

popliteal angle the angle formed at the knee when the thigh of the supine infant is flexed on the chest and the leg is extended by pressure behind the ankle.

position attitude or posture assumed to achieve comfort or purpose.

positive signs of pregnancy indications that confirm the presence of pregnancy.

posterior back or dorsal surface of a body or body part.

posterior fontanelle small triangular area between the occipital and parietal bones of the skull; generally closed by 8–12 weeks of life.

postmature infant a newborn that is overly developed or that is more than 42 gestational weeks of age.

postnatal occurring after birth.

postnatal period period from 28 days following birth to 11 months of age.

postpartum after childbirth or delivery.

precipitate delivery (1) unduly rapid progression of labor, one that lasts less than three hours; (2) a delivery in which no physician is in attendance.

precocious teeth small unrooted teeth found in the newborn.

preeclampsia toxemia of pregnancy, characterized by hypertension, albuminuria, and edema. See also *eclampsia.*

pre-embryonic stage the first 14 days of human development; also called *stage of the ovum.*

pregnancy the condition of having a developing embryo or fetus in the body after fertilization of the female egg by the male sperm.

premature infant any infant born before 38 weeks' gestation.

premonitory serving as a warning.

prenatal before birth.

prepuce a covering or fold of skin.

preparatory phase of labor the latent phase of labor.

presentation see *lie.*

presenting part the fetal part present in or on the cervical os.

pressure edema accumulation of excessive fluid,

primarily in the lower extremities. In obstetrics, caused by pressure of the pregnant uterus on the larger veins.

presumptive signs of pregnancy symptoms that suggest pregnancy but that do not confirm it, such as cessation of menses, quickening, Chadwick's sign, and morning sickness.

preterm infant see *premature infant.*

priapism persistent abnormal erection of the penis, usually occurring without sexual desire and accompanied by pain and tenderness.

primigravida a woman who is pregnant for the first time.

primipara a woman who has given birth to her first child (past the point of viability), whether or not that child is living or was alive at birth.

primordial original or primitive; being the simplest form of development.

probable signs of pregnancy manifestations that strongly suggest the likelihood of pregnancy, such as a positive pregnancy test, enlarging abdomen, and positive Goodell's, Hegar's, and Braxton Hicks signs.

proband someone who comes to the attention of a genetic investigator because of the occurrence of an inherited trait; propositus.

progesterone a hormone produced by the corpus luteum, adrenal cortex, and placenta whose function it is to stimulate proliferation of the endometrium to facilitate growth of the embryo.

projectile vomiting emesis that appears to have been propelled out of the mouth by extreme force.

prolactin a hormone secreted by the anterior pituitary that stimulates and sustains lactation in mammals.

prolan see *human chorionic gonadotropin (HCG).*

prolapsed cord umbilical cord that becomes trapped in the vagina before the fetus is delivered.

promontory of the sacrum projecting eminence or process of the sacrum corresponding to the junction of the sacrum and L5.

prophylactic pertaining to a preventive measure or to a measure used to ward off a disease or event.

propositus the first to present a particular trait that triggers a genetic investigation.

proteinuria the presence of an excessive amount of serum protein in the urine.

pseudocyesis a condition in which the woman has symptoms of pregnancy but in which hormonal pregnancy tests are negative; false pregnancy.

pseudomenstruation blood-tinged mucus from the vagina in the newborn female infant; caused by withdrawal of maternal hormones that were present during pregnancy.

pseudopregnancy see *pseudocyesis.*

pseudoprematurity see *intrauterine growth retardation (IUGR).*

psychologic miscarriage maternal lack of love for the infant; emotional detachment.

psychoprophylaxis psychophysical training aimed at preparing the expectant parents to cope with the processes of labor and to avoid concentration on the discomforts associated with childbirth.

puberty the period of time during which the secondary sexual characteristics develop and the ability to procreate is attained.

pubic pertaining to the pubes or pubis.

pudendal block injection of an anesthetizing agent at the pudendal nerve to produce numbness of the external genitals and the lower one-third of the vagina to facilitate childbirth and permit episiotomy if necessary.

pudendum the external genitals of humans.

puerperal sepsis infection of the reproductive organs caused by unsterile childbirth conditions; also called *childbed fever* and *puerperal fever.*

puerperium the period or state of confinement after completion of the third stage of labor until involution of the uterus is complete, usually six weeks.

pustule a small, raised, sharply circumscribed lesion filled with purulent material; less than 1 cm in size.

quickening the first fetal movements felt by the mother, usually between 16 and 18 weeks' gestation.

rabbit test see *Friedman's test.*

radium insertion introduction of a radium rod or device into the cervix or uterus to destroy cancer cells.

rales an abnormal respiratory sound heard usually with the aid of a stethoscope; caused by air passing through fluid in the alveoli and terminal bronchioles.

RDS see *hyaline membrane disease.*

recessive trait a trait that is expressed only when no dominant genes are present.

recoil to spring back; to return to a starting point; for example, to return to a position of flexion after involuntary extension.

rectocele herniation of part of the rectum into the vagina.

reflex an involuntary response.

relaxin a water-soluble protein secreted by the corpus luteum that causes relaxation of the symphysis and cervical dilatation.

residual urine urine left in the bladder after voiding.

respiratory distress syndrome see *hyaline membrane disease.*

restitution in obstetrics, turning the fetal presenting part either right or left after it has fully exited the birth canal so that the spine is once again in a straight line.

resuscitation restoration of life or consciousness by means of artificial respiration and cardiac massage.

retained placenta placenta that fails to be expelled after childbirth because of adherence or incarceration.

retraction to be drawn up or back.

retroflexion of the uterus the bending back of the body of the uterus toward the cervix, resulting in a sharp angle at the point of bending.

retrolental fibroplasia formation of fibrotic tissue behind the lens; associated with retinal detachment and arrested eye growth, seen with hyperoxemia in premature infants.

retroversion of the uterus the turning backward of the entire uterus in relation to the pelvic area.

Rh factor antigens present on the surface of blood cells that make the blood cell incompatible with blood cells that do not have the antigen.

rhonchi coarse, abnormal auscultatory sounds made by the passage of air over mucous plugs.

rhythm method the timing of sexual intercourse to avoid the fertile time associated with ovulation.

ribonucleic acid (RNA) the complex protein responsible for transfering genetic information within a cell.

ripe being in a state of optimal readiness or consistency.

Ritgen maneuver a procedure used to control delivery of the head.

role a cluster of interpersonal behaviors, attitudes, and activities associated with an individual in a certain situation or position.

rooming-in unit a hospital unit where the infant can reside in the same room with his mother after delivery and during their postpartal stay.

rooting reflex an infant's tendency to turn his head and open his lips to suck when one side of his mouth or his cheek is touched.

rotation turning of the fetal head as it follows the pelvic curves during childbirth.

Rubin's test tubal insufflation with a gas, usually carbon dioxide, to test the patency of the tubes or to clear small obstructions.

sacroiliac the joints or articulation between the sacrum and ilium and their associated ligaments.

sacrum five fused vertebras that form a triangle of bone just beneath the lumbar vertebras and between the hip bones.

saddle block anesthesia sensory and motor anesthesia of the buttocks, perineum, and inner aspects of the thighs, produced by spinal or entrathecal injection of an anesthetic agent at approximately L3–L5.

sagittal suture band of connective tissue that separates the parietal bones and extends anteriorly and posteriorly.

salpingo-oophorectomy surgical removal of a fallopian tube and an ovary.

scalines eczema on the cheeks, behind the ears, and on the popliteal and antecubital areas.

Scanzoni's maneuver rotation of the presenting fetal head from a posterior position to an anterior position through double forceps application.

scaphoid abdomen abdomen with a sunken interior wall, giving it a small, empty appearance.

scarf sign the position of the elbow when the hand of a supine infant is drawn across to the other shoulder until it meets resistance.

Schultze's mechanism delivery of the placenta with the shiny or fetal surface presenting first.

sclerema patchy or generalized progressive hardening of subcutaneous fat in infants; lesions are cold, yellow, and very firm.

sebaceous glands oil-secreting glands in the skin.

seborrhea dermatus see *cradle cap.*

secondary areola increased area of pigmentation surrounding the areola that occurs during pregnancy as a result of hormonal influences; becomes apparent at about the third month.

second stage of labor stage lasting from complete dilatation of the cervix to expulsion of the fetus.

secundines see *afterbirth.*

segmentation the process of division of the fertilized ovum into many cells before differentiation into layers.

semen thick whitish fluid ejaculated by the male during orgasm and containing the spermatozoa and their nutrients.

sensitization initial exposure to a substance that results in an immune response.

septic abortion a serious uterine infection that occurs most commonly after a criminal abortion.

sex chromatin see *Barr body.*

sex chromosomes the X and Y chromosomes, which are responsible for sex determination.

sex-limited trait a characteristic that is expressed in only one sex.

sex-linked trait a characteristic that is determined by genes on the X chromosome.

simian line a single palmar crease frequently found in children with Down's syndrome.

singleton pregnancy with a single fetus.

small for gestational age (SGA) inadequate weight or growth for gestational age; birth weight below the 10th percentile.

sole creases lines caused by folds covering the underpart of the foot. Distribution and number of creases contribute to determining gestational age.

souffle a soft blowing sound made by blood turbulence in the vessels.

spermatogenesis process by which mature spermatozoa are formed, during which chromosome number is reduced by half.

spermatozoa mature sperm cells of the male animal produced by the testes.

sphincter muscle a ringlike band of muscle fibers that constricts or closes a passage or orifice.

spina bifida occulta a defect in the vertebras of the spinal column without protrusion of neural components; may be completely asymptomatic.

spontaneous abortion abortion that occurs naturally; a *miscarriage.*

square window the angle formed at the wrist when the infant's hand is flexed toward the ventral forearm.

startle reflex see *Moro reflex.*

station relationship of the presenting fetal part to an imaginary line drawn between the pelvic ischial spines.

stepled palate high palate that rises to an angle instead of the more normal round shape.

sterility inability to conceive or to produce offspring.

stillbirth the delivery of a dead infant.

strabismus an eye condition in which the visual axis does not converge on a desired object; incoordinate action of the extrinsic ocular muscles.

striae gravidarum stretch marks; shiny reddish lines that appear on the abdomen, breasts, thighs, and buttocks of pregnant women as a result of stretching the skin.

Sturge-Weber syndrome syndrome of unknown etiology characterized by flat facial hemangiomata and meningeal hemangiomata with seizures.

subinvolution failure of a part to return to its

normal size after functional enlargement, such as failure of the uterus to return to normal size after pregnancy.

subluxation incomplete or partial dislocation.

subtotal hysterectomy removal of the fundus and body of the uterus, leaving the cervical stump.

succedaneum see *caput succedaneum.*

sucking reflex the infant's tendency to suck on any object placed in his mouth.

superfecundation successive fertilization of two or more ova during the same menstrual cycle as the result of more than one act of intercourse.

superfetation fertilization and development of an ovum while a developing fetus is already in the uterus.

supernumerary nipples excess number of nipples, varying from small pink spots to normal size and pigmentation, usually present along an imaginary line from midclavicle to groin.

surfactant a surface-active mixture of lipoproteins secreted in the alveoli and air passages that reduces surface tension of pulmonary fluids and contributes to the elasticity of pulmonary tissue.

suture fibrous connection of opposed joint surfaces, as in the skull. Also, the uniting of edges of a wound.

symphysis pubis fibrocartilagenous joint between the pelvic bones in the midline.

syndactyly malformation of the fingers or toes in which there may be webbing or complete fusion of two or more digits.

tachycardia abnormally rapid heart rate.

tachypnea excessively rapid respirations.

talipes equinovarus congenital defect of the foot with changes in the ligament and tendons consisting chiefly of contractures and anomalous insertions. The forefoot is adducted and supine and there is inversion of the heel and fixed plantar flexion of the foot. Also known as *clubfoot.*

telangiectatic nevi small clusters of pink-red spots appearing on the nape of the neck and around the eyes of infants; localized areas of capillary dilatation. Also referred to as *stork bites.*

teratogen a nongenetic factor that can produce malformations of the fetus.

term infant a live born infant of 38–42 weeks' gestation.

testes the male gonads, in which sperm and testosterone are produced.

testosterone the male hormone; responsible for the development of secondary male characteristics.

tetralogy of Fallot a combination of four congenital anomalies that together make up a specific cardiac syndrome.

therapeutic abortion medically induced termination of pregnancy when a malformed fetus is suspected or when the mother's health is in jeopardy.

thermogenesis the production of heat, especially within the body.

thermal neutral environment an environment that provides for minimal heat loss or expenditure.

third stage of labor the time from delivery of the fetus to the time when the placenta has been completely expelled.

threatened abortion a condition in which discharge of the fertilized ovum is threatened by bleeding from the vagina, which may be accompanied by cervical dilatation.

thromboembolus thrombotic material or clot carried by the bloodstream from one site to another vessel, causing obstruction.

thrombophlebitis inflammation of a vein associated with thrombus formation.

thrush a fungus infection of the oral mucous membranes caused by *Candida albicans.* Most often seen in infants; characterized by white plaques.

toco, tokos combined word form designating childbirth.

tocodynamometer external device that can be used to estimate uterine contraction pressures during labor.

tongue tie abnormally short frenulum of the tongue that limits its motion.

tonic neck reflex postural reflex seen in the newborn. When the supine infant's head is turned to one side, the arm and leg on that side extend while the extremities on the opposite side flex; also called the *fencing position.*

torticollis contracted neck muscles, producing a twisting and contraction of the head toward the affected side; wryneck.

total hysterectomy removal of the entire uterus, including the cervix, leaving the ovaries and fallopian tubes.

toxemia a group of pathologic conditions, essentially metabolic disturbances, occurring in pregnant women and manifested by preeclampsia and eclampsia.

tracheoesphageal fistula a congenital anomaly in which there is a communication between the trachea and the esophagus.

traditional family a family type that draws its strength from the autocratic and authoritarian patriarchal line.

transition the period during labor when the cervix becomes approximately 8 cm dilated, contractions are very strong, and the patient may feel that she cannot go on.

translocation the occurrence of a chromosome segment at an abnormal site.

Treacher-Collins syndrome mandibulofacial dysostosis.

Trichomonas vaginalis a parasitic protozoan that may cause inflammation of the vagina characterized by itching and burning of vulvar tissue and by white, frothy discharge.

trimester three months, or one-third of the gestational time for pregnancy.

trisomy the presence of three homologous chromosomes rather than the normal two.

trophoblast the outer layer of the blastoderm that will eventually establish the nutrient relationship with the uterine endometrium.

tubal ligation see *ligation.*

Turner's syndrome a number of anomalies that occur when a female has only one X chromosome; characteristics include short stature, little sexual differentiation, webbing of the neck with a low posterior hairline, and congenital cardiac anomalies.

transverse lie a lie in which the fetus is positioned cross-wise in the uterus.

twins two offspring produced by the same pregnancy. See also *dizygotic twins; monozygotic twins.*

umbilical cord the structure connecting the placenta to the umbilicus of the fetus and through which nutrients from the mother are exchanged for wastes from the fetus.

umbilical vasculitis inflammation of the umbilical cord and its contents.

umbilicus see *navel.*

urachus a canal connecting the fetal bladder with the allantois; at birth it collapses and becomes mostly fibrotic, forming the median umbilical ligament.

urinary meatus external opening of the urethra.

uterine souffle a soft sound made by the blood within the arteries of a gravid uterus.

uterine tetany prolonged or continuous uterine contractions.

uterine tubes see *fallopian tubes.*

uterus hollow muscular organ in which the fertilized ovum is implanted and in which the developing fetus is nourished until birth.

vagina the musculomembranous tube or passageway located between the external genitals and the uterus of the female.

valgus bent outward.

variable expressivity the differences in severity of a trait produced by the same gene in different individuals.

varicose veins permanently distended veins.

vasectomy surgical removal of a portion of the vas deferens (ductus deferens) to produce infertility.

venous referring to veins or to unoxygenated blood.

vernix caseosa a protective cheeselike whitish substance made up of sebum and desquamated epithelial cells that is present on the fetal skin.

version a change of position, usually to alter the presenting fetal part and facilitate delivery.

vertex the top or crown of the head.

vesical blastoderm a stage in the development of the mammalian embryo consisting of a hollow sphere of cells enclosing a cavity.

vesicular composed of or relating to small saclike structures filled with fluid.

vestibule a space or cavity at the entrance to a canal.

viable capable of living.

villi short vascular processes or protrusions appearing on some membranes. See also *chorionic villi.*

vulva the external structure of the female genitals, lying below the mons veneris.

vulvectomy surgical removal of the vulva.

Waardenburg's syndrome a congenital syndrome transmitted as an autosomal recessive trait and characterized by cochlear deafness, wide bridge of the nose, lateral displacement of the medial canthi, confluent eyebrows, eyes of different colors, white eyelashes, white forelock, and leukodermia.

Wharton's jelly yellow-white gelatinous material surrounding the vessels of the umbilical cord.

witch's milk whitish secretion from the infant's mammary glands for approximately seven days after delivery; caused by influence of the mother's hormones.

womb see *uterus.*

xanthoma yellow-white plaque on the skin as a result of lipid deposition.

X chromosome female sex chromosome.

X linkage genes located on the X chromosome.

Y chromosome male sex chromosome.

zona pellucida transparent inner layer surrounding an ovum.

zygote a fertilized egg.

INDEX